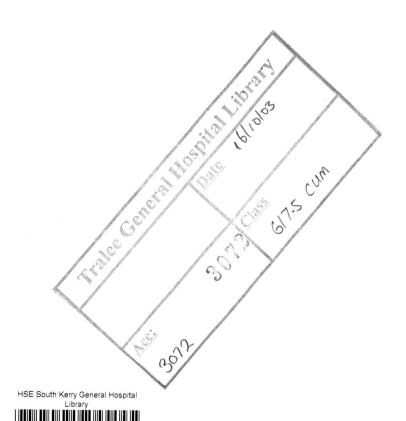

OTOLARYNGOLOGY HEAD AND NECK SURGERY

OTOLARYNGOLOGY—HEAD AND NECK SURGERY

VOLUME ONE
Part One: General Considerations in Head and Neck
Charles W. Cummings, editor
Paul W. Flint, associate editor
Part Two: Face
Charles J. Krause, editor
J. Regan Thomas, associate editor

VOLUME TWO
Part Three: Nose
Charles J. Krause, editor
J. Regan Thomas, associate editor
Part Four: Paranasal Sinuses
Charles J. Krause, editor
J. Regan Thomas, associate editor
Part Five: Salivary Glands
David E. Schuller, editor
K. Thomas Robbins, associate editor
Part Six: Oral Cavity/Oropharynx/Nasopharynx
David E. Schuller, editor
K. Thomas Robbins, associate editor

VOLUME THREE
Part Seven: Neck
David E. Schuller, editor
K. Thomas Robbins, associate editor
Part Eight: Larynx/Hypopharynx, Trachea/Bronchus and Esophagus
John M. Fredrickson, editor
Bruce H. Haughey, associate editor
Part Nine: Thyroid/Parathyroid
John M. Fredrickson, editor
Bruce H. Haughey, associate editor

VOLUME FOUR
Part Ten: Ear and Cranial Base
Lee A. Harker, editor
Part Eleven: Vestibular System
Lee A. Harker, editor
Part Twelve: Facial Nerve
Lee A. Harker, editor
Part Thirteen: Auditory System
Lee A. Harker, editor
Part Fourteen: External Ear
Lee A. Harker, editor
Part Fifteen: Eustachian Tube, Middle Ear, and Mastoid
Lee A. Harker, editor
Part Sixteen: Inner Ear
Lee A. Harker, editor
Part Seventeen: Skull Base
Lee A. Harker, editor

VOLUME FIVE
Pediatric Otolaryngology
Mark A. Richardson, editor

VOLUME ONE

OTOLARYNGOLOGY HEAD & NECK SURGERY

THIRD EDITION

EDITED BY

Charles W. Cummings, M.D.
Andelot Professor and Chairman
Department of Otolaryngology-Head and Neck Surgery
Johns Hopkins University School of Medicine
Baltimore, Maryland

John M. Fredrickson, M.D.
Lindburg Professor and Head
Department of Otolaryngology
Washington University School of Medicine
St. Louis, Missouri

Lee A. Harker, M.D.
Deputy Director
Boys Town National Research Hospital
Vice Chairman
Department of Otolaryngology and Human Communication
Creighton University School of Medicine
Omaha, Nebraska

Charles J. Krause, M.D.
Professor
Department of Otolaryngology-Head and Neck Surgery
University of Michigan Medical School
Ann Arbor, Michigan

David E. Schuller, M.D.
Professor and Chairman
Department of Otolaryngology
Director, Arthur G. James Cancer Hospital and Research Institute
Co-Director, Comprehensive Cancer Center
The Ohio State University
Columbus, Ohio

Mark A. Richardson
Vice Chairman
Department of Otolaryngology-Head and Neck Surgery
Johns Hopkins University School of Medicine
Baltimore, Maryland

with 333 contributors
with 4061 illustrations, including 18 color plates

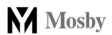 Mosby

St. Louis Baltimore Boston Carlsbad Chicago Minneapolis New York Philadelphia Portland
London Milan Sydney Tokyo Toronto

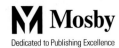

Publisher: Geoff Greenwood
Editor: Robert Hurley
Developmental Editor: Lauranne Billus
Associate Developmental Editor: Marla Sussman
Editorial Assistant: Jori Matison

Project Managers: Christopher Baumle, David Orzechowski
Senior Production Editor: Stacy M. Loonstyn
Production Editor: Susie Coladonato
Designer: Carolyn O'Brien
Manufacturing Manager: William A. Winneberger, Jr.

Third Edition
Copyright © 1998 by Mosby–Year Book, Inc.
Previous editions copyrighted 1986, 1993

Printed in the United States of America
Composition by Maryland Composition
Printing/binding by Maple Vail Book Manufacturing Group

Mosby–Year Book, Inc.
11830 Westline Industrial Drive
St. Louis, Missouri 63146

Library of Congress Cataloging-in-Publication Data

Otolaryngology—head and neck surgery / edited by Charles W. Cummings.
— 3rd ed.
    p.   cm.
  Includes bibliographical references and index.
  Contents: v. 1. General considerations in head and neck, face /
[edited by] Charles W. Cummings, Charles J. Krause — v. 2. Nose,
paranasal sinuses, salivary glands, oral
cavity/oropharynx/nasopharynx / [edited by] Charles J. Krause, David
E. Schuller — v. 3. Neck, larynx/hypopharynx, trachea/bronchus and
esophagus, thyroid/parathyroid / [edited by] David E. Schuller, John
M. Fredrickson — v. 4. General (ear and cranial base), vestibular
system, facial nerve, auditory system, external ear, eustachian
tube, middle ear, and mastoid, inner ear, skull base / [edited by]
Lee A. Harker — v. 5. Pediatric otolaryngology / [edited by] Mark
A. Richardson.
    ISBN 0-8151-2136-9 (set)
    1. Otolaryngology, Operative. 2. Head—Surgery. 3. Neck—
Surgery. I. Cummings, Charles W. (Charles William), 1935– .
    [DNLM: 1. Otorhinolaryngologic Diseases—surgery. WV 168 088
1998]
RF51.086   1998
617.5′ 1059—DC21
DNLM/DLC
for Library of Congress   98-2986
                                                        CIP

Figures 1, 2A, 2C, 3, 5 through 20, 22 through 26, 28, 29, and 31 in Chapter 56 are used with permission from Som PM, Curtin HD: *Head and neck imaging*, ed 3, St Louis, 1996, Mosby.

97 98 99 00 01 / 9 8 7 6 5 4 3 2 1

Associate Editors

Paul W. Flint, M.D.
Associate Professor
Department of Otolaryngology-Head and Neck Surgery
Johns Hopkins University School of Medicine
Baltimore, Maryland

Bruce H. Haughey, M.B., Ch.B.
Associate Professor
Department of Otolaryngology-Head and Neck Surgery
Washington University School of Medicine
Director
Division of Head and Neck Surgical Oncology
Barnes-Jewish Hospital
St. Louis Children's Hospital
St. Louis, Missouri

K. Thomas Robbins, M.D.
Professor and Chairman
Department of Otolaryngology-Head and Neck Surgery
University of Tennessee College of Medicine
Director
Head and Neck Oncology Program
Memphis, Tennessee

J. Regan Thomas, M.D.
Professor and Chairman
Department of Otolaryngology-Head and Neck Surgery
St. Louis University School of Medicine
Director
The Facial Plastic Surgery Center
St. Louis, Missouri

Contributors

Paul J. Abbas, Ph.D.
Professor
University of Iowa
Iowa City, Iowa

George L. Adams, M.D., F.A.C.S.
Professor and Head
Department of Otolaryngology
University of Minnesota
Minneapolis, Minnesota

David Albert, M.B., B.S., F.R.C.S.
Pediatric Otolaryngologist
Hospital for Sick Children
London, United Kingdom

James Alex, M.D.
Assistant Professor
Section of Otolaryngology
Director
Division of Facial Plastic and Reconstructive Surgery
Yale University School of Medicine
New Haven, Connecticut

Eugene L. Alford, M.D., F.A.C.S.
Assistant Professor
Department of Otorhinolaryngology
Baylor College of Medicine
Department of Dermatology and Division of Plastic Surgery
The Methodist Hospital and St. Luke's Hospital
Houston, Texas

Carl M. Allen, D.D.S., M.S.D.
Professor
Oral and Maxillofacial Pathology
Ohio State University
College of Dentistry
Columbus, Ohio

Mário Andrea, M.D., Ph.D.
Head and Chairman
Department of Otolaryngology
Faculty of Medicine
Lisbon, Portugal

Edward L. Applebaum, M.D.
Professor and Department Head
Department of Otolaryngology-Head and Neck Surgery
University of Illinois at Chicago
Chief of Service
Department of Otolaryngology-Head and Neck Surgery
University of Illinois Eye and Infirmary
Chicago, Illinois

Richard L. Arden, M.D., F.A.C.S.
Assistant Professor
Department of Otolaryngology-Head and Neck Surgery
Wayne State University
Detroit, Michigan

William B. Armstrong, M.D.
Adjunct Associate Professor
Department of Otolaryngology-Head and Neck Surgery
University of California, Irvine, College of Medicine
Orange, California

Moisés A. Arriaga, M.D., F.A.C.S.
Adjunct Associate Professor of Surgery
Otorhinolaryngology and Neurosurgery
Director
Hearing and Balance Center
Allegheny University of the Health Sciences
Associate Clinical Professor of Otolaryngology
University of Pittsburgh School of Medicine
Pittsburgh, Pennsylvania

H. Alexander Arts, M.D.
Assistant Professor
Division of Otology/Neurotology
Department of Otolaryngology-Head and Neck Surgery
University of Michigan
Ann Arbor, Michigan

Douglas Backous, M.D.
Otology, Neurotology and Skull Base Surgery
Virginia Mason Medical Center
Seattle, Washington

Shan R. Baker, M.D.
Professor of Otolaryngology
Chief, Division of Facial Plastic Surgery
University of Michigan Medical School
Ann Arbor, Michigan

Thomas Balkany, M.D., F.A.C.S., F.A.A.P.
Hotchkiss Professor and Vice-Chair
Department of Otolaryngology
Professor
Department of Neurological Surgery and Pediatrics
University of Miami School of Medicine
Director
University of Miami Ear Institute
Miami, Florida

Robert W. Baloh, M.D.
Professor of Neurology and Surgery (Head and Neck)
UCLA School of Medicine
Los Angeles, California

Fuad M. Baroody, M.D.
Assistant Professor of Otolaryngology-Head and Neck
Surgery and Pediatrics
University of Chicago, Pritzker School Of Medicine
Chicago, Illinois

Robert W. Bastian, M.D.
Associate Professor of Otolaryngology
Loyola University of Chicago Stritch School of Medicine
Chicago, Illinois

John G. Batsakis, M.D.
Professor and Chairman
Department of Pathology
University of Texas M.D. Anderson Cancer Center
Houston, Texas

Carol A. Bauer, M.D.
Assistant Professor
Division of Otolaryngology-Head and Neck Surgery
Southern Illinois University School of Medicine
Springfield, Illinois

Daniel G. Becker, M.D.
Instructor
Department of Otolaryngology
University of Pennsylvania
Philadelphia, Pennsylvania

Ferdinand F. Becker, M.D.
Clinical Assistant Professor
University of Florida College of Medicine
Medical Director
Facial Plastic Surgery Center, Inc.
Vero Beach, Florida

G. Jan Beekhuis, M.D.
Clinical Professor
Department of Otolaryngology
Wayne State University School of Medicine
Detroit, Michigan

Bruce Benjamin, F.R.A.C.S., D.L.O., F.A.A.P.
Clinical Professor
Department of Otolaryngology
University of Sydney
Royal Alexandra Hospital for Children
Royal North Shore Hospital
Sydney, Australia

Joseph E. Berg, M.D.
Fellow
Division of Plastic and Reconstructive Surgery
University of Missouri
Kansas City, Missouri

Carol M. Bier-Laning, M.D.
Assistant Professor
Department of Otorhinolaryngology
University of Texas Southwestern Medical Center
Dallas, Texas

James Blaugrund, M.D.
Instructor
Department of Otolaryngology-Head and Neck Surgery
Johns Hopkins University School of Medicine
Baltimore, Maryland

Andrew Blitzer, M.D., D.D.S.
Professor of Clinical Otolaryngology
Columbia University College of Physicians and Surgeons
Director
New York Center for Voice and Swallowing Disorders
New York, New York

George Gordon Blozis, D.D.S., M.S.
Professor Emeritus
Ohio State University College of Dentistry
Consultant
Dayton Virginia Medical Center
Columbus Children's Hospital
Columbus, Ohio

Charles D. Bluestone, M.D.
Eberly Professor of Pediatric Otolaryngology
University of Pittsburgh School of Medicine
Director of Pediatric Otolaryngology
Children's Hospital of Pittsburgh
Pittsburgh, Pennsylvania

Derald E. Brackmann, M.D.
Clinical Professor
Otolaryngology/Head and Neck Surgery and Neurosurgery
University of Southern California School of Medicine
President
House Ear Clinic, Inc.
Los Angeles, California

Gregory H. Branham, M.D., F.A.C.S.
Associate Professor
Department of Otolaryngology-Head and Neck Surgery
St. Louis University School of Medicine
St. Louis, Missouri

Mitchell F. Brin, M.D.
Associate Professor
Department of Neurology
Director
Division of Movement Disorders
Mt. Sinai Medical Center
New York, New York

Kenneth B. Briskin, M.D.
Attending Surgeon
Crozer-Chester Memorial Hospital
Riddle Memorial Hospital
Chester, Pennsylvania

Patrick E. Brookhouser, M.D.
Father Flanagan Professor and Chairman
Department of Otolaryngology and Human
    Communication
Creighton University School of Medicine
Director
Boys Town National Research Hospital
Omaha, Nebraska

Allan C. D. Brown, M.B., Ch.B., F.R.C.A.
Associate Professor
Departments of Anesthesiology and Otorhinolaryngology-
    Head and Neck Surgery
University of Michigan Medical School
Director
The Difficult Airway Clinic
University of Michigan Medical Center
Ann Arbor, Michigan

Karla Brown, M.D.
Fellow
Boston Children's Hospital
Harvard Medical Center
Boston, Massachusetts

Mark T. Brown, M.D.
Assistant Professor
Department of Otolaryngology-Head and Neck Surgery
Johns Hopkins University School of Medicine
Baltimore, Maryland

Orval E. Brown M.D.
Associate Professor
University of Texas Southwestern Medical Center at Dallas
Children's Medical Center of Dallas
Dallas, Texas

J. Dale Browne, M.D., F.A.C.S
Assistant Professor Of Otolaryngology
Bowman Gary School of Medicine of Wake Forest
    University
Winston-Salem, North Carolina

Daniel Buchbinder, M.D.
Associate Professor
Department of Oral, Maxillo-Facial Surgery and
    Otolaryngology
Mt. Sinai School of Medicine
Chief of Oral Maxillo-Facial Surgery
Mt. Sinai Medical Center
New York, New York

Robert M. Bumsted, M.D.
Professor
Department of Otolaryngology and Bronchoesophagology
Rush Medical College
Chicago, Illinois

Michael Cannito, Ph.D., CCC-SLP
Associate Professor
School of Audiology and Speech-Language Pathology
University of Memphis
Adjunct Associate Professor
Department of Otolaryngology-Head and Neck Surgery
University of Tennessee College of Medicine
Memphis, Tennessee

Roy D. Carlson, M.D.
Senior Clinical Instructor
Department of Otolaryngology
Temple University School of Medicine
Philadelphia, Pennsylvania
Memorial Hospital of Burlington County
Mt. Holly, New Jersey

Alan B. Carr, D.M.D., M.S.
Associate Professor
Director
Department of Maxillofacial Prosthetics
Ohio State University College of Dentistry
A.G. James Cancer Hospital and Research Institute
Columbus, Ohio

Roy R. Casiano, M.D.
Associate Professor
Department of Otolaryngology
University of Miami School of Medicine
Director
Center for Sinus and Voice Disorders
Sylvester Comprehensive Cancer Center
Miami, Florida

Sujana S. Chandrasekhar, M.D.
Assistant Professor of Clinical Surgery
University of Medicine and Dentistry of New Jersey-
    New Jersey Medical School
Director of Otology/Neurotology
University of Medicine and Dentistry of New Jersey-
    University Hospital
Newark, New Jersey

Mack L. Cheney, M.D.
Assistant Professor
Harvard Medical School
Director
Facial Plastic and Reconstructive Surgery
Massachusetts Eye and Ear Infirmary
Boston, Massachusetts

Sukgi S. Choi, M.D.
Assistant Professor
Department of Otolaryngology and Pediatrics
George Washington University
Children's National Medical Center
Washington, D.C.

Richard A. Chole, M.D., Ph.D.
Lindburg Professor and Head
Department of Otolaryngology-Head and Neck Surgery
Washington University School of Medicine
St. Louis, Missouri

Moo-Jin Choo, M.D.
Fellow
Department of Otolaryngology
University of California, Davis, Medical Center
Sacramento, California

James M. Chow, M.D.
Associate Professor
Loyola University
Loyola University Medical Center
Maywood, Illinois

John E. Clemons, M.D.
Clinic Instructor
University of Wisconsin
Madison, Wisconsin
Gundersen Lutheran Medical Center
LaCrosse, Wisconsin

Ross A. Clevens, M.D.
Director
The Center for Facial Cosmetic Surgery
Melbourne and Palm Bay, Florida

Lanny Garth Close, M.D.
Howard W. Smith Professor and Chairman
Department of Otolaryngology-Head and Neck Surgery
Columbia University College of Physicians and Surgeons
Director
Department of Otolaryngology-Head and Neck Surgery
Columbia Presbyterian Medical Center
New York, New York

D. Thane Cody, II, M.D.
Fellow in Head and Neck Oncologic and Microvascular
    Surgery
Department of Otolaryngology-Head and Neck Surgery
University of Iowa
Iowa City, Iowa

Noel L. Cohen, M.D.
Professor and Chairman
Department of Otolaryngology
New York University Hospital and Bellevue Hospital
New York, New York

Newton Coker, M.D.
Clinical Professor
Bobby R. Alford Department of Otorhinolaryngology and
    Communicative Sciences
Baylor College of Medicine
Director
Texas Center for Hearing and Balance
Houston, Texas

Jeffrey J. Colton, M.D.
Clinical Assistant Professor
Department of Otolaryngology
University of Michigan, Ann Arbor
Henry Ford Hospital
Detroit, Michigan

Philippe Contencin, M.D.
University of Paris
Hopital St. Vincent-De-Paul
Paris, France

Cheryl S. Cotter, M.D.
Fellow
Department of Pediatric Otolaryngology
Harvard Medical School
Boston Children's Hospital
Boston, Massachusetts

Robin T. Cotton, M.D.
Professor
Department of Otolaryngology and Maxillofacial Surgery
University of Cincinnati College of Medicine
Director
Department of Otolaryngology and Maxillofacial Surgery
Children's Hospital Medical Center
Cincinnati, Ohio

Marion E. Couch, M.D., Ph.D.
Assistant Professor
Johns Hopkins Hospital
Baltimore, Maryland

Mark S. Courey, M.D.
Assistant Professor
Department of Otolaryngology
Vanderbilt University
Medical Director
Vanderbilt Voice Center
St. Thomas Medical Center
Nashville, Tennessee

Roger L. Crumley, M.D.
Professor and Chairman
Department of Otolaryngology
University of California, Irvine, Medical Center
Orange, California

Bernard J. Cummings, M.B., Ch.B
Professor and Chair
Department of Radiation Oncology
University of Toronto
Chief
Department of Radiation Oncology
Princess Margaret Hospital
Toronto, Ontario, Canada

Charles W. Cummings, M.D.
Andelot Professor and Chairman
Department of Otolaryngology-Head and Neck Surgery
Johns Hopkins University School of Medicine
Baltimore, Maryland

Robert W. Dalley, M.D.
Associate Professor
Department of Radiology
University of Washington Medical Center
Seattle, Washington

Terence M. Davidson, M.D.
Professor
Department of Head and Neck Surgery
Associate Dean for Continuing Medical Education
University of California, San Diego, School of Medicine
San Diego, California

Larry E. Davis, M.D.
Professor of Neurology and Microbiology
University of New Mexico School of Medicine
Chief
Neurology Service
Albuquerque Veterans Administration Medical Center
Albuquerque, New Mexico

Antonio De La Cruz, M.D.
Clinical Professor
Department of Otolaryngology-Head and Neck Surgery
University of Southern California
Director of Education
House Ear Institute
Los Angeles, California

Steven R. DeMeester, M.D.
Assistant Professor
Department of Cardiothoracic Surgery
University of Southern California University Hospital
Los Angeles, California

Lawrence W. DeSanto, M.D.
Professor and Chairman Emeritus
Department of Otolaryngology-Head and Neck Surgery
Mayo Clinic
Scottsdale, Arizona

Leigh Anne Dew, M.D.
Resident Physician
University of Utah
Salt Lake City, Utah

Oscar Dias, M.D., Ph.D.
Assistant Professor
Department of Otolaryngology
Faculty of Medicine
Lisbon, Portugal

Robert A. Dobie, M.D.
Chairman and Thomas Walthall Folbre Professor
Department of Otolaryngology-Head and Neck Surgery
University of Texas Health Science Center
San Antonio, Texas

Timothy D. Doerr, M.D.
Department of Otolaryngology-Head and Neck Surgery
Wayne State University School of Medicine
Detroit, Michigan

Larry G. Duckert, M.D., Ph.D.
Professor
Department of Otolaryngology-Head and Neck Surgery
University of Washington School of Medicine
University of Washington Medical Center
Seattle, Washington

Newton O. Duncan, III, M.D.
Clinical Assistant Professor
Departments of Otorhinolaryngology and Pediatrics
Baylor College of Medicine
Co-Director
Texas Pediatric Otolaryngology Center
Houston, Texas

David W. Eisele, M.D.
Associate Professor
Department of Otolaryngology-Head and Neck Surgery
Johns Hopkins University School of Medicine
Director
Division of Head and Neck Surgery
Johns Hopkins Hospital
Baltimore, Maryland

Charles N. Ellis, M.D.
Professor and Associate Chair
Department of Dermatology
University of Michigan Medical School
Chief
Dermatology Service
Veterans Affairs Medical Center
Ann Arbor, Michigan

Jane M. Emanuel, M.D., F.A.C.S.
Assistant Professor
Department of Otolaryngology and Human Communication
Creighton University School of Medicine
Staff Otolaryngologist
Boys Town National Research Hospital
Omaha, Nebraska

Emily J. Erbelding, M.D., M.P.H.
Assistant Professor
Johns Hopkins University School of Medicine
Baltimore, Maryland

Ramon M. Esclamado, M.D.
Associate Professor
Department of Otolaryngology
Director
Division of Head and Neck Surgery
The Cleveland Clinic
Cleveland, Ohio

David N.F. Fairbanks, M.D.
Clinical Professor
Department of Otolaryngology
George Washington University School of Medicine
Sibley Memorial Hospital
Washington, D.C.

Michael L. Farrell, M.B.B.S., F.R.A.C.S.
Visiting Medical Officer
St. George Hospital
Liverpool Hospital
Sydney, New South Wales, Australia

Edward H. Farrior, M.D.
Clinical Associate Professor
University of South Florida
Tampa, Florida

Richard T. Farrior, M.D., F.A.C.S.
Clinical Professor
University of South Florida School of Medicine
Tampa, Florida
Clinical Professor
University of Florida School of Medicine
Gainesville, Florida

Willard E. Fee, Jr., M.D.
Edward C. and Amy H. Sewall Professor and Chairman
Stanford University Medical Center
Stanford, California

Berrylin J. Ferguson, M.D.
Assistant Professor
Department of Otolaryngology
University of Pittsburgh School of Medicine
Director
Sino-Nasal Disorders and Allergies
University of Pittsburgh Medical Center
Pittsburgh, Pennsylvania

Paul W. Flint, M.D.
Associate Professor
Department of Otolaryngology-Head and Neck Surgery
Johns Hopkins University School of Medicine
Baltimore, Maryland

Arlene A. Forastiere, M.D.
Associate Professor
Department of Medical Oncology
Johns Hopkins University
Baltimore, Maryland

L. Arick Forrest, M.D.
Assistant Professor
Department of Otolaryngology
Ohio State University
University Hospital Clinic
Columbus, Ohio

James W. Forsen, Jr., M.D.
Instructor
Pediatric Otolaryngology
Washington University School of Medicine
St. Louis, Missouri

Howard W. Francis, M.D.
Assistant Professor
Johns Hopkins University
Assistant Chief of Service
Johns Hopkins Hospital
Baltimore, Maryland

John M. Fredrickson, M.D.
Lindburg Professor and Head
Department of Otolaryngology
Washington University School of Medicine
Director
Implantable Hearing Aid Development Program
St. Louis, Missouri

John L. Frodel, M.D.
Associate Professor and Director
Division of Facial Plastic Surgery
Department of Otolaryngology-Head and Neck Surgery
John Hopkins University School of Medicine
Baltimore, Maryland

Nabil S. Fuleihan, M.D.
Chairman
Department of Otolaryngology-Head and Neck Surgery
Boston University Medical Center
Boston, Massachusetts

Ruth Gaare, J.D., M.P.H.
Academic Program Director
The Bioethics Institute
Johns Hopkins University
Baltimore, Maryland

Bruce J. Gantz, M.D.
Professor and Head
Department of Otolaryngology-Head and Neck Surgery
University of Iowa College of Medicine
Iowa City, Iowa

C. Gaelyn Garrett, M.D.
Assistant Professor
Department of Otolaryngology
Vanderbilt University Medical Center
Nashville, Tennessee

George A. Gates, M.D.
Professor
Department of Otolaryngology-Head and Neck Surgery
University of Washington School of Medicine
Director
Virginia Merrill Bloedel Hearing Research Center
Seattle, Washington

Scott M. Gayner, M.D.
Instructor in Otorhinolaryngology
Mayo Clinic
Rochester, Minnesota

Eric M. Genden, M.D.
St. Louis, Missouri

Douglas A. Girod, M.D.
Assistant Professor and Vice Chairman
Chief
Department of Otolaryngology
Veteran's Administration Medical Center
Kansas City, Missouri

Harvey S. Glazer, M.D.
Professor of Radiology
Washington University School of Medicine
St. Louis, Missouri

Jack L. Gluckman, M.D.
Professor and Chairman
Department of Otolaryngology-Head and Neck Surgery
University of Cincinnati
Cincinnati, Ohio

George S. Goding, Jr., M.D.
Associate Professor
University of Minnesota
Minneapolis Veterans Administration Medical Center
Minneapolis, Minnesota

W. Jarrard Goodwin, Jr., M.D., F.A.C.S.
Sylvester Professor and Chairman
Department of Otolaryngology
University of Miami School of Medicine
Director
Sylvester Comprehensive Cancer Center
University of Miami Hospitals and Clinics
Jackson Memorial Hospital
Miami, Florida

Michael P. Gorga, Ph.D.
Professor
Department of Otolaryngology and Human Communication
Creighton University School of Medicine
Director
Clinical Sensory Physiology Laboratory
Boys Town National Research Hospital
Omaha, Nebraska

H. Devon Graham, III, M.D., F.A.C.S.
Clinical Assistant Professor
Department of Otolaryngology-Head and Neck Surgery
Tulane University School of Medicine
New Orleans, Louisiana

Daniel O. Graney, M.D.
Associate Professor
Department of Biological Structure
University of Washington School of Medicine
Seattle, Washington

Steven D. Gray, M.D.
Associate Professor
University of Utah School Of Medicine
Primary Children's Medical Center
Alta View Hospital
Salt Lake City, Utah

William C. Gray, M.D.
Associate Professor
Department of Otolaryngology-Head and Neck Surgery
University of Maryland School of Medicine
Baltimore, Maryland

Roy C. Grekin, M.D.
Assistant Professor
Department of Dermatology
University of Michigan Medical School
Ann Arbor, Michigan

Andrew J. Griffith, M.D., Ph.D.
Chief Resident
Department of Otolaryngology-Head and Neck Surgery
University of Michigan Hospitals
Ann Arbor, Michigan

Kenneth M. Grundfast, M.D.
Professor of Otolaryngology and Pediatrics
Georgetown University School of Medicine
Washington, D.C.

Jerry Thomas Guy, M.D.
Clinical Professor of Medicine
Ohio State University
Director of Oncology
Park Medical Center
Regional Oncology Center at Park
Columbus, Ohio

Joseph Haddad, Jr., M.D.
Associate Professor and Vice Chairman
Department of Otolaryngology-Head and Neck Surgery
Columbia University College of Physicians and Surgeons
Director
Pediatric Otolaryngology-Head and Neck Surgery
Babies and Children's Hospital
New York, New York

Jeffrey R. Haller, M.D.
Assistant Professor
Division of Otolaryngology
University of Utah School of Medicine
Salt Lake City, Utah

Ronald C. Hamaker, M.D.
Physician
Head and Neck Surgery Associates
Indianapolis, Indiana

Ehab Y. Hanna, M.D.
Assistant Professor
Department of Otolaryngology-Head and Neck Surgery
University of Arkansas for Medical Science
Little Rock, Arkansas

Lee A. Harker, M.D.
Deputy Director
Boys Town National Research Hospital
Vice Chairman
Department of Otolaryngology and Human
    Communication
Creigton University School of Medicine
Omaha, Nebraska

Stephen G. Harner, M.D.
Professor of Otolaryngology
Mayo Medical School
Consultant, Department of Otolaryngology
Mayo Clinic
Rochester, Minnesota

Jeffrey P. Harris, M.D., Ph.D.
Chief of the Division of Head and Neck Surgery
University of California
San Diego, California

Donald F.N. Harrison, M.D., M.S., Ph.D., F.R.C.S.
Emeritus Professor
Departments of Laryngology and Otology
University of London
Royal National ENT Hospital
London, England

Bruce H. Haughey, M.B., Ch.B.
Associate Professor
Department of Otolaryngology
Washington University School of Medicine
Director
Division of Head and Neck Surgical Oncology
Barnes-Jewish Hospital
St. Louis Children's Hospital
St. Louis, Missouri

Gerald B. Healy, M.D.
Professor of Otology and Laryngology
Harvard Medical School
Otolaryngologist-in-Chief, Surgeon-in-Chief
Children's Hospital
Boston, Massachusetts

Arden K. Hegtvedt, D.D.S.
Assistant Professor
Department of Oral and Maxillofacial Surgery
Ohio State University
Columbus, Ohio

Jay P. Heiken, M.D.
Professor
Department of Radiology
Director
Abdominal Imaging
Co-Director
Body Computed Tomography
Mallinckrodt Institute of Radiology
Washington University School of Medicine
St. Louis, Missouri

David A. Hendrick, M.D.
Clinical Instructor
Veterans Administration Hospital
Denver, Colorado
Private Practice
Vail, Colorado

Hajime Hirose, M.D., D.M.Sc.
Professor
Department of Otolaryngology
School of Allied Health Sciences
Kitasato University and Univeristy Hospital
Sagamihara, Japan

William E. Hitselberger, M.D.
Neurosurgeon
St. Vincent's Hospital
Los Angeles, California

Henry T. Hoffman, M.D.
Associate Professor
Department of Otolaryngology
University of Iowa College of Medicine
Iowa City, Iowa

Lauren D. Holinger, M.D., F.A.C.S, F.A.A.P.
Professor
Department of Otolaryngology
Northwestern University School of Medicine
Head
Pediatric Otolaryngology
Children's Memorial Hospital
Chicago, Illinois

David B. Hom, M.D., F.A.C.S
Assistant Professor
Division of Facial Plastic and Reconstructive Surgery
Department of Otolaryngology-Head and Neck Surgery
University of Minnesota School of Medicine
Associate Physician
Department of Otoalryngology-Head and Neck Surgery
Facial Plastic Surgery
Hennepin County Medical Center
Minneapolis, Minnesota

Vicente Honrubia, M.D.
Professor and Director of Research
Division of Head and Neck Surgery
The Center of the Health Sciences
University of California
Los Angeles, California

John W. House, M.D.
Clinical Professor
Department of Otolaryngology
University of Southern California School of Medicine
House Ear Clinic
Los Angeles, California

Andrew F. Inglis, Jr., M.D.
Associate Professor
Department of Otolaryngology
University of Washington
Children's Hospital and Medical Center
Seattle, Washington

Robert K. Jackler, M.D.
Professor of Otolaryngology and Neurological Surgery
University of California Medical Center
San Francisco, California

John R. Jacobs, M.D.
Professor
Department of Otolaryngology and Radiation Therapy
Wayne State University School of Medicine
Director
Head and Neck Cancer Program
Karmanos Cancer Center
Detroit, Michigan

Ivo P. Janecka, M.D., F.A.C.S.
Director, Longwood Skull Base Program
Departments of Otolaryngology, Neurosurgery and Plastic
   Surgery
Harvard Medical School
Boston, Massachusetts

Pawel J. Jastreboff, M.D.
Professor
Department of Surgery and Physiology
University of Maryland School of Medicine
Director
University of Maryland Tinnitus and Hyperacusis Center
Baltimore, Maryland

Virginia W. Jenison, M.A.
Clinical Instructor
Department of Otolaryngology-Head and Neck Surgery
Washington University School of Medicine
St. Louis, Missouri

Herman Jenkins, M.D.
Professor
Baylor College of Medicine
Houston, Texas

Calvin M. Johnson, Jr., M.D.
Director
Hedgewood Surgical Center
New Orleans, Louisiana

Jonas T. Johnson, M.D.
Professor and Vice Chairman
Department of Otolaryngology
Director
Division of Head and Neck Oncology and Immunology
University of Pittsburgh School of Medicine
Pittsburgh, Pennsylvania

Timothy M. Johnson, M.D.
Assistant Professor
Department of Dermatology, Otolaryngology, Surgery
University of Michigan
Director
Cutaneous Surgery and Oncology Unit
Ann Arbor, Michigan

Kim Richard Jones, M.D., Ph.D.
Assistant Professor
Division of Otolaryngology-Head and Neck Surgery
University of North Carolina School of Medicine
University of North Carolina Hospitals
Chapel Hill, North Carolina

Sheldon S. Kabaker, M.D., F.A.C.S.
Associate Clinical Professor
Division of Facial Plastic Surgery
Department of Otolaryngology
University of California
San Francisco, California

Joel C. Kahane, M.D.
Professor
Director
Anatomical Sciences Laboratory
School of Audiology and Speech-Language Pathology
University of Memphis
Memphis, Tennessee

Michael Kaliner, M.D.
Clinical Professor
George Washington University School of Medicine
Medical Director
Institute of Asthma and Allergy
Washington Hospital/George Washington University
Washington, D.C.

William J. Kane, M.D.
Assistant Professor
Department of Plastic and Reconstructive Surgery
Mayo Clinic
Rochester, Minnesota

Dan H. Kelly, Ph.D.
Associate Professor
Department of Otolaryngology-Head and Neck Surgery
University of Cincinnati College of Medicine
Voice Pathologist
Barrett Cancer Center
ENT Voice Center
Cincinnati, Ohio

Eugene B. Kern, M.D.
Professor
Department of Otorhinolaryngologic Surgery
Endicott Professor of Medicine
Mayo Medical School
Mayo Clinic
Rochester, Minnesota

Robert C. Kern, M.D.
Assistant Professor
Northwestern Medical School
Northwestern Memorial Hospital
Chicago, Illinois

Maurice Morad Khosh, M.D.
Assistant Clinical Professor
Department of Otolaryngology-Head and Neck Surgery
Columbia University School of Medicine
St. Luke's/Roosevelt Hospital Center
New York, New York

S. Khosla, M.D.
Resident
Department of Otolaryngology
Washington University School of Medicine
St. Louis, Missouri

Paul R. Kileny, Ph.D.
Professor
Department of Otolaryngology
University of Michigan Medical School
Director
Audiology and Electrophysiology
University of Michigan Health Systems
Ann Arbor, Michigan

Sam E. Kinney, M.D.
Clinical Associate Professor
Department of Otolaryngology-Head and Neck Surgery
Case Western Reserve University
Head
Section of Otology and Neurotology
Cleveland Clinic Foundation
Cleveland, Ohio

Wayne Martin Koch, M.D.
Associate Professor
Department of Otolaryngology-Head and Neck Surgery
Johns Hopkins University and Hospital
Baltimore, Maryland

James A. Koufman, M.D.
Director
Center for Voice Disorders
Professor
Department of Otolaryngology
Bowman Gray School of Medicine
Wake Forest University Medical Center
Winston-Salem, North Carolina

Frederick K. Kozak, M.D., F.R.C.S.C.
Assistant Professor
University of British Columbia
Pediatric Otolaryngologist
B.C. Children's Hospital
Vancouver, British Columbia, Canada

Eric H. Kraut, M.D.
Professor of Medicine
Ohio State University
Arthur James Cancer Hospital Research Institute
Columbus, Ohio

Dario Kunar, M.D.
Instructor
Department of Otolaryngology-Head and Neck Surgery
Johns Hopkins University School of Medicine
Baltimore, Maryland

Ollivier Laccourreye, M.D.
Department of Otolaryngology-Head and Neck Surgery
Laennec Hospital
University of Rene-Descartes
Paris, France

Paul R. Lambert, M.D.
Professor, Director
Division of Otolaryngology-Neurology
Department Otolaryngology-Head and Neck Surgery
University of Virginia Medical Center
Richmond, Virginia

George E. Laramore, M.D., Ph.D.
Professor
Department of Radiation Oncology
University of Washington
Vice Chairman
Department of Radiation Oncology
University Medical Center
Seattle, Washington

Peter E. Larsen, D.D.S.
Associate Professor
Oral and Maxillofacial Surgery
Ohio State University
College of Dentistry
Columbus, Ohio

Daniel M. Laskin, D.D.S., M.S.
Professor and Chairman
Department Oral and Maxillofacial Surgery
Medical College of Virginia
Virginia Commonwealth University
Director
Temporomandibular Joint and Facial Pain Research Center
Richmond, Virginia

Richard E. Latchaw, M.D.
Professor
Department of Radiology and Neurosurgery
Chief, Interventional Neuroradiology Section
University of Miami School of Medicine
Miami, Florida

Susanna Leighton, B.Sc., F.R.C.S. (Orl)
Pediatric Otolaryngologist
Hospital for Sick Children
London, England

Donald Leopold, M.D.
Associate Professor
Johns Hopkins University
Department of Otolaryngology-Head and Neck Surgery
Baltimore, Maryland

Greg R. Licameli, M.D.
Assistant Professor
Director of Pediatric Otolaryngology
Department of Otolaryngology-Head and Neck Surgery
University of Illinois at Chicago
Chicago, Illinois

William H. Liggett, Jr., M.D., D.M.D., D.M.S.C.
Senior Clinical Fellow in Medical Oncology
Johns Hopkins School of Medicine
Baltimore, Maryland

Raleigh E. Lingeman, M.D.
Betty Morgan Professor
Department of Otolaryngology-Head and Neck Surgery
Indiana University School of Medicine
Indianapolis, Indiana

Neal M. Lofchy M.D., F.R.C.S.C.
Clinical Instructor
Rush Medical College
Rush-Presbyterian-St. Luke's Medical Center
Chicago, Illinois

Jeri Logemann, Ph.D.
Ralph and Jean Sundin Professor
Department of Communication Sciences and Disorders
Professor
Departments of Head and Neck Surgery and
  Neurology and Dental Prosthetics
Northwestern University Medical School
Director
Speech, Voice and Swallowing Service
Northwestern Memorial Hospital
Chicago, Illinois

Brenda L. Lonsbury-Martin, Ph.D.
Chandler Professor
Director of Research
Department of Otolaryngology Research Laboratories
University of Miami Ear Institute
University of Miami School of Medicine
Miami, Florida

Rodney P. Lusk, M.D.
Associate Professor
Department of Otolaryngology
Washington University School of Medicine
Otolaryngologist-in-Chief
St. Louis Children's Hospital
St. Louis, Missouri

Joseph P. Lynch, III, M.D.
Professor
Department of Internal Medicine
Division of Pulmonary and Critical Care Medicine
University of Michigan Medical Center
Ann Arbor, Michigan

Anna Lysakowski, Ph.D.
Assistant Professor
Department of Anatomy and Cell Biology
University of Illinois
Chicago, Illinois

Richard L. Mabry, M.D.
Professor
Department of Otorhinolaryngology
University of Texas Southwestern Medical Center
Dallas, Texas

Michael R. Macdonald, M.D., F.R.C.S.C.
Chief
Division of Head and Neck Surgery
Alameda County Hospital
Oakland, California
Director
Aesthetic Surgery Center
San Francisco, California

Eileen M. Mahoney, M.C., U.S.A., M.D.
Pediatric Staff
Otolaryngology Section
Brook Army Medical Center
Fort Sam
Houston, Texas

Robert H. Maisel, M.D.
Professor
Department of Otolaryngology
University of Minnesota
Chief
Department of Otolaryngology-Head and Neck Surgery
Facial Plastic Surgery
Hennepin County Medical Center
Minneapolis, Minnesota

Patrizia Mancini, M.D.
Policlinico Umberto
Ear Nose and Throat Department
University "La Sapienza"
Rome, Italy

Lee M. Mandel, M.D.
Co-Director
Head and Neck-Facial Plastic Surgery Associates of South
  Florida
Plantation, Florida

Scott C. Manning, M.D.
Associate Professor
Department of Otolaryngology-Head and Neck Surgery
University of Washington School of Medicine
Chief, Pediatric Otolaryngology-Head and Neck Surgery
Children's Hospital and Medical Center
Seattle, Washington

Lawrence J. Marentette, M.D.
Associate Professor
Director
Cranial Base Program
Department of Otolaryngology
University of Michigan
Ann Arbor, Michigan

James E. Marks, M.D.
Radiation Oncologist
Missouri Baptist Medical Center
St. Louis, Missouri

Bernard R. Marsh, M.D.
Professor
Department of Otolaryngology-Head and Neck Surgery
Johns Hopkins University
Johns Hopkins Hospital
Baltimore, Maryland

Michael Marsh, M.D.
The Holt-Krock Clinic
Ear, Nose and Throat
Fort Smith, Arkansas

Glen K. Martin, Ph.D.
Professor
Department of Otolaryngology
University of Miami Ear Institute
Miami, Florida

Robert H. Mathog, M.D.
Professor and Chairman
Wayne State University
Harper Hospital
Detroit, Michigan

Douglas E. Mattox, M.D.
Professor and Head
Department of Otolaryngology-Head and Neck Surgery
Emory University
Atlanta, Georgia

Ernest L. Mazzaferri, M.D., F.A.C.P.
Professor and Chairman
Ohio State University
Columbus, Ohio

Thomas V. McCaffrey, M.D., Ph.D.
Professor
Mayo Medical School
Consultant
Department of Otorhinolaryngology
Mayo Clinic
Rochester, Minnesota

Robert A. McCrea, Ph.D.
Associate Professor
Department of Pharmacological and Physiological Sciences
University of Chicago
Chicago, Illinois

Timothy M. McCulloch, M.D.
Associate Professor
Department of Otolaryngology-Head and Neck Surgery
University of Iowa College of Medicine
Iowa City, Iowa

Thomas J. McDonald, M.D., M.S., F.A.C.S., F.R.C.S. Irel.
Professor
Department of Otolaryngology
Mayo Medical School
Chairman
Department of Otorhinolaryngology
Mayo Clinic and Foundation
Rochester, Minnesota

John T. McElveen, Jr., M.D.
Head
Otology-Neurotology
Carolina Ear and Hearing Clinic
Director
Carolina Ear Research Institute
Raleigh Community Hospital
Rex Hospital
Wake Medical Center
Raleigh, North Carolina

Trevor J.I. McGill, M.D.
Associate Professor
Department of Otolaryngology
Harvard Medical School
Clinical Director of Otolaryngology
The Children's Hospital
Boston, Massachusetts

W. Frederick McGuirt, Sr., M.D.
Professor
Department of Otolaryngology
Bowman Gray School of Medicine
Wake Forest University
Winston-Salem, North Carolina

Christine M. Menapace, M.A.
U.S. Clinical Manager
Symphonix Devices, Inc.
San Jose, California

Saumil N. Merchant, M.D.
Assistant Professor
Department of Otology and Laryngology
Harvard Medical School
Massachusetts Eye and Ear Infirmary
Boston, Massachusetts

Charles A. Miller, Ph.D.
Assistant Research Scientist
Department of Otolaryngology-Head and Neck Surgery
University of Iowa
Iowa City, Iowa

Lloyd B. Minor, M.D.
Associate Professor
Department of Otolaryngology-Head and Neck Surgery
Johns Hopkins University
School of Medicine
Baltimore, Maryland

Mahmood Moosa, M.D.
Clinical Fellow In Endocrinology
Ohio State University, College of Medicine
Ohio State University Medical Center
Columbus, Ohio

Jeffrey Morray, M.D.
Professor
Department of Anesthesiology and Pediatrics
University of Washington School of Medicine
Director
Department of Anesthesia and Critical Care
Children's Hospital and Medical Center
Seattle, Washington

Michael R. Morris, M.D., F.A.C.S.
Staff Otolaryngologist
Moore Regional Hospital
Pinehurst Surgical Clinic
Pinehurst, North Carolina

John B. Mulliken, M.D.
Associate Professor of Surgery
Harvard Medical School
Director
Craniofacial Center
Division of Plastic Surgery
The Children's Hospital
Boston, Massachusetts

Craig S. Murakami, M.D.
Associate Professor
Department of Otolaryngology/Head and Neck Surgery
University of Washington School of Medicine
Seattle, Washington

Alan D. Murray, M.D.
Assistant Professor
Department of Otorhinolaryngology
University of Texas Southwestern Medical Center
Attending Physician
Children's Medical Center of Dallas
Dallas, Texas

Charles M. Myer, III, M.D.
Professor
Department of Otolaryngology and Maxillofacial Surgery
University of Cincinnati College of Medicine
Professor
Department of Otolaryngology and Maxillofacial Surgery
Children's Hospital Medical Center
Cincinnati, Ohio

Eugene N. Myers, M.D.
Professor and Chairman
Department of Otolaryngology
University of Pittsburgh School of Medicine
University of Pittsburgh Medical Center
Pittsburgh, Pennsylvania

Robert M. Naclerio, M.D.
Professor and Chief
Otolaryngology-Head and Neck Surgery
University of Chicago Pritzker School of Medicine
Chicago, Illinois

Joseph B. Nadol, Jr., M.D.
Walter Augustus Lecompte Professor and Chairman
Department of Otology and Laryngology
Harvard Medical School
Chief of Otolaryngology
Massachusetts Eye and Ear Infirmary
Boston, Massachusetts

Philippe Narcy, M.D.
Professeur of Otorhinology
Universite Paris VII
Chief
Department of Pediatric Otorhinolaryngology
Hopital Robert Debre
Paris, France

Julian Nedzelski, M.D., F.A.C.S. (C)
Otolaryngologist in Chief
Sunnybrook Health Science Centre
Professor and Chairman
Department of Otolaryngology
University of Toronto
Toronto, Ontario, Canada

H. Bryan Neel, III, M.D., Ph.D.
Professor and Past Chairman
Mayo Medical School
Consultant
Mayo Clinic
Rochester, Minnesota

John Niparko, M.D.
Professor
Department of Otolaryngology-Head and Neck Surgery
Director of Otology/ Neurotology
Johns Hopkins University School of Medicine
Baltimore, Maryland

Daniel W. Nuss, M.D., F.A.C.S.
Professor and Chairman
Department of Otolaryngology-Head and Neck Surgery
Louisiana State University School of Medicine
New Orleans, Louisiana

Rick M. Odland, M.D, Ph.D., F.A.C.S.
Assistant Professor
Division of Facial, Plastic and Reconstructive Surgery
Department of Otolaryngology-Head and Neck Surgery
University of Minnesota School of Medicine
Hennepin County Medical Center
Minneapolis, Minnesota

Michael J. O'Leary, M.D.
Assistant Clinical Professor of Surgery
Uniformed Services University of the Health Sciences
Chief
Neurotology/Skull Base Surgery Division
Department of Otolaryngology
Navy Medical Center
San Diego, California

Patrick J. Oliverio, M.D.
Instructor
Department of Diagnostic Radiology and Neuroradiology
Johns Hopkins Medical Institution
Staff Neuroradiologist
Radiological Consultants Association
Fairmount, Wisconsin

Bert W. O'Malley, Jr., M.D.
Associate Professor
Department of Otolaryngology-Head and Neck Surgery
Department of Oncology
Johns Hopkins University School of Medicine
Baltimore, Maryland

Lisa A. Orloff, M.D.
Associate Professor of Surgery
University of California, San Diego, Medical Center
San Diego, California

Rosemary J. Orr, M.D.
Clinical Associate Professor
University of Washington
Associate Clinical Director of Operating Room
Children's Hospital Medical Center
Seattle, Washington

Robert H. Ossoff, D.M.D., M.D.
Guy M. Maness Professor and Chairman
Associate Vice Chancellor for Health Affairs
Chief of Staff
Vanderbilt University Hospital
Executive Medical Director
Vanderbilt Voice Center
Nashville, Tennessee

Steven Otto, M.A.
Audiologist and Coordinator
Brain Stem Implant Project
House Ear Institute
Los Angeles, California

John F. Pallanch, M.D., M.S.
The Midlands Clinic
Sioux City, Iowa

William R. Panje, M.D.
Professor and Director
Head and Neck Reconstruction and Skull Base Surgery
Rush-Presbyterian-St. Luke's Medical Center
Chicago, Illinois

Stephen S. Park, M.D., F.A.C.S.
Director
Division of Facial, Plastic and Reconstructive Surgery
Department of Otolaryngology-Head and Neck Surgery
University of Virginia
Charlottesville, Virginia

Carl Patow, M.D., M.P.H., F.A.C.S.
Associate Professor
Johns Hopkins School of Medicine
Baltimore, Maryland

G. Alexander Patterson, M.D.
Joseph C. Bancroft Professor of Surgery
Washington University School of Medicine
Barnes-Jewish Hospital
St. Louis, Missouri

Larry J. Peterson, D.D.S.
Professor
Department of Oral-Maxillofacial Surgery
Ohio State University
Ohio State University Hospitals
Columbus, Ohio

Guy I. Petruzzelli, M.D., Ph.D.
Assistant Professor
Department of Otolaryngology-Head and Neck Surgery
Loyola University Hospital/Medical Center
Maywood, Illinois

Jay F. Piccirillo, M.D.
Assistant Professor
Department of Otolaryngology
Washington University School of Medicine
Barnes-Jewish Hospital
St. Louis, Missouri

Catherine A. Picken, M.D., F.A.C.S.
Assistant Professor
Department of Otolaryngology-Head and Neck Surgery
Georgetown University Medical Center
Washington Hospital Center
Washington, D.C.

Judy Pinborough-Zimmerman, Ph.D.
Adjunct Faculty
Department of Communicative Disorders
University of Utah
Program Director
Child Development Clinic
Utah Department of Health
Salt Lake City, Utah

Jennifer Parker Porter, M.D.
Resident
Department of Otorhinolaryngology
Baylor College of Medicine
Houston, Texas

Gregory N. Postma, M.D.
Assistant Professor
Department of Otolaryngology
Center for Voice Disorders of Wake Forest University
North Carolina Baptist Hospital
Winston-Salem, North Carolina

William P. Potsic, M.D.
Professor of Otorhinolaryngology Head and Neck Surgery
University of Pennsylvania School of Medicine
Director
Pediatric Otolaryngology and Human Communication
Children's Hospital of Philadelphia
Philadelphia, Pennsylvania

Frederic A. Pugliano, M.D.
Resident Physician
Washington University
Resident Physician
Barnes Hospital
St. Louis, Missouri

Vito C. Quatela, M.D.
Associate Professor
University of Rochester School of Medicine and Dentistry
Clinical Instructor
Strong Memorial Hospital Medical Center
Rochester, New York

Leslie E. Quint, M.D.
Department of Radiology
University of Michigan Medical Center
Ann Arbor, Michigan

C. Rose Rabinov, M.D.
Fellow
Department of Facial Plastic and Reconstructive Surgery
University of California, Irvine
Orange, California

Gordon D. Raphael, M.D.
Associate Clinical Professor
George Washington University School of Medicine
Washington, D.C.

Christopher Rassekh, M.D.
Assistant Professor
Department of Otolaryngology-Head and Neck Surgery
University of Texas Medical School at Galveston
Galveston, Texas

Elie E. Rebeiz, M.D.
Associate Professor
Tufts University School of Medicine
Director
Head and Neck Surgery
Tufts-New England Medical Center
Boston, Massachusetts

Lou Reinisch, Ph.D.
Assistant Professor and Director of Laser Research
Department of Otolaryngology
Vanderbilt University Medical Center
Nashville, Tennessee

Bradford D. Ress, M.D.
Chief Resident
Department of Otolaryngology
University of Miami School of Medicine
Miami, Florida

Dale H. Rice, M.D.
Tiber/Alpert Professor and Chair
Department of Otolaryngology-Head and Neck Surgery,
University of Southern California School of Medicine
Los Angeles, California

Brock D. Ridenour, M.D.
Assistant Professor and Director
Facial Plastic Surgery Division
Washington University School of Medicine
Barnes-Jewish Hospital
St. Louis, Missouri

K. Thomas Robbins, M.D., F.R.C.S.C., F.A.C.S.
Professor and Chairman
Department of Otolaryngology-Head and Neck Surgery
University of Tennessee, Memphis College of Medicine
Director
Head and Neck Oncology Program
Memphis, Tennessee

William D. Robertson, M.D.
Professor
Department of Radiology
University of Washington Medical Center
Seattle, Washington

Robert A. Robinson, M.D., Ph.D.
Professor
Department of Pathology
University of Iowa College of Medicine
Iowa City, Iowa

J. Thomas Roland, Jr., M.D.
Assistant Professor
Department of Otolaryngology
New York University School of Medicine
Bellevue Hospital
Manhattan VA Medical Center
New York, New York

Anne M. Rompalo, M.D.
Associate Professor
Johns Hopkins University School of Medicine
Johns Hopkins Hospital
Baltimore, Maryland

Richard M. Rosenfeld, M.D., M.P.H.
Associate Professor
Department of Otolaryngology
SUNY Health Science Center at Brooklyn
Director of Pediatric Otolaryngology
University Hospital Brooklyn and The Long Island College
   Hospital
Brooklyn, New York

Jay T. Rubinstein, M.D., Ph.D.
Assistant Professor
Department of Otolaryngology-Head and Neck Surgery
   and Physiology and Biophysics
University of Iowa
Iowa City, Iowa

Stephen J. Salzer, M.D.
Clinical Instructor in Surgery
Department of Otolaryngology
Yale University School of Medicine
New Haven, Connecticut

Peter A. Santi, Ph.D.
Professor
Departments of Otolaryngology and Neuroscience
University of Minnesota
Minneapolis, Minnesota

Clarence T. Sasaki, M.D.
Charles W. Ohse Professor
Yale School of Medicine
New Haven, Connecticut

Gordon H. Sasaki, M.D.
Chief, Plastic Surgery Section
St. Luke Medical Center
Pasadena, California

Steven D. Schaefer, M.D.
Professor and Chair
Department of Otolaryngology
New York Medical College
Chair
Department of Otolaryngology
New York Eye and Ear Infirmary and Affiliated Hospitals
Valhalla, New York

David Arthur Schessel, M.D., Ph.D.
Assistant Professor
Department of Otolaryngology and Neurosurgery
George Washington University
Assistant Professor
George Washington University Hospital
Washington, D.C.

David E. Schuller, M.D.
Professor and Chairman
Department of Otolaryngology
The Ohio State University
Director
Arthur G. James Cancer Hospital and Research Institute
Columbus, Ohio

Timothy A. Scott, M.D.
Private Practice
John Muir Hospital
Walnut Creek, California

Roy B. Sessions, M.D.
Professor and Chairman,
Department Otolaryngology-Head and Neck Surgery
Georgetown University
Washington, D.C.

Larry R. Severeid, M.D.
Clinical Assistant Professor
University of Wisconsin-Madison Medical School
Gunderson Clinic
LaCrosse, Wisconsin

Robert V. Shannon, Ph.D.
Head
Department of Auditory Implants and Perception
House Ear Institute
Los Angeles, California

Stanley M. Shapshay M.D., F.A.C.S.
Professor
Department Otolaryngology-Head and Neck Surgery
Tufts University School of Medicine
Otolaryngologist-in-Chief (Chairman)
Tufts-New England Medical Center
Boston, Massachusetts

Pramod K. Sharma, M.D.
Oncologic Surgery Fellow
Department of Otolaryngology
Ohio State University Medical Center
Columbus, Ohio

Clough Shelton, M.D., F.A.C.S.
Associate Professor
University of Utah, School of Medicine
Salt Lake City, Utah

Neil T. Shepard, Ph.D.
Associate Professor
Department of Otolaryngology
University of Michigan Medical School
Director
Vestibular Testing Center
University of Michigan Hospital and Clinics
Ann Arbor, Michigan

David A. Sherris, M.D.
Assistant Professor
Mayo Medical School
Senior Associate Consultant
Mayo Clinic
Rochester, Minnesota

Kevin A. Shumrick, M.D.
Associate Professor
Department of Clinical Otolaryngology
University of Cincinnati College of Medicine
Director
Division of Facial Plastic and Maxillofacial Trauma
University Hospital
Cincinnati, Ohio

Kathleen C.Y. Sie, M.D.
Assistant Professor
Department of Otolaryngology-Head and Neck Surgery
University of Washington School of Medicine
Children's Hospital and Medical Center
Seattle, Washington

Robert W. Seibert, M.D.
Professor
Department of Otolaryngology-Head and Neck Surgery
University of Arkansas for Medical Sciences
Chief, Pediatric Otolaryngology
Arkansas Children's Hospital
Little Rock, Arkansas

Marilyn J. Siegel, M.D.
Professor
Department of Radiology and Pediatrics
Washington University School of Medicine
St. Louis, Missouri

Patricia Silva, M.D.
Clinical Assistant Professor
Department of Radiology
University of Miami School of Medicine
Miami, Florida

Jonas Singer, M.D.
Visiting Professor
Mallinckrudt Institute of Radiology, St. Louis Program
Alton Memorial Hospital
Alton, Illinois

Margaret W. Skinner, Ph.D.
Professor
Director of Adult Cochlear Implant Program
Department of Otolaryngology-Head and Neck Surgery
Washington University School of Medicine
St. Louis, Missouri

Richard J.H. Smith, M.D.
Professor and Vice-Chairman
Department of Otolaryngology-Head and Neck Surgery
University of Iowa College of Medicine
Head
Division of Pediatric Otolaryngology
Director
Molecular Otolaryngology Research Laboratories
Iowa City, Iowa

Gordon B. Snow, M.D.
Professor and Chairman
Department of Otolaryngology-Head and Neck Surgery
Free University Hospital
Amsterdam, Netherlands

Robert C. Sprecher, M.D.
Assistant Professor
Departments of Otolaryngology and Pediatrics
Rainbow Babies and Children's Hospital
Case Western Reserve University
Cleveland, Ohio

Steven J. Staller, Ph.D.
Clinical Studies Manager
Cochlear Corporation
Englewood, Colorado

Robert B. Stanley, Jr., M.D., D.D.S.
Professor
Department of Otolaryngology-Head and Neck Surgery
University of Washington School of Medicine
Chief
Department of Otolaryngology-Head and Neck Surgery
Harborview Medical Center
Seattle, Washington

Patricia G. Stelmachowicz, Ph.D.
Professor
Department of Otolaryngology and Human Communication
Creighton University School of Medicine
Director, Audiological Services
Boys Town National Research Hospital
Omaha, Nebraska

Laura M. Sterni, M.D.
Fellow
Division of Pediatric Pulmonary
Johns Hopkins Children's Center
Baltimore, Maryland

Susan Strauss, M.D.
Assistant Professor
University of Washington
Children's Regional Hospital and Medical Center
Seattle, Washington

Barbara S. Stroer, M.A.
Assistant Professor
Department of Communication Disorders
Fontbonne College
St. Louis, Missouri
Coordinator of Audiology Services
St. Joseph Institute for the Deaf
Chesterfield, Missouri

James Y. Suen, M.D.
Professor and Chairman
Department of Otolaryngology-Head and Neck Surgery
University of Arkansas for Medical Sciences
University Hospital of Arkansas
Little, Arkansas

Gordon W. Summers, D.M.D, M.D.
Department of Otolaryngology-Head and Neck Surgery
Providence Medical Center
Portland, Oregon

Neil A. Swanson, M.D.
Professor and Chair
Department of Dermatology
Professor
Department of Otolaryngology-Head and Neck Surgery
Oregon Health Sciences University
Portland VA Medical Center
Lagacy Emmanuel Medical Center
St. Vincent's Hospital
Portland, Oregon

Jonathan M. Sykes, M.D.
Associate Professor
Facial Plastic Surgery
Department of Otolaryngology/Head and Neck Surgery
University of California, Davis, Medical Center
Sacramento, California

M. Eugene Tardy, Jr., M.D.
Professor
Department of Clinical Otolaryngology
Director, Division of Facial Plastic Surgery
University of Illinois College of Medicine
Chicago, Illinois

Steven A. Telian, M.D.
Associate Professor
University of Michigan Medical Center
Ann Arbor, Michigan

Fred F. Telischi, M.D.
Assistant Professor
Department of Otolaryngology
University of Miami Ear Institute
Miami, Florida

Jeffrey E. Terrell, M.D.
Assistant Professor
University of Michigan Medical Center
Ann Arbor, Michigan

Stanley E. Thawley, M.D.
Associate Professor
Department of Otolaryngology
Washington University School of Medicine
Chief Adult Division Department of Otolaryngology
Barnes-Jewish Hospital
St. Louis, Missouri

J. Regan Thomas, M.D.
Professor and Chairman
Department of Otolaryngology-Head and Neck Surgery
St. Louis University School of Medicine
Director
The Facial Plastic Surgery Center
St. Louis, Missouri

James N. Thompson, M.D.
Dean
Wake Forest University
Bowman Gray School of Medicine
North Carolina Baptist Hospital
Winston-Salem, North Carolina

R. David Tomlinson, Ph.D.
Associate Professor
Departments of Otolaryngology, Physiology, and Medicine
University of Toronto
Toronto, Ontario, Canada

Dean M. Toriumi, M.D.
Associate Professor
Division of Facial Plastic and Reconstructive Surgery
Department of Otolaryngology-Head and Neck Surgery
University of Illinois College of Medicine
Chicago, Illinois

Joseph B. Travers, Ph.D.
Associate Professor
Department of Oral Biology
Ohio State University College of Dentistry
Columbus, Ohio

David E. Tunkel, M.D.
Associate Professor
Department of Otolaryngology-Head and Neck Surgery
    and Pediatrics
Johns Hopkins University School of Medicine
Director
Division of Pediatric Otolaryngology
Johns Hopkins Hospital and Outpatient Center
Baltimore, Maryland

Mark L. Urken, M.D., F.A.C.S.
Professor and Chairman
Mt. Sinai School of Medicine
Mt. Sinai Medical Center
New York, New York

Thierry Van Den Abbeele, M.D.
Chef de Clinique
Faculte de Medecine Bichat
Assistant
Service D'or Pediatrique
Hopital Robert Debre
Paris, France

Isaäc van der Waal, D.D.S., Ph.D.
Head
Department of Oral Maxillofacial Surgery Pathology
Professor
Department of Oral Pathology
Hospital of the Free University
Amsterdam, Netherlands

Mark A. Varvares, M.D.
Instructor
Department of Otolaryngology and Laryngology
Harvard Medical School
Massachusetts Eye and Ear Infirmary
Boston, Massachusetts

David L. Walner, M.D.
Assistant Professor
Rush-Presbyterian St. Luke's Medical Center
Chicago, Illinois

Harrison G. Weed, M.D.
Assistant Professor
Department of Internal Medicine
Ohio State University College of Medicine
Arthur G. James Cancer Hospital and Research Institute
Columbus, Ohio

Mark S. Weinberger, M.D.
Clinical Instructor
University of Illinois at Chicago
Fellow
Facial Plastic and Reconstructive Surgery
University of Illinois Eye and Ear Infirmary
Chicago, Illinois

Gregory S. Weinstein, M.D.
Assistant Professor
Department of Otorhinolaryngology-Head and Neck
    Surgery
University of Pennsylvania
Philadelphia, Pennsylvania

Ralph F. Wetmore, M.D.
Associate Professor
Department of Otorhinolaryngology-Head and Neck Surgery
University of Pennsylvania School of Medicine
Children's Hospital Of Philadelphia
Philadelphia, Pennsylvania

Ernest A. Weymuller, Jr., M.D.
Professor and Chairman
Department Otolaryngology-Head and Neck Surgery
University of Washington School of Medicine
Seattle, Washington

Brian J. Wiatrak, M.D.
Associate Professor
Department of Surgery and Pediatrics
University of Alabama School of Medicine
Chief of Pediatric Otolaryngology
Children's Hospital of Alabama
Birmingham, Alabama

Gregory J. Wiet, M.S., M.D.
Fellow
Department of Pediatric Otolaryngology
University of Arkansas for Medical Sciences
Arkansas Children's Hospital
Little Rock, Arkansas

Ewain P. Wilson, M.B., B.Ch.
Assistant Professor
Director, Head and Neck Surgical Oncology
West Virginia University School of Medicine
Morgantown, West Virginia

Franz J. Wippold, II, M.D.
Associate Professor
Mallinckrodt Institute of Radiology
Washington University School of Medicine
Barnes-Jewish Hospital
St. Louis Children's Hospital
St. Louis, Missouri

Gregory T. Wolf, M.D.
Professor and Chair
Department of Otolaryngology
University of Michigan Medical School
Ann Arbor, Michigan

Gayle Ellen Woodson, M.D., F.A.C.S., F.R.C.S.C.
Professor
Department of Otolaryngology-Head and Neck Surgery
Director
Voice Disorder Clinic
University of Tennessee
Memphis, Tennessee

Audie L. Woolley, M.D.
Assistant Professor
Division of Otolaryngology-Head and Neck Surgery
University of Alabama School of Medicine
Birmingham, Alabama

Eiji Yanagisawa, M.D.
Clinical Professor
Department of Otolaryngology
Yale University School of Medicine
New Haven, Connecticut

Charles D. Yingling, Ph.D.
Director
Neurophysiologic Monitoring Service
University of California San Francisco Medical Center
San Francisco, California

Christine Yoshinaga-Itano, Ph.D.
Associate Professor
Department of Speech, Language, and Hearing Sciences
University of Colorado, Boulder
Boulder, Colorado

George H. Zalzal, M.D.
Associate Professor
Department of Otolaryngology and Pediatrics
George Washington University
Chairman
Department of Otolaryngology
Children's National Medical Center
Washington, D.C.

David S. Zee, M.D.
Departments of Neurology, Otolaryngology-Head and Neck
Surgery and Ophthalmology
Johns Hopkins University School of Medicine
Baltimore, Maryland

S. James Zinreich, M.D.
Associate Professor
Johns Hopkins Medical Institution
Baltimore, Maryland

Teresa A. Zwolan, Ph.D.
Director and Assistant
Cochlear Implant Program
Research Scientist
University of Michigan Medical Center
Ann Arbor, Michigan

Preface

Otolaryngology—Head and Neck Surgery was created to fill the needs for a contemporary, definitive textbook on the specialty of otolaryngology-head and neck surgery. The scope of the third edition is a testimonial to the tremendous expansion of knowledge in this specialty. Our desire is to record this expansion in a retrievable fashion so that these volumes become indispensable reference works. The third edition builds on the success of the past two editions. The reader will note new algorithms and boxed lists which serve to enhance learning.

The field of otolaryngology-head and neck surgery is represented in all of its diversity; the extensive interrelationship of its various components provided the skeleton for the table of contents. These volumes are intended as a detailed reference text and not as a surgical atlas: a definitive work, not an introductory overview. It is designed for residents and practitioners alike. We hope that our quest to document significant and up-to-date information in the specialty has been successful.

Another of our goals throughout the pages of this text-book is to acknowledge all those who have contributed to the specialty. Since significant medical expertise has no geographic boundaries, there are contributors from countries all over the world. Recognizing the unique aspects of pediatric otolaryngology-head and neck surgery, the editors have created an additional volume edited by Mark A. Richardson. This freestanding resource meets the global criteria of the comprehensive textbook.

To ensure continuity at the editorship level, Drs. Paul Flint, Bruce Haughey, K. Thomas Robbins, and J. Regan Thomas have assumed associate editorship roles in this expanded effort. It is hoped that the ecumenicism which combines the effort of all the contributors will further the excellence of those now associated with otolaryngology-head and neck surgery and provide the foundation for continued progress by the generations to follow. This third edition builds on the success of the first two. It is more comprehensive, is of broader scope, and continues the tradition established 11 years ago.

Acknowledgments

The editors of these volumes wish to acknowledge the individuals who have contributed immeasurably to the successful completion of our task; most specifically, the contributors to these many pages. These authors were specifically selected by the editorial board to ensure the presence of the most contemporary thinking on their respective topics. The expertise of all of these individuals provides for this book's infinite potential.

In addition, we wish to thank all the employees at Mosby–Year Book, Inc. This is a truly first rate organization. Special mention should be made of the efforts of Robert Hurley and Lauranne Billus for this current edition as well as those of Anne Patterson and Carol Trumbold, so instrumental in the past success. Most certainly those who contributed time, words, and expertise to this edition should be thanked collectively as well as individually.

Acknowledgments

I would like to acknowledge my father for enabling me to survive comfortably during my seemingly endless years of education. As well, my wife, Jane, and my family who have recognized the importance of and supported the mission that resulted in, this resource for Otolaryngology Head and Neck Surgery. I would also like to acknowledge the students and residents who are a constant source of motivation and the patients who served as the fuel that energized this project. Through their coping with illness we are constantly aware that our search for resolution of illness must continue.

Charles W. Cummings

Once again, it has been great fun working with my co-editors. As this is my last contribution as co-editor, I will miss the fellowship which has grown over the years. I thank the authors for their excellent work and our Mosby colleagues for their diligence and professionalism. Foremost, I thank my partner, Alix, and with love, I dedicate my contribution to her and our children, Kristin, Lisa, and Erik.

John M. Fredrickson

Scientific knowledge is fleeting; part of what we know today is true, and part soon will be disproven or rendered obsolete. Galen was as right in his day as we are today. The authors of volume four have done a superb job of expressing today's knowledge. I thank them for that and for responding to my suggestions and prodding. Thanks are also extended to Dr. Patrick Brookhouser at Boy's Town National Research Hospital for his encouragement and support. My contribution to this volume is dedicated with love to my wife, Jill, my mother, my late father, and to Elizabeth, Robert, and Alexa.

Lee A. Harker

I would like to dedicate my contribution to these volumes to my wife, Barbara, and our children, Sharon, John, and Ann, for their encouragement and support throughout this lengthy endeavor; and to my parents, William and Ruby Krause, who committed so much more of their lives to their children. I would like to thank my administrative secretary, Linda Edberg Diebold, for her effort, her patience, and the very considerable skill with which she assisted on this project.

Charles J. Krause

It has been a special opportunity to continue to be involved with the original authors who have demonstrated tremendous dedication to maintaining the highest standards for this textbook. All of the students, residents, fellows, and patients certainly provide a strong motivation to be actively involved in life-long learning activities. But Carole, Becky, and Mike have continued to be my strongest supporters. My involvement is dedicated to them as an expression of my love as well as to my parents, Daniel and Elsie, who instilled in me the enjoyment of learning. I would also like to express appreciation for the excellent support and patience provided by Debra O. Parker, administrator of our head and neck oncology program, as we jointly worked to meet the numerous deadlines.

David E. Schuller

This volume represents the cooperative efforts of many who we think have created a sum greater than any of its component parts. My special thanks go to the senior editors, Drs. Cummings, Fredrickson, Harker, Krause, and Schuller for the opportunity to participate in their reference work in otolaryngology and their guidance in editorship. Also, the individual contributors who have provided so much time and work to produce this volume and without whom it would not exist. The editorial staff, including Bob Hurley, Lauranne Billus, Marla Sussman, Jori Matison, Susie Coladonato, and Stacy Loonstyn who kept me and the volume on track. Especially my wife Ellen, daughters Caroline and Abigail, who are a never ending source of inspiration and support, and my mother and father who enabled me to pursue medicine and otolaryngology as a career.

Mark A. Richardson

Table of Contents

PART ONE

GENERAL CONSIDERATIONS IN HEAD AND NECK

Chapter 1

History and Physical Examination

Marion E. Couch

It is a privilege to be a physician requested to evaluate a person and render an opinion and diagnosis. The importance of an accurate, detailed history cannot be overemphasized because it is the framework on which the otolaryngologist places all available information, building toward an accurate diagnosis and management plan. Without this, the evaluation may be incomplete and the diagnosis flawed. Unnecessary testing may ensue, and, at the minimum, a delay in management may result. In the worst scenario, a misdiagnosis may occur. Therefore, the energy expended in obtaining a complete history is always worthwhile.

In addition to the challenge of obtaining a comprehensive history, the otolaryngologist is faced with examining the complex anatomy of the head and neck region. There are many different examination techniques to learn and much specialized equipment to use. It may take years to master the fundamentals of a complete head and neck examination. Even experienced otolaryngologists are continually modifying and refining their techniques to better examine patients.

Finally, the otolaryngologist should be efficient, and often this means politely directing the questions in the interview to avoid rambling answers from the patients that may contribute little to the history. The same efficiency is helpful when examining patients. The time saved by proficient examination of regions unrelated to the patients' problem will allow for a more careful and thorough examination of the problem area.

GATHERING A PATIENT HISTORY

Many physicians will mail a detailed and directed questionnaire to their patients before their office visit. This has multiple advantages. First, it enables patients to accurately record the symptoms they are experiencing and to chronicle the history of their problems. In addition, the names of all their medications and the correct dosages and any drug allergies can be listed. Addresses and telephone numbers that are difficult to recall, such as those of their primary care or referring physician, can be listed for later use. Some patients with special communicative disorders, such as those with laryngectomies, tracheostomies, or spastic dysphonia, may appreciate the opportunity to relay information without lengthy verbal discussions. For these reasons, the otolaryngologist is better able to efficiently gather important information even before the patient has arrived in the office. This information also may allow a preliminary differential diagnosis to be formulated in certain patients.

It also is helpful to request that previous medical records pertaining to the patient's current problem be sent to the office before the visit. The primary care physician, referring physician, patient, or a family member often can assist in obtaining these records. If previous operations have been performed, operative reports can be important sources of information. In addition, pertinent radiographic imaging is helpful to obtain for review. Reports of computed tomography (CT) or magnetic resonance imaging (MRI) scans are valuable but cannot substitute for actual review of the imaging by the otolaryngologist. For head and neck cancer patients, any pathologic slide specimens from past biopsies should be sent to the pathology department for review so that a second opinion may be rendered. This is especially true when patients are referred with an unusual pathologic diagnosis. Finally, laboratory values can provide much information and should be carefully reviewed.

The questionnaire, although valuable, is no substitute for a thoughtful and thorough interview with the patient. The chief complaint should be addressed by determining duration, intensity, location, frequency, factors that make the problem worse or better, any past therapy, and related symptoms. Whether the complaint is vertigo, pain, sinusitis, hearing loss, allergies, or a neck mass, the approach should entail asking many of the same basic questions followed by more specific ones designed to elucidate the full scope of the problem.

A discussion of the patient's medical history not only leads to a better understanding of the patient, but it often reveals pertinent information to the otolaryngologist. For instance, a patient with an otitis externa who also is diabetic requires a higher level of concern for malignant otitis externa, and this may be reflected in the management plan. If the patient requires surgery, complete knowledge of the patient's medical problems is necessary before the operative procedure. Easy bruising and prolonged bleeding, pulmonary disease, or coronary artery disease are obvious examples of medical issues that should be addressed before surgery. However, what about the patient with cervical spine stenosis and intermittent limb paresis? Any manipulation of the cervical spine intraoperatively could have serious ramifications. Therefore, it is essential to elicit a complete medical history because requesting the proper preoperative evaluations and consultations can only be done if this information is known.

The surgical history is equally valuable. All the past operations of the head and neck area are important to note, including surgery for past facial trauma, cosmetic facial plastic surgery, otologic surgery, and any head and neck surgery for neoplasm, although full disclosure of all past operations may be critical. For example, the choice of a free flap may depend on whether a patient has had previous abdominal surgery with incisions that would have transected the flap pedicle. If any patient goes to surgery, it is essential to know if a patient has had previous adverse reactions to anesthetic agents or had a difficult intubation.

Obviously, any known drug allergies and side effects are critical to note prominently in the medical chart. True allergies should be distinguished from side effects because an effective antibiotic may be needlessly avoided when the patient has previously experienced common side effects such as gastrointestinal discomfort, which can be safely managed. In addition, all medications and current dosages should be accurately recorded. Often, it is valuable to inquire whether the patient has been compliant with the medication regimen that was prescribed because it is important to consider the doses that the patient actually is receiving. For instance, nasal steroids should be used daily and are not as effective when used intermittently. Therefore, a poor response may be solely a result of subtherapeutic levels of the medication.

After this, it often is advantageous to assess for risk factors associated with certain disease states. Tobacco use is important to note. It is helpful to specifically ask about cigarette, cigar, and chewing tobacco consumption—either current or past use. Patients being assessed for head and neck cancer may deny tobacco use if only asked if they smoke cigarettes, although they may have extensively used cigars or chewed "snuff." Alcohol consumption also is occasionally difficult to quantitate unless the interviewer asks direct questions regarding frequency, choice of beverage, and duration of use. Recreational drug use should be addressed, as should risk factors for communicable diseases such as the human immunodeficiency virus (HIV) and hepatitis virus. For patients being assessed for hearing loss, major risk factors such as exposure to machinery, loud music, or gunfire should be discussed. Finally, past irradiation (implants, external beam, or by mouth) and dosage (either high- or low-dose) should be ascertained. A history of accidental radiation exposure also is important to document.

The social history should not be overlooked because it may often reveal more occult risk factors for many diseases. For instance, a retired steel worker may have an extensive history of inhaling environmental toxins, whereas a World War II veteran may have noise-induced hearing loss from his or her military service. Family history often is equally revealing, and asking patients questions about their familial history of such conditions as hearing loss, congenital defects, atopy, or cancer may uncover useful information that they had not previously considered.

Finally, a review of systems is part of every comprehensive history. This review includes changes in the patient's respiratory, neurologic, cardiac, endocrine, psychiatric, gastrointestinal, urogenital, cutaneous skin, or musculoskeletal systems. The otolaryngologist often may derive more insight into the patient's problem by inquiring about constitutional changes such as weight loss or gain, fatigue, heat or cold intolerance, rashes, and the like (Box 1-1).

PHYSICAL EXAMINATION

It is imperative to develop an approach to the head and neck examination that allows the patient to feel comfortable while the physician performs a complete and comprehensive evaluation. Many of the techniques used by the otolaryngologist, such as fiberoptic nasopharyngolaryngoscopy, may leave a patient feeling alienated if not done correctly, with a sensitivity to the patient's emotions. Even allowing inspection of one's oral cavity or nares requires a certain amount of trust by the patient. Thus, it is essential to establish a rapport with a patient before proceeding with the examination. At the same time, the physician should be confident and comfortable with a standard routine examination that allows systematic examination of every patient so that nothing is forgotten or overlooked.

A word of caution is necessary. The head and neck examination should only be done with the examiner wearing gloves and, in most instances, protective eye covering. Universal precautions are mandatory in today's practice of medicine.

Box 1-1. History

Introduce yourself
　Review
　　Questionnaire
　　Medical records
　　Radiographic imaging
　　Laboratory values
　　Pathology specimens
Inquire about chief complaints
　Location
　Duration
　Characteristics
Medical history
Surgical history
Allergies
Medications
Risk factors
　Tobacco, alcohol
Social history
Family history
Review of systems
　Respiratory
　Neurologic
　Cardiac
　Endocrine
　Psychiatric
　Gastrointestinal
　Urogenital
　Skin
　Musculoskeletal

Table 1-1. AAQ-HNS facial nerve grading system

Grade	Facial movement
I. Normal	Normal facial function at all times
II. Mild dysfunction	Forehead: moderate-to-good function
	Eye: complete closure
	Mouth: slight asymmetry
III. Moderate dysfunction	Forehead: slight-to-moderate movement
	Eye: complete closure with effort
	Mouth: slightly weak with maximum effort
IV. Moderately severe dysfunction	Forehead: none
	Eye: incomplete closure
	Mouth: asymmetric with maximum effort
V. Severe dysfunction	Forehead: none
	Eye: incomplete closure
	Mouth: slight movement
VI. Total paralysis	No movement

Therefore, routine hand-washing and wearing gloves should be incorporated into the examination ritual. This has the added benefit of showing the patient that the examiner is concerned about not transmitting any diseases, which builds trust between the patient and physician.

General appearance

Much information can be obtained by first assessing the general behavior and appearance of the patient. For instance, the patient's affect may suggest possible depression, anxiety, or even alcoholic intoxication. Psychotic behavior in the office may be a result of many factors but may indicate profound hypothyroidism in head and neck cancer patients. Astute observation of the patient's appearance is equally important. Tar-stained fingernails, teeth, or moustache are harbingers for heavy tobacco consumption. Even the gait of patients as they enter or leave the office may reveal information. Neurologic impairments, especially involving the cerebellum, may affect the patient's ability to navigate into the room.

Facies

After assessing the patient's overall appearance, the face should be analyzed for facial asymmetry by positioning the head squarely in front of the examiner. This simple step may yield subtle but important information. For instance, in patients considering facial plastic surgery, a hemifacial microsomia may affect the final outcome, and this should be discussed before the operation. In addition, a paretic facial nerve always is a serious finding that can be detected by observing the tone of the underlying facial musculature and overlying facial skin. Facial wrinkles are more prominent when the facial nerve is functioning. Other maneuvers to assess facial nerve function include having the patient broadly smile, wrinkle the nose, and close the eyes tightly. For patients recovering from facial nerve paralysis, the AAQ-HNS Facial Nerve Grading System is a respected standard for reporting gradations of nerve function (Table 1-1).

Facial skeleton

The facial skeleton then should be carefully palpated for bony deformities. This is especially true in patients with recent facial trauma. The periorbital rims may be irregular as a result of fractures involving the zygomatic arches or orbital floor. The dorsum of the nose may be displaced as a result of a comminuted nasal fracture. After evaluation of the facial skeleton, the regions overlying the paranasal sinuses may be firmly palpated or tapped for tenderness, which may be present during an episode of sinusitis.

Evaluation of the temporomandibular joint (TMJ) is convenient to perform at this point in the examination. By having the examiner place three fingers over the TMJ region, which is anterior to the external auditory canal, anteromedial dislocation (caused by the action of the lateral pterygoid muscle) or clicking of the joint can be ascertained. The patient should open and close the jaw to assist in evaluating this synovial joint.

Parotid

Masses in the parotid may be benign or malignant neoplasms of the parotid, cysts, inflammatory masses, or lymph node metastasis from other areas. The tail of the parotid extends to the region lateral and inferior to the angle of the mandible. This is a common site for parotid masses to reside. The parotid–preauricular and retroauricular lymph nodes also should be systematically assessed in every patient. By facing the patient and placing both hands behind the ears before palpating the preauricular nodes, the often-neglected retroauricular nodes will not be missed.

Skin

Skin covering the face and neck should be examined, and suspicious lesions should be noted. The external auricles often receive sun exposure and are at risk for developing the skin malignancies such as basal cell and squamous cell carcinomas. The scalp should be examined for hidden skin lesions, such as melanoma, basal cell carcinoma, or squamous cell carcinoma. All moles should be inspected for irregular borders, heterogeneous color, ulcerations, and satellite lesions.

Neck

The neck, an integral part of the complete otolaryngology examination, is best approached by palpating it while visualizing the underlying structures (Fig. 1-1). The midline structures such as the trachea and larynx can be easily located and then palpated for deviation or crepitus. If there is a thyroid cartilage fracture, tenderness and crepitus may be present. In thick, short necks, the ''signet ring'' cricoid cartilage is a good landmark to use for orientation. The hyoid bone can

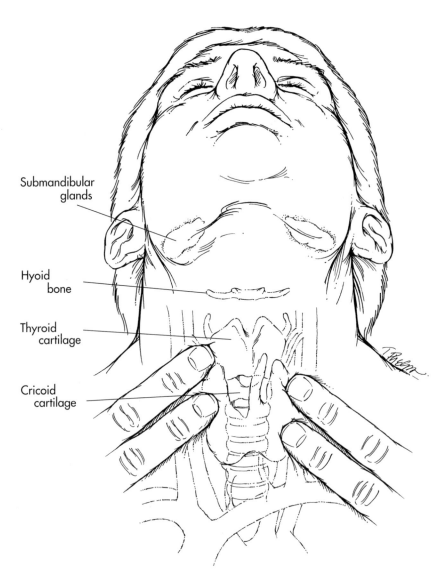

Submandibular glands

Hyoid bone

Thyroid cartilage

Cricoid cartilage

Fig. 1-1. Basic anatomy of the anterior neck. Visualize structures while performing neck examination.

be inspected and palpated by gently rocking it back and forth.

Thyroid gland

Traveling more inferior in the neck, the thyroid gland, which resides below the cricoid cartilage, should be examined by standing behind the patient and placing both hands on the paratracheal area near the cricoid cartilage. Having the patient swallow or drink a sip of water often helps better delineate the thyroid lobes by having the trachea rise and fall. Pressing firmly in one tracheal groove allows the contents of the other side to be more easily distinguished by gentle palpation. Nodules or cystic structures should be carefully noted and evaluated, often by fine-needle aspiration. Adjacent adenopathy also should be carefully assessed.

Adenopathy

After this, palpation of the supraclavicular area, from the paratracheal grooves posteriorly to the sternocleidomastoid muscle to the trapezius muscle, will help detect masses or enlarged lymph nodes, which are worrisome for metastasis from sources such as the abdomen, breast, or lung. Proceeding more superiorly, the area inferior to the angle of the mandible houses the carotid arteries and often has many lymph nodes, either ''shoddy'' and indistinct or firm. Palpable nodes always should be noted and may need evaluation with either fine-needle aspiration or radiologic imaging when observation is not appropriate. The carotid artery, often mistaken for a prominent node, can be assessed for the presence of bruits. The entire jugulodigastric chain of lymph nodes merits careful inspection by outlining the sternocleidomastoid muscle and palpating the soft tissue anterior and posterior to it. The submandibular and submental regions are palpated by determining the outline of the glands and any masses present. It often is difficult to distinguish masses from the normal architecture of the submandibular gland, and therefore, bimanual palpation of this area using a gloved finger in the floor of the mouth is helpful.

Triangles of the neck

It is helpful to define the neck in terms of triangles when communicating the location of physical findings (Fig. 1-2). The sternocleidomastoid muscle divides the neck into a posterior triangle, whose boundaries are the trapezius, clavicle, and sternocleidomastoid muscles, and an anterior triangle, which is bordered by the sternohyoid, digastric, and sternocleidomastoid muscles. These triangles are further divided into smaller triangles. The posterior triangle houses the supraclavicular and the occipital triangles. The anterior triangle then may be divided into the submandibular, carotid, and muscular triangles.

Lymph node regions

Another classification system for neck masses uses the lymph node regions, which is especially useful for head and neck surgeons when depicting the location of adenopathy

(Fig. 1-3). Level IA is the submental triangle, and level IB is the submandibular triangle. The upper third of the jugulodigastric chain is level II, whereas the middle and lower third represent levels III and IV, respectively. More specifically, the jugulodigastric lymph nodes from the skull base to the hyoid bone are located in level II. Level III extends from the hyoid bone to the cricoid cartilage, and level IV includes the lymph nodes located from the cricoid to the clavicle. Level V is the posterior triangle, which includes the spinal accessory and supraclavicular nodes. The prethyroid nodes are contained in level VI, whereas the tracheoesophageal nodes are in level VII. The parotid–preauricular, retroauricular, and suboccipital regions often are designated as the P, R, and S regions.

Ears

Auricles

The postauricular region, which is frequently overlooked, often has many hidden physical findings. For instance, well-healed surgical incisions signify previous otologic procedures have been performed. In children, the postauricular mastoid area may harbor important clues that a mastoiditis with a subperiosteal abscess has developed. The erythema and edema may cause the entire auricle to be pushed down outward, away from the temporal bone, obliterating the postauricular sulcus. Finally, in patients with head trauma, postauricular ecchymosis, or Battle's sign, suggests that a temporal bone fracture may have occurred.

The area anterior to the pinna, at the root of the helix, may house preauricular pits or sinuses, which may become infected. The external auricles also may reflect abnormalities or congenital malformations, including canal atresia, accessory auricles, microtia, and prominent protruding ''bat ears.'' The outer ears may have edema with weeping, crusting otorrhea, which may signify an infection is present. Psoriasis of the auricle or external auditory canal with its attendant flaking, dry skin, and edema is another common finding.

Careful inspection of the auricles may reveal conditions that mandate prompt management. For instance, an auricular hematoma, with a hematoma separating the perichondrium from the underlying anterior auricular cartilage, will present as a swollen auricle with distortion of the normal external anatomy. If not surgically drained, a deformed ''cauliflower ear'' may result. Another important diagnosis is that of carcinoma of the auricle. Because early diagnosis is important, all suspicious lesions or masses should be judiciously biopsied or cultured. A maculopapular rash on the auricle and the external auditory canal in patients with facial nerve paralysis most likely is a result of herpes zoster oticus or Ramsey-Hunt syndrome. Finally, an erythematous painful pinna may represent many entities, such as perichondritis, relapsing polychondritis, Wegener's granulomatosis, or chronic discoid lupus erythematosus.

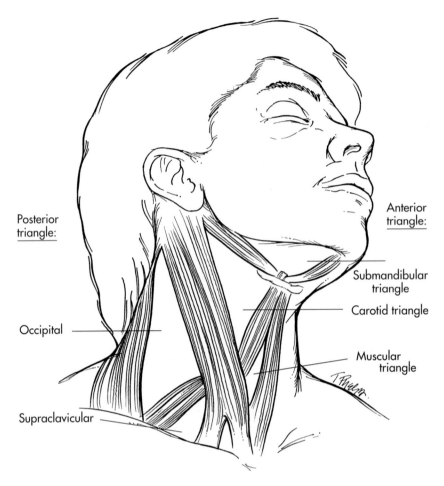

Fig. 1-2. Triangles of the neck. The anterior triangle is divided from the posterior triangle by the sternocleidomastoid muscle.

Metabolic disorders also may have manifestations that affect the auricles. Patients with gout may have tophus on the pinna that will exude a chalky white substance if squeezed. Ochronosis is an inherited disorder of homogentisic acid that will cause the cartilage of the auricles to blacken. These examples of various diseases and syndromes illustrate the importance of examining the auricles on a routine basis.

External auditory canal

The outer third (approximately 11 mm) of the auditory canal is cartilaginous, and the adnexa of the skin contains many sebaceous and apocrine glands that produce cerumen. Hair follicles also are present. The inner two thirds (approximately 24 mm) of the canal is osseous and has only a thin layer of skin overlying the bone. Cerumen is commonly found accumulating in the canal, often obstructing it. When removing cerumen, remember two points. The canal is well supplied with sensory fibers: CN V3, the auricular branch of CN X, C3, and CN VII. Second, the canal curves in an S-shape toward the nose. To visualize the ear canal, gently grasp the pinna and elevate it upward and backward. This

will open the external auditory canal opening and allow atraumatic insertion of the otoscopic speculum. Cerumen impaction may be removed with many techniques, such as careful curetting, gentle suctioning, or irrigation with warm water.

An otitis externa, or "swimmer's ear," is a painful condition with an edematous, often weeping external canal. If severe, the entire canal may be so edematous and inflamed that it closes, making inspection of the tympanic membrane difficult. Gently tugging on the auricle is painful for many patients. The periauricular lymph nodes may be tender and enlarged. If the patient is immunocompromised or diabetic, the canal should be carefully inspected for the presence of granulation tissue at the junction of the cartilaginous and bony junction. This may signify that a malignant otitis externa is present, which, as an osteomyelitis of the temporal bone, requires aggressive management, including prompt intravenous antibiotics.

In older patients, atrophy of the external auditory canal skin is frequently seen and may be associated with psoriasis or eczema of the canal. If patients attempt to sooth an itch

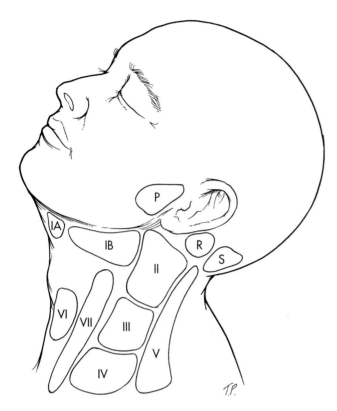

Fig. 1-3. Lymph node regions of the neck.

with foreign objects such as keys, hair pins, or cotton-tipped swabs, scabs or areas of ecchymosis may be present in the posterior canal wall.

Children are most likely to inset foreign bodies into the ear canal. Although most objects will lodge lateral to the narrowest part of the canal, the isthmus, some will be found in the anterior recess by the tympanic membrane, making it especially difficult to visualize with an otoscope, so have patients turn their head to view this area. In adults, cotton plugs are commonly lodged and often are impacted against the tympanic membrane. In patients of all ages, insects may find their way into the canal. Instilling the canal with alcohol or lidocaine is effective in killing this particularly annoying foreign body. A combination of suctioning, alligator forceps, and irrigation frequently is needed to remove foreign body objects. An operating microscope allows excellent visualization and enables the physician to use both hands to manipulate the instruments needed to remove the object.

Otorrhea is commonly seen in the external auditory canal. The characteristics of the aural discharge may reveal the etiology of the otorrhea. For instance, mucoid drainage is associated with a middle ear chronic suppurative otitis media because only the middle ear has mucus glands. In these patients, a tympanic membrane perforation should be present to allow the mucoid otorrhea to escape. Foul-smelling otorrhea may be caused by chronic suppurative otitis media with a cholesteatoma. Bloody, mucopurulent otorrhea frequently is

seen in patients with acute otitis media, trauma, or carcinoma of the ear. Otorrhea with a watery component may signify a cerebrospinal fluid leak or eczema of the canal. Black spores in the otorrhea may be present in a fungal otitis externa caused by *Aspergillus* species. Gentle suctioning is used to clean the canal and to inspect it thoroughly.

In patients with head trauma, a temporal bone fracture is important to recognize. Bloody otorrhea in conjuction with an external canal laceration or hemotympanium are very serious findings. Longitudinal fractures often involve the external canal. Because longitudinal fractures may be bilateral, careful inspection of both canals is essential.

Tympanic membrane

To view the tympanic membranes, the correct otoscope speculum size is used to allow a seal of the ear canal. With pressure from the pneumatic bulb, the tympanic membrane will move back and forth if the middle ear space is well aerated. Perforations and middle ear effusions are common causes for nonmobile tympanic membranes.

The tympanic membrane is oval, not round, and has a depressed central part called the *umbo*, wherein the handle of the malleus attaches to the membrane. The lateral process of the malleus is located in the superior anterior region and is seen as a prominent bony point in atelectatic membranes. Superior to this process is the pars flaccida, wherein the tympanic membrane lacks the radial and circular fibers present in the pars tensa, which is the remainder of the ear drum. This superior flaccid area is critical to examine carefully because retraction pockets may develop here, which may develop into cholesteatomas. In congenital cholesteatomas, often diagnosed in young children, the tympanic membrane is intact, and a white mass is seen in the anterior superior quadrant. Acquired cholesteatomas in adults are different in that they often are in the posterior superior quadrant and are associated with retraction pockets, chronic otitis media with purulent otorrhea, and tympanic membrane perforations.

To assess the middle ear for effusions, use the tympanic membrane as a window that allows a view of the middle ear structures (Fig. 1-4). Effusions may be clear (serous), cloudy with infection present, or bloody. When the patient performs a Valsalva maneuver, actual bubbles may form in the effusion.

Hearing assessment

Tuning fork tests, usually done with a 512-Hz fork, allow one to distinguish between sensorineural and conductive hearing loss (Table 1-2). They also may be used to confirm the audiogram, which may give spurious results because of poor fitting earphones or variations in equipment or personnel. Be sure to conduct all tests in a quiet room without background noise. Also, be certain that the external auditory canal is not blocked with cerumen.

The Weber test is performed by placing the vibrating tuning fork in the center of the patient's forehead or at the

Table 1-2. Tuning fork testing

Begin with 512-Hz fork, then include 256- and 1024-Hz forks

Weber	Place tuning fork in center of patient's forehead. Ask patient if sound is louder on one side or is heard midline.		
	Weber "negative"	Weber right	Weber left
Patient response	"Sound is midline"	"Sound is louder on right"	"Sound is louder on left"
Interpretation	Bone-conducted sound equal in both ears	Unilateral right conductive hearing loss; unilateral left sensorineural hearing loss	Unilateral left conductive hearing loss; unilateral right sensorineural hearing loss
Rinne	Place tuning fork lateral to ear canal, then place it firmly on mastoid process. Ask patient if sound is louder by canal or on mastoid bone.		
	Rinne "positive"	Rinne "negative"	Rinne "equal"
Patient response	"Sound louder when fork by canal"	"Sound louder when fork on mastoid process"	"Sound equal"
Interpretation	Air conduction louder than bone conduction; normal	Bone conduction louder than air conduction; conductive hearing loss	Air and bone conduction equal

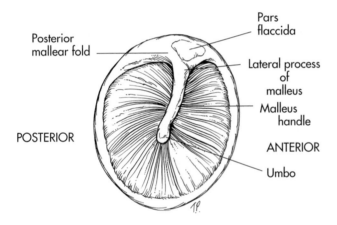

Fig. 1-4. The tympanic membrane.

Pars flaccida

Posterior mallear fold

Lateral process of malleus

Malleus handle

POSTERIOR

ANTERIOR

Umbo

bridge of the nose. If the patient has difficulty with these locations, the mandible or front teeth may be used, however, the patient then should tightly clench his or her teeth. The patient then is asked if the sound is louder in one ear or is heard midline. The sound waves should be transmitted equally well to both ears through the skull bone. A unilateral sensorineural hearing loss will cause the sound to lateralize to the ear with the better cochlear function. However, a unilateral conductive hearing loss will cause the Weber test to lateralize to the side with the conductive loss because the cochlea is intact bilaterally and because bone conduction causes the sound to be better heard in the ear with the conductive loss (because there is less background noise detected through air conduction). Interestingly, a midline Weber result is referred to as "negative." "Weber right" and "Weber left" refer to the direction the sound lateralized.

To compare air conduction with bone conduction, perform the Rinne test. The 512-Hz tuning fork is placed by the ear canal and then on the mastoid process. The patient determines whether the sound is louder when the tuning fork is by the canal (air conduction) or on the mastoid bone (bone conduction). A "positive test" result is air conduction louder than bone conduction. A conductive hearing loss will make bone conduction louder than air conduction, and this is called "Rinne negative." When the air and bone conduction are equal, it is called "Rinne equal."

The Schwabach test compares the patient's hearing with the examiner's and uses multiple tuning forks such as the 256-, 512-, 1024-, and 2048-Hz forks. The stem of the vibrating tuning fork is placed on the mastoid process of the patient and then is placed on the mastoid of the physician. This is done, alternating between the two participants, until one can no longer hear the tuning fork. Of course, this test assumes that the examiner has normal hearing. If the patient hears the sound as long as the physician, the result is "Schwabach normal." If the patient hears the sound longer than the physician, it is called "Schwabach prolonged," and this may indicate a conductive hearing loss for the patient. If the patient hears the sound for less time, it is called "Schwabach shortened" and is consistent with sensorineural hearing loss for the patient.

Oral cavity

The boundaries of the oral cavity extend from the skin–vermillion junction of the lips, hard palate, anterior two thirds of the tongue, buccal membranes, upper and lower alveolar ridge, and retromolar trigone to the floor of the mouth. This region may be best seen by having the otolaryngologist use a well-directed headlight and a tongue depressor in each gloved hand. The lips should be carefully inspected and may have ulcers present that may be caused by herpes simplex virus, syphilis, or carcinoma. Remember that lip squamous cell carcinoma is more common on the lower lip. The commissures may have fissuring, which is seen in angular stomatitis or cheilosis. When the fissures and cracking are present on the mid-portion of the lips, this may be cheilitis.

The occlusion of the teeth and the general condition of the alveolar ridges, including the gums and teeth, should be noted. The tongue, especially the lateral surfaces where carcinomas are most common, should be inspected for induration or ulcerative lesions. Gently grabbing the anterior tongue with a gauze sponge allows the examiner to move the anterior tongue from side to side. By having the patient lift the tongue toward the hard palate, the floor of mouth and Wharton's ducts (associated with submandibular glands) can be viewed. Pooling of carcinogens in the saliva on the floor of the mouth has been postulated to cause this area to have a high incidence of carcinoma in the oral cavity. Be sure to palpate the floor of mouth using a bimanual approach with one gloved hand in the mouth.

The buccal membranes should be inspected for white plaques that may represent oral thrush, if easily scraped off with a tongue blade, or leukoplakia, which cannot be removed. More worrisome for a precancerous condition is erythroplakia; therefore, all red lesions and most white lesions should be judiciously biopsied for cancer or carcinoma *in situ*. While examining the buccal membranes, note the location of the parotid duct, or Stenson's duct, as it opens near the second upper molar. Small yellow spots in the buccal mucosa are sebaceous glands, commonly referred to as *Fordyce spots*, and are not abnormal. Aphthous ulcers, or the common canker sore, are painful white ulcers that can be on any part of the mucosa but are commonly present on the buccal membrane.

The hard palate may have a bony outgrowth known as a *torus palatinus*. These midline bony deformities are benign and should not be biopsied, although growths that are not in the midline should be more carefully evaluated as possible cancerous lesions.

Oropharynx

The oropharynx includes the posterior third of the tongue, anterior and posterior tonsillar pillars, the soft palate, the lateral and posterior pharyngeal wall, the soft palate, and the vallecula (Fig. 1-5). It is best visualized using a headlight and two tongue depressors. A dental mirror is instrumental in viewing the vallecula and the posterior pharyngeal wall, which often are obscured. Using a gloved finger to examine the base of tongue or tonsil may reveal indurated areas that may be appropriate for biopsy for neoplasm. The patient should be aware of the possibility that gagging may ensue when this is done. In patients with especially strong gag reflexes, a fiberoptic examination may be necessary to fully assess the base of tongue, posterior pharyngeal wall, and vallecula. By carefully passing the flexible fiberoptic endo-

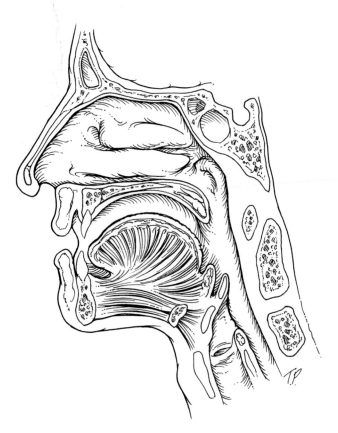

Fig. 1-5. The oropharynx, which includes the posterior third of the tongue, soft palate, tonsillar pillars (anterior and posterior), lateral and posterior pharyngeal wall, and vallecula.

scope through the anesthetized nose, the interaction of the soft palate and tongue base during swallowing also may be viewed. The uvula should be inspected because a bifid structure may signify a submucosal cleft palate is present. In addition, an inflamed large uvula may mean the uvula is traumatized during the night if the patient snores heavily. Small carcinomas or papilloma lesions also may be present, so careful palpation may be indicated.

The size of the tonsils usually is denoted as $1+$, $2+$, $3+$, or $4+$ (for "kissing tonsils" that meet in the midline). The tonsils and the base of tongue may contribute to upper airway obstruction, especially if the soft palate and uvula extend posteriorly. Therefore, the oropharyngeal aperture should be carefully assessed in each patient. Tonsillitis, caused by either bacterial or viral sources such as group A streptococcus or mononucleosis, often presents with an exudate covering the cryptic tonsils. A culture of the exudate should be taken because of the importance of diagnosing and managing a streptococcal tonsillitis. Tonsilliths are a common cause for a foreign body sensation in the back of the throat. These yellow or white concretions in the tonsillar crypts are not caused by food trapping or infection, but they often cause the patient to have halitosis and should be removed with a cotton-tipped swab.

Larynx and hypopharynx

The larynx often is subdivided into the supraglottis, glottis, and subglottis. The supraglottic area includes the epiglottis, the aryepiglottic folds, the false vocal cords, and the ventricles. The inferior floor of the ventricle, the true vocal folds, and the arytenoids comprise the glottis. The subglottis region generally is considered to begin 5 to 10 mm below the free edge of the true vocal fold and to extend to the inferior margin of the cricoid cartilage, although this is somewhat controversial (Fig. 1-6).

The hypopharynx can be challenging to understand. It extends from the superior edge of the hyoid bone to the inferior aspect of the cricoid cartilage by the cricopharyngeus muscle. It connects the oropharynx with the esophagus. Three areas comprise this region: the pyriform sinuses, posterior hypopharyngeal wall, and the postcricoid area. This area, rich in lymphatics, may harbor tumors that often are detected only in an advanced stage. Thus, early detection of these relatively "silent" carcinomas is important and should not be missed.

The examiner should not only detect anatomic abnormalities but should observe how the larynx and hypopharynx are functioning to allow the patient to have adequate airway, vocalization, and swallow function. It is not enough to survey the larynx for lesions and assess the true vocal fold function. For example, the patient with a normal-appearing larynx may have decreased laryngeal sensation with resultant aspiration and may need further diagnostic and therapeutic evaluation. Therefore, important information can be obtained if the physician carefully assesses the anatomic and functional aspects of this complex area.

Correct positioning of patients increases their comfort while maximizing the examiner's view of the larynx. The legs should be uncrossed and placed firmly on the footrest. The back should be straight with the hips planted firmly against the chair. Patients, while leaning slightly forward from the waist, should place their chin upward so that the examiner's light source is illuminating the oropharynx well. After discussing the examination procedure with the patient, the patient's tongue is pulled forward by the examiner, who uses a gauze sponge between the thumb and index finger. This allows the physician's long middle finger to retract the patient's upper lip superiorly. A warm dental mirror (to prevent fogging) is placed in the oropharynx and elevates the uvula and soft palate to view the larynx (Fig. 1-7). The patient with a strong gag reflex may benefit from a small spray of local anesthetic to help suppress the reflex.

There are some maneuvers that will allow better visualization of the larynx and its related structures. Panting, quiet breathing, and phonating with a high-pitched *E* aid in assessing true vocal fold function.

The epiglottis should be crisp and whitish. An erythematous, edematous epiglottis may signify epiglottitis, a serious infection or inflammation that mandates consideration of airway control. The petiole of the epiglottis is a peaked structure on the laryngeal surface of the epiglottis above the anterior commissure of the true vocal folds. It may be confused for a cyst or mass but is a normal prominence. Irregular

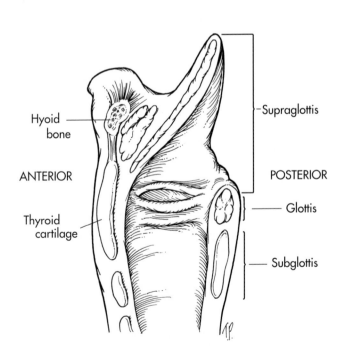

Fig. 1-6. The larynx.

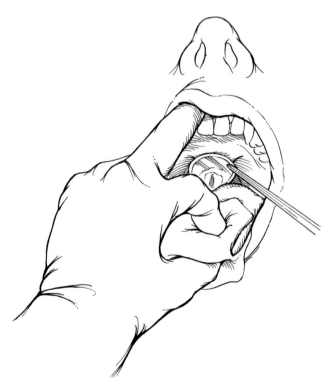

Fig. 1-7. The laryngeal examination.

mucosal lesions may be carcinomas and require further evaluation.

In the posterior glottis, movement of the arytenoids allows determination of true vocal fold mobility. The interarytenoid mucosa may be edematous or erythematous, sometimes representing gastroesophageal reflux laryngitis. The mucosa over the arytenoids may be erythematous as a result of rheumatoid arthritis or as a result of recent intubation trauma. Posterior glottic webs or scars also may be present.

The true vocal folds should have translucent white, crisp borders that meet each other. Edema of the folds that extends for the entire fold length often is caused by Reinke's edema, seen in tobacco users. Actual polypoid degeneration of the vocal cord with obstructing polyps may occasionally be seen in patients and may be a result of tobacco use or hypothyroidism. Ulcerative or exophytic lesions deserve further investigation, usually requiring operative direct laryngoscopy. True vocal fold paralysis and subtle gaps present between the folds during cord adduction should be noted.

During abduction of the cords, the subglottic area may be viewed. A prominent cricoid cartilage, seen inferiorly to the anterior commissure, may be mistaken for a subglottic stenosis. It is difficult to fully inspect the subglottic area in the office setting. Any concerns about subglottic inflammatory swelling, masses, or stenosis should be addressed in an operative setting or with radiographic imaging.

Flexible endoscopy

Perhaps the best technique to evaluate the function of the larynx uses the flexible fiberoptic nasopharyngolaryngoscope. In conjunction with a strong light source, this allows a more complete evaluation of the structures of the larynx than a mirror examination.

A topical decongestant and anesthetic spray usually is applied to the nares, and the patient is asked to gently sniff these nose sprays. One percent pontocaine and 2% lidocaine are commonly used as topical anesthetics. Another way to administer anesthesia is to carefully apply a viscous 2% lidocaine solution to the nares with a cotton-tipped applicator. It is important to allow time for these topical agents to anesthetize the nasal mucosa, and while the physician is waiting, the scope can be prepared. The focus ring is used to get the brightest possible image. Often there is a small amount of residue at the end of the fiberoptic scope, and this can be carefully removed using either a pencil eraser or an alcohol swab. If the image is not clear when the scope is out of the nose, it will not allow for a useful image when the fiberoptic scope has been passed through the nares. Once the best possible focus has been obtained, a small amount of water-soluble lubricant should be applied approximately 1 cm from the tip of the scope. This is to prevent breakage of the fiberoptic component of the scope while it is passed through the nose.

The laryngoscope then is gently passed along the floor of the nose, and with the instrument tip held above the epiglottis, the larynx may be viewed. Pooling of secretions in the pyriform sinuses is abnormal and is common in patients with decreased laryngeal sensation, neurologic impairment, or tumors. Saliva freely flowing in and out of the true cords is another indication of decreased laryngeal function. In some patients, having patients inhale and hold their breath often aids in viewing the pyriform sinuses. Asking the patient to cough and swallow and then viewing the residual saliva or phlegm also is helpful. The flexible fiberoptic examination enables the patient to freely phonate, unlike with the mirror examination, and the true vocal folds may be assessed by moving the instrument tip into the laryngeal vestibule for closer inspection.

Rigid telescopic examination with 70°, 90°, and 110° telescopes is performed in a similar fashion to the mirror examination. It permits photographic documentation of the laryngeal examination. In patients with trismus, this is better tolerated than the mirror examination, and a minimal amount of local anesthetic usually is necessary.

Nose

Anterior rhinoscopy, using a headlight and nasal speculum allows assessment of the nasal septum and inferior turbinates. The speculum should be directed laterally to avoid touching the sensitive septum with the metal edges. The point wherein numerous small branches of the external and internal carotid arteries meet, or Kesselbach's plexus, is the most common site for epistaxis; prominent vessels in this area should be noted. Anterior septal deviations and bony spurs often are evident. The characteristics of the mucosa of the inferior turbinate may range from the boggy, edematous, pale mucosa seen in those with allergic rhinitis to the erythematous, edematous mucosa seen in those with sinusitis.

Rhinorrhea often reveals important clinical information. Clear mucus often is associated with allergic rhinitis or chronic vasomotor rhinitis. Yellow or green mucopurulence is common with sinusitis. Clear watery rhinorrhea may represent spinal fluid and may indicate a cerebrospinal fluid leak.

Nasal endoscopy using rigid endoscopes allows thorough examination of even the most posterior portions of the nasal cavity. After applying a local anesthetic to the nares, either lidocaine or pontocaine spray or topical 4% cocaine, the rigid 0° endoscope may be passed into the nose along the floor of the nasal vault. The septum, inferior turbinate, and eustachian tube orifices in the nasopharynx may be seen this way. Often, at this time, it is necessary to spray a decongestant to shrink the nasal mucosa. It is helpful to attempt to view the nasal anatomy in the native state and after the decongestant so that the effect of the decongestant may be seen. After inspecting both sides, the endoscope is placed above the inferior turbinate to view the middle turbinate. Accessory ostia from the maxillary sinus often are present, especially in patients with chronic sinusitis. These openings into the lateral nasal wall often are mistaken for the true maxillary ostium.

Nasopharynx

The nasopharynx extends from the skull base to the soft palate. This is a challenging area to examine, but with the available technology, there are many ways to approach this region. The technique used often will depend on the anatomy of the patient. In the patient with a high posterior soft palate and small tongue base, an otolaryngologist with a headlight may use a small dental mirror to visualize the nasopharynx. By having the patient sit upright in the chair, the physician may firmly pull the tongue forward while opening the mouth to place the mirror just posterior to the soft palate. In a manner analogous to that used to view the larynx with a mirror, the structures in the nasopharynx will be seen when the mirror is oriented upward.

Another method uses a fiberoptic nasopharyngoscope, which allows excellent visualization of this area. After anesthetizing the nares with either topical cocaine (on pledgets) or applying lidocaine spray, many otolaryngologists will spray the nares with a decongestant. The flexible fiberoptic scope then is gently passed along the floor of the nostril beneath the inferior turbinate. The eustachian tube orifice, torus tubarius, and fossa of Rosenmueller should be inspected on each side. This may be accomplished by using the hand control to turn the tip of the scope from side to side. The midline also should be inspected for any masses, ulcerations, or bleeding areas. Rigid endoscopes offer good visualization also, although the ability to view both sides of the nasopharynx often means passing the endoscope through each nostril. The endoscopes have various angles, such as 70°, 90°, and 110°.

Arguably, the best view of all may be obtained using a 90° rigid scope in the oropharynx. By advancing the rigid scope through the mouth and by placing the beveled edge posterior to the soft palate, the nasopharynx may be seen in its entirety. Both sides of the nasopharynx may be compared for symmetry using this technique.

Whereas children will have adenoid tissue present, adults should not have much adenoid tissue remaining in this area. Thus, adenoid tissue should not be a cause of nasal or eustachian tube obstruction in adults. One possible exception is patients with HIV infections, who may manifest adenoid hypertrophy as part of their disease. Nonetheless, adults with an otitis media, especially unilateral in nature, should have their nasopharynx inspected for possible nasopharyngeal masses. If present, it is important to diagnose nasopharyngeal carcinomas, which are most common lateral to the eustachian tube orifice in the fossa of Rosenmueller. In young male patients, nasopharyngeal angiofibromas are locally aggressive, but histologically benign masses that are most commonly present in the posterior choana or nasopharynx. These masses should not be missed. Another malignancy to consider is non-Hodgkin's lymphoma. Cysts in the superior portion of the nasopharynx may represent a benign Tornwaldt cyst or a malignant craniopharyngioma.

Table 1-3. Neurologic examination

Cranial nerves	Tests
I	Sense of smell to several substances
	Do not use ammonia (common chemical sense caused by CN V stimulation)
II	Visual acuity
	Visual fields
	Inspect optic fundi
III	Extraocular movements in six fields of gaze
IV	Pupillary reaction to light
V	Palpate temporal and masseter muscles
	Patient should clench teeth
	Test forehead, cheeks, jaw for pain, temperature and light (cotton) touch
	Corneal reflex (blinking in response to cotton touching the cornea)
VI	Near reaction to light
	Ptosis of upper eyelids
VII	Symmetry of face in repose
	Raise eyebrows, frown, close eyes tightly, smile, puff out cheeks
VIII	Auditory—Tuning fork tests for hearing
	Vestibular—Nystagmus on lateral gaze; Hallpike-Dix test; headshaking; Caloric testing; Frenzel lenses
IX, X	Hoarseness
	True vocal cord mobility
	Gag reflex (CN IX or X)
	Movement of soft palate and pharynx
XI	Shrug shoulders against examiner's hand (trapezius muscle)
	Turn head against examiner's hand (sternocleidomastoid muscle)
XII	Stick tongue out
	Tongue deviates toward side of lesion
	Tongue atrophy, fasciculations

NEUROLOGIC EXAMINATION

Table 1-3 outlines the basics of a neurologic examination appropriate for most head and neck patients. Certainly, patients presenting with vertigo or disequilibrium require a highly specialized neurologic examination, but that is beyond the scope of this chapter. Much valuable clinical information can be obtained with an evaluation of the cranial nerves.

CONCLUSION

This chapter serves as an outline for approaching the head and neck examination. There are many ways to perform the examination and to take the patient's history. This chapter is not meant as an exhaustive review of all the examination techniques available, and the order in which the head and neck regions are examined can be changed to suit the physician. Remember to be consistently thorough with each patient. Developing a competently performed, routine examination increases the probability of discovering important clinical information.

Chapter 2

The Preoperative Evaluation

James Blaugrund
Dario Kunar

Preoperative evaluation of surgical patients is, in its broadest sense, an extension of the diagnostic process. The surgeon should strive to determine the extent of disease; prove the necessity of surgery or clearly demonstrate its benefit to the patient; optimize the choice of surgical procedure; and minimize the risk to the patient by defining concomitant health problems and instituting appropriate therapy or precautionary measures. Integral to each of these goals is an appreciation of the ideal set forth in the Hippocratic Oath—Above all else, do no harm. It is the surgeon's responsibility to ensure that an appropriate patient assessment has been completed prior to entering the surgical suite. Surgical complications can often be avoided by recognizing the physiologic limitations of the patient preoperatively. Documentation of findings, decision making, and discussion between surgeon and patient regarding surgical risks and benefits have become medicolegal imperatives.

GENERAL CONSIDERATIONS

The patient presenting with an otolaryngologic disease process that requires surgical management must be evaluated by both general and specialty-specific criteria. As with the initial patient evaluation, preoperative assessment relies heavily on a careful history and physical examination. Special attention should be given to the patient's past medical and surgical history. A thorough review of systems helps to identify the conditions and risk factors that may complicate the perioperative course. Information should be elicited regarding the cardiovascular, pulmonary, renal, gastrointestinal, endocrine, hematologic, neurologic, immune, musculoskeletal, integumentary, and psychiatric systems. Additional testing, prophylactic measures, and behavioral modification prior to surgery can then be implemented to maximize the

surgical outcome. In addition, the patient's prior anesthetic record provides invaluable insight into issues such as airway management and overall tolerance of general, regional, local, or neuroleptic anesthesia. A social history can often be extremely beneficial as well, providing a means of anticipating postoperative needs and circumventing some prolonged admissions. Any significant issues should be raised with the departmental or hospital social worker, preferably prior to surgery. Lastly, it is important to elicit a detailed list of current medications and allergies.

In uncomplicated cases, the history and physical examination are followed by routine screening tests. Blood is drawn for a complete blood count (CBC), serum electrolytes, blood urea nitrogen (BUN), creatinine, glucose, and a clotting profile to rule out a wide range of possible occult abnormalities. In patients over 40 years of age or in those with pertinent past medical histories, chest radiography and electrocardiography (ECG) are performed. Additionally, women of childbearing age should undergo pregnancy testing.

When the need arises, consultation with appropriate specialties should be sought quickly. The consultant should be clearly informed about the nature of the proposed procedure and should be asked to comment specifically on the relative safety of performing the procedure with respect to concomitant disease processes. In cases complicated by many medical problems or in those in which the establishment of a safe airway is an issue, the authors advise close consultation with the anesthesia team to avoid undue delay, cancellation of the procedure, or an undesirable outcome.

Increasingly, the primary care physician conducts the preoperative evaluation. This phenomenon has become particularly prevalent in the managed care environment. Although a good internist can often facilitate the preoperative process, it is imperative to have copies of all laboratory results, radiographs, and pertinent tests available for review prior to surgery. Additional studies should be ordered by the surgeon as deemed necessary.

CONSENT

Although a detailed discussion of the legal ramifications of informed consent is beyond the scope of this chapter, the ethical ideal deserves consideration. A thorough and candid explanation of the procedure, its risks, and the probable outcomes has become an integral part of the preoperative process. More and more patients now come to their physician prepared to ask in-depth questions and expecting to receive detailed answers. The relationship that develops between the surgeon and patient at this time often does more to prevent litigation in the unfortunate circumstance of maloccurrence than any legal document detailing the ''risks and benefits.''

ALLERGY

The surgeon must guard against anaphylactic reactions in all patients. The crux of this process is to have the patient identify any untoward reactions to medications, foods, or other materials. In most instances, many of the drug ''reactions'' quoted by patients do not represent true allergic phenomena. Instead, they are simply medicinal side effects. Nonetheless, these reactions require thorough documentation and avoidance in the perioperative period.

Anaphylaxis is triggered by antigen-specific immunoglobulin E (IgE) antibody crosslinking at the mast cell surface. Subsequent mast cell degranulation releases potent inflammatory agents, vasoactive substances, and proteases, all of which mediate the shock reaction. The patient may develop urticaria, profound hypotension, tachycardia, bronchoconstriction, and airway-compromising edema of the mucosal surfaces of the upper aerodigestive tract. Even in intubated patients, rapid oxygen desaturation is often a prominent feature. As the reaction progresses, cardiac arrest can ensue despite maximal resuscitative efforts. Given the potential morbidity and mortality of anaphylactic reactions, the otolaryngologist must identify all allergens in the preoperative phase.

The incidence of serious adverse reactions to penicillin is about 1%. It is widely believed that there is a 10% to 15% chance that patients who manifest these reactions also react adversely to cephalosporins. The authors frequently administer intravenous cephalosporins intraoperatively, and the safety of their use in patients allergic to penicillin often comes into question. Based on empiric observations at the authors' institution, it is believed that unless these patients have had a history of significant atopy or penicillin-induced urticaria, mucosal edema, or anaphylaxis, they can be given cephalosporins with relative impunity. Anaphylactic reactions to cephalosporins in true penicillin-allergic patients are probably less than 2%. Moreover, cephalosporins cause their own independent hypersensitivity reactions; the notion of cross-reactivity with penicillin on skin testing seems to stem from data obtained in the 1970s, in which contamination of cephalosporins with penicillin was subsequently proven. Finally, if a serious penicillin allergy is evident, alternative antibiotics such as clindamycin may be substituted for the cephalosporins.

Mucosal absorption of latex protein allergens from the surgeon's gloves can rapidly incite anaphylactic shock in patients who are highly sensitive to latex. In fact, the authors have recently witnessed this dramatic reaction in the operating room. In preparation for surgery, a healthy, young patient was intubated, arterial and venous catheters were placed, and a Foley catheter was inserted. All procedures were performed by physicians and technicians wearing standard latex gloves. Shortly thereafter, the patient became profoundly hypotensive and hypoxic. Resuscitation was initiated and, after ruling out all other likely etiologies, the diagnosis of latex allergy was entertained. The patient was subsequently managed with latex-free products and, fortunately, survived a near catastrophe. The patient later recalled developing orofacial edema when he inflated balloons, and that rubber gloves would cause pruritus of his hands. Subsequent serum testing confirmed his latex allergy. It should be noted that about 7% to 10% of healthcare workers regularly exposed to latex and 28% to 67% of children with spina bifida demonstrate positive skin tests to latex proteins. Preoperatively, if a patient gives a history suspicious for latex allergy, it should be investigated prior to surgery; if the allergy is documented, perioperative precautions to avoid latex exposure must be instituted at all costs.

Similarly, patients with allergic or adverse reactions to soybean or eggs may react to propofol, a ubiquitous induction agent. Protamine and intravenous contrast agents can potentially provoke hypersensitivity responses in patients with known shellfish or other fish allergies. Although rare, some patients may have allergic reactions to ester types of local anesthetics such as cocaine, procaine, and tetracaine.

Finally, if the suspicion of allergy or adverse reaction exists, the best course of action is to avoid use of the potential offending agent altogether during surgery. If this is not feasible for some reason, then the surgeon and anesthesiologist should plan on premedicating the patient with systemic steroids, histamine antagonists, and even bronchodilators and should be prepared to deal with the potential worst-case scenario of anaphylactic shock.

SYSTEMS

Cardiovascular

Cardiovascular complications are the most common cause of perioperative mortality. Specifically, there is an almost 50% mortality rate associated with perioperative myocardial infarction. Meticulous review of the cardiovascular system is of utmost importance in determining a patient's surgical candidacy, especially for those who will require a general anesthetic. Risk factors for a perioperative cardiovascular complication include jugular venous distention, third heart sounds, recent myocardial infarction (MI) (within 6 months), nonsinus heart rhythm, frequent premature ventricular contractions (>5 per minute), over 70 years of age, valvular aortic stenosis, previous vascular or thoracic surgery, and poor overall medical status. Emergency surgery poses an additional risk for cardiovascular complications. In the head and neck oncology patient population, the high incidence of tobacco and alcohol abuse leads to a relatively high incidence of coronary artery disease, cardiomyopathy, and peripheral vascular disease.

The otolaryngologist should obtain a history of previous MIs, angina, angioplasty or bypass surgery, congestive heart failure (CHF) or dyspnea on exertion, hypertension, general exercise tolerance, paroxysmal nocturnal dyspnea, claudication, stroke or transient ischemic attack (TIA), syncope, palpitations or other arrhythmias, as well as known anatomic or auscultative cardiac anomalies. The presence or suspicion of coronary artery disease, heart failure, untreated hypertension, or significant peripheral vascular disease should prompt a specific anesthesiology or cardiology consultation before surgery. This evaluation would include an assessment of the electrocardiogram as well as possible exercise or chemical stress testing, echocardiography, and cardiac catheterization as indicated. The result of this consultation should determine the surgical and anesthetic risk and should optimize the patient's preoperative cardiovascular status. Furthermore, specific intraoperative and postoperative physiologic (e.g., invasive monitors) and pharmacologic precautionary measures should be delineated, as should the level of postoperative observation.

In general, patients are maintained on their antihypertensive, antianginal, and antiarrhythmic regimens up to the time of surgery. Certain medications such as diuretics and digoxin may be withheld at the discretion of the anesthesiologist or cardiologist. Preoperatively, serum electrolytes and antiarrhythmic levels should be checked and adjusted as necessary. Coagulation studies (prothrombin time [PT]/partial thromboplastin time [PTT]) and platelet quantification are routinely obtained in patients with the above-mentioned risk factors because significant bleeding can lead to major perioperative cardiovascular complications. A relatively current chest radiograph is considered essential in this high-risk group.

Preoperatively, the otolaryngologist must be aware of the types of procedures that may have specific cardiovascular ramifications. For instance, the intravascular volume loading that occurs during and after free flap surgery, through use of agents such as dextran and Hespan (Hetastarch, Dupont Pharma, Wilmington, Delaware), can have a significant impact on patients with a history of congestive heart failure, poor ventricular function, or atrial fibrillation. Furthermore, the fall in hematocrit often seen with the use of these agents can potentially induce coronary ischemia. Patients with pros-

thetic valves and those with a history of rheumatic fever, endocarditis, congenital heart defects, mitral valve prolapse with regurgitation, or hypertrophic cardiomyopathy should receive prophylactic antibiotics at the time of surgery. Such prophylaxis is especially important during procedures performed on the oral cavity and upper aerodigestive tract as well as dealing with surgical drainage of head and neck infections, in which the risk of hematogenous bacterial seeding is high. For low-risk procedures, intravenous ampicillin, 2 g given 30 minutes prior to surgery followed by 1 g 6 hours later, is sufficient prophylaxis. In high-risk procedures, intravenous gentamicin, 1.5 mg/kg, and intravenous ampicillin, 2 g, are administered 30 minutes before surgery, followed by the same doses of each 8 hours later. Patients with pacemakers or implanted defibrillators and those with mitral valve prolapse without regurgitation do not require endocarditis prophylaxis.

Airway, carotid, and vagus nerve manipulation can induce bradycardia and hypotension. Agents such as lidocaine, epinephrine, and cocaine, which are frequently used in sinonasal surgery, can trigger undesirable cardiovascular events. Injury to the cervical sympathetic chain may precipitate postural hypotension postoperatively. Finally, the surgeon must also be cognizant of the fact that a unipolar electrocautery device can reprogram a pacemaker during surgery.

Respiratory

Postoperative pulmonary complications are considered the second most common cause of perioperative mortality. This is not surprising when considering the effects of general anesthesia and surgery on pulmonary performance. Atelectasis and ventilation/perfusion mismatch occur secondary to a number of factors, including the use of anesthetic agents and positive pressure ventilation as well as supine positioning. Anesthetic agents, barbiturates, and opioids tend to diminish the ventilatory response to hypercarbia and hypoxia. Endotracheal intubation bypasses the warming and humidifying effects of the upper airway, leading to impaired ciliary function, thickened secretions, and subsequent decreased resistance to infection. Furthermore, postoperative pain substantially affects a patient's ability to cough, especially following thoracic or abdominal procedures (e.g., chest myocutaneous flap, gastric pull up, percutaneous endoscopic gastrostomy (PEG), rectus free-flap, iliac crest bone graft). Because of their attenuated respiratory reserve, patients with chronic pulmonary disease are much more likely to suffer postoperative pulmonary complications than are healthy patients. For instance, heavy smokers have a threefold increase in the risk of postoperative pulmonary complications when compared with nonsmokers. Hence it is imperative to identify these patients during the preoperative evaluation.

Specifically, a positive history of asthma, chronic obstructive pulmonary disease (COPD), emphysema, tobacco abuse, pneumonia, pulmonary edema, pulmonary fibrosis, or adult respiratory distress syndrome (ARDS) requires heightened attention prior to surgery. The prior treatment of these lung problems, including the number of hospitalizations and emergency room visits; the use of medications like steroids, antibiotics, and bronchodilators; and the need for intubation or chronic oxygen therapy should be addressed. The otolaryngologist should obtain an estimate of the patient's dyspnea, exercise limitation, cough, hemoptysis, and sputum production. Factors that exacerbate chronic lung disease must be identified. Once again, it is of paramount importance to investigate the tolerance of previous anesthetics in this high-risk group. Coexisting cardiac and renal disease such as CHF and chronic renal failure also impact heavily on pulmonary function. Pulmonary hypertension and cor pulmonale secondary to obstructive sleep apnea, cystic fibrosis, muscular dystrophy, emphysema, or kyphoscoliosis further complicate anesthetic management. Congenital diseases affecting the lungs such as cystic fibrosis and Kartagener's syndrome (rare) present the challenge of perioperative clearance of secretions.

On physical examination, the clinician should be attuned to the patient's body habitus and general appearance. Obesity, kyphoscoliosis, and pregnancy can all predispose to poor ventilation, atelectasis, and hypoxemia. Cachectic patients are more likely to develop postoperative pneumonia. It should be noted that clubbing and cyanosis, although suggestive, are not reliable indicators of chronic pulmonary disease. The patient's respiratory rate is determined, and the presence of accessory muscle use, nasal flaring, diaphoresis, or stridor should be documented. Auscultation that reveals wheezing, rhonchi, diminished breath sounds, crackles, rales, and altered inspiratory:expiratory time ratios should raise the suspicion of pulmonary compromise.

In patients with pulmonary disease, preoperative posteroanterior and lateral chest radiography is mandatory, because findings will often direct modification of the anesthetic technique used during surgery. Arterial blood gas (ABG) testing on room air is also indicated. Patients with an arterial oxygen tension less than 60 mm Hg or an arterial carbon dioxide tension greater than 50 mm Hg are more likely to have postoperative pulmonary complications. Serial ABG determinations can also assess the overall efficacy of preoperative medical and respiratory therapy. As with chest radiography, preoperative ABG levels also provide a baseline for postoperative comparison. Preoperative pulmonary function tests such as spirometry and flow–volume loops are quite helpful. A quantitative measure of ventilatory function can also be used to assess the efficacy of both preoperative and surgical interventions. Spirometry can be used to differentiate restrictive from obstructive lung disease as well as to predict perioperative morbidity from pulmonary complications. Generally, a forced expiratory volume in 1 second: forced vital capacity ratio of less than 75% is considered abnormal, whereas a ratio of less than 50% carries a significant risk of perioperative pulmonary complications. Preoperative flow–volume loops can distinguish among fixed (e.g.,

goiter), variable extrathoracic (e.g., unilateral vocal cord paralysis), and variable intrathoracic (e.g., tracheal mass) airway obstructions.

The preoperative management of otolaryngology patients with significant pulmonary disease is vital and should follow the recommendations of a pulmonologist. Smokers are advised to cease smoking for at least a week prior to surgery. Known airway irritants and triggers of bronchospasm should be avoided as much as possible. The patient should be well hydrated and should breathe warm, humidified air or oxygen. Chest physiotherapy aimed at increasing lung volumes and clearing secretions is instituted. This includes coughing and deep breathing exercises, incentive spirometry, and chest percussion with postural drainage. It is not advisable to operate on a patient with an acute exacerbation of pulmonary disease or with an acute pulmonary infection. Acute infections should be cleared with antibiotics and chest physiotherapy prior to elective surgery. Prophylactic antibiotics in noninfected patients are not recommended for fear of selecting out resistant organisms. Finally, the medical regimen, including the use of inhaled β-adrenergic agonists, cromolyn, and steroids (inhaled or systemic), must be optimized. Serum levels of theophylline, if used, should be therapeutic.

Renal

The preoperative identification and evaluation of renal problems is also imperative. Any significant electrolyte abnormalities uncovered during the routine screening of healthy patients should be corrected preoperatively, and surgery should be delayed if additional medical evaluation is warranted. Preexisting renal disease is a major risk factor for the development of acute tubular necrosis both during and after surgery. Renal failure, whether acute or chronic, influences the types, dosages, and intervals of perioperative drugs and anesthetics. An oliguric or anuric condition requires judicious fluid management, especially in patients with cardiorespiratory compromise. Furthermore, chronic renal failure (CRF) is often associated with anemia, platelet dysfunction, and coagulopathy. Electrolyte abnormalities, particularly hyperkalemia, can lead to arrhythmias, especially in the setting of the chronic metabolic acidosis that often accompanies CRF. Hypertension and accelerated atherosclerosis resulting from CRF are risk factors for developing myocardial ischemia intraoperatively. Blunted sympathetic responses may predispose to hypotensive episodes during administration of anesthesia. The otolaryngologist must also be wary of the potential for injury to demineralized bones during patient positioning. An impaired immune system can contribute to poor wound healing and postoperative infection. Finally, because patients with CRF have often received blood transfusions, they are at increased risk of carrying blood-borne pathogens such as hepatitis B and C.

The possible causes of renal disease, including hypertension, diabetes, nephrolithiasis, glomerulonephritis, polycystic disease, lupus, polyarteritis nodosa, Goodpasture's or

Wegener's syndromes, trauma, or previous surgical or anesthetic insults, should be elicited. The symptoms of polyuria, polydipsia, fatigue, dyspnea, dysuria, hematuria, oliguria or anuria, and peripheral edema are recorded, as is a complete listing of all medications taken by the patient.

In dialyzed patients, it is important to document the dialysis schedule. A nephrologist should assist with the preoperative evaluation and should optimize the patient's fluid status and electrolytes prior to surgery. A nephrologist should also be available to help manage these issues postoperatively, especially when major head and neck, skull-base, or neurotologic surgery, which may require large volumes of fluids or blood transfusions intraoperatively, is planned.

Preoperative testing on patients with significant renal disease routinely includes ECG, chest radiography, electrolytes and chemistry panel, CBC, PT/PTT, platelet counts, and bleeding times. In addition to a nephrologic consultation, patients with significant renal disease should also receive a preoperative anesthesiology consultation, and, if indicated, further evaluation by a cardiologist.

A history of benign prostatic hypertrophy or prostate cancer, with or without surgery, may predict a difficult urinary tract catheterization intraoperatively. Finally, elective surgery should not be performed on patients with acute genitourinary tract infections because the potential for urosepsis can be increased by the transient immunosuppression associated with general anesthesia.

HEPATIC DISORDERS

Preoperative evaluation of patients with suspected or clinically evident liver failure should begin with a history eliciting the details of hepatotoxic drug therapy, jaundice, blood transfusion, upper gastrointestinal bleeding, and previous surgery and anesthesia. The physical should include examination for hepatomegaly, splenomegaly, ascites, jaundice, asterixis, and encephalopathy. The list of blood tests is fairly extensive and includes hematocrit, platelet count, bilirubin, electrolytes, creatinine, BUN, serum protein, PT/PTT, serum aminotransferases, alkaline phosphatase, and lactate dehydrogenase. A viral hepatitis screen can be obtained as well. Of note, patients with moderate to severe chronic alcoholic hepatitis may present with relatively normal-appearing liver function tests and coagulation parameters; these patients are at risk for perioperative liver failure. In the last few years, at least four patients under the authors' care ultimately succumbed to complications of liver failure following surgery.

Cirrhosis and portal hypertension have wide-ranging systemic manifestations. Arterial vasodilation and collateralization leads to decreased peripheral vascular resistance and an increased cardiac output. This hyperdynamic state can occur even in the face of alcoholic cardiomyopathy. The responsiveness of the cardiovascular system to sympathetic discharge and administration of catechols is also reduced, likely secondary to increased serum glucagon levels. Cardiac output can be reduced by the use of propranolol, which has been advocated by some as a treatment for esophageal varices. By decreasing cardiac output, flow through the portal system and the esophageal variceal collaterals is diminished. Additionally, there is likely a selective splanchnic vasoconstriction. Once initiated, β-blockade cannot be stopped easily because of a significant rebound effect.

Renal sequelae vary with the severity of liver disease from mild sodium retention to acute failure associated with the hepatorenal syndrome. Diuretics given to decrease ascites can often lead to intravascular hypovolemia, azotemia, hyponatremia, and encephalopathy. Fluid management in the perioperative period should be followed closely and dialysis instituted as needed for acute renal failure.

From a hematologic standpoint, patients with cirrhosis often have an increased 2,3-diphosphoglycerate level in their erythrocytes causing a shift to the right of the oxyhemoglobin dissociation curve. Clinically, this results in a lower oxygen saturation. This situation is further compounded by the frequent finding of anemia. Additionally, significant thrombocytopenia and coagulopathy may be encountered. The preoperative use of appropriate blood products can lead to short-term correction of hematologic abnormalities, but the prognosis in these patients remains poor.

Encephalopathy stems from insufficient hepatic elimination of nitrogenous compounds. Although measurements of BUN and serum ammonia levels are useful, they do not always correlate with the degree of encephalopathy. Treatment includes hemostasis, antibiotics, meticulous fluid management, low-protein diet, and lactulose.

ENDOCRINE DISORDERS

Thyroid

Symptoms of hyperthyroidism include weight loss, diarrhea, skeletal muscle weakness, warm, moist skin, heat intolerance, and nervousness. Laboratory test results may demonstrate hypercalcemia, thrombocytopenia, and mild anemia. Elderly patients also can present with heart failure, atrial fibrillation, or other dysrhythmias. The term *thyroid storm* refers to a life-threatening exacerbation of hyperthyroidism that results in severe tachycardia and hypertension.

Treatment of hyperthyroidism attempts to establish a euthyroid state and to ameliorate systemic symptoms. Propylthiouracil inhibits both thyroid hormone synthesis and the peripheral conversion of T4 to T3. Complete clinical response may take up to 8 weeks, during which the dosage may need to be tailored to prevent hypothyroidism. Potassium iodide (Lugol's solution), which works by inhibiting iodide organification, can be added to the medical regimen. In patients with sympathetic hyperactivity, β-blockers have been used effectively. Propranolol has the added benefit of decreasing T4-to-T3 conversion. It should not be used in patients with CHF secondary to poor left ventricular function or bronchospasm because it will exacerbate both of these conditions. Ideally, medical therapy should prepare a mildly thyrotoxic patient for surgery within 7 to 14 days. If the need for emergency surgery arises, intravenous propranolol or esmolol can be administered and titrated to keep the heart rate below 90 bpm. Other medications that can be used include reserpine and guanethidine, which deplete catechol stores, and glucocorticoids, which decrease both thyroid hormone secretion and T4-to-T3 conversion. Radioactive iodine also can be used effectively to obliterate thyroid function but should not be given to women of childbearing years.

The symptoms of hypothyroidism result from inadequate circulating levels of T4 and T3 and include lethargy, cognitive impairment, and cold intolerance. Clinical findings may include bradycardia, hypotension, hypothermia, hypoventilation, and hyponatremia. There is no evidence to suggest that patients with mild to moderate hypothyroidism are at increased risk for anesthetic complications, but all elective surgery patients should be treated with thyroid hormone replacement prior to surgery. Severe hypothyroidism resulting in myxedema coma is a medical emergency and is associated with a high mortality rate. Intravenous infusion of T3 or T4 and glucocorticoids should be combined with ventilatory support and temperature control as needed.

Parathyroid

The prevalence of primary hyperparathyroidism increases with age. Sixty percent to 70% of patients with primary hyperparathyroidism present initially with nephrolithiasis secondary to hypercalcemia, and 90% are found to have benign parathyroid adenomas. Hyperparathyroidism secondary to hyperplasia occurs in association with medullary thyroid cancer and pheochromocytoma in multiple endocrine neoplasia (MEN) type IIA and, more rarely, with malignancy. In humoral hypercalcemia of malignancy, nonendocrine tumors have been demonstrated to secrete a parathyroid hormone–like protein. Secondary hyperparathyroidism usually results from chronic renal disease. The hypocalcemia and hyperphosphatemia associated with this condition lead to increased parathyroid hormone production and, over time, to parathyroid hyperplasia. Tertiary hyperparathyroidism occurs when the CRF is rapidly corrected as in renal transplantation.

In addition to nephrolithiasis, signs and symptoms of hypercalcemia include polyuria, polydipsia, skeletal muscle weakness, epigastric discomfort, peptic ulceration, and constipation. Radiographs may show significant bone resorption in 10% to 15% of patients. Depression, confusion, and psychosis also may be associated with marked elevations in serum calcium levels.

Immediate treatment of hypercalcemia usually combines sodium diuresis with a loop diuretic and rehydration with normal saline as needed. This becomes urgent once the serum calcium levels rise above 15 g/dl. Several medications can be used to decrease serum calcium levels. Etidronate inhibits abnormal bone resorption. The cytotoxic agent mithramycin inhibits parathyroid hormone–induced osteo-

cytoclastic activity but is associated with significant side effects, and calcitonin works transiently again by direct inhibition of osteoclast activity. Hemodialysis can also be used in the appropriate patient population.

The most common cause of hypoparathyroidism is iatrogenic. Thyroid and parathyroid surgery occasionally results in the inadvertent removal of all parathyroid tissue. Ablation of parathyroid tissue can also occur after major head and neck surgery and postoperative radiation therapy. Symptoms include tetany, perioral and digital paresthesias, muscle spasm, and seizures. Chvostek's sign (facial nerve hyperactivity elicited by tapping over the common trunk of the nerve as it passes through the parotid gland) and Trousseau's sign (finger and wrist spasm after inflation of a blood pressure cuff for several minutes) are clinically important indicators of latent hypercalcemia. Treatment is with calcium supplementation and vitamin D analogs.

Adrenal

Adrenal gland hyperactivity can result from a pituitary adenoma, a corticotropin hormone (ACTH)-producing nonendocrine tumor, or a primary adrenal neoplasm. Symptoms include truncal obesity, proximal muscle wasting, "moon" facies, and changes in behavior that vary from emotional lability to frank psychosis. Diagnosis is made through the dexamethasone suppression test, and treatment is adrenalectomy or hypophysectomy. It is important to regulate blood pressure and serum glucose levels and to normalize intravascular volume and electrolytes. Primary aldosteronism (Conn's syndrome) results in increased renal tubular exchange of sodium for potassium and hydrogen ions. This leads to hypokalemia, skeletal muscle weakness, fatigue, and acidosis. The aldosterone antagonist spironolactone should be used if the patient requires diuresis.

Idiopathic primary adrenal insufficiency (Addison's disease) results in both glucocorticoid and mineralocorticoid deficiencies. Symptoms include asthenia, weight loss, anorexia, abdominal pain, nausea, vomiting, diarrhea, constipation, hypotension, and hyperpigmentation. Hyperpigmentation is caused by overproduction of ACTH and β-lipotropin, which leads to melanocyte proliferation. Measurement of plasma cortisol levels 30 and 60 minutes after intravenous administration of ACTH, 250 mg, aids in diagnosis. Patients with primary adrenal insufficiency demonstrate no response. Glucocorticoid replacement is required on a twice-daily basis and should be increased with stress. Mineralocorticoid therapy can be given once daily. Of note, patients treated for more than 3 weeks with exogenous glucocorticoids for any medical condition should be assumed to have suppression of their adrenal–pituitary axis and should be treated with stress-dose steroids perioperatively.

Pheochromocytoma is a tumor of the adrenal medulla that secretes both epinephrine and norepinephrine. Five percent of these tumors are inherited in an autosomal dominant fashion as part of a multiple endocrine neoplasia syndrome.

Symptoms include hypertension (which is often episodic), headache, palpitations, tremor, and profuse sweating. Preoperative treatment begins with phenoxybenzamine, a long-acting α-blocker, or prazosin at least 10 days prior to surgery. A β-blocker is added only after the establishment of α-blockade to avoid unopposed β-mediated vasoconstriction. Acute hypertensive crises can be managed with nitroprusside or phentolamine.

Diabetes mellitus

Diabetes is a disorder of carbohydrate metabolism that results in a wide range of systemic manifestations. It is the most common endocrine abnormality found in surgical patients and can be characterized as either insulin-dependent (type I or juvenile onset) or non-insulin–dependent (type II). Hyperglycemia may result from a variety of etiologies that affect insulin production and function. Management techniques seek to avoid hypoglycemia and maintain high normal serum glucose levels throughout the perioperative period. These goals are often difficult to maintain, however, because infection, stress, exogenous steroids, and variations in carbohydrate intake can all cause wide fluctuations in serum glucose levels. Close monitoring is mandatory, with correction of hyperglycemia using a sliding scale for insulin dosage or continuous intravenous infusion in more severe cases. Fluid management should focus on maintaining hydration and electrolyte balance.

HEMATOLOGIC DISORDERS

A history of easy bruising or excessive bleeding with prior surgery should raise suspicion of a possible hematologic diathesis. A significant number of patients will also present on anticoagulative therapy for coexisting medical conditions. It is therefore important for the surgeon to recognize and treat the diagnosis and therapy of the more common hematologic disorders, both congenital and acquired.

After a careful history, the physician should obtain laboratory studies. PT, PTT, and platelet count are included in the routine preoperative screen. PT evaluates both the extrinsic and the final common pathways. Included in the extrinsic pathway are the vitamin K–dependent factors II, VII, IX, and X, which are inhibited by warfarin. Conversely, heparin inhibits thrombin and factors IXa, Xa, and XIa, elements of the intrinsic clotting pathway. PTT measures the effectiveness of the intrinsic and final common pathways. Relative to the normal population, some patients may demonstrate significant variation in the quantitative levels of certain factors in the absence of clinically relevant clotting abnormalities. Thrombocytopenia or platelet dysfunction can also lead to derangements in coagulation. A standard CBC includes a platelet count, which should be greater than 50,000 to 70,000 before surgery. The ivy bleeding time, a clinical test of platelet function, should be between 3 and 8 minutes. Fibrin split products may also be measured to help determine the diagnosis of disseminated intravascular coagulation.

Congenital

Congenital deficiencies of hemostasis affect up to 1% of the population. Fortunately, the majority of these deficiencies are clinically mild. Two of the more serious deficiencies involve factor VIII, which is a complex of two subunits, factor VIII:C and factor VIII:von Willebrand's factor. Sex-linked recessive transmission of defects in the quantity and quality of factor VIII:C leads to hemophilia A. Because of its short half-life, perioperative management of factor VIII:C requires infusion of cryoprecipitate every 8 hours. Historically, these patients have had a high incidence of hepatitis and HIV due to the administration of pooled blood products. Improved screening of blood products and recombinant deoxyribonucleic acid (DNA) technology have markedly diminished this problem.

von Willebrand's disease has a milder presentation than hemophilia A; bleeding tends to be mucosal rather than visceral. There are three subtypes. Types I and II represent quantitative and qualitative deficiencies, respectively, and are passed by autosomal dominant transmission. Type I also is characterized by low levels of factor VIII:C. Much rarer and transmitted as an autosomal recessive gene, type III von Willebrand's disease presents with symptoms similar to those of hemophilia A. Because of the longer half-life of factor VIII:von Willebrand's factor, patients with type II von Willebrand's disease can be transfused with cryoprecipitate up to 24 hours before surgery, with repeat infusions every 24 to 48 hours. Patients with type I von Willebrand's disease require additional transfusion just prior to surgery in order to boost factor VIII:C levels and normalize bleeding time.

Patients with hemophilia, von Willebrand's disease, and other less common congenital hemostatic anomalies should be followed perioperatively by a hematologist. Correction of factor deficiencies should be instituted in a timely fashion, and patients should be monitored closely for any evidence of bleeding.

Anticoagulants

Warfarin, heparin, and aspirin have become commonly used medications in the medical arsenal. Conditions such as atrial fibrillation, deep vein thrombosis, pulmonary embolism, and heart valve replacement are routinely treated initially with heparin, followed by warfarin on an outpatient basis. This therapy markedly decreases the incidence of thromboembolic events and, when appropriately monitored, only slightly increases the risk of hemorrhagic complications. Aspirin is widely used both as an analgesic and as prophylaxis for coronary artery disease. Patients taking any of these medications need careful evaluation to assess the severity of the condition necessitating anticoagulation. The benefit of surgery relative to the risk of normalizing coagulation should be clearly established with both the patient and the physician prescribing the anticoagulant.

Warfarin should be stopped at least 3 days prior to surgery

depending on liver function. Patients who have been determined to be at high risk for thromboembolism should be admitted for heparinization prior to surgery. The infusion rate can then be adjusted to maintain the PTT in a therapeutic range. Discontinuation of heparin approximately 6 hours before surgery should provide adequate time for reversal of anticoagulation. In emergency situations, warfarin can be reversed with vitamin K in approximately 6 hours and more quickly with the infusion of fresh frozen plasma (FFP). Heparin can be reversed with protamine or FFP. Of note, a heparin rebound phenomenon in which anticoagulative effects are reestablished can occur up to 24 hours after the use of protamine. Anticoagulative therapy can be reinstituted soon after surgery if necessary. Most surgeons, however, prefer to wait several days unless contraindicated. It is often helpful to discuss the timing of postoperative therapy with the hematologist prior to surgery.

Aspirin, an irreversible inhibitor of platelet function, leads to prolonged bleeding time. There is no strong evidence to link aspirin therapy with excessive intraoperative bleeding. However, the theoretical risk that aspirin and other nonsteroidal antiinflammatory medications present leads most surgeons to request that their patients stop taking these medications up to 2 weeks prior to surgery to allow the platelet population to turn over.

Liver failure

Patients with liver failure can present with several hematologic abnormalities. Bleeding from esophageal varices secondary to portal hypertension can lead to anemia. Hypersplenism and alcoholic bone marrow suppression can result in serious thrombocytopenia. An elevated PT may indicate a deficiency in the vitamin K-dependent factors of the extrinsic clotting pathway as well as factors I, V, and XI, which are also produced in the liver. Lastly, as liver failure progresses, excessive fibrinolysis may occur. All of these hematologic sequelae of hepatic failure increase the risk of operative morbidity and mortality. Preoperative management should attempt to correct anemia and thrombocytopenia as indicated and replenish deficient clotting factors with FFP. Fluid management may prove to be a difficult issue.

Another less common cause of PT elevation is the intestinal sterilization syndrome in which intestinal flora, a major source of vitamin K, are eradicated by prolonged doses of antibiotics in patients unable to obtain vitamin K from other sources. Reversal occurs rapidly with vitamin K therapy.

Thrombocytopenia

A decrease in platelet count can occur as a result of a variety of medical conditions, including massive transfusion, liver failure, disseminated intravascular coagulation, aplastic anemia, hematologic malignancy, and idiopathic thrombocytopenic purpura. With the increasing use of chemotherapeutics for a variety of malignancies, the prevalence of iatrogenic thrombocytopenia has risen. Preoperatively, the

platelet count should be greater than 50,000; at levels below 20,000, spontaneous bleeding may occur. Additionally, any indication of platelet dysfunction should be evaluated with a bleeding time. Severe azotemia secondary to renal failure may lead to platelet dysfunction (uremic platelet syndrome). Dialysis should be performed as necessary.

Correction of thrombocytopenia with platelet transfusion should preferably come from human leukocyte antigen–matched donors, particularly in patients who have received prior platelet transfusions and may be sensitized. One unit of platelets contains approximately 5.5×10^{11} platelets. One unit per 10 kg of body weight is a good initial dose. The platelets should be infused rapidly just prior to surgery.

Hemaglobinopathies

Of the more than 300 hemaglobinopathies, sickle cell disease and thalassemia are by far the most common. Approximately 10% of blacks in the United States carry the gene for sickle cell anemia. The heterozygous state imparts no real anesthetic risk. There are significant clinical manifestations to the 1 in 400 blacks who are homozygous for hemoglobin S. The genetic mutation results in the substitution of valine for glutamic acid in the sixth position of the β-chain of the hemoglobin molecule, leading to alterations in the shape of erythrocytes when the hemoglobin deoxygenates. The propensity for sickling directly relates to the quantity of hemoglobin S. Clinical findings include anemia and chronic hemolysis. Infarction of multiple organ systems can occur secondary to vessel occlusion. Most patients die by 30 years of age as a result of complications of their disease.

Treatment consists of preventive measures. Oxygenation and hydration help maintain tissue perfusion. Transfusion prior to surgical procedures decreases the concentration of erythrocytes carrying hemoglobin S, thereby lowering the chance of sickling.

There are multiple types of thalassemia, each caused by genetic mutations in one of the subunits of the hemoglobin molecule. Symptoms vary on the severity of the mutation. Patients with the most severe form, β-thalassemia major, are transfusion dependent, which often leads to iron toxicity. Other thalassemias cause only mild hemolytic anemia. If transfusion dependency exists, the patient should be screened carefully for hepatic and cardiac sequelae of iron toxicity.

NEUROLOGIC

A solid, working familiarity with the cranial nerves is intrinsic to the specialty of otolaryngology. Numerous pathologic processes, both benign and malignant, as well as traumatic injuries have the potential for cranial nerve and intracranial involvement. In the preoperative setting, therefore, the otolaryngologist is obliged to perform a thorough neurologic examination and review of the neurologic system. A cursory search for symptoms of visual loss, diplopia, anosmia, facial pain and tics, headaches, paresthesias and hypoesthesias, facial paralysis or paresis, dysequilibrium, hearing loss, dysphagia, hoarseness, and tongue deviation or fasciculations forms a basis of the neurologic history. A more specific review can then be tailored based on the presenting complaint and physical findings. Recognition of constellations of signs and symptoms, as seen in Horner's syndrome, is useful in establishing a diagnosis.

Confirmation of neurologic deficits can be made using various examinations and tests such as audiometry, electronystagmography, electromyography, cine-esophagography, videostroboscopy, and fiberoptic laryngoscopy. For medicolegal reasons, it is critical to document all neurologic abnormalities. It is important to distinguish peripheral from central lesions, and computed tomography (CT) or magnetic resonance imaging (MRI) is often helpful in this regard. Frequently, neurologic consultation is sought in the setting of subtle findings or confusing or paradoxic findings and for evaluation of possible nonotolaryngologic etiologies of certain complaints such as headache and dysequilibrium. During preoperative counseling of the patient, the surgeon must be aware of the potential for nerve injury or sacrifice and must communicate the possible sequelae of these actions to the patient.

If present, a history of seizures should be outlined with respect to the type, pattern, and frequency of epilepsy as well as the current anticonvulsant medications in use and their side effects. Phenytoin therapy can lead to poor dentition and anemia, whereas treatment with carbamazepine can cause hepatic dysfunction, hyponatremia, thrombocytopenia, and leukopenia, all of which represent concerns for the surgeon and anesthesiologist. Preoperative CBC, liver function tests, and coagulation studies are thus advised. Anesthetic agents such as enflurane, propofol, and lidocaine have the potential to precipitate convulsant activity, depending on their doses. In general, antiseizure medications must be at therapeutic serum levels and should be continued up to and including the day of surgery.

Symptomatic autonomic dysfunction can contribute to intraoperative hypotension. It may be necessary to augment intravascular volume preoperatively through increasing dietary salt intake, maximizing hydration, and administering fludrocortisone.

Additional considerations must be taken into account in patients with upper motor neuron diseases, such as amyotrophic lateral sclerosis, or lower motor neuron processes affecting cranial nerve nuclei in the brainstem. In either case, the otolaryngologist may be confronted with bulbar symptoms such as dysphagia, dysphonia, and inefficient mastication. As bulbar impairment progresses, the risk of aspiration increases significantly. When respiratory muscles are affected, the patient is likely to have dyspnea, intolerance to lying flat, and an ineffective cough. Coupled with aspiration, these factors put the patient at considerable surgical risk for pulmonary complications. Hence, if surgery is necessary for these patients, preoperative evaluation should include a pulmonary workup (including chest radiography, pulmonary function tests, ABG analysis) and consultation. A video study of swallowing function may also be indicated. Finally, the patient's neurologist should be closely involved in the decision making (i.e., whether to proceed with surgery).

Parkinsonism presents the challenges of excessive salivation and bronchial secretions, gastroesophageal reflux, obstructive and central sleep apnea, and autonomic insufficiency, all of which predispose to difficult airway and blood pressure management in the perioperative period. Dopaminergic medications should be administered up to the time of surgery in order to avoid the potentially fatal neuroleptic malignant syndrome. Medications such as phenothiazines, metoclopromide, and other antidopaminergics should be avoided. Preoperatively, the patient's pulmonary function and autonomic stability should be investigated.

If clinically indicated, patients with multiple sclerosis should also undergo full pulmonary evaluation preoperatively, because these patients can present with poor respiratory and bulbar function. The presence of contractures can limit patient positioning on the operating table. In addition, prior to surgery, the patient must be free of infection because pyrexia can exacerbate the conduction block in demyelinated neurons.

Otolaryngologists often must manage patients with facial trauma and head injury, usually in the acute care setting. Preoperative evaluation should be guided by the ABC's of resuscitation. Emergency situations predisposing to loss of the airway or cardiovascular collapse must be addressed immediately. Additionally, once stabilized, a thorough neurosurgical or neurologic assessment is required prior to elective fixation of injuries such as facial fractures.

Preoperative management of patients with any of the other remaining neurologic disorders is not discussed here. Evaluation in these patients should be focused primarily on airway, cardiopulmonary, and neurologic issues, as well as any other coexisting medical problems that may compromise anesthetic outcome.

Finally, for medicolegal reasons, an estimation of the mental status of all patients should be documented preoperatively.

THE GERIATRIC PATIENT

The elderly represent the fastest growing segment of the U.S. population. Twenty-five percent to 33% of all surgeries are currently performed on individuals over 65 years of age, and this percentage is likely to increase in the next decade as the "baby boom" generation reaches retirement age. A greater likelihood of comorbid conditions exists with increasing age. In addition, physiologic reserve is often compromised. Preoperative assessment in this population should take these considerations into account and weigh the benefit of the procedure against the often increased risks in this population. Consultation with the anesthesia service facilitates planning for high-risk elderly patients.

Approximately 50% of all postoperative deaths in the elderly occur secondary to cardiovascular events. Severe cardiac disease should be treated prior to any elective procedure and should be weighed against the benefit of any more urgent procedure. If surgery is required, cardiac precautions should be instituted. Patients with physical evidence or a history of peripheral vascular disease should be evaluated for carotid artery stenosis. If a critical stenosis is identified, carotid endarterectomy should be performed to any elective procedure that requires a general anesthetic. The risk of a cerebrovascular accident should be considered when evaluating patients for more urgent procedures. In vasculopathic patients requiring free-flap reconstruction after major head and neck resection, examination of both recipient and donor vessels should be performed prior to surgery to minimize complications and assist in the appropriate choice of reconstructive options.

From a respiratory standpoint, increasing age leads to loss of lung compliance, stiffening of the chest wall, and atrophy of respiratory muscles. In many otolaryngology procedures, the risk of intraoperative or postoperative aspiration and postobstructive pulmonary edema must also be considered. Patients with borderline pulmonary function may not tolerate even mild respiratory complications. The function of all the organ systems diminishes with age, necessitating a thorough preoperative evaluation to maximize patient safety in the elderly population.

CONCLUSION

This chapter has provided a brief overview of the preoperative evaluation. Disturbances in one organ system often have repercussions for other systems, and so an interdisciplinary approach involving the otolaryngologist, anesthesiologist, internist, and specialized consultants is often warranted. The authors have chosen to emphasize the physiologic aspects of the evaluation. This is not intended to overshadow the importance of gaining insight into a patient's psychosocial preparedness, which often requires the help of family members, social workers, psychiatrists, and support groups as well as a keen sense of intuition on the part of the surgeon. Furthermore, preoperative teaching provides a means to reinforce postoperative expectations and coping mechanisms. Finally, it must be reiterated that the responsibility of ensuring an appropriate preoperative evaluation lies with the surgeon and that the expediency of this process should be in keeping with the best interest of the patient.

SUGGESTED READINGS

Adkins Jr RB: *Preoperative assessment of the elderly patient.* In Cameron JL, editor: *Current surgical therapy,* St Louis, 1992, Mosby.

Buckley FP: *Anesthesia and obesity and gastrointestinal disorders.* In Barash PG, Cullen BF, Stoelting RK, editors: *Clinical anesthesia,* Philadelphia, 1989, JB Lippincott.

Curzen N: *Patients with permanent pacemakers in situ.* In Goldstone JC, Pollard BJ, editors: *Handbook of clinical anesthesia,* New York, 1996, Churchill Livingstone.

Davies W: *Coronary artery disease.* In Goldstone JC, Pollard BJ, editors: *Handbook of clinical anesthesia,* New York, 1996, Churchill Livingstone.

Ellison N: *Hemostasis and hemotherapy.* In Barash PG, Cullen BF, Stoelting RK, editors: *Clinical anesthesia,* Philadelphia, 1989, JB Lippincott.

Gelman S: *Anesthesia and the liver.* In Barash PG, Cullen BF, Stoelting RK, editors: *Clinical anesthesia,* Philadelphia, 1989, JB Lippincott.

Goldstone JC: *COPD and anesthesia.* In Goldstone JC, Pollard BJ, editors: *Handbook of clinical anesthesia,* New York, 1996, Churchill Livingstone.

Graf G, Rosenbaum S: *Anesthesia and the endocrine system.* In Barash PG, Cullen BF, Stoelting RK, editors: *Clinical anesthesia,* Philadelphia, 1989, JB Lippincott.

Hirsch NP, Smith M: *Central nervous system.* In Goldstone JC, Pollard BJ, editors: *Handbook of clinical anesthesia,* New York, 1996, Churchill Livingstone.

Hurford WE: *Specific considerations with pulmonary disease.* In Firestone LL, Lebowitz PW, Cook CE, editors: *Clinical anesthesia procedures of the Massachusetts General Hospital,* ed 3, Boston/Toronto, 1988, Little, Brown.

Kovatsis PG: *Specific considerations with renal disease.* In Davidson JK, Eckhardt III WF, Perese DA, editors: *Clinical anesthesia procedures of the Massachusetts General Hospital,* ed 4, Boston/Toronto/London, 1993, Little, Brown.

Long TJ: *General preanesthetic evaluation.* In Davidson JK, Eckhardt III WF, Perese DA, editors: *Clinical anesthesia procedures of the Massachusetts General Hospital,* ed 4, Boston/Toronto/London, 1993, Little, Brown.

Morgan C: *Cardiovascular disease, general considerations.* In Goldstone JC, Pollard BJ, editors: *Handbook of clinical anesthesia,* New York, 1996, Churchill Livingstone.

Rotter S: *Specific considerations with cardiac disease.* In Davidson JK, Eckhardt III WF, Perese DA, editors: *Clinical anesthesia procedures of the Massachusetts General Hospital,* ed 4, Boston/Toronto/London, 1993, Little, Brown.

Strang T, Tupper-Carey D: *Allergic reaction.* In Goldstone JC, Pollard BJ, editors: *Handbook of clinical anesthesia,* New York, 1996, Churchill Livingstone.

Sussman GL, Beezhold DH: Allergy to latex rubber, *Ann Intern Med* 122: 43, 1995.

Vandam LD, Desai SP: *Evaluation of the patient and preoperative preparation.* In Barash PG, Cullen BF, Stoelting RK, editors: *Clinical anesthesia,* Philadelphia, 1989, JB Lippincott.

Chapter 3

Overview of Diagnostic Imaging of the Head and Neck

Robert W. Dalley
William D. Robertson
Patrick J. Oliverio
S. James Zinreich

Diagnostic medical imaging has changed medical and surgical diagnosis in ways never imagined. Every area of clinical medicine has been affected in a profound way. Medical imaging specialists are able, through their consultations, to assist the otolaryngologist in a variety of ways, including providing primary diagnosis, confirming a clinical impression, evaluating regional anatomy, assessing response to treatment, and assisting in definitive treatment of patients.

Neuroradiologists are subspecialty trained diagnostic radiologists who specialize in the imaging of the head and neck, skull base, temporal bone, brain, and spine. They are the primary imaging consultants for otolaryngologists.

This chapter will provide an introduction and overview of modern head and neck imaging for the otolaryngologist. The various imaging modalities available will be discussed. Imaging strategies for various regions and clinical questions will be reviewed. The basic approach to the radiologist's image acquisition and interpretation will be described so that the referring physician will gain a measure of understanding of this field. This is intended to maximize the usefulness of diagnostic imaging in the care of patients.

The scope of head and neck imaging is too broad a topic to be covered in one chapter. The authors intend to provide the clinician with an outline and brief synopsis of the field. There are definitive textbooks for each area of head and neck imaging.[14,48,50,54]

AVAILABLE IMAGING MODALITIES

Conventional radiography

Since the discovery of the x-ray, it has been used in imaging the head and neck region. The traditional projections obtained with conventional radiography that are applicable to head and neck imaging include the following.

Views of the facial bones and sinuses include the lateral view, Caldwell view, Waters view, and submentovertex (SMV or base) view. The lateral view will show the frontal, maxillary, and sphenoid sinus. It is best obtained 5° off the true lateral position to avoid superimposition of the posterior walls of the maxillary sinuses. The Caldwell view displays the frontal sinuses and posterior ethmoid air cells. It is obtained in the posteroanterior (PA) projection with 15° of caudal angulation of the x-ray beam. The Waters view can show the maxillary sinuses, anterior ethmoid air cells, and orbital floors. It is obtained in the PA projection with the neck in 33° of extension. The SMV view can show the sphenoid sinuses and the anterior and posterior walls of the frontal sinuses. It is obtained in the anteroposterior (AP) projection with the head in 90° of extension.

Views of the neck AP and lateral views of the neck exposed for soft-tissue detail are useful to evaluate the overall contour of the soft tissues of the neck. These are essentially the same projections used in the evaluation of cervical traumas, but they are not exposed for bone detail.

Cervical spine imaging The complete plain film assessment of the cervical spine requires an AP, lateral, RAO and LAO oblique views, and an open mouth AP view of the upper cervical spine to visualize the odontoid process of the second cervical vertebral body. Specialized views such as the "swimmer's" or Twining view or "pillar" views can be used as needed. A "swimmer's" view is used to identify the lower cervical vertebral bodies when they cannot be seen from a routine lateral view. The "pillar" view is used to visualize the cervical articular masses *en face.*

Temporal bone imaging There are several accepted projections for visualizing portions of the temporal bone, including the Schuller projection, a lateral view of the mastoid obtained with 30° of cephalocaudad angulation. The Stenvers projection is an oblique projection of the petrous bone obtained with the patient's head slightly flexed and rotated 45° toward the side opposite the one under study. The beam is angulated 14°. The transorbital projection is a frontal projection of the mastoids and petrous bones. Conventional imaging of the temporal bone has largely been replaced by computed tomography (CT) scanning.

Computed Tomography

CT was developed for clinical use in the mid-1970s by Hounsfield. CT uses a tightly collimated x-ray beam that is differentially absorbed by the various body tissues to generate highly detailed cross-sectional images. The degree of attenuation of the x-ray photons is assigned a numeric readout. These units of attenuation are known as Hounsfield units (HU) and generally range from -1000 HU to $+1000$ HU. Water is assigned a value of 0 HU.

To create images, CT uses complex mathematical reconstruction algorithms. Bone disease and bone trauma are best visualized with a bone detail algorithm (Fig. 3-1). The raw data generated from the scan can be used in any number of ways. Images from a given reconstruction algorithm can be displayed in various ways to highlight differences in attenuation of different structures. In CT scanning, *window width* refers to the range of attenuation values in HU that make up the gray scale for a given image. The *window level* refers to the center HU value for that given window width. There are standard window width and level settings used for various types of CT scans.

Computed tomography image display

Multiple options for displaying the image (adjusting the window level and width parameters on the imaging console) and recording it permanently on radiographic film are available. Each pixel (picture element) of the CT image is given a density value. Water has been assigned a value of 0 on this scale developed by Hounsfield, fat is approximately -80 to -100 HU. Calcium and bone are in the 100 to 400 HU range, and most fluids are in the 0 to 30 HU range. The window level is simply the midpoint of the densities chosen for display. The range of densities chosen above and below the window level define the window width. A narrow window width of 80 HU and a level of $+40$ HU is frequently used for brain imaging because it centers the density at the common density of brain tissue and displays only those densities 40 HU greater than and 40 HU less than the window level. Thus any density greater than $+80$ HU will be displayed as white, and any density less than 0 will be displayed as black on the gray scale. Any intermediate density will be spread out evenly along the gray scale. For imaging of the soft tissues of the head and neck, a window level of approximately 40 to 70 HU is usually chosen, at a midpoint approximately equal to the density of muscle. The window width frequently is in the 250 to 400 HU range, thus displaying a wider range of densities including calcification, intravenous contrast, muscle, and fat to best advantage. For imaging bony structures such as paranasal sinuses and temporal bone, window levels from 0 to $+400$ HU and a wide window width of 2000 to 4000 HU may be chosen. The reason for a wide bone window width is that a wide range of densities ranging from cortical bone (approximately $+1000$ HU) down to gas (-1000 HU) need to be displayed on the same image. However, structures of intermediate density between bone and gas occupy a narrow range on the gray scale at this window width and are poorly discriminated (appear washed-out) on these settings. The terminology commonly used to describe the previously mentioned windows includes soft-tissue windows (window width of 250 to 400 HU) and bone windows (2000 to 4000 HU).

It is important to understand that these display windows are completely independent of the mathematical imaging algorithm chosen for creation of the image. In other words, an image created by a soft-tissue algorithm can be displayed with soft tissue and bone window widths (Fig. 3-1 *A, C*). Conversely, the image may be computer reconstructed using a bone algorithm and displayed with either soft tissue or bone window width (Fig. 3-1 *B, D*). To optimize the imaging of the soft tissue lesion and the adjacent bone, a soft-tissue and a bone algorithm may be used, generating images with the appropriate soft-tissue and bone windows (see also Fig. 3-10 *A, C*).

Patient cooperation

Patient cooperation is necessary to obtain optimal image quality. The patient is instructed not to swallow and to stop breathing or to maintain quiet breathing during each slice acquisition to minimize motion artifact from the adjacent airway and pharyngeal structures. Occasionally, provocative maneuvers such as blowing through a small straw or using a cheek-puffing (modified Valsalva) maneuver to distend the hypopharynx or phonating to assess vocal cord movement may be necessary (Figs. 3-2 and 3-3).

CT scanners have evolved over time such that the most advanced scanners now scan in a "helical" fashion, in which the scanner uses a slip-ring technique. This allows the table to move as the scan is performed, resulting in complete volumes of tissue being imaged with skipping tissue between

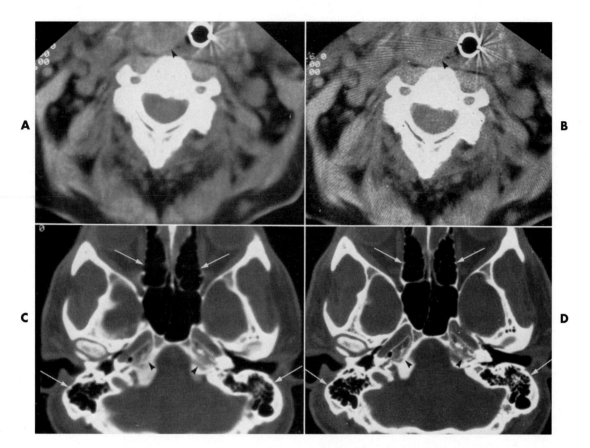

Fig. 3-1. Comparison of various computed tomography algorithms and windows. **A,** Soft-tissue algorithm and, **B,** bone algorithm images of a laryngeal hematoma *(arrowheads)* using soft-tissue windows (350 HU width). The bone algorithm image has much more grainy appearance, whereas the standard algorithm gives a more pleasant smoothed image. **C,** Soft-tissue algorithm and, **D,** bone algorithm images of the skull base using bone windows (4000 HU width). Note improved sharpness of petrous apex trabeculae *(arrowheads)* and bony walls of mastoid and ethmoid sinus air cells *(arrows).*

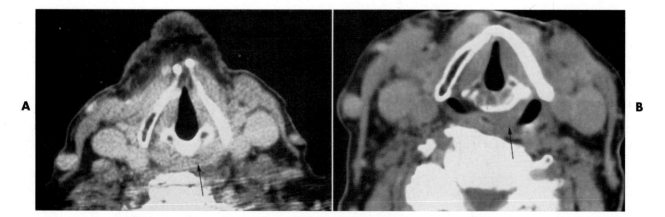

Fig. 3-2. Larynx without and with modified Valsalva maneuver. **A,** Axial contrast-enhanced computed tomography (CECT) performed during quiet breathing does not allow discrimination of retro-cricoid carcinoma *(arrow)* because posterior pharyngeal wall is collapsed against mass. **B,** Axial CECT in the same patient (a few minutes later) obtained with modified Valsalva maneuver causes distension of now air-filled hypopharynx, permitting tumor detection *(arrow).*

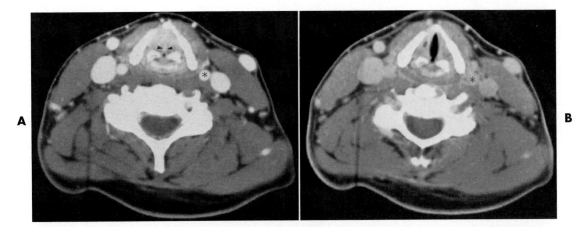

Fig. 3-3. Axial contrast-enhancing computed tomography during breath holding and while phonating. **A,** This axial computed tomography, obtained during breath holding, shows true vocal cords adducting and approximating eachother *(arrowheads)*. Note superb high-contrast density in common carotid artery *(asterisk)* and jugular veins. **B,** Phonating "eeee" causes vocal cords to partially adduct into paramedian position. Note the contrast density has significantly decreased in common carotid artery *(asterisk)* and jugular veins in this delayed image, obtained well after contrast infusion had finished.

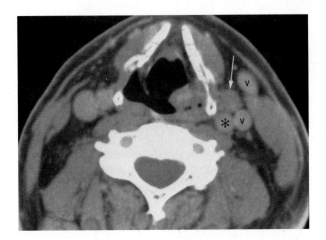

Fig. 3-4. Contrast-enhancing computed tomography (CECT) with suboptimal contrast infusion. This axial CECT of a patient with left piriform sinus tumor was obtained with insufficient contrast infusion, resulting in poor discrimination of common carotid artery *(asterisk)* and jugular vein *(v)* from isodense adjacent metastatic lymph node *(arrow)*. Inadequate contrast infusion also reduces likelihood of identifying focal defect in nodal metastasis.

slices. Currently CT scanners can obtain slices 1- or 1.5-mm thick. These levels of precision are of value in evaluating the temporal bone.

Contrast enhancement often is used to opacify blood vessels and to identify regions of abnormal tissue as identified by abnormal enhancement patterns (Fig. 3-4). As it relates to head and neck imaging, contrast is particularly useful in CT scans of the neck and orbits. Contrast often is not needed in evaluation of the temporal bones, although it can be necessary on occasion. CT of the facial bones and paranasal sinuses usually does not require intravenous contrast.

As a brief review, the radiation exposure (dose) that a patient receives is known as the *radiation absorbed dose*. This radiation absorbed dose is a measure of the total radiation energy absorbed by the tissues, and it is expressed in an SI unit known as the Gray (Gy). One Gy is the amount of radiation needed to deposit the energy of 1 Joule (J) in 1 kg of tissue (1 Gy = 1 J/kg). Formerly, the unit used to express radiation absorbed dose was the rad (1 rad = amount of radiation needed to deposit the energy of 100 ergs in 1 g of tissue). The conversion of rads to Gy is: 1 Gy = 100 rad.

Radiation dose equivalent is a more useful term as it considers the "quality factor" (Q) of the radiation involved (radiation dose equivalent = radiation absorbed dose × Q). The quality factor considers the varying biologic activity of various types of ionizing radiation. For x-rays, the Q = 1. Thus, when discussing diagnostic x-rays, the radiation dose equivalent equals radiation absorbed dose. The SI unit for the radiation dose equivalent is the Sievert (Sv). The former unit was the rem. In summary, 1 Gy = 1 SV, and 1 Sv = 100 rem.

Radiation dose equivalent depends on the kVp and mAs of the exposure. For a given kVp, radiation dose equivalent varies linearly with the mAs. At 125 kVp, the radiation dose equivalent for a CT slice is approximately 1.1 to 1.2 cSv/100 mAs (1.1 to 1.2 rem/100 mAs). The actual dose will vary from machine to machine. Table 3-1 illustrates the dose can be reduced by the use of low mAs technique when possible.

In contiguous CT imaging, the dose to the region scanned is approximately equal to the per slice dose. The dose will be slightly lower if a gap is maintained between slices, and it will be slightly higher if there is overlap between slices.

The effective dose equivalent was developed as a means

Table 3-1. Relative radiation dose for sinus CT (using 125 kVp)

mAs	Radiation dose equivalent
450	4.95–5.40 cSv (4.95–5.40 rem)
240	2.64–2.88 cSv (2.64–2.88 rem)
160	1.76–1.92 cSv (1.76–1.92 rem)
80	0.88–0.96 cSv (0.88–0.96 rem)

From Zinreich S: Imaging of inflammatory sinus disease, *Otolaryngol Clin North Am* 26:535, 1993.

Table 3-2. Estimated effective dose equivalent of common examinations

Examination	Effective dose equivalent
Sinus series, four views	7.0 mrem
Chest, PA and lateral	7.2 mrem
Kidneys and upper bladder	8.7 mrem
Lumbar spine, five views	125.1 mrem
CT, brain*	112.0 mrem
CT, sinus (160 mAs)†	51.2 mrem
CT, sinus (80 mAs)‡	25.6 mrem

From Zinreich S: Imaging of inflammatory sinus disease, *Otolaryngol Clin North Am* 26:535, 1993; and Zinreich S, Abidin M, Kennedy D: Cross-sectional imaging of the nasal cavity and paranasal sinuses, *Operative Techniques Otolaryngol Head Neck Surg* 1:93, 1990.

* 120 kVp, 240 mAs, 10-mm slice thickness, contiguous.

† 125 kVp, 160 mAs, 3-mm slice thickness, contiguous.

‡ 125 kVp, 80 mAs, 3-mm slice thickness, contiguous.

of representing the fraction of the total stochastic risk of fatal cancers and chromosomal abnormalities resulting from the irradiation of a particular organ or tissue when the body is uniformly irradiated. A system of weighting is used to consider the individual sensitivity of the body's major tissues and organs. A full discussion of this is beyond the scope of this introductory chapter. Suffice it to say that for a given examination, the effective dose to the patient is less than the dose (radiation dose equivalent) received by the area under examination. A list of common radiographic procedures and their effective dose equivalents is seen in Table 3-2.

Magnetic resonance imaging

Magnetic resonance imaging (MRI) is an imaging modality that uses the response of biologic tissues to an applied and changing magnetic field to generate images. It is not possible to completely describe the principles of MRI in an introductory chapter of all head and neck imaging. A brief summary of MRI follows.

There are two types of magnets that are used to perform clinical MRIs: permanent magnets and superconducting magnets. Permanent magnets do not require continual input of energy to maintain the magnetic field. They are composed of large magnetic metallic elements set up to generate a uniform magnetic field between components. Superconducting magnets are electromagnets usually composed of niobium–titanium wire. They require input of energy to start them, but once they are up to strength, they are maintained in a superconductive state by means of an encasing system of liquid nitrogen and liquid helium shells.

The earth has a magnetic field strength of 0.5 Gauss (G). The tesla (T) is another unit of magnetic strength that is related to G by the equation 1 T = 10,000 G. Clinical MRI units usually operate at magnetic field strengths of between 0.3 and 1.5 T. Small bore research scanners of strengths of 4.0 T are in use.

There are many available MR pulse sequences available to generate images. The most common pulse sequence in MRI is the spin–echo technique.

MRI is one of the most active areas of development and research within diagnostic radiology. MRI derives signal from hydrogen protons most abundant in tissue fat and water, by placing them in a high magnetic field. This tends to align the spinning protons in the direction of the magnetic field. Radio frequency pulses are transmitted into the subject to excite the spinning protons, changing their orientation with respect to the magnetic field. As the protons realign with the magnetic field, they lose energy and give off signal, which is measured and reconstructed by the MR scanner into an image. The quality of MRI depends on a high signal-to-noise ratio, which improves image contrast and spatial resolution.[15] In general, the higher the field strength of the magnet, the higher the signal-to-noise ratio. Thus MRI scanners with field strengths of 0.5 to 2.0 T are commonly used for imaging.

Surface coils significantly improve the quality of head and neck imaging by increasing the signal-to-noise ratio. A surface coil is a receiving antenna for the radio frequency signal that is emitted from the imaging subject after the initial radio frequency stimulation. The standard head coil is usually adequate for studying head and neck disease above the angle of the mandible. A head coil allows imaging of the adjacent brain and orbits, an advantage when head and neck lesions extend intracranially. Neck coils cover a larger area from the skull base to the clavicles and come in various configurations, for example, volume neck coil, anterior neck coil, 5-inch flat coil placed over the anterior neck, and bilateral temporomandibular joint (TMJ) coil. Slice thickness on MRI is most commonly 5 mm, with 3-mm sections used for smaller regions of interest. However, a thinner slice has a smaller signal-to-noise ratio. Occasionally, 1- to 2-mm sections may be needed for small structures (e.g., facial nerve), requiring a volume acquisition technique. The number of slices is limited in MRI (as opposed to CT) by the specific sequence used, ranging from six to eight slices with a short TI inversion recovery technique up to 14 to 18 slices with a T2-weighted sequence; volume acquisition techniques will allow 60 or more thin slices.

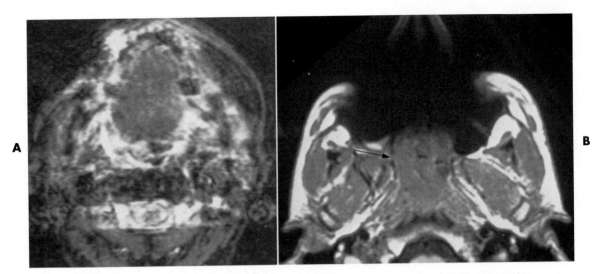

Fig. 3-5. Magnetic resonance imaging artifacts. **A,** Motion during axial short T1 inversion recovery sequence caused significant degradation of image with anatomic distortion and mismapping of signal intensity. **B,** Metallic dental braces cause artifacts distorting anterior facial structures in this T1-weighted image of a boy with juvenile angiofibroma filling nasal cavity *(arrow)* and nasopharynx. Anterior maxilla and portion of nose have been distorted.

Magnetic resonance imaging artifacts

Motion artifact, chemical shift artifact, dental work (amalgam, implants, braces, etc.), and eyelid mascara degrade MRIs (Fig. 3-5). Motion artifact becomes more prominent with increased field strength, increased length of individual pulse sequences, and the total length of the imaging study. A typical imaging sequence may last from 2 to 8 minutes. To limit motion artifact, sequences less than 4 minutes are preferred, and the patient should be instructed not to swallow and to breath shallowly and quietly.

Chemical shift artifact arises from the differences in resonance frequencies of water and fat protons. The result is an exaggerated interface (spatial mismapping) in areas where fat abuts structures containing predominantly water protons such as the posterior globe or a mass. Chemical shift artifact may produce the appearance of a pseudocapsule around a lesion or cause obscuration of a small-diameter structure such as the optic nerve. Chemical shift artifact may be identified by a bright band on one side of the structure and a black band on the opposite side. This is usually most noticeable on T1-weighted images (T1WIs).

Metallic artifact from dental work varies in severity depending on amount and composition of the metal in the mouth, as well as the pulse sequence and field strength of the MRI scanner. Most dental amalgam causes mild distortion to the local magnetic field, resulting in a mild dropout of signal around the involved teeth. Extensive dental work, metallic implants, and braces may cause more severe distortion of the image, precluding visualization of the maxilla, mandible, and floor of the mouth. Mascara containing metallic compounds can also cause localized signal loss in the anterior orbit and globe.

Magnetic resonance imaging pulse sequences

Numerous pulse sequences are available on clinical MRI units; the details of the physics of MRI may be found in most radiology/MRI textbooks.[7] Commonly used imaging protocols include T1-weighted, spin (proton) density, T2-weighted, gadolinium-enhanced T1-weighted, fat-suppressed, and gradient echo imaging; magnetic resonance angiography is infrequently obtained (Figs. 3-6 and 3-7). The abbreviations used to identify sequence parameters on hard copy film or in journal articles are repetition time (TR), echo time (TE), and inversion time (TI) and are measured in milliseconds. The following description of pulse sequences is presented to assist the clinician in identifying and understanding the commonly performed sequences and in determining their respective use in the head and neck.

T1-weighted images. T1-weighted (short TR) sequences (Figs. 3-6, *A* and 3-7, *A*) use a short TR (500 to 700 ms) and a short TE (15 to 40 ms). T1-weighted imaging is the fundamental head and neck sequence because it provides excellent soft tissue contrast with a superior display of anatomy, a high signal-to-noise ratio, and a relatively short imaging time (2 to 5 minutes), minimizing motion artifacts. Fat is high signal intensity (bright or white) on T1WIs and provides natural contrast in the head and neck. Air, rapid blood flow, bone, and fluid-filled structures (e.g., vitreous and cerebrospinal fluid [CSF]) are low signal intensity (dark or black) on T1WIs. Muscle is low to intermediate in signal intensity on T1WIs. The inherent high contrast of fat relative to adjacent structures allows excellent delineation of the muscles, globe, blood vessels, and mass lesions that border on fat. Surrounding bone is black, except for the enclosed bone marrow (e.g., sphenoid wing, mandible, and thyroid

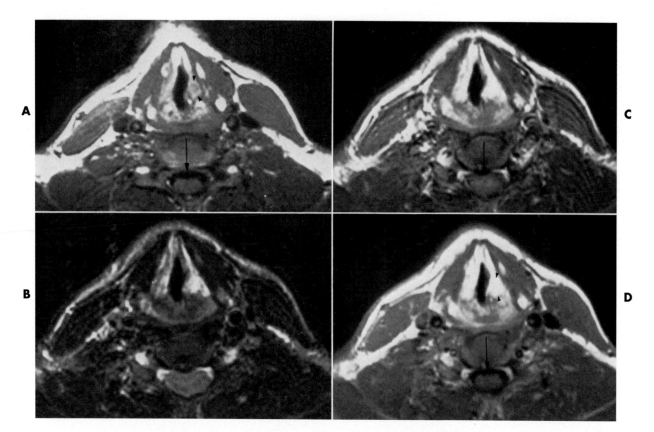

Fig. 3-6. Common magnetic resonance imaging pulse sequences without fat suppression. **A,** Axial T1-weighted image (T1WI) of left glottic tumor *(arrowheads)*, which is intermediate in signal intensity and thickens true cord. Note cerebrospinal fluid (CSF) surrounding spinal cord *(arrow)* is black, indicating that this is a T1WI. **B,** Spin density–weighted image also reveals high signal intensity (caused by increased water content) of vocal cord tumor. CSF is now isointense to spinal cord *(arrow)*, indicating this is a spin density sequence. **C,** T2-weighted image demonstrates high signal intensity mass clearly demarcated against dark background of fat and muscle. **D,** Postgadolinium T1WI shows enhancement of cord tumor *(arrowheads)*. CSF remains black *(arrow)*.

cartilage), which is bright from fat within the marrow. The aerated paranasal sinuses are black, whereas retained mucous or mass lesions are of low to intermediate signal intensity. Most head and neck mass lesions will show a low-to-intermediate signal intensity on T1WIs. Fewer slices are available with a short TR compared with a long TR sequence. (To quickly identify a T1WI: fat is white, CSF and vitreous are black, and nasal mucosa is low signal.)

Spin (proton) density-weighted images. Spin density-weighted sequences (also known as proton density, balanced, or mixed sequences) use a long TR (2000 to 4000 ms) and a short TE (20 to 40 ms). Spin density images (Fig. 3-6, *B*) show air and bone as low signal intensity and fluid-containing structures and muscles as intermediate signal intensity, with fat remaining moderately high in signal intensity but somewhat decreased in signal from T1WI. A solid mass or fluid-filled lesion with a high protein content will demonstrate moderate-to-high signal intensity, which may improve its visibility relative to muscle but may obscure it relative to the adjacent fat. Paranasal sinus inflammation typically appears very bright on spin density images. (To

quickly identify a spin density image: CSF and vitreous are intermediate in signal.)

T2-weighted images. T2-weighted images (Fig. 3-6, *C*) use a long TR (2000 to 4000 ms) and a long TE (50 to 90 ms) and are sometimes referred to as long TR/long TE images. Note that spin density and T2WI are acquired simultaneously from a single sequence that produces two sets of images with the same TR but different TEs; for example, spin density = 2000/30 and T2WI = 2000/80. T2WIs are most useful for highlighting pathologic lesions. T2WIs show the vitreous and CSF as high signal intensity (bright) relative to the low-to-intermediate signal intensity of head and neck fat and muscle. Fat loses signal intensity with increased T2 weighting. Most head and neck masses are higher signal intensity on a T2WI compared with their low-to-intermediate signal intensity on T1WI. The combination of the T1WI and T2WI is often useful for characterizing fluid-containing structures, solid components, and hemorrhage. Bone, rapid vascular flow, calcium, hemosiderin, and air-containing sinuses are black. Inflammatory sinus disease and normal airway mucosa appear very bright. (To quickly identify a

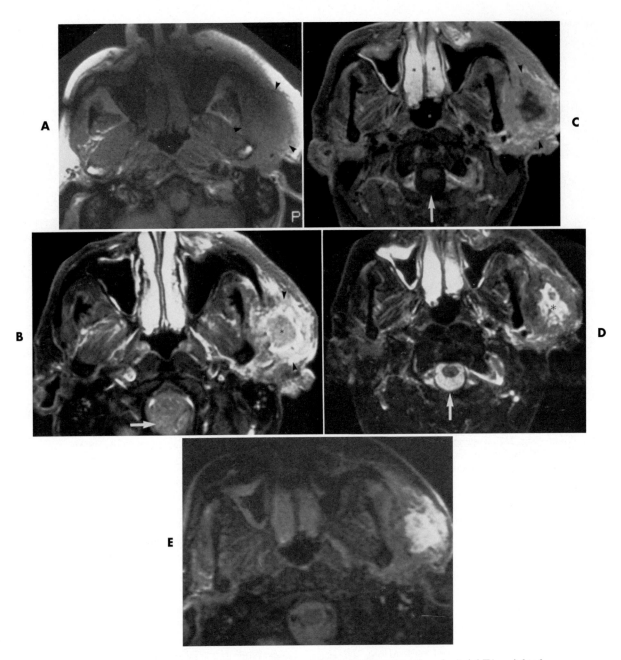

Fig. 3-7. Magnetic resonance imaging pulse sequences with fat suppression. **A,** Axial T1-weighted image (T1WI) without contrast in a patient with squamous cell cancer shows poorly defined mass in left parotid gland *(arrowheads)*. Suboptimal signal in image is the result of signal drop-off at the edge of the anterior neck surface coil. **B,** Axial postgadolinium T1WI with fat saturation has adequate suppression of subcutaneous fat (compared with **A**) and enhancement of tumor *(arrowheads)*. Center of mass enhances less and likely is necrotic. Cerebrospinal fluid (CSF) is black *(arrow)*, indicating a T1WI. Note marked enhancement of inferior turbinates *(asterisks)* compared with precontrast T1WI. **C,** Axial postgadolinium spin density image with fat saturation shows high signal in mass *(arrowheads)* with lower-intensity necrotic center *(asterisk)*. Fat signal is suppressed and image is similar to **B**; CSF is isointense with spinal cord indicating use of a spin density sequence. Turbinates are very bright. **D,** Axial T2-weighted image with fat saturation demonstrates nearly ideal fat suppression, almost as good as short T1 inversion recovery (STIR) sequence. Necrotic or cystic center of mass *(asterisk)* and CSF *(arrow)* have become very bright. **E,** On this axial STIR image with excellent fat suppression, margin and center of mass are bright.

T2WI: CSF, vitreous, and nasal mucosa are white. Fat is low to intermediate in signal.)

Gadolinium enhancement. Paramagnetic gadolinium compounds are commonly used in central nervous system (CNS) imaging for lesion enhancement. Gadolinium is used in conjunction with T1WI sequences (gadolinium shortens the T1), and with the dose used it has little effect on T2WI. The advantages of gadolinium enhancement are increased lesion conspicuity and improved delineation of the margins of a mass relative to the lower signal of muscle, bone, vessel, or globe.[9] However, gadolinium enhancement (without concomitant fat suppression) has had limited usefulness within the head and neck, as well as in the orbit, because of the large amount of fat present within these regions (Fig. 3-6, *D*). Following gadolinium injection the signal increases within a lesion, often obscuring the lesion within the adjacent high signal intensity fat.[40] Therefore for head and neck imaging, gadolinium is optimally used with specific fat suppression techniques that turn fat dark or black (see below). Gadolinium enhances normal structures including nasal and pharyngeal mucosa, lymphoid tissue in Waldeyer's ring, extraocular muscles, and slow-flowing blood in veins, all of which may appear surprisingly bright, especially if combined with fat suppression techniques. (To quickly identify a gadolinium-enhanced T1WI: nasal mucosa is white, fat is white, and CSF and vitreous are black. Also look for Gd-DTPA or Magnevist [Berlex] printed directly on the image or on adhesive study labels.)

Fat suppression methods. Several sequences have been developed that suppress fat signal intensity. T2WIs, short TI inversion recovery (STIR), spectral presaturation inversion recovery (SPIR), and chemical shift selective presaturation (fat saturation) are some of the more common clinically available methods of fat suppression. One advantage of fat suppression is reduction or elimination of chemical shift artifacts by removing fat signal from the image while preserving water signal. Additionally, some fat suppression techniques take advantage of gadolinium enhancement by eliminating the surrounding high intensity signal from fat while retaining the high intensity enhancement produced by gadolinium. Most pathologic lesions have increased water content, and gadolinium exerts its paramagnetic effects while in solution in blood vessels and in the increased extracellular fluid of the lesion, but gadolinium does not enhance fat.

1. T2WIs provide a moderate degree of fat suppression and discrimination of fat from water protons, yet enough fat signal persists to obscure some head and neck inflammatory and neoplastic lesions, especially lymph nodes. This sequence may be used before or after gadolinium and, because of the long TR used, yields the highest number of slices.
2. STIR (Fig. 3-7, *E*) is superior to T2WI for suppressing fat signal. The inversion time (e.g., TI = 140 ms) is individually "tuned" for each patient to place fat at the null point of signal intensity and thus eliminates

fat signal by turning it completely black. STIR images show the mucosa, vitreous, and CSF as very high signal intensity.[2] Most mass lesions in the head and neck will have similar high signal intensity on STIR and T2WI. The disadvantage of STIR is image degradation secondary to a decreased signal-to-noise ratio, an increased susceptibility to motion artifacts, and increased scan time. It is inadvisable to perform STIR after gadolinium administration because the gadolinium can result in a "paradoxical" signal loss (rather than enhancement) by shortening the T1; the longer the T1 of a structure, the brighter it becomes on STIR. STIR is often limited to six to eight slices, making full neck evaluation difficult, unless a concatenated technique is used, which increases slices acquired but requires a doubling of scan time. (To quickly identify a STIR image: fat is almost completely black; CSF, vitreous, and mucosa are white. A TI time is listed with the TR and TE times on the image.)

3. Chemical shift selective presaturation sequences (Fig. 3-7, *B*) used with a spin–echo technique (Chem-Sat, General Electric) or with an inversion recovery technique (SPIR, Phillips) selectively suppress either water or fat signal, but fat saturation (suppression) is the most clinically useful technique. (Note that for the remainder of this chapter the terms *fat suppression* and *fat saturation* are used interchangeably and refer to chemical shift selective presaturation techniques.) T1-weighted fat saturation sequences take full advantage of gadolinium enhancement. A gadolinium-enhancing lesion within the head and neck retains its high signal intensity and is not obscured, because fat is suppressed to become low-to-intermediate signal intensity. Enhancing masses within the head and neck and orbit are particularly well imaged with this technique.[28] The disadvantages of fat saturation sequences are that non–gadolinium-enhancing lesions may be less well discriminated, that these sequences are more susceptible to artifacts, and that nonuniform fat suppression occurs. Also, two to three fewer slices are acquired compared with T1WI, unless the TR time is lengthened. (To quickly identify a gadolinium-enhanced T1WI with fat saturation: mucosa and small veins are white, fat is low to intermediate intensity, and CSF and vitreous are black.) Fat saturation can optimize long TR (spin density and T2WI) sequences (Fig. 3-7, *C, D*). The advantage occurs when the spin density image is performed after gadolinium, since moderate T1-shortening effects by gadolinium occur with this sequence. Most lesions and vascular structures will show a mild degree of enhancement, with an image almost equivalent with a postgadolinium fat saturation T1WI. Fat-saturated T2WIs provide excellent fat suppression almost equivalent to STIR, optimizing the high signal from normal structures and le-

sions that are high in water content contrasted against a black background of fat.

Gradient echo techniques. Numerous new and faster gradient echo sequences are available that have a variety of applications. Gradient echo scans have a very short TR (30 to 70 ms), a very short TE (5 to 15 ms), and a flip angle of less than 90°. They have a variety of proprietary acronyms including GRASS, MPGR, and SPGR (General Electric) and FLASH and FISP (Siemens). Gradient echo sequences take advantage of the phenomenon of flow-related enhancement; that is, any rapidly flowing blood will appear extremely bright. These sequences are useful for localizing normal vessels, detecting obstruction of flow in compressed or thrombosed vessels, or showing vascular lesions that have tubular, linear, or tortuous bright signal representing regions of rapid blood flow (Fig. 3-8). Gradient echo sequences may be obtained faster than conventional spin–echo techniques, although their increased susceptibility to motion artifact decreases the benefits of a short scan time. Gradient echo techniques also permit volume; that is, three-dimensional versus two-dimensional acquisition of images, allowing computer workstation reconstruction of any imaging plane at any desired thickness with increased spatial resolution. The disadvantage of gradient echo sequences is the increased magnetic susceptibility artifact from bone or air, thus limiting their role near the skull base or paranasal sinuses. (To quickly identify a gradient echo image: arteries and often veins are white; fat, CSF, vitreous, and mucosa may have variable signal intensities depending on the technique used.)

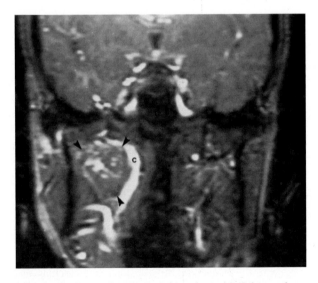

Fig. 3-8. Gradient echo sequence in patient with right vagal paraganglioma. Coronal multiplanar gradient echo image demonstrates mass *(arrowheads)* displacing internal carotid artery *(c)* medially. Arterial blood flow is very high in signal intensity in medially displaced internal carotid artery, as well as within feeding vessels deep inside mass.

Magnetic resonance angiography. Magnetic resonance angiography is a technique that takes advantage of phase or time-of-flight differences in flowing blood relative to motionless structures and selectively produces images of structures with rapid blood flow. Two- and three-dimensional images of normal vessels and vascular lesions can be generated. At present magnetic resonance angiography does not equal the spatial resolution of conventional angiography, but the technology is in rapid evolution. Early experience in the head and neck indicates magnetic resonance angiography will be useful for evaluating vascular compression and vessel patency and for characterization of vascular masses and malformations.[37]

Magnetic resonance imaging disadvantages

Several disadvantages of MRI of the head and neck bear consideration. MRI frequently requires 45 to 90 minutes of scanning time, during which time the patient must remain motionless, a process difficult for a sick patient to accomplish. Motion artifacts are more frequently encountered than with CT, although dental artifacts may be less problematic. Although no known harmful effects during pregnancy have been demonstrated, at most institutions MRI is used sparingly during the first trimester. (MRI avoids the use of ionizing radiation, and no harmful effects have been shown with its use at current field strengths.) Absolute contraindications to MRI include patients with cardiac pacemakers, cochlear implants, and ferromagnetic intracranial aneurysm clips. Those patients at risk for metallic orbital foreign bodies should be screened with plain films or CT before MRI. Generally, ocular prostheses and ossicular implants are safe. Unfortunately, MRI is also the most expensive of all the imaging modalities.

Ultrasound

High-resolution diagnostic ultrasound uses the properties of reflected high-frequency sound waves to produce cross-sectional images, obtainable in almost any plane. The transducer, a high-frequency 5- or 10-MHz probe, scans over the skin surface of the region of interest. Fat has a moderate degree of internal echoes (echogenicity). Skeletal muscle is less echogenic than fat. A solid mass has well-defined margins and variable echogenicity but is usually less echogenic than fat. A cyst has few, if any, internal echoes, a strongly echogenic back wall, and strong through-transmission of sound behind the cyst. Both calcium and bone are strongly echogenic, thus obscuring adjacent structures by an acoustic shadow. Ultrasound has no known harmful effects and no contraindications. High-resolution ultrasound is quick and accurate; further, it is relatively inexpensive compared with CT or MRI.

Nuclear medicine

Scintigraphy has several applications in the head and neck. In salivary gland imaging technetium-99m (^{99m}Tc)-pertechnetate imaging may be useful for assessing salivary gland function in autoimmune and inflammatory disease of the salivary glands. If the salivary glands are obstructed, the degree of obstruction as well as the follow-up of obstruction after treatment can be assessed. In evaluating neoplasms of the salivary glands the findings of the ^{99m}Tc-pertechnetate scan are almost pathognomonic of Warthin's tumor and oncocytoma. Spatial resolution is approximately limited to 1.5 cm, so accurate localization of the mass within the gland is difficult. Single photon emission computed tomography (SPECT) may be useful in some cases.

Techniques of thyroid imaging and thyroid therapy are described in several textbooks.[33,53] Many centers use I-123 to obtain a thyroid update determination, and ^{99m}Tc-pertechnetate is used to obtain whole gland images. It is these images that determine if thyroid nodules are "hot" or "cold." I-131 is used for therapy of hyperthyroidism and in follow-up to detect and treat residual, recurrent, and metastatic thyroid cancers.

Medullary carcinoma of the thyroid is difficult to visualize, but ^{99m}Tc-DmSA has been used. More recently, In-111 pentetreotide has been used with some success.

Identification of parathyroid adenomas has been done for

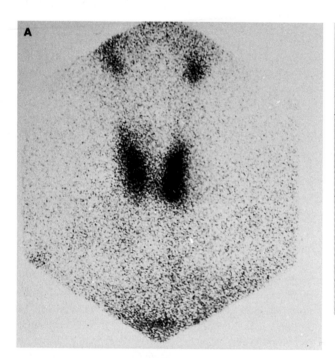

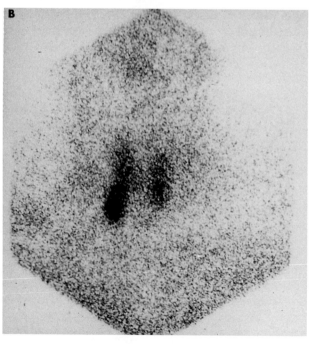

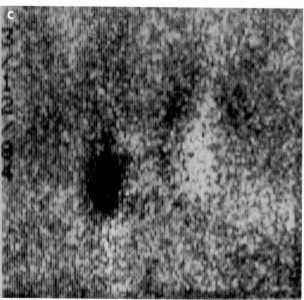

Fig. 3-9. A, Technetinum-99m (^{99m}Tc)-pertechnetate scintigraphy in a patient with suspected parathyroid adenoma is essentially normal. **B,** Corresponding Tl-201 scintigraphy reveals an apparent area of increased uptake adjacent to the lower pole of the right lobe. **C,** Subtraction of the ^{99m}Tc-pertechnetate study from the Tl-201 study confirms the presence of a parathyroid adenoma.

several years with a subtraction technique using ^{99m}Tc-pertechnetate and Tl-201 (Fig. 3-9). The basis of this test is that thallium is taken up by thyroid tissue and parathyroid tissue. ^{99m}Tc-pertechnetate is taken up only by thyroid tissue. Therefore, the subtraction of the ^{99m}Tc-pertechnetate image from the thallium-201 image should leave only parathyroid tissue. The sensitivity of this technique is believed to be excellent for lesions over 1 g. Sensitivity decreases with smaller lesions, and the subtraction technique can be hampered by patient motion. Lately, ^{99m}Tc-sestamibi has been used to identify parathyroid adenomas. A single radiopharmaceutical double-phase protocol is the most recent improvement in identification of parathyroid adenomas.

CSF leaks can be detected with ^{111}In DTPA placed into the subarachnoid space. This technique is described and illustrated in Chapter 63.

Three-dimensional reconstruction techniques

Image data from either CT or MRI can be processed to create three-dimensional reconstructions, but a separate computer workstation with appropriate imaging software is necessary. CT data are loaded as a stack of contiguous two-dimensional slices that defines the scanned volume. Reconstructions are created either from choosing a specific range of densities for display or by manually tracing the outline of the desired structure. Magnetic resonance data for image analysis are best acquired using a ''volume acquisition'' method, in which data are acquired as a complete three-dimensional block rather than as individual slices. Because volume acquisition takes longer, gradient echo techniques are usually required to reduce the imaging time. Once acquired, the data are displayed in any desired plane and, by selecting a range of signal intensities or by tracing specific structures with a cursor, three-dimensional surface models are created.

The utility of three-dimensional reconstruction is best appreciated with craniofacial reconstructions.[17,32] Contiguous 1- to 2-mm noncontrast CT axial sections are processed on the workstation to obtain a three-dimensional model of the bone surfaces. Directly visualizing the three-dimensional relationships of the facial structures aids surgical planning. Three-dimensional models of the face and orbital structures are useful for teaching medical students, residents, and anatomy students. To date, the spatial resolution of CT is superior to MRI in the head and neck for displaying bony relationships. However, MRI provides a superior display of transcranial soft-tissue structures, such as the entire visual pathway, and has better tissue contrast resolution than CT. Thus CT and MRI will likely have complementary roles in three-dimensional image display.

APPLICATIONS OF CT, MRI, AND ULTRASOUND IN THE HEAD AND NECK

Each anatomic region requires a different imaging approach to optimize the detection and characterization of the structure or lesion of interest. The following is a description of the indications for using CT, MRI, or ultrasound in specific head and neck regions, plus a general imaging approach relevant to each anatomic region in terms of imaging planes, slice thickness, contrast agents, and pulse sequences. Whenever possible CT and MRI are performed before biopsy or resection of lesions because the resulting edema may obscure the true margins of a mass.

Application of computed tomography by head and neck region

Suprahyoid neck

Suprahyoid neck CT is often performed for simultaneous evaluation of the deep extent of mucosal-based tumors and to evaluate associated metastatic disease to the cervical lymph node chains. To cover the region from the skull base down to the root of the neck, contiguous axial 3- to 5-mm sections from the bottom of the sella down to the hyoid bone, followed by 3- to 5-mm sections at 5-mm intervals from the hyoid bone down to the sternal notch (thoracic inlet), are required. Because streak artifacts from dental fillings frequently obscure the oropharynx and nasopharynx, it is usually necessary to obtain additional angled sections to assess the pharynx directly posterior to the dental work (Fig. 3-10). Direct coronal 3- to 5-mm images are very useful in defining craniocaudal relationships in lesions of the oral cavity and facial bones. The use of intravenous contrast is critical for adequate performance and interpretation of this study, especially the axial sections. Optimally, contrast is continuously infused during the entire scanning sequence so that a high concentration of intravascular (both arterial and venous) contrast allows differentiation of vessels (see Figs. 3-3 and 3-4) from other higher density structures such as lymph nodes and muscle. Otherwise, determination of vascular invasion, compression, and discrimination of vessels from nodes and small muscle bundles can be extremely difficult. Contrast is best administered with a mechanical pump infusion (although a drip infusion technique may also be effective) giving a single dose (40 g iodine) up to a double dose (80 g iodine) of contrast. Frequently, only a soft-tissue algorithm is necessary with each slice photographed with both soft-tissue and bone windows. However, sections of the skull base and mandible may need reconstruction using a bone algorithm if a suspicion of bone erosion or destruction by tumor or inflammation exists. Direct coronal images are advantageous when assessing lesions of the tongue, floor of mouth, retromolar trigone, mandible, or skull base.

Cervical lymphadenopathy

Lymph node CT evaluation is concomitantly performed during CT investigation of most suprahyoid and infrahyoid tumors or inflammation. Axial 3- to 5-mm slices must extend from the skull base to the clavicles to encompass the many node chains that extend the length of the neck. As mentioned above, the quality of lymph node assessment depends very much on the success of achieving a high concentration of

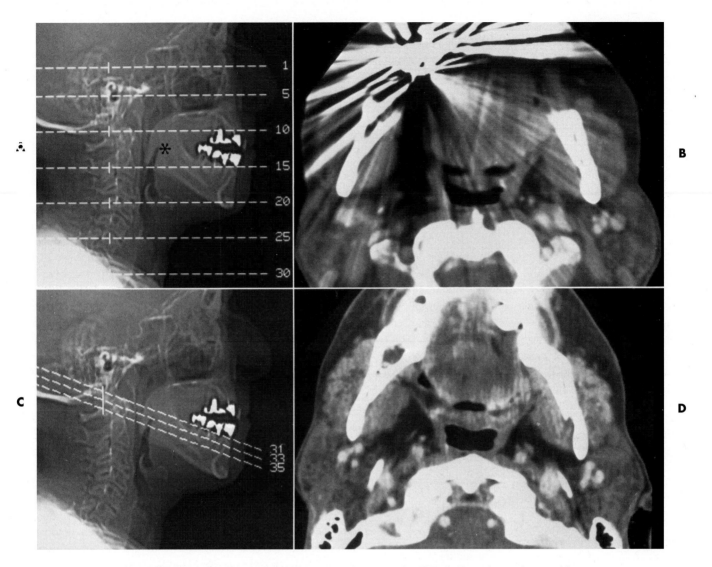

Fig. 3-10. Avoiding dental artifacts on computed tomography (CT). **A,** Lateral scout image without angulation of CT gantry (dotted lines represent selected axial images) in a patient with numerous metallic densities in teeth from dental work. Posterior tongue *(asterisk)* and soft palate lie directly posterior to metal. **B,** Axial contrast-enhanced computed tomography (CECT) at level of dental work is uninterpretable because of numerous streak artifacts caused by metallic fillings and crowns. **C,** Scout view depicting additional slices with CT gantry angled to avoid dental work. **D,** Angled axial CECT at the same level as **B** shows significant improvement in image quality of posterior tongue and oropharynx.

contrast in the arterial and venous structures of the neck; otherwise, nodes and vessels may appear remarkably similar.

Postoperative neck

Imaging the postoperative neck uses the same techniques as the suprahyoid/infrahyoid neck. Thinner sections or supplemental coronal images in the region of suspected recurrence may be required.

Salivary glands

Salivary gland CT is most frequently performed with the axial plane parallel to the infraorbitomeatal line and can be used for assessment of both the parotid and the submandibular gland. However, dental amalgam can cause significant streak artifacts that obscure the parotid or submandibular gland parenchyma. If the dental work is identified on the lateral scout view (scanogram), dental artifacts can usually be avoided if an oblique semiaxial projection is chosen with the scanner gantry angled in a negative direction (between a coronal and an axial plane), thus avoiding the teeth. This plane has the advantage of visualizing both parotid and submandibular glands in the same slice and is parallel to the posterior belly of the digastric muscle.[55] The direct coronal projection may yield additional anatomic information for evaluating both the parotid and the submandibular glands and avoids creating dental artifacts through the parotid gland, but the dental artifacts may still compromise visualization of the submandibular duct and gland. A slice thickness of 3 to 5 mm is generally adequate for evaluating the gland parenchyma. Occasionally, supplemental 1- to 2-mm slices are required for evaluating smaller lesions.

With the current generation of high-resolution scanners, noncontrast computed tomography (NCCT) may suffice for the salivary glands. However, contrast-enhanced computed tomography (CECT) is preferable to NCCT in most cases because CECT maximizes the tissue contrast resolution between a salivary lesion and the adjacent normal gland, fat, and muscle.[10,47] CECT is also essential for assessment of salivary tumor metastases to the lymph node chains of the neck. A normal parotid gland is a relatively fatty structure with a density intermediate between the low-density facial fat and the higher-density adjacent masseter muscle. However, the parotid gland has a wide variation in normal density and may have increased density approaching that of muscle in children and adults or in patients with chronic inflammation. The submandibular gland normally has density just slightly less than skeletal muscle and lymph nodes. In those occasional cases in which the gland parenchyma is similar to muscle in density, either MRI, CECT, or even CT sialography (CTS) may be necessary to discriminate the margins of a suspected mass from the surrounding glandular tissue.

Sialography and computed tomography sialography

Conventional sialography remains the best radiographic method for evaluating ductal anatomy in obstructive, inflammatory, and autoimmune salivary gland diseases. Supplemental CTS may be performed when routine sialography shows an unexpected mass lesion or in the infrequent situation when NCCT (or CECT) shows a dense, enlarged gland in which a mass is suspected but not clearly demarcated. CTS is unnecessary in most salivary tumor cases because of the much improved capabilities and thin sections of the high-resolution third- and fourth-generation CT scanners compared with early-generation scanners. However, MRI may be the preferred alternative method of studying dense salivary glands. CTS may be obtained at the time of intraductal injection of fat-soluble or water-soluble contrast or after a routine sialogram (the gland may be reinjected during the CT with the catheter left in place). The plane of study is the same as that used for NCCT and should be similarly angled to avoid dental filling artifacts. The use of concentrated sialographic contrast material may cause significant streak artifacts if too much contrast collects in dilated ducts, acini, or large pools, all of which can obscure smaller masses in the gland. For optimal CTS, the injection is extended into the acinar phase to maximize parenchymal opacification and thereby silhouette mass lesions within the parenchyma.[16]

Larynx and infrahyoid neck

Laryngeal and infrahyoid neck CT is most commonly requested to evaluate squamous cell carcinoma of the larynx or hypopharynx, associated cervical lymph node metastasis, trauma, and inflammation. Thus axial imaging from the angle of the mandible down to the sternal notch is required to survey the lymphatic chains and infrahyoid neck, using 3- to 5-mm contiguous sections and intravenous contrast infusion. However, the fine detail of the larynx and vocal cords requires thinner contiguous sections of 2 to 3 mm. When assessing the true vocal cords and the arytenoid cartilages, 1- to 1.5-mm contiguous sections may occasionally be necessary to get adequate spatial resolution. Sections through the vocal cords are optimally obtained parallel to the plane of the cords by angling the scanner gantry parallel to the plane of the hyoid bone or the closest adjacent cervical disk space. Because assessment of vocal cord mobility is important in staging glottic carcinoma, various provocative techniques may facilitate laryngeal imaging in those cases where the vocal cords are obscured on physical examination. Quiet breathing places the cords in a partially abducted position. By having the patient blow through a straw or do a modified Valsalva maneuver (puffing out the cheeks) the hypopharynx and supraglottic larynx can be distended, allowing better separation of the aryepiglottic folds from the hypopharynx, while simultaneously abducting the cords (see Fig. 3-3). The vocal cords can be assessed by phonating ("eeee"), which causes the cords to adduct and move to a paramedian position (see Fig. 3-3). Breath holding will also adduct the vocal cords, close the glottis, and significantly reduce motion artifacts. By scanning the larynx twice, once to adduct and a second time (sections limited to the glottis) to abduct the vocal cords, the radiologist can assess vocal cord motion and identify fixation. Intravascular contrast should be given to differentiate vascular structures from adjacent nodes and muscles and to assess tumor margins. Evaluation of laryngeal trauma may not require intravenous contrast. Bone windows are helpful for assessing cartilage fractures or tumor erosion. In a cooperative patient with a flexible neck it may be possible to obtain direct coronal images to assess the configuration of the true and false vocal cords, yielding similar information to that obtained by conventional AP tomography of the larynx.

Thyroid and parathyroid glands

Thyroid gland CT is performed in the same manner as the scanning of the larynx. The indication for performing CT arises when physical examination, ultrasound, or a nuclear medicine study suggests an unusually large or fixed mass. CT can help determine the extent of invasion and compression of adjacent structures in the larynx, hypopharynx, and mediastinum. The 3- to 5-mm sections are obtained from the hyoid bone to the top of the aortic arch to cover potential sites of ectopic thyroid and parathyroid tissue. Although the normal thyroid is hyperdense because of its natural iodine content on NCCT, a CECT is preferred for this study. The normal thyroid enhances intensely on CECT, with most mass lesions of the thyroid enhancing less. The parathyroids are rarely imaged primarily by CT because nuclear medicine and ultrasound techniques are excellent procedures for localizing these small glands.

Paranasal sinuses

Paranasal sinus CT can be approached in several ways depending on the anticipated disease process. Plain films may be used as the initial screening device for evaluating sinusitis or facial trauma. Once a mass or inflammatory lesion is detected within the sinuses, CT is the method of choice for further evaluation. A better substitute for the plain film sinus series is a screening axial sinus NCCT (Fig. 3-11, *A*), which gives superior information on specific sinus involvement by inflammatory processes as well as better delineation of bony sclerosis or destruction. One method is to use 5-mm thick sections obtained at 10-mm intervals (5-mm gap), which can cover the entire paranasal sinuses with six to eight slices. Using a bone algorithm and photographing using bone windows, an accurate assessment of the presence or absence of sinus disease can be made. Another advantage of using the axial plane rather than the coronal plane for screening the sinuses is the inclusion of the mastoid air cells and middle ear, which can be another source of infection in a patient with a fever of unknown origin.

When endoscopic sinus surgery is anticipated, direct coronal NCCT imaging of the sinuses is mandatory for preoperative evaluation of the extent of sinus disease, to detect anatomic variants, and for planning the surgical approach (Fig. 3-11, *B*). This study is done with thin sections ranging from 2 to 3 mm of thickness. Five-millimeter slice thickness is frequently suboptimal, causing volume averaging of small structures and obscuring the fine details of ostiomeatal anatomy. Coronal imaging may be performed with the neck extended in either the prone or the supine position. An advantage of the prone position is that free fluid in the maxillary sinus layers dependently in the inferior portion of the sinus. In the supine position, fluid and mucus layer superiorly at the maxillary sinus ostium and may cause confusion with inflammatory mucosal thickening. Frequently, only the bone algorithm with its edge enhancement properties is needed for evaluating the detailed anatomy of the ostiomeatal complex. Contrast-enhanced sinus CT is usually not necessary for routine sinusitis, although when severe nasal polyposis is suspected, contrast may be useful to demonstrate the characteristic "cascading" appearance of the enhancing polyps or to characterize an associated mucocele. A soft-tissue algorithm with soft-tissue windows may be useful when using CECT for intracranial complications from sinus inflammatory processes. A nasal decongestant may be used to help decrease normal but asymmetric nasal mucosa congestion (normal nasal mucosal cycle) from a mucosal-based mass.

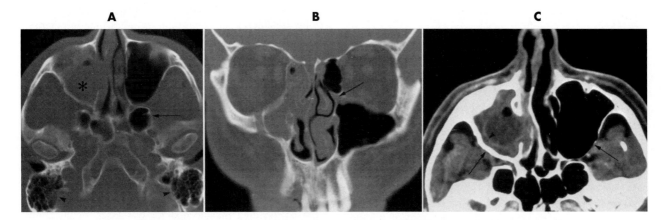

Fig. 3-11. Computed tomography in evaluation of sinusitis. **A,** Axial 5-mm sinus screening noncontrast computed tomography (NCCT) using bone algorithm and bone windows in a patient with chronic right maxillary sinusitis. Excellent bony detail is obtained of both maxillary sinuses (posterior wall thickening and sclerosis are present on right) and mastoids. Clear discrimination of soft-tissue opacification of right maxillary sinus *(asterisk)* is achieved compared with normal air-filled left maxillary sinus. Pneumatized pterygoid process *(arrow)* is an extension of sphenoid sinus pneumatization. **B,** Coronal 3-mm NCCT with bone algorithm and bone windows in same patient clearly demonstrates mucosal thickening and opacification of right maxillary and ethmoid sinuses, and left maxillary infundibulum *(arrow)*. Sharp anatomic detail of bony architecture and the use of coronal plane are essential for preoperative planning before endoscopic sinus surgery. **C,** Axial 3-mm contrast-enhanced computed tomography with soft tissue algorithm and soft tissue windows exaggerates right maxillary sinus posterior wall thickness *(arrows)*. Thickened mucosa has thin rim of enhancement along its luminal margin *(arrowhead)*. Combination of bony sclerosis and mucosal thickening is often seen in chronic sinusitis.

The assessment of sinus tumors requires the most detailed imaging. Both axial CECT and coronal CECT with 3-mm sections are used to precisely determine the extent of sinus tumor spread into adjacent compartments including the anterior and middle cranial fossa, orbit, and parapharyngeal space. For an optimal study, both soft-tissue and bone algorithms are used, allowing differentiation of the soft tissue component as well as evaluating subtle bony destruction (Fig. 3-11, *A*, *C*). The coronal plane is best for evaluating the cribriform plate. CECT is used to maximize the enhancement characteristics of the tumor and differentiate it from adjacent soft-tissue structures. In some cases it may be necessary to extend the axial sections beyond the sinuses to include the cervical lymph node chains of the neck. If this is the case, a constant infusion technique is performed, scanning from the sternal notch up to the top of the paranasal sinuses, followed by the coronal images through the paranasal sinuses. This permits the optimal concentration of intravascular contrast to be obtained in the lower neck to distinguish vessels from lymph nodes.

Facial trauma

Facial trauma CT characterizes fractures and facial soft tissue injury very well. Both axial NCCT and coronal NCCT are obtained to optimally determine the three-dimensional relationships of fracture fragments. Scanning may be performed with either 3-mm sections in both planes or, alternatively, contiguous 1.5-mm sections with coronal reformatted images when the patient cannot tolerate the coronal position because of other trauma or cervical spine instability. However, reformatted images are frequently degraded by motion artifact, and spatial resolution is usually unsatisfactory unless thin sections are used. Bone algorithm is preferred; images are photographed with bone and soft-tissue windows. Soft-tissue algorithm for assessing orbital and facial soft-tissue injury is optional and requires additional image reconstruction time. Three-dimensional reconstructions may help the surgeon plan facial restoration.

Temporal bone and skull base

In the past, evaluation of the skull base and temporal bones was principally performed using plain films and conventional tomography performed in the AP and lateral projections to assess bone destruction and mastoid or middle ear opacification. Tomograms are now rarely done or needed. The development of CT has completely eliminated the need for tomography in this region since the spatial and contrast resolution is superior; also, overlapping structures do not degrade the CT image. CT of the temporal bones requires imaging, preferably in two planes, using thin sections. Contiguous 1- to 1.5-mm sections are frequently obtained in the axial and the direct coronal planes. In some cases if the need for reformatted images is anticipated, scanning in the axial plane with a 0.5-mm overlap may optimize reformatted coronal and sagittal images. In general, intravenous contrast is not necessary for temporal bone imaging,

although vascular tumors or squamous cell carcinoma invading the temporal bone may require the use of intravenous contrast plus supplemental soft-tissue algorithms to best image the extracranial and intracranial soft-tissue component of the lesion. However, bone algorithm with bone windows is used in all temporal bone imaging. CECT of other lesions of the skull base proper may require both axial and coronal 3-mm sections. Bone and soft-tissue algorithms are necessary for assessing skull base tumor spread.

Application of magnetic resonance imaging by head and neck region

Suprahyoid neck

MRI is ideally suited for imaging the suprahyoid neck (including nasopharynx, oropharynx, oral cavity, and tongue). Surface oils that improve signal detection may be used for imaging this area. The standard head coil will permit visualization of the suprahyoid neck structures caudally down to approximately the level of the inferior margin of the mandible and floor of mouth. For imaging the oral cavity, floor of mouth, submandibular space, and cervical lymph node chains, a head coil will not suffice. Either an anterior or volume neck coil is needed to visualize the entire neck from the skull base to the thoracic inlet (from dura to pleura). Several pulse sequences and imaging planes using 5-mm thick sections are required to adequately assess the deep and superficial structures of the neck. (Implicit in this discussion of MRI technique for all areas of the head and neck is the fact that a sagittal T1WI is obtained as the initial sequence in all of the authors' studies and is used primarily as a scout view for the proper positioning in other imaging planes, as well as for anatomic information.) A precontrast axial T1WI and often a coronal T1WI are required to optimally assess fat planes in the neck. Fat provides an excellent white background from which muscle and fascial planes, bone, sinus, and vascular structures can easily be discriminated. The coronal plane is particularly useful for visualizing the relationships of the suprahyoid neck structures to the skull base and also for delineating the anatomy of the tongue and floor of mouth. A T2WI, usually obtained in the axial plane, is required to detect structures with a long T2 (e.g., water, tumors, edema, proteinaceous cysts) that appear brighter than the background muscle and fat (fat loses signal intensity with increased T2 weighting). Postgadolinium T1WIs with fat saturation (suppression) in the axial and coronal plane are frequently helpful to discriminate the enhancing margins of a lesion or to detect perineural spread of tumor. The T2WI may also be combined with fat suppression and gadolinium usage to optimize the information obtained by this more time-consuming long TR sequence.

Lymphadenopathy

Before the widespread use of gadolinium and fat suppression techniques, MRI was often less sensitive and less specific than CT in detecting cervical lymph node metastases.

However, improved MRI scanner technology, gadolinium enhancement, and fat suppression sequences have allowed considerable progress toward that goal. Also, the MRI detection of carotid artery invasion by extracapsular spread of tumor from nodes is often superior to CECT. Controversy still exists in defining the role of MRI in cervical lymph node imaging. Prospective studies of MRI in head and neck tumor and node staging are planned.

An anterior or volume neck coil using 5-mm thick sections with a small 1- to 2-mm interslice gap is necessary to encompass the entire lymph node chains throughout the neck from the skull base to the clavicles within the imaging field of view. The axial plane is frequently used, but the full craniocaudal extent of nodal disease is often better appreciated on coronal and sagittal views. Because the primary tumor is being scanned concomitantly, a choice between pulse sequences for characterizing both the lymph nodes and primary lesion must be made, yet with a minimum number of sequences (shortening the total scan time). Although most of the following sequences are quite sensitive for detecting adenopathy, few of them are specific in discriminating malignant metastatic nodes from reactive (inflammatory) adenopathy. The detection of cervical lymphadenopathy with MRI may be accomplished with (in decreasing order of sensitivity) a STIR sequence, a fat saturation T2WI, a fat saturation postgadolinium T1WI, a conventional T2WI, or a precontrast T1WI. Although STIR is the most sensitive sequence, it also yields the fewest slices, making full nodal evaluation problematic. However, a fat saturation T1WI can be obtained in a much shorter time than either a STIR or T2WI, and the fat saturation T1WI promises improved MRI specificity in metastatic node differentiation from inflammatory disease. The significance of a ring-enhancing node on MRI should be analogous to ring enhancement of a metastatic node seen with the current gold standard, CECT.

Salivary glands

MRI of the parotid gland can be accomplished with a standard head coil using 3- to 5-mm slices but at the risk of excluding a portion of the submandibular gland that lies at the edge of the usable field of view. A volume neck coil is the better coil for imaging both parotid and submandibular glands within the same field of view, especially if a malignancy is suspected and cervical lymph node metastases are sought lower in the neck. A smaller TMJ coil may be necessary for evaluation of perineural tumor spread along with facial nerve into the mastoid segment of the facial nerve canal. As discussed previously in assessing the suprahyoid neck (in which the salivary glands also reside) the MRI sequences that are most suited to salivary imaging include axial or coronal precontrast T1WI or both, axial and coronal fat saturation postgadolinium T1WI, axial T2WI (precontrast or postgadolinium with fat saturation), and often an axial or coronal STIR (for lymph node detection). T1WIs allow for detection of a low-intensity mass within the high-

intensity background of a fatty parotid gland or for assessment of the adjacent fat planes.[10] The fat saturation postgadolinium T1WI is used for detecting the margins of a mass within a less fatty parotid or submandibular gland, for detecting extension beyond the margins of the gland, and especially for detecting perineural tumor spread along the fifth and seventh cranial nerves (best appreciated in the coronal plane). T2WIs are useful for localizing a tumor with a high water content or one with cystic or necrotic areas.[47]

Larynx and infrahyoid neck

The larynx and infrahyoid neck require either an anterior or a volume neck coil, preferably using no thicker than 3-mm sections for the larynx. The field of view should include the area from the inferior margin of the mandible to the clavicles. Although the larynx can be examined well by both axial CECT and MRI, laryngeal MRI has a higher proportion of suboptimal studies. Laryngeal MRI is more susceptible to motion artifacts than MRI of other regions of the neck because of a combination of swallowing, breathing, and vascular pulsation from the adjacent common carotid arteries. A brief training session instructing the patient how to minimize swallowing and breathing artifacts may significantly improve results if it is done immediately before scanning. Additionally, shorter pulse sequences (i.e., T1WI) are more likely to be free of swallowing artifacts. Precontrast axial and coronal T1WIs are essential to assess the paralaryngeal (paraglottic) fat planes; the coronal plane, angled parallel to the airway, is especially useful for determining transglottic tumor spread.[52] Fat saturation postgadolinium T1WIs in the axial and coronal planes are best for detecting lesion margins, invasion of adjacent cartilage, and associated malignant nodes. T2WI in the axial plane may help detect moderately increased tumor signal and improve detection of high signal cystic or necrotic neck lesions. The longer T2WI and STIR sequences are more prone to motion artifacts and are occasionally suboptimal in quality.

Thyroid and parathyroid glands

The same techniques and slice thickness as those of the larynx are used for the thyroid and parathyroid glands. The field of view may need lower centering to include the upper mediastinum and ensure complete evaluation of the inferior extent of a thyroid tumor or an ectopic parathyroid gland. Coronal and sagittal views aid understanding of the craniocaudal extent of the lesion relative to the aortic arch, great vessels, and mediastinum; this information is especially useful to the surgeon. Although MRI may detect an unsuspected thyroid or parathyroid lesion during routine neck or cervical spine imaging, MRI is less frequently used for primary evaluation of these lesions because of the cost of the study and susceptibility to motion artifacts. The normal thyroid gland will enhance mildly on both gadolinium-enhanced MRI and CECT. A solid mass in the thyroid or parathyroid is usually low intensity on T1WI and high signal on T2WI, and it may enhance with gadolinium. Cystic lesions are bright on T2WI.

Paranasal sinuses

Sinus MRI is primarily indicated for evaluating sinus tumors (and occasionally inflammatory disease such as a mucocele) and may be accomplished with a standard head coil, using 3- to 5-mm slices. The principal value of MRI over CT for sinus tumors is the ability of MRI to distinguish between tumor and obstructed sinus secretions and to predict the true extent of the tumor. A precontrast sagittal, axial, or coronal T1WI will provide a good demonstration of the sinuses, nasal cavity, cribriform plate, masticator and parapharyngeal spaces, and orbits. T1WI may differentiate hydrated from viscous sinus secretions; secretions are low signal when hydrated or fluid-like and are intermediate to high signal when viscous and desiccated. Coronal T2WIs or axial T2WIs (either pregadolinium, or postgadolinium with fat saturation) are useful for detecting inflammatory sinus secretions, which are high signal when hydrated or fluid and are low signal when viscous and desiccated. However, tumors tend to be intermediate in signal on T2WI. Because fat is not present to any significant degree in the paranasal sinuses, a STIR sequence frequently adds little over a T2WI and is unnecessary. Sagittal, coronal, or axial fat saturation T1WI is recommended to better define the sinus tumor margins when the tumor extends directly or by perineural spread beyond the sinus into the anterior cranial fossa, orbit, parapharyngeal space, or pterygopalatine fossa. The sagittal and coronal planes are very helpful for evaluating cribriform plate extension; the coronal and axial planes are best for orbital, cavernous sinus, pterygopalatine fossa, and parapharyngeal space spread.

Temporal bone

MRI has significantly improved the detection of internal auditory canal (IAC), facial nerve canal, and jugular foramen lesions. Gadolinium-enhanced MRI has eliminated the need for air-contrast CT cisternography to detect a small intracanalicular acoustic schwannoma. MRI is useful, in combination with CT, for assessing expansile or destructive lesions of the temporal bone and external auditory canal. A standard head coil is adequate for most temporal bone lesions, but a smaller 5- to 10-cm TMJ coil may be needed for evaluating the mastoid and parotid segments of the facial nerve. The small size of the temporal bone structures and their respective lesions requires high spatial resolution images, which may be accomplished by using thinner slices of 0.5 to 3 mm (preferably without an interslice gap), smaller surface coils (higher signal-to-noise ratio), volume acquisition, or T1WI (higher signal-to-noise ratio). Precontrast T1WI in the sagittal and axial planes is useful for defining anatomy and for detection of high-signal lesions such as fat, methemoglobin, and viscous or proteinaceous cysts. Postgadolinium T1WIs (without or with fat saturation) in the axial and coronal planes are essential for detecting small enhancing lesions and determining the extent of larger lesions. In fact, for routine evaluation of a suspected acoustic schwannoma only a post-

gadolinium axial and coronal T1WI study may be required. T2WIs are frequently unnecessary for IAC tumors but may be helpful when brainstem ischemic or demyelinating disease, meningioma, blood products, proteinaceous secretions, or a large destructive tumor is suspected or is being further evaluated after a preliminary temporal bone CT. A facial nerve lesion in the mastoid segment of the facial nerve canal is best evaluated for proximal and distal extension using a TMJ coil with sagittal and coronal pregadolinium and postgadolinium T1WIs.

Skull base

MRI may be indicated for primary lesions of the skull base or for intracranial and extracranial lesions that secondarily involve the skull base. A standard head coil using 3- to 5-mm slices images this region well. Pregadolinium sagittal, axial, and/or coronal T1WI allows for assessment of the fat planes of the suprahyoid neck and detection of high-signal intensity blood breakdown products, proteinaceous fluids, or fat within the lesion. Postgadolinium axial and coronal (occasionally sagittal) fat saturation T1WIs are excellent for determining the extent of an enhancing lesion above, below, and within the skull base. T2WI in the axial or coronal plane may be helpful for detecting a high-signal lesion. STIR images usually give similar information to T2WIs in the skull base and may not be necessary.

Ultrasound applications in the head and neck

High-resolution ultrasound evaluation of the suprahyoid neck, salivary glands, and infrahyoid neck is limited to the more superficial neck structures because of the impediment to sound transmission caused by the highly reflective facial bones, mandible, mastoid tip, and air within the oral cavity and pharynx. The ultrasound technique, using a high-frequency, 5- to 10-MHz probe and multiple imaging planes, is similar for all these regions. A small superficial lesion is best seen with a high-frequency probe, whereas a larger and deeper lesion may require a lower frequency probe. Color flow Doppler technique may help differentiate vascular structures from a cystic or solid lesion. Head and neck ultrasound is performed less frequently in North America than in Europe, perhaps because of the common availability of CT in North America and the perception of the greater accuracy of CT. Head and neck ultrasound has no role as a staging modality for skull base and sinus neoplasms.

Suprahyoid neck

Ultrasound may be used for the assessment of tumors of the floor of the mouth, anterior two thirds of the tongue, malignant adenopathy, and invasion of the carotid artery and jugular vein. The deep structures centered around the parapharyngeal space are inadequately assessed by this technique and are better investigated by CT and MRI. Ultrasound can assess tumor extent in the floor of the mouth and tongue but has limitations: The mandible obscures the pterygoid muscles; pharyngeal air hides the posterior pharyngeal wall and epiglottis.[18] Ultrasound excels in differentiating cystic from solid masses; a cyst has few internal echoes, a strongly echogenic back wall, and strong through-transmission of sound, whereas a solid mass has many internal echoes and no additional through-transmission.

Metastatic lymphadenopathy

Ultrasound is very sensitive for detecting metastatic involvement of the lower two thirds of the internal jugular, spinal accessory, submental, and submandibular nodes. Its accuracy may exceed CT for detecting enlarged lymph nodes, but ultrasound does not reliably differentiate large reactive nodes from metastatic nodes.[24] The upper one third of the internal jugular, retropharyngeal, and tracheoesophageal groove nodes are poorly evaluated because of obscuration by bone or airway structures. Ultrasound may be the best method (possibly better than MRI or CT) for determining the presence of tumor invasion of the common or internal carotid artery and internal jugular vein by adjacent primary tumor or extracapsular spread from metastatic nodes. Invasion of the carotid artery is characterized by loss of the echogenic fascial plane between the vessel wall and the tumor.

Salivary glands

Ultrasound has indications for both inflammatory and neoplastic disease. It may detect salivary duct stones as small as 2 mm. An obstructed dilated duct may appear as a tubular cystic structure. An abscess may be detected and drained under ultrasound guidance during the acute stage of sialadenitis, a time during which sialography is contraindicated. A mass in the superficial parotid gland is easily assessed by ultrasound, but the deep lobe of the parotid gland is obscured by the mandible, styloid process, and mastoid tip. Ultrasound is also very sensitive for a mass in the submandibular gland. Although ultrasound can determine the sharpness of margins of the lesion (well-defined margins usually indicate a benign mass and infiltrative margins suggest malignancy), an aggressive neoplasm or inflammatory process extending beyond the margins of the gland is better evaluated by MRI or CECT because the deep landmarks are more easily demonstrated with MRI or CECT.

Infrahyoid neck

Ultrasound using a high-frequency transducer is usually the first imaging modality for evaluating superficially located thyroid gland and parathyroid gland masses because it is relatively inexpensive and easily performed. In the infrahyoid neck, ultrasound is not used for the larynx, retropharyngeal space, or thoracic inlet because overlying cartilage, airway structures, sternum, and clavicles cause acoustic shadows that may obscure lesions. The right, left, and pyramidal lobes may be evaluated by scanning in the axial, sagittal, and oblique planes. A thyroid mass and highly echogenic calcification are easily assessed. A parathyroid adenoma is readily evaluated if its location is cranial to the sternum. Ultrasound-guided fine needle biopsy of a thyroid or para-

thyroid mass is possible at the time of scanning. Large cystic and solid masses of the infrahyoid neck may be differentiated by ultrasound. Lymphoma of the neck may appear weakly echogenic, sometimes simulating a cyst.

PRINCIPLES OF IMAGE INTERPRETATION

Strategy for image interpretation and differential diagnosis

This section is included to aid the beginning surgeon or oncologist in developing a basic strategy for image interpretation. Normally, the radiologist chooses and supervises the appropriate imaging study, evaluates and interprets the images, and communicates its significance to the referring physician. However, frequent dialogue between the referring physician and the radiologist will significantly improve interpretation of the imaging study. Accurately interpreting an imaging study of the head and neck requires a systematic method of observation, a knowledge of the complex anatomy, spaces, and pathophysiology, and an understanding of imaging principles. The differential diagnosis of lesions of the head and neck requires a systematic approach as well. One such diagnostic imaging process is summarized below:

1. Obtain clinical data: age, sex, history, physical findings.
2. Survey the films for all abnormalities and summarize these findings.
3. Compartmentalize the lesion.
4. Interpret the chronicity and aggressiveness of the observations: acute or chronic, nonaggressive or aggressive, benign or malignant.
5. Develop a differential diagnosis. Use pathologic categories: congenital, inflammatory, tumor, trauma, vascular. Use clinical and radiographic information to narrow the choices and arrive at the most appropriate diagnosis.

By using such a strategy it is unlikely that important findings will be missed because all the images have been evaluated. This may be done by looking at all the anatomic spaces on each slice and proceeding sequentially through all the slices; alternatively each anatomic space can be evaluated on serial slices, followed by the next anatomic space, and so on. Characterizing a lesion requires specific observations: location, anatomic space of the epicenter, size, definition of margins, extent of spread in each direction, invasion of adjacent compartments, involvement of neurovascular structures, enhancement pattern, cysts, calcification, density, signal intensity, echogenicity, hemorrhage, and lymphadenopathy. Next, summarizing the findings helps to tie them together into a logical pattern. Compartmentalizing a lesion is the last step in the observational process and requires placing the epicenter or site of origin of the lesion in a specific anatomic space, although some lesions may be multicompartmental. The origin of a lesion is limited by the types of tissue that reside in each specific space. An example of such a summary would be, "A 35-year-old male has a cystic, nonenhancing mass in the sublingual space.'' A frequent cause of misdiagnosis is the failure to make all the observations first; interpretation and differential diagnosis of the lesion are the final steps.

The interpretation of the significance of a lesion uses both its radiologic and clinical features; for example, inflammatory (edema; abscess cavity; fever), nonaggressive (remodeling of bone; slow progression of symptoms), aggressive (destruction of bone; rapid progression), benign neoplastic (well-defined margins; displacement of adjacent structures; nonpainful), malignant (poorly defined margins; invasion and destruction of adjacent structures; pain and neuropathies), or cystic (low-density center with a thin rim of enhancement; fluctuant). The differential diagnosis is narrowed by further refining the interpretation, ''A 35-year-old male has an asymptomatic cystic, nonenhancing mass in the sublingual space that appears chronic and nonaggressive.'' With knowledge of the relevant clinical findings, the proper differential diagnosis, which is specific for each anatomic space, can then be constructed and limited to one (or at least a few) possible pathologic causes. In this example, a ranula would be the most likely consideration.

IMAGING ANATOMY, SITE-SPECIFIC LESIONS, AND PSEUDOTUMORS OF HEAD AND NECK

Spaces of suprahyoid neck

The traditional approach to radiographic interpretation of the head and neck region has been to follow a surgical compartmental approach: nasopharynx, oropharynx, oral cavity, pharynx, and larynx. The nasopharynx extends vertically from the skull base to the soft palate; the oropharynx encompasses the area from the soft palate/hard palate to the hyoid bone. The oral cavity is located anterior to the oropharynx. Below the hyoid bone reside the larynx anteriorly and the hypopharynx more posteriorly. With the advent of cross-sectional imaging in radiology, first with CT and later with MRI, the radiologic interpretive approach changed from a pattern based on surgical compartmental anatomy to one dependent on fascial spaces. However, a combination of the two interpretive approaches, for example, parapharyngeal space at the nasopharyngeal level (with the compartmental designation serving as a modifier) may be more helpful in precisely defining a lesion location.

The head and neck region, the anatomic territory that extends from the skull base to the thoracic inlet, is best and most conveniently divided into the suprahyoid and infrahyoid neck with the hyoid bone serving as the divisional point.[26] Figures 3-12 through 3-14 demonstrate normal cross-sectional CT and MRI anatomy of the suprahyoid neck. The suprahyoid neck may be divided into a series of fascial spaces based on the division and layers of the superficial and deep cervical fascia. The superficial cervical fascia surrounds the face and neck, providing a fatty layer on which the skin is able to slide. The underlying deep cervical fascia is separated into three distinct layers: superficial (investing) layer, middle (visceral) layer, and deep (prevertebral) layer. (Space limitations and the complexity of the fascial spaces do not allow for a detailed description or explanation of the deep cervical fascia.) Although not usually visualized on CT or MRI, these fascial layers divide the suprahyoid neck into distinct anatomic and surgically defined spaces:

1. Parapharyngeal space (PPS)
2. Pharyngeal mucosal space (PMS)
3. Parotid space (PS)
4. Carotid space (CS)
5. Masticator space (MS)
6. Retropharyngeal space (RPS)
7. Prevertebral space (PVS)
8. Oral cavity (OC)
9. Sublingual space (SLS)
10. Submandibular space (SMS)

Inflammatory and neoplastic disease, the major pathophysiologic processes of the head and neck territory, tend to grow and spread in the boundaries and confines of these fascial spaces.[5] Nevertheless, this approach based on the use of fascial anatomy allows delineation of specific anatomic spaces, with identification of disease-specific lesions for each of these spaces. As a consequence, a more accurate differential diagnosis and resulting final diagnosis are attained.

Parapharyngeal space

The crucial anatomic center point to understanding suprahyoid anatomy is the parapharyngeal space (PPS); this fibrofatty fascial space extends from the skull base to the level of the hyoid bone and serves as a marker space around which the remaining fascial spaces are arranged. It contains fat, portions of the third division of cranial nerve V, the internal maxillary artery, the ascending pharyngeal artery, and the pterygoid venous plexus. In the axial plane, this space has a triangular configuration and demonstrates bilateral symmetry. In the coronal plane the PPS has an hourglass shape, thicker at the skull base and hyoid level and thinner in the midsuprahyoid neck.

The PPS is clearly defined and located on both the axial and coronal planes with both CT and MRI.[43] With the former technique, the predominant fat content serves as a low-density marker between the medial muscles of deglutition found in the pharyngeal mucosal space and the muscles of mastication, located more laterally. With MRI the PPS has a bright signal intensity on T1WI (the scanning sequence that best highlights fat and muscle tissue differences); with longer TR times and more T2 weighting this fatty space becomes less intense in signal.

Because this space is the epicenter around which the other fascial spaces are arranged, it serves as a potential marker or pivotal space. By noting the position and direction of displacement of the PPS, one can determine the epicenter

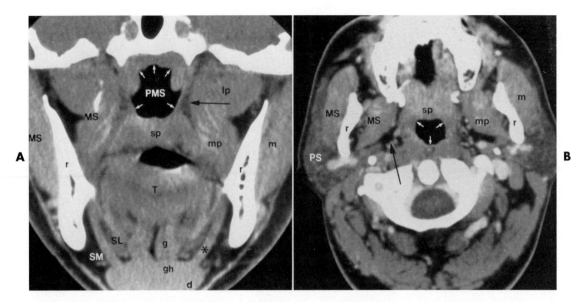

Fig. 3-12. The normal computed tomography anatomy of suprahyoid neck. **A,** Coronal contrast-enhanced computed tomography (CECT) and, **B,** axial CECT demonstrate low-fat density of the parapharyngeal space *(arrow).* Note its central position as a marker space. The following structures can be identified: anterior belly of digastric muscle *(d),* genioglossus muscle *(g),* geniohyoid muscle *(gh),* lateral pterygoid muscle *(lp),* masseter muscle *(m),* medial pterygoid muscle *(mp),* masticator space *(MS),* mylohyoid muscle *(asterisk),* nasopharyngeal mucosal space *(PMS, small arrows),* parotid space *(PS),* ramus of mandible *(r),* sublingual space *(SL),* submandibular space *(SM),* soft palate *(sp),* and intrinsic tongue musculature *(T).*

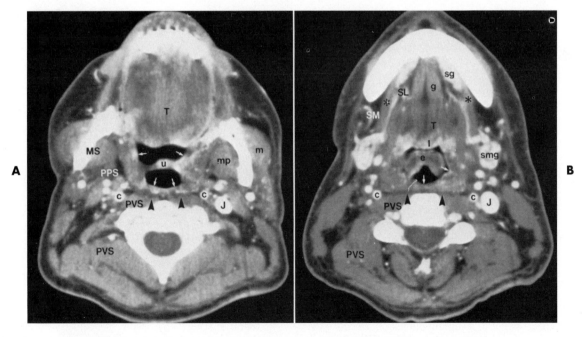

Fig. 3-13. The normal computed tomography anatomy of sublingual space, submandibular space, and oral cavity. **A,** Axial contrast-enhanced computed tomography at superior and, **B,** inferior tongue levels, respectively. Note the following structures: internal carotid *(c),* epiglottis *(e),* genioglossus muscle *(g),* jugular vein *(J),* lingual tonsil *(l),* masseter muscle *(m),* medial pterygoid muscle *(mp),* masticator space *(MS),* mylohyoid muscle *(asterisk),* pharyngeal mucosal space of oropharynx *(small arrows),* prevertebral space *(PVS),* retropharyngeal space *(arrowheads),* sublingual space *(SL),* submandibular space *(SM),* submandibular gland *(smg),* intrinsic musculature of tongue *(T),* and uvula of soft palate *(u).*

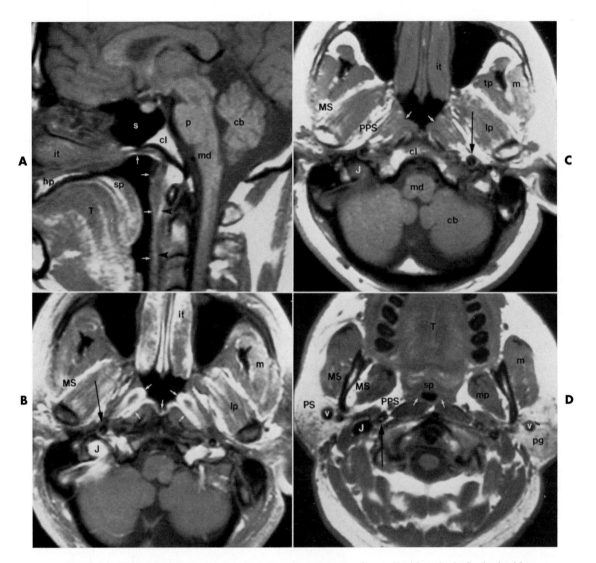

Fig. 3-14. The normal magnetic resonance imaging anatomy of suprahyoid neck. **A,** Sagittal midline noncontrast T1-weighted image (T1WI). **B,** Axial noncontrast T1WI at the level of jugular foramen. **C,** Axial postgadolinium T1WI at the same level of **B** demonstrates enhancement of nasopharyngeal mucosa and jugular veins. **D,** Axial noncontrast T1WI at the level of C2 vertebral body and midtongue demonstrates high signal intensity of parapharyngeal space fat. The following structures are labelled: cerebellum *(cb)*, clivus *(cl)*, hard palate *(hp)*, internal carotid artery *(arrow)*, inferior turbinates *(it)*, jugular vein *(J)*, lateral pterygoid muscle *(lp)*, masseter muscle *(m)*, medulla *(md)*, masticator space *(MS)*, nasopharyngeal mucosal space *(small arrows)*, pons *(p)*, parotid gland *(pg)*, parapharyngeal space *(PPS)*, parotid space *(PS)*, retropharyngeal space *(arrowheads)*, sphenoid sinus *(s)*, soft palate *(sp)*, intrinsic musculature of tongue *(T)*, temporalis muscle *(tp)*, and retromandibular vein *(v)*.

and fascial space origin of a suprahyoid lesion. Because the PPS contains few structures from which lesions arise, most lesions found in this space have spread here secondarily from an adjacent fascial space.[44]

The fascial spaces that are centered about the parapharyngeal space include the pharyngeal mucosal space (PMS), the carotid space (CS), the parotid space (PS), the masticator space (MS), the retropharyngeal space (RPS), and the pre-

vertebral space (PVS). Each space has well-defined anatomic boundaries, contains major structures of importance, and gives rise to pathologic processes that are site selective for that space. For consideration of pathologic processes in each fascial space, it is convenient to use the following outline: congenital, inflammatory, neoplastic (benign and malignant), pseudolesions, and miscellaneous. This approach, using these few disease categories, elicits most of the major lesions to be found in the head and neck, and is used in the following discussion of suprahyoid and infrahyoid lesions.

Pharyngeal mucosal space

The PMS lies medial to the PPS and anterior to the PVS. It encompasses the mucosal surfaces of the inner boundaries of the nasopharynx and oropharynx and includes lymphoid (adenoidal) tissue, minor salivary glands, portions of the constrictor muscles, and muscles of deglutition; the medial portion of the eustachian tube passes through it. These structures lie medial to or on the airway side of the buccopharyngeal fascia; this fascial structure may be seen on MRI as a band of low signal intensity. On CECT or gadolinium-enhanced MRI studies, the overlying pharyngeal mucosa enhances.

The PMS extends from the skull base to the lower margin of the cricoid cartilage, extending into the upper portion of the infrahyoid neck. It encompasses the nasopharynx, oropharynx, and portions of the hypopharynx. Lesions in this space displace the PPS laterally.

In general, caution is used when interpreting the mucosal surfaces of the pharynx, oral cavity, and larynx. The normal mucosa is high signal on T2WI and STIR and enhances on postgadolinium T1WI (and with CECT); it may be confused with a superficial mucosal-based malignancy. Likewise, a small superficial mucosal-based tumor may be indistinguishable from the adjacent normal mucosa. The direct clinical examination of the mucosal surfaces is still superior to cross-sectional CT or MR imaging in detecting superficial tumor; however, both CT and MRI excel in detecting submucosal tumor and deep invasion. Mucosal irregularity and slight asymmetry are common, especially near the fossa of Rosenmüller (the lateral pharyngeal recesses of the nasopharynx), and care is taken in ascribing abnormality. Repeat studies with a modified Valsalva maneuver to distend the airway may be helpful. Involvement of the submucosal muscles and adjacent deep structures, such as the PPS, will confirm the presence of a suspected neoplastic mucosal lesion. Lymphoid (adenoidal) tissue is often hypertrophic and prominent, especially in children and young adolescents, and may encroach on the airway. On CT lymphoid tissue is isodense to muscle; with MRI it has a similar intensity to muscle on T1WI but has a bright signal on T2WI. It lies superficial to the buccopharyngeal fascia and is relatively homogeneous.

Inflammatory lesions of the PPS include pharyngitis, abscess (especially tonsillar abscess), and postinflammatory retention cysts (Fig. 3-15). Benign mixed salivary tumor is the most common benign neoplasm.

A Thornwaldt cyst is a common congenital lesion of the midline posterior nasopharyngeal mucosa and only rarely becomes secondarily infected. It is very bright on long TR sequences on MRI.

Squamous cell carcinoma (SCC), the most common tumor of the upper aerodigestive tract, originates from the PMS; the majority of lesions arise from squamous epithe-

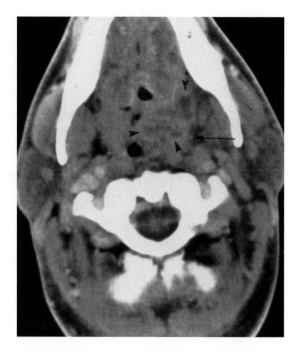

Fig. 3-15. Tonsillar abscess. Axial contrast-enhanced computed tomography demonstrates low-density left tonsillar lesion *(arrowheads)* with thin peripheral rim enhancement. The left tonsil is increased in size. Partially effaced left parapharyngeal space *(arrow)* is lateral in position.

lium in the region of the lateral pharyngeal recess (Figs. 3-16 and 3-17). Small submucosal lesions may be missed on the clinical examination but may be detected with cross-sectional imaging. Involvement of the adjacent musculofascial spaces confirms the presence of a mucosal lesion. It may become large and lead to extensive invasion and destruction of the neighboring fascial spaces or extend medially to involve the PPS. With CT, SCC demonstrates inhomogeneous lesion enhancement, commonly with extension into adjacent spaces. With MRI it is of intermediate intensity on T1WI and high intensity on T2WI and enhances after gadolinium infusion.[39] It may cause serous otitis media and mastoid cell opacification because of dysfunction of the eustachian tube from invasion or mass effect. Extension superior to the skull base is common; the foramen lacerum, foramen ovale, carotid canal, jugular foramen, and clivus may be affected. Perineural tumor spread along cranial motor nerve V is common and its presence should be diligently sought, especially if there is unilateral atrophy of the muscles of mastication innervated by the mandibular division of the fifth cranial nerve. Inferiorly, nasopharyngeal SCC may extend to involve the soft palate, tonsillar pillars, and nasal cavity. Asymptomatic cervical adenopathy with involvement of the superior internal jugular and spinal accessory lymph node chains is the presenting mode in over 50% of patients. Lymph nodes are usually considered positive when over 1.5 cm in diameter; an enhancing lymph node rim with necrotic low-density center on CECT indicates neoplastic involvement. On MRI lymph nodes have bright signal intensity on

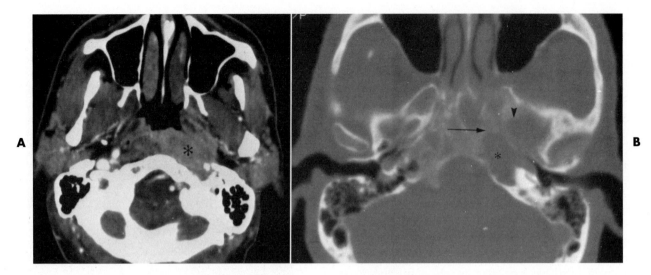

Fig. 3-16. Nasopharyngeal carcinoma. **A,** Axial contrast-enhanced computed tomography (CECT) demonstrates enhancing lesion *(asterisk)* involving pharyngeal mucosa space, retropharyngeal spaces, and prevertebral space; tumor abuts skull base. **B,** Axial CECT image with bone settings at the level of the skull base demonstrates lytic destructive lesion involving anteromedial left petrous bone *(asterisk)*, medial portion of greater sphenoid wing *(arrowhead)*, and adjacent clivus *(arrow)*.

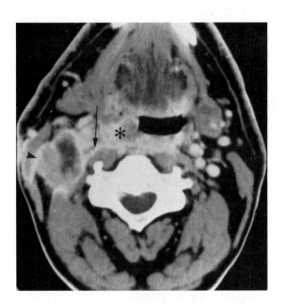

Fig. 3-17. Squamous cell carcinoma of oropharynx. Axial contrast-enhanced computed tomography demonstrates mixed-density enhancing lesion *(asterisk)* in right oropharynx. The tumor has extended posterolaterally to surround carotid vessels *(arrow)*. Enhancing lymph node *(arrowhead)* with low-density necrotic center is noted posterior to carotid space, lying just beneath sternocleidomastoid muscle. Enhancement of the adjacent sternocleidomastoid muscle indicates muscle invasion.

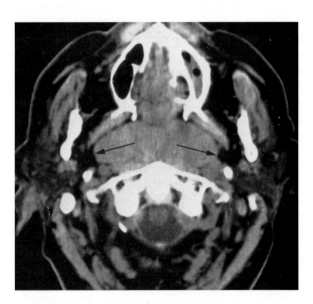

Fig. 3-18. Nasopharyngeal lymphoma. Axial non-contrast computed tomography demonstrates large homogeneous pharyngeal mucosal space with nasopharyngeal mass lesion, displacing prevertebral and retropharyngeal spaces posteriorly. The lesion bulges into parapharyngeal space bilaterally *(arrows)*.

T2WI; on T1WI postgadolinium administration, lymph node enhancement may be seen.

The extensive lymphoid tissue in this space is a source for development of non-Hodgkin's lymphoma (Fig. 3-18). Both SCC and lymphoma may have extensive lymph node involvement; the nodes associated with SCC commonly have necrotic centers whereas those of lymphoma are usually noncavitary and homogeneous. Malignant minor salivary gland tumors also occur in this space. The above three malignant lesions are difficult to separate radiologically.

Parotid space

The PS, the home of the parotid gland and the extracranial portion of the facial nerve, lies lateral to both the PPS and the CS and posterior to the masticator space. It extends superiorly from the level of the midsquamous temporal bone to the angle of the mandible inferiorly. It contains the parotid gland, multiple lymph nodes (within and outside the parotid gland parenchyma), the facial nerve, the retromandibular vein, and branches of the external carotid artery. The parotid gland overlies the posterior portion of the masseter muscle; its deep retromandibular portion lies posterior to the mandible and lateral to the PPS and the CS. The posterior belly of the digastric muscle separates the PS from the CS.

Because of its high fat content, especially in the adult, the parotid gland parenchyma is frequently low density on CT but may vary and approach muscle density. It is high intensity on T1WI (slightly less than subcutaneous fat) and has decreased intensity on T2WI but often retains its bright T2 signal intensity relative to muscle. The retromandibular vein lies just posterior to the lateral margin of the mandibular ramus. The diagonal course of the facial nerve, paralleling a line drawn from the stylomastoid foramen to a point just lateral to the retromandibular vein, divides the parotid gland into superficial and deep portions. Although this is not a true anatomic division, it is useful for surgical planning. The facial nerve may be seen on some MRI studies. Its course must be considered and determined when removal of deep parotid lobe lesions is planned.

Lesions in the parotid space are usually surrounded by parotid gland tissue and are better defined with MRI than CT.[49] With NCCT, lesions are usually isodense to the normal gland or increased density; with MRI, lesions are muscle intensity on T1WI and usually hyperintense to normal parotid gland on T2WI.[41] When small, parotid lesions tend to be homogeneous; with increase in lesion size areas of hemorrhage, necrosis, and calcification may develop. If the lesion extends or originates from the deep portion of the gland, it displaces the PPS medially and occasionally anteriorly. Large lesions in the parotid gland proper will cause widening of the stylomandibular notch, the space between the posterior border of the mandible and the styloid process; comparison to the contralateral side will make subtle widening of this space evident.[25] Deep lobe lesions, if large, may displace the carotid artery posteriorly. Benign lesions as a general rule are usually well defined; malignant lesions have indistinct margins and may invade adjacent structures. Lesions in the PPS or CS may extend laterally into the parotid space, mimicking a parotid lesion clinically.

Congenital lesions of the PS include hemangioma, lymphangioma, and first and second branchial cleft cyst, the latter presenting as a cystic-appearing lesion with smooth walls.[27] Enhancing margins of the cyst indicate it is secondarily infected. Inflammatory disease may present as diffuse swelling or as a localized abscess; infection of the adjacent skull base is best demonstrated with CT. Infection may occur secondary to calculus disease.

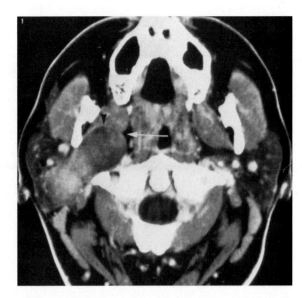

Fig. 3-19. Benign pleomorphic adenoma of the right parotid gland. Axial contrast-enhanced computed tomography demonstrates dumbbell-shaped tumor with enhancement of its superficial portion; its deep portion is predominantly low density. Parapharyngeal space is displaced medially *(arrow).* The lateral pterygoid muscle is indented and lies anteriorly *(arrowhead).* The lesion has displaced ramus of mandible anteriorly.

Calculi are also best demonstrated by sialography as intraluminal filling defects or by CT because of its tenfold higher sensitivity over plain films for detecting calcified calculi. Sialadenitis, autoimmune disease, and strictures are still best evaluated by conventional sialography, which best demonstrates ductal anatomy. Chronic sialadenitis will cause the affected parotid gland CT density to approach that of muscle; this appears as lower parotid gland signal on T1WI and brighter signal on T2WI than that of the contralateral parotid gland. Autoimmune diseases such as Sjögren's syndrome demonstrate bilateral parotid enlargement. Bilateral gland enlargement by benign lymphoepithelial cysts is seen in acquired immunodeficiency syndrome.

Benign pleomorphic adenoma (benign mixed tumor), the most common benign neoplasm of the parotid gland, is well defined and demonstrates variable degrees of contrast enhancement (Fig. 3-19). It is usually ovoid in configuration and may involve either the superficial or deep lobe of the parotid gland or less commonly both. Rarely, benign mixed tumors may arise from salivary rest tissue medial to the deep lobe and have a fat border on both their medial and lateral margins. Calcification is occasionally seen within the tumor. The tumor is hypointense on T1WI and hyperintense on T2WI. Both the superficial and deep lobes of the parotid gland may be involved, leading to a dumbbell configuration of the mass and associated widening of the stylomandibular notch.

Malignant lesions include mucoepidermoid carcinoma, adenoid cystic carcinoma, acinic cell carcinoma, and malig-

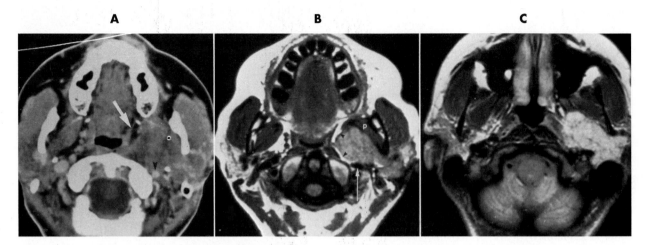

Fig. 3-20. Acinic cell tumor of left parotid gland. **A,** Axial contrast-enhanced computed tomography at level of C1 and C2 demonstrates inhomogeneous irregular mass lesion involving both superficial and deep portions of the left parotid gland. Lesion displaces parapharyngeal space anteriorly and medially *(arrow)*. Stylomandibular distance is increased. Areas of patchy enhancement are noted around periphery and throughout lesion. Lesion has displaced carotid artery posteriorly *(arrowhead)*. **B,** Axial T1-weighted image demonstrates superior contrast resolution of magnetic resonance imaging. Both superficial and deep portions of lesion are well outlined. The margin of the lesion can be separated from lateral pterygoid muscle *(p)*, which is displaced anteriorly and laterally. PPS *(arrowheads)*, indicated by its high-intensity fat, is displaced medially. The flow void marks the site of left carotid artery *(arrow)*. **C,** Axial spin density magnetic resonance imaging image at the level of the skull base demonstrates well-defined lesion of increased signal intensity. Involvement of both superficial and deep lobes is well delineated.

nant mixed tumor (Fig. 3-20). High-grade malignant lesions have infiltrative borders. MRI is superior to CT for showing lesion margins and extent. Because of the abundant lymph node tissue within the parotid gland, lymph node involvement may be seen with non-Hodgkin's lymphoma, and metastatic involvement may be seen with SCC and malignant melanoma. Basal cell carcinoma of the adjacent ear and cheek may metastasize to the parotid lymph nodes.

Carotid space

The CS, the space of vessels, nerves, and lymph nodes, lies posterior to the PPS, lateral to the retropharyngeal space, anterolateral to the prevertebral spaces, and medial to the PS and styloid process. The posterior belly of the digastric muscle separates the CS from the parotid space. The CS is formed from portions of all three layers of the deep cervical fascia. The CS extends from the temporal bone and base of the skull superiorly to the mediastinum inferiorly.[19] It contains the common carotid artery, its major divisions, the internal and external carotid artery, the jugular vein, cranial nerves IX to XII, sympathetic plexus, and lymph nodes. The jugular vein lies lateral and posterior to the carotid artery; the vagus nerve lies in the posterior groove between the two vessels. Cranial nerves IX, XI, and XII migrate to the anteromedial portion of the CS lower in the neck. Lesions of the CS displace the PPS anteriorly and, if large, may remodel the styloid process, displacing it anterolaterally.

Infection of the CS occurs most commonly secondary to

spread of infection from adjacent fascial spaces. Reactive inflammatory lymph nodes, which are characteristically homogeneous and less than 1 cm in size, may be seen in any portion along the carotid space and be seen with such varied infectious processes as sinusitis, infectious mononucleosis, and tuberculosis. Suppurative lymph nodes may have low-density centers and may not be distinguished from malignant lymph nodes; clusters or groups of lymph nodes lumped into large masses are not uncommon. Cellulitis causes a loss of normal soft-tissue planes; abscesses are characterized by focal fluid collections with enhancing margins.

On CECT, normal blood vessels demonstrate contrast enhancement; with dynamic CECT a wash-in phase (early visualization of contrast) may be demonstrated within normal vessels and within the feeding or draining vessels of a mass, which further indicates the vascular etiology of a lesion. On MRI, blood vessels appear as circular or linear areas of flow void, because of flow of fast-moving blood. Turbulent or slow flow may lead to areas of mixed signal intensity. Vessel ectasia, dissection, aneurysm, pseudoaneurysm, and thrombosis may be diagnosed readily with either cross-sectional imaging technique. Assessment of adjacent sectional images will demonstrate a tubular configuration to the lesion. An ectatic carotid artery or an asymmetrically enlarged jugular vein may present clinically as a lateral neck mass but is readily discernible radiologically. The right jugular vein is usually larger than the left and at times may be several times larger than the left, reflecting its greater venous drainage

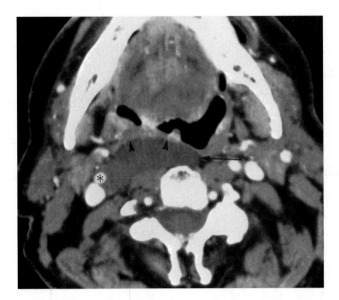

Fig. 3-21. Left carotid space and retropharyngeal space ganglio-neuroma. Axial contrast-enhanced computed tomography at the level of midtongue demonstrates a C- or sausage-shaped, well-defined, low-density lesion in anteromedial portion of left carotid space. The lesion partially encases the left carotid artery *(asterisk)* and displaces it posterolaterally. It extends medially into the left retropharyngeal space *(arrow)*. Parapharyngeal space has been displaced laterally. Pharyngeal mucosal space *(arrowheads)* lies anterior to lesion.

from the brain. Thrombosis, either arterial or venous in nature, appears as a linear or tubular intraluminal filling defect with or without associated mass effect on CECT because the vasa vasorum of the vessel wall enhances in a ring-like fashion.[1] Subacute thrombosis or vessel wall hemorrhage secondary to dissection or trauma will yield a bright signal on T1WI because of the T1 shortening effects of paramagnetic methemoglobin, a blood breakdown product.

Most mass lesions originating in the CS are of neoplastic origin. Most neurogenic tumors are schwannomas (Fig. 3-21). A schwannoma arises from Schwann cells that form the covering of nerves and most commonly originate from the vagus nerve and less commonly from the sympathetic plexus. A neurofibroma contains mixed neural and Schwann cell elements and arises from the peripheral nerves. Neurofibromas are rare and when present usually are multiple and part of neurofibromatosis, type two. Both tumors are well defined with CT with either tumor having a low-density component because of fat infiltration. On CECT neurofibromas demonstrate variable degrees of enhancement; on MRI they have a similar appearance. On both CT and MRI most neural tumors have similar density and intensity characteristics to salivary gland tumors and often may not be differentiated. Neural tumors may have dense enhancement and simulate paragangliomas. On angiography, neuromas characteristically are hypovascular in contrast to paragangliomas, which are hypervascular. Neurogenic lesions arise pos-

terior to the internal carotid artery and thus cause anterior displacement of the latter.

Paragangliomas, lesions developing from neural crest cell derivatives, may arise in the jugular foramen (glomus jugulare), along the course of the vagus nerve (glomus vagale), or at the carotid bifurcation (carotid body tumor) (Figs. 3-22 and 3-23). Paragangliomas are multiple in up to 5% of patients. The lesion is ovoid with smooth margins. Because of its marked hypervascularity, it is densely enhancing on CT; angiography reveals a very vascular tumor with dense capillary staining. At the skull base, it erodes the jugular spine and causes permeative bone erosion of the jugular foramen in contradistinction to a schwannoma, which causes a smooth expansion with intact cortical margins. A jugular foramen paraganglioma may extend into the temporal bone or infiltrate through the skull base, presenting as a posterior fossa mass. In the midneck a paraganglioma causes characteristic displacement of the carotid artery anteriorly and the jugular vein posterolaterally. At the carotid bifurcation a lesion causes splaying of the internal and external carotid arteries. On MRI it is recognized by its hypervascularity characterized by multiple areas of signal void and flow-related enhancement from enlarged feeding and draining vessels.[35]

Lymph node involvement in the CS may be seen most commonly with metastases from SCC or as part of a general involvement by non-Hodgkin's lymphoma. Lymph node involvement may be the initial manifestation of squamous cell carcinoma. Extracapsular spread of disease may occur; complete encasement of the carotid artery (carotid fixation) may indicate inoperability. However, the carotid artery may be sacrificed at operation if the patient successfully tolerates a carotid balloon occlusion test. Metastatic lymph nodes are characteristically inhomogeneous, especially after contrast enhancement.

Masticator space

The MS, the space of the muscles of mastication and the posterior portion of the mandibular ramus, lies anterior to the PS and is separated from the muscles of deglutition in the pharyngeal mucosal space by the PPS.[11] It contains the masseter, temporalis, and medial and lateral pterygoid muscles, motor branch of the third division of cranial nerve V, inferior alveolar nerve (sensory second division of cranial nerve V), internal maxillary artery and its branches, pterygoid venous plexus, and the ramus and posterior body of the mandible. It includes the temporal fossa (suprazygomatic MS) superiorly, encompasses the zygomatic arch, and extends inferiorly to include the infratemporal fossa and structures on both sides of the mandible. A mass in the MS displaces the PPS posteriorly and medially.

Infection (cellulitis, abscess, osteomyelitis) may involve the mandible or the muscles of mastication; extension through the skull base or involvement of the suprazygomatic masticator space may occur and should be ruled out (Fig.

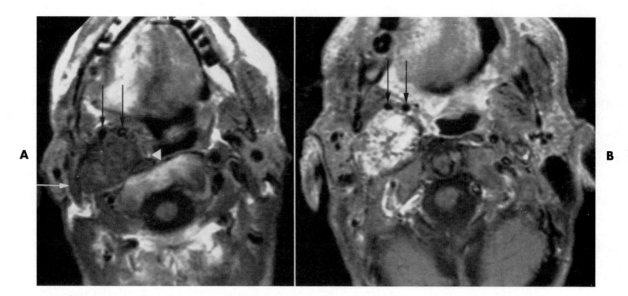

Fig. 3-22. Glomus vagale (paraganglioma) of right carotid space. **A,** Axial T1-weighted image (T1WI) at the level of C2 demonstrates mixed-density, predominantly low-density lesion involving posterior aspect of left carotid space. The lesion displaces the posterior belly of digastric muscle laterally *(white arrow)* and internal and external carotid arteries anteriorly *(black arrows)*. Parapharyngeal fat is displaced medially *(arrowhead)*. The lesion bulges into medial aspect of airway. The small areas of punctate low intensity noted along the margin and in the anterior portion of the lesion represent tumor vessel flow voids. **B,** Axial T1WI at the same level postgadolinium injection demonstrates dense patchy enhancement of lesion. Again noted are multiple punctate vascular flow voids within the lesion and around periphery. Carotid vessels *(arrows)* are noted overlying anterior lesion margin.

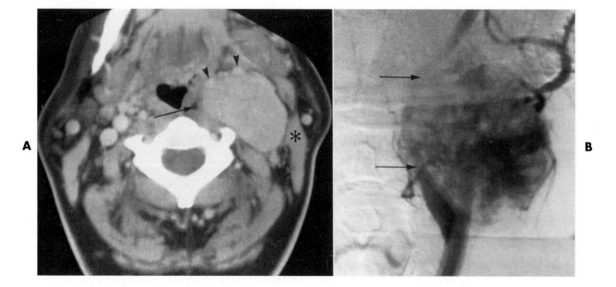

Fig. 3-23. Glomus vagale of left carotid space. **A,** Axial contrast-enhanced computed tomography at the level of midtongue demonstrates relatively homogeneous, well-defined enhancing lesion in the left carotid space. Carotid vessels lie on anteromedial margin of lesion *(arrowhead)*. Parapharyngeal space is displaced medially *(arrow)*. The lesion lies deep to sternocleidomastoid muscle *(asterisk)*. **B,** Anteroposterior digital subtraction angiogram demonstrates densely vascular staining tumor displacing internal carotid artery medially *(arrows)*. Vascularity and dense tumor stain indicate the lesion is paraganglioma.

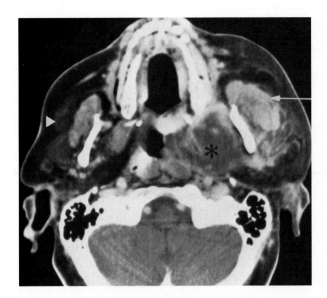

Fig. 3-24. Left masticator space abscess. Axial contrast-enhanced computed tomography at the level of superior alveolar ridge demonstrates low-density lesion *(asterisk)* in medial aspect of left masticator space, involving left lateral pterygoid muscle. The abscess is surrounded by a rim of irregular enhancement. Edema has infiltrated and obscured parapharyngeal space. Left masseter muscle *(arrow)* is thickened and edema is present in soft tissue planes, lateral to masseter muscle and in buccal space anteriorly. Note the accessory parotid gland overlying right masseter muscle *(arrowhead)*.

3-24). Abscesses commonly arise from an odontogenic focus or from poor dentition. The bone changes of osteomyelitis are best demonstrated with CT.

Benign lesions include hemangioma and lymphangioma (Fig. 3-25). Nasopharyngeal angiofibroma, a tumor of young adolescent males, arises in the pterygopalatine fossa and commonly extends into the masticator space (Fig. 3-26). Primary bone neoplasms may arise from the mandible; chondrosarcoma and osteosarcoma present with chondroid calcification and new bone formation, respectively. The bone lesion is characteristically muscle intense on T1WI and hyperintense with T2WI; postgadolinium T1WI demonstrates extensive enhancement. An infiltrating mass with mandibular destruction may be indistinguishable from metastatic disease. Non-Hodgkin's lymphoma may present with bone involvement, with a soft tissue mass, or as a lymph node mass. SCC presents as an infiltrating mass and occurs secondary to extension from a neighboring fascial space (Fig. 3-27). Perineural spread of tumor is common in the MS; the fifth nerve should be assessed for thickening and enhancement along its course as it passes from the brainstem to the cavernous sinus, through the foramen ovale, and eventually below the skull base as it passes inferiorly to innervate the individual muscles of mastication (Fig. 3-28). The foramen ovale may be increased in size and tumor may be found within the cavernous sinus. Tumor involvement of the inferior alveolar nerve may cause erosion, irregular enlargement, or destruction of the inferior alveolar canal of the mandible.[3]

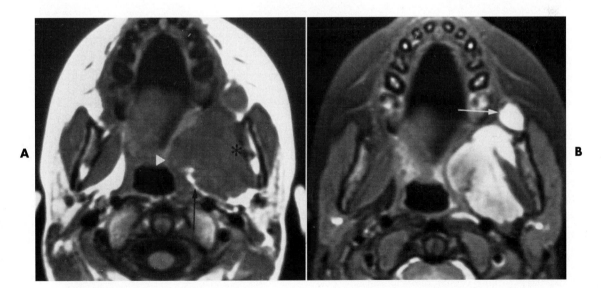

Fig. 3-25. Lymphangioma of left masticator space. **A,** Axial T1-weighted image at the level of the base of the tongue and tonsillar region of oropharynx demonstrates inhomogeneous low-density soft tissue mass involving left lateral pterygoid muscle *(asterisk)*. It displaces parapharyngeal space medially and anteriorly *(arrow)*. The mass extends to the anterior medial wall of the left oropharynx *(arrowhead)*. **B,** Axial spin density image with fat suppression demonstrates a lesion with bright signal intensity. The lesion margins are now better defined; the lesion can now be separated from the lateral pterygoid muscle. The lesion abuts anteromedial wall of oropharynx. Anteriorly, the lesion extends into buccal space *(arrow)*, anterior to cortical margin of mandible.

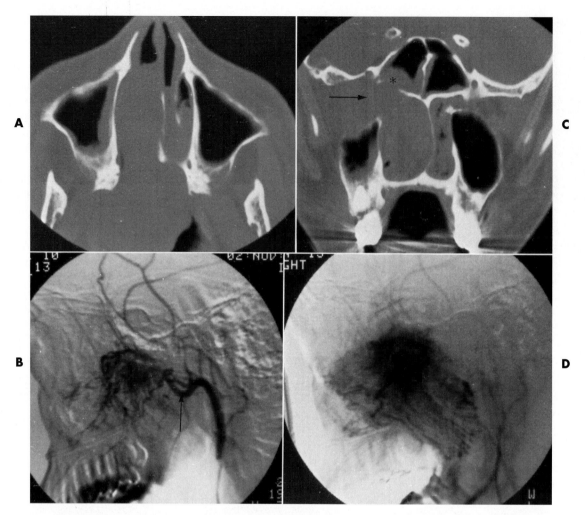

Fig. 3-26. Nasopharyngeal angiofibroma. **A,** Axial noncontrast computed tomography (NCCT) demonstrates homogeneous soft tissue mass enlarging right nasal aperture; a large component of the tumor projects posteriorly into the nasopharynx and oropharynx. **B,** Coronal NCCT also demonstrates complete opacification and expansion of right nasal aperture by soft tissue mass; the tumor extends into and widens right infraorbital fissure *(arrow)*. The tumor *(asterisk)*, having destroyed right floor, is present in sphenoid sinus. **C** and **D,** Lateral subtraction angiograms (early arterial and capillary phase) demonstrate vascular mass in nasopharynx and nasal aperture. Internal maxillary artery *(arrow)* gives rise to leash of tumor vessels; dense tumor stain is noted in capillary phase.

Pseudotumors may mislead the unwary. An accessory parotid gland overlying the anterior border of the masseter muscle or asymmetric enlargement of the parotid gland may simulate tumor. In both situations the parotid gland variant retains MRI signal characteristics identical to the normal parotid gland. Hypertrophy of the masseter muscle may occur secondary to teeth grinding, mimic a mass lesion, or be bilateral. If the fifth cranial nerve is injured or invaded by tumor resulting in denervation of the muscles, ipsilateral atrophy of the muscles of mastication and fat infiltration ensue; the normal contralateral muscle group may be incorrectly considered enlarged and misinterpreted as tumor involvement.

Retropharyngeal space

The RPS, a potential space between the middle and deep layers of the deep cervical fascia, lies posterior to the pharyngeal mucosal space, anterior to the PVS, and medial to the carotid space. It extends from the skull base superiorly to the T3 level of the upper mediastinum inferiorly.[13] Its importance derives from its potential to serve as a passageway for infection to spread among the head, neck, and mediastinum. Its contents are fat and lymph nodes, the principal nodes being the nodes of Rouvier (the classical lateral retropharyngeal nodes) and the medial retropharyngeal nodes. This nodal group is commonly involved in children, and up to 1

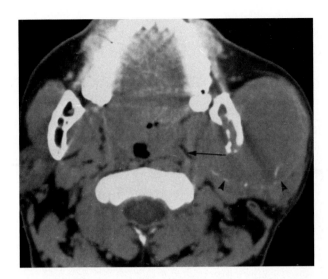

Fig. 3-27. Squamous cell carcinoma (SCC) of mandibular ramus. Axial contrast-enhanced computed tomography at the level of C2 demonstrates large soft tissue tumor destroying the central portion and medial margin of the left mandibular ramus with extension of soft tissue tumor into masseter and lateral pterygoid muscles. Parapharyngeal space has been displaced medially *(arrow)*. Thin rim of circular enhancement is noted posteriorly and laterally *(arrowheads)*.

cm in size is considered normal; but a node over 5 mm is viewed with suspicion in an adult.

A mass lesion in the RPS will displace the PPS anterolaterally. Infection, either pharyngitis or tonsillitis, may give RPS lymph node involvement. Diffuse cellulitis or abscess may occur, the latter usually secondary to infection of the pharyngeal mucosal space or prevertebral space. Infection or mass in the lateral alar portion of the infrahyoid RPS may have a "bow-tie" appearance on axial imaging (Fig. 3-29). SCC may invade the RPS directly or may present solely with lymph node involvement; the pattern is one of inhomogeneous enhancement, commonly with necrotic low-density centers. With non-Hodgkin's lymphoma, lymph nodes are homogeneous and multiple, commonly involving more than one of the fascial spaces.

Prevertebral space

The PVS, also defined by the deep layers of the deep cervical fascia, is divided into anterior and posterior compartments. The former encompasses the anterior cervical vertebral bodies, extending from one transverse process to another; the posterior compartment surrounds the posterior spinal elements. The PVS contains the prevertebral, scalene, and paraspinal muscles, the brachial plexus, the phrenic nerve, the vertebral body, and the vertebral artery and vein. Similar to the anatomy of the RPS, the PVS extends from the skull base superiorly to the mediastinum inferiorly.

The PVS lies directly posterior to the RPS and posteromedial to the carotid space. An anterior compartment PVS mass causes thickening of the prevertebral muscles and displaces the prevertebral muscles and the PPS anteriorly. A mass in the posterior compartment of the PVS displaces the paraspinous musculature and the posterior cervical space fat laterally, away from the posterior elements of the spine. Infection and malignant disease, the common disease processes of the PVS, usually involve the vertebral body.

Infection, including tuberculosis and bacterial pathogens, characteristically involves the vertebral body as well as the adjacent intervertebral disk space. Benign processes, although much less common, include chordoma, osteochondroma, aneurysmal bone cyst, giant cell tumor, and plexiform neurofibroma. Malignant disease processes include metastatic disease, leukemia, lymphoma, and direct invasion by SCC. Vertebral body destruction with associated soft tissue mass may be seen; the spinal canal and dural sac may be compromised.

Oral cavity

The oral cavity, the space of the anterior two thirds of the tongue and the floor of the mouth, lies below the hard palate, medial to the superior and inferior alveolar ridge and teeth, anterior to the oropharynx, and superior to the mylohyoid muscle, the muscle stretching between the inferomedial margins of the mandible. The oral cavity is separated from the oropharynx posteriorly by the circumvallate papillae, tonsillar pillars, and soft palate. The oral cavity includes the oral tongue (the anterior two thirds of the tongue), whereas the oropharynx contains the base of the tongue (the posterior one third of the tongue), the soft palate, the tonsils, and the posterior pharyngeal wall.

The oral cavity can be divided into two major spaces, the sublingual space (SLS) and the submandibular space (SMS). The mylohyoid muscle, which constitutes the floor of the mouth, is the boundary marker between these two spaces. Other areas of the oral cavity include the floor of the mouth, oral tongue, hard palate, buccal mucosa, upper alveolar ridge, lower alveolar ridge, retromolar trigone, and lip; assessment of these regions is also needed.

Most masses in the oral cavity and oropharynx are amenable to direct clinical assessment; mucosal lesions are readily visualized. The purpose of sectional imaging is to evaluate the degree of submucosal involvement. The majority of neoplasms of the oral cavity are readily detected on clinical examination; SCC accounts for approximately 90% of oral cavity and oropharyngeal neoplasms (Figs. 3-30 through 3-32). Cross-sectional imaging has an important role to play in estimation of tumor size, identification of tumor invasion, and assessment of nodal metastasis.

Congenital lesions include lingual thyroid and cystic lesions (epidermoid, dermoid, and teratoid cysts). Most infections of the oral cavity are dental in origin. Dental infections anterior to the second molar tend to involve the sublingual space and lie superior to the mylohyoid muscle; infections of the posterior molars usually involve the SMS and lie inferior to the mylohyoid muscle. Knowledge of which space is involved is crucial to plan adequate surgical drainage.

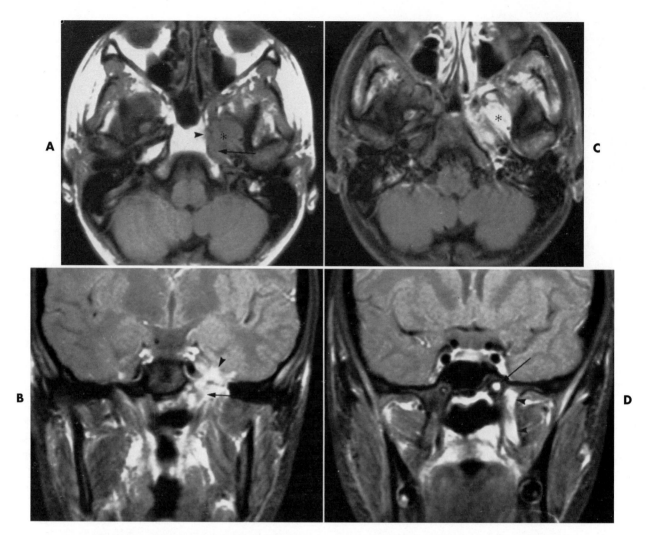

Fig. 3-28. Adenoid cystic carcinoma of masticator space invading left skull base. **A,** T1-weighted image (T1WI) magnetic resonance imaging demonstrates low-density, well-defined lesion *(asterisk)* abutting the lateral border of the clivus and destroying the medial apex of the left petrous temporal bone *(arrow)*. Lateral cortical margin of clivus has been eroded *(arrowhead)*. **B,** Axial postgadolinium fat-suppressed T1WI demonstrates diffuse patchy enhancement of the left middle fossa lesion *(asterisk)*. On this sequence, normal high signal intensity of fat has been suppressed. **C,** Coronal postgadolinium fat-suppressed spin density image demonstrates enhancing tumor *(arrowhead)* below the skull base with extension through the foramen ovale into the left middle fossa *(arrow)*. **D,** Coronal spin density with fat suppression postgadolinium infusion demonstrates enhancing tumor in expanded vidian canal *(arrow)* and pterygoid fossa *(arrowheads)*.

Sublingual space

The SLS is located in the anterior tongue, lateral to the intrinsic muscles of the tongue (genioglossus and geniohyoid) and superior and medial to the mylohyoid muscle. Anteriorly, it extends to the genu of the mandible, and posteriorly, it connects freely with the SMS at the posterior margin of the mylohyoid muscle. It contains the anterior portion of the hyoglossus muscle, the lingual nerve (sensory division of cranial nerve V), the chorda tympani branch of cranial nerve VII, the lingual artery and vein, the deep portion of the submandibular glands and ducts, and the sublingual glands and ducts.

Congenital lesions of the sublingual space include epidermoid, dermoid, lymphangioma, and hemangioma. Lingual thyroid tissue will result if there is failure of normal descent of developing thyroid tissue from the base of the tongue into the lower neck. On CT the lingual thyroid is midline in the posterior portion of the tongue and demonstrates dense contrast enhancement; nuclear medicine thyroid scans demonstrate functioning thyroid tissue.

Cellulitis and abscess may occur secondary to dental or mandibular infections or arise as a consequence of calculus disease of either the submandibular or sublingual glands. Abscess is characterized by central areas of low density with or without boundary enhancement (Fig. 3-33). As with parotid

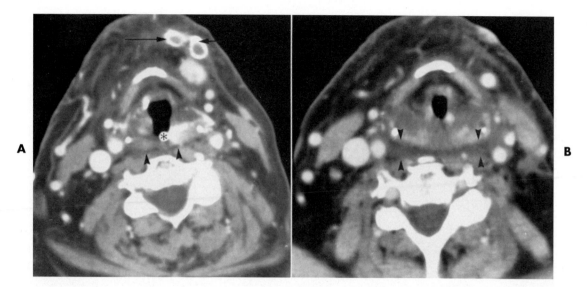

Fig. 3-29. Retropharyngeal space (RPS) edema and abscess. **A,** Axial contrast-enhanced computed tomography (CECT) at the level of the superior margin of hyoid bone demonstrates nasogastric tube *(asterisk)* in the posterior wall of the oropharyngeal airway and mild thickening of the lateral wall of the larynx. RPS is normal *(arrowhead)*. Two lymph nodes *(arrows)* with rim enhancement lie anterior to the left submandibular gland. **B,** Repeat axial CECT at the same level 6 months later demonstrates a well-defined ''bow-tie'' appearance of edema in RPS *(arrowheads)*.

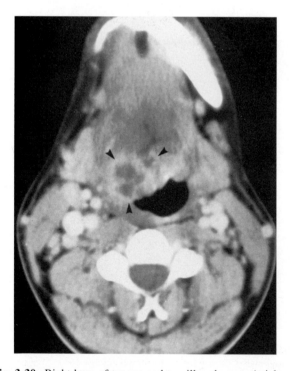

Fig. 3-30. Right base of tongue and tonsillar abscess. Axial contrast-enhanced computed tomography of suprahyoid neck demonstrates inhomogeneous mixed low-density enhancing mass *(arrowheads)* in the base of the tongue and in the right tonsillar region. Low-density area of lesion indicates pus within the abscess.

gland calculi, CT readily identifies calcified stones and demonstrates bone destruction and sequestra of mandibular osteomyelitis. Ranula, a postinflammatory retention cyst of the sublingual gland, presents as a cystic low-density lesion. As it enlarges, it extends posteriorly and inferiorly into the submandibular space, where it is referred to as a ''diving ranula'' (Fig. 3-34).

SCC, the most common malignancy of the SLS, may spread from the oropharynx, oral cavity, alveolar ridge, or anterior portion of the tongue. A mass with irregular areas of enhancement, ulceration, central necrosis, and lymph node involvement is characteristic; normal fat planes may be obscured. Tumor spread across the midline of the tongue, along the lingual or mandibular nerve, or invasion of the cortex or medulla of the mandible is an important finding that alters treatment planning.

Submandibular space

The SMS lies inferior and lateral to the SLS; it is located inferior to the mylohyoid bone and superior to the hyoid bone. It contains the anterior belly of the digastric muscle, fat, submandibular and submental lymph nodes, the superficial portion of the submandibular gland, the inferior portion of the hypoglossal nerve, and the facial artery and vein.

Congenital lesions are not uncommon and include second branchial cleft cyst, thyroglossal duct cyst, and cystic hygroma (lymphangioma). Branchial cleft cyst occurs most commonly at the angle of the mandible, posterior to the submandibular gland, anterior to the sternocleidomastoid muscle, and anterolateral to the carotid space (Fig. 3-35). It

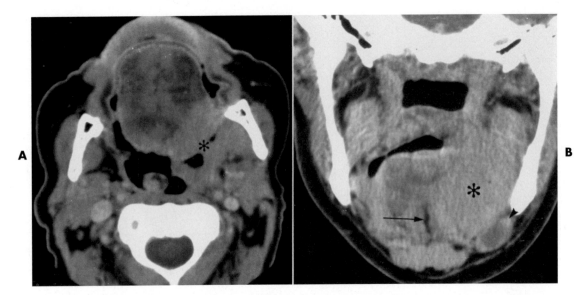

Fig. 3-31. Squamous cell carcinoma of the base of tongue and the floor of the mouth. **A,** Axial contrast-enhanced computed tomography (CECT) at the level of midtongue demonstrates homogeneous lesion *(asterisk),* isodense relative to the muscles of mastication, involving lateral and posterior margins of the left side of tongue, left lateral pterygoid muscle, and tonsillar region of oropharynx. **B,** Coronal CECT demonstrates homogeneous mass involving lateral portion of tongue, extending from the floor of mouth inferiorly to the tonsillar region superiorly *(asterisk).* Midline septum *(arrow)* of tongue is displaced laterally. Necrotic lymph node *(arrowhead)* lies inferior to tongue.

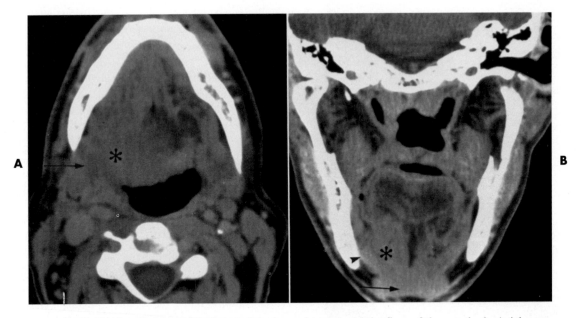

Fig. 3-32. Non-Hodgkin's lymphoma of the base of tongue and the floor of the mouth. **A,** Axial contrast-enhanced computed tomography (CECT) at the midlevel of the tongue demonstrates enlargement of the right side of tongue by homogeneous mass lesion *(asterisk),* isodense to normal tongue musculature; submandibular space *(arrow),* located more laterally, is also involved. **B,** Coronal CECT demonstrates homogeneous involvement of the right inferior lateral base of tongue *(asterisk),* mylohyoid muscle *(arrowhead),* and floor of mouth. Lesion lies above anterior belly of digastric muscle *(arrow).* Homogeneous nature of lesion favors lymphoma.

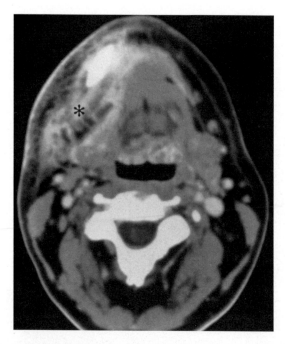

Fig. 3-33. Submandibular abscess and cellulitis. Axial contrast-enhanced computed tomography demonstrates mixed low-density and enhancing lesion *(asterisk)* involving right submandibular space (SMS). Abscess displaces midline structures of tongue to the left. Edema extends laterally from SMS into overlying soft tissues; fat is of increased density because of infiltration by edema.

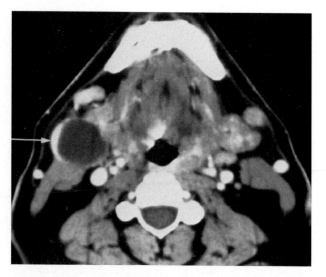

Fig. 3-35. Infected branchial cleft cyst. Axial contrast-enhanced computed tomography at midlevel of tongue and base of the mandible demonstrates well-defined, low-density lesion in lateral portion of submandibular space lying anterior to the right sternocleidomastoid. A thin rim of peripheral enhancement is noted anteriorly and medially; the lateral wall demonstrates thick enhancement *(arrow)*. Location favors the second branchial cleft cyst. Enhancement of the cyst wall indicates that it is infected.

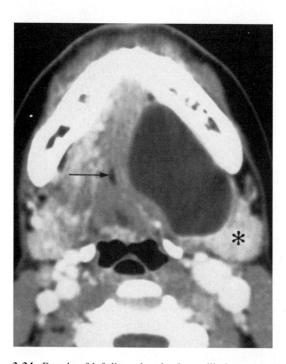

Fig. 3-34. Ranula of left lingual and submandibular space. Axial contrast-enhanced computed tomography at the level of body of mandible demonstrates large, low-density lesion with well-defined margins involving both sublingual and submandibular space. Lesion displaces midline tongue structures *(arrow)* to the right. Submandibular gland is displaced posteriorly and laterally *(asterisk)*.

may have an associated fistula or sinus tract. Thyroglossal duct cysts are midline in location and are found anywhere from the tongue base to the midportion of the thyroid gland. Cystic hygroma, a malformation of lymphatic channels, is a multilocular fluid density lesion that may involve both the SLS and SMS in the adult.

Ranula, a retention cyst of the sublingual gland, commonly extends into and may predominantly involve the SMS; it is unilocular in configuration. Its tail of origin should be carefully searched for in the SLS because this will aid in establishing its origin and diagnosis.

Benign tumors include benign mixed cell tumor, lipoma, dermoid, and epidermoid. Most malignant disease represents secondary submandibular and submental nodal involvement, commonly from SCC of the oral cavity and face. Multiple enlarged lymph node involvement may be seen with non-Hodgkin's lymphoma.

Spaces of infrahyoid neck

The infrahyoid neck extends superiorly to the hyoid bone and inferiorly to the clavicles and contains the following spaces:

1. Infrahyoid RPS
2. Infrahyoid PVS
3. Anterior and posterior (lateral) cervical spaces
4. Hypopharyngeal mucosal space (PMS)
5. Visceral space and larynx
6. CS

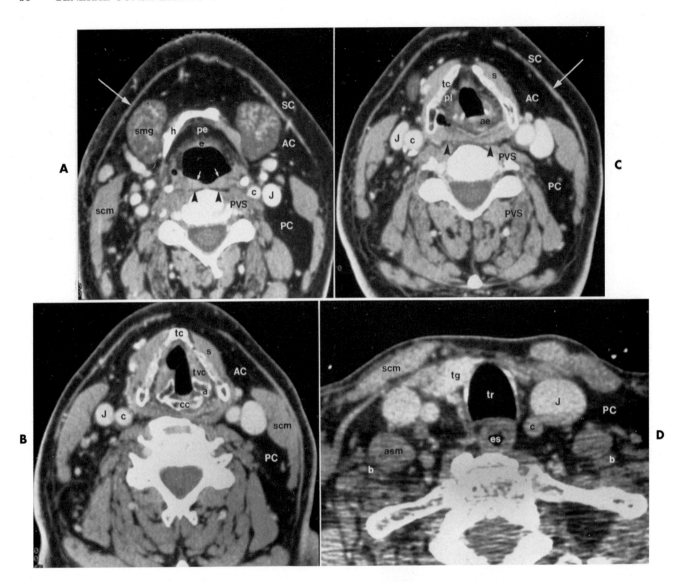

Fig. 3-36. Normal axial contrast-enhanced computed tomography (CECT) anatomy of infrahyoid neck. CECT obtained at, **A,** hyoid bone; **B,** false vocal cord; **C,** true vocal cord; and **D,** thyroid gland levels. (Streaky densities in superficial fat of right neck area in **A** and **B** from prior radiation of right parotid mass.) Note the following structures: arytenoid cartilage *(a)*, anterior cervical space *(AC)*, aryepiglottic fold *(ae)*, anterior scalene muscle *(asm)*, brachial plexus *(b)*, carotid artery *(c)*, cricoid cartilage *(cc)*, epiglottis *(e)*, esophagus *(es)*, hyoid bone *(h)*, jugular vein *(J)*, posterior cervical space *(PC)*, preepiglottic fat *(pe)*, paralaryngeal fat *(pl)*, prevertebral space *(PVS)*, pharyngeal mucosal space *(small arrows)*, platysma muscle *(large arrow)*, retropharyngeal space *(arrowheads)*, strap muscle *(s)*, superficial cervical space *(SC)*, sternocleidomastoid muscle *(scm)*, submandibular gland *(smg)*, thyroid cartilage *(tc)*, thyroid gland *(tg)*, trachea *(tr)*, and true vocal cord *(tvc)*.

Normal cross-sectional anatomy of the infrahyoid neck is presented in Figs. 3-36 through 3-38. The PPS ends at the hyoid bone and does not continue into the infrahyoid neck. The mucosal, carotid, retropharyngeal, prevertebral, and posterior cervical spaces are all continuous superiorly with the suprahyoid neck and extend inferiorly to the thoracic inlet.[45] These spaces are discussed in more detail under the suprahyoid neck section, except for the posterior cervical space, which is described below. Lesions may secondarily invade the structures of the infrahyoid neck from the cranial margin (submandibular, parapharyngeal, carotid, retropharyngeal, and oropharyngeal mucosal spaces), posterior margin (prevertebral space and vertebrae), and inferior margin (mediastinum and chest wall).

Infrahyoid retropharyngeal space

The infrahyoid RPS, a potential space containing a thin layer of fat and no lymph nodes, is bounded by the middle layer of deep cervical fascia anteriorly, the alar fascia of the carotid sheath laterally, and the deep layer of deep cervical

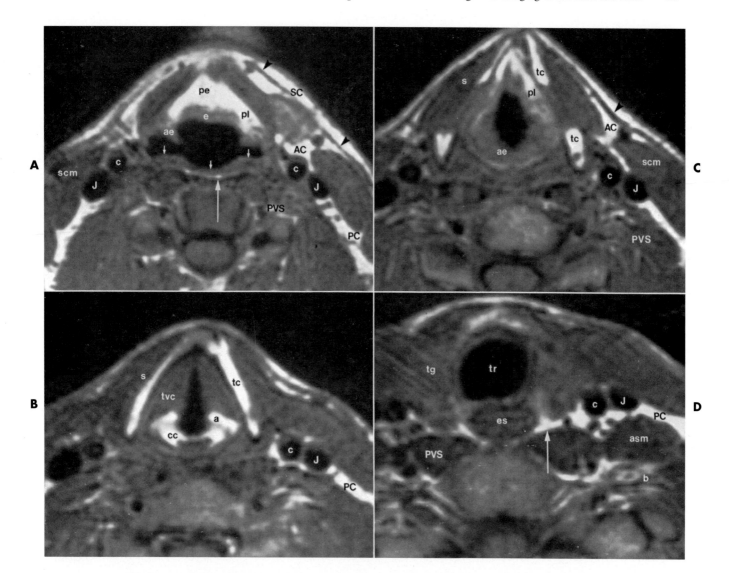

Fig. 3-37. Normal axial magnetic resonance anatomy of infrahyoid neck. Noncontrast T1-weighted images obtained at, **A,** hyoid bone; **B,** false vocal cord; **C,** true vocal cord; and **D,** thyroid gland levels. The following structures are labelled: arytenoid cartilage *(a)*, anterior cervical space *(AC)*, aryepiglottic fold *(ae)*, anterior scalene muscle *(asm)*, branchial plexus *(b)*, carotid artery *(c)*, cricoid cartilage *(cc)*, epiglottis *(e)*, esophagus *(es)*, jugular vein *(J)*, posterior cervical space *(PC)*, preepiglottic fat *(pe)*, paralaryngeal fat *(pl)*, prevertebral space *(PVS)*, pharyngeal mucosal space *(small arrows)*, platysma muscle *(arrowheads)*, retropharyngeal space *(large arrow)*, strap muscle *(s)*, superficial cervical space *(SC)*, sternocleidomastoid muscle *(scm)*, thyroid cartilage *(tc)*, thyroid gland *(tg)*, trachea *(tr)*, and true vocal cord *(tvc)*.

fascia posteriorly.[12] Unlike the suprahyoid RPS, which contains both fat and lymph nodes, the infrahyoid RPS only contains fat. On CT and MRI the normal infrahyoid RPS is an inconsistently demonstrated fat stripe overlying the anterior margin of the longus colli muscles, nestled between the two carotid sheaths.

The infrahyoid RPS may be involved by processes arising from tissues within this space, but more commonly it is affected by external invasion from the adjacent spaces. Lesions within this space have a characteristic "bow-tie" configuration and lie anterior to the longus colli muscles (Fig. 3-39).

Lipomas and lymphangiomas are two low-density congenital lesions arising primarily in or secondarily extending into the infrahyoid RPS. Inflammation of this space may arise from pharyngeal mucosal laceration, discitis, or osteomyelitis from the PVS or from infections tracking in through the posterior cervical space. Gas in this space suggests laceration of the pharynx, larynx, or trachea, pneumomediastinum, or the presence of gas-forming organisms (Fig. 3-40). Edema from inflammation in an adjacent space may track into the RPS and occasionally mimic a true fluid collection or abscess. Neoplasms arising in the hypopharyngeal MS, CS,

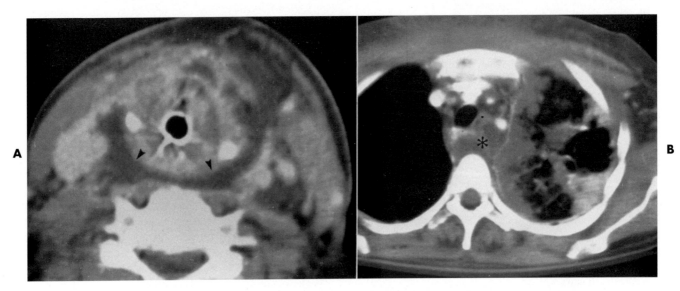

Fig. 3-38. Normal sagittal and coronal magnetic resonance of infrahyoid neck. **A,** Sagittal T1-weighted image (T1WI) and, **B,** coronal T1WI obtained through the larynx. Note the following structures: cricoid cartilage *(cc)*, epiglottis *(e)*, false vocal cord *(asterisk)*, pharyngeal mucosal space *(small arrows)*, preepiglottic fat *(pe)*, paralaryngeal fat *(pl)*, retropharyngeal space *(arrowheads)*, strap muscle *(s)*, superficial cervical space *(SC)*, submandibular gland *(smg)*, trachea *(tr)*, and true vocal cord *(tvc)*.

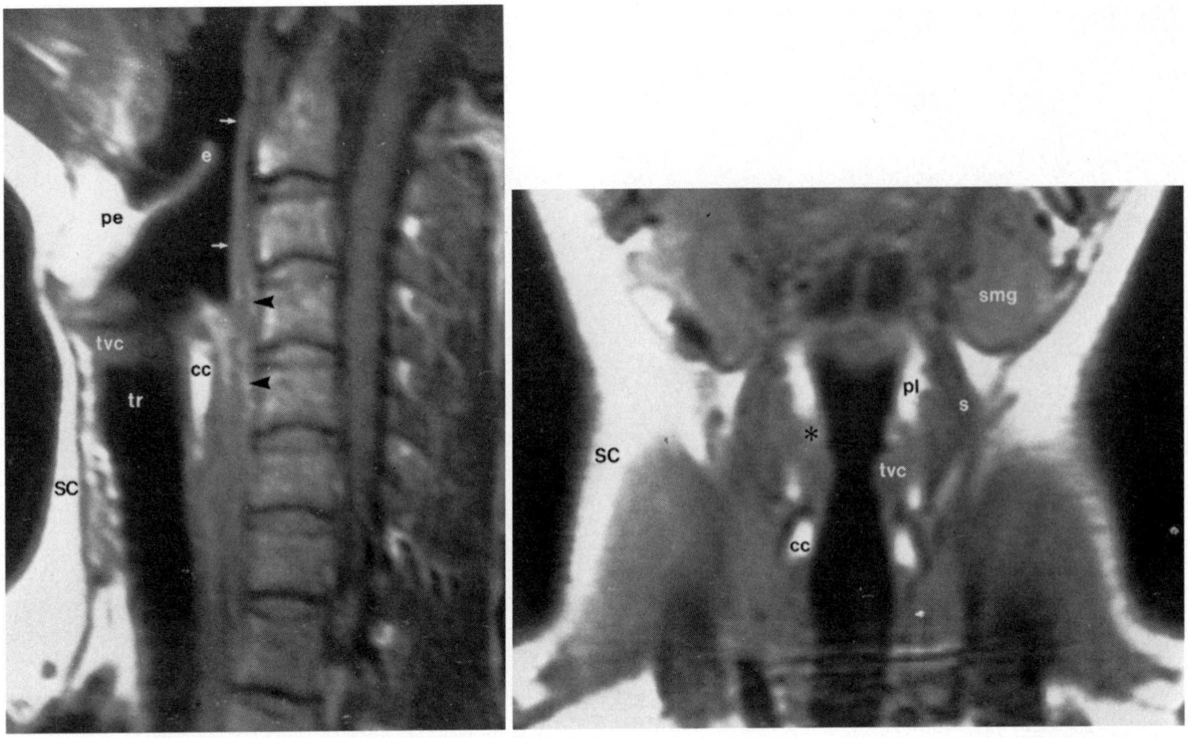

Fig. 3-39. Infrahyoid retropharyngeal space and visceral space abscess. **A,** An axial contrast-enhanced computed tomography at level of false vocal cords demonstrates low-density abscess in retropharyngeal space *(arrowheads)* creating a "bow-tie" configuration. The abscess extends laterally to the left posterior cervical space and anteriorly into the visceral and anterior cervical spaces. **B,** Communication between retropharyngeal space and mediastinum is well demonstrated by cephalad extension of this mediastinal abscess *(asterisk)* posterior to the trachea.

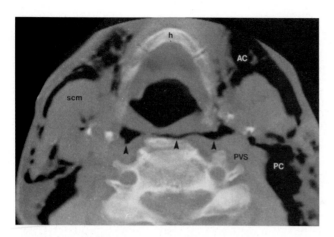

Fig. 3-40. Axial non-contrast computed tomography of subcutaneous emphysema highlighting cervical spaces. Gas from a pneumonomediastinum has dissected into anterior cervical space *(AC)*, posterior cervical space *(PC)*, and retropharyngeal space *(arrowheads)*. Note the ''bow-tie'' pattern of retropharyngeal space. Other labelled structures include hyoid bone *(h)*, sternocleidomastoid muscle *(scm)*, and prevertebral space *(PVS)*.

posterior thyroid gland, and larynx may involve the RPS. Extracapsular spread of internal jugular and spinal accessory metastatic nodes, as well as recurrent visceral space neoplasms, occasionally may invade the RPS. One common pseudomass that indents into this space is a tortuous common or internal carotid artery, usually seen in the middle-aged and elderly populations.

Infrahyoid prevertebral space

The infrahyoid PVS continues superiorly into the suprahyoid PVS and inferiorly to the mediastinum. This space is susceptible to the same pathologic processes as the suprahyoid component, which include inflammatory and infectious processes (arthritis, discitis, osteomyelitis), as well as neoplasms arising in the spinal canal, brachial plexus, paraspinous musculature, or vertebral bodies (Fig. 3-41).

Anterior and posterior cervical (lateral cervical) spaces

The posterior cervical (lateral cervical) space corresponds to the posterior triangle and is a fibrofatty layer containing the internal jugular, spinal accessory, and transverse cervical lymph node chains, as well as the spinal accessory and phrenic nerves. The posterior cervical space is limited by the sternocleidomastoid muscle and investing layer of deep cervical fascia anterolaterally, the carotid sheath anteriorly, and the prevertebral fascia posteromedially. It extends superiorly from the mastoid process and skull base down to the first rib and clavicles inferiorly.[36] Thus a small portion of the posterior cervical space extends into the suprahyoid neck, with the majority occupying the infrahyoid neck.

A transspatial lesion (lymphangioma, plexiform neurofibroma, lipoma, hemangioma) may invade two or more anatomic compartments, without respect for fascial boundaries.[56] Congenital lesions of the posterior cervical space include a second branchial cleft cyst, which tends to lie along the anterior margin of the sternocleidomastoid muscle, and a lymphangioma or cystic hygroma (Fig. 3-42). Both lesions are CSF density on CT, low intensity on T1WI, high intensity on T2WI, and may ring-enhance if secondarily infected. Inflammation may enter this space from cutaneous lesions or from abscessed lymph nodes. Benign neoplasms include neurogenic tumors (plexiform neurofibroma, schwannoma), a lipoma, or a hemangioma. Malignant neoplasms in the posterior cervical space are most commonly metastatic to the spinal accessory or internal jugular lymph nodes, with SCC representing the largest group of both primary and secondary tumors involving this space. Less commonly, sarcomas such as liposarcoma, leiomyosarcoma, or malignant fibrous histiocytoma arise here. Normal structures such as the scalene muscles, poorly opacified vessels on CT, and high-signal, flow-related enhancement in vessels on MRI may be misinterpreted as a pseudomass. Denervation atrophy of the sternocleidomastoid muscle or other neck muscles may occasionally cause an incorrect interpretation of the contralateral (normal-sized) muscles as representing masses.

Hypopharyngeal mucosal space

The hypopharyngeal mucosal space forms the walls of the hypopharynx and includes the continuation of the pharyngeal mucosal space below the hyoid bone posteriorly, the piriform sinuses laterally, the aryepiglottic folds and epiglottis anteriorly, and the cricopharyngeus muscle inferiorly. The hypopharyngeal mucosal space, piriform sinuses, and aryepiglottic folds are frequently challenging to evaluate on CECT and MRI because they are relatively thin membranous spaces that are normally collapsed together when the pharynx is relaxed. A modified Valsalva maneuver is usually required to distend the hypopharynx enough to obtain adequate imaging (see Fig. 3-2).

As with the suprahyoid pharyngeal mucosal space, caution must be exercised in assigning abnormality to this space since redundancy of the mucosa and incomplete distension may mimic tumor. Foreign bodies, inflammation, and SCC are the most common lesions in this space. Inflammation may cause ulceration or swelling of the mucosa, with gas or a ring-enhancing fluid collection suggesting the diagnosis; reactive lymph nodes are common. The best indicator of hypopharyngeal malignancy is a bulky mass with invasion and destruction of submucosal and deep structures including the retropharyngeal space, aryepiglottic folds, cricoid cartilage and larynx, as well as associated necrotic lymph nodes (Fig. 3-43).

Visceral space and larynx

The visceral space, corresponding to the muscular triangle, is confined by the middle layer of deep cervical fascia with the anterior fascial layer splitting around the thyroid

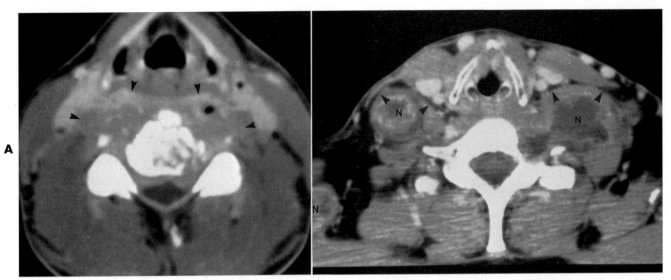

Fig. 3-41. Prevertebral space (PVS) lesions. **A,** Axial contrast-enhanced computed tomography (CECT) of prevertebral abscess extending anteriorly from C5-6 discitis. Anterolateral margins of abscess *(arrowheads)* displace pharyngeal mucosa and posterior cervical spaces anteriorly. A small amount of gas is present in the abscess on the left. **B,** Axial CECT of bilateral plexiform neurofibromas *(N)* arising from brachial plexus in PVS shows anterior displacement of fat in the posterior cervical spaces *(arrowheads)*.

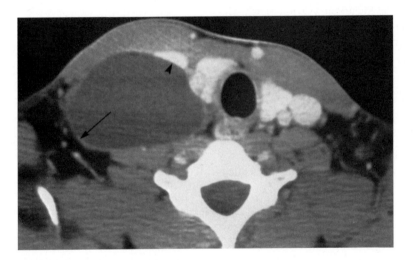

Fig. 3-42. Posterior cervical space lymphangioma. Contrast-enhanced computed tomography reveals homogeneous, bright, low-density mass with sharp margins displacing posterior cervical space fat *(arrow)* posterolaterally and internal jugular vein *(arrowhead)* anteriorly.

gland. The visceral space contains the larynx, trachea, hypopharynx, esophagus, parathyroid glands, thyroid gland, recurrent laryngeal nerve, and tracheoesophageal lymph nodes.[4] The superior margin is the hyoid bone, and the inferior border is the mediastinum. The skeleton of the larynx includes the thyroid, cricoid, arytenoid, cuneiform, and corniculate cartilages. These cartilages may reveal a variable degree of calcification or ossification; these findings progress with age. Ligaments from the stylohyoid and stylothyroid muscles frequently calcify. Knowledge of the normal

patterns of calcification is helpful for distinguishing opaque foreign bodies, such as chicken bones, from normal structures on plain films or CT.

Larynx. The hyoid bone supports the laryngeal skeleton and is occasionally fractured in blunt trauma or destroyed by neoplasms. Fractures of the laryngeal skeleton appear on CT as linear lucencies, often with displacement or distortion of the cartilage. A fracture is best appreciated (on bone windows) in well-ossified cartilage, but its identification is more challenging in noncalcified cartilage requiring the use of

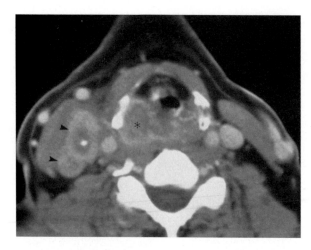

Fig. 3-43. Piriform sinus squamous cell carcinomas. Axial contrast-enhanced computed tomography shows mildly enhancing mass in the right piriform sinus *(asterisk)* displacing aryepiglottic fold anteromedially. Focal defects in the internal jugular and spinal accessory nodes *(arrowheads)* indicate metastatic tumor spread; calcification is noted in the internal jugular node.

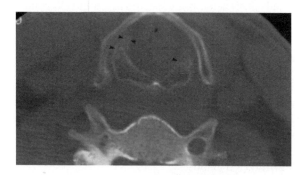

Fig. 3-44. Laryngeal trauma. Axial non-contrast computed tomography at the level of cricothyroid articulation shows laterally displaced cricoid ring *(arrowheads)* fracture and subglottic hematoma obstructing the airway.

a narrower window width and careful scrutiny of cartilage configuration. Laryngeal trauma may result in hematomas of the aryepiglottic folds, false cords, true cords, or subglottis and may potentially compromise the airway (Fig. 3-44). Adjacent subcutaneous emphysema may result from trauma to the laryngopharyngeal mucosa, from a penetrating injury to the neck, or from upward dissection from the chest wall or mediastinum.

Laryngoceles are formed by increased intraglottic pressure (e.g., horn players, glass blowers) or from obstruction of the laryngeal ventricle and its distal appendix by inflammatory or neoplastic lesions (Fig. 3-45). An internal laryngocele tracks superiorly within the paralaryngeal (paraglottic) fat, is air- or fluid-filled (obstructed laryngocele), and causes variable compromise of the supraglottic larynx. A mixed (external) laryngocele extends further superolaterally, piercing the thyrohyoid membrane, and may present as a neck

mass. A mucocele (mucous retention cyst) of the supraglottic laryngeal mucosa may be indistinguishable from an obstructed internal laryngocele. Inflammation of the supraglottic larynx may lead to epiglottitis, thickening the epiglottis and aryepiglottic folds, and compromising the airway (Fig. 3-46).

Apart from routine evaluation of adenopathy from suprahyoid neck and sinus tumors, laryngeal and hypopharyngeal SCC is the most common indication for imaging the infrahyoid neck. Because both CECT and MRI are relatively insensitive to superficial mucosal-based lesions, knowledge of the physical examination findings and specific locations of concern is mandatory to facilitate lesion localization and characterization. Findings that help identify SCC of the superficial mucosa of the larynx or pharynx are a mass, mucosal irregularity or asymmetry, and ulceration. Fat planes in the laryngopharynx are critical for determining the extent of deep invasion or inflammation. The fat in the preepiglottic space, epiglottis, and aryepiglottic folds and paralaryngeal fat of the supraglottic larynx are major landmarks that are easily identified on axial CT and MRI. Coronal T1WIs are particularly useful for evaluating the configuration of the airway and for determining the craniocaudal margins of a supraglottic, glottic, infraglottic, or transglottic lesion because the vertically oriented paralaryngeal fat plane terminates inferiorly at the true vocal cords (thyroarytenoid muscle). A lesion becomes transglottic when the fat interface between the thyroarytenoid muscle (true vocal cord) and the paralaryngeal fat (false vocal cord) is eliminated, indicating the tumor has crossed the laryngeal ventricle (Fig. 3-47, *A*). The anterior commissure should be less than 1-mm thick; greater thickness in this area represents tumor spread from the anterior margin of one cord to another. A diagnosis of vocal cord fixation may be made when the involved cord remains paramedian during quiet breathing or with a modified Valsalva maneuver (Fig. 3-47, *B*).

Cartilage invasion or destruction by aggressive infections or tumors is an important part of staging and is often difficult to predict on CECT or MRI when the cartilage is incompletely calcified. If the cartilage has ossified, CECT and MRI are relatively sensitive for detecting cartilage erosion. MRI using a combination of T1WI, T2WI, and postgadolinium fat saturation T1WI may be more sensitive than CECT to invasion of the central layer of the thyroid cartilage, especially if the cartilage has ossified and the central fatty marrow has been locally replaced by invading tumor. The best indicator of cartilage invasion is the presence of tumor on the external margin of the cartilage in the strap muscles (Fig. 3-48).

Thyroid gland. The thyroid gland lies within the anterior leaves of the middle layer of deep cervical fascia (within the visceral space) anterior and lateral to the thyroid, cricoid, and upper tracheal cartilages. It consists of the lateral thyroid lobes, isthmus, and pyramidal lobe. Normal iodine content of the thyroid gland makes it higher density than

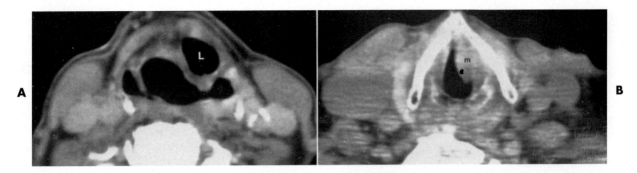

Fig. 3-45. Laryngocele. **A,** Axial contrast-enhanced computed tomography (CECT) at the level of thyrohyoid membrane demonstrates air-filled internal laryngocele *(L)* displacing preepiglottic fat and aryepiglottic fold. Note that it is separated from piriform sinus by aryepiglottic fold. **B,** Axial CECT at the true cord level reveals the cause of laryngocele—an obstructing transglottic carcinoma *(m).*

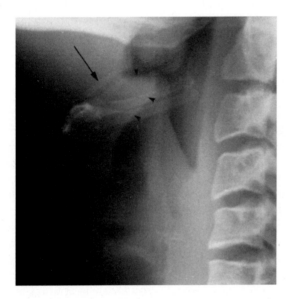

Fig. 3-46. Epiglottitis. Lateral plain film of the neck demonstrates swollen epiglottis *(arrowheads)* and aryepiglottic folds. The lower portion of stylohyoid ligament *(arrow)* has ossified bilaterally.

muscle on NCCT. The gland is normally homogeneous with enhancement on both CECT and MRI, but internal inhomogeneity from calcification, goiter, colloid cyst, or a solid mass is occasionally encountered on routine neck imaging. When physical examination, ultrasound, or thyroid scintigraphy raises the suspicion of a thyroid carcinoma or thyroid lymphoma, CECT or MRI may be used for further characterization, especially if it is a low thoracic inlet thyroid or parathyroid mass.

Absence of the thyroid gland at the level of the thyroid cartilage should redirect attention to the tongue for an ectopic lingual thyroid gland (Fig. 3-49). A thyroglossal duct cyst is a remnant of the embryonic thyroglossal duct and may occur anywhere along its migratory path from the foramen cecum in the tongue to the pyramidal lobe, although most occur just inferior to the hyoid bone (Fig. 3-50). Inflammatory thyroiditis may enlarge the thyroid gland. Benign enlargement may also result from colloid cysts and goiters. Thyroid calcification is nonspecific and occurs in goiters as well as in benign thyroid adenomas. Primary malignancies of the thyroid include papillary, follicular, mixed, and anaplastic carcinomas, as well as non-Hodgkin's lymphoma, all of which may have a similar imaging appearance (Fig. 3-51). Indistinct margins of a thyroid mass, infiltration of adjacent tissues, and necrotic lymph nodes are all indications of thyroid malignancy. Metastasis to the thyroid gland more commonly arises from extracapsular spread of SCC in adjacent nodes than from hematogenous deposits.

Parathyroid glands. The parathyroid glands are usually four to six in number and underlie the posterior surface of the thyroid gland. Because they are quite small, normal parathyroid glands are frequently not visualized on routine neck imaging. An ectopic parathyroid gland may occur in the mediastinum (Fig. 3-52). A parathyroid adenoma is usually a discrete mass lying deep to the thyroid lobes. Occasionally, an adenoma may be detected on routine CT or MRI as a nodular, enhancing mass that may be differentiated from lymph nodes by its location posterior to the thyroid gland.

Lymphadenopathy

Lymph node anatomy and classification

The nodes of the superficial triangles of the neck are organized by major lymphatic chains. The traditional classification of lymph nodes of the head and neck includes 10 groups: lateral cervical, anterior cervical, submandibular, submental, sublingual, parotid, facial, mastoid, and occipital. The lateral cervical chains are further subdivided into the deep and superficial chains. The deep lateral cervical chain includes the internal jugular, spinal accessory, and transverse cervical (supraclavicular) nodes; the superficial lateral cervical chain consists of the external jugular nodes. The anterior

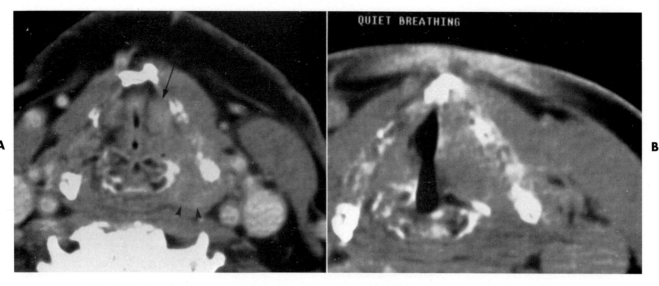

Fig. 3-47. Transglottic laryngeal squamous cell carcinoma with vocal cord fixation. **A,** True vocal cords are adducted on axial contrast-enhanced computed tomography (CECT) obtained during breath holding, with tumor extending anteriorly and superiorly from the left true cord into adjacent paralaryngeal fat *(arrow)* and posteriorly into cricoarytenoid joint *(arrowheads)*. Anterior corner of calcified left arytenoid cartilage *(asterisk)* has been eroded by the tumor. **B,** Repeat axial CECT, performed during quiet breathing, reveals fixation of the left true cord in midline; right cord is partially abducted.

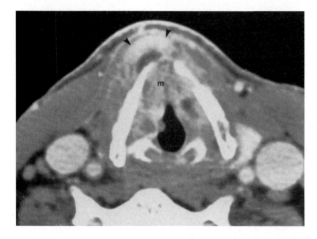

Fig. 3-48. Transglottic squamous cell carcinoma with cartilage invasion. Axial CECT at the true vocal cord level shows enhancing mass *(m)* originating in the left vocal cord, crossing anterior commissure, and invading anterior third of the right cord. The tumor has invaded through anterior thyroid cartilage and displaces thyroid strap muscles anteriorly *(arrowheads)*.

cervical (juxtavisceral) group contains the prelaryngeal (Delphian), pretracheal, prethyroid, and lateral tracheal (tracheoesophageal or paratracheal) nodes.[46] The cervical lymph node chains are found throughout several of the spaces of the neck:

1. Posterior cervical space: spinal accessory, transverse cervical, and internal jugular (posterior to the internal jugular vein) nodes

2. Carotid space: internal jugular nodes (anterior to the internal jugular vein posterior margin)
3. Submandibular space: submandibular and submental nodes
4. Parotid space: parotid nodes
5. Suprahyoid retropharyngeal space: medial and lateral retropharyngeal nodes
6. Visceral space: prelaryngeal, prethyroid, pretracheal, and tracheoesophageal nodes
7. Subcutaneous tissues of the scalp and face: occipital, mastoid, and facial nodes

A condensation of this nomenclature into seven groups with Roman numerals (levels I to VII) has been proposed and is a useful shorthand for node documentation and statistical analysis. Because this latter classification is not standard at all institutions, to prevent confusion its use should be agreed to by the head and neck surgeons, radiation therapists, oncologists, and radiologists. Level I combines the submandibular and submental lymph nodes. Levels II to IV divide the internal jugular chain roughly into thirds, using landmarks that are easily recognizable on cross-sectional imaging. Level II is the jugular-digastric group of internal jugular nodes from the skull base down to the hyoid bone (approximately the level of the common carotid bifurcation). Level III is the supraomohyoid internal jugular chain from the hyoid bone to the cricoid cartilage (approximately the level of the omohyoid muscle). Level IV includes the infraomohyoid internal jugular nodes from the cricoid to the clavicles. Level V combines the spinal accessory and transverse cervical (supracla-

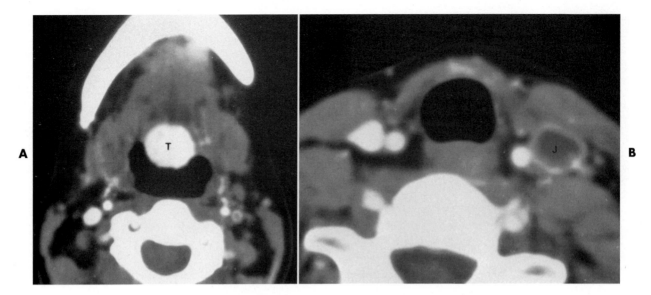

Fig. 3-49. Lingual thyroid gland. **A,** Densely enhancing mass of ectopic thyroid tissue *(T)* bulges posteriorly from tongue at level of the foramen cecum on axial contrast-enhanced computed tomography. **B,** CECT at upper tracheal level reveals thyroid gland is absent from its normal location. Note pseudotumor of thrombosed internal jugular vein *(J)* mimicking ring-enhancing node metastasis.

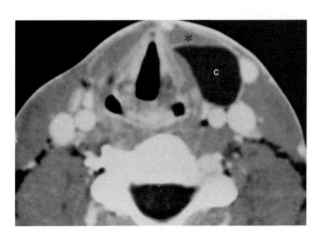

Fig. 3-50. Thyroglossal duct cyst. Low-density thyroglossal duct cyst *(c)* elevates thyroid strap muscles *(asterisk)* and laterally displaces sternocleidomastoid muscle in this axial contrast-enhanced computed tomography.

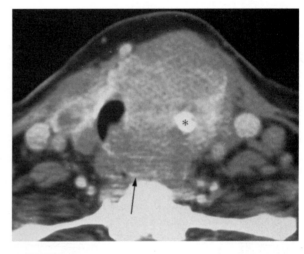

Fig. 3-51. Thyroid follicular carcinoma. Axial contrast-enhanced computed tomography just below cricoid shows large mass with nodular calcification *(asterisk)* displacing trachea to the right and distorting the airway; posteriorly it has invaded retropharyngeal space *(arrow)*.

vicular) nodes from the skull base to the clavicles. Separation of internal jugular nodes from the spinal accessory nodes on cross-sectional imaging may be difficult, especially in the suprahyoid neck, because these two chains converge at the skull base. A somewhat arbitrary distinction between these chains is made using the posterior margin of the internal jugular vein as the dividing line on axial imaging; any nodes anterior to this line are defined as internal jugular nodes, and those posterior to this margin are called spinal accessory nodes. Level VI contains the prethyroid nodes. Level VII

consists of the tracheoesophageal nodes. The retropharyngeal nodes are not included in this classification and are mentioned separately.

Lymph nodes: normal and pathologic

CECT remains the gold standard for detecting and classifying cervical lymphadenopathy as benign or malignant. The important considerations in radiographic lymph node detection and characterization are location, size, number, cluster-

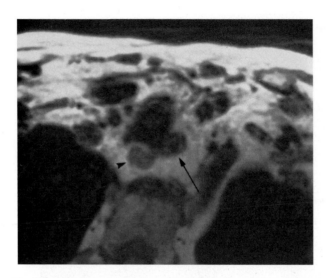

Fig. 3-52. Parathyroid adenoma. Retrotracheal ectopic parathyroid adenoma *(arrowhead)* looks similar to adjacent normal esophagus *(arrow)* on axial T1-weighted image.

ing, enhancement pattern, calcification, sharpness of margins, and invasion or displacement of adjacent structures. First the nodes must be detected and localized to a specific nodal chain or level using one of the conventions for labeling node regions discussed previously. Node involvement is described as unilateral or bilateral and in terms of the specific level(s) or chain(s) affected.

Inflammatory (reactive) lymph nodes on CECT tend to be less than 10 mm (rarely larger than 20 mm), have central hilar or mild homogeneous enhancement, and have well-defined margins (Fig. 3-53). Node margins should remain sharp in reactive adenopathy, except in cases with large abscessed nodes that elicit an inflammatory reaction in the adjacent fat, obscuring the node margins (Fig. 3-54). Calcification is a common finding in previously infected or healed nodes and frequently occurs in tuberculosis or bacterial infections. Multiple nodes may be present, but they tend not to cluster. On MRI these reactive nodes are enlarged and have well-defined margins on all sequences. They are muscle intensity on T1WI, enhance moderately and homogeneously on postgadolinium fat-suppressed T1WI, and are bright on T2WI and STIR.

The correlation of lymph node size with sensitivity and specificity in predicting malignant metastasis has been performed for different neck regions in patients with head and neck carcinoma, allowing more appropriate size criteria for distinguishing normal from abnormal lymph nodes.[46] Although CT can readily detect lymph node enlargement, it has also proven capable of accurately diagnosing metastases in "normal size" nodes from head and neck primary SCC. The upper range of normal for cervical lymph node size is between 5 and 10 mm, with the jugular digastric node ranging up to 15 mm. The exceptions are the submandibular and submental nodes, which are usually abnormal if larger than

5 mm, and the retropharyngeal nodes when greater than 10 mm in children or greater than 5 mm in adults. Generally, cervical nodes larger than 10 to 15 mm are potentially malignant and nodes smaller than this are considered reactive or inflammatory. Nodes larger than 20 mm are frequently malignant because the average size of a clinically positive metastatic node is 21 mm by physical examination and 20 mm by CT. Clinically occult neck disease occurs in 15% to 40% of patients with head and neck SCC; clinically occult nodes average 12 mm (Fig. 3-55). Studies comparing clinical and CT staging of nodal metastases have shown that physical examination of the neck has an accuracy of 70% to 82% compared with 87% to 93% for CT. In patients with no nodal disease on examination, CT is likely to upstage an N0 neck to N1 in 20% to 46% and upstage clinical staging of the neck between 5% and 67% overall. CT may downstage the clinical neck examination in 3% to 36% of cases.[8,31]

The enhancement pattern on CT is very helpful, but not infallible, in distinguishing inflammatory nodes from metastatic nodes. Node detection is improved by performing CECT with a constant infusion technique. The presence of a focal defect (central low density) or peripheral enhancement is characteristic of malignancy even in normal-sized nodes less than 15 mm. A focal defect in an enlarged node is a strong indication of a necrotic node metastasis, although tuberculosis or an abscessed node may mimic this appearance. Central dense or linear enhancement of the hilum of an enlarged node without ring enhancement is usually a distinguishing sign of a reactive node. Nodes larger than 20 to 40 mm without central necrosis often indicate lymphoma or sarcoidosis (Fig. 3-56). Treated lymphomatous nodes may have dystrophic calcification, and rarely, calcium matrix-forming tumors (osteosarcoma, chondrosarcoma) may have radiodense metastases. When margins of an enlarged node with central necrosis are indistinct, extracapsular penetration of the tumor through the node capsule has likely occurred (Fig. 3-57). This sign may decrease the 5-year survival by 50%. The number of nodes involved is important; multiple nodes suggest a more widespread inflammatory or neoplastic process. Clustering of multiple nodes, sometimes into a seemingly single, complex mass, suggests malignancy and may be palpable as a single large mass. Round rather than bean-shaped nodes, clusters of nodes, and indistinct margins suggest malignancy but are less specific than size greater than 15 mm, ring enhancement, or focal defect.

MRI of malignant adenopathy has both advantages and limitations compared with CECT. Malignant nodes appear as muscle intensity on T1WI, may show ring enhancement on postgadolinium fat-suppressed T1WI, are very bright on STIR, and are usually bright on T2WI (although necrosis may give both high and low signal on long TR sequences) (Fig. 3-58). Fat-suppressed long TR sequences will diminish background fat signal, further improving detection. The STIR image is superior to CECT in sensitivity for any enlarged lymph node but is nonspecific for metastases. MRI

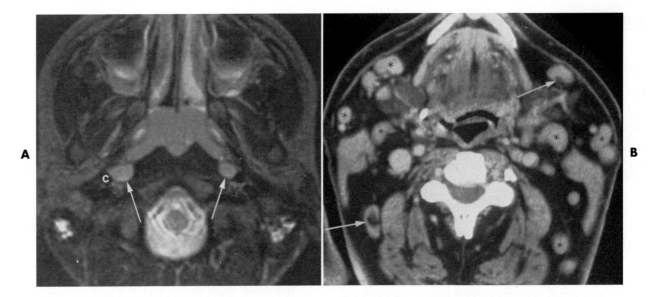

Fig. 3-53. Normal lymph node anatomy. **A,** In this 8-year-old child, normal lateral retropharyngeal nodes *(arrows)* lie medial to internal carotid arteries *(c)* and demonstrate moderately high signal on T2-weighted images. High-signal adenoidal tissue is commonly prominent at this age. **B,** Multiple mildly enlarged nodes *(asterisks)* are present in submandibular, anterior jugular, internal jugular, and spinal accessory lymphatic chains on this contrast-enhanced computed tomography. Note eccentric fatty hilum *(arrows)* in two nodes, a potential pitfall in diagnosis of focal defect in metastatic node.

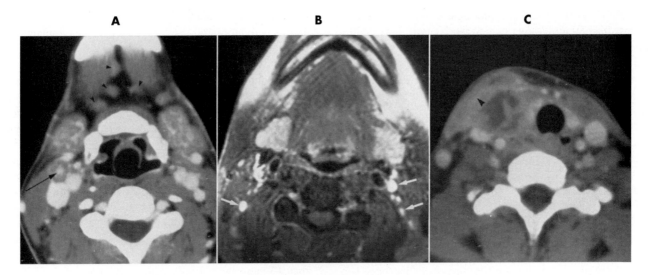

Fig. 3-54. Reactive and inflammatory lymph nodes on contrast-enhanced computed tomography (CECT) and magnetic resonance imaging. **A,** Axial CECT of hyperplastic nodes in a patient with acquired immunodeficiency syndrome-related complex displays multiple submental nodes *(arrowheads)* and enlarged internal jugular node with central hilar enhancement *(arrow).* **B,** Small, normal, or reactive lymph nodes *(arrows)* enhance on this fat saturation postgadolinium T1-weighted image. **C,** Axial CECT of tuberculous nodal mass (scrofula) with peripheral enhancement and invasion of sternocleidomastoid muscle *(arrowhead)* is difficult to distinguish from the cluster of metastatic nodes.

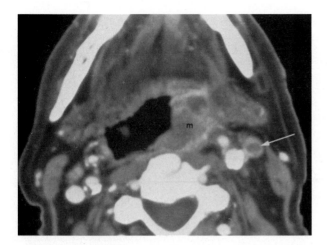

Fig. 3-55. Metastatic node on contrast-enhanced computed tomography (CECT). Axial CECT in a patient with left piriform sinus squamous cell carcinoma *(m)* and "normal-sized" 9-mm node *(arrow)* with focal defect (ring enhancement with "necrotic" center) diagnostic of metastasis.

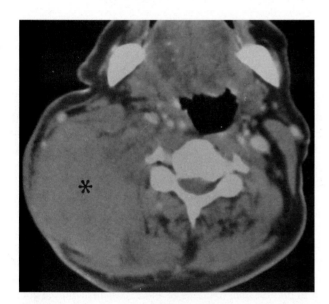

Fig. 3-56. Node involvement by non-Hodgkin's lymphoma. Axial contrast-enhanced computed tomography shows very large, homogeneous spinal accessory node *(asterisk)* invading both skin and prevertebral space paraspinous musculature. The absence of central necrosis or focal defects in a mass this large is suggestive but not diagnostic of lymphoma.

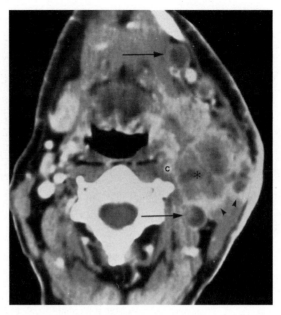

Fig. 3-57. Extracapsular spread in multiple nodes in a patient with tonsillar squamous cell carcinoma (SCC). Left submandibular and spinal accessory node metastases *(arrows)* have typical ring enhancement and central low density on axial contrast-enhanced computed tomography. The large cluster of metastatic nodes *(asterisk)* in left internal jugular chain shows central low-density focal defects. Note poorly defined infiltrative margins of this mass of nodes characteristic of extracapsular tumor spread; tumor is invading sternocleidomastoid muscle *(arrowheads)* posterolaterally and prevertebral space medially. About 40% of the left internal carotid artery *(c)* circumference is surrounded by tumor, which may still allow surgical preservation of the carotid artery.

and CECT rely on the same criteria of size, clustering, margin sharpness, and shape for characterization of abnormal nodes. The specificity of ring enhancement on CECT is the main advantage of CT for diagnosis of metastases. The same finding of ring enhancement on postgadolinium fat-suppressed T1WI likely represents focal tumor or central necrosis as well. Otherwise, the other MRI sequences described above are nonspecific. MRI may better demonstrate invasion of adjacent structures, especially muscles, than does CECT.

With extracapsular spread, adjacent fat, bone, cartilage, and muscle are commonly compressed or invaded. Secondary invasion of adjacent structures and anatomic spaces by aggressive lymph node lesions may develop in the carotid sheath structures, skull base, PVS and vertebrae, and mandible. The superficial nodes may invade adjacent muscle and skin. Internal jugular and spinal accessory nodes may invade the carotid, parapharyngeal fat, prevertebral, and infrahyoid visceral spaces. Parotid nodes may violate the surrounding parotid parenchyma, skin, masticator space, and parapharyngeal space. Suprahyoid retropharyngeal nodes may extend laterally into the CS, posteriorly into the PVS, anteriorly into the mucosal space, and superiorly into the skull base. The tracheoesophageal nodes may involve the common carotid artery and the internal jugular vein in the CS, the recurrent laryngeal nerve, the visceral space structures of the larynx and thyroid, and the mediastinum.

Invasion of the carotid artery carries a poor prognosis with local recurrence rate of 46% and a distant metastatic rate of 56% to 68%. For patients with tumor involving the carotid artery, the 5-year survival rate decreases to 7%, and the mean survival decreases to less than 1 year. Prolonged survival is possible if the involved carotid artery is resected.

A **B** **C**

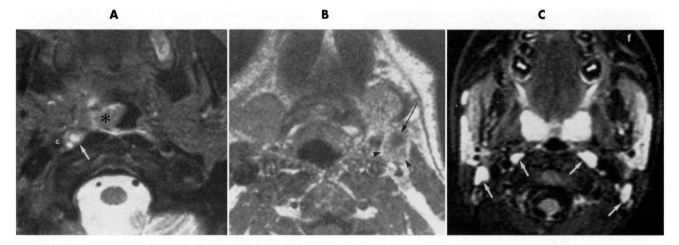

Fig. 3-58. Metastatic nodes and focal defects on magnetic resonance imaging. **A,** Axial T2-weighted image at soft palate level depicts high-signal intensity right tonsillar squamous cell carcinoma (SCC) *(asterisk)*. A 10-mm metastatic lateral retropharyngeal node of Rouvier with a high-signal intensity central defect *(arrow)* lies medial to internal carotid artery *(c)*. **B,** Left jugular digastric node *(arrowheads)* with low-signal intensity focal defect *(arrow)* on gadolinium-enhanced T1-weighted image is analogous to focal defect seen with metastases on contrast-enhanced computed tomography. **C,** Axial short T1 inversion recovery (STIR) image achieves excellent fat suppression of subcutaneous fat *(f)*. Metastatic neuroblastoma is demonstrated in bright internal jugular and spinal accessory nodes *(arrows)*. Note bright appearance of normal tonsillar and parotid gland tissues on STIR.

Detection of carotid artery invasion by MRI may be more accurate than ultrasound. The best imaging modality among CECT, MRI, or ultrasound for evaluating carotid fixation remains controversial.[30] Surprisingly, criteria for carotid invasion are not well established in the literature. CT and MRI criteria, based on the work of Picus in aortic invasion by esophageal carcinoma, include effacement of the fascial plane surrounding greater than 25% of the vessel circumference.[38] More recent criteria suggest a very high likelihood of fixation exists if tumor involves three fourths or more of the circumference of the carotid and if nodal extracapsular penetration has occurred (see Fig. 3-57). Ultrasonography is a potentially valuable adjunctive technique capable of demonstrating invasion of the common and internal carotid artery, as well as the internal jugular vein.

SINUSES AND SKULL BASE

Nose and paranasal sinuses

The sinonasal region can be divided into three major regions: the sinuses, the ostiomeatal complex, and the nasal cavity. The paranasal sinuses are mucosal-lined, air-filled cavities that are named after the bones of the face in which they develop. This mucosa is prone to both inflammatory and neoplastic disease. The frontal, maxillary, ethmoid, and sphenoid sinuses all drain through ostia into the nasal cavity. The frontal, maxillary, anterior ethmoid, and middle ethmoid sinuses drain into the semilunar hiatus under the middle turbinate. This area represents the ostiomeatal complex or unit; a small lesion here can cause obstruction to multiple sinus

ostia. The posterior ethmoids and sphenoid sinus drain under the superior turbinate or sphenoethmoidal recess. The nasal cavity extends from the nares anteriorly to the choana posteriorly and from the hard palate inferiorly to the cribriform plate superiorly. The midline nasal septum, lateral turbinates, and maxillary and ethmoid sinuses form the walls.

The compartments adjacent to the sinuses that are at risk for invasion by aggressive inflammatory or neoplastic processes include the anterior cranial fossa, orbits, cavernous sinus (from the sphenoid sinus), MS, pterygopalatine (pterygomaxillary) fossa, oral cavity, and anterior soft tissues of the face. These compartments are carefully viewed for dural or brain invasion, optic nerve and extraocular muscle compromise, perineural spread into the skull base, or direct extension into the deep compartments of the suprahyoid neck and oral structures. Involvement of any one of these secondary compartments can significantly alter treatment planning and surgical approach.

Paranasal sinuses

Congenital and developmental anomalies of the sinonasal cavities are sought on all CT examinations. Common anatomic variants include pneumatization or paradoxical curvature of the turbinates, deviated septum, sinus hypoplasia, and Haller air cells (Fig. 3-59). Sinus underdevelopment may range from aplasia to hypoplasia. Pneumatization implies sinus development has occurred; aeration indicates that the pneumatized portion of the sinus is air-filled. Mucosal thickening or opacification signifies the pneumatized section is

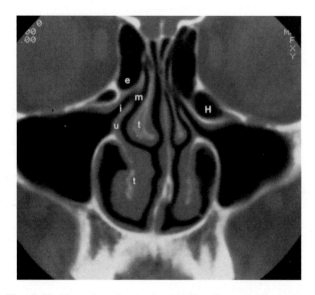

Fig. 3-59. Normal ostiomeatal complex. Coronal non-contrast computed tomography demonstrates ostiomeatal complex to the best advantage. Normal mucociliary drainage is from maxillary sinus up through infundibulum *(i)* and maxillary sinus ostium into middle meatus *(m)*. Ethmoid bulla *(e)* and uncinate process *(u)* form lateral and medial walls of infundibulum, respectively. Normal anatomic variant of a Haller air cell *(H)* underlying orbit causes mild narrowing of the left infundibulum; smaller Haller cell is present on the right. Note mildly asymmetric mucosa of turbinates *(t)*, which is part of normal nasal cycle.

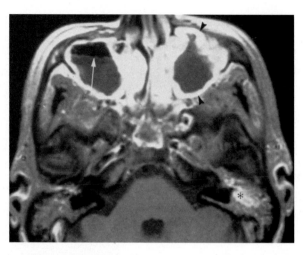

Fig. 3-60. Acute and chronic sinusitis. Postgadolinium fat saturation T1-weighted image demonstrates air-fluid level *(arrow)* in right maxillary sinus and is diagnostic of acute sinusitis (superimposed on chronic sinusitis). Left maxillary sinus is filled with low-intensity secretions and has a peripheral ring of enhancing inflamed mucosa *(arrowheads)* typical of chronic sinusitis. Mastoid air cells and left middle ear cavity *(asterisk)*, which normally appear black, are filled with enhancing inflammatory tissue.

filled with soft-tissue inflammation or fluid. Either hypoplasia or the reactive new bone formation (chronic inflammation) may cause thickening and sclerosis of the sinus walls.

In general, evaluation of the paranasal sinuses involves assessment of two components: (1) the sinus contents (including the mucosa) and (2) the bony walls. Normal sinus mucosa is very thin and not seen on CT or MRI, and the bone is normally thin and delicate in the posterior maxillary, ethmoid, and sphenoid sinuses. CT or MRI readily reveals the presence of a normally aerated sinus, mucosal thickening (chronic sinusitis, retention cysts, or polyps), an air-fluid level (acute sinusitis, intubation, and trauma), or complete opacification (mucocele, trauma, and acute or chronic sinusitis) (Fig. 3-60). The normally delicate posterolateral maxillary sinus wall is a much better indicator of bony sclerosis than the anterior wall; the normally thick anterior wall of the maxillary (and frontal) sinus may range from 1 to 3 mm (see Fig. 3-11 *A, C*). Beginning observers frequently forget to assess the bone for important clues such as thickening and sclerosis (chronic sinusitis or hypoplasia), fractures, remodeling (slowly expanding mucocele or neoplasm), or destruction (malignancy or aggressive infection such as mucormycosis).

Deciding which portion of the opacified sinus, sinuses, or nasal cavity contains tumor and which contains obstructed mucous secretions is clinically important with a sinus or

nasal tumor. The question is more problematic with NCCT or CECT because tumor and sinus secretions are frequently similar in density, and both the tumor and the mucosa may enhance; however, MRI is usually much more informative (Fig. 3-61). Evaluation of this problem requires a knowledge of signal intensity patterns of tumor versus mucus. Sinonasal tumors tend to be low-to-intermediate signal intensity on T1WI and intermediate signal intensity on T2WI, although minor salivary tumors and adenoid cystic carcinoma may be of high signal intensity.[42] The highly cellular aggressive neoplasms tend to have a lower water content and are less bright on T2WI. Tumors enhance moderately and, more or less, uniformly with gadolinium. Sinus secretions are complex in their patterns. Hydrated, nonviscous mucus is low intensity on T1WI and high intensity on T2WI. Desiccated, viscous mucus tends to be high intensity on T1WI and low-to-intermediate intensity on T2WI. Extremely desiccated mucus may lack signal intensity on T1WI or T2WI, simulating bone or air. Both an obstructed sinus and an expansile mucocele frequently have two or more layers of mucus in a concentric ring pattern with the most desiccated, viscous secretions located centrally. The peripheral mucosa of an obstructed sinus enhances in chronic sinusitis or with a pyomucocele but does not enhance with a simple mucocele. The presence of tumor versus obstructed secretion is best solved by comparing the respective change in signal intensity of

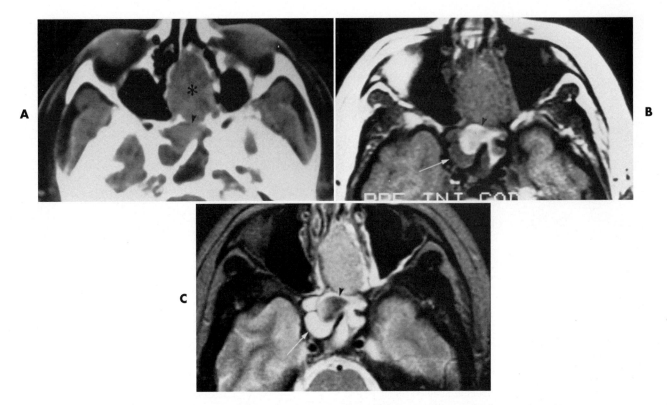

Fig. 3-61. Comparison of computed tomography and magnetic resonance imaging for separating sinonasal small cell tumor from sphenoid pyomucocele. **A,** Axial contrast-enhanced computed tomography shows a mildly enhancing mass *(asterisk)* in the left posterior nasal cavity and ethmoids, which appears to extend into the sphenoid sinus. Sphenoid sinus contents actually represent two different viscosities of mucus, with higher density mucus anteriorly *(arrowhead)* correlating with most desiccated or viscous mucus. **B,** Axial noncontrast T1-weighted image demonstrates intermediate-signal nasal tumor. Anterior, high-signal, viscous mucus *(arrowhead)* in the sphenoid sinus is clearly discriminated from nasal tumor anteriorly and from low-signal hydrated mucus *(arrow)* posteriorly. **C,** On axial noncontrast T2-weighted image, nasal tumor signal is intermediate, similar to the brain. Anterior viscous mucus *(arrowhead)* in sphenoid sinus has reversed signal to become low intensity, whereas hydrated mucus *(arrow)* posteriorly has now become very bright.

each component on the T1WI, T2WI, and postgadolinium T1WI and is rarely answered by a single sequence; a minimum of a T1WI and a T2WI is required.

Ostiomeatal complex

The ostiomeatal complex has become an area of active radiologic and pathophysiologic investigation with the development of endoscopic sinus surgery for inflammatory sinus disease. Coronal thin section NCCT is the best means of demonstrating the anatomy of this area (see Fig. 3-59). Pertinent observations include (1) the individual's sinonasal anatomy and the presence of any anatomic variants (hypoplastic maxillary sinus, concha bullosa, agger nasi air cells, Haller air cells, deviated septum, deviated uncinate process, prominent ethmoid bulla, paradoxical curvature of the middle turbinate), (2) the location of obstructed air cells, (3) the extent of the chronic or acute sinus disease and whether this pattern is consistent with obstruction of the ostiomeatal complex, and (4) the presence of any prior surgical alterations (Caldwell-Luc, internal

or external ethmoidectomy, uncinatectomy, etc.). Ostiomeatal complex obstruction may result from anatomic compression, mucosal inflammation, polyps, benign neoplasms, and SCCA. Mucoceles, indicated by sinus expansion and low-density mucus on CECT or by concentric rings of variably desiccated mucus in an expanded sinus on MRI, are a complication of chronic sinus obstruction (Fig. 3-62). A mucocele only shows peripheral enhancement when it is infected and is then called a pyomucocele.

Nasal cavity

The nasal cavity is occasionally the site of symptomatic disease. Anatomic variants include choanal atresia, concha bullosa, paradoxical curvature of the middle turbinate, wide nasal cavity from a hypoplastic maxillary sinus, and septal deviation. The nasal mucosa of the turbinates may be asymmetric in thickness because of the normal nasal cycle or the presence of polyps or inflammation. Obstruction of the ostiomeatal complex and other sinuses may occur with benign

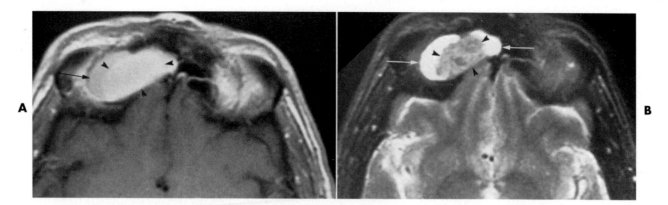

Fig. 3-62. Simple mucocele on magnetic resonance imaging. **A,** Frontal mucocele on axial T1-weighted image expands right frontal sinus and has very high-signal central viscous or desiccated component *(arrowheads)* and lower-intensity peripheral concentric ring of less viscous mucus *(arrow)*. **B,** Axial T2-weighted image reversal of signal intensities in concentric rings, with peripheral hydrated mucus *(arrow)* becoming bright and central viscous mucus *(arrowheads)* losing signal.

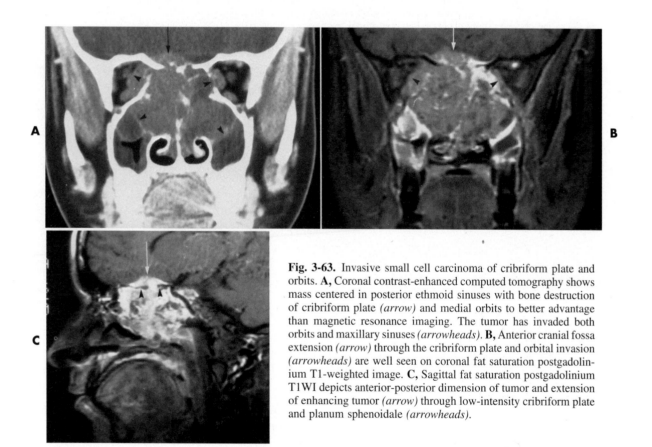

Fig. 3-63. Invasive small cell carcinoma of cribriform plate and orbits. **A,** Coronal contrast-enhanced computed tomography shows mass centered in posterior ethmoid sinuses with bone destruction of cribriform plate *(arrow)* and medial orbits to better advantage than magnetic resonance imaging. The tumor has invaded both orbits and maxillary sinuses *(arrowheads)*. **B,** Anterior cranial fossa extension *(arrow)* through the cribriform plate and orbital invasion *(arrowheads)* are well seen on coronal fat saturation postgadolinium T1-weighted image. **C,** Sagittal fat saturation postgadolinium T1WI depicts anterior-posterior dimension of tumor and extension of enhancing tumor *(arrow)* through low-intensity cribriform plate and planum sphenoidale *(arrowheads)*.

(antrochoanal polyp, neural tumors, inverting papilloma) or malignant (SCC, adenocarcinoma, adenoid cystic carcinoma) tumors (Fig. 3-63). If a nasal mass is present, the extent of the mass within the nasal cavity, adjacent sinuses, or orbits or involvement of the cribriform plate may be determined by coronal CECT or sagittal and coronal MRI because this may affect the surgical approach and postoperative therapy.

Facial trauma

Facial trauma is briefly included here because of the intimate relationship of the facial bones and sinuses. Thin-section axial and direct coronal NCCT is the ideal method for determining the full extent of facial trauma. One strategy for evaluating the extent of sinus trauma is to visually trace each bony outline on consecutive slices in both imaging planes, looking

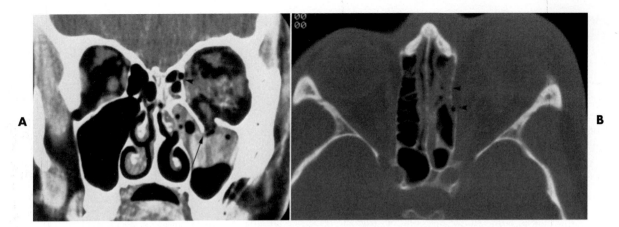

Fig. 3-64. Medial and lateral orbital blowout fractures. **A,** Coronal noncontrast computed tomography (NCCT) with soft-tissue windows shows orbital blowout fracture with displacement of floor *(arrow)*, distortion of inferior rectus, and herniation of orbital fat through orbital floor defect. Both intraconal hemorrhage and high-density maxillary sinus hemorrhagic air-fluid level are well demonstrated on these windows. Medial orbital blowout fracture *(arrowhead)* is suspected as well. **B,** Axial NCCT using bone windows shows opacified left anterior ethmoid air cells that help direct the observer to the displaced medial orbital fracture *(arrowheads)*.

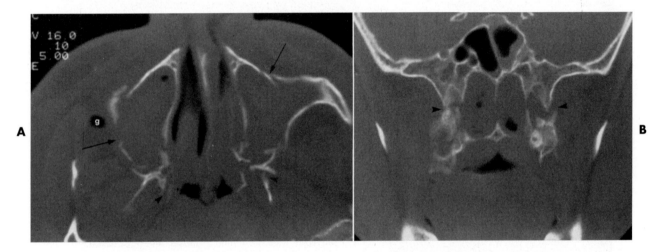

Fig. 3-65. Facial fractures. **A,** Bilateral Le Fort type II fractures of maxillary sinus anterior and posterior walls *(arrows)* and pterygoid plates *(arrowheads)* appear as discontinuities or lucencies of the bone on this 3-mm axial noncontrast computed tomography (NCCT). Indirect signs of facial fracture are opacified maxillary sinuses, gas *(g)* in right buccal fat pad, and premalar facial swelling. **B,** Coronal NCCT clearly demonstrates bilateral pterygoid plate fractures *(arrowheads)*.

for fractures, normal fissures and canals, and displacements. However, the quickest way to locate sinus fractures is to search for indirect signs of fracture (Fig. 3-64): an air-fluid level, complete opacification of a sinus with blood, and the presence of gas outside the sinus (pneumocephalus, subcutaneous emphysema, infratemporal fossa, or orbital gas). Identification of the fractures allows determination of fracture classification: nasal, orbital blowout, trimalar or tripod, Le Fort (I, II, III, and complex), or nasoethmoid complex fracture (Fig. 3-65). Assessment is made of the extent of soft-tissue trauma, particularly the orbital soft tissues of the lens, globe, extraocular muscles, and optic nerve. Displaced orbital floor

fractures may entrap fat or the extraocular muscles and result in enophthalmos or dysfunction of ocular motility.

Skull base

Anatomically, the skull base can be divided into the anterior, middle, and posterior fossae. The lesser and greater wings of the sphenoid bone divide the anterior fossa from the middle fossa while the petrous pyramid and mastoid portions of the temporal bone divide the middle and posterior fossae. The parietal and occipital lobes of the brain do not directly contact the skull base.

The skull base is formed from five bones: frontal, ethmoid, temporal, sphenoid, and occipital; the frontal and temporal bones are paired. Each of these bones can be subdivided into component bones; for example, the occipital bone has basioccipital, condylar, and squamosal portions. The skull base has its longest diameter in the AP plane, extending from the region of the crista galli to the posterior margin of the foramen magnum posteriorly. It is the thinnest in its superior-inferior direction, ranging between 3 and 5 mm in most areas with the exception of the much thicker petrous temporal bone.

With CT the skull base may be imaged using the axial or the coronal plane (only a modified coronal plane is possible because of limited gantry tilt). The coronal plane is excellent for delineating the superior inferior extent of a lesion. CT gives excellent visualization of bone detail, especially when bone algorithm techniques are used. In addition to the axial plane, MRI allows imaging both in a true coronal plane and in the sagittal plane, the latter especially useful for the study of midline lesions (e.g., chordoma). MRI also yields improved lesion contrast and conspicuity and more accurate delineation of lesion extent.

Using an anatomic approach skull base lesions may be classified as anterior, middle, or posterior fossa and a unique differential then developed for the medial and lateral portions of each fossa. Lesions may also be categorized as primary, those arising within the skull base itself and secondary, those extending down from the cranial cavity above (endocranial lesions) or growing up from below (exocranial lesions). Endocranial masses are extracerebral and intracerebral lesions, whereas the exocranial lesions are secondary to extension superiorly from a disease process of the orbit, suprahyoid head and neck, cervical spine, and prevertebral muscles.

The skull base contains multiple foramina that allow the exit of cranial nerves and inflow and outflow of arteries and veins. These foramina also provide an access route for disease processes to spread from the cranial cavity to the infracalvarial structures and vice versa.[5] MRI performed after gadolinium infusion and with the use of fat suppression techniques allows sensitive detection of perineural spread, most readily seen with involvement of the fifth and seventh cranial nerves.[29]

Skull base fractures are readily detected with CT using thin slice sections and re-formation techniques. Sinus air-fluid levels, sinus opacification, and clouding of the temporal bones may herald the presence of a fracture. Similarly, sinus opacification and fracture location may indicate the site of a CSF leak.

Inflammatory skull base lesions are now less common. Osteitis is seen as sclerosis of bone margins. Osteomyelitis usually involves all three skull tables and is characterized by irregular serpiginous lytic areas, occasionally with areas of bone sequestration present.

The osseous changes of neoplastic disease may be erosive, infiltrative, expansive, lytic, sclerotic, or of mixed density. Primary skull neoplastic lesions are uncommon; benign conditions include osteoma, chondroma, giant cell tumor, cholesterol granuloma, and aneurysmal bone cyst (Fig. 3-66). Osteosarcoma, chondrosarcoma, fibrosarcoma, and rarely Ewing's sarcoma and lymphoma are examples of malignant lesions. Metastatic lesions are more common than primary skull base lesions and frequently have an associated soft-tissue component (Fig. 3-67). Osteoblastic metastases are most commonly caused by carcinoma of the prostate or breast; sclerotic changes may be seen occasionally in lymphoma (Fig. 3-68). Lytic lesions are more common than osteoblastic findings and are usually secondary to carcinoma of the lung, breast, kidney, or colon.

Intracerebral neoplastic processes may have associated osseous changes. Cerebral gliomas rarely cause local bone erosion or expansion; however, optic gliomas may cause expansion of the optic canal. Neuromas (nerve sheath tumors) may cause smooth expansion of skull base foramina: internal auditory canal (cranial nerve VIII), jugular foramen (cranial nerves IX, X, and XI), hypoglossal canal (cranial nerve XII), and lateral wall clivus and foramen rotundum (cranial nerve V). Paragangliomas cause irregular erosive changes in the skull base foramina (Fig. 3-69). A meningioma is often heralded by hyperostosis (bone sclerosis), especially common with a lesion of the middle fossa involving either the greater or lesser sphenoid wing. Chordoma, a tumor of notochordal remnants, typically causes destruction of the clivus (basisphenoid and basiocciput), typically with associated soft-tissue mass and calcification.[34,51] Erosion of the sella floor and sella expansion are characteristic of pituitary adenomas.

Temporal bone

Determination of temporal bone abnormality requires assessment of the external ear, middle ear, mastoid air cells, petrous apex, inner ear, IAC, facial nerve canal, and vascular compartment (jugular foramen and carotid canal). The adjacent compartments into which an aggressive temporal bone lesion can spread, or from which a lesion can invade the temporal bone include cerebellopontine angle (meningioma, acoustic schwannoma), middle cranial fossa (geniculate schwannoma, cholesteatoma), jugular foramen (schwannoma, paraganglioma, glomus tumor), skull base and clivus (chordoma), carotid space (aneurysm, schwannoma), parotid space (adenoid cystic carcinoma), and soft tissues of the external ear and scalp (SCC).

For the external ear and external auditory canal (EAC) the search for abnormality may be accomplished with either high-resolution CT or MRI. Abnormal development (external ear hypoplasia, fibrous or bony EAC atresia), soft tissue opacification (cerumen, EAC cholesteatoma, SCC), bone erosion (EAC cholesteatoma, mucormycosis, squamous cell carcinoma), bone formation (exostoses), or scutum erosion (par flaccida cholesteatoma) can easily be detected and their extent defined by CT. MRI may add additional information on soft-tissue involvement below the skull base or on infiltration of the auricle and scalp.

The middle ear is best evaluated with high-resolution CT. Ossicular chain anomalies (fusion, dislocation, prosthesis,

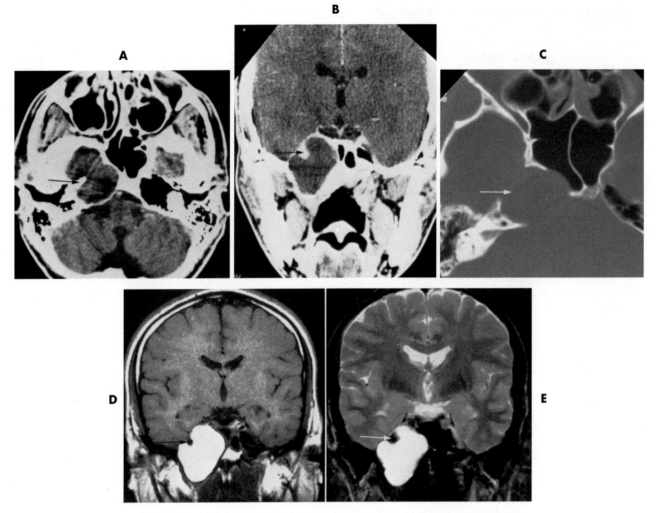

Fig. 3-66. Cholesterol granuloma. **A,** and **B,** Axial and coronal contrast-enhanced computed tomography (CECT) images demonstrate expansile lesion of the right petrous apex and greater wing of sphenoid. Lesion is homogeneously low density in nature. Displaced right internal carotid artery *(arrows)* lies in the lateral aspect of the lesion. **C,** Axial CECT bone algorithm image using bone windows demonstrates truncation of anteromedial portion of the right petrous temporal bone *(arrow)* and adjacent posterolateral portion of the sphenoid bone. The lesion bulges into the right sphenoid sinus. **D** and **E,** Coronal T1-weighted image and T2-weighted image demonstrate lesion that is high intensity on both sequences, consistent with methemoglobin. Right internal carotid artery is noted in midlateral portion of lesion *(arrow)*. The lesion extends above and below skull base and invaginates into sphenoid sinus.

stapedial foot-plate sclerosis), air-fluid level (trauma, acute otitis media), soft-tissue opacification (acute or chronic otitis media, cholesteatoma, trauma, chronic endotracheal or nasogastric intubation), and tympanic membrane thickening (otitis media) may all be characterized (Fig. 3-70). The radiographic approach to the mastoid air cells and petrous apex is similar to that of the paranasal sinuses and consists of the evaluation of the mastoid and petrous apex soft-tissue contents and the bony walls. Assessment is made of development or pneumatization of these regions (pneumatization or opacification by soft tissue), the bony septae and walls (hypoplasia or sclerosis from chronic otomastoiditis), the

margins of the mastoid or petrous apex (expanded by a primary or secondary cholesteatoma [Fig. 3-71] or a cholesterol granuloma), bone destruction (SCC, malignant fibrous histiocytoma, glomus tumor). MRI may complement CT for assessment of larger petrous apex or mastoid masses. A normal unpneumatized, fatty (marrow-filled) petrous apex is high signal on T1WI and low signal on T2WI, but a cholesterol granuloma is high signal on T1WI and T2WI from the methemoglobin (see Fig. 3-66). Mucus in an air cell is low intensity on T1WI, is very high intensity on T2WI, and enhances mildly with gadolinium. A primary cholesteatoma is similar to CSF in intensity, appearing low intensity on T1WI

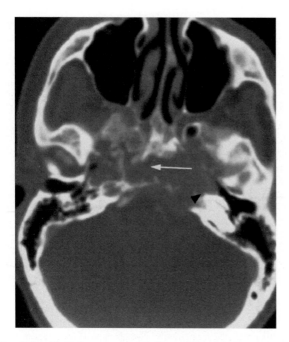

Fig. 3-67. Skull base metastasis from adenocarcinoma of the breast. Axial noncontrast computed tomography demonstrates metastatic tumor infiltrating and destroying majority of middle fossa; clivus *(arrow)* and anteromedial left temporal bone *(arrowhead)* are especially affected.

A saccular vestibule is one of the more common congenital anomalies. A cochlea with less than 2½ to 2¾ turns represents a Mondini malformation (Fig. 3-72). The basal turn of the cochlea and round window may be identified on both axial and coronal CT images. The horizontal (lateral) semicircular canal cortex may be eroded by a cholesteatoma. The oval window and foot plate of the stapes are thickened in stapedial otosclerosis, and the ring of the otic capsule is demineralized in labyrinthine otosclerosis (otospongiosis). The entire petrous bone may be abnormally low density with dysplasias such as osteogenesis imperfecta or sclerotic in osteopetrosis and Paget's disease. Inflammatory or neoplastic lesions may involve the cochlea and vestibule without obvious bony changes on CT; however, MRI with gadolinium-enhanced T1WI may show an enhancing lesion.

The IAC and facial nerve canals are best evaluated by high-resolution CT for bony detail and by gadolinium-enhanced MRI for the soft-tissue abnormality. On CT the findings might include widening (acoustic schwannoma, surgery) or narrowing (bone dysplasia, hyperostosis from a meningioma) of the IAC. The facial nerve canal may be traced along its entire course in both axial and coronal planes for areas of erosion (facial neuroma, paraganglioma, hemangioma) or abnormal position (anterior location of mastoid segment with EAC atresia). Gadolinium-enhanced MRI is the modality of choice for evaluating the seventh and eighth cranial nerves within the IAC and temporal bone (schwannomas of the facial nerve, of the vestibular nerve, or within the cochlea) or for demonstrating seventh cranial nerve inflammation (Bell's palsy) (Figs. 3-73 and 3-74). Note that the facial nerves may normally enhance mildly and usually symmetrically within the facial nerve canal; asymmetric enhancement is more likely to be abnormal.

and moderately high signal on T2WI, and does not enhance with gadolinium. Postoperative findings encountered on CT and MRI include metallic ossicular prostheses, cochlear implants, and various types of mastoidectomies.

The inner ear structures are best assessed by high-resolution CT with attention to anatomic variants and bone density.

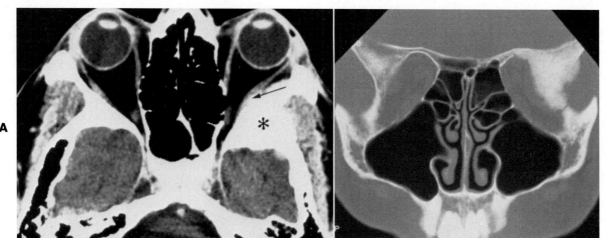

Fig. 3-68. Metastatic prostate carcinoma to left orbit. **A,** Axial contrast-enhanced computed tomography (CECT) demonstrates sclerotic metastasis of posterolateral margin of left orbit *(asterisk)*. Small soft tissue component *(arrow)* lies deep to hyperostosis, displacing the lateral rectus muscle medially. **B,** Coronal CECT with bone settings demonstrates marked sclerotic reaction of superior lateral portion of the left orbit; intraorbital volume is decreased.

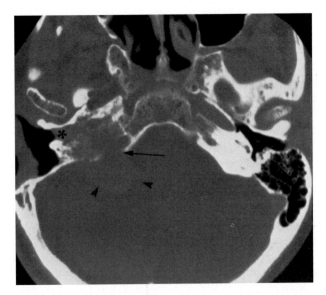

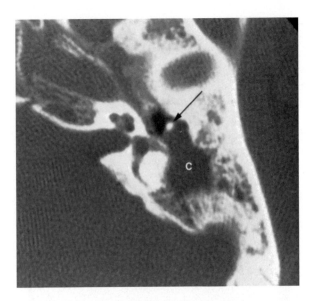

Fig. 3-69. Glomus tumor (paraganglioma) of the right petrous temporal bone. Axial contrast-enhanced computed tomography with bone windows demonstrates infiltrative destructive lesion of the middle and superior portions of the right petrous temporal bone *(arrow)*. Poorly defined margin of lesion is characteristic of glomus tumor. Soft-tissue mass *(arrowheads)* is noted in the right cerebellopontine angle cistern and in the inferior portion of the right middle ear cavity *(asterisk)*. Previous right mastoidectomy has been performed.

Fig. 3-71. Pars flaccida cholesteatoma. Middle ear cholesteatoma *(c)* expands mastoid antrum and epitympanic recess on axial noncontrast computed tomography. The absence of incus and soft tissue abutting the head of malleus *(arrow)* confirm ossicular erosion.

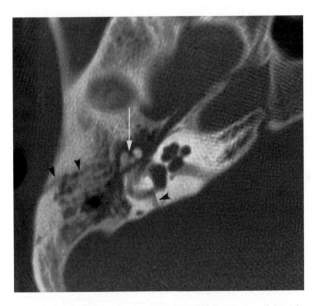

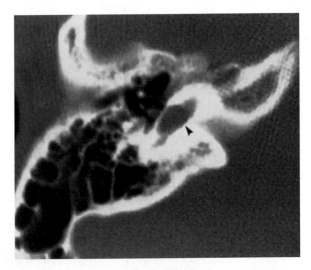

Fig. 3-70. Transverse petrous fracture with ossicular dislocation. High-resolution 1.5-mm noncontrast computed tomography using bone algorithm and bone windows shows a transverse petrous fracture *(arrowheads)* extending through mastoid bone and semicircular canals. Ossicular dislocation of the head of malleus from its articulation with fractured body of incus *(arrow)* is seen; middle ear opacification also confirms presence of temporal bone trauma.

Fig. 3-72. Mondini malformation. Saccular combined vestibule and cochlea *(arrowhead)* reveal a severe form of Mondini malformation on axial noncontrast computed tomography.

POSTOPERATIVE NECK AND FACE

A preoperative CECT or MRI is extremely helpful for interpreting the postoperative neck, skull base, or face for sites of concern and potential tumor recurrence. Likewise, a baseline CECT or MRI 3 to 6 months after surgery and radiation further improves the ability of imaging to detect posttreatment tumor recurrence. The posterior cervical space is the most frequently altered neck space, and part or all of its contents may be resected for staging and treatment of head and neck carcinoma; note is made of missing structures.[20] A radical neck dissection (Fig. 3-75, *A*) removes the sternocleidomastoid muscle, internal jugular vein, regional lymph nodes, and most of the fibrofatty tissue that comprises this space. Modified radical, functional, and supraomohyoid neck dissections remove less.

The oral cavity and face also are affected by surgery. Facial trauma is frequently treated by internal fixation with metallic screws and plates. Internal fixation also is per-

formed as part of composite reactions where the mandible is split or when the mandible is partially resected for invasion by tumor. Metal wires, screws, and plates may cause artifacts obscuring sites of posttraumatic CSF leak or potential tumor recurrence. Sinus and palate tumors may require resection of the maxilla, palate, orbital walls and soft tissue, and cribriform plate. The fat, muscle, or bone contained in free flaps, myocutaneous flaps, and osteocutaneous flaps placed in the surgical cavity further complicates image interpretation (Fig. 3-75, *B*). Laryngeal surgery may remove part or all of the laryngeal skeleton, often with placement of a tracheostomy. The remaining soft tissues of the collapsed visceral space are difficult to accurately evaluate.

Radiotherapy frequently causes an edematous pattern, characterized on CT by a streaky increase in density of the subcutaneous, parapharyngeal, and posterior cervical space fat planes (Fig. 3-76, *A*); on MRI it may have increased signal on T2WI. The mucosal space of the pharynx and larynx may also develop swelling and edema, appearing as diffuse mucosal thickening and enhancement on CECT, while MRI may show high signal on long TR sequences and on gadolinium-enhanced T1WI (Fig. 3-76, *B*). Postradiation edema, particularly of the larynx and pharynx, may mimic recurrent neoplasm for as long as 6 months to 7 years after radiotherapy.[21] Finally, treated lymph nodes may decrease in size or totally disappear, leaving a ''dirty fat'' appearance.

Recurrent tumor spread often produces strands or nodules of soft-tissue density within or replacing the normal fat

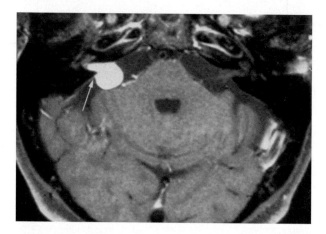

Fig. 3-73. Acoustic schwannoma. Axial fat saturation postgadolinium T1-weighted image demonstrates brightly enhancing right cerebellopontine angle mass with intracanalicular (characteristic of acoustic schwannoma) and extracanalicular components. Note the acute angle that the mass makes with petrous ridge *(arrow)*.

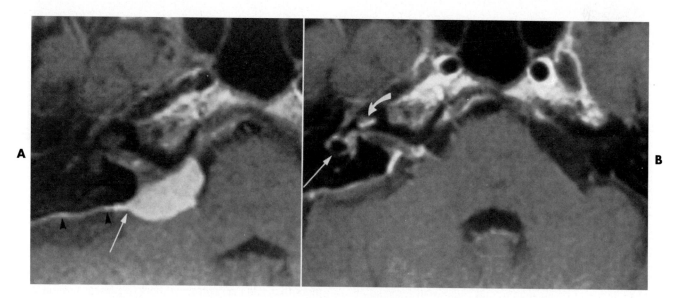

Fig. 3-74. Magnetic resonance imaging (MRI) of internal auditory canal (IAC) and facial nerve. **A,** Axial postgadolinium T1-weighted image shows broad-based brightly enhancing meningioma overlying IAC. Note its obtuse angle *(arrow)* with petrous ridge and dural ''tail'' extending posteriorly *(arrowhead)*, which are characteristic of meningioma. **B,** In the same patient as in **A,** postoperative labyrinthitis has developed on this follow-up axial postgadolinium T1-weighted images. Abnormal enhancement of vestibule, semicircular canals *(straight arrow)*, and cochlea *(curved arrow)* are new findings (which can only be observed by gadolinium-enhanced MRI).

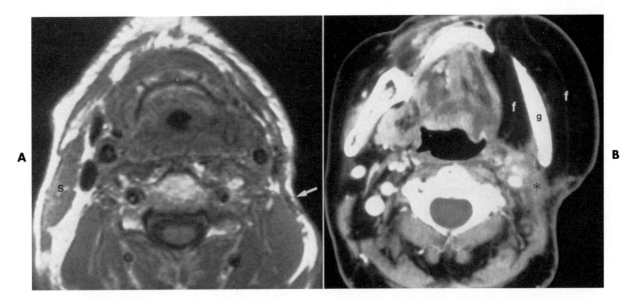

Fig. 3-75. Postoperative appearance of neck. **A,** Axial T1-weighted image demonstrates prior left neck dissection *(arrow)* with removal of sternocleidomastoid muscle *(s)* and posterior cervical space fat. **B,** Patient with osteocutaneous flap, with thick fat *(f)* on deep and external margins of mandibular graft *(g)*, has developed deep recurrent tumor *(asterisk)* around carotid sheath.

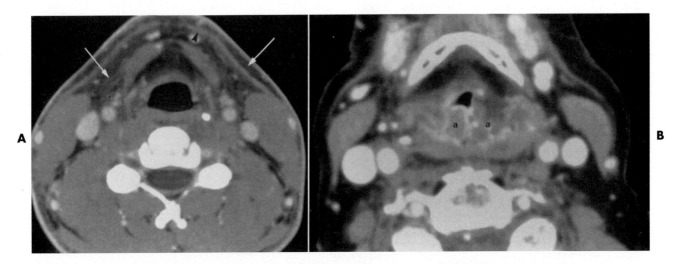

Fig. 3-76. Radiation changes in neck. **A,** Axial contrast-enhanced computed tomography (CECT) demonstrates streaky densities in fat throughout superficial cervical and anterior cervical spaces *(arrows)* and thickening of platysma muscle *(arrowhead)*. **B,** Different patient who had radiation therapy for glottic carcinoma has developed thickening of epiglottis and aryepiglottic folds *(a)* on axial CECT. This finding may persist for many months after therapy.

planes. However, CECT has difficulty detecting small (<1 cm) or mucosal-based tumors and reliably differentiating between recurrent carcinoma and fibrosis or edema. A new bulky, ring-enhancing mass, local tissue invasion, or further bone destruction is a strong sign of recurrent tumor. MRI is reportedly capable of distinguishing tumor from radiation-induced fibrosis in some cases. Posttreatment fibrosis or scarring is similar to or lower than muscle in signal on all sequences (particularly on T2WI), is usually linear, is not mass-like, and may enhance mildly in a linear fashion. MRI is superior to CT (particularly NCCT) in discrimination of recurrent tumor from muscle and vascular structures. In the posttreatment neck, gadolinium-enhanced MRI may have the potential to identify tumor recurrence and allow separation of tumor from fibrosis because recurrent tumor may ring-enhance, a pattern not seen with scar.

REFERENCES

1. Albertyn LE, Alcock MK: Diagnosis of internal jugular vein thrombosis, *Radiology* 162:505, 1987.
2. Atlas SW and others: STIR MR imaging of the orbit, *Am J Neuroradiol* 9:969, 1988.
3. Ator GA and others: Evaluation of mandibular tumor invasion with magnetic resonance imaging, *Arch Otolaryngol Head Neck Surg* 116:454, 1990.
4. Babbel RW, Smoker WRK, Harnsberger HR: The visceral space: the unique infrahyoid space, *Semin Ultra CT MR* 12:1991.
5. Batsakis JG: *Tumors of the head and neck: clinical and pathological considerations.* Baltimore, 1979, Williams & Wilkins.
6. Bluemm R: Direct sagittal (positional) computed tomography of the head, *Neuroradiology* 22:199, 1982.
7. Brant-Zawadzki M: *Magnetic resonance imaging principles: the bare necessities.* In Brant-Zawadzki M, Norman D, editors: *Magnetic resonance imaging of the central nervous system,* New York, 1987, Raven Press.
8. Close LG and others: Computed tomographic evaluation of regional lymph node involvement in cancer of the oral cavity and oropharynx, *Head Neck* 11:309, 1989.
9. Crawford SC and others: The role of gadolinium-DTPA in the evaluation of extracranial head and neck mass lesions, *Radiol Clin North Am* 27:219, 1989.
10. Curtin HD: Assessment of salivary gland pathology, *Otolaryngol Clin North Am* 21:547, 1988.
11. Curtin HD: Separation of the masticator space from the parapharyngeal space, *Radiology* 163:195, 1987.
12. Davis WL, Smoker WRK, Harnsberger HR: The normal and diseased infrahyoid retropharyngeal, danger, and prevertebral spaces, *Semin Ultra CT MR* 12:241, 1991.
13. Davis WL and others: Retropharyngeal space: evaluation of normal anatomy and diseases with CT and MR imaging, *Radiology* 174:59, 1990.
14. Delblasio AM, editor: *Maxillofacial imaging,* Philadelphia, 1990, WB Saunders.
15. Elliot DO: Magnetic resonance imaging fundamentals and system performance, *Radiol Clin North Am* 25:409, 1987.
16. Evers K and others: CT sialography: utilising acinar filling, *Br J Radiol* 58:839, 1985.
17. Fishman EK and others: Three-dimensional reconstruction of the human body, *Am J Roentgenol* 150:1419, 1988.
18. Fruehwald FX: Clinical examination, CT and US in tongue cancer staging, *Eur J Radiol* 8:236, 1988.
19. Fruin ME, Smoker WRK, Harnsberger HR: The carotid space of the infrahyoid neck, *Semin Ultra CT MR* 12:224, 1991.
20. Glazer HS and others: Neck neoplasms: MR imaging. II. Posttreatment evaluation, *Radiology* 160:349, 1986.
21. Glazer HS and others: Radiation fibrosis: differentiation from recurrent tumor by MR imaging, *Radiology* 156:721, 1985.
22. Gordon BM and others: Parathyroid imaging with Tc-99m sestamibi, *Am J Roentgenol* 167:1563, 1996.
23. Grossman RI, Yousem DM: *Neuroradiology, the requisites,* St Louis, 1994, Mosby.
24. Hajek PC and others: Lymph nodes of the neck: evaluation with US, *Radiology* 158:739, 1986.
25. Harnsberger HR: CT and MRI of masses of the deep face, *Curr Probl Diagn Radiol* 16:141, 1987.
26. Harnsberger HR: *Head and neck imaging: handbooks in radiology,* Chicago, 1990, Mosby.
27. Harnsberger HR and others: Branchial cleft anomalies and their mimics: CT evaluation, *Radiology* 152:739, 1984.
28. Hendrix LE and others: MR imaging of optic nerve lesions: value of gadopentetate dimeglumine and fat-suppression technique, *Am J Neuroradiol* 11:749, 1990.
29. Laine FJ and others: Perineural tumor extension through the foramen ovale: evaluation with MR imaging, *Radiology* 174:65, 1990.
30. Langman AW and others: Radiologic assessment of tumor and the carotid artery: correlation of magnetic resonance imaging, ultrasound, and computed tomography with surgical findings, *Head Neck* 11:443, 1989.
31. Mancuso AA, Dillon WP: The neck, *Radiol Clin North Am* 27:407, 1989.
32. Marentette LJ, Maisel RH: Three-dimensional CT reconstruction in midfacial surgery, *Otolaryngol Head Neck Surg* 98:48, 1988.
33. Mettler FA, Gulberteau MJ: *Essentials of nuclear medicine imaging,* ed 3, Philadelphia, 1991, WB Saunders.
34. Moore T, Ganti SR, Lindfors KK: CT appearance of clival chordomas, *J Comput Assist Tomogr* 10:34, 1986.
35. Olsen WL and others: MR imaging of paragangliomas, *Am J Roentgenol* 148:201, 1987.
36. Parker GD, Harnsberger HR, Smoker WRK: The anterior and posterior cervical spaces, *Semin Ultra CT MR* 12:257, 1991.
37. Pernicone JR and others: Three-dimensional phase-contrast MR angiography in the head and neck: preliminary report, *Am J Neuroradiol* 11:457, 1990.
38. Picus D and others: Computed tomography in the staging of esophageal carcinoma, *Radiology* 146:433, 1983.
39. Rafto SE, Gefter WB: MRI of the upper aerodigestive tract and neck, *Radiol Clin North Am* 26:547, 1988.
40. Robinson JD and others: Extracranial lesions of the head and neck: preliminary experience with Gd-DTPA-enhanced MR imaging, *Radiology* 172:165, 1989.
41. Schwartz JD and others: MR imaging of parotid mass lesions: attempts at histopathological differentiation, *J Comput Assist Tomogr* 13:789, 1989.
42. Shapiro MD, Som PM: MRI of the paranasal sinuses and nasal cavity, *Radiol Clin North Am* 27:447, 1989.
43. Silver AJ and others: CT of the nasopharynx and related spaces. I. Anatomy, *Radiology* 147:725, 1983.
44. Silver AJ and others: CT of the nasopharynx and related spaces. II. Pathology, *Radiology* 147:733, 1983.
45. Smoker WRK: Normal anatomy of the infrahyoid neck: an overview, *Semin Ultra CT MR* 12:192, 1991.
46. Som PM: Lymph nodes of the neck, *Radiology* 165:593, 1987.
47. Som PM: *Salivary glands.* In Som PM, Bergeron RT, editors: *Head and neck imaging,* St Louis, 1990, Mosby.
48. Som PM, Curtin HD, editors: *Head and neck imaging,* ed 3, St Louis, 1996, Mosby.
49. Som PM and others: Benign and malignant parotid pleomorphic adenomas: CT and MR studies, *J Comput Assist Tomogr* 12:65, 1988.
50. Swartz JD, Harnsberger HR: *Imaging of the temporal bone,* ed 2, 1992, Thieme Medical Publishers.
51. Sze G and others: Chordoma: MR imaging, *Radiology* 166:187, 1988.
52. Teresi LM, Lufkin RB, Hanafee WN: Magnetic resonance imaging of the larynx, *Radiol Clin North Am* 27:393, 1989.
53. Thrall JH, Ziessman HA: *Nuclear medicine, the requisites,* St Louis, 1995, Mosby.
54. Valvassori GE, Mafee MF, Carter BL: *Imaging of the head and neck,* 1995, Thieme Medical Publishers.
55. van den Akker HP: Diagnostic imaging in salivary gland disease, *Oral Surg Oral Med Oral Pathol* 66:625, 1988.
56. Vogelzang P, Harnsberger HR, Smoker WRK: Multispatial and transpatial diseases of the extracranial head and neck, *Semin Ultra CT MR* 12:274, 1991.

Chapter 4

Biophysiology and Clinical Considerations in Radiotherapy

George E. Laramore

The use of ionizing radiation in medicine dates back almost to the very date of its discovery. In 1895, Wilhelm Roentgen discovered x-rays, and 3 years later, Pierre and Marie Curie announced that they had isolated radium from pitchblende. The first documented radiation biology experiment was performed inadvertently at about this time when Antoine Becquerel developed a "burn" on his chest from carrying a vial of radium salt in his vest pocket. It soon became apparent that this newly discovered entity—radiation—had the ability to affect profound biologic change. The public embraced this new agent, and it was touted as a cure for almost every ailment known to humans. The results of these early clinical trials are not well documented, but it is probably safe to assume that most were not very successful. However, the first "cure" of a malignant neoplasm achieved with ionizing radiation was reported in 1899.[10]

During the early 1900s, most clinical radiotherapy was done by surgeons who used it as another form of cautery. Radiation was used in large doses to produce a "tissue slough" and the adverse side effects associated with its early use still color the attitudes many physicians have toward radiotherapy. Used properly, ionizing radiation produces selective modifications of cells through subtle changes introduced into deoxyribonucleic acid (DNA) and other cellular elements. Special training is required to understand these effects and how to best use them in clinical settings. From this need, radiation oncology has emerged as a separate medical specialty.

The capabilities of the radiation oncologist have increased in keeping with advancing technology. Initially, only low-energy x-rays were available, and these were capable of treating only superficial tumors, without causing severe side effects to the intervening healthy tissues. High-energy linear accelerators were then developed for research purposes and soon were used to produce "megavoltage" x-rays for medical use in a few large centers, although the "megavoltage" era in radiotherapy really began with the use of γ-ray beams from ^{60}Co sources. Now compact linear accelerators are used routinely in radiotherapy departments. Similarly, research into nuclear physics made it possible to produce many artificial radioisotopes that have had application in medicine; the field is no longer restricted to ^{226}Ra as it was in the past. Also, specialized, high-dose rate brachytherapy devices have been developed, which reduce the duration of the implant and simplify the radiation protection problem. Investigations in new areas such as particle beam radiotherapy, radiation protecting agents, hypoxic cell sensitizers, chemotherapy–radiotherapy combination treatments, and hyperthermia are taking place today and have the potential for changing the field of radiotherapy as much in the future as it has been changed in the past.

The purpose of this chapter is to provide the clinician with an overview of the basic principles of physics and biophysiology that underlie modern radiotherapy. Limitations of space necessitate the presentation of the overall picture only, rather than a detailed chronologic account of the development of the field. Topics will be covered in a manner that assumes no previous expertise on the part of the reader. The references cited will be representative and illustrative in nature rather than comprehensive.

BASIC OVERVIEW OF PHYSICS

Conventional types of radiation

Radiotherapy is performed most commonly using high-energy photons or "quanta" of electromagnetic radiation. The electromagnetic spectrum is a continuum with radiowaves 10 to 1000 m in length lying at one end and energetic cosmic rays 10^{-12} cm in length lying at the other end. The γ-rays produced from a ^{60}Co source are about 1.3 million electron volts (MeV) in energy, which corresponds to a wavelength of 10^{-10} cm. Energies of 3 to 5 electron volts (eV) are needed to break chemical bonds, and this typically requires photons shorter than 10^{-4} cm. Microwaves used for heating purposes are less energetic than this and act by exciting bending and rotational modes in molecules (e.g., H_2O).

High-energy photons used in radiotherapy initially interact in matter (i.e., tissue) to produce high-energy electrons by one of three principal processes: photoelectric effect, Compton scattering, or pair production. In the photoelectric effect, a photon excites a tightly bound, inner-shell electron and is completely annihilated. This process scales like Z^3/E^3 per gram of material, where Z is the "effective" nuclear charge of the material, and E is the photon energy. This process is most important for photon energies in the range of 10 to 50 kiloelectron volts (keV), which is the range typically used in diagnostic radiology. The higher effective "Z" of bone relative to soft tissue causes it to show up well on diagnostic films.

The Compton effect is most important in the 500 keV to 10 MeV range of photon energies used in therapy. It scales like Z^0 per gram of material and decreases in a complex way with increasing energy. Physically, a photon can be thought of as transferring a part of its energy to a loosely bound outer electron and emerging at a lower energy and longer wavelength. Within this energy range, all tissues absorb photons at about the same rate on a gram-for-gram basis. This is important for therapeutic purposes, such as when managing soft-tissue tumors adjacent to bone. On films exposed with megavoltage x-rays, the distinction between bone and soft tissue is lost.

Pair production refers to a high-energy photon being annihilated in the strong electromagnetic field of an atomic nucleus and producing an electron–positron pair. The threshold energy for this process is 1.02 MeV. It scales like Z per gram of material and increases with increasing photon energy. For a 10 MeV photon, this accounts for about 28% of the total absorption cross-section in tissue. Other processes also can take place at higher photon energies.

Once one of these primary processes has occurred, a high-energy electron is produced, which creates secondary ionization events as it travels through tissue. Typically, about 34 eV of energy is lost for each ion pair that is produced. The resulting ionization clusters are relatively isolated on a scale of typical cellular distances. Most of the events involve water molecules in the cell cytoplasm, and their reaction products initiate complex sequences of chemical reactions that generally involve free radicals. The biologic properties of different megavoltage photon beams are equivalent per unit of energy deposited.

Radiation doses are specified in terms of the energy deposited in a unit quantity of material. In the past, the conventional dose unit was the *rad*, which was equivalent to 100 ergs being deposited per gram of material. More recently, an international commission[58] has agreed that radiation doses should be specified in terms of *gray* (Gy), which corresponds to 1 joule being deposited per kilogram of material. The older literature will have radiation doses specified in terms of rad, whereas the newer literature will have the doses specified in terms of Gy. Doses in this chapter will be specified in terms of the latter unit. Numerically, doses in rad can be converted to equivalent doses in Gy by dividing by 100 (i.e., 100 rad = 1 Gy).

Typical depth–dose curves for photon beams used in the therapy of head and neck cancers are shown in the upper panel of Figure 4-1. The plots are for the dose along the central axis for a 10 cm × 10 cm field size. The energy of the beam is specified by the energy to which the incident electron beam is accelerated before impacting the target and actually producing the x-rays. The x-ray beam is a continuum with the maximum energy equal to that of the electron beam. To express that a range of x-ray energies is produced, the term *MV* is used rather than *MeV*. Appropriate filtering elements also are used to "harden" and "shape" the beam, but for most practical purposes, at a given source-axis distance (SAD), the beams from given energy linear accelerators are essentially equivalent. The three curves have the same general shape but vary somewhat in specific details. Note that they do not start out at their maximum value, but rather there is a build-up region, which occurs because the initial, high-energy electrons produced by the photon beam are directed primarily in the forward direction. The number of these electrons increases with depth until a distance equal to the average electronic path length is reached. The deposited dose is low at the surface and then increases to a maximum, after which it decreases with depth because of attenuation of the radiation field. The distance of the dose maximum from the surface is referred to as *Dmax*. It varies from 1.2 cm for the 4 MV (80 cm SAD) beam, to 1.3 cm for the 6 MV (100 cm-SAD) beam, and to 3 cm for the 15 MV (100 cm SAD) beam. The skin and subcutaneous tissues are spared within this build-up region, enabling the delivery of

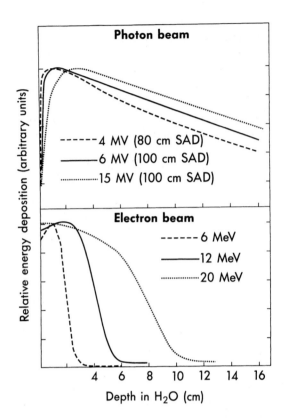

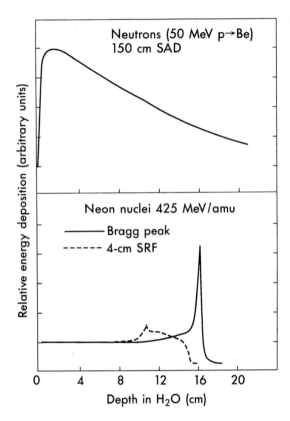

Fig. 4-1. Typical depth–dose curves for megavoltage photon and electron beams commonly used in the therapy of head and neck cancers. The upper panel shows curves for 10 cm × 10 cm fields for a 4-MV (80-cm SAD) linear accelerator (*dashed line*), a 6-MV (100-cm SAD) linear accelerator (*solid line*), and a 15-MV (100-cm SAD) linear accelerator (*dotted line*). The lower panel shows depth–dose curves for 10 cm × 10 cm fields for 6-MeV (*dashed line*), 12-MeV (*solid line*), and 20-MeV (*dotted line*) electron energies.

Fig. 4-2. The upper panel shows a typical depth–dose curve for a neutron beam used in therapy. It is for a 10 cm × 10 cm field size and was generated from a 50-MeV p → Be reaction at 150 cm SAD. The lower panel shows the pure Bragg curve (*solid line*) for a neon ion beam of energy 425 MeV/amu and the resulting curve (*dotted line*) when a 4-cm spiral ridge filter (SRF) is used to broaden the beam for therapy. The data in the lower panel are from the BEVALAC facility at the Donner Laboratories.

a higher dose of radiation to a deeper tumor. Higher energy photon beams can be used with even greater values of Dmax, but these have increased usefulness for the more deeply seated tumors of the thorax, abdomen, or pelvis.

Alternatively, the high-energy electron beam produced by the linear accelerator can be used directly in patient treatments. Typical depth–dose curves for various electron energies are shown in the lower panel of Figure 4-1. Note that these beams typically penetrate a given distance and then fall off rapidly. There is a slight amount of skin sparing for the 6 MeV beam but not for the others. These beams are useful for treating skin cancers, tumors of the buccal mucosa, or even superficial tumors of the oral cavity, provided that appropriate applicator cones are used.[55] Optimal treatment of a given lesion may require some combination of electron and photon beams,[50] and this in turn requires the services of a comprehensive radiation treatment facility. Megavoltage electron beams have the same biologic properties as megavoltage photon beams for an equivalent dose of absorbed radiation.

Particle radiation

In the strictest sense, the electron beams used in conventional radiotherapy facilities are a type of "particle" radiation, but this section will be devoted to the heavier charged particles (e.g., protons, α-particles, heavy ions, π-mesons, and fast neutrons) used experimentally at a small number of radiotherapy centers throughout the world. These particles are of special interest because of their different radiobiologic properties or their better depth–dose characteristics, which allow for higher tumor doses without causing a commensurate increase in the dose to the surrounding healthy tissues.

The particle for which there has been the greatest amount of clinical work to date is the fast neutron. A depth–dose curve for a beam from the cyclotron facility at the University of Washington is shown in the upper panel of Figure 4-2. Note that this is similar in general appearance to the photon beam curves in Figure 4-1. Fast neutrons are of clinical interest because of their radiobiologic properties, which occur because of the much greater amount of energy they deposit when they go through tissue. Neutrons are neutral particles and interact with the atomic nuclei, producing "heavy" charged particles such as protons, α-particles, or nuclear fragments that in turn create a dense chain of ionization events as they go through tissue. The distribution of these secondary particles depends on the energy spectrum of the neutron beam, and hence the biologic properties of the beam strongly depend on its energy spectrum. Neutrons used in therapy generally are produced by accelerating charged particles, such as protons or deuterons, and impacting them on a beryllium target. To a first approximation, the beam can be specified by indicating the charged particle that is accelerated, the energy of the particle when it impacts the target, and the distance between the target and the treatment axis (SAD). The curve in Figure 4-2, for example, is for a 10 cm × 10 cm field for a beam produced by accelerating a stream of protons to 50 MeV and impacting them on a beryllium target of a thickness that absorbs about 50% of the beam energy. It has approximately the same penetration characteristics as the photon beam from a 6 MV linear accelerator. Most often, cyclotrons are used to accelerate the charged particle beams, but special linear accelerators can be used.

Neutrons also are produced using deuterium–tritium (DT) generating tubes that yield a quasimonoenergetic beam of 14 or 15 MeV neutrons. Although the cost of systems using the DT reaction is lower than cyclotron-based systems, their lower neutron output makes them less suitable for therapy. Although once popular, such DT systems now are used for clinical purposes only in a few centers in Europe. Neutrons in the energy range most commonly used in therapy deposit most of their energy via a "knock-on" reaction, whereby a hydrogen nucleus is impacted, producing a recoil proton. This process is more efficient in tissues that contain a greater quantity of hydrogen, such as adipose or nerve tissue, and is less efficient in bone. Compared with muscle, the absorption can vary by ± 10%.[7] Typically, the recoil fragments produced by therapy neutron beams deposit 50 to 100 times more energy than the electrons created by megavoltage photon beams. The energy deposited by a radiation beam is characterized by its linear energy transfer (LET) spectrum. The primary high-energy electrons produced by megavoltage photons have LETs in the range of 0.2 to 2 keV per micron traversed, whereas the recoil protons produced by fast neutrons have LETs in the range of 20 to 100 keV per micron. It is this difference in LETs that results in the special radiobiologic properties discussed in the next section.

There also is considerable interest in using the charged particle beams directly for therapeutic purposes, which generally requires beams of much higher energy than those used to produce neutrons. The lighter particles, such as protons and α-particles, are of interest because of their extremely favorable depth–dose characteristics. The radiobiologic properties of these beams are similar to those of conventional photon or electron beams. In the United States, proton beam radiotherapy is carried out at the Massachusetts General Hospital using a Harvard University cyclotron and at a dedi-

cated clinical facility at Loma Linda, California. Heavy charged particles combine the favorable depth–dose properties of the proton and α-particle beams with the favorable biologic properties of the neutron beams. Energies are on the order of several hundred MeV per nucleon rather than the few MeV per nucleon for the recoil fragments produced by neutrons. These highly energetic particles do not deposit much energy in tissue until they reach the end of their path, where they are moving slowly. Hence, they do not produce much radiation damage in the intervening tissues.

The lower panel of Figure 4-2 shows a "pure" Bragg peak for a neon beam (solid line) and for its spread form (dotted line). These data are from the BEVALAC facility at the Donner Laboratories in Berkeley, California. Note the high ratio of the energy deposited at the peak compared with that deposited at shallower depths for the unspread beam. The Bragg peak itself is narrow, and so it must either be "scanned" across a tumor while its penetration depth is being varied, or it must be spread out by passing it through appropriate filters. The dotted curve shows the result after the beam is passed through a 4 cm spiral ridge filter (SRF). Note that this lowers the peak-to-plateau ratio of energy deposition, and at the same time, it broadens the trailing edge of the peak. Clearly, both are undesirable for therapeutic purposes, although the dose of radiation deposited along the initial portion of the path is still lower than that deposited across the spread peak, which represents an advantage over the other types of radiation discussed thus far in this chapter. The broadening of the trailing edge of the peak occurs because of fragmentation of the neon nuclei in the filter, and this does not occur with protons or α-particles. Thus, the spread peaks for the latter two particles have somewhat better localization than the curve shown here. A more sophisticated approach is to use true three-dimensional scanning, which changes the particle energy as the beam is swept across the target. Currently, heavy ion radiotherapy is available only at the Heavy Ion Medical Accelerator (HIMAC) facility in Chiba, Japan.

Another type of charged particle that has been used in radiotherapy is the π-meson. The π-meson is a subatomic particle produced by accelerating protons to energies of 400 to 800 MeV and then impacting them into an appropriate target. Magnetic fields are then used to focus the resulting π-mesons into a beam that can be used for therapy. The π-meson is much lighter than the other charged particles discussed in this section, being only 273 times the mass of the electron (the proton, for example, is 1836 times the mass of the electron). Like the other charged particles, it does not lose much energy until it is near the end of its path, resulting in a "Bragg-peak" type of energy deposition curve. When it stops, an atomic nucleus "captures" it and then explodes into massive charged fragments that deposit considerable energy in a very localized region. Neutrons also are produced in this process, and they deposit their energy throughout a somewhat greater volume. The biologic properties of a π-

meson beam are complex because of the large number of processes involved, but in a crude sense, they can be thought of as behaving like a mixture of low-LET and high-LET radiation.

FUNDAMENTALS OF RADIOBIOLOGY

Cell killing by radiation

Within the cell, there are certain key "targets" that must be affected by the radiation before the cell is killed. The nuclear DNA is probably the most critical target, but other elements, such as the nuclear membrane and mitochondria, also may be important. When any form of radiation interacts with the cell material, there is some probability that one or more of the key target areas will be directly affected. This is the "direct" mechanism of action. Conversely, the radiation interaction may be with some other element such as a molecule in the cell's cytoplasm, and the loss of this molecule may not be critical to the cell's continued function. The reaction products may be capable of damaging the critical targets, provided that they can diffuse to them and interact before being converted to nontoxic elements by other chemical interactions (for the OH radical produced by the interaction of radiation with H_2O in the cell, the diffusion distance is about 2 nm). This is the "indirect" mechanism of action. All forms of radiation interact by both mechanisms, but because of the smaller amount of energy deposited by low-LET radiation, it primarily interacts through the "indirect" mechanism. High-LET radiation kills a significant fraction of cells via the "direct" mechanism. Comparing the biologic effects of low- and high-LET radiation provides a way of studying the results of these two processes.

Perhaps the simplest biologic experiment imaginable is simply to irradiate a colony of cells with different amounts of a given type of radiation and see how many are alive and able to reproduce afterward. This is done by plating the cells out on a new growth medium and counting the resulting colonies. This assays for a reproductive viability that is the quantity of paramount importance in tumor control. The radiation is given in a single dose, and the cells are plated out immediately.

A plot of the surviving fraction of cells as a function of the radiation dose is shown in Figure 4-3. By convention, the surviving cell fraction is plotted on a logarithmic scale, and the radiation dose is plotted on a linear scale. This curve is representative of most mammalian cells. Consider the solid curve, which represents the survival data. Note that there are two distinct regions to the curve. There is an initial region for low radiation doses, where the slope of the curve is shallow. In this region, small incremental changes in the amount of radiation are not very effective at increasing the number of cells that are killed. This is called the *shoulder* region, and its width is characterized by the parameter D_q. It is the distance along the dose axis at a surviving fraction of unity between the abscissa and the point where the extra-

polated linear portion of the curve is intersected. It is a measure of the ability of the cells to repair small amounts of radiation damage.

At higher doses of radiation, the curve becomes a straight line on a semilog plot. Its slope is characterized by D_o, which is the incremental dose change required to reduce the surviving cell fraction to 1/e of its value. The steeper the slope in this region, the smaller is the value of D_o and the more radiosensitive is the cell line. When extrapolated back to a zero radiation dose, it intersects the abscissa at a value N. A curve of this type can be modeled using the equation

$$S = 1 - [1 - \exp(-D/D_o)]^N$$

where S is the surviving fraction, D is the radiation dose, and N and D_o are as indicated in the figure. In target theory, N can be thought of as the number of distinct targets in the cell that should receive one radiation "hit" before the cell is inactivated. Other parameters also can be introduced into the analysis by requiring more than one radiation "hit" to

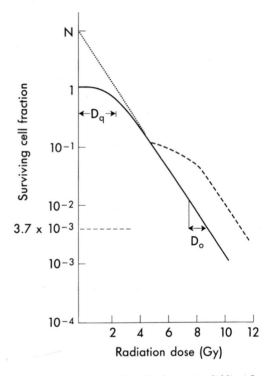

Fig. 4-3. A representative cell survival curve *(solid line)* for mammalian cells exposed to single doses of radiation. The surviving cell fraction is plotted on a logarithmic scale, and the radiation dose is plotted on a linear scale. D_q characterizes the width of the shoulder region, which in target theory also may be characterized by the extrapolation number, N. D_o characterizes the slope of the "straight line" portion of the curve. The *dotted line* shows the extrapolation of the linear portion of the curve back to the abscissa. The *dashed line* shows the regeneration of the cell survival curve if, after giving a certain amount of radiation, 6 to 8 hours are allowed to pass before additional radiation is given. (Redrawn from Hall EJ: *Radiobiology for the radiologist,* Philadelphia, 1994, JB Lippincott.)

inactivate a given target, but such refinements are beyond the scope of this overview. Radiobiologic data also can be analyzed using a linear–quadratic model of the form

$$S = \exp(-\alpha D - \beta D^2)$$

where α and β are simply parameters used to fit the curve over some restricted dose range.[35] Large $\beta : \alpha$ ratios correspond to curves with large shoulder regions. There is one final point to note from Figure 4-3. If 5 Gy are given, resulting in a 10% cell survival, and then 6 to 8 hours pass before giving additional radiation, the shoulder region of the survival curve is regenerated as shown by the dashed curve. During the waiting period, the cells have recovered most of their original ability to recover from small doses of radiation. This is called *sublethal damage repair.*

The basic features of the cell survival curves can be qualitatively understood in terms of DNA repair processes as outlined in Figure 4-4. The complementary strands of the helix are represented by the parallel straight lines, and the base pairings between the strands are represented by the open circles and dots that link the lines. In the upper panel, a photon schematically interacts with one strand of the DNA, which could either be via the direct or the indirect mechanism, with the particular nature of the damage event being irrelevant to the present discussion. What is important is that only one strand of the DNA is affected. Most cells contain repair enzymes that can excise the damaged portion and then, using the information on the complementary strand, can resynthesize the damaged portion. This is what is taking place in the shoulder region of the cell survival curve. If small amounts of radiation are given, there is a likelihood that many cells will experience only one damage event that can

be repaired in this manner, although when larger amounts of radiation are given, a situation as shown in the lower panel occurs. Now many of the cells experience multiple damage events, and there is increased probability that some cells will have damage to both strands of the DNA. When the cell attempts to repair the radiation damage, a portion of both strands is excised, and a portion of the genetic information is lost. If this information loss occurs in a "silent" region of the DNA, the cell continues to live. If the information loss occurs in a key area of the genome, then the cell ultimately dies. This is the situation that occurs in the straight portion of the cell survival curve.

Relative biologic effectiveness and oxygen enhancement ratio

High-LET radiation deposits so much energy as it goes through the cell that radiation damage events are clustered closely in space and time, which means that if one strand of the DNA is damaged, there is a high probability that the other strand also will be damaged. Thus, the situation as shown in the lower panel of Figure 4-4 occurs, with an increasing portion of the radiation damage being irreparable. As the LET of the radiation is increased, expect to see the shoulder of the cell survival curve decrease (i.e., $D_q \rightarrow 0$) and the slope of the straight portion of the curve become steeper (i.e., $D_o \rightarrow 0$). This effect is shown in Figure 4-5, which shows survival curves for human kidney cells exposed to 250 kVp x-rays, 15 MeV neutrons from a DT generator, and 4 MeV α-particles. The LET of the radiation increases as indicated, and the curves change as expected.

Because the shapes of the cell survival curves shown in

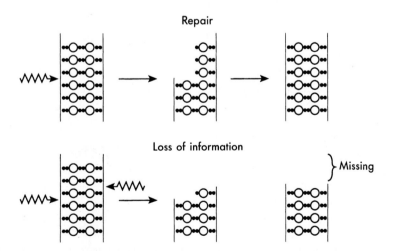

Fig. 4-4. Schematic illustration of the interaction of radiation with cellular deoxyribonucleic acid (DNA). In the upper portion, the radiation interacts with one strand of the DNA, and using the appropriate repair enzymes, the cell can excise the damaged portion and resynthesize the affected region using the genetic information on the complementary strand. In the lower portion, the radiation interacts with both strands of the DNA. When the cell attempts to repair the radiation damage, genetic information is lost.

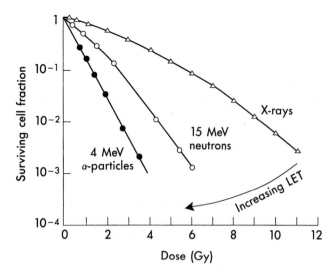

Fig. 4-5. Survival curves for cultured human cells exposed to radiation having different linear energy transfers (LETs). The *triangles* indicate data for 250 kVp x-rays, the *open circles* indicate data for 15 MeV neutrons from a DT reaction, and the *closed circles* indicate data for 4 MeV α-particles. Note that with increasing LET, the shoulder on the curve decreases, and the slope of the straight portion increases. (Redrawn from Hall EJ: *Radiobiology for the radiologist,* Philadelphia, 1994, JB Lippincott; original data from Broerse JJ, Bardensen GW, van Kersen GR: *Int J Radiat Biol* 13: 559, 1967.)

Figure 4-5 differ according to the type of radiation used, it is difficult to define biologically equivalent doses for therapeutic purposes. Consider the neutron and the x-ray curves, for example. If one chooses as an endpoint the amount of radiation required to kill 99% of the cells, this requires about 9.3 Gy of x-rays but only about 4.2 Gy of neutrons. Hence on a physical dose basis, the neutrons are more effective, and a relative biologic effectiveness (RBE) of 9.3/4.2 = 2.2 can be defined. If one chooses as an endpoint the amount of radiation required to kill 50% of the cells, then the respective doses are 2.8 Gy of x-rays and 1.1 Gy of neutrons for an RBE of 2.5. This situation illustrates a general phenomenon: because of the increased shoulder on the cell survival curves for low-LET radiation, the RBE for neutrons and other high-LET radiation increases with lower dose increments. The change is greatest for cell lines that have the largest shoulders on the low-LET curves (e.g., gut, nerve tissue) and is smallest for cell lines having small shoulders (e.g., bone marrow, germ cells).[30] In the early days of neutron radiotherapy, workers did not appreciate the dependence of the RBE on dose size and tissue type, which led to a high incidence of treatment-related complications. These effects now are being considered, and the incidence of complications is much lower.

Previously in this chapter, it was noted that low-LET radiation primarily killed cells through the "indirect" mechanism, which involved the radiation interacting with molecules in the cell cytoplasm. The sequence of chemical reactions that can take place is complex, but at some point, a free radical generally is involved. A free radical is a chemical species that contains an unpaired electron and is highly reactive. Oxygen acts to stabilize the free radicals, thus allowing them to diffuse to the DNA or other target regions where they react chemically to produce damage. An obvious question is how great an oxygen concentration is required. Experiments have been performed on many species of bacteria, yeasts, and mammalian cells; the overall conclusions are summarized in Figure 4-6, which shows the relative radiosensitivity as a function of the oxygen concentration in Torr (1 Torr = 1 mm Hg). Note that the radiosensitivity does not change much until the oxygen concentration decreases below about 20 Torr, and then it decreases fairly rapidly. At essentially 0 Torr, the cells are 2.5 to 3.0 times less radiosensitive than they are on the flat portion of the curve. Healthy tissues of the body are at oxygen concentrations between that of arterial and venous blood—between 40 to 100 Torr—and so are on the radiosensitive portion of the curve. However, large tumors tend to outgrow their blood supply and develop regions of necrosis surrounded by cells in a very hypoxic state. These tumor cells lie on the radioresistant portion of the curve, and this is thought to be one reason why large tumors are not as well controlled by radiotherapy as small ones.

One way of avoiding this problem is to use a mode of radiotherapy that is not as dependent on the presence of oxygen for cell killing. One possibility is to use high-LET radiation, for which the "direct" mechanism of cell killing is more important. Figure 4-7 shows cell survival curves for human kidney cells irradiated in well-oxygenated (open circles) and hypoxic (closed circles) conditions. If a 90% cell kill is chosen as the endpoint, then for 250 kVp x-rays, it takes 2.5 times as much radiation to kill hypoxic cells as it does when they are well oxygenated. The oxygen enhancement ratio (OER) is 2.5. As the LET of the radiation increases—going to 15 MeV neutrons from a DT reaction and then to 4 MeV α-particles, and finally to 2.5 MeV α-particles—the OER decreases to 1. This shows the effect of the increasing importance of the "direct" mechanism as the LET of the radiation increases. In general, the OER decreases with increasing LET until a value of 1 is reached, for a LET of about 150 keV/micron.

Cell cycle effects

Cycling mammalian cells proliferate by undergoing mitotic divisions. To define terms, take mitosis or M phase as a starting point. After this comes a "resting" phase, G_1, before the cell starts undergoing DNA synthesis. After DNA synthesis (S), there is another "resting" phase, G_2, before the cell again enters mitosis. Although it is well recognized that many chemotherapeutic agents act at specific points along the cell cycle, it is not commonly appreciated that cells vary in their degree of radiosensitivity according to their position in the cell cycle. Synchronously dividing cell populations are needed in experiments that measure this effect.

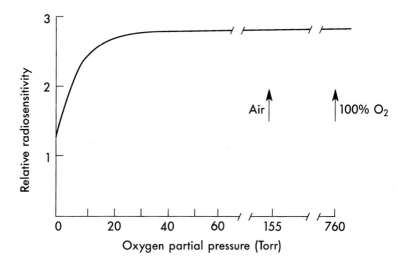

Fig. 4-6. Plot of relative radiosensitivity of cells as a function of the oxygen concentration in Torr. Well-oxygenated cells are 2.5 to 3.0 times more sensitive than their hypoxic counterparts. Oxygen concentrations for room air and 100% O_2 at 1 atmosphere of pressure are indicated by the arrows. This curve is schematic and is not meant to represent any particular cell line.

One way of producing such a cell population is to exploit the fact that at the time of mitosis, many cells growing in monolayers attached to the surface of culture containers will take on a spherical shape and become loosely attached to the vessel wall. If the container is subjected to a gentle shaking motion, these cells will become detached and float to the surface of the growth medium where they can be collected. These cells can then be inoculated into a fresh growth medium, wherein they will grow in synchrony through several cell cycles. Radiobiologic experiments can be performed on these cells at different times after "shake-off," and they can be caught at different points along the cycle.

The result of radiosensitivity measurements for typical mammalian cells is shown in Figure 4-8. Relative radioresistance is shown along the abscissa as a function of position along the cell cycle. The position of the cells along the cycle is shown at the top of the figure. The cells are radiosensitive early in the M phase but become more resistant toward the end of this phase. They are resistant in the early G_1 phase but then become more sensitive in the late G_1 and early S phases. They then become sensitive again in the late G_2 and M phases. Cell lines vary in the time they require to go through the cycle, but this is mostly caused by different lengths of the G_1 phase. The exact mechanisms underlying this change in radiosensitivity are not clear, but it is interesting to note that at the beginning of mitosis, the DNA in the chromosomes aggregates into a discrete state, whereas in the late S phase, the DNA content of the cell has doubled. These points in the cycle correspond, respectively, to the points of maximum and minimum radiosensitivity. Other variations in radiosensitivity may correlate with different amounts of sulfhydryl compounds in the cell. Sulfhydryl

compounds act as free radical scavengers and so act to protect the cell from the "indirect" effects of radiation.

Figure 4-9 shows specific cell survival curves for Chinese hamster ovary cells at different points along the cell cycle.[22,23,42] The open symbols are for cells exposed to γ-rays from a ^{60}Co source, and the closed symbols are for cells exposed to a fast neutron beam. Note that for each form of radiation there is the same type of variation along the cell cycle, but the degree of variation is about a factor of 4 less for the neutron beam. OERs are about the same for different points along the cycle, so this represents an effect apart from this.

Many tumor systems contain an appreciable fraction of cells in a noncycling or G_o phase. Radiation damage to cells in this phase cannot be monitored until the cells are recruited back into the cycle and until it can be seen whether they produce viable progeny. Noncycling cells can be produced in the laboratory by allowing them to grow in a medium until some key nutrient is exhausted. Cell proliferation then stops, and if the cells are kept in this suboptimal medium, the number of cells remains constant. Such cells are said to be in the plateau phase of growth[29] and are mostly in the G_o phase. These cells can be irradiated and then can either be immediately inoculated into fresh growth medium or can be incubated for a period in the suboptimal medium before the inoculation takes place. Once they are placed in the fresh growth medium, they return to their normal cycling mode, although the cell survival curve varies depending on whether they have been incubated for a time before being placed in the fresh medium.

This effect is shown in Figure 4-10. The circular data points indicate cells treated with ^{60}Co radiation, and for a

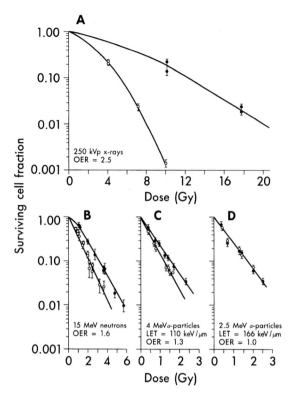

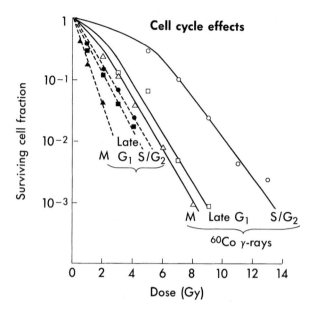

Fig. 4-7. Cell survival curves for human kidney cells irradiated during hypoxic and well-oxygenated conditions for radiation beams having different LET values. The *open circles* represent the well-oxygenated cells, and the *closed circles* represent the hypoxic cells. **A,** 250 kVp x-rays; **B,** 15 MeV neutrons from a DT generator; **C,** 4 MeV α-particles; and **D,** 2.5 MeV α-particles. Values of the oxygen enhancement ratio (OER) are indicated in the respective panels. The OER decreases as the LET increases. (Redrawn from Hall EJ: *Radiobiology for the radiologist,* Philadelphia, 1994, JB Lippincott; original data from Broerse JJ, Bardensen GW, van Kersen GR: *Int J Radiat Biol* 13:559, 1967.)

Fig. 4-9. Cell survival curves for synchronously dividing Chinese hamster ovary cells at different points along the cell cycle. The *open symbols* indicate cells irradiated with ^{60}Co γ-rays, and the *closed symbols* indicate cells irradiated with a 50 MeV D→Be neutron beam from the TAMVEC facility. The circles represent cells in late S and early G_2; the squares represent cells in late G_1; and the triangles represent cells in mitosis. (Redrawn from Gragg RL and others: *Radiat Res* 76:283, 1978; and Meyn RE, personal communication, 1984.)

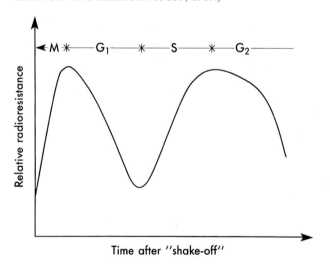

Fig. 4-8. Schematic illustration of the variation in the radiosensitivity of mammalian cells with their position along the cell cycle. The abscissa shows relative radioresistance as a function of time after ''shake-off.'' The relative position along the cell cycle is indicated along the top of the curve. The curve is schematic and not meant to represent any particular cell line.

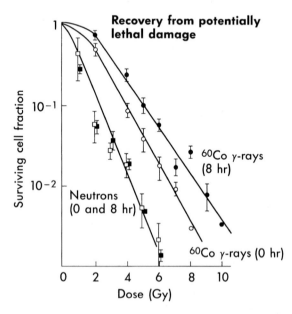

Fig. 4-10. Potentially lethal damage repair for Chinese hamster ovary cells irradiated in the plateau phase. The circular data points correspond to cells irradiated with ^{60}Co photons, and the square data points correspond to cells irradiated with a 50 MeV D→Be neutron beam from the TAMVEC facility. The *open symbols* indicate cells plated out immediately, and the *closed symbols* represent cells plated out after an 8-hour delay. Surviving cell fraction is plotted along the abscissa as a function of the radiation dose. (Redrawn from Gragg RL, Humphrey RM, Meyn RE: *Radiat Res* 71: 461, 1977.)

given dose of radiation, there are more surviving cells after an 8-hour delay than if the cells immediately started cycling. This effect is called *potentially lethal damage repair* because the effect of the radiation damage depends on what happens to the cell after the irradiation. The dose is only "potentially" but not necessarily lethal to the cell because the cell can repair itself before reentering the mitotic cycle where it is expressed. The square data points are for cells irradiated with 50 MeV D→Be neutrons. For high-LET radiation, potentially lethal damage cannot be repaired (or can be repaired only to a limited extent), a fact that may be important in certain clinical settings.

THERAPEUTIC WINDOW CONCEPT

Dose–response curves for tumor control and normal tissue damage are sigmoidal in shape. Whether radiation can safely control a given tumor depends on the relative positions of these two curves. Dose–response curves for a "radiosen-

sitive" tumor are shown in Figure 4-11. Here, giving a therapeutic dose of radiation results in a 95% probability of tumor control and only a 5% probability of normal tissue complication. There is a large gap between the two curves—that is, there is a wide "therapeutic window." This should be contrasted with the situation shown in Figure 4-12 for a "radio-resistant" tumor. In this situation, a dose of radiation that would result in a 95% probability of tumor control would result in an unacceptably high probability of normal tissue damage. Giving doses that are within the limits of normal tissue tolerance would yield only a low likelihood of tumor control, and the separation between the two curves is narrow. Clearly, the concept of a therapeutic window depends on the radiobiologic properties of the tumor and the healthy tissue in the irradiated volume.

In general, local control of tumors can be improved by better dose localization, which means moving higher on the tumor-response curve without moving higher on the normal

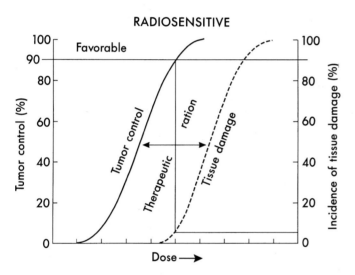

Fig. 4-11. Dose–response curves for tumor control *(solid line)* and for healthy tissue damage *(dashed line)* for a "radiosensitive" tumor. This corresponds to a wide "therapeutic window," in that doses that yield a high probability of tumor control have a low probability of causing healthy tissue damage.

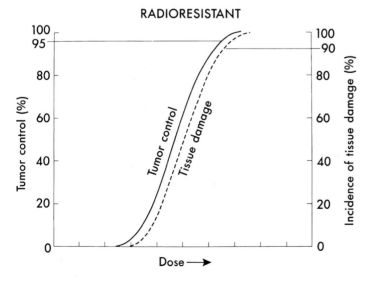

Fig. 4-12. Dose–response curves for tumor control *(solid line)* and for healthy tissue damage *(dashed line)* for a "radioresistant" tumor. This corresponds to a narrow "therapeutic window," in that doses that yield a high probability of tumor control have a high probability of causing healthy tissue damage.

tissue complication curve, or by exploiting some intrinsic difference in the properties of the tumor and normal tissues, which effectively widens the gap between the two curves. Three-dimensional treatment planning and delivery, brachytherapy, intraoperative radiotherapy, and the use of charged particle radiation are examples of the former approach; the use of high-LET radiation, altered fractionation schedules, radiosensitization agents, and radioprotective agents are examples of the latter.

CLINICAL CORRELATION

Fractionated radiotherapy

The intent of clinical radiotherapy is to sterilize tumors and at the same time to avoid untoward damage to the healthy tissues in the treatment volume. To accomplish this goal, fractionated schemes of delivering radiotherapy have evolved over time. The tumor and the healthy tissue consist of heterogeneous populations in regard to the position of the cells in the cycle. In addition, the tumor may have an appreciable fraction of its cells in a hypoxic state. Figure 4-13 shows what happens when such a mixture of cells is irradiated with equal-dose fractions of magnitude D. The

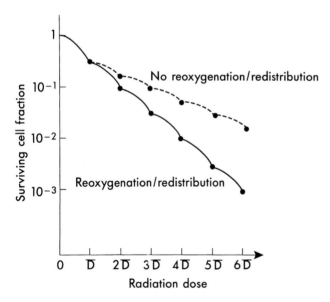

Fig. 4-13. Illustration of the effects of fractionated radiotherapy on a heterogeneous cell population. Surviving cell fraction is plotted along the abscissa as a function of the radiation dose. The dose is given in increments, $\overline{D}$, with the time interval between successive doses being long enough to allow for sublethal damage repair. The initial dose increment kills a greater fraction of well-oxygenated cells than it does their hypoxic counterparts. It also preferentially kills those cells in the radiosensitive phases of the cell cycle. The *solid curve* indicates when the remaining cells reoxygenate and redistribute along the cell cycle before the next radiation dose is given. The *dashed curve* indicates when there is no reoxygenation or redistribution, and successive radiation doses are delivered to a more radioresistant cell population. The figure is schematic and is not meant to represent any particular cell line.

first dose increment preferentially kills the cells that are well oxygenated and are in radiosensitive portions of the cell cycle. If several hours pass before delivering the next dose increment, during this period, there is repair of sublethal damage. With the killing of a substantial number of cells, there is less competition for the available oxygen, hence some of the formerly hypoxic cells can reoxygenate. Also, some of the cells can proceed along the cell cycle and thus be in a more radiosensitive phase when the next dose of radiation is delivered. Assuming that both effects occur, the result is the solid curve shown in Figure 4-13. If there is no reoxygenation or redistribution throughout the cell cycle, then the result is the dotted curve, which shows less cell kill because the remaining cells are in a radioresistant state. These are not the only effects: there is continued cell division and regrowth during the time interval between radiation fractions. These tumor repopulation kinetics have not been considered in Figure 4-13. To maximize the cell kill, it is important that the size of the dose fractions be greater than D_q—the width of the shoulder region of the single fraction cell survival curve.

These effects are known as the four Rs of radiotherapy: (1) repair (of sublethal damage), (2) redistribution (across the cell cycle), (3) repopulation, and (4) reoxygenation. Fractionated radiotherapy has evolved to exploit the differences in these effects between tumors and healthy tissues. With few exceptions, radiotherapy works not because tumors are intrinsically more radiosensitive than normal tissue (i.e., a smaller value of D_o, but because normal tissues are better at repair and repopulation.

Time–dose considerations are important in estimating the effect of a given total radiation dose. If the dose were given in a single fraction, then the healthy tissues would experience more cell killing than if it were given in a fractionated manner. This difference occurs because single fractions allow no opportunity for sublethal damage repair. In general, smaller total radiation doses given over shorter total treatment times produce the same normal tissue effects as larger total radiation doses given over longer time intervals. The classic measurements that illustrate this point are the isoeffect measurements on skin that were made by Strandquist.[49] He showed that the isoeffect lines for various degrees of skin damage and for curing skin cancer were straight when plotted on a log-log scale of total dose versus time. Moreover, the lines appeared to have the same slope (i.e., were parallel). The required dose to produce a given effect was proportional to time to the 0.33 power. Ellis[17] extended this concept to clinical radiotherapy by allocating a portion of the exponent 0.33 to the overall treatment time, T, and a portion to the number of fractions, N. He defined the nominal standard dose (NSD) by

$$\text{NSD} = \frac{D_t}{T^{0.11}N^{0.24}}$$

where D_t is the total radiation dose. The exponents in this expression are for skin and no doubt vary for other tissues.

The linear–quadratic model discussed previously in this chapter provides another way of comparing the biologic effectiveness of different radiation schedules. Assuming that there are ''n'' separated doses of radiation of magnitude, ''D,'' the cumulative biologic effect of the treatments can be given by

$$E = nD(\alpha + \beta D) = \alpha D_t\left(1 + \frac{D}{\alpha/\beta}\right)$$

where D_t is the total dose of radiation. Dividing through by α the following is obtained

$$\frac{E}{\alpha} = D_t\left(1 + \frac{D}{\alpha/\beta}\right)$$

where E/α is the biologically effective dose. For purposes of comparing radiation schedules, $\alpha/\beta = 3$ can be used for late-responding tissues, and $\alpha/\beta = 10$ can be used for early-responding tissues (i.e., acute effects). It is also possible to modify this expression to crudely account for tumor proliferation during the radiation course.[30]

Altered fractionation schedules

The highly fractionated radiotherapy schemes used today are the result of many years of clinical experience, but radiobiologic considerations may provide guidance for their future improvement. For example, acute radiation side effects such as mucositis and pharyngeal edema are caused by changes in tissues that are composed of rapidly proliferating cells. Late effects, such as subcutaneous fibrosis, vascular damage, radiation necrosis, and spinal cord injury, are caused by changes in tissues composed of more slowly proliferating cells. Radiobiologic measurements indicate that for low-LET radiation, the tissues experiencing late effects are characterized by cell survival curves having large shoulders.[57] It is the late effects that ultimately limit the total dose that can be delivered in the treatment of head and neck cancer. Hence, a logical approach would be to give smaller radiation treatment fractions so as not to exceed the shoulder on the ''late effects'' tissue curves and then give a higher total dose, which, it is hoped, would result in greater tumor control. This would effectively widen the therapeutic window. Note that the assumption is implicitly made that the tumor will behave like the rapidly proliferating healthy tissues and thus will not have a large shoulder on its cell survival curve. To avoid too great a prolongation of the overall treatment time and hence allowing tumor repopulation kinetics to dominate, multiple daily fractions should be given. A sufficient time interval (generally ≥ 6 hours) should elapse between the multiple daily treatments to allow for adequate repair of sublethal and potentially lethal damage in the healthy tissues.

Hyperfractionation refers to giving multiple daily doses of radiation of such a size that the overall treatment time is about the same as for conventionally fractionated course of once-a-day radiotherapy. Several randomized clinical trials recently have been completed using the hyperfractionation approach. The European Organization for Radiation Therapy in Cancer (EORTC) reported on a trial comparing a ''standard'' radiation schedule of 2 Gy-fractions, once-a-day treatment to 70 Gy versus a hyperfractionation schedule of 1.15 Gy-fractions given twice daily to 80.5 Gy.[32] A total of 356 patients with oropharyngeal lesions were studied. At the 5-year endpoint, the local control rates were 59% versus 40% ($P = 0.02$) in favor of the hyperfractionation arm. There was a suggestion of improved survival for the hyperfractionation arm, but this did not achieve statistical significance ($P = 0.08$). There was no increase in complications on the hyperfractionation arm, which agrees with the basic radiobiologic concepts discussed in a preceding section of this chapter. In the United States, comparative, hyperfractionation studies have been conducted that indicate the potential for improved local control for more advanced head and neck tumors.[45] The Radiation Therapy Oncology Group (RTOG) has conducted a dose-searching study to determine the maximum dose that could safely be given for patients with head and neck cancers.[11] Patients were randomized to receive either 67.2, 72, 76.8, or 81.6 Gy at 1.2 Gy given twice daily. A preliminary analysis based on 479 patients suggested an improvement in local tumor control at 2 years with increasing radiation doses for the lowest three dose arms: 25% versus 37% versus 42% ($P = 0.08$). No survival differences were noted, and the incidence of major late complications was the same at all three dose levels. Data analysis is still pending for the 81.6 Gy arm. A phase III clinical trial comparing hyperfractionation versus conventional fractionation for head and neck cancers is currently underway.

Accelerated fractionation refers to giving multiple daily doses of such a size that the overall treatment time is shortened relative to that of conventional radiotherapy. This may have a potential advantage for overcoming repopulation effects in rapidly proliferating tumors.[51] Wang has used such a schema in the treatment of advanced head and neck tumors.[54,56] He uses 1.6 Gy fractions twice daily, which is too high a total daily dose for patients to tolerate without a planned treatment interruption to allow for repopulation and recovery of the mucosa. No randomized trials have been conducted using this schema, but a comparison with historical controls indicates a possible benefit.

One of the more extreme accelerated schedules is the continuous hyperfractionated accelerated radiotherapy treatment (CHART) regimen.[14] This regimen consists of giving three daily radiation treatments of 1.5 Gy each to a total dose of 54 Gy without giving any weekend breaks. As might be expected, acute radiation reactions have been severe, but of more concern was the fact that there were two incidences of cervical myelitis. A comparative analysis with similar patient groups seems to show an improvement in local control, but as yet there have been no randomized studies with this regimen.

Another version of accelerated radiation that attempts to

limit the healthy tissue acute reactions is the concomitant "boost" regimen proposed by Ang and others, which delivers the accelerated portion of the radiation only during the last phase of treatment.[1] In this approach, the volume of tissue receiving the twice-daily treatments is limited to the primary target volume, and no breaks in treatment are given. There is a further theoretic advantage in that the accelerated portion of the radiation is given at a time when the proliferation rate has been increased for the tumor and the healthy tissues. The RTOG is currently carrying out a randomized trial using this approach as one arm of the study.

The altered fractionation approaches discussed previously have their rationale in the basic radiobiology of tumor and healthy tissue response. They all incorporate at least a 6-hour interval between sequential radiation treatments to allow for repair of sublethal and potentially lethal damage in the irradiated healthy tissues. Other types of "hybrid" schemes have been reported in the context of phase I trials involving small patient numbers. Although conceptually attractive, nonstandard radiation schemes have inherent toxicities and should be used with caution in nonprotocol settings. Late morbidity and efficacy data are still accumulating.

Brachytherapy

Many radioactive isotopes are used in modern radiotherapy practice. Although radium needles are still used as implants in certain head and neck tumors, the trend now is toward afterloading techniques using ^{192}Ir sources. These sources produce a lower-energy γ-ray, thus simplifying the radiation protection requirements associated with routine patient care. These sources are left in place for a specified time and then are removed. Alternatively, permanent implants using ^{198}Au and ^{125}I can be used. These implants deliver their total radiation dose over the effective lifetime of the radioactive material.

One obvious advantage to using implants for a portion of the planned radiotherapy is better dose localization, which results in less radiation damage to the healthy tissue surrounding the tumor. Another advantage is the relatively prolonged time over which the radiation is delivered. External beam radiation is given at the rate of 1.5 to 2.0 Gy per minute. A typical ^{192}Ir implant delivers its dose at the rate of 0.4 to 0.8 Gy per hour. This can be thought of as "continuous" fractionation, and it allows for healthy tissue repair and reoxygenation of the tumor throughout the time course of the implant. A typical ^{125}I implant delivers its dose at an even slower rate. Often high total doses in the range of 100 to 200 Gy are given, but one half of the total dose is given during the first 60-day half-life, one fourth of the total dose is given during the next 60-day half-life, and so on. The actual radiobiology of such extremely low dose rates is somewhat uncertain.

More recently, high-dose rate remote afterloading devices have been developed. These devices push a single, high-activity ^{192}Ir source through a set of interstitial catheters, and a computer program controls the source dwell time at various points throughout the implant. Typically, about 3.0 to 3.5 Gy is given to a distance of about 1 cm from the periphery of the catheters each treatment, and two daily treatments are given about 6 hours apart. Each treatment takes about 15 to 30 minutes, depending on the strength of the radioactive source and the complexity of the implant. There are approximate guidelines to determine how a radiation dose delivered in this manner corresponds to the more familiar doses delivered via low-dose rate implants,[5,52] but long-term late effects data are still being accrued. Because these treatments are given in a shielded area in the radiation oncology department, no radioactive material is left in the catheters when patients return to their room, and the radiation protection problem is greatly reduced.

Intraoperative radiotherapy

During the past several decades, there has been increasing interest in Japan and in the United States in radiotherapy directly administered to the exposed tumor bed at the time of surgery. Intraoperative radiotherapy (IORT) is given as a single, large fraction using either orthovoltage x-rays or megavoltage electrons. In this approach, it is often possible to move critical structures outside the radiation fields, and the surgeon can aid in identifying the areas at highest risk for residual tumor. A few institutions have dedicated equipment in operating rooms, but the majority of facilities offering IORT transport patients from the operating room to a sterilized unit in the radiation oncology center where the radiation actually is delivered.

Because the biologic effectiveness of a single large dose of radiation is much greater than if the same amount of radiation was given in multiple increments, the total dose given intraoperatively should be reduced compared with that given in a course of fractionated radiotherapy. Most of the IORT experience is for tumors of the abdomen and pelvis, but some general guidelines can be given regarding the tolerance of certain classes of normal structures of importance in the head and neck region. Major blood vessels tolerate single doses in the range of 20 to 25 Gy, whereas damage to peripheral nerves has been noted at doses higher than 20 Gy.[36] Tumor hypoxia may be a greater problem when the radiation dose is given in a single increment because there is no time for reoxygenation to take place. High electron affinic radiation sensitizers, such as misonidazole or SR-2508, may play a role in future IORT study protocols. Similarly, tumor redistribution kinetics do not have time to operate during IORT, and thus tumor cells in radioresistant parts of the cell cycle may be preferentially spared with this technique.

IORT probably can best be used in patients in whom there is a limited number of well-defined sites at high risk for microscopic residual disease. Possible indications are (1) tumor fixation to the carotid artery or deep structures of the neck, (2) "close" margins because of the necessity to preserve vital structures, or (3) tumor extending to bony structures such as the base of the skull, spinal column, sternum, or clavicle.

High-linear energy transfer radiation

Most clinical data on the use of high-LET radiation in the management of head and neck tumors are for fast neutrons. This will be the topic of this section.

Squamous cell carcinomas

The usefulness of fast neutron radiotherapy in the treatment of squamous cell carcinomas of the head and neck is a subject of considerable controversy. The first reported work dates back to the 1940s when Stone and others conducted a series of clinical studies using an early cyclotron at Berkeley.[48] A total of 249 patients were treated, and about half of these patients had head and neck tumors. Although many dramatic tumor responses were reported, the late complication rate was unacceptably high. Interest in fast neutron radiotherapy waned until the late 1950s when a better understanding of fast neutron radiobiology indicated that most of Stone's patients had inadvertently received extremely high doses of radiation. Investigation of fast neutron radiotherapy then began at Hammersmith Hospital, and an early report noted dramatic tumor response again, but this time with a more acceptable complication rate.[8] Unfortunately, other trials in Europe and the United States failed to confirm this benefit.[15,16,24,27] They showed no improvement in either local control at the primary site or in survival rates with neutron radiation, although they seemed to show improved local control for clinically positive neck nodes—45% versus 26%, $P = 0.004$.[25,27] This fact can be qualitatively understood in terms of the basic radiation biology of these tumors. Battermann and others measured the response rates of pulmonary metastases from various tumor histologies using fast neutrons and conventional photon irradiation.[3] They found that the RBE for squamous cell tumors was about the same as for the normal tissue side effects (RBE—3.0 to 3.8), so a therapeutic gain would not necessarily be expected if some other factor such as tumor hypoxia was not a problem and if OER effects would come into play. Guichard and others[28] have demonstrated in animal models that metastatic lymph nodes often have a greater fraction of hypoxic cells than primary tumors of equal size. Measurements of oxygen partial pressure in humans show that hypoxic regions within cervical lymph node metastases constitute approximately 20% of their volume.[21] Hence, it may be that tumor hypoxia in enlarged cervical lymph nodes, and not at the primary tumor site, accounts for the clinical observations reported thus far. In an attempt to resolve this matter, the RTOG undertook yet another randomized trial to study squamous cell tumors of the head and neck. The sophisticated treatment techniques now possible with modern neutron radiotherapy facilities were used, but unfortunately no particular benefit was noted for fast neutron radiotherapy for those with squamous cell tumors.[40]

Tumors that recur after initial radiotherapeutic or after surgical treatment represent another situation wherein high-LET radiotherapy may offer some benefits over conventional radiotherapy. Such recurrences may derive from clones of cells exhibiting a resistance to conventional photon irradiation. Further, the initial treatment may have compromised the vascularity, and the recurrent tumors may have a greater degree of hypoxia than tumors treated *de novo*. Two nonrandomized clinical trials support this hypothesis. Fermi Laboratories reported an 85% initial response rate, a 45% complete response rate, and an ultimate local control rate of 35% in 20 patients irradiated with neutrons for squamous cell carcinoma recurrent in regions that had received previous photon irradiation.[46] A report from Hammersmith on nine similar patients showed an 89% complete remission rate and a 56% local control rate at 1 year.[18] The rate of major treatment complications was about 25%.

Salivary gland malignancies

Based on the radiobiologic data of Battermann and others, salivary gland tumors exhibit high RBEs for neutron irradiation.[3] They found an RBE of 8 for fractionated neutron radiation of acinic cell carcinoma metastatic to lung, which would indicate a large therapeutic gain factor in using neutrons to treat this tumor system. Phase II clinical trials and a randomized phase III study support this conclusion.

The randomized trial and the historical series are summarized in Table 4-1.[26,37] The data in this table are for patients treated for gross disease—either *de novo* or for tumor recurrent after surgery. Patients with microscopic residual disease after a surgical resection are not included. Although the number of patients in the randomized trial is small, the difference in the local control rates at 2 years is statistically significant ($P = 0.005$). The rates of complete tumor clearance in the cervical lymph nodes were six of seven (86%) for the neutron group and one of four (25%) for the photon group. There was an association between improved local control and survival rate at 2 years—62% for the neutron group versus 25% for the photon group ($P = 0.1$). Given the dramatic differences between the two groups of patients and historical control data that closely paralleled the trial results, it was

Table 4-1. Local control rates for salivary gland tumors treated definitively with radiotherapy

Photon radiation		
Historical data	61/254	24%
Randomized trial	2/12	17%
Neutron radiation		
Historical data	194/289	67%
Randomized trial	9/13	67%

The appropriate references are in the papers by Laramore and Griffin and others. (Laramore GE: *Int J Radiat Oncol Biol Phys* 13:1421, 1987 and Griffin TW and others: *Int J Radiat Oncol Biol Phys* 15:1085, 1988; by permission Pergamon Press.)

thought to be unethical to continue the trial further. Ten-year data on this study recently have been published that continue to show improved local and regional control in the neutron group (56% versus 17%, $P = 0.009$) but no difference in survival rate.[39] The lack of correlation between improved local and regional control and survival rate was a result of distant metastases, which became of greater importance on the neutron arm because of a reduction in deaths caused by local disease. Neutron facilities now consider fast neutron radiation the treatment of choice for patients with either inoperable lesions or with gross residual disease after surgery. Salivary gland tumors constitute a diverse spectrum of histologies, and the fact that the number of patients in the randomized trial is small can certainly be criticized in this respect. Analysis of the historical series seems to indicate that all histologies of salivary gland tumors respond equally well to fast neutron treatments. There also was no apparent difference between major and minor salivary gland tumors. Given the rarity of these tumors and the current opinions of the radiotherapy community, it is unlikely that the randomized trial will be repeated, although data from larger patient series with longer follow-up times will continue to be of interest.

Charged particle radiotherapy

The use of "heavy" charged particles in radiotherapy allows the delivery of high radiation doses to tumors without causing much damage to the healthy intervening tissue. In terms of the curves in Figure 4-12, this enables work to be done at comparatively low doses on the healthy tissue side effects curve and at high doses on the tumor-response curve. The trailing edge of the Bragg peak for protons and α-particles decreases very rapidly because there are no fragmentation effects. With such beams, it is possible to deliver very high doses to the target volume with millimeter precision. In certain patients, such as those with juxtaspinal cord tumors, some head and neck sarcomas, and cordomas of the clivus, these beams often are the only way of delivering curative doses of radiation without causing life-threatening complications. Local control rates using this approach are excellent.[2,4,33] These beams also are used in the treatment of ocular melanomas, wherein they allow eradication of the tumor and preservation of vision at the same time. A study is currently underway comparing this approach for ocular melanoma with ^{60}Co plaque therapy.

Hyperthermia and radiotherapy

Hyperthermia refers to the use of elevated temperatures in an attempt to control tumors. In killing cells with heat alone, the temperature to which the tissue is increased and the exposure time at that temperature are the critical factors. There are at least three basic mechanisms that have been proposed in heat-induced cell death: (1) altered membrane permeability, (2) microtubule breakdown, and (3) enhance-ment of antigen expression or antigen–antibody complexation.

A marked synergy has been shown between hyperthermia and ionizing radiation. Tissue culture experiments show that the cytotoxic effects of these two modalities are additive in the G_1 phase of the cell cycle but are synergistic in late S phase. This may be a result of inhibition of DNA repair by heat shock proteins or by alterations of cellular membrane structures important in the repair process. Hyperthermia also seems to inhibit repair of potentially lethal damage in G_0 phase cells. A low pH renders cells more sensitive to heat, and in tumors, a low pH generally is associated with hypoxic cells. Hence, hyperthermia could potentially help to eradicate the fraction of cells most resistant to conventional photon irradiation.

The most significant impediment to a thorough study of hyperthermia is the inability to deliver and monitor thermal dosages in clinical trials. Methods of delivery include radiofrequency heating, use of microwaves, and ultrasound. In most patients, the resulting temperature profiles are highly inhomogenous, making it difficult to address fundamental issues such as the optimal sequencing of the two modalities. Although the relatively superficial tumors of the head and neck are easier to heat than more deeply seated tumors located elsewhere in the body, interest in the approach is waning because of lack of any documented clinical benefit.

Radiosensitizers and radioprotectors

Radiosensitizers are chemical agents that potentiate the effects of radiation. They should, ideally, be nontoxic in themselves. The basic idea is to increase the effect of the radiation on tumor cells but not on healthy tissue and thus "separate" the two dose–response curves. Hence, these agents should exploit some key differences between the two tissues. The halogenated pyrimidines such as 5-bromodeoxyuridine (BUdR) are preferentially incorporated into the DNA of rapidly proliferating cells in place of thymidine. After their incorporation, the cells are able to repair radiation damage to a lesser degree. The application of these agents for head and neck cancer may be limited because the oral mucosa is a rapidly cycling tissue and also is sensitized. High electron-affinic hypoxic cell sensitizers, such as misonidazole and SR-2508, preferentially sensitize hypoxic cells, which should be more common in tumors than in healthy tissue. Many studies using misonidazole have been done; the results are mixed. A review by Dische[13] showed that misonidazole was beneficial in only five of 33 clinical trials involving various tumor sites.

More recently, several randomized trials using misonidazole have been done. As noted in the preceding section on altered fractionation, the EORTC conducted a trial combining misonidazole with an altered fractionation regimen and found no improvement in either local control or survival rate compared with a course of standard fractionation radiotherapy.[53] A randomized trial was conducted in Denmark to evaluate the effect of adding misonidazole to two different split-course radiotherapy regimens.[43] A total of 626 patients was entered into the study. There was no difference in overall local control rates with the addition of misonidazole (37% versus 34%), but a subset analysis showed a benefit for the patients with pharyngeal lesions. The preirradiation hemoglobin level also was found to be of prognostic importance. The RTOG performed a trial of 298 patients, evaluating the addition of misonidazole to a "standard" course of radiotherapy.[19,20] There were no significant differences in either local control or survival rate, and subset analysis failed to reproduce the results of the Danish group with respect to either pharyngeal primaries or pretreatment hemoglobin levels.

A problem with the use of misonidazole as a hypoxic cell radiosensitizer relates to peripheral neuropathy, which is its principal toxicity. This limits the amount of radiosensitizer that can be used, and it may be that insufficient amounts have been used in the clinical trials reported to date. New agents, such as SR-2508 and Ro-03-8799, are more efficient radiosensitizers than misonidazole, and clinical trials using these agents may be more adequate tests of the radiosensitization concept.

Another approach to widening the therapeutic window is to shift the normal tissue-response curve to the right without changing the position of the tumor-response curve via the use of agents that selectively "protect" the healthy tissues in the radiation field. The radioprotective agent studied most extensively thus far is a thiophosphate derivative of cysteine known as *WR-2721*. This compound probably protects cells by neutralizing intracellular free radicals before they can interact with the key target areas. Clinical work shows that it protects the bone marrow during hemibody irradiation.[9] It is known that WR-2721 preferentially concentrates in the salivary glands, and thus it may be advantageous in reducing the xerostomia that often is a result of the radiotherapeutic treatment of head and neck cancer. New and more effective agents are being developed.

CHEMOTHERAPY AND RADIOTHERAPY COMBINATIONS

There are two basic intents to the addition of chemotherapy to the treatment regimen for those with head and neck cancer: (1) there is potentially a synergistic effect with radiotherapy by the chemotherapy altering the radiobiologic parameters "α," "β," and the effective tumor doubling time, and (2) the chemotherapy may be effective at eradicating micrometastases, thus reducing the incidence of distant metastases. By far, the most data have been accumulated on the sequential addition of chemotherapy to the regimen. To date, there has been no consistent, overall improvement in local and regional control or survival rate, although there have been several large, randomized studies that have shown a reduction in the incidence of distant metastases even though the basic intent of these studies was different. The

Intergroup Study 0034 investigated the effect of adding sequential chemotherapy after surgery and before radiotherapy for patients with operable tumors.[38] The Head and Neck Contracts study compared three arms—one with standard therapy consisting of surgery and postoperative radiotherapy, one with induction chemotherapy before standard therapy, and one arm with induction chemotherapy followed by standard therapy followed by maintenance chemotherapy.[31,34] A Southwest Oncology Group study[47] investigated the use of induction chemotherapy before surgery, and the Veterans Administration laryngeal study[12] investigated using the response to induction chemotherapy as a predictor of radioresponsiveness. The Padua, Italy, study compared the effect of four cycles of neoadjuvant chemotherapy plus radiation with radiation alone for patients with inoperable tumors.[44] The common finding in all these studies was a reduction in the overall incidence of distant metastases for the patients on the chemotherapy arm (in the case of the Head and Neck Contracts study, it was only for the group on the maintenance chemotherapy arm). Because distant failure is not the main cause of death for patients with squamous cell tumors of the head and neck, there was, in general, no improvement in overall survival rate. The Padua, Italy, study was the only one of the five that also showed an improvement in local and regional control and survival rate. The data are consistent with some modest efficacy of current chemotherapeutic agents for this class of tumors.

Currently, there is more interest in using chemotherapy concomitantly with radiotherapy, which has greater potential for giving a synergistic rather than an additive effect but also is associated with increased acute toxicity. Large scale, randomized clinical trials using this approach are only now being done. An early success of this approach is Intergroup Study (IG0099) for locally advanced nasopharyngeal cancer that has been stopped early because an interim analysis showed a statistically significant advantage to the experimental arm. In the experimental arm, patients were given concomitant chemotherapy consisting of cisplatinum at 100 mg/m^2 every 3 weeks along with radiotherapy followed by four cycles of consolidation chemotherapy with cisplatinum and 5-fluorouracil. In the control arm, patients were treated with standard fractionated radiotherapy. At the time of closure, median progression-free survival rate was 52 months on the experimental arm versus 13 months ($P < 0.0001$) on the control arm and respective absolute survival rates were "median not yet reached" versus 30 months ($P = 0.0007$). Nasopharyngeal cancer is unique among head and neck cancers in many respects, and the extension of this approach to other head and neck sites must await the results of other clinical trials.

REFERENCES

1. Ang KK and others: Concomitant boost radiotherapy schedules in the treatment of carcinoma of the oropharynx and nasopharynx, *Int J Radiat Oncol Biol Phys* 19:1339, 1990.
2. Auston-Seymour and others: Fractionated proton radiation therapy of

chordoma and low grade chondrosarcoma of the base of skull, *J Neurosurg* 70:13, 1989.

3. Battermann JJ and others: Observations on pulmonary metastases in patients after single doses and multiple fractions of fast neutrons and cobalt-60 gamma rays, *Eur J Cancer* 17:539, 1981.

4. Berson AM and others: Charged particle irradiation of chordoma and chondrosarcoma of the base of skull and cervical spine: the Lawrence Berkeley Laboratory experience, *Int J Radiat Oncol Biol Phys* 15:559, 1988.

5. Brenner DJ, Hall EJ: Conditions for the equivalence of continuous to pulsed low dose rate brachytherapy, *Int J Radiat Oncol Biol Phys* 20:181, 1991.

6. Broerse JJ, Barendsen GW, van Kersen GR: Survival of cultured human cells after irradiation with fast neutrons of different energies in hypoxic and oxygenated conditions, *Int J Radiat Biol* 13:559, 1967.

7. Catterall M, Bewley DK: *Fast neutrons in the treatment of cancer,* London, 1979, Academic Press.

8. Catterall M, Bewley DK, Sutherland I: Second report on a randomized clinical trial of fast neutrons compared with X- or gamma ray in treatment of advanced cancers of the head and neck, *BMJ* 1:1942, 1977.

9. Constine LS and others: Protection by WR 2721 of human bone marrow function following irradiation, *Int J Radiat Oncol Biol Phys* 12:1505, 1986.

10. Coutard H: Principles of x-ray therapy of malignant disease, *Lancet* 2:1, 1934.

11. Cox JD and others: Dose-response for local control with hyperfractionated radiation therapy in advanced carcinomas of the upper aerodigestive tracts: preliminary report of Radiation Therapy Oncology Group protocol 83-13, *Int J Radiat Oncol Biol Phys* 18:515, 1990.

12. Department of Veterans Affairs Laryngeal Cancer Study Group: Induction chemotherapy plus radiation compared with surgery plus radiation in patients with advanced laryngeal cancer, *N Engl J Med* 324:1685, 1991.

13. Dische S: Chemical sensitizers for hypoxic cells: a decade of experience in clinical radiotherapy, *Radiother Oncol* 3:97, 1985.

14. Dische S, Saunders MI: The rationale for continuous, hyperfractionated radiotherapy (CHART), *Int J Radiat Oncol Biol Phys* 19:1317, 1990.

15. Duncan W and others: Fast neutrons in the treatment of head and neck cancers: the results of a multi-centre randomly controlled trial, *Radiother Oncol* 2:293, 1984.

16. Duncan W and others: Fast neutron therapy for squamous cell carcinoma in the head and neck region: results of a randomized trial, *Int J Radiat Oncol Biol Phys* 13:171, 1987.

17. Ellis F: *Fractionation in radiotherapy.* In Delly T, Wood C, editors: *Modern trends in radiotherapy,* vol 1, London, 1967, Butterworth.

18. Errington RD, Catterall M: Re-irradiation of advanced tumors of the head and neck with fast neutrons, *Int J Radiat Oncol Biol Phys* 12:191, 1986.

19. Fazekas J and others: Failure of misonidazole-sensitized radiotherapy to impact upon outcome among stage III-IV squamous cancers of the head and neck, *Int J Radiat Oncol Biol Phys* 13:1155, 1987.

20. Fazekas JT and others: The role of hemoglobin concentration in the outcome of misonidazole-sensitized radiotherapy of head and neck cancers: based on RTOG trial 79-15, *Int J Radiat Oncol Biol Phys* 17:1177, 1989.

21. Gatenby RA and others: Oxygen distribution in squamous cell carcinomas and its relationship to outcome of radiation therapy, *Int J Radiat Oncol Biol Phys* 14:831, 1988.

22. Gragg RL, Humphrey RM, Meyn RE: The response of Chinese hamster ovary cells to fast-neutron radiotherapy beams II: sublethal and potentially lethal damage recovery capabilities, *Radiat Res* 71:461, 1977.

23. Gragg RL and others: The response of Chinese hamster ovary cells to fast neutron radiotherapy beams III: variation in relative biological effectiveness with position in the cell cycle, *Radiat Res* 76:283, 1978.

24. Griffin TW and others: Fast neutron radiation therapy for unresectable squamous cell carcinomas of the head and neck: the results of a randomized RTOG study, *Int J Radiat Oncol Biol Phys* 10:2217, 1984.

25. Griffin TW and others: Fast neutron irradiation of metastatic cervical adenopathy: the results of a randomized RTOG study, *Int J Radiat Oncol Biol Phys* 9:1267, 1983.

26. Griffin TW and others: Neutron vs photon irradiation of inoperable salivary gland tumors: results of an RTOG-MRC cooperative randomized study, *Int J Radiat Oncol Biol Phys* 15:1085, 1988.

27. Griffin TW and others: Mixed neutron/photon irradiation of unresectable squamous cell carcinomas of the head and neck: the final report of a randomized trial, *Int J Radiat Oncol Biol Phys* 17:959, 1989.

28. Guichard M and others: Radiosensitivity of lymph node metastases versus initial subcutaneous tumors in nude mice, *Radiat Res* 78:278, 1979.

29. Hahn GM, Little JB: Plateau phase cultures of mammalian cells, *Curr Top Radiat Res Q* 8:39, 1972.

30. Hall EJ: *Radiobiology for the radiologist,* Philadelphia, 1994, JB Lippincott.

31. Head and Neck Contracts Program: Adjuvant chemotherapy for advanced head and neck squamous carcinoma: final report of the Head and Neck Contracts Program, *Cancer* 60:301, 1987.

32. Horiot J and others: Hyperfraction versus conventional fractionation in oropharyngeal cancer: final analysis of a randomized trial of the EORTC cooperative group of radiotherapy, *Radiother Oncol* 25:231, 1993.

33. Hug EB and others: Locally challenging osteo- and chondrogenic tumors of the axial skeleton: results of combined proton and photon radiation therapy using three-dimensional treatment planning, *Int J Radiat Oncol Biol Phys* 31:467, 1995.

34. Jacobs C, Makuch R: Efficacy of adjuvant chemotherapy for patients with resectable head and neck cancer: a subset analysis of the Head and Neck Contracts Program, *J Clin Oncol* 8:838, 1990.

35. Kellerer AM, Rossi HH: RBE and the primary mechanism of radiation action, *Radiat Res* 47:15, 1971.

36. Kinsella TJ and others: Tolerance of peripheral nerve to intraoperative radiotherapy (IORT): clinical and experimental studies, *Int J Radiat Oncol Biol Phys* 11:1579, 1985.

37. Laramore GE: Fast neutron radiotherapy for inoperable salivary gland tumors: is it the treatment of choice? *Int J Radiat Oncol Biol Phys* 13:1421, 1987.

38. Laramore GE and others: Adjuvant chemotherapy for resectable squamous cell carcinomas of the head and neck: report of Intergroup Study 0034, *Int J Radiat Oncol Biol Phys* 23:705, 1992.

39. Laramore GE and others: Neutron versus photon irradiation for unresectable salivary gland tumors: final report of an RTOG-MRC randomized clinical trial, *Int J Radiat Oncol Biol Phys* 27:235, 1993.

40. Maor MH and others: Fast neutron therapy in advanced head and neck cancer: a collaborative international randomized trial, *Int J Radiat Oncol Biol Phys* 32:599, 1995.

41. Marcial VA and others: Hyperfractionated photon radiation therapy in the treatment of advanced squamous cell carcinoma of the oral cavity, pharynx, larynx, and sinuses, using radiation therapy as the only planned modality: preliminary report by the Radiation Therapy Oncology Group (RTOG), *Int J Radiat Oncol Biol Phys* 13:41, 1987.

42. Meyn RE: Personal communication, 1984.

43. Overgaard J and others: Misonidazole combined with split course radiotherapy in the treatment of invasive carcinoma of the larynx and pharynx: report from the DAHANCA study, *Int J Radiat Oncol Biol Phys* 15:1065, 1989.

44. Paccagnella A and others: Phase III trial of initial chemotherapy in stage III or IV head and neck cancers: a study of the Gruppo di Studia sui Tumorii della Testa e del Collo, *J Natl Cancer Inst* 86:265, 1994.

45. Parsons JT and others: Hyperfractionation for head and neck cancer, *Int J Radiat Oncol Biol Phys* 14:649, 1988.

46. Saroja JR and others: Re-irradiation of locally recurrent tumors with fast neutrons, *Int J Radiat Oncol Biol Phys* 15:115, 1988.
47. Schuller DE and others: Preoperative chemotherapy in advanced resectable head and neck cancer: final report of the Southwest Oncology Group, *Laryngoscope* 98:1205, 1988.
48. Stone RS: Neutron therapy and specific ionization, *Am J Roentgenol* 59:771, 1948.
49. Strandquist M: Studien uber die Kumulative urkung der roentgenstrahlen bei fractionerung, *Acta Radiol (Stock)* 55(suppl):1, 1944.
50. Tapley ND: *Electron beam.* In Fletcher GH, editor: *Textbook of radiotherapy*, ed 3, Philadelphia, 1980, Lea & Febiger.
51. Thames HD and others: Accelerated fractionation vs. hyperfractionation: rationales for several treatments per day, *Int J Radiat Oncol Biol Phys* 9:127, 1983.
52. Visser AG, van den Aardweg GJMJ, Levendag PC: Pulsed dose rate and fractionated high dose rate brachytherapy: choice of brachytherapy schedules to replace low dose rate treatments, *Int J Radiat Oncol Biol Phys* 34:497, 1996.
53. van der Bogaert V and others: Early results of the EORTC randomized clinical trial on multiple fractions per day (MFD) and misonidazole in advanced head and neck cancer, *Int J Radiat Oncol Biol Phys* 12:587, 1986.
54. Wang CC: Local control of oropharyngeal carcinoma after two accelerated hyperfraction radiation therapy schemes, *Int J Radiat Oncol Biol Phys* 14:1143, 1988.
55. Wang CC, Doppkes KP, Biggs PJ: Intra-oral cone radiation therapy for selected carcinomas of the oral cavity, *Int J Radiat Oncol Biol Phys* 9:1185, 1983.
56. Wang CC, Suite HD, Blitzer PH: Twice-a-day radiation therapy for supraglottic carcinoma, *Int J Radiat Oncol Biol Phys* 12:3, 1986.
57. Withers HR, Thames HD, Peters LJ: Biological basis for high RBE values for late effects of neutron irradiation, *Int J Radiat Oncol Biol Phys* 8:2071, 1982.
58. Wyckoff HO, Allisy A, Liden K: The new special names of SI units in the field of ionizing radiations, *Phys Med Biol* 20:1029, 1975.

SUGGESTED READINGS

Hendee WR: *Medical radiation physics: roentgenology, nuclear medicine, and ultrasound*, ed 2, Chicago, 1979, Mosby.
Johns HE, Cunningham JR: *The physics of radiology*, ed 4, Springfield, Ill, 1983, Charles C Thomas.
Laramore GE: *Radiation therapy of head and neck cancer*, Berlin, 1989, Springer-Verlag.
Meyn RE, Withers HR: *Radiation biology in cancer research*, New York, 1979, Raven Press.
Pizzarello DJ: *Radiation biology*, Boca Raton, 1982, CRC Press.

Chapter 5

Current Concepts in Antibiotic Therapy

Emily J. Erbelding
Anne M. Rompalo

With the availability of an increasing array of antibiotic agents, the approach to antimicrobial therapy is becoming complex. Increasing cost pressures in this era of managed medical care and new patterns of antibiotic resistance among clinical isolates make this area a challenging one for the continuing education of any practitioner. This chapter will discuss the principles of antibiotic selection and summarize the general features of the more common antibiotics that may be useful in the treatment of head and neck infections.

APPROACH TO ANTIBIOTIC CHOICE

Ideally, the chosen drug will be inexpensive, have a narrow spectrum of activity covering only the bacteria involved in the process, and be safe (Table 5-1). Antibiotic therapy can be targeted most easily when a bacterial infection has been defined by laboratory culture. For example, penicillin is prescribed for a patient presenting with pharyngitis whose throat culture grows *Streptococcus pyogenes*, or a combination of ceftazidime and tobramycin is prescribed to a diabetic patient whose mastoid bone fragment grows *Pseudomonas aeruginosa* sensitive to these agents. Gram's stain of drainage from infected tissue often provides valuable information quickly before culture results are available. Much more commonly in clinical practice, laboratory tests are not done, but a clinical diagnosis is made based on the presenting history and physical findings. If these support the diagnosis of bacterial infection, antibiotics are chosen to target the organisms usually responsible for the process. Knowledge of local bacterial resistance patterns, such as rates of penicillin-resistant pneumococcus in the community, may influence antibiotic

choice. Pharmacologic properties of different agents and their ability to penetrate physical compartments, such as the vitreous humor or the central nervous system, also will impact on antibiotic selection.

Most bacterial infections are treated with a course of a single antibiotic agent, although there are situations that call for combinations of antibiotics rather than monotherapy. Two or more antibiotics used together serve to cover a broader spectrum of organisms and may be an appropriate choice in a patient with a polymicrobial infection. Some combinations of antibiotics, such as penicillins and aminoglycosides, act synergistically (provide greater bacterial killing together than if the effect of each separately were added together) and are used together to enhance bacteriocidal effect. Combinations also may prevent the emergence of resistant organisms during the course of therapy, as in the treatment of tuberculosis.

The question of how long to continue antibiotic therapy is often asked of the infectious disease consultant. For some deep-seated infections, such as endocarditis or acute osteomyelitis, clinical trials lasting 4 to 6 weeks and documenting high response rates have defined the standard duration of therapy. For other infections, the recommended duration of antibiotics is defined by the response of the host. For example, in the treatment of pneumococcal pneumonia, antibiotics are continued for 3 to 5 days after the patient defervesces.

The cause of apparent treatment failure with antibiotics often is difficult to define. If the diagnosis was made presumptively, persistent fever can occur during the course of therapy because the initial diagnosis was incorrect or be-

Table 5-1. Commonly used antibiotics and their spectrum of activity

Antibiotic	Spectrum of antimicrobial activity	Common clinical indications
Penicillins		
Penicillin G	Most streptococci, anaerobic mouth flora, most pneumococci, *Actinomycosis*	Streptococcal pharyngitis, pneumococcal pneumonia, dental infections
Ampicillin, amoxicillin	Most streptococci, nonlactamase-producing *H. influenzae*, and *M. catarrhalis*, some *E. coli*, *L. monocytogenes*	Otitis media, acute sinusitis
Nafcillin, oxacillin	*S. aureus*	Cellulitis, deep infections due to sensitive *S. aureus*
Piperacillin, ticarcillin	Most streptococci, many *P. aeruginosa*, some Enterobacteriaceae	Infections due to susceptible *P. aeruginosa* (in combination with second agent)
Amoxicillin-clavulanate, ampicillin-sulbactam	As with amoxicillin/ampicillin, along with *H. influenzae*, *S. aureus*, and anaerobes	Sinusitis, bronchitis, infected diabetic foot ulcer
Ticarcillin-clavulanate, piperacillin-tazobactam	As with piperacillin/ticarcillin, along with *S. aureus* and anaerobes	Nosocomial pneumonia
Cephalosporins		
Cefazolin, cephalothin	Most streptococci (except the enterococci), staphylococci, some Enterobacteriaceae	Cellulitis
Cefuroxime	Most streptococci, *H. influenzae, M. catarrhalis*	Community-acquired pneumonia
Cefoxitan, cefotetan	Most streptococci, many Enterobacteriaceae, most anaerobes including some *B. fragilis*	Prophylaxis for colorectal surgery, treatment of mild abdominal infections
Cefotaxime, ceftriaxone, ceftizoxime	Streptococci, staphylococci, *Neisseria sp.*, most Enterobacteriaceae	Empiric therapy for bacterial meningitis, community-acquired pneumonia
Ceftazidime, cefoperazone	Most Enterobacteriaceae, many *P. aeruginosa*	Nosocomial pneumonia
Cefepime	Streptococci, Staphylococci, Enterobacteriaceae, many *P. aeruginosa*	Nosocomial pneumonia
Erythromycin	Most streptococci, many staphylococci, *Bordetella pertussis, Legionella* sp., *M. pneumoniae, Corynebacterium diphtheriae*	Community-acquired pneumonia, pharyngitis
Trimethoprim-sulfamethoxazole	*H. influenzae, M. catarrhalis*, many Enterobacteriaceae, many streptococci	Otitis media, acute sinusitis, exacerbation of chronic bronchitis
Ciprofloxacin, ofloxicin	Many Staphylococci, some Streptococci, Enterobacteriaceae, many *P. aeruginosa*	Pyelonephritis, malignant otitis externa due to *P. aeruginosa*
Aminoglycosides	Enterobacteriaceae, many *P. aeruginosa*	With ceftazidime as combination therapy for *P. aeruginosa* infections
Vancomycin	Streptococci, Staphylococci	Methicillin-resistant *S. aureus* infections

cause the organisms targeted in antibiotic selection were not the true pathogens. An abscess needing surgical drainage or a retained foreign body causing a nidus of infection can cause antibiotic failure, even if antibiotic selection was appropriate. Bacterial superinfection with a resistant organism, often occurring in hospitalized patients, can lead to treatment failure. An infection may be effectively controlled, but the antibiotic agent itself may cause fevers as a manifestation of an adverse drug reaction. Lastly, patient noncompliance with medication may explain apparent antibiotic failure if the prescribed therapy is oral.

PENICILLIN

Drugs of the penicillin class kill susceptible bacteria by inhibiting cell wall synthesis. Penicillin binds to specific bacterial proteins involved in the transpeptidation step that forms cross-links during bacterial cell wall synthesis. Resistance to these agents occurs by either the production of hydrolyzing enzymes (penicillinases or β-lactamases) or by altered affinity of the penicillin-binding proteins involved in cell wall synthesis.

The natural penicillins were the first available for clinical use, but resistance has now developed among many species of bacteria that were previously susceptible to these agents. Penicillin G remains the drug of choice for infections caused by *Streptococcus pyogenes, S. agalactiae Neisseria meningitidis,* anaerobic mouth flora, actinomycosis, and treponemes. Increasing levels of penicillin resistance among *S. pneumoniae* isolates in some communities have limited its usefulness in managing this organism unless laboratory susceptibility data demonstrate sensitivity. Penicillin V, the oral form of natural penicillin, resists destruction at gastric pH and is well absorbed. Repository penicillin preparations, such as procaine penicillin G and benzathine penicillin G, are slowly released after intramuscular injection, and low but persistent serum concentrations are maintained.

The penicillinase-resistant penicillin group includes methicillin, nafcillin, oxacillin, and dicloxacillin. They are used primarily in the treatment of infections caused by *Staphylococcus aureus*. They should not be used to treat infections known to be caused by streptococci, enterococci, anaerobic bacteria, or *Neisseria* species.

The aminopenicillins include ampicillin and amoxicillin. These agents possess enhanced activity against gram-negative organisms, such as species of *Hemophilus, Proteus,* and *Escherichia coli,* which do not produce β-lactamases. Any organisms testing susceptible to penicillin G also should be susceptible to the aminopenicillins. There are no major differences between ampicillin and amoxicillin in their spectrum of antimicrobial activity, but amoxicillin is better absorbed from the gastrointestinal tract.

The extended spectrum penicillins include agents with carboxy- or ureido- substitutions and provide the best coverage of all agents in the penicillin family against gram-negative bacilli and anaerobes. Ticarcillin and carbenicillin are active against *Streptococcus* sp. and against those strains of *E. coli, P. mirabilis,* and *Hemophilus influenzae* that do not produce β-lactamases. Mezlocillin, piperacillin, and azlocillin provide better coverage than ticarcillin and carbenicillin against *P. aeruginosa*.

Clavulanate, sulbactam, and tazobactam are β-lactam compounds with little inherent antimicrobial activity but that bind irreversibly to β-lactamases and inactivate them. Combining these compounds with β-lactam antibiotics enhances antimicrobial activity against β-lactamase–producing organisms and creates an agent suitable for treating polymicrobial infections. Amoxicillin-clavulanate, ampicillin-sulbactam, and piperacillin-tazobactam combinations retain the activity of the penicillin drug compound, but have extended activity against *S. aureus*, β-lactamase–producing gram-negative bacilli, and anaerobic bacteria. The addition of a β-lactamase inhibitor does not confer added benefit over that of the parent compound alone for activity against organisms that do not produce resistance through β-lactamase production, such as *P. aeruginosa* and methicillin-resistant *S. aureus*.

CEPHALOSPORINS

The cephalosporins, like penicillin, are modifications of naturally occurring antibacterial compounds. They have a β-lactam ring attached to a dihydrothiazine ring. Similar to penicillin, chemical substitutions on these rings alter antimicrobial susceptibility and pharmacologic properties. The drugs act by binding to penicillin-binding proteins to block cross-linking of the peptidoglycan wall. The cephalosporins are classified into four ''generations'' based on timing of release and antimicrobial effects. As a general rule, activity

against gram-positive organisms decreases from first generation cephalosporins to third generation cephalosporins, and activity against gram-negative organisms increases. Fourth generation cephalosporins are either recently available or still investigational. They provide excellent coverage against gram-negative bacilli and retain excellent activity against gram-positive organisms. None of the cephalosporins provide coverage against enterococci, methicillin-resistant staphylococci, or *Listeria monocytogenes*.

The first generation cephalosporins include cephalothin and cefazolin (both used parenterally) and cephalexin, cephradine, and cefadroxil (used orally). All are effective agents against community-acquired infections caused by streptococci and staphylococci, but they provide unreliable coverage against gram-negative organisms that are commonly involved in infections of the respiratory or urinary tract.

The second generation cephalosporins possess, as a group, expanded coverage against gram-negative bacilli compared with first generation cephalosporins. Cefuroxime remains stable in the presence of many β-lactamases, thus providing good coverage against *H. influenzae* and other agents of community-acquired respiratory tract infections. Cefoxitan provides activity against many anaerobic organisms including *Bacteroides fragilis*; thus it, along with other members of its class effective against anaerobes (cefotetan, cemetazole), is a suitable choice for the treatment of moderately severe abdominal or pelvic infections.

The third generation cephalosporins possess enhanced coverage against gram-negative bacteria. Cefotaxime, ceftriaxone, and ceftizoxime provide similar coverage against the same spectrum of bacteria and are useful for the treatment of serious infections caused by gram-negative bacteria. They all maintain good coverage against gram-positive organisms including *S. pneumoniae*, and all can penetrate the central nervous system reliably, thus providing good empiric coverage for the presumptive treatment of bacterial meningitis. They all have excellent activity against most strains of *E. coli, Klebsiella, Enterobacter, Hemophilus, Citrobacter,* and *Serratia* species. Ceftriaxone has the unique feature among the group of a long serum half-life. It can be administered at 12- to 24-hour dosing intervals and often is used when outpatient treatment of a serious infection is deemed appropriate.

Cefixime and cefpodoxime proaxetil are orally administered third generation cephalosporins. They are highly effective agents against *S. pneumoniae, H. influenzae,* and many of the *Enterobacteriaceae*. They possess only modest activity against staphylococci.

Cefoperazone and ceftazidime are the third generation cephalosporins that have activity against *P. aeruginosa*. They are less reliable than other members of this class against gram-positive bacteria, particularly *Staphylococcus* species. Of the two agents, ceftazidime has greater activity against *Pseudomonas* and penetrates the central nervous system well, making it an effective therapy for meningitis caused by susceptible gram-negative species.

Cefepime is a newly available parenteral agent classified into a proposed class called *fourth generation* cephalosporins, distinct from third generation agents because they provide exceptionally broad antibacterial coverage. Cefepime has very good activity against streptococci, *S. aureus, H. influenzae*, and gram-negative bacilli, including many strains of *P. aeruginosa*. It resists degradation by β-lactamases produced by some Enterobacteriaceae that cause resistance to third generation cephalosporins. This drug, along with other investigational agents in this class, will play a role in the treatment of nosocomially acquired mixed infections, especially those involving resistant gram-negative bacilli.

OTHER BETA-LACTAM COMPOUNDS

Imipenem and aztreonam are part of the β-lactam family and work against bacteria by inhibiting wall synthesis through a similar mechanism. Imipenem is structurally classified in the family known as *carbapenems*. It is highly active against gram-positive, gram-negative, and anaerobic bacteria and has one of the broadest activity spectra of any antibiotic. It is not effective against *Enterococcus faecium, Legionella,* methicillin-resistant *S. aureus,* and many coagulase-negative staphylococci. Cilastatin is added to the active drug to inhibit degradation of imipenem by the renal tubules and to preserve antibiotic effect. Imipenem-cilastatin is used for the treatment of serious polymicrobial infections, including those with resistant organisms.

Aztreonam is a monobactam agent that has activity only against gram-negative organisms. It is effective against most *Enterobacteriaceae, H. influenzae,* and many species of *P. aeruginosa.* Because of its relatively narrow spectrum of activity, it is rarely chosen when presumptive intravenous antibiotic therapy is indicated.

MACROLIDES

Erythromycin is a bacteriostatic antibiotic in the macrolide group that works by binding to the 50S subunit of bacterial ribosomes. It is one of the safest antibiotics available. It has good activity against *S. pyogenes, Staphylococcus* sp., and commonly is chosen to treat gram-positive infections when β-lactam antibiotics are contraindicated because of a history of an adverse reaction. It also is effective against many agents of atypical pneumonia syndrome and is the drug of choice for the treatment of legionellosis. Historically, erythromycin has shown good activity against most isolates of *S. pneumoniae* in the United States, but an increasing rate of resistant clinical isolates has been reported in many areas.

Extended spectrum macrolides have recently become available. Azithromycin is an azalide modification of erythromycin, but with better gastrointestinal absorption and a very long half-life. Its activity against gram-negative bacteria, including those that are common respiratory tract pathogens such as *H. influenza* and *M. catarrhalis*, is enhanced over that of erythromycin. It is an effective choice in treating sinusitis and otitis media. Azithromycin also possesses good activity against the agents of atypical pneumonia, including *Mycoplasma pneumoniae* and *Chlamydia pneumoniae*. Clarithromycin offers better activity against gram-positive bacteria compared with erythromycin and azithromycin. Both agents are suitable choices in the treatment of community-acquired pneumonia.

TRIMETHOPRIM-SULFAMETHOXAZOLE

The combination of trimethoprim and sulfamethoxazole acts in synergy to inhibit folinic acid metabolism of bacteria and inhibit their growth. Because the two drugs act at different steps in metabolism, resistance is less likely to evolve than when sulfa agents are used separately. Mammalian cells lack these synthetic enzymes and use dietary folate; thus, they are not susceptible to inhibition by these agents. The combination drug has a relatively broad spectrum of activity and is active against many species of streptococci, staphylococci, and gram-negative bacilli. They have no activity against anaerobes. Because these drugs have traditionally been effective against bacterial pathogens in the respiratory tract (*S. pneumoniae, H. influenzae, M. catarrhalis*) and are unaffected by β-lactamase production, the combination agent is a good choice for the treatment of exacerbations of chronic bronchitis, sinusitis, and otitis media. This agent is ineffective therapy in the treatment of odontofacial infections because it lacks anaerobic activity. Trimethoprim-sulfamethoxazole also is a common choice in the treatment of urinary tract infections and is a first-line choice against infections caused by *Pneumocystis carinii* and *Nocardia.*

Although *S. pneumoniae* has traditionally been susceptible to trimethoprim-sulfamethoxazole, the prevalence of resistance to this combination agent is high in many communities and may limit its effectiveness in treating upper respiratory tract infections.

QUINOLONES

Fluoroquinolones are a relatively new class of antibiotics available since the 1980s. They are bactericidal and interfere with deoxyribonucleic acid (DNA) gyrase, an enzyme essential in the superhelical twisting of the chromosome required in bacterial replication. Bacterial resistance to fluoroquinolones occurs by an alteration in DNA gyrase or by changes in outer membrane porins, which allow drug transport into the cell. Three agents of this class are currently marketed in the United States: norfloxacin is available orally, and ciprofloxacin and ofloxacin are available for oral and parenteral use. Ciprofloxacin and ofloxacin are well absorbed and achieve excellent tissue levels; thus, they are suitable for the management of moderately severe infections on an outpatient basis. Fluoroquinolones are active against gram-negative bacilli and cocci, including *N. gonorrhoeae, H. influenzae, M. catarrhalis*, the Enterobacteriaceae, and many species of *P. aeruginosa.* They also are active against many strains of *Staphylococcus* sp., but they have no activity against anaerobes.

Although ciprofloxacin and ofloxacin provide excellent coverage against common gram-negative respiratory pathogens, they have not proven themselves to be reliable against *S. pneumoniae* and are not recommended as a first-line agent for community-acquired infections of the respiratory tract. They are most useful in the treatment of urinary tract infections, including pyelonephritis and prostatitis. They also are effective in the treatment of enteroinvasive diarrhea, chronic osteomyelitis, and in soft-tissue infections involving gram-negative bacilli, such as diabetic foot ulcers or infected decubital ulcers. Invasive otitis externa in diabetic patients caused by sensitive strains of *P. aeruginosa* responds to oral ciprofloxacin, 750 mg, given twice daily for 6 weeks.

MISCELLANEOUS ANTIBIOTICS

Vancomycin is a glycopeptide that acts by inhibiting cell wall synthesis. Its spectrum of activity is limited to gram-positive bacteria. It is the drug of choice in the treatment of methicillin-resistant *S. aureus* and coagulase-negative *Staphylococcus* sp., and resistant diphtheroids and penicillin-resistant pneumococci.

Clindamycin works by binding to the 50S ribosomal subunit of bacteria and by inhibiting protein synthesis. It is effective in the treatment of infections caused by streptococci (except enterococcus), many staphylococci, and anaerobes, including many strains of *B. fragilis*. It is often useful in the treatment of gram-positive bacterial infections in patients who are unable to take β-lactam antibiotics and in the treatment of anaerobic respiratory tract infections.

Metronidazole is a bactericidal agent useful in the treatment of anaerobic bacterial infections and infections caused by some protozoa. The agent has no effect against gram-positive or gram-negative aerobes. It is useful in the treatment of severe anaerobic infections in which *B. fragilis* may play a role, brain abscesses, and also protozoal infections such as that by *G. lamblia*.

Chloramphenicol is one of the oldest available antibiotics. Despite its broad spectrum of activity and its relatively low cost, it is not widely used in the United States because of the rare but irreversible adverse event of aplastic anemia. It is bacteriostatic and interferes with protein synthesis by binding to the 50S ribosomal subunit. It is effective therapy against anaerobes, most gram-positive organisms, and rickettsiae. Although it penetrates into the central nervous system well and provides coverage against many of the agents of bacterial meningitis, clinical trials have shown that it is inferior when compared with cephalosporins, and these agents are now preferred in meningitis therapy.

ANTIVIRAL AGENTS

Acyclovir is a nucleoside analog that is effective in the treatment of infection caused by viruses of the herpes family. It is a prototype drug in its class. Acyclovir is activated after three phosphorylation steps, first by viral thymidine kinases and then by cellular kinases. The active metabolite of the drug, acyclovir triphosphate, inhibits replication of susceptible viruses by inhibiting viral DNA polymerase. Oral acyclovir is used in the management of symptomatic outbreaks of herpes labialis and genital herpes in hosts with normal immunity. Intravenous acyclovir is recommended for serious infections caused by herpesvirus infections in hosts with compromised immunity or in the management of life-threatening infections such as herpes encephalitis. Acyclovir has been shown to decrease viral shedding, time to lesion healing, and the formation of new lesions caused by herpes simplex virus, but it does not prevent future recurrences. High dose (800 mg, 5 times daily) oral acyclovir is effective in the treatment of herpes zoster and zoster ophthalmicus. It reduces the duration of symptoms in primary infections due to varicella-zoster virus if therapy is begun within 24 hours of the onset of rash. Topical forms of acyclovir are available, but they do not affect the development of new herpes lesions and are not considered as effective as systemic therapy.

Valaciclovir is an ester prodrug form of acyclovir that is more bioavailable than acyclovir. After absorption, it is hydrolyzed to acyclovir and therefore confers no extra benefit in treating acyclovir-resistant viral strains. Famciclovir is the ester prodrug of penciclovir, a nucleoside analog that is similar in structure to acyclovir and undergoes phosphorylation to an active intracellular metabolite in a similar manner. Valaciclovir and famciclovir are approved for the treatment of herpes zoster infections.

ANTIFUNGAL AGENTS

Amphotericin B is one of the oldest antifungal agents and, given intravenously, is the mainstay for treatment of invasive fungal infections. It is a polyene compound that binds avidly to ergosterol of fungal cell membranes to cause leakage and cell death. After administration, it is distributed throughout the body but accumulates predominantly in the liver and lungs and then is slowly released from tissue stores for weeks after administration. Toxicities include bone marrow suppression and renal impairment. Oral amphotericin solution is available for the treatment of thrush. A liposomal amphotericin formulation is available for targeted drug delivery in patients who either cannot tolerate the standard formulation or are at high risk for amphotericin-related toxicity.

Ketoconazole, fluconazole, and itraconazole are azole agents that are available for the oral therapy of fungal infections. Fluconazole and ketoconazole also are available intravenously. They are effective in treating oral candidal infections and may be useful in the treatment of some deeper infections. Fluconazole is reliably absorbed and is used for the treatment of systemic cryptococcosis in patients with acquired immunodeficiency syndrome (AIDS). Other topical agents effective for the treatment of oral candidiasis include clotrimazole and nystatin.

THE IMMUNOCOMPROMISED HOST

In this era of AIDS and of increasing success maintaining solid organ transplantations and treating malignancies, a large proportion of hospitalized patients may have compromised immune systems. Specific host abnormalities predisposing to bacterial infection include (1) neutropenia, such as that after chemotherapy, or qualitative defects in neutrophil function; (2) defects in humoral immunity with either complement defects or impaired antibody formation, such as that observed in patients with multiple myeloma; and (3) specific defects in cell-mediated immunity, such as that observed in organ transplantation patients on immunosuppressive regimens or in those with AIDS. Some of these conditions uniquely predispose to certain types of infections, and guidelines exist for presumptive antibiotic therapy, but the list of possible etiologic agents is usually broad enough in the compromised host that pursuing a specific microbiologic diagnosis through invasive measures is warranted. Because many of these conditions also lead to an impaired inflammatory response, physical signs indicating inflammation (meningismus, or erythema and fluctuance at an abscess site) are often absent, even with an established infection, in the setting of immunocompromise.

Neutropenia after cancer chemotherapy is one of the commonest immune defects encountered and is one with some guidelines established for antibiotic management in those with suspected infection. A patient with fever and absolute neutropenia (a neutrophil count below 500/mm^3) should be thoroughly examined for any suggestion of infection and then begun on presumptive antibiotic therapy. Bacteremia with gram-negative organisms (including *P. aeruginosa*) is a common cause of fever in the early period of neutropenia and may lead to rapid clinical deterioration. Thus, initial antibiotic therapy should always provide good gram-negative coverage that includes activity against *P. aeruginosa*. In some institutions, gram-positive bacteria also are a common cause of early fever in the neutropenic host, especially in patients with an indwelling intravenous catheter, and vancomycin therapy directed against common pathogens associated with line infections (coagulase-negative *Staphylococcus* species) also is added initially. For the patient who has persistent fevers (more than 5 to 7 days) on broad spectrum antibiotic therapy, empiric antifungal coverage with amphotericin B is recommended.

SUGGESTED READINGS

Anonymous: Azithromycin and clarithromycin, *Med Lett Drugs Ther* 34: 45, 1992.

Anonymous: Ciprofloxacin, *Med Lett Drugs Ther* 30:11, 1988.

Anonymous: The choice of antibacterial drugs, *Med Lett Drugs Ther* 34: 49, 1992.

Anonymous: Famciclovir for herpes zoster, *Med Lett Drugs Ther* 36:97, 1994.

Anonymous: Ofloxacin, *Med Lett Drugs Ther* 30:75, 1991.

Bartlett JG: *Pocket book of infectious disease therapy*, ed 7, Baltimore, 1996, Williams & Wilkins.

Easterbrook P, Wood MJ: Successors to acyclovir, *J Antimicrob Chemother* 34:307, 1994.

Hill MK, Sanders CV: Principles of antimicrobial therapy for head and neck infections, *Med Clin North Am* 66:57, 1988.

Lonks JR, Medeiros AA: The growing threat of antibiotic-resistant *Streptococcus pneumoniae, Med Clin North Am* 79:523, 1995.

Mandell GL, Douglas RG Jr, Bennett JE: *Principles and practice of infectious diseases*, ed 4, New York, 1995, Churchill Livingstone.

Pizzo PA: Management of fever in patients with cancer and treatment-induced neutropenia, *N Engl J Med* 328:1323, 1993.

Sand MA, Kapusnik-Uner JE, Mandell GL: *Chemotherapy of microbial diseases.* Section XI in *Goodman and Gilman's the pharmacologic basis of therapeutics*, ed 8, New York, 1990, Pergamon Press.

Schreiber JR, Jacobs MR: Antibiotic-resistant pneumococci, *Pediatr Clin North Am* 42:519, 1995.

Chapter 6

Chemotherapy for Head and Neck Cancer

William H. Liggett, Jr.
Arlene A. Forastiere

The otolaryngologist frequently cares for patients with head and neck cancer who will receive chemotherapy as part of their treatment (Table 6-1). These patients usually have metastatic or locally advanced disease that is not amenable to curative therapy with surgery or radiation. Many have previously undergone surgery and radiotherapy. Chemotherapy also is indicated for those with advanced carcinomas of the larynx as part of primary curative treatment when voice preservation is desired. Chemotherapy also may be used in experimental protocols as primary therapy or combined with radiotherapy (chemoradiation) for patients with a high risk of relapse. The majority of the malignancies encountered are squamous carcinomas, with salivary gland cancers the next most common histology. Melanomas and sarcomas also are seen in the head and neck, although they are much rarer.

To evaluate the appropriate use of chemotherapy for these patients, the surgeon should be familiar with the following: (1) the principles of clinical trials, (2) the proper doses and expected toxic reactions of specific chemotherapeutic agents, (3) the basic principles of combination chemotherapy and combined modality programs, and (4) the standard use and experimental approaches of chemotherapy for head and neck squamous cancers and salivary gland tumors.

PRINCIPLES OF CLINICAL TRIALS

The efficacy of chemotherapy or combined modality programs is investigated through clinical trials.[190] To evaluate the use of a particular treatment, clinicians establish at the onset the parameters to be evaluated: object response rate, survival, disease-free survival or duration of response, and toxicity. The parameters of interest for a specific trial design are defined before the initiation of study and analyzed at the completion of the study. The primary endpoint depends on the nature of the clinical trial or phase of testing.

The evaluation of chemotherapeutic agents occurs in three steps or phases. The goals of phase I trials are to determine the toxic effects associated with a new drug and to establish the highest dose of the drug that can be safely administered. Patients with different tumor types refractory to conventional chemotherapy are enrolled. The purpose of phase II trials is to determine if a drug or drug combination tested in patients with the same tumor type has enough activity to warrant further testing in a comparative trial. The primary endpoint is response rate. Phase III trials are randomized comparisons of two or more treatment options, often comparing a standard treatment to a new or more complex therapy. Response rate, disease-free survival, or response duration and survival are primary endpoints. The determination of sample size, patient entry criteria, and the follow-up evaluation and monitoring of patients are critical for a valid interpretation of a phase III trial.[161]

Standard definitions exist for the various endpoints in clinical trials that allow objective reporting of results. Definitions of response are complete, partial, minor, stable, and progressive disease (Box 6-1). The most meaningful response in terms of prolongation of survival is the attainment of a complete response in which no tumor is detectable after a thorough examination. By convention, a partial response indicates that the disease has regressed by at least 50% as determined by serial bidimensional measurements and that

Table 6-1. Chemotherapeutic agents with activity in head and neck cancers

Agent	Mechanism	Toxicity
Alkylators		
Cyclophosphamide	DNA cross-linker	Neutropenia, nausea, cystitis
Ifosfamide	DNA cross-linker	Myelosuppression, cystitis, confusion, alopecia
Antimetabolities		
Methotrexate	Binds dihydrofolate reductase	Mucositis, myelosuppression
5-Fluorouracil	Inhibits thymidylate synthetase	Mucositis, myelosuppression, diarrhea
Antibodies		
Bleomycin	Scission of DNA	Pulmonary fibrosis, rash, mucositis
Adriamycin	DNA intercalator	Cardiotoxicity, mucositis, myelosuppression, alopecia
Vinca Alkaloids		
Vincristine	Mitotic arrest	Neurotoxicity, myelosuppression, alopecia
Vinblastine	Mitotic arrest	Neurotoxicity, myelosuppression, alopecia
Miscellaneous		
Cisplatin	DNA intercalator	Nephrotoxicity, vomiting, ototoxicity, neuropathy
Carboplatin	DNA intercalator	Myelosuppression
Taxanes		
Paclitaxel	Microtubule stabilizer	Myelosuppression, neuropathy
Docetaxel	Microtubule stabilizer	Edema, neutropenia, neuropathy

---

Box 6-1. Criteria for response

Complete response	Complete disappearance of all evidence of tumor for at least 4 weeks.
Partial response	Disease regression by at least 50% of the sum of the product of the perpendicular diameters of all measurable tumor for at least 4 weeks. No simultaneous increase in the size of any lesion or appearance of new lesions may occur.
Minor response	Regression by less than 50% of the sum of the products of the perpendicular diameters of all measurable lesions.
Stable disease	No appreciable change in dimensions of all evaluable lesions.
Progressive disease	Increase in the size of any detectable lesions by at least 25% or the appearance of new lesions.

---

no new lesions have appeared elsewhere for a period of at least 4 weeks. The response rate represents the number of complete and partial responders. Minor response or stable disease usually is of little value.

Once a study is completed, there are several ways to compute response rate. In calculating the fraction of responders, the numerator should always be the number of patients who qualify in a particular response category, but the denominator often varies from study to study. Some investigators compute response rate using all patients entered into a study, whereas others evaluate response rates after eliminating early death or patients failing to receive a specific number of cycles of treatment. The latter method of computing a response rate results in a much larger value than the former.

Survival usually is calculated from date of study entry until date of death. Disease-free survival is calculated from study entry until disease progression or from achievement of complete response until disease progression. Duration of response is calculated from response date until date of disease progression. Toxicity should be strictly defined for every study before initiation. The National Cancer Institute has developed a comprehensive set of standardized drug-induced toxicity criteria. Using a 0 to 4 grading scale, toxicity to each organ system can be objectively assessed. All toxic reactions should be reported in detail in the final results.

In planning a clinical trial, particularly a phase III trial, having comparable patients in each group is critical. This requirement often is accomplished by randomization with stratification for important prognostic variables. Prognostic variables are those factors known to influence response, regardless of treatment. One of the more well-known, important prognostic variables is the Karnofsky Performance Status. In 1948, a 0 to 100 performance scale was devised by

---

Box 6-2. Performance status

ECOG, SWOG, Zubrid Scales

0 Fully active, able to carry on all predisease performance without restriction

1 Restricted in physical strenuous activity but ambulatory and able to do work of a light or sedentary nature, e.g., light housework, office work

2 Ambulatory and capable of all selfcare but unable to do any work activities; up and about more than 50% of waking hours

3 Capable of only limited selfcare, confined to bed or chair more than 50% of waking hours

4 Completely disabled. Cannot do any selfcare; totally confined to bed or chair

5 Dead

Karnofsky Scale

100 Normal, no complaints, no evidence of disease

90 Able to carry on normal activity; minor signs or symptoms

80 Normal activity with effort; some signs or symptoms of disease

70 Cares for self; unable to do normal activity or active work

60 Requires occasional assistance, but is able to care for most needs

50 Requires considerable assistance and frequent medical care

40 Disabled, requires special care and assistance

30 Severely disabled, hospitalization indicated; death not imminent

20 Very sick, hospitalization and active support treatment necessary

10 Moribund, fatal process, progressing rapidly

0 Dead

ECOG—Eastern Cooperative Oncology Group; SWOG—Southwestern Oncology Group

David Karnofsky to describe a patient's functional ability. This scale is used today interchangeably with a 0 to 5 point scale (Box 6-2) adapted by several cooperative groups. Performance status is an established prognostic variable that directly correlates with response to chemotherapy. Those patients with a performance status greater than 2 or less than 50% are poor candidates for phase II and III clinical trials and are poor candidates for chemotherapy with palliative intent. These patients usually have a large tumor burden, are malnourished, and have a very short survival time regardless of treatment. By definition, they are nonambulatory for more than 50% of their waking hours and require special care and assistance. If a trial is randomized but not stratified for performance status, a large number of patients with poor Karnofsky Performance Status could be randomized to one of the treatment groups and make it appear less efficacious than a second, when it actually may be equal or better. Important prognostic variables should be defined at the onset of a study and analyzed in the results.

It is important in designing and drawing conclusions from trials to note whether the trial is prospectively randomized with concurrent controls or is a clinical trial with historical controls. Proponents of the randomized trial believe that one is more certain of equality between the two groups by a concurrent randomization process.[190] This will reduce the bias of selecting controls from a historical pool and also will reduce the problem of improvements in management or changes in treating physicians with time.

SQUAMOUS CELL CARCINOMA

Overview of current concepts

Before 1970, chemotherapy had a limited role in the management of squamous cell cancer of the head and neck in community practice and at academic centers. In part, this was because of the paucity of available drugs with documented antitumor activity for this disease. The only drug with clearly established activity, used worldwide, was the folic acid analog methotrexate. Many other drugs had been tested, although the assessment criteria used to define response were not uniform. Hence, the reported response rates were unreliable, representing an accumulation of observations of any degree of tumor regression. In contrast, during the past two decades, a rigid system has been applied to the testing of potentially useful drugs. There now are clearly defined parameters for the objective evaluation of response and survival time and statistical guidelines for the design of clinical research trials to establish efficacy or to show improvement compared with standard therapies.

The serendipitous identification of the metal compound cisdiamine-dichloroplatinum (II) (cisplatinum) as a potential anticancer agent by Rosenberg[173] in 1968 spurred clinical research efforts to test new agents and combination chemotherapy regimens for the palliation of patients with locally recurrent and metastatic head and neck cancer. Several highly effective chemotherapy regimens were identified and then incorporated into a combined modality approach to treating the newly diagnosed patient. The goal was to improve survival time. It became clear that chemotherapy administered before definitive surgery or radiotherapy could result in rapid regression of tumor in the majority of patients without increasing the morbidity of subsequent surgery or radiation. Further, a proportion of the responding patients would have no evidence of tumor in the resected specimen. This increased the possibility of altering the standard surgical approach at some sites to preserve organ function. In addition to investigative trials using chemotherapy before definitive local therapy, traditional adjuvant chemotherapy administered after surgical resection and chemotherapy used as a radiosensitizer concomitant with radiotherapy have been under active investigation.

Prognostic factors

Many chemotherapy trials have been analyzed to determine factors that would predict response to chemotherapy and prolonged survival time. Because squamous cell cancer of the head and neck is a heterogeneous disease, each factor should be evaluated in the context of multiple primary sites. Most single-institution trials have only modest numbers of patients and therefore lack the statistical confidence to draw firm conclusions. For patients with recurrent disease, poor prognostic factors are a low performance status, poor nutrition, a large tumor burden, and extensive previous radiotherapy and surgery.[13] In these circumstances, any response to chemotherapy is likely to be marginal and brief without impact on overall survival time. However, it seems clear that survival time may be prolonged in patients who achieve a complete response to chemotherapy. These patients in general have a good performance status; they are not malnourished and have not received previous chemotherapy for recurrent disease.

For the newly diagnosed patient treated with induction chemotherapy, the most consistent prognostic factor for overall response and complete response is T and N stage. There is a significant correlation between tumor size and response, with lower response rates observed in T4 and N3 stage disease in particular.[38,70,103] The importance of primary site as a prognostic factor for response to chemotherapy is unclear. One investigator, in an analysis of 208 patients, reported that cancers within the oral cavity and nasopharynx were significantly associated with high response rates.[105] Nasopharynx cancer was found significant in two other trials.[6,70] The pattern of failure for patients with nasopharyngeal carcinoma also is different from that of other sites with metastatic sites assuming a larger proportion. Besides nasopharyngeal carcinoma, most trials have failed to demonstrate differences by site, which may be because of inadequate patient numbers and ineffective chemotherapy regimens.

Because of the importance of performance status as a predictor of outcome for the recurrent disease patient, induction chemotherapy trials have excluded patients with poor performance status (<50% on the Karnofsky scale). Within the range of 50% to 100%, no differences have been observed. Tumor differentiation does not appear to be a predictive factor in studies that have used cisplatin-based combination chemotherapy regimens. It is well established that overall survival time correlates with performance status, T and N stage, primary site,[5,70,103] and extracapsular extension of tumor.[119,192] The survival time of patients with cancers of the nasopharynx and larynx is longer than those with oral cavity and hypopharyngeal primary cancers after other factors are corrected for in multivariate analyses of patients receiving induction chemotherapy.

The application of biologic factors, such as DNA content,[68] immunologic status, and circulating immune complexes,[185] to predict response and survival outcome is under investigation. Evidence exists that DNA ploidy and DNA content can predict for survival and disease-free survival times.[212,239] Molecular markers (such as *p53* and *p16*) that act as predictors for response and survival time also are under investigation.[22,23]

CHEMOTHERAPY FOR PALLIATION

Systemic management of recurrent head and neck cancer is a major concern because 30% to 50% of patients diagnosed this year will die with recurrent local and regional disease within 5 years. Distant metastases will be present clinically in 20% to 40% of patients, but occult disease determined at autopsy may be present in up to 60%.[128] The primary goal of conventional chemotherapy used for palliation should be to prolong survival time. Patients with locally advanced or disseminated recurrent squamous cell carcinomas of the head and neck have a median survival time of 6 months, and 20% survive 1 year. Chemotherapy has not yet altered these statistics, although it has been useful in palliation. One often hears that pain relief can be achieved with chemotherapy, but this should not constitute the sole reason for treatment. Small amounts of tumor regression may be associated with a transient diminution of pain, although the aggressive use of a variety of available oral analgesics (tablet and elixir preparations) is a much more rational approach to pain management.

Single agents

The response rate (complete and partial) of recurrent or metastatic squamous cell cancer to commonly used agents is provided in Table 6-2. In general, about one third of patients respond. The majority are partial responses, with less than 5% of patients achieving a complete response. Response duration is brief, on the order of 2 to 4 months, and the median survival time is 6 months.

Methotrexate

Methotrexate is a folic acid analog that is S-phase specific. Its mechanism of action involves binding to the enzyme dihydrofolate reductase, which blocks the reduction of dihydrofolate to tetrahydrofolic acid. Tetrahydrofolic acid is necessary for the synthesis of thymidylic acid and purine synthesis. This then interrupts the synthesis of DNA, RNA, and protein. The cytostatic effects of methotrexate can be circumvented by the administration of reduced folates, such as leucovorin, which can be converted to the tetrahydrofolate coenzyme required for purine biosynthesis. The therapeutic index of methotrexate can be increased if leucovorin is administered at intervals after methotrexate is given. This results from a selective rescue of nonmalignant cells and forms the basis for the use of high doses of methotrexate followed by leucovorin to ameliorate methotrexate toxicity to healthy cells. Cancer cells may lack transport sites for leucovorin

Table 6-2. Activity of single agent chemotherapy

Agent	Dosing schedule	Response/rate (%)
Methotrexate	40–50 mg/m^2 weekly	30
Cisplatin	80–120 mg/m^2 every 3–4 weeks	33
Carboplatin	400 mg/m^2 every 4 weeks	24
Paclitaxel	135–200 mg/m^2 every 3–4 weeks	38
Docetaxel	75 mg/m^2 every 3 weeks	38
Ifosfamide	1.5–2.5 g/m^2 every 4 weeks	26
Bleomycin	15 mg/m^2 twice weekly	18
5-Fluorouracil	500 mg/m^2 weekly	15

and are subject to the lethal effects of methotrexate. Mechanisms for resistance to methotrexate include selection of cells with decreased transport of methotrexate into cells and increased dihydrofolate reductase activity.

Methotrexate can be administered by intramuscular injection or subcutaneous, intravenous, or oral routes. Weekly or biweekly administration is the preferred schedule. A conventional dose of intravenous methotrexate is 40 to 60 mg/m^2 weekly. When higher doses of methotrexate are used, they may be in the moderate-dose range (250 to 500 mg/m^2, intravenous) or the high-dose range (5 to 10 g/m^2). These are both followed by leucovorin rescue, usually beginning at 24 hours and continuing until the plasma methotrexate level is less than 10^{-8} mol/l. At this dose range, the toxicity for patients with normal renal function usually is limited to mild stomatitis and myelosuppression. More severe, life-threatening reactions consisting of confluent mucositis, pancytopenia, liver function abnormalities, and an exfoliative maculopapular rash occur rarely and require intensive medical support. Renal dysfunction may occur with high-dose methotrexate administration because of precipitation of the drug, especially in an acid urine. Hydration and alkalinization of the urine before and after methotrexate administration can reduce the risk.

Methotrexate is the most widely used drug for management of squamous cancers of the head and neck and is the standard to which new agents or combinations often are compared. Therapy with this drug is relatively nontoxic, inexpensive, and convenient. Response rates to conventional doses vary between 8% and 50%, averaging 30%.[17] Weekly treatment, if tolerable, is superior to twice monthly or monthly treatments. Levitt and others[134] have shown *in vitro* that when moderate-to-high doses of methotrexate are used with leucovorin rescue, an enhanced therapeutic index results from the high intracellular levels of drug associated with selective rescue of healthy tissue. The initial results of pilot trials of moderate- or high-dose methotrexate suggested improvement in response rates for those with head and neck cancers. However, there is no evidence of improved responses to the higher dose of drug, as much as 5000 mg, from prospective randomized trials comparing conventional

with moderate- or high-dose methotrexate with or without leucovorin rescue.[223,238]

Cisplatin

Cisplatin is an inorganic metal coordination complex with major antitumor activity in a number of diseases. The drug behaves as a bifunctional alkylating agent binding to DNA to cause interstrand and intrastrand cross-linking. Cisplatin also binds to nuclear and cytoplasmic proteins. Resistance is believed to develop through increased metabolic inactivation. Cisplatin is administered by the intravenous route and requires aggressive hydration and diuresis to prevent renal tubular damage. A dose of 80 to 120 mg/m^2 every 3 or 4 weeks is the usual dose given by intravenous infusion with mannitol diuresis[102] or by 24-hour infusion.[114] The drug is not schedule-dependent, although it has been shown that 5-day continuous infusion increases exposure to the active platinum species when compared with bolus dosing.[81]

The major toxic reaction is renal dysfunction, manifested by an increase in serum creatinine levels or a decrease in creatinine clearance. The peak serum creatinine level occurs at 1 or 2 weeks and returns to baseline by 3 or 4 weeks. An increase in serum creatinine level to 2 mg/dl has been noted in up to 20% of patients in several series. This drug should not be used in patients with a creatinine clearance below 40 ml/min. Nausea and vomiting are almost universal. Ototoxicity can occur, usually in the 4000 to 8000 Hz range. It tends to be dose-related and cumulative and may be permanent. Hematologic toxicity, including neutropenia and thrombocytopenia, is mild, with a nadir at 2 weeks. Anemia is common and appears to be a result of bone marrow suppression; rarely patients manifest an acute hemolytic anemia. Hypomagnesemia can occur in part because of renal wasting. A peripheral neuropathy—predominantly sensory—occurs and is related to cumulative cisplatin dosage. Ototoxicity and peripheral neuropathy are common toxicities when the cumulative cisplatin dose approaches or exceeds 600 mg/m^2. These toxicities preclude long-term management with cisplatin in chemotherapy responders and dose intensification. This led to a search for analogs with similar efficacy but a different spectrum of toxicity.

Cisplatin has the same response rate as methotrexate, approximately 30%, with some reported complete responses and a duration of response of approximately 4 months.[114,236] Two controlled trials comparing methotrexate with cisplatin found no difference in response rate or survival time between the two but only different toxicities.[94,107] Advantages of cisplatin over methotrexate are its relatively rapid response rate and the fact that it needs to be given only once every 3 or 4 weeks, although methotrexate is more convenient because it can be given on an outpatient basis, whereas the higher doses of cisplatin require hospitalization. Cisplatin has been studied at different doses to determine if a dose–response effect exists. In a comparison of 60 mg/m^2 and 120 mg/m^2, Veronesi and others[218] found no difference in response rates.

Forastiere and others[78] conducted a pilot trial evaluating 200 mg/m^2 and observed a 73% response rate or double that expected with conventional dosing. Although this suggested benefit from the higher dose, ototoxicity and neurotoxicity occurred frequently and limited treatment duration.

Carboplatin

More than one dozen derivatives of cisplatin have been evaluated for clinical development. Of these, carboplatin (cis-diamine-cyclobutane dicarboxylato-platinum II) was the first to become widely available. Carboplatin appears to have a mechanism of action similar to the parent compound, but it has a different toxicity profile. The dose-limiting toxicity is myelosuppression, primarily leukopenia and thrombocytopenia, which should be considered when carboplatin is combined with other myelosuppressing agents. Renal toxicity, ototoxicity, and neurotoxicity are rare, and the emetogenic potential of carboplatin is less. The drug can be administered in the outpatient setting without the need for hydration. Based on pharmacokinetic parameters, an intravenous dose of 400 mg/m^2 is considered the equivalent in potency to 100 mg/m^2 of cisplatin and can be safely administered to patients with creatinine clearance of 60 mg/ml or more. For patients with poor renal function, carboplatin dose should be calculated using the Calvert[30] or Egorin[64] formulae, which account for delayed renal excretion leading to increased drug exposure.

Carboplatin has a 24% response rate in phase II trials in patients with recurrent squamous cell cancer of the head and neck. It does not appear to be as active as cisplatin; one comparative trial in patients with untreated disease has documented an inferior outcome for carboplatin.[10] Thus, carboplatin should be reserved for patients who are not candidates for cisplatin therapy because of renal impairment or preexisting peripheral neuropathy. Carboplatin can be administered in the outpatient setting and requires no prehydration. The major toxicity caused by carboplatin is myelosuppression, which limits the total dose that can be given and the frequency of drug administration. The availability of colony-stimulating factors that can lessen the degree and duration of myelosuppression may provide a new avenue for clinical investigations with this agent.

Taxanes

The taxanes are a new class of compounds that include paclitaxel (taxol) and docetaxel (taxotere). These drugs act by stabilizing microtubules by binding to the β-subunit of tubulin, thereby inhibiting microtubule depolymerization, which results in a cell cycle arrest at G$_2$. Preclinical studies showed that the taxanes were active against a variety of solid tumors and that prolonged infusions were more effective.[86,95,168,220] Trials of head and neck cancer patients have shown response rates of approximately 30% to 40%.[33,63,77,80,208]

Paclitaxel has been dosed at 135 to 250 mg/m^2 given over 3 or 24 hours, and docetaxel has been given at 60 to 100 mg/m^2 by bolus injection every 3 weeks. The major toxicity is neutropenia particularly with high doses, and infection is the chief concern. Growth factors such as GM-CSF and G-CSF often are used to shorten the neutropenic nadir duration and hopefully lessen the risk of infection.[174] Given this risk, only patients with good performance status should be treated with high doses (200 to 250 mg/m^2). Patients with poor performance status should receive lower doses, starting at 135 mg/m^2, and escalate the dose, depending on individual toxicity. Paclitaxel has been given over several schedules, and the optimal dosing schedule is being investigated. Docetaxel is a semisynthetic agent and may be more effective than paclitaxel. In two small phase II studies, response rates of 32% and 50% were observed.[34,63]

Ifosfamide

Ifosfamide is structurally related to cyclophosphamide (to be discussed) and has a similar mechanism of action, leading to DNA interstrand and intrastand cross-linking that disrupts DNA replication. It is activated by hepatic p-450 mixed-function oxidase, and its metabolites are excreted in the urine. Ifosfamide in total doses of 7 to 10 g/m^2 usually is administered as a 5-day continuous infusion or over 3 to 5 days in equally divided doses. The drug is repeated at 3 or 4 week intervals. Sodium mercaptoethane sulfonate (MESNA) is a thiol compound that should be administered concomitantly with ifosfamide to limit urothelial toxicity. The total daily dose of MESNA should equal the daily dose of ifosfamide. It may be administered as a continuous infusion or in five divided doses given every 4 hours starting 30 minutes before ifosfamide is administered each day. Patients need to be well hydrated before drug administration. The major dose-limiting toxicity is hemorrhagic cystitis, although with the use of MESNA, myelosuppression, nausea, vomiting, and hyponatremia are more frequent toxicities. Central nervous system toxicities, which include cerebellar dysfunction, seizures, confusion, and lethargy, occur in up to 30% of patients treated with doses of 8 to 10 g/m^2 over 5 days. Early phase II results with this drug are promising with reported response rates ranging from 6% to 43% with a median of 26%.*

Bleomycin

Bleomycin (Blenoxane) is an antineoplastic antibiotic that binds to DNA and produces DNA strand breaks by generating oxygen free-radicals. The conventional dose of bleomycin is 10 to 20 units/m^2 once or twice weekly given intramuscularly or intravenously. It also may be given by a continuous 24-hour infusion over 5 or 7 days at a dose of 10 units/m^2 each 24 hours. The major disposition of bleomycin is via the kidneys. It is important that the dose of bleomycin be reduced if the level of serum creatinine is abnormal.

---

* Refs. 27, 35, 111, 125, 145, 219.

A 50% dose reduction is recommended for a creatinine clearance of 15 to 30 ml/min, and a 75% reduction is recommended if the creatinine clearance is below 15 ml/min. Approximately half of the patients receiving this drug will develop fever or chills during the first 24 hours, which can be reduced with the use of antipyretics. A rare complication is an anaphylactic reaction. It has been recommended that a dose of 1 unit be given several hours before the first dose of bleomycin. Alopecia can occur, particularly with the higher dosage of drug. Skin toxicity, including erythema, thickening, and hyperpigmentation, is common. Patients may develop stomatitis, which necessitates discontinuing a prolonged infusion.

Pulmonary toxicity is potentially one of the most serious complications of bleomycin administration. Patients may develop pneumonitis, a dry cough, and rales. Pulmonary function tests most commonly show a decreased carbon monoxide diffusion capacity. Pulmonary fibrosis with associated hypoxia and restrictive lung disease can result. Bleomycin pulmonary toxicity is more common in elderly patients, in patients who have had previous lung irradiation, and in patients who have had a total dose higher than 200 units. Patients should be closely monitored with serial tests of diffusion capacity when the cumulative dose exceeds 150 units. Giving the drug by continuous infusion may lessen pulmonary toxicity.[230]

Bleomycin has undergone testing using an intermittent bolus dosing schedule with response rates of 18%. A pharmacokinetic advantage may be achieved by continuous infusion because both agents have a short plasma half-life. Bleomycin is most frequently used combined with other agents.

5-Fluorouracil

5-Fluorouracil (5-FU) is a fluorinated pyrimidine similar to uracil. 5-FU competes for the enzyme thymidylate synthetase by displacing uracil, which in turn inhibits the formation of thymidine, an essential factor in DNA synthesis. The conventional intravenous dose of 5-FU is 10 to 15 mg/kg weekly. An alternate method of delivery is a loading dose of 400 to 500 mg/m^2 daily for 5 days, followed by a weekly intravenous dose of 400 to 500 mg/m^2. It is recommended that no more than 800 mg be given as a single bolus. The therapeutic index of 5-FU may be enhanced by giving it by continuous infusion, which allows delivery of up to 1 g/m^2/day for 5 days repeated every 3 or 4 weeks, without enhanced toxicity. Continuous infusion of 5-FU has been studied primarily in patients with adenocarcinomas of the gastrointestinal tract. However, the results of one randomized trial in head and neck cancer patients comparing bolus and continuous infusion of 5-FU showed improved response rates with continuous infusion.[124] 5-FU toxic reactions include myelosuppression with neutropenia and thrombocytopenia occurring at 1 or 2 weeks. Nausea, vomiting, and diarrhea may occur, and stomatitis is common with higher doses. Patients may develop alopecia, hyperpigmentation, or a maculopapular rash. 5-FU is most commonly used in combination with other drugs. In patients with head and neck carcinomas, treatment with 5-FU can produce response rates of 15%, thus it usually is used in combination with other agents, particularly cisplatin.[8,162]

Other Single Agents with Activity in Head and Neck Cancer

Several other chemotherapeutic agents were reported to have response rates in excess of 15% for patients with recurrent disease. They include adriamycin, cyclophosphamide, hydroxyurea, and vinblastine.[9] Several of these are only marginally effective as single agents for recurrent disease, although when used in combinations or in patients with no previous treatment, they may be more efficacious. These agents will be discussed.

Cyclophosphamide

Cyclophosphamide is activated in the liver by microsomal enzymes. Its major mechanism of action is cross-linking DNA strands, preventing further division. Cyclophosphamide can be given orally or intravenously. When given intravenously, it usually is given as a single dose of 500 to 1500 mg/m^2 repeated every 3 or 4 weeks. It can be given daily at 60 to 120 mg/m^2 but should be adjusted according to blood count results. It is important to hydrate patients well before and after giving cyclophosphamide. Drugs that stimulate liver enzymes, such as barbiturates, should be avoided, or the cyclophosphamide dose should be modified. After an intravenous dose, bone marrow suppression, predominantly neutropenia, can occur in 1 or 2 weeks, with a recovery at 2 or 3 weeks. Many patients have some degree of nausea and vomiting. Alopecia and ridging of the nails can occur. Azoospermia and cessation of menses, often with permanent infertility, can occur with most alkylating agents.

Acute hemorrhagic cystitis occurs most commonly in patients who are poorly hydrated. It is recommended that patients drink at least 2 quarts of fluid per day while taking cyclophosphamide. Toxicity may occur as microscopic hematuria or gross bleeding. This can eventually result in a fibrotic bladder, and a few cases of bladder carcinoma have been described in patients who have received cyclophosphamide.

Adriamycin

Adriamycin (doxorubicin) is an anthracycline derivative that intercalates between nucleotide pairs in DNA to interfere with nuclei acid synthesis. This drug is given intravenously, usually at doses of 60 to 90 mg/m^2 every 3 weeks. Alternate schedules that are associated with much lower risk of cardiac toxicity include doses of 20 to 30 mg/m^2 daily for 3 days repeated every 3 weeks, low doses given weekly, or prolonged infusions.[16] The urine may be red for 1 or 2 days after adriamycin treatment.

If adriamycin infiltrates subcutaneous tissue, it can cause

severe necrosis of skin and subcutaneous tissue. The drug causes alopecia, which can be decreased by using scalp hypothermia. Stomatitis, nausea, vomiting, and diarrhea are common. Adriamycin, like actinomycin D, can cause radiation recall in patients who have had previous radiotherapy. The drug also can cause neutropenia and thrombocytopenia with a nadir at 1 or 2 weeks and a return to normal values by 3 weeks.[18]

The most dose-limiting toxic effect of adriamycin is cardiac toxicity, which manifests as a cardiomyopathy,[228] leading to congestive heart failure in approximately 10% of patients who receive a cumulative dose greater than 550 mg/m^2. Other predisposing factors include age, previous cardiac irradiation, other cardiotoxic chemotherapeutic agents, and a previous history of heart disease. Many methods of observing patients have been used, including endomyocardial biopsy. Radionuclide ejection fraction is a relatively easy and accurate way to determine the amount of damage to the heart from adriamycin.

Vinca alkaloids

Vinblastine and vincristine are vinca alkaloids and act by disrupting microtubular spindle formation, causing mitotic arrest. Vinblastine (Velban) can be given weekly at 5 mg/m^2, or it may be given by continuous infusion over several days. The major toxic reactions are myelosuppression, alopecia, and myalgias. Vincristine (Oncovin) usually is given at 1.0 to 1.5 mg/m^2 once or twice monthly. It is recommended for adults that a single dose not exceed 2 mg. The drug is neurotoxic, which is most commonly manifested as a sensory motor peripheral neuropathy or hoarseness that will progress if the drug is not discontinued. Most patients will experience constipation, and they should take stool softeners with the drug. Vincristine causes alopecia, but it has almost no myelosuppressive effects.

Hydroxyurea

Hydroxyurea (Hydrea) inhibits ribonucleotide reductase, interfering with the conversion of ribonucleotide to deoxyribonucleotide and causing inhibition of DNA synthesis. The drug is given orally, usually in an intermittent regimen of 80 mg/kg every third day. The major toxic responses are neutropenia and thrombocytopenia, so that the dose should be reduced or delayed if the leukocyte count decreases to less than 25,000/mm^3 or the platelet count decreases to less than 1,000,000/mm^3. The nadir occurs approximately 10 days after starting the drug. Nausea and diarrhea are common. Stomatitis can occur, particularly if there is concurrent irradiation. Patients also may develop a maculopapular rash.

New single agents

Many new drugs are being investigated for their activity in patients with head and neck cancer in phase I and II studies. Topotecan is a topoisomerase I inhibitor that had activity in one small phase II study.[170] Response rates of 25% were

observed and have led to further evaluation by two large cooperative groups—the Southwestern Oncology Group (SWOG) and the Eastern Cooperative Oncology Group (ECOG). Results of these trials are pending.

Gemcitabine is a pyrimidine antimetabolite that may have antitumor activity in patients with head and neck carcinomas. This agent is converted to an active triphosphate metabolite, which is then incorporated into DNA and terminates transcription. Early phase II results have demonstrated only modest activity with response rates of 18%.[34]

Vinorelbine is a semisynthetic vinca alkaloid with dramatically less neurotoxicity than other agents of its class. Early studies have demonstrated response rates of 22%.[90,207] Finally, analogs of methotrexate have been evaluated for response in small series. Trimetrexate, edatrexate, and piritrexim are active in squamous cell carcinomas of the head and neck but offer no advantage over methotrexate.[53,169,178,213,226]

COMBINATION CHEMOTHERAPY FOR RECURRENT DISEASE

In an effort to improve response rates and hopefully survival time, combination chemotherapy was developed. Many combination chemotherapy regimens have been evaluated in phase II trials in a few patients with recurrent head and neck cancer. Often, the results indicate a high response rate that suggests improvement over that expected from single agent methotrexate or cisplatin. However, the median duration of response ranges from 2 to 6 months, and no one has yet documented improved survival time over single-agent chemotherapy. Many of the regimens are complex, often with additional toxic effects.

Only through large comparative trials with patients randomized and stratified for prognostic variables can it be determined if therapeutic benefit exists with combination chemotherapy. The results of 12 trials comparing combination chemotherapy to single-agent cisplatin or methotrexate are shown in Table 6-3. Some of the studies had small numbers of patients and lacked balance between treatment groups for prognostic factors such as performance status and extent of previous treatment. However, four large multiinstitutional trials that were well designed with respect to prognostic factors showed a significant difference in response rates between the combination treatment and the single-agent control arm.[40,76,83,116,222]

The ECOG compared an outpatient regimen of cisplatin, bleomycin, and methotrexate to weekly methotrexate.[222] The response to single agent therapy with methotrexate was 35%, and to the combination 48%, a significant improvement (P = 0.04). However, toxicity was greater for the combination with no difference in survival time.

The SWOG reported a comparison of cisplatin and 5-FU and carboplatin and 5-FU to weekly methotrexate.[76,83] The response rates for the three arms were 32%, 21%, and 10%, respectively. There was a significant difference comparing

Table 6-3. Randomized trials of chemotherapy for recurrent head and neck cancer

Author	Regimens	CR + PR (%)	Survival (months)
Davis and Kessler, 1979[50]	PMB	11	
	P	13	
Jacobs, 1983[115]	PM	33	6.3
	P	18	6.9
Drelichman, 1983[60]	P		
	Vb	41	5.6
	M	33	4.0
Vogl, 1985[222]	PMB	48	5.6
	M	35	5.6
Morton, 1985[155]	PB	24	4.0
	P	13	4.2
	B	14	2.8
	No chemotherapy		2.1
*Williams, 1986[235]	PVbB	23	6.8
	M	16	7.2
Campbell, 1987[31]	PF	19	2.7
	PM	40	8.7
	P	31	5.3
	M	33	6.7
Eisenberger, 1989[65]	CM	25	6
	M	25	6
Liverpool Study, 1990[139]	P	14	6
	PF	12	6
	M	6	2
	PM	11	6
Forastiere, 1992[83]	PF	32	6.6
	CF	21	5.0
	M	10	5.6
Jacobs, 1992[116]	PF	32	5.5
	P	17	5.0
	F	13	6.1
Clavel, 1994[40]	PMBVb	34	7.0
	PF	31	7.0
	P	15	7.0

Reprinted with permission from *Tumors of the nasal cavity and paranasal sinuses, nasopharynx, oral cavity, and oropharynx.* In Schantz SP, Harrison LB, Forastive AA: *Cancer—principles and practice of oncology,* ed 5, Philadelphia, 1997, Lippincott-Raven.
CR—Complete response; PR—Partial response; P—Cisplatin; M—Methotrexate; B—Bleomycin; Vb—Vinblastine; C—Carboplatin; F—5-Fluorouracil.

the cisplatin combination with methotrexate ($P < 0.001$); the difference between the response to the carboplatin combination and the response to methotrexate approached statistical significance ($P = 0.05$). The cisplatin and 5-FU arm was associated with significantly more toxicity than methotrexate; carboplatin and 5-FU were intermediate in toxicity. Despite these findings, the median survival times were not different, varying between 4.7 and 6.6 months.

The third study to show a difference in response rates compared the combination of cisplatin and 5-FU with each drug used alone.[116] The response rate to the combination was 40% compared with 18% for cisplatin and 15% for con-

tinuous infusion 5-FU ($P < 0.01$). Although the median survival times were not different, an analysis of patients surviving longer than 9 months showed a 40% survival rate for the combination treatment group compared with 27% and 24% for the single-drug treatments ($P < 0.05$).

The latter two trials also are of interest in the similar response rates observed for cisplatin and 5-FU, which were administered using the same dose and schedule in both studies. Cisplatin and 5-FU is a commonly used drug regimen for the treatment of patients with head and neck cancer for palliation and in combined modality programs. Response rates to this combination reported from small phase II trials in patients with recurrent disease range from 11% to 79%.[214] The results of these two large multiinstitutional trials have served to establish a response rate of 32% that can be expected from the cisplatin and 5-FU combination in patients with recurrent head and neck cancer.

Clavel and others[40] also observed significant differences between combination chemotherapy and single agents. They found significant differences in response rate for two cisplatin-containing combinations compared with single agent methotrexate, 34%, 31%, and 15%, respectively. These data corroborate the work of Vogl, Jacobs, and Forastiere.

Two comparative trials listed in Table 6-3 showed significant differences in median survival time.[31,155] Morton and others[155] compared the combination of cisplatin and bleomycin to each single agent and to a no-treatment control arm. The response rate to each of the three chemotherapy arms was low, although the two cisplatin arms had median survival times of 4.0 and 4.2 months, which was improved over a 2.1-month survival time for the no treatment arm. In the four-arm trial reported by Campbell and others,[31] survival time was significantly longer for single-agent cisplatin compared with methotrexate, and there was no advantage for the combination treatments. Both of these trials had small numbers of patients and were unevenly balanced for prognostic factors, which serves to decrease the reliability of the statistical interpretation. Thus, from these randomized trials, it appears that higher response rates can be achieved with some combination chemotherapy regimens. Toxicity is more severe, and overall survival time as measured by median survival time is not improved. However, one study did find that a significantly greater proportion of patients treated with cisplatin and 5-FU lived longer than 9 months when compared with those receiving single-agent therapy. The patients who are more likely to be in the subset showing improvement have a better performance status.

As for other sites, the most effective combinations for treating those with nasopharyngeal carcinoma are cisplatin-based regimens. Higher complete and partial response rates than those from other sites have been reported in several phase II trials.* A few long-term disease-free survivors have been seen with cisplatin-based combinations.[21,39,73] French

* Refs. 21, 39, 45, 52, 73, 90.

investigators have formed a collaborative group to study nasopharyngeal cancer. They have reported a series of studies evaluating cisplatin combination chemotherapy. Their regimen of cisplatin, bleomycin, and 5-FU resulted in a 20% complete response rate and an 86% overall response rate. Four patients with metastatic disease were long-term disease-free survivors for 52 to 58 months.[21,48,143] In their series, 131 patients with metastatic nasopharyngeal carcinoma were treated between 1985 and 1991. Ten percent of this group were long-term disease-free survivors. Thus, this disease entity shows a unique chemosensitivity even in patients with either bone or visual metastasis.[73] Browman and Cronin[25] summarized all of the available data regarding combination therapy by use of a metaanalysis. They analyzed all randomized trials published between 1990 and 1992 and concluded that cisplatin was the most effective single agent. Further, they found that the combination cisplatin and 5-FU was more efficacious than any single agent or other reported combinations. The combination of cisplatin and 5-FU is the gold standard to which all new combinations should be compared. Response rates achieved with this combination are approximately 32%, and the complete response rate ranges from 5% to 15%. Given these low response rates, one of the goals of clinical trials is to find new single agents and new combinations that may be more effective. Patients with locally advanced or metastatic disease should be considered for trials in an effort to improve on these statistics. Patients who have undergone previous surgery and radiation with good performance status and no previous chemotherapy are the best candidates to test new treatment protocols.

COMBINED MODALITY THERAPY

Although surgery and radiotherapy cure a high percentage of patients with early-stage squamous cell carcinoma of the head and neck, conventional treatment will not cure the majority of those with advanced disease. Because treatment for recurrent disease with chemotherapy is far from satisfactory, much effort has been directed toward improvements in the primary treatment program by using combined modality therapy. To this end, three general approaches have been undertaken: (1) induction also known as neoadjuvant therapy where chemotherapy is given before surgery or radiation; (2) chemoradiation where chemotherapy is given simultaneous with radiation to enhance its effect; and (3) adjuvant therapy where chemotherapy is given after surgery or radiation in an effort to decrease metastatic disease burden.

Induction chemotherapy

Theoretically, treating with chemotherapy before surgery or radiation has several advantages. Neoadjuvant chemotherapy allows for the delivery of drugs to the best possible host in terms of medical condition, which leads to increased compliance and better tolerance of therapy. Chemotherapy when given first can reduce tumor burden and downstage patients, resulting in the preservation of organ function by obviating the need for surgery. Further, induction therapy can reduce metastatic seeds and eliminate problems with poor vascularity that often occur after surgery or radiation, thus reducing a potential pharmacologic sanctuary.

One of the first uses of induction chemotherapy involved methotrexate with leucovorin rescue given twice before surgery.[204] It was reported that 77% of patients had some tumor shrinkage, although by strict criteria of tumor response (greater than 50% in all sites), the response rate was only 20%. Although it could not be concluded that the result was better than with surgery alone, no increased incidence of postoperative complications occurred. Many other studies followed using single agent methotrexate and bleomycin. The complete response rate was approximately 5% in these studies.

With the introduction of cisplatin into clinical trials in the mid-1970s, combination therapy consisted of cisplatin followed by a 5- to 7-day continuous infusion of bleomycin. Early series[108,165] reported overall response rates of 71% to 76% with a 20% complete response rate. Other investigators added vinblastine, vincristine, or methotrexate to the two-drug combination with similar results.[9] An alternate and probably more effective regimen tested in the 1980s at Wayne State University is cisplatin (100 mg/m^2) followed by a 5-day infusion of 5-FU (1 g/m^2 per day by continuous infusion).[172] In phase II trials, this regimen was associated with as high as a 93% overall response rate and a 54% complete response rate when three cycles were administered. Although the toxicity from cisplatin is the same, 5-FU appears to be better tolerated than bleomycin, without the associated allergic phenomena or lung toxicity.

Ensley and others[66,67] from Wayne State University have reported a high complete response rate using five or six courses of cisplatin and 5-FU alternating with methotrexate, leucovorin, and 5-FU. In one study, the complete response rate was 65% in 31 patients completing the protocol, although toxicity was formidable, and approximately one third of patients withdrew from the study early. Despite the potential for improvement in response rate, the feasibility of this approach has yet to be demonstrated.

Investigators at the Dana Farber Cancer Center[61] and at the University of Chicago[225] have used leucovorin to biochemically modulate the cytotoxic effects of 5-FU. Leucovorin results in an increase in intracellular-reduced folate levels and inhibition of thymidylate synthase.[152] Dreyfuss and others[61] administered cisplatin, 5-FU, and high-dose leucovorin (500 mg/m^2), all by continuous infusion, over 6 days to 35 patients with local regionally advanced head and neck cancer. The overall response rate was 80%, and 66% had a complete response by clinical assessment. A pathologic complete response was documented in 14 of 19 patients (74%). Moderate-to-severe mucositis occurred in the majority of patients, although with dosage adjustment, the regimen was tolerable and acceptable to patients. Vokes and others[225] treated 31 patients with similar disease with a less intensive cisplatin, 5-FU, and leucovorin regimen. Leucovorin was administered orally in a dose of 100 mg every 4 hours during the 5-day infusion of 5-FU. After two courses, the overall response rate in 29 evaluable patients was 90%, and the complete response rate was 30%.

Since the early 1980s, the many uncontrolled trials of induction chemotherapy before surgery or radiotherapy have shown that this approach is feasible for those with locally advanced disease and does not add to the morbidity of subsequent definitive local treatment.[130,196] With the cisplatin plus 5-FU regimen, response can be expected in 80% to 90% of patients with, on average, a 40% complete response rate. Approximately two thirds of complete responses by clinical examination will be confirmed pathologically. Response to induction chemotherapy correlates with response to subsequent radiotherapy.[69,92,110] Thus patients who are resistant to cisplatin-based induction chemotherapy have a high likelihood of not responding to radiotherapy. Large randomized trials that consider all the important prognostic variables and have long-term follow-up periods are necessary to draw conclusions regarding disease-free survival and overall survival benefit.[82] The results of 17 randomized controlled trials of induction chemotherapy before surgery or radiotherapy or both have been published.

Three of the most important trials are listed in Table 6-4, The Head and Neck Contracts program,[103] the SWOG trial,[180] and the Veterans Affairs Laryngeal Cancer Study Group trial,[221] were large multiinstitutional randomized studies. The patients had advanced resectable head and neck cancer, and the treatment arms were well balanced to T, N stage, and primary site. The Head and Neck Contracts program randomized patients to one of three treatments: (1) surgery followed by radiation, (2) induction chemotherapy with one cycle of cisplatin plus bleomycin followed by surgery and radiation, or (3) induction chemotherapy, surgery, radiation, and maintenance chemotherapy with cisplatin for 6 months. The 5-year survival rates were 35%, 37%, and 45%, respectively, for the three regimens; the differences were not significant. However, the time to development of distant metastases and the frequency of distant metastases as a site of first recurrence were significantly less in patients in the maintenance chemotherapy arm compared with the other two groups. On subgroup analysis, there was a significant difference in disease-free survival time for patients receiving maintenance chemotherapy for oral cavity primary tumors and for N1 or N2 disease.[117] In retrospect, it is not surprising that this trial did not show any improvement in overall survival time because only one cycle of cisplatin and bleomycin was administered before surgery, resulting in a low response rate of 37%.

The SWOG[180] randomized patients to receive either three cycles of cisplatin, bleomycin, methotrexate, and vincristine before surgery and radiotherapy or standard treatment with surgery and radiotherapy. The median survival time was 30 months for patients in the standard treatment arm compared with 18 months for the induction chemotherapy arm. The distant metastatic rate was 49% with standard treatment and 28% with induction chemotherapy. Although differences in survival time and pattern of recurrence are striking, statistical significance was not reached. This trial fell short of its accrual goals and had a high rate of noncompliance, with only 56% of patients randomized to induction chemotherapy completing the treatment per protocol.

The most encouraging data to emerge from induction chemotherapy trials are in the area of organ preservation (see the section on organ preservation). The Veterans Affairs Laryngeal Cancer Study Group[221] completed a randomized trial in patients with resectable stage III and IV squamous cell cancer of the larynx. Patients were randomized to receive standard therapy with total laryngectomy and postoperative radiotherapy or to receive a maximum of three cycles of cisplatin and 5-FU chemotherapy followed by radiotherapy. Surgery was reserved to salvage patients with persistent or recurrent disease. If patients did not have at least a partial response at the primary site after two cycles of chemotherapy, they underwent immediate surgery. The complete and partial response rate after two cycles of chemotherapy was 85%, and after three cycles was 98%. The pathologically confirmed complete response rate at the primary site was 64%. At a median follow-up period of 33 months, there was no significant difference in survival time. However, the patterns of relapse differed: recurrence at the primary site was 2% with surgery versus 12% with chemotherapy ($P = 0.0005$); regional node recurrence rates were similar ($P = 0.305$); distant metastases were 17% with surgery versus 11% with chemotherapy ($P = 0.016$); rate of second primary malignancies was 6% with surgery versus 2% with chemotherapy ($P = 0.029$). After 3 years of follow-up, 66% of surviving patients in the induction chemotherapy treatment group had a preserved, functional larynx. Similar results were reported by the EORTC comparing cisplatin and 5-FU induction chemotherapy followed by radiotherapy to laryngopharyngectomy and radiation in patients with locally advanced cancer of the hypopharynx. No survival time differences were observed, and 28% of patients were alive with a functional larynx. The larynx preservation rate was 42% at 3 years, considering only deaths from local disease as failure.[133]

None of the listed trials in Table 6-4 has demonstrated a survival benefit from induction chemotherapy. Two trials showed an improvement in survival time for chemotherapy-treated patients after subset analysis. Paccagnella and others[156,157] in a large Italian study observed an improvement in local control, metastatic rate, and survival time for inoperable patients. In a follow-up study to the Head and Neck Contracts Program, Jacobs and others reported an improvement in survival time for the subgroup with oral cavity primaries and limited nodal disease. In terms of patterns of

Table 6-4. Randomized trials of neoadjuvant chemotherapy before surgery or radiotherapy

Author	Regimen	Sites	Number of patients	Operability	Survival benefit	Other outcomes
HN Contracts (1987, 1990)[103]	PB	OC,L,HP	443	O	For N_2 disease in subset analysis	Disease in distant metastases
Carugati (1988)[32]	PB ± M	OC,OP,L	120	O	None	
Toohill (1987)[210]	PF	OC,OP,HP,NP	60	O + I	None	
Jaulerry (1992)[118]	PFV	OC,OP,HP,L	108	NS	None	
	PBVM		100	NS	None	
Szpirglas (1987)[201]	DVcBP	OC,OP	114	I	None	
Mazeron (1992)[148]	PFBM	OC,OP	107	O + I	None	
Martin (1990, 1995)[146,147]	PF	OC,OP,HP,L	75	O + I	None	
Schuller (1988)[180]	PBMF	OC,OP,HP,L	158	O	None	Decrease in distant metastases
VA Study (1991)[221]	PF	L	332	O	None	Larynx preserved in 64% at 2 years
						Decrease in distant metastases
Paccagnella (1994)[157]	PF	OC,OP,HP	237	O + I	For inoperable patients in subset analysis	Decrease in distant metastases; improved L-R control for inoperable patients only
Depondt (1993)[55]	CF	OC,OP,HP,L	324	O	None	
DiBlasio (1994)[57]	PF	NS	69	O	Significantly worse with chemotherapy	Larynx preserved in 42% at 3 years
Hasegawa (1994)[100]	PF	OC,OP,HP,L	50	O	None	
Chan (1995)[36]	PF	HP	82	NA	None	
Eschwege (1995)[72]	BEP	NP	339	NA	Significant improvement	
Dalley (1995)[49]	PF	HP	91	O	Survival at 7 years	
Lefebvre (1996)[133]	PF	HP	202	O	Statistically equivalent survival	Decrease in distant metastases

Reprinted with permission from *Tumors of the nasal cavity and parnasal sinuses, nasopharynx, oral cavity, and oropharynx.* In Schantz SP, Harrison LB, Forastive AA: *Cancer—principles and practice of oncology,* ed 5, Philadelphia, 1997, Lippincott-Raven.
P—Cisplatin; B—Bleomycin, OC—Oral cavity; L—Larynx; HP—Hypopharynx; O—Operable; M—Methotrexate; OP—Oropharynx; F—5-fluorouracil; NP—Nashopharynx; I–Inoperable; V—Vinblastine; Vc—Vincristine; L-R—Locoregional; C—Carboplatin; NS—Not specified; NA—Not applicable; E—Epirubicin.

failure, five trials showed a decrease in the rate of distant metastasis.[116,133,157,180]

These trials have helped to clarify many issues. First the overall response rates range from 60% to 90% with complete response rates of 20% to 50%. Survival time is improved in patients with a complete response compared with nonresponders, and pathologic complete response can be seen in 30% to 70%. Second, response to chemotherapy predicts for response to radiotherapy. Patients who fail to respond to chemotherapy do not respond to radiation. Third, neoadjuvant chemotherapy does not increase either surgical or radiotherapy complication rates. Fourth, the most critical prognostic factors for response are TN stage and type of chemotherapy. Biologic behavior appears to differ per site. Fifth, although no benefit in overall survival time has yet been shown, a significant reduction in the rate of distant metastases has been observed. Finally, organ preservation and improved quality of life can result with induction chemotherapy. For patients with advanced laryngeal cancer who would require a total laryngectomy, the available data indicate that laryngeal function can be preserved in two thirds without jeopardizing survival time.

Neoadjuvant chemotherapy has been used to manage advanced nasopharyngeal carcinoma similarly to other sites. To date, two randomized prospective trials have been conducted. The International Nasopharyngeal Study Group[113] randomized 339 patients to receive three cycles of bleomycin, epirubicin, and cisplatin chemotherapy followed by radiotherapy to radiotherapy alone in high risk for relapse patients (i.e., N_2, N_3 disease). At a median follow-up period of 49 months, there was a significant difference in disease-free survival time, 42% versus 29% at 4 years, $P = 0.006$, in favor of the chemotherapy arm. No difference in overall survival time was observed, 50% versus 42%, although median survival time was superior for the chemotherapy and radiation arm compared with radiation alone, 50 and 37 months, respectively.

In the second study, Chan and others[36] randomized 82

patients to receive either radiotherapy alone or two cycles of cisplatin and 5-FU followed by radiotherapy. These patients had tumors 4 cm or large or N_3 nodal disease. The overall response rate to chemotherapy was 81%, and this increased to 100% after radiation versus 95% for radiation alone. However, at a median follow-up period of 28.5 months, 2-year survival and disease-free survival time were not significantly altered by the addition of chemotherapy. This lack of difference may be accounted for partly by the less intensive nature of the chemotherapy with the 5-FU being given at 1000 cy/m^2/day over 3 days.

Concurrent radiotherapy and chemotherapy

Concurrent radiotherapy and chemotherapy have been used primarily in patients with unresectable disease to improve local and regional control. The major drugs with efficacy for this tumor type and *in vitro* evidence of radiation enhancement capability have been tested as single agents since the 1960s. The theoretic rationale and mechanism for the interaction between cytotoxic drugs and radiation that results in additive or synergistic enhancement have been reviewed in detail.[87,194,202] This biologic phenomenon rests on several mechanisms. These include (1) inhibition of DNA repair, (2) redistribution of cells in sensitive phases of the cell cycle, and (3) promoting oxygenation of anoxic tissues. The net effect is to improve cellular cytotoxicity.[225] Most of the single agents used to treat patients with head and neck cancer have been combined with radiation.

Nearly all reported trials of concomitant chemotherapy and radiotherapy have noted enhanced acute radiation-induced toxicity, primarily mucosal, which often has resulted in dose reductions and lengthy interruptions in radiation without evidence of survival benefit. Thus, in combining these two treatment modalities, it is essential that toxicity not preclude the use of chemotherapy and radiation in the optimal dose and schedule.

Single agents and radiotherapy

For an outline of randomized trials of simultaneous single agent chemotherapy with radiotherapy versus radiotherapy, see Table 6-5.

Methotrexate plus radiotherapy. Methotrexate can produce an S-phase block of the cell cycle, resulting in accumulation of cells in the G1 phase and causing increased radiosensitivity.[14] In one early study, 96 patients with inoperable disease were randomized to receive radiotherapy alone or radiation preceded by intravenous methotrexate.[126] The complete response rate was the same in both groups, as was the 3-year survival rate. However, the incidence of mucositis increased in those patients who received chemotherapy. A second large study of patients with stage III and IV squamous cell carcinoma, similar to the previous study, again showed no difference in the 3-year survival rate, although the rate of distant metastases was only 19% in patients who received chemotherapy plus radiation compared

with 33% of patients who received radiotherapy alone.[142] The Radiation Therapy Oncology Group (RTOG) randomized 712 patients to radiotherapy alone or radiation plus pretreatment methotrexate.[74] No difference occurred in survival time between the treatment groups, and more patients failed to complete irradiation in the combined therapy group. In a randomized study published by Condit and others,[42] there was no improvement in survival time in the combined group. In another study, Gupta[96] observed an improvement in survival time and better control of the primary tumor. This was especially true for those with oropharyngeal tumors. Thus three randomized series with adequate patient numbers showed negative results, and a fourth study showed improved survival time.

Hydroxyurea plus radiotherapy. Hydroxyurea kills cells in the S-phase and synchronizes cells into the more radiosensitive G_1 phase. Despite good theoretic activity, three randomized trials have shown no advantage of hydroxyurea in addition to radiotherapy. In one series, 12 patients with advanced cancer were randomized to radiation alone or with hydroxyurea (80 mg/kg biweekly).[195] The complete response rate at the primary site was 40% in both groups, but survival time was inferior in the combination group. In addition, distant metastases developed in 23% of patients receiving combined treatment as compared with 8% receiving irradiation alone. Another study of 40 patients comparing radiotherapy alone or with hydroxyurea (80 mg/kg three times per week) showed no difference in complete response rate or survival times, but it did show a 40% incidence of mucositis in the combined group.[167]

Bleomycin plus radiotherapy. Bleomycin and irradiation have been studied *in vitro*, and the enhanced effects are believed to be caused by interference with cellular repair after irradiation. Nine randomized trials have compared radiotherapy alone with radiation plus bleomycin. The first series included 227 patients with advanced oropharyngeal carcinomas.[29] Bleomycin was given at 15 mg twice weekly for 5 weeks. No difference in response rate or survival time was noted, and bleomycin was not well tolerated, causing a significant amount of mucositis. The results were unchanged in a recent update of this trial.[71] Similar results were reported by Vermund and others.[217] In contrast, a third large series,[184] from India, included patients with advanced buccal mucosa cancers and compared radiotherapy given alone with radiation plus bleomycin (10 to 15 mg three times per week for 6 weeks). The complete response rate in the radiotherapy group was 21% compared with 77% in the combined therapy group.

An improvement in disease-free survival time, local and regional control, and complete response rate, but not overall survival time, was reported by Fu and others.[88] In this Northern California Oncology Group trial, patients received either radiotherapy alone or radiation with bleomycin (5 mg twice weekly) followed by 16 weeks of maintenance bleomycin and methotrexate. The complete response rates were 45%

Table 6-5. Randomized trials of simultaneous single agent chemotherapy with radiotherapy versus radiotherapy

Investigations	Chemotherapy	Number of patients	Response rate	Survival benefit
Richards (1969)[167]	HU	40	Yes	NR
Stefani (1971)[195]	HU	150	No	No
Hussey (1975)[112]	HU	42	No	No
Condit (1968)[42]	MTX	40	Yes	NR
Gupta (1987)[96]	MTX	313	Yes	Yes
Kapstad (1978)[121]	Bleomycin	29	Yes	NR
Shanta (1980)[183]	Bleomycin	157	No	Yes
Morita (1980)[153]	Bleomycin	45 (tongue)	No	No
Scandolaro (1982)[177]	Bleomycin	30	No	No
Parvinen (1985)[159]	Bleomycin	46	NR	No
Shetty (1985)[186]	Bleomycin	38	No	No
Vermund (1985)[217]	Bleomycin	222	Yes	No
Fu (1987)[88]	Bleomycin	104	No	Yes-DFS
Eschwege (1988)[71]	Bleomycin	199	NR	No
Shigematsu (1971)[188]	5-FU	63	Yes	Yes-DFS
Lo (1976)[140]	5-FU	163	Yes	Yes
Browman (1993)[26]	5-FU	175	Yes	No
Weissberg (1989)[231]	Mitomycin-C	117	Yes	Yes
Haselow (1990)[101]	CDDP	319	Yes	NR

Reprinted with permission from *Tumors of the nasal cavity and paranasal sinuses, nasopharynx, oral cavity, and oropharynx.* In Schantz SP, Harrison LB, Forastive AA: *Cancer—principles and practice of oncology,* ed 5, Philadelphia, 1997, Lippincott-Raven.
HU—hydroxyurea; MTX—methotrexate; 5-FU—5-fluorouracil; DFS—disease-free survival; CDDP—cisplatin.

with radiotherapy alone and 67% for the combined treatment ($P = 0.056$). The 2-year local and regional control rate was significantly improved with the addition of bleomycin, 26% versus 64% ($P = 0.001$). The incidence of distant metastases as a site of failure was similar in both treatment groups, indicating that the bleomycin and methotrexate maintenance regimen was ineffective in controlling micrometastatic disease. In this trial, in contrast to the others reported, the dose of bleomycin used with radiotherapy was well tolerated. A significant reduction in radiation dose or treatment delays did not occur as a result of enhancement of acute radiation toxicity.

Nine randomized trials of bleomycin and radiation have been completed. Only three of these showed a response benefit.[88,121,183]

5-Fluorouracil plus radiotherapy. Several early trials indicated that 5-FU was an active radiosensitizer for patients with head and neck cancer. Three randomized trials have been published. Lo and others[140] randomized 134 patients with advanced head and neck cancer to radiotherapy with or without 5-FU (10 mg/kg per day for 3 days, 5 mg/kg per day for 4 days, 5 mg/m^2 three times per week). The 5-year survival rate for radiation alone was 14%, and for combined treatment, it was 32%. This improvement in survival time occurred for patients with primary lesions in the tongue or tonsil only. In another study, Shigematsu[188] used intraarterial 5-FU with radiotherapy to treat patients with maxillary sinus carcinoma and observed an improvement in disease-free survival time. Browman[26] randomized patients

to infusional 5-FU and radiation to radiation alone and observed a higher complete response rate but no change in survival time.

Mitomycin and radiotherapy. Mitomycin is an antibiotic that during hypoxic conditions is enzymatically reduced to form an active alkylating species.[175] It is selectively toxic to hypoxic cells. Therefore, because hypoxic cells within tumors have reduced sensitivity to the effects of radiation, it has been hypothesized that combined treatment could improve the therapeutic ratio.[171] This concept was tested by Weissberg and others[231] in a randomized trial by treating 120 patients with advanced head and neck cancer with radiotherapy alone or with radiation with mitomycin (15 mg/m^2). Disease-free survival time at 5 years was 49% for the radiotherapy alone patients and 75% for those treated with mitomycin ($P < 0.07$). Local and regional control rates were significantly improved with administration of mitomycin, 55% versus 75% ($P < 0.01$). There was no difference in the incidence of distant metastases or overall survival time between treatment groups.

Cisplatin and radiotherapy. The exact mechanism of interaction between cisplatin and radiation is not known. Hypoxic and aerobic cell sensitization and the inhibition of cellular repair processes for sublethally damaged cells contribute to the effects observed in *in vitro* systems.[56] In a phase II trial, the RTOG administered cisplatin (100 mg/m^2) every 3 weeks to 124 patients with locally advanced, unresectable head and neck cancer.[6] Sixty percent of patients completed the combined treatment per protocol, and 69% of all patients achieved a complete response. Separate analysis of the disease-free and overall survival times for those with nasopharynx and nonnasopharynx primary sites with more than 5 years of follow-up have been published.[7,144] A comparison to RTOG patients treated with radiotherapy alone suggested improvement in survival time for the combined treatment.

Wheeler and others[233] piloted high-dose cisplatin (200 mg/m^2) every 4 weeks with concurrent radiotherapy in 18 patients with unresectable disease and observed complete responses in 94%. The median survival time was 23 months with 56% and 41% alive and disease-free at 1 and 2 years, respectively. A high rate of distant relapse was observed. Only one randomized trial has been conducted to evaluate concomitant cisplatin and radiotherapy.[101] Through the Head and Neck Intergroup mechanism, 371 patients with unresectable local regional squamous cell head and neck cancer were randomized to receive radiotherapy alone or radiation plus weekly low-dose cisplatin, 20 mg/m^2.

There was a significant difference in overall response rate (complete and partial), 59% for those receiving radiation alone and 73% for those receiving the combined treatment ($P = 0.007$). However, there was no significant difference in complete response or survival time. The lack of survival benefit may be because of the low total dose of cisplatin received, only 120 to 140 mg/m^2 over the 6 to 8 weeks of radiation treatment.

Concomitant chemotherapy and radiotherapy have been useful for the treatment of patients with nasopharyngeal carcinoma. A small group of patients were treated with cisplatin and radiotherapy by Al-Sarraf and others.[7] Local control and survival time were improved in comparison to historical controls. A head and neck intergroup trial closed in November 1995 showed promising results for the combined approach in this disease.[11] In this study, patients received either radiotherapy alone or cisplatin (100 mg/m^2 days 1, 22, and 43) during radiotherapy followed by adjuvant chemotherapy with cisplatin and 5-FU (three cycles). Analysis of 138 randomized patients revealed significant differences in 2-year survival time (80% versus 55%) and progression-free survival time (52 months versus 13 months) favoring the chemotherapy group. This exciting result has now changed the standard of care for those with nasopharyngeal carcinoma in the United States. Patients with stage III or IV disease should be treated with concomitant chemoradiotherapy followed by adjuvant chemotherapy.

Randomized trials of single agents and radiotherapy have shown improved survival time with methotrexate, bleomycin, and 5-FU.[140,184] Improved disease-free survival but not overall survival time has been shown in two other trials with use of bleomycin and mitomycin.[88,231] Because mucosal toxicity is enhanced with these regimens and because overall survival time, although improved, remains poor, none of these regimens has become a standard therapy. The exciting results of the intergroup trial using concurrent cisplatin in

patients with locally advanced nasopharyngeal cancer cannot be generalized to other sites but will form a basis for further investigation.

The favorable results from concurrent cisplatin and radiotherapy followed by adjuvant chemotherapy establish this as a standard management approach for locally advanced nasopharyngeal cancer in the United States.

Multiple agents and radiotherapy

Combining several drugs with radiation will enhance acute toxicity, which may be severe. Therefore, investigators have piloted trials designed with split-course radiation to allow for healthy tissue recovery. Most of these studies are limited to patients with stage III and IV locally advanced unresectable squamous cell cancer and have improved survival time as the primary goal. These regimens alternate chemotherapy and radiotherapy or use split-course radiotherapy to maximize tumor cell kill and minimize tissue toxicity. For those with head and neck cancer, protracted radiation results in decreased local control rates because of accelerated repopulation of cancer cells that survive the initial insult.[12,158] Thus, alternating two non–cross-resistant agents may potentially eliminate not only tumor cell repopulation but primary drug resistance.

Early phase I and II studies have used infusional 5-FU as originally reported by Byfield and others,[28] adding cisplatin[1,205] or hydroxyurea[224] with concurrent split-course single daily fraction radiation. Alternatively, cisplatin and fluorouracil with leucovorin modulation have been combined with split-course accelerated radiotherapy.[232] Several studies with long follow-up periods reported promising survival and response data but also severe toxicity.[3,98,205,227,232]

Mature data were reported by Taylor and others[205] using cisplatin plus continuous infusion 5-FU and radiotherapy and alternating 1 week of treatment with 1 week of rest. The median survival time for 53 patients with a median follow-up period in excess of 4 years was 37 months. The complete response rate was 55%. The total dose received of radiation and 5-FU but not cisplatin correlated with outcome. Local control was poorest in stage IV patients with N3 disease.

Although these pilot trials all report encouraging data for improved survival time, randomized trials that use radiotherapy alone as the control are needed before these approaches can be recommended outside the research setting. Data from six randomized trials are shown in Table 6-6. The South-East Cooperative Oncology Group (SECOG)[193] compared alternating with sequential chemotherapy and radiotherapy. The chemotherapy selected was vincristine, bleomycin, and methotrexate with a further randomization to inclusion of 5-FU or not. Survival rates were lower than observed in a previous pilot trial, and a significant improvement in disease-free survival time was observed on subset analysis for larynx primaries managed with the alternating schedule. The alternating regimen was associated with a higher frequency of severe mucosal reactions.

Table 6-6. Randomized trials of concomitant or alternating combination chemotherapy and radiation

Author (Ref)	Treatment	Number of patients	Survival	Other outcomes
Keane (1993)[123]	Concurrent MMC + F/RT	104	NS	
	RT	105		
Merlano (1992)[151]	Alternating PF/RT	80	Significant increase	Significant improvement in CR + L-R control with PFS/RT
	RT	77		
Taylor (1994)[206]	Concurrent PF/RT	108	NS	Significant improvement L-R control for $T_{3-4}N_2$ subset with PFS/RT
	Sequential PF → RT	107		
Adelstein (1990b)[2]	Concurrent PF/RT	24	NS	Significant improvement in DFS with concurrent PFS/RT
	Sequential PF → RT	24		
Merlano (1991)[149]	Alternating VBM/RT	61	Significant increase	Significant increase in CR and PFS with concurrent VBM/RT
	Sequential VBM → RT	55		
SECOG (1986)[193]	Concurrent VBM ± F/RT	136	NS	DFS improved for larynx with concurrent VBM ± F/RT
	Sequential VBM ± F → RT	131		

Reprinted with permission from *Tumors of the nasal cavity and paranasal sinuses, nasopharynx, oral cavity, and oropharynx.* In Schantz SP, Harrison LB, Forastive AA: *Cancer—principles and practice of oncology*, ed 5, Philadelphia, 1997, Lippincott-Raven.
MMC—Mitomycin C; F—5-fluorouracil; RT—Radiotherapy; NS—Not significant; PFS—Progress-free survival; CR—Complete response; DFS—Disease-free survival; SECOG—South East Cooperative Oncology Group; P—Cisplatin; V—Vinblastine; B—Bleomycin; M—Methotrexate; L-R—Locoregional.

Merlano and others[149] published the final report of a randomized comparison of alternating and sequential chemotherapy (vinblastine, bleomycin, methotrexate) and radiotherapy followed by surgical salvage if feasible. Four courses of chemotherapy were alternated with three courses of radiotherapy (20 Gy each). All patients had unresectable stage III or IV squamous cell cancer. The complete response rate before and after surgical intervention and the overall survival time at 4 years were significantly superior for patients receiving concomitant treatment. Severe mucosal toxicity was observed in 30.5% of patients in the alternating regimen compared with only 6% of those receiving chemotherapy before radiotherapy. The results of a follow-up trial reported by Merlano and others[149,150] showed a significant difference in relapse-free and overall survival time for patients treated with alternating cisplatin plus 5-FU and radiotherapy compared with radiotherapy alone. All patients had unresectable locally advanced squamous cell cancer of the head and neck.

In a small randomized trial, Adelstein and others[2] compared simultaneous cisplatin plus 5-FU and radiotherapy to sequential treatment. Patients with stage II, III, or IV, either resectable and unresectable disease, were eligible. In the simultaneous treatment, patients were evaluated for surgery after chemotherapy and 30 Gy. Complete responders and those with unresectable disease continued treatment with chemotherapy and radiotherapy. In the sequential treatment, surgical evaluation occurred after three cycles of chemotherapy and before radiotherapy. The results with follow-up period ranging 9 to 41 months showed a significant difference in disease free-survival but not overall survival time. At this

point in follow-up, 18 of 48 patients were complete responders and had not required surgery.

Finally, Taylor,[206] similarly to Adelstein and others,[3] compared cisplatin plus 5-FU and concomitant radiotherapy with sequential treatment. They found a significant improvement in local and regional control on subset analysis for patients with T3–T4 N0 and T1–T2 N2 diseases receiving concomitant treatment.

The results of these trials indicate that improved disease-free and overall survival times are possible for patients with locally advanced squamous cell head and neck cancer using alternating or concomitant chemotherapy and radiotherapy. Well-designed clinical trials are needed to determine optimal chemotherapy and radiotherapy schedules. Randomized trials are currently in progress to help clarify these issues.

Adjuvant chemotherapy

Adjuvant chemotherapy after primary surgery has been shown to be effective in patients with breast cancer and osteogenic sarcoma. To date, three randomized trials have been designed to address this question in those with head and neck cancer. Adjuvant chemotherapy has several potential advantages over neoadjuvant treatment. With adjuvant treatment, surgery is not delayed, and a patient with resectable disease can undergo surgery sooner. Secondly, neoadjuvant therapy can blur the margins of disease, making the degree of surgical resection less obvious. Finally, neoadjuvant therapy, if successful, can lead to symptom abatement, resulting in patient refusal of surgery afterward.

Through the Head and Neck Intergroup mechanism, a large multiinstitutional trial was conducted to test whether the addition of chemotherapy to surgery and radiotherapy prolonged survival time or altered the pattern of recurrence.[132] Patients with stage III or IV squamous cell carcinoma of the oral cavity, oropharynx, or larynx and those with stage II, III, or IV of the hypopharynx who had negative pathologic margins of resection were eligible.

Randomization was to immediate postoperative radiotherapy or to three cycles of cisplatin plus 5-FU chemotherapy followed by radiotherapy. A preliminary analysis of the 503 patients randomized has shown no significant difference in disease-free survival time, overall survival time, and local and regional control. However, there was a significantly lower rate of distant metastases as a site of failure ($P = 0.016$) at any time for patients treated with adjuvant chemotherapy. Perhaps more important was the finding that a high-risk subset of patients (those with extracapsular extension, carcinoma *in situ*, or close surgical margins) appears to benefit from adjuvant chemotherapy with increased survival time and local control that approached statistical confidence when compared with those receiving radiation alone.

Two trials testing induction chemotherapy added maintenance chemotherapy to one treatment group and observed differences in outcome. The Head and Neck Contracts Program[103] trial of one course of cisplatin and bleomycin induction chemotherapy before surgery and radiation included 6 months of maintenance chemotherapy in one of the three treatment arms. There was a significant decrease in the distant metastatic rate observed for those patients. Ervin and others[70] randomized patients showing a response to cisplatin, bleomycin, and methotrexate induction chemotherapy to receive three additional cycles or observation after definitive surgery and radiotherapy. The 3-year disease-free survival time for patients receiving maintenance chemotherapy was 88% compared with 57% for the controls ($P = 0.03$). In a phase II pilot, Johnson and others[119] treated 42 patients with extracapsular spread of tumor in cervical lymph node metastases with 6 months of methotrexate and 5-FU after resection and radiotherapy. The 2-year disease-free survival rate was 66%, which was improved from an expected control rate of 38% based on historical experience.

Considered together, the results of these five trials indicate that adjuvant chemotherapy can affect micrometastatic disease and decrease the rate of distant recurrence. The data also suggest that disease-free survival time may be improved. The major impediment to successfully conducting adjuvant or maintenance chemotherapy trials in patients with head and neck cancer is patient noncompliance. The morbidity of the primary treatment, combined with the medical and social situations of this group of patients, makes classical adjuvant chemotherapy unacceptable or not feasible in many patients. In addition, there appears to be no role for adjuvant chemotherapy in low-risk patients, although high-risk patients may benefit.

ORGAN PRESERVATION

Many squamous cell cancers of the head and neck are diagnosed at a late stage. Stage III and IV tumors often necessitate extensive or radical surgery that can alter function. Problems with radical surgery include loss of speech, loss of swallowing function, or disfigurement without a concomitant improvement in survival time. Therefore, preservation of function has become one of the major challenges of the 1990s. A role for combined modality treatment in preserving organ function already has been noted for laryngeal preservation as in the V.A. larynx study. In this study, neoadjuvant chemotherapy followed by radiotherapy was more successful in preserving voice function compared with surgery without a loss in survival time.

Neoadjuvant chemotherapy has been used to preserve organ function for patients with hypopharyngeal, laryngeal, and oropharyngeal cancers. Several nonrandomized studies have been completed using cisplatin-based chemotherapy. In these studies, patients were required to have achieved either a partial or complete response to go on to conventional radiotherapy. Nonresponders then went on to radical surgery. In these pilot studies, there were no survival differences between the surgical groups and the groups that avoided surgery, suggesting that quality of life may be improved without worsening survival.*

In addition to the V.A. larynx study,[221] one other large randomized study has been completed. This study[133] was done in Europe by the European Organization for Research and Treatment of Cancer (EORTC) beginning in 1990 and compared a larynx-preserving therapy (induction chemotherapy plus radiation) with conventional surgery plus postoperative radiation. The design of the EORTC study was similar to the V.A. larynx study, as patients were randomized to either treatment, and patients receiving induction chemotherapy received cisplatin plus 5-FU. After two cycles of chemotherapy, only responders (i.e., partial or complete responders) received a third cycle. Patients achieving a complete response then received definitive radiotherapy. Nonresponding patients or those with partial response underwent conventional surgery followed by postoperative radiation.

As in the V.A. study, the overall survival data were not different between the two arms, and the median duration of survival time was longer for the chemotherapy arm. Local failures occurred more commonly in the chemotherapy arm, but the distant metastatic rate was lower. In both studies, a large number of patients were enrolled, and of the surviving patients, a significant percentage were able to retain their larynx. These exciting results are changing the standard of care for patients with advanced laryngeal cancer and suggest that this approach may be feasible for other sites. Patients with stage III or IV laryngeal or hypopharyngeal carcinomas should now be given the option of organ preservation therapy (chemotherapy and radiotherapy). Further, patients with ad-

* Refs. 51, 54, 91, 122, 129, 131, 160, 164, 189.

vanced carcinomas of the oropharynx and oral cavity should be enrolled in organ-preservation trials to assess the effectiveness of this therapy versus standard care.

INTRAARTERIAL CHEMOTHERAPY

Poor response to chemotherapy after surgery or radiotherapy may be caused by impaired drug delivery into the region. Intraarterial chemotherapy has been used in attempts to overcome this for almost three decades. The rationale for intraarterial therapy is based on the steep dose–response curve exhibited by most cytotoxic drugs.[84] Maximum cell kill occurs when the tumor exposure to a high concentration of drug is optimized. Drug toxicity also follows a steep curve. Therefore, regional drug delivery has the potential to increase tumor drug exposure and reduce systemic exposure that affects critical healthy tissues.[37,41] The principal determinant of a drug's therapeutic advantage is the ratio of total body clearance to the regional exchange rate.

Several factors should be considered in choosing a drug for intraarterial delivery: (1) drug concentration, not time of exposure, is the major factor in cell killing; (2) the drug should be deactivated in the systemic circulation; (3) there should be a high tissue extraction; and (4) a drug should not require activation in the liver.

Intraarterial cisplatin has been shown to be effective and relatively nontoxic in patients with several solid tumors. Pharmocakinetic studies have shown a regional increase in plasma and tissue platinum concentrations in the infused area. Several studies indicate significant palliation in patients with head and neck squamous cancers in whom irradiation and surgery failed to eradicate the tumor. A response rate of 87% using intraarterial 5-FU, methotrexate, and bleomycin was reported by Donegan and Harris.[59] Tumor regression lasted up to 13 months. Intraarterial methotrexate and bleomycin have been used before irradiation for patients with advanced head and neck cancer, with a 28% partial response rate.[240] Intraarterial cisplatin given before surgery or radiation has produced responses in the 70% to 80% range.[93,154]

One of the major drawbacks of intraarterial therapy is catheter-related complications: air and plaque emboli, sepsis, and patient immobility during chemotherapy administration. These problems have been overcome by the introduction of an implantable infusion pump.[15] This system has been used successfully in treating patients with recurrent head and neck cancer with continuous infusion of dichloromethotrexate and fluorodoxyuridine.[79,234]

One primary site for which intraarterial chemotherapy has been more extensively studied is paranasal sinus cancer. Japanese investigators have favored cannulation of the superficial temporal artery and infusion of 5-FU integrated with surgery and radiotherapy.[176,187] More recently, investigators in the United States have evaluated superselective arterial catheterization and short-term intraarterial chemotherapy to debulk locally advanced resectable and unresectable paranasal sinus carcinoma. This approach minimizes

potential toxic effects to adjacent healthy tissues. Dimery[58] reported evaluating intraarterial cisplatin and bleomycin by this technique combined with intravenous 5-FU. A complete response rate of 23% was achieved in those receiving the chemotherapy alone. After surgery or radiotherapy, 63% of patients were disease-free, and 61% were spared orbital exenteration.

Although intraarterial therapy has several theoretic advantages over systemic chemotherapy, it has not been established as a superior approach. Most series contain small numbers of selected patients. This therapy should not be viewed as a standard of care by the community, but further investigation appears warranted.

SALIVARY GLAND CANCERS

Cancers of the salivary gland represent approximately 3% of all neoplasms in the head and neck region. The majority originate in the parotid gland. Despite optimal treatment with surgery and postoperative radiotherapy, patients with advanced salivary gland cancers have a poor prognosis, with survival times ranging from 0% to 32% at 10 years. Survival time varies with histology, with 10-year survival rates of 96% reported for low-grade mucoepidermoid carcinoma and 29% reported for adenoid cystic carcinoma.[85] Probability of recurrence also varies with site. Local or distal recurrence occurs in up to 66% of patients with cancers of major salivary glands and in up to 92% of patients with cancers of the minor salivary glands.[43] Reasons for recurrence include failure of local control and spread of disease to distant sites, particularly the lung.

Chemotherapy in the management of salivary gland cancers has been used mainly for the treatment of patients with recurrent disease. Because of the relatively small number of patients, trials often contain few patients with a variety of histologic findings. Many reports document single cases, leaving uncertainty as to the number of patients who may have been treated. Suen and Johns[200] showed that response to chemotherapy varies with histologic findings. They also found that response varies with site recurrence, with local and regional disease having a higher response rate than distal disease. In addition, patients without previous radiotherapy had a better response to chemotherapy. Drawing conclusions from most series is difficult because they usually include a group of patients treated for many years with a variety of combinations and single agents. In addition, some cancers with distal spread, such as adenoid cystic carcinoma, can grow at such a slow rate that responses and impact on survival time are difficult to interpret.

Suen and Johns[200] reported large series of patients treated at their institutions and at others in an attempt to define the best single agents or combinations of drugs for salivary gland cancers of specific histologic categories. For those with adenoid cystic carcinoma, the best single agents are cisplatin, 5-FU, and doxorubicin (Table 6-7). Cisplatin has been re-

Table 6-7. Combination chemotherapy for salivary gland cancer

Histology	Author	Chemotherapy	Number of patients	Response (CR and PR) (%)
Adenoid cystic carcinoma	Posner, 1982[163]	Adriamycin + cyclophosphamide	5	40
	Dreyfuss, 1987[62]	Cisplatin + adriamycin + cyclophosphamide	9	33
	Venook, 1987[215]	Cisplatin + adriamycin + 5-FU	9	22
	Triozzi, 1987[211]	Cyclophosphamide + vincristine + 5-FU	8	25
	Creagan, 1988[47]	4 cisplatin-based regimens	11	18
Adenocarcinoma	Alberts, 1981[4]	Cisplatin + adriamycin + cyclophosphamide	3	100
	Dreyfuss, 1987[62]		4	75
	Creagan, 1988[47]	4 cisplatin-based regimens	14	43
	Venook, 1987[215]	Cisplatin + adriamycin + 5-FU	3	100
Mucoepidermoid carcinoma	Posner, 1982[163]	Cisplatin + bleomycin + methotrexate	3	67
	Venook, 1987[215]	Cisplatin + adriamycin + 5-FU	4	25
	Creagan, 1988[47]	4 cisplatin-based regimens	7	14

CR—Complete response; PR—Partial response.

ported to have a complete response rate of 29% and an overall response rate of 64% in 14 treated patients.[179,200] Complete responses lasted from 7 to 18 months. 5-FU has been reported to have a partial response rate of 46% in 13 patients.[120,203] Adriamycin was noted to have a response rate of 13% in seven patients.[166,216] Methotrexate, vincristine, and cyclophosphamide appear to have little activity for adenoid cystic carcinoma. The combination of adriamycin and cyclophosphamide has been used in five patients with a 40% partial response rate.[163] Because of poor prognosis of patients with advanced disease and the activity of cisplatin, Sessions and others[181] treated four patients with intraarterial cisplatin before further therapy. All patients had some tumor shrinkage, but only two had a partial response. There was minimal toxicity.

Very few studies of single-agent chemotherapy for mucoepidermoid carcinoma exist. Several of the studies were done before the widespread use of cisplatin, and data on its use as a single agent for the management of this carcinoma are not available. Methotrexate has been used in four patients, with one achieving a complete response and one having a partial response. Posner and others[163] used two different combinations for recurrent mucoepidermoid carcinoma. Two of three patients responded to a combination of cisplatin, bleomycin, and methotrexate. Three patients failed to respond to a combination of cyclophosphamide and adriamycin. Further studies need to be done to determine the most active agents for mucoepidermoid carcinoma.

Only scattered reports of the use of chemotherapy for the other salivary gland cancers exist. The combination of adriamycin, cisplatin, and cyclophosphamide achieved one complete response and two partial responses in three treated patients with adenocarcinoma.[4] The small numbers of patients in each series preclude firm conclusions regarding the true level of antitumor activity of these drugs. However, the data provide an indication of which drugs are reasonable to choose for single-agent or combination chemotherapy. Creagan and others[47] reported the results of cisplatin-based chemotherapy in 34 patients with locally recurrent or metastatic cancers originating from the salivary gland or contiguous structures (see Table 6-7). Most patients received cyclophosphamide or mitomycin, plus adriamycin and cisplatin combination chemotherapy. A 38% response rate was observed, listing a median of 7 months. The median survival time was 18 months for responders to chemotherapy and 15 months for nonresponders. Thus, response to treatment did not appear to confer a survival advantage. Dreyfuss and others[62] also evaluated cyclophosphamide, adriamycin, and cisplatin in a series of 13 patients (nine with adenoid cystic carcinoma and four with adenocarcinoma), observing responses in 46% (three complete and three partial responses).

In another combination chemotherapy trial, Venook and others[215] treated 17 patients with advanced or recurrent salivary cancer with cisplatin, adriamycin, and 5-FU. Thirty-five percent of patients responded to chemotherapy. In this small series, response rate was not influenced by the extent of previous treatment.

In conclusion, cisplatin, adriamycin, and 5-FU or cyclophosphamide appear to be the most active agents and combinations for those with adenoid cystic carcinoma and adenocarcinoma. The most active agents for the other cancers have not been defined. Whether combination chemotherapy can improve survival time in patients with recurrent disease is not clear. In some patients with recurrent disease, particularly adenoid cystic carcinoma, the pace of disease can be so slow that patients often do not need to be treated with chemotherapy for a prolonged period. This slow growth rate in some patients may be one of the factors accounting for the poor response to chemotherapy. New agents need to be evaluated in adequate numbers of patients to determine activity with statistical confidence. One such trial is in progress in the ECOG. The taxane derivative paclitaxel (Taxol) is being studied in cohorts of patients with adenoid cystic, mucoepidermoid, and adenocarcinoma of the salivary gland origin in this multicenter trial. Studies of adjuvant chemotherapy in the disease have not been undertaken because of the small numbers of patients and relatively ineffective chemotherapy. Clearly, collaborative efforts by many investigators will be necessary before conclusions can be drawn concerning the use of chemotherapy for salivary gland cancers.

CHEMOPREVENTION OF HEAD AND NECK CANCER

Chemoprevention is defined as the administration of pharmacologic agents to inhibit the events occurring during the multistep process of carcinogenesis or the reversal of a premalignant condition. The biology of carcinogenesis leading to upper aerodigestive tract malignancies is not well understood. Tumor formation is believed to be a multistep process involving biochemical and molecular changes that result in dysregulated differentiation and proliferation.[75] Chromosomal alterations and mutations of specific oncogenes are associated with epithelial cancers.[99,237] Investigators studying various genomic, proliferation, and differentiation biomarkers have found alterations in specific markers (keratin, involucrin, transglutaminase) during the process of abnormal squamous differentiation. These biomarkers may be useful as intermediate end points in future chemoprevention trials.[136] Our understanding of the biology of carcinogenesis for head and neck cancer and other aerodigestive tract tumors is expected to rapidly expand in the next decade.

Chemoprevention is particularly relevant to patients who are curatively treated for an early stage head and neck squamous cell cancer. It is recognized that second primary malignancies develop at a constant rate of 3% to 4% per year in these patients.[44,135] The explanation for this risk is based on the concept of field cancerization first formulated in the 1950s.[191,199] Repeated exposure of the entire epithelial surface to carcinogens, such as tobacco and alcohol, can lead to the development of multiple sites of premalignant and malignant change. The ability of retinoids and carotenoids to affect epithelial growth and differentiation is supported by *in vitro*, animal, and epidemiologic studies.[20] Although the exact mechanism by which retinoids inhibit carcinogenesis is not known, retinoids have been shown to modify genomic expression at the level of messenger RNA synthesis and to regulate transcription of specific genes.[141,229] Clinically, retinoids and carotenoids have been used to prevent malignant transformation of dysplastic leukoplakia lesions. Most recently, retinoids have been studied in the prevention of second primary cancers. Retinoids are the synthetic and natural analogs of vitamin A. β-carotene is the major source of vitamin A in the diet.

The major limitation in the use of retinoids is the associated toxicity. Acute toxicity includes dryness of conjunctival and oral mucous membranes, cheilitis, skin desquamation, hypertriglyceridemia, bone tenderness, arthralgias, and myalgias. Chronic toxicities include hepatotoxicity and bone remodeling.[104] These compounds are teratogenic, causing multiple malformations. Because of these toxicities, a number of retinoids have been synthesized. Four used clinically are vitamin A or retinol; β-all-transretinoic acid or retinoid; 13-cis retinoic acid or isotretinoin; and an aromatic ethyl ester derivative, etretinate.[104] In contrast to the retinoids, the major toxicity of the carotenoids is yellowing of the skin. Other compounds that may have use in chemoprevention based mainly on *in vitro* and animal data are α-tocopherol (vitamin E), selenium, and N-acetyl cysteine. The latter compound is a precursor of intracellular glutathione that enhances its antioxidant activity as a free radical scavenger. N-acetyl cysteine is nontoxic and currently under investigation in Europe for the prevention of second malignancies in patients with a previous head and neck or lung carcinoma.[24,104]

Studies with retinoids and carotenoids in patients with leukoplakia are listed in Table 6-8. Stich and others[197,198] reported two trials conducted in India and the Philippines in betel nut chewers. In one placebo-controlled trial, β-carotene was compared with β-carotene plus vitamin A. Complete response was observed in 3% of the placebo patients, in 15% of β-carotene–treated patients, and in 28% of those taking the combination. These patients demonstrated significant suppression of micronuclei expression and index of DNA damage on serial cytologic examinations. In a subsequent study, patients were randomized to placebo or twice the dose of vitamin A (200,000 IU/week) received in the first trial. A 57% complete response rate was observed with total suppression of the development of new leukoplakic lesions. In the placebo group, the complete response rate was 3%, and there was a 21% rate of new lesion formation.[198] In a small pilot study, Garewal and others[89] observed a 71% complete and partial response rate in 24 patients treated with β-carotene. There was no significant toxicity. The preliminary results of a fourth study[209] showed only a 27% response rate, although the dose of β-carotene was higher. Other investigators reported complete and partial response rates ranging from 60% to 100% with 13-cis retinoic acid.[127,182]

These results led Hong and others[106] to conduct a randomized placebo-controlled trial of 13-cis retinoic acid (1 or 2 mg/kg/day) in oral leukoplakia with dysplastic change. All patients were assessed with pretreatment and posttreatment biopsies. Patients were treated for 3 months and observed for 6 months. There was a highly significant difference in response rate, 67% versus 10%, comparing the treated with the placebo group. Histologic reversal of dysplastic change was documented in 54%. Unfortunately, after stopping treatment, the relapse rate was high within 2 or 3 months, and the regimen was associated with considerable toxicity. In a follow-up trial,[137] 56 patients received 13-cis

Table 6-8. Results of randomized chemoprevention trials in the head and neck

Study	Design	Number of patients	Intervention and dose	Results
Oral premalignancy				
Hong and others, 1986[106]	Induction	44	Isotretinoin (2 mg/kg/d)	Positive
Lippman and others, 1993[138]	Maintenance	70	Isotretinoin (0.5 mg/kg/d)	Positive
Stich and others, 1988[198]	Induction	65	Vitamin A (200,000 IU/wk)	Positive
Han and others, 1990[97]	Induction	61	Retinamide (40 mg/d)	Positive
Costa and others, 1994[46]	Maintenance	153	Fenretinide (200 mg/d)	Positive
Previous cancer				
Hong and others, 1990[109]	Adjuvant	103	Isotretinoin (50 to 100 mg/m^2/d)	Positive
Bolla and others, 1994[19]	Adjuvant	316	Etretinate (50 mg/d; 25 mg/d)	Negative

Reprinted with permission from Lippman and others: Strategies for chemoprevention study of premalignancy and second primary tumors in the head and neck, *Curr Opin Oncol* 7:234, 1995.

retinoic acid (1.5 mg/kg/day) for 3 months, followed by randomization to low-dose 13-cis retinoic acid (0.5 mg/kg/day) or β-carotene maintenance therapy. cis-Retinoic acid proved superior in maintaining remissions and had an acceptable level of toxicity in this low dosage.

Most recently, Hong and others[109] reported the results of using 13-cis retinoic acid to prevent second primary malignancies in patients with squamous cell cancer of the head and neck rendered disease-free with surgery and radiotherapy. This placebo-controlled chemoprevention trial randomized 103 patients to receive high-dose 13-cis retinoic acid (50 to 100 mg/m^2/day) or placebo for 1 year. At a median follow-up period of 32 months, second primary tumors had developed in 4% of those receiving retinoic acid compared with 24% of the placebo group ($P = 0.005$). The results of this trial have led to the initiation of two multiinstitutional confirmatory trials in the United States; two chemoprevention trials are in progress in Europe.[24] In the United States, the North Central Cancer Treatment Group and ECOG are randomizing patients with stage I and II squamous cancers of the head and neck rendered disease-free with surgery or radiotherapy to placebo or low-dose 13-cis retinoic acid (0.15 mg/kg/day) for 2 years. Patients should be randomized within 35 days of definitive local therapy. The MD Anderson Cancer Center and Radiation Therapy Oncology Group are conducting a placebo-controlled trial for the same patient group testing a higher dose of cis-retinoic acid, 30 mg/day, for the first year with dose reduction, if toxicity occurs, in years 2 and 3. Patients may enter the study if disease-free between 16 weeks and 3 years after their primary treatment.

These trials along with those ongoing in Europe should establish the benefits and risks of these particular retinoids in the prevention of second cancers in these patients. Etretinate and isotretinoin (13-cis retinoic acid) are commercially available for other indications. Their use in patients with oral premalignant lesions or in patients with curatively treated early-stage head and neck cancer is not recommended outside an investigational research trial. These agents are associated with considerable toxicity; moreover, the minimal effective dose and duration of treatment are not known. Less toxic retinoids or combinations of retinoids and carotenoids may prove to be more effective, but this can only be determined through carefully designed clinical and laboratory investigations.

SUMMARY

Tumors of various histologic types occur in the head and neck. Excluding the thyroid, approximately 80% are squamous cell carcinomas. Data evaluating the impact of chemotherapy on survival time, particularly for combined modality treatments, are limited to this common histologic type where patient numbers are available for randomized comparative trials. Phase I, II, and III studies in patients with locally recurrent or metastatic disease have shown that chemotherapy can produce response rates of 30% to 40%, and combination chemotherapy is more effective than single agents. These response rates, however, have a brief duration and thus, in general, have not prolonged survival time. Thus, chemotherapy for these patients is palliative. An exception to this is for patients with tumors of the nasopharynx in whom higher response rates and a small proportion of long-term disease-free survivors are observed. Prognostic factors have been identified that should be used by the physician to select patients most likely to benefit from palliative treatment.

In the newly diagnosed patient with locally advanced disease, high response rates have been achieved with induction chemotherapy. Improved curability, however, has not been shown. A more important role for chemotherapy may be to preserve organ function at selected sites. Two large multicenter randomized trials were successfully conducted to preserve laryngeal function. A proportion of patients with re-

CANCER OF THE HEAD AND NECK

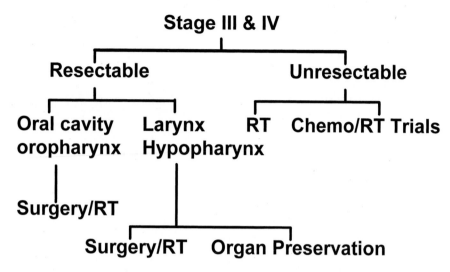

Fig. 6-1. Management of late-stage squamous cell carcinomas of the head and neck.

sected disease at high risk for recurrence treated with chemotherapy in the adjuvant setting may achieve improvement in survival time. This needs to be confirmed, and multicenter trials are in progress. Chemotherapy concurrent with radiotherapy has improved local control and survival time in selected series. The increase in toxicity associated with these regimens should be carefully considered when selecting patients for this combined treatment. Chemotherapy for those with parotid cancers has been studied only for recurrent disease. Response rates are low, and impact on survival time has not been demonstrated.

Figure 6-1 shows an algorithm for management of late stage (locally advanced) squamous cell carcinomas of the head and neck. Patients with earlier stage disease (i.e., stage I or II) should receive conventional therapy with either surgery or radiotherapy or both. Patients with stage III or IV disease can be divided into those with resectable or unresectable disease. Those with unresectable disease should be treated with either radiotherapy or entered into a combined chemoradiation treatment program. Those with stage III disease may benefit the most from combination treatment as part of a clinical trial. Patients with metastatic disease should receive chemotherapy with palliative intent if they exhibit good performance status.

Patients with resectable disease can be further divided by site. Those with primary oral cavity or oropharynx tumors would be best served by surgery followed by radiation, whereas patients with larynx or hypopharyngeal tumors can receive conventional therapy or be offered neoadjuvant chemotherapy followed by radiation in an organ preservation approach.

Chemoprevention will continue to be an important area

of research in the coming decade. One randomized trial has shown a decreased rate of second primary tumors in patients with curatively treated upper aerodigestive tract primary tumors. Confirmatory trials are in progress in the United States and Europe.

The management of head and neck cancer has become multidisciplinary. The identification of effective chemotherapeutic agents and their integration into the initial curative therapy of head and neck cancer has the potential to improve survival time and preserve organ function. Through well-designed and executed clinical trials, coupled with basic research of the biology of upper aerodigestive tract tumors, further advances in the management and prevention of these cancers can be achieved.

REFERENCES

1. Adelstein DJ and others: Long-term results after chemo-radiotherapy for locally confined squamous cell head and neck, *Am J Clin Oncol* 13:440, 1990.
2. Adelstein DJ and others: Simultaneous versus sequential combined technique for squamous cell head and neck cancer, *Cancer* 65:1685, 1990.
3. Adelstein DJ and others: Concurrent radiation therapy and chemotherapy for locally unresectable squamous cell head and neck cancer. An Eastern Cooperative Oncology Group pilot study, *J Clin Oncol* 11: 2136, 1993.
4. Alberts DS and others: Adriamycin, cis-platinum, cyclosphosphamide combination chemotherapy for advanced carcinoma of the parotid gland, *Cancer* 47:645, 1981.
5. Al-Sarraf M and others: *Adjuvant chemotherapy for patients with locally advanced head and neck cancer: RTOG and Wayne State University experiences.* In Salmon SE, editor: *Adjuvant therapy of cancer,* vol 5, Philadelphia, 1987, Grune & Stratton.
6. Al-Sarraf M and others: Concurrent radiotherapy and chemotherapy with cisplatin in inoperable squamous cell carcinoma of the head and neck, *Cancer* 59:259, 1987.

7. Al-Sarraf M and others: Chemoradiotherapy in patients with locally advanced nasopharyngeal carcinoma: a Radiation Therapy Oncology Group study, *J Clin Oncol* 8:1342, 1990.

8. Al-Sarraf M: Chemotherapeutic management of head and neck cancer, *Cancer Metast Rev* 6:191, 1987.

9. Al-Sarraf M: Head and neck cancer: chemotherapy concepts, *Semin Oncol* 15:70, 1988.

10. Al-Sarraf M: *Management strategies in head and neck cancer: the role of carboplatin.* In Bunns PA Jr and others, editors: *Current perspectives and future directions*, Philadelphia, 1990, WB Saunders.

11. Al-Sarraf M and others: Superiority of chemoradiotherapy vs radiotherapy in patients with locally advanced nasopharyngeal cancer. Preliminary results of intergroup (0099) (SWOG 8892, RTOG 8817, ECOG 2388) randomized study, *Proc Am Soc Clin Oncol* 15, 1996 (abstract).

12. Amdur RJ and others: Split-course versus continuous-course irradiation in the postoperative setting for squamous cell carcinoma of the head and neck, *Int J Radiat Oncol Biol* 17:279, 1989.

13. Amer MH and others: Factors that affect response to chemotherapy and survival of patients with advanced head and neck cancer, *Cancer* 43:2202, 1979.

14. Bagshaw MA, Doggett RLS: A clinical study of chemical radiosensitization, *Front Radiat Ther Oncol* 4:164, 1969.

15. Baker SR and others: Intraarterial infusion chemotherapy for head and neck cancer using a totally implantable infusion pump, *Head Neck Surg* 4:118, 1981.

16. Benjamin RS and others: *Adriamycin cardiac toxicity: an assessment of approaches to cardiac monitoring and cardioprotection.* In Hacker MP, Lazo LS, Tritton TR, editors: *Organ directed toxicities of anticancer drugs*, Boston, 1988, Martinus Nijhoff.

17. Bertino JR, Mosher MB, DeConti RC: Chemotherapy of cancer of the head and neck, *Cancer* 31:1141, 1973.

18. Blum RH: An overview of studies with adriamycin (NSC-123127) in the United States, *Cancer Chemother Rep* 6:247, 1975.

19. Bolla M and others: Prevention of second primary tumours with etretinate in squamous cell carcinoma of the oral cavity and oropharynx. Results of a multicentric double-blind randomized study, *Eur J Cancer* 30A:767, 1994.

20. Boone CW, Kelloff GJ, Malone WE: Identification of candidate cancer chemopreventive agents and their evaluation in animal models and human clinical trials: a review, *Cancer Res* 50:2, 1990.

21. Boussen H and others: Chemotherapy of metastatic and/or recurrent undifferentiated nasopharyngeal carcinoma with cisplatin, bleomycin, and fluorouracil, *J Clin Oncol* 9:1675, 1991.

22. Boyle JO and others: The incidence of p53 mutations increases with progression of head and neck cancer, *Cancer Res* 53:4477, 1993.

23. Brennan JA and others: Molecular assessment of histopathologic staging in squamous cell carcinoma of the head and neck, *N Engl J Med* 332(26):1787, 1995.

24. Briggs RJS, Forastiere AA: Isotretinoin for prevention of second squamous cell carcinoma of the head and neck, *Otolaryngol Head Neck Surg* 105:752, 1991.

25. Browman GP, Cronin L: Standard chemotherapy in squamous cell head and neck cancer: what we have learned from randomized trials, *Semin Oncol* 21:311, 1994.

26. Browman GP and others: Placebo-controlled randomized trial of iv infusional 5-fluorouracil concurrent with standard radiotherapy in stage III and IV head and neck cancer, *Proc Am Soc Clin Oncol* 12: 891, 1993.

27. Buesa JM and others: Phase II trial of ifosfamide in recurrent and metastatic head and neck cancer, *Ann Oncol* 2:151, 1991.

28. Byfield JE and others: Phase I and II trial of 5-day infused 5-fluorouracil and radiation in advanced cancer of the head and neck, *J Clin Oncol* 2:406, 1984.

29. Cachin Y and others: Preliminary results of a randomized EORTC study comparing radiotherapy and concomitant bleomycin to radio-therapy alone in epidermoid carcinomas of the oropharynx, *Eur J Cancer* 13:1389, 1977.

30. Calvert AH: Dose optimization of carboplatin in adults, *Anticancer Res* 14(6A):2273, 1994.

31. Campbell JB and others: A randomized phase III trial of cisplatinum, methotrexate, cisplatin + methotrexate, and cisplatinum + 5-fluorouracil in end-stage head and neck cancer, *Acta Otolaryngol* 103:519, 1987.

32. Carugati A, Pradier R, de la Torre A: Combination chemotherapy pre-radical treatment for head and neck squamous cell carcinoma, *Proc Am Soc Clin Oncol* 7:152, 1988.

33. Catimel G and others: A phase II study of gemcytabine (LY188011) in patients with advanced squamous cell carcinoma of the head and neck, *Ann Oncol* 5:543, 1994.

34. Catimel G and others: Docetaxel (Taxotere): an active drug for the treatment of patients with advanced squamous cell carcinoma of the head and neck, *Ann Oncol* 5:533, 1994.

35. Cervellino JC and others: Ifosfamide and MESNA for the treatment of advanced squamous cell head and neck cancer, *Oncology* 48:89, 1991.

36. Chan ATC and others: A prospective randomized study of chemotherapy adjunctive to definitive radiotherapy in advanced nasopharyngeal carcinoma, *Int J Radiat Oncol Biol Phys* 33:761, 1995.

37. Chen HG, Gross JF: Intraarterial infusion of anticancer drugs: theoretic aspects of drug delivery and review of responses, *Cancer Treat Rep* 64:31, 1980.

38. Choksi AJ, Dimery IW, Hong WK: Adjuvant chemotherapy of head and neck cancer: the past, the present, and the future, *Semin Oncol* 15(suppl 3):45, 1988.

39. Choo R, Tannock I: Chemotherapy for recurrent or metastatic carcinoma of the nasopharynx. A review of the Princess Margaret Hospital experience, *Cancer* 68:2120, 1991.

40. Clavel M and others: Randomized comparison of cisplatin, methotrexate, bleomycin, and vincristine (CABO) versus cisplatin and 5-fluorouracil (CF) versus cisplatin (C) in recurrent or metastatic squamous cell carcinoma of the head and neck, *Ann Oncol* 5:521, 1994.

41. Collins JM: Pharmacologic rationale for regional drug delivery, *J Clin Oncol* 2:498, 1984.

42. Condit PT: Treatment of carcinoma with radiation therapy and methotrexate, *MO Med* 65:832, 1968.

43. Conley J, Dingman DL: Adenoid cystic carcinoma in the head and neck (cylindroma), *Arch Otolaryngol* 100:81, 1974.

44. Cooper JS and others: Second malignancies in patients who have head and neck cancer: incidence, effect on survival and implications based on RTOG experience, *Int J Radiat Oncol Biol Phys* 17:449, 1989.

45. Cortes EP and others: Chemotherapy for head and neck cancer relapsing after chemotherapy, *Cancer* 47:1966, 1981.

46. Costa A and others: Prospects of chemoprevention of human cancers with the synthetic retinoid fenretinide, *Cancer Res* 54:2032, 1994.

47. Creagan ET and others: Cisplatin-based chemotherapy for neoplasms arising from salivary glands and contiguous structures in the head and neck, *Cancer* 62:2313, 1988.

48. Cvitkovic E and others: 5-fluorouracil (5FU), mitomycin (M), epirubicin (E), cisplatin (P) in recurrent and/or metastatic undifferentiated nasopharyngeal carcinoma (UCNT), *Proc Am Soc Clin Oncol* 10:200, 1991 (abstract).

49. Dalley D and others: The value of chemotherapy prior to definitive local therapy in patients with locally advanced squamous cell carcinoma of the head and neck, *Proc Am Soc Clin Oncol* 14:297, 1995.

50. Davis D, Kessler W: Randomized comparison of cisdiaminedichloroplatinum versus cisdiaminedichloroplatinum, methotrexate and bleomycin in recurrent squamous cell carcinoma of the head and neck, *Cancer Chemother Pharmacol* 3:57, 1979.

51. de Andres L and others: Function preservation in stage III squamous laryngeal carcinoma: results with an induction chemotherapy protocol, *Laryngoscope* 105:822, 1995.

52. Decker DA and others: Chemotherapy for nasopharyngeal carcinoma: a ten year experience, *Cancer* 52:602, 1983.

53. Degardin M and others: Phase II piritrexim study in recurrent and/or metastatic head and neck cancer, *Proc Am Soc Clin Oncol* 11:244, 1992.

54. Demard F and others: Induction chemotherapy for larynx preservation in laryngeal and hypopharyngeal cancers. In Johnson JT, Didolkar MS, editors: *Head and neck cancer*, vol 3, Amsterdam, 1993, Excerpta Medica.

55. Depondt J and others: Neoadjuvant chemotherapy with carboplatin/5-fluorouracil in head and neck cancer, *Oncology* (suppl 50):23, 1993.

56. Dewit L: Combined treatment of radiation and cisdiaminedichloroplatinum (II): a review of experimental and clinical data, *Int J Radiat Oncol Biol Phys* 13:403, 1987.

57. Di Blasio B and others: A prospective randomized trial in resectable head and neck carcinoma: loco-regional treatment with and without neoadjuvant chemotherapy, *Proc Am Soc Clin Oncol* 13:279, 1994 (abstract).

58. Dimery IW and others: Neoadjuvant therapy of advanced paranasal sinus carcinoma with combined intraarterial and systemic chemotherapy. Presented at the Third International Head and Neck Oncology Research Conference, Las Vegas, Sept 26–28, 1990 (abstract 8.5).

59. Donegan WL, Harris HS: Factors influencing the success of arterial infusion chemotherapy for cancer of the head and neck, *Am J Surg* 123:549, 1972.

60. Drelichman A, Cummings G, Al-Sarraf M: A randomized trial of the combination of cis-platinum, oncovin and bleomycin (COB) versus methotrexate in patients with advanced squamous cell carcinoma of the head and neck, *Cancer* 52:399, 1983.

61. Dreyfuss AI and others: Continuous infusion high-dose leucovorin with 5-fluorouracil and cisplatin for untreated stage IV carcinoma of the head and neck, *Ann Int Med* 112:167, 1990.

62. Dreyfuss AI and others: Cyclophosphamide, doxorubicin, and cisplatin combination chemotherapy for advanced carcinomas of salivary gland origin, *Cancer* 60:2869, 1987.

63. Dreyfuss AI and others: Doxetaxel (Taxotere): an active drug for squamous cell carcinoma of the head and neck, *J Clin Oncol* 14:1672, 1996.

64. Egorin MJ and others: Prospective validation of a pharmacologically based dosing scheme for the cis-diamminedi-chloroplatinum (II) analogue diaminecyclobutanedicarboxylatoplatinum, *Cancer Res* 45:6502, 1985.

65. Eisenberger M and others: A comparison of carboplatin plus methotrexate versus methotrexate alone in patients with recurrent and metastatic head and neck cancer, *J Clin Oncol* 7:1341, 1989.

66. Ensley JF and others: An intensive five course, alternating combination chemotherapy induction regimen used in patients with advanced, unresectable head and neck cancer, *J Clin Oncol* 6:1147, 1988.

67. Ensley JF and others: An intensive six course alternating induction regimen for patients with advanced squamous cell cancers of the head and neck: a Wayne State University and Southwest Oncology Group pilot study, *Proc Am Soc Clin Oncol* 10:205(A-682), 1991.

68. Ensley JF and others: Cellular DNA content parameters in untreated and recurrent squamous cell cancers of the head and neck, *Cytometry* 10:334, 1989.

69. Ensley JF and others: Correlation between response to cisplatinum-combination chemotherapy and subsequent radiotherapy in previously untreated patients with advanced squamous cell cancers of the head and neck, *Cancer* 54:811, 1984.

70. Ervin TJ and others: An analysis of induction and adjuvant chemotherapy in the multidisciplinary treatment of squamous cell carcinoma of the head and neck, *J Clin Oncol* 5:10, 1987.

71. Eschwege F and others: Ten-year results of randomized trial comparing radiotherapy and concomitant bleomycin to radiotherapy alone in epidermoid carcinomas of the oropharynx: experience of the European Organization for Research and Treatment of Cancer, *NCI Monogr* 6:275, 1988.

72. Eschwege F and others: Randomized multicentric international phase III trial of neoadjuvant chemotherapy with bleomycin, epirubicin, cisplatin, followed by radiotherapy versus radiotherapy alone in undifferentiated carcinoma of naso-pharyngeal type: preliminary results, *Int J Radiat Oncol Biol Phys* 82(suppl):192, 1995.

73. Fandi A and others: Nasopharyngeal cancer: epidemiology, staging, and treatment, *Semin Oncol* 21:382, 1994.

74. Fazekas JT, Sommer C, Kramer S: Adjuvant intravenous methotrexate or definitive radiotherapy alone for advanced squamous cancers of the oral cavity, oropharynx, supraglottic larynx or hypopharynx, *Int J Radiat Oncol Biol Phys* 6:533, 1980.

75. Fearon ER, Vogelstein B: A genetic model for colorectal tumorigenesis, *Cell* 61:759, 1990.

76. Forastiere AA: *Carboplatin plus 5-fluorouracil trials in advanced head and neck cancer.* In Bunn PA and others, editors: *Carboplatin (JM-8): current perspectives and future directions,* Philadelphia, 1990, WB Saunders.

77. Forastiere AA: *Head and neck malignancies.* In McGuire WP, Rowinsky EK, editors: *Paclitaxel in cancer treatment,* New York, 1995, Marcel Dekker.

78. Forastiere AA and others: High-dose cisplatin in advanced head and neck cancer, *Cancer Chemother Pharmacol* 19:155, 1987.

79. Forastiere AA and others: Intraarterial cisplatin and FUDR in advanced malignancies confined to the head and neck, *J Clin Oncol* 5:1601, 1987.

80. Forastiere AA: Paclitaxel (taxol) for the treatment of head and neck cancer, *Semin Oncol* (suppl 21):49, 1994.

81. Forastiere AA and others: Pharmacokinetic and toxicity evaluation of 5-day continuous infusion versus intermittent bolus cisdiaminedichloroplatinum (II) in head and neck cancer patients, *Cancer Res* 48:3869, 1988.

82. Forastiere AA: Randomized trials of induction chemotherapy: a critical review, *Hematol/Oncol Clin North Am* 5:725, 1991.

83. Forastiere AA and others: Randomized comparison of cisplatin and 5-fluorouracil versus carboplatin + 5-FU versus methotrexate in advanced squamous cell carcinoma of the head and neck, *J Clin Oncol* 10:1245, 1992.

84. Frei E III, Canellos GP: A critical factor in cancer chemotherapy, *Am J Med* 69:583, 1980.

85. Friedman M and others: Malignant tumors of the major salivary glands, *Otolaryngol Clin North Am* 19:625, 1986.

86. Fromes Y and others: Differential effects of taxol or taxotere on tau and MAP2 containing microtubules, *Proc AACR* 33:551, 1992.

87. Fu KK: Biological basis for the interaction of chemotherapeutic agents and radiation therapy, *Cancer* 55:2123, 1985.

88. Fu KK and others: Combined radiotherapy and chemotherapy with bleomycin and methotrexate for advanced inoperable head and neck cancer: update of a Northern California Oncology group randomized trial, *J Clin Oncol* 5:1410, 1987.

89. Garewal HS and others: Response of oral leukoplakia to beta-carotene, *J Clin Oncol* 8:1715, 1990.

90. Gebbia V and others: Chemotherapeutic treatment of recurrent and/or metastatic nasopharyngeal carcinoma: a retrospective analysis of 40 cases, *Br J Cancer* 68:191, 1993.

91. Giglio R and others: Organ preservation (LP) in resectable stage III and IV epidermoid carcinoma of the larynx (LC) with sequential chemotherapy (CT) + radiation therapy (RT), *Proc Am Soc Clin Oncol* 12:282, 1993 (abstract).

92. Glick JH and others: The adjuvant treatment of inoperable stage III and IV epidermoid carcinoma of the head and neck with platinum and bleomycin infusions prior to definitive radiotherapy, *Cancer* 46:1919, 1980.

93. Grigoleto G and others: Intra-arterial cisplatin in head and neck cancer: a phase I-II study, *Proc Am Soc Clin Oncol* 23:198, 1982.

94. Grose WE and others: Comparison of methotrexate and cisplatin for patients with advanced squamous cell carcinoma of the head and neck region: a Southwest Oncology Group study, *Cancer Treat Rep* 69: 577, 1985.

95. Gueritte-Voegelein F and others: Relationships between the structure of taxol analogues and their antimitotic activity, *J Med Chem* 34:992, 1991.

96. Gupta NK, Pointon RCS, Wilkinson PM: A randomized clinical trial to contract radiotherapy with radiotherapy and methotrexate given synchronously in head and neck cancer, *Clin Radiol* 38:575, 1987.

97. Han J and others: Evaluation of N-4-(hydroxycarbophenyl) retinamide as a cancer prevention agent and as a cancer chemotherapeutic agent, *In Vivo* 4:153, 1990.

98. Haraf DJ and others: Survival and analysis of failure following hydroxyurea, 5-fluorouracil, and concomitant radiation therapy in poor prognosis head and neck cancer, *Am J Clin Oncol* 14:419, 1991.

99. Harris CC and others: *Aberrations of growth and differentiation pathways during neoplastic transformation of human epithelial cells.* In Kakunaga T and others, editors: *Cell differentiation, genes and cancer,* New York, 1988, Oxford University Press.

100. Hasegawa Y and others: A randomized trial in resectable head and neck carcinoma: loco-regional treatment with and without neoadjuvant chemotherapy, *Proc Am Soc Clin Oncol* 13:286, 1994 (abstract).

101. Haselow RE and others: *Radiation alone versus radiation plus weekly low-dose cis-platinum in unresectable cancer of the head and neck.* In Fee WE Jr and others, editors: *Head and neck cancer,* vol 2, Philadelphia, 1990, Mosby.

102. Hayes DM and others: High-dose cis-platinum diaminedichloride: amelioration of renal toxicity by mannitol diuresis, *Cancer* 39:1372, 1977.

103. Head and Neck Contracts Program: Adjuvant chemotherapy for advanced head and neck squamous carcinoma, *Cancer* 60:301, 1987.

104. Heyne KE, Lippman SM, Hong WK: Chemoprevention in head and neck cancer, *Hematol Oncol Clin North Am* 5:783, 1991.

105. Hill BT, Price LA: *The significance of primary site in assessing chemotherapy response and survival in advanced squamous cell carcinomas of the head and neck treated with initial combination chemotherapy without cisplatin: analysis at nine years.* In Salmon S, editor: *Adjuvant therapy of cancer,* vol 5, Philadelphia, 1987, Grune & Stratton.

106. Hong WK and others: 13-cis retinoic acid in the treatment of oral leukoplakia, *N Engl J Med* 315:1501, 1986.

107. Hong WK and others: A prospective randomized trial of methotrexate versus cisplatin in the treatment of recurrent squamous cell carcinoma of the head and neck, *Cancer* 52:206, 1983.

108. Hong WK and others: Induction chemotherapy in advanced squamous head and neck carcinoma with high-dose cis-platinum and bleomycin infusion, *Cancer* 44:19, 1979.

109. Hong WK and others: Prevention of second primary tumors with isotretinoin in squamous cell carcinoma of the head and neck, *N Engl J Med* 323:795, 1990.

110. Hong WK and others: Sequential response patterns to chemotherapy and radiotherapy in head and neck cancer: potential impact to treatment in advanced laryngeal cancer, *Prog Clin Oncol Res* 201:191, 1985.

111. Huber MH and others: A phase II study of ifosfamide in recurrent squamous cell carcinoma of the head and neck, *Am J Clin Oncol* 19: 379, 1996.

112. Hussey D, Abrams J: Combined therapy in advanced head and neck cancer with hydroxyurea and radiotherapy, *Prog Clin Cancer* 6:79, 1975.

113. International Nasopharynx Cancer Study Group: VUMCA I Trial: preliminary results of a randomized trial comparing neoadjuvant chemotherapy (cisplatin, epirubicin, bleomycin) plus radiotherapy vs. radiotherapy alone in stage IV ($\geq$ N2, M0) undifferentiated nasopha-

ryngeal carcinoma: a positive effect on progression-free survival, *Int J Rad Oncol Biol Phys* 35:463, 1996.

114. Jacobs C and others: 24-hour infusion of cis-platinum in head and neck cancers, *Cancer* 42:2135, 1978.

115. Jacobs C and others: A randomized phase III study of cisplatin with or without methotrexate for recurrent squamous cell carcinoma of the head and neck: a Northern California Oncology Group study, *Cancer* 52:1563, 1983.

116. Jacobs C and others: A phase III randomized study comparing cisplatin and fluorouracil as single agents and in combination for advanced squamous cell carcinoma of the head and neck, *J Clin Oncol* 10:257, 1992.

117. Jacobs C, Makuch R: Efficacy of adjuvant chemotherapy for patients with resectable head and neck cancer: a subset analysis of the Head and Neck Contracts Program, *J Clin Oncol* 8:838, 1990.

118. Jaulerry C and others: Induction chemotherapy in advanced head and neck tumors: results of two randomized trials, *Int J Radiat Oncol Biol Phys* 23:483, 1992.

119. Johnson JT and others: Adjuvant chemotherapy for high-risk squamous cell carcinoma of the head and neck, *J Clin Oncol* 5:456, 1987.

120. Johnson RO and others: Infusion of 5-fluorouracil in cylindroma treatment, *Arch Otolaryngol* 79:625, 1964.

121. Kapstad B and others: Combined preoperative treatment with cobalt and bleomycin in patients with head and neck carcinoma: a controlled clinical study, *Int J Radiat Oncol Biol Phys* 4:85, 1978.

122. Karp DD and others: Larynx preservation using induction chemotherapy plus radiation therapy as an alternative to laryngectomy in advanced head and neck cancer, *Am J Clin Oncol* 14:273, 1991.

123. Keane TJ and others: A randomized trial of radiation therapy compared to split course radiation therapy combined with mitomycin and 5-fluorouracil as initial treatment for advanced laryngeal and hypopharyngeal squamous carcinoma, *Int J Radiat Oncol Biol Phys* 25: 613, 1993.

124. Kish JA and others: A randomized trial of cisplatin (CACP) + 5-fluorouracil (5-Fu) infusion and CACP + 5-Fu bolus for recurrent and advanced squamous cell carcinoma of the head and neck, *Cancer* 56:2740, 1985.

125. Kish JA and others: Activity of ifosfamide (NSC-109724) in recurrent head and neck cancer patients, *Proc Am Assoc Cancer Res* 31:190, 1990 (abstract).

126. Knowlton AH and others: Methotrexate and radiation therapy in the treatment of advanced head and neck tumors, *Radiology* 116:709, 1975.

127. Koch H: Biochemical treatment of precancerous oral lesions: the effectiveness of various analogues of retinoic acid, *J Maxillofac Surg* 6:59, 1978.

128. Kotwall C and others: Metastatic patterns in squamous cell cancer of the head and neck, *Am J Surg* 154:439, 1987.

129. Kraus DH and others: Larynx preservation with combined chemotherapy and radiation therapy in advanced hypopharynx cancer, *Otolaryngol Head Neck Surg* 111:31, 1994.

130. Kun LE and others: A randomized study of adjuvant chemotherapy for cancer of the upper aerodigestive tract, *Int J Radiat Oncol Biol Phys* 12:173, 1986.

131. Laccourreye O and others: *Preservation of the larynx following neoadjuvant chemotherapy: a preliminary report.* In Banzet P and others, editors: *Neoadjuvant chemotherapy,* Paris, 1991, Springer-Verlag.

132. Laramore G and others: Adjuvant chemotherapy for resectable squamous cell carcinomas of the head and neck: report on Intergroup study 0034, *Int J Radiat Oncol Biol Phys* 23:705, 1992.

133. Lefebvre JL and others: Larynx preservation in hypopharynx and lateral epilarynx cancer: preliminary results of EORTC randomized phase III trial 24891, *J Natl Cancer Inst* 88:890, 1996.

134. Levitt M and others: Improved therapeutic index of methotrexate with leucovorin rescue, *Cancer Res* 33:1729, 1973.

135. Licciardello JT, Spitz MR, Hong WK: Multiple primary cancer in

patients with cancer of the head and neck: second cancer of the head and neck, esophagus, and lung, *Int J Radiat Oncol Biol Phys* 17:467, 1989.

136. Lippman SM and others: Biomarkers as intermediate end points in chemoprevention trials, *J Natl Cancer Inst* 82:555, 1990.

137. Lippman SM and others: Low-dose 13-cis-retinoic acid maintains remission in oral premalignancy: more effective than b-carotene in randomized trial, *Proc Am Soc Clin Oncol* 9:59, 1990 (abstract).

138. Lippman SM and others: Comparison of low-dose isotretinoin with beta-carotene to prevent oral carcinogenesis, *N Engl J Med* 328:15, 1993.

139. Liverpool Head and Neck Oncology Group: A phase III randomized trial of cisplatinum, methotrexate, cisplatinum + methotrexate and cisplatinum + 5-FU in end stage squamous cell carcinoma of the head and neck, *Br J Cancer* 61:311, 1990.

140. Lo TCM and others: Combined radiation therapy and 5-fluorouracil for advanced squamous cell carcinoma of the oral cavity and oropharynx: a randomized study, *Am J Roentgenol* 126:229, 1976.

141. Lotan R: Effects of vitamin A and its analogs (retinoids) on normal and neoplastic cells, *Biochem Biophys Acta* 605:33, 1980.

142. Lustig RA, Demare PA, Kramer S: Adjuvant methotrexate in the radio-chemotherapeutic management of advanced tumors of the head and neck, *Cancer* 37:2703, 1976.

143. Mahjoubi R and others: Metastatic undifferentiated carcinoma of nasopharyngeal type treated with bleomycin (B), epirubicin (E), and cisplatin (C): Final report, *Proc Am Soc Clin Oncol* 11:240, 1992 (abstract).

144. Marcial VA and others: Concomitant cisplatin chemotherapy and radiotherapy in advanced mucosal squamous cell carcinoma of the head and neck: long-term results of the Radiation Therapy Oncology Group study 81-17, *Cancer* 66:1861, 1990.

145. Martin M and others: Ifosfamide in advanced epidermoid head and neck cancer, *Cancer Chemother Pharmacol* 31:340, 1993.

146. Martin M and others: Randomized study of 5-fluorouracil and cisplatin as neoadjuvant therapy in head and neck cancer: a preliminary report, *Int J Radiat Oncol Biol Phys* 19:973, 1990.

147. Martin M and others: A randomized prospective study of CDDP and 5-FU as neoadjuvant chemotherapy in head and neck cancer: a final report, *Proc Am Soc Clin Oncol* 14:294, 1995.

148. Mazeron JJ and others: Induction chemotherapy in head and neck cancer: results of a phase III trial, *Head Neck* 14:85, 1992.

149. Merlano M and others: Combined chemotherapy and radiation therapy in advanced inoperable squamous cell carcinoma of the head and neck, *Cancer* 67:915, 1991.

150. Merlano M and others: Five-year update of a randomized trial of alternating radiotherapy and chemotherapy compared with radiotherapy alone in treatment of unresectable squamous cell carcinoma of the head and neck, *J Natl Cancer Inst* 88:58, 1996.

151. Merlano M and others: Treatment of advanced squamous-cell carcinoma of the head and neck with alternating chemotherapy and radiotherapy, *N Engl J Med* 327:1115, 1992.

152. Moran RG: Leucovorin enhancement of the effects of fluoropyrimidines on thymidylate synthase, *Cancer* 63(suppl):1008, 1989.

153. Morita K: Clinical significance of radiation therapy combined with chemotherapy, *Strahlentherapie* 156:228, 1980.

154. Mortimer JE and others: Feasibility and efficacy of weekly intraarterial cisplatin in locally advanced (stage III and IV) head and neck cancers, *J Clin Oncol* 6:969, 1988.

155. Morton RP and others: Cisplatinum and bleomycin for advanced or recurrent squamous cell carcinoma of the head and neck: a randomized factorial phase III controlled trial, *Cancer Chemother Pharmacol* 15: 283, 1985.

156. Paccagnella A and others: Chemotherapy before locoregional treatment in stage III & IV head and neck cancer: intermediate results of an ongoing randomized phase III trial. AGSTIC study, *Proc Am Soc Clin Oncol* 9:173, 1990.

157. Paccagnella A and others: A phase III trial of initial chemotherapy in stage III or IV head and neck cancer. A study by the gruppo di studio sui tumori della testa e del collo, *J Natl Cancer Inst* 86:265, 1994.

158. Pajak TF and others: Elapsed treatment days—a critical item for radiotherapy quality control review in head and neck trials: RTOG report, *Int J Radiat Oncol Biol Phys* 20:13, 1991.

159. Parvinen LM and others: Combined bleomycin treatment and radiation therapy in squamous cell carcinoma of the head and neck region, *Acta Radiol Oncol* 24:487, 1985.

160. Pfister DG and others: Larynx preservation with combined chemotherapy and radiation therapy in advanced but resectable head and neck cancer, *J Clin Oncol* 9:850, 1991.

161. Piantadosi S: Principles of clinical trial design, *Semin Oncol* 15:423, 1988.

162. Pinto HA, Jacobs CJ: Chemotherapy for recurrent and metastatic head and neck cancer, *Hematol Oncol Clin North Am* 5:667, 1991.

163. Posner MR and others: Chemotherapy of advanced salivary gland neoplasms, *Cancer* 50:2261, 1982.

164. Price LA, Hill BR: Larynx preservation after initial chemotherapy plus radiation therapy as opposed to surgical intervention with or without radiation therapy in previously untreated advanced head and neck cancer: final analysis, *Proc Am Soc Clin Oncol* 11:244, 1992, (abstract).

165. Randolph VL and others: Combination therapy of advanced head and neck cancer: induction of remissions with diaminedichloroplatinum (II) bleomycin and radiation therapy, *Cancer* 41:460, 1978.

166. Rentschler R, Burgess MA, Byers R: Chemotherapy of malignant major salivary gland neoplasms, *Cancer* 40:619, 1977.

167. Richards GJ Jr, Chambers RG: Hydroxyurea: a radiosensitizer in the treatment of neoplasms of the head and neck, *Am J Roentgenol* 105: 555, 1969.

168. Ringel I, Horwitz SB: Studies with RP 56976 (taxotere): a semisynthetic analog of taxol, *J Natl Cancer Inst* 83:288, 1991.

169. Roberts F: Trimetrexate as a single agent in patients with advanced head and neck cancer, *Semin Oncol* 15:22, 1988.

170. Roberts F and others: Phase II study of topotecan in advanced head and neck cancer: identification of an active new agent, *Proc Am Soc Clin Oncol* 13:281, 1994.

171. Rockwell S, Sartorelli AC: *Mitomycin C and radiation*. In Hill B, Bellamy A, editors: *The interactions between antitumor drugs and radiation*, Boca Raton, Fl, 1989, CRC Press.

172. Rooney M and others: Improved complete response rate and survival in advanced head and neck cancer after three-course induction therapy with 120-hour 5-FU infusion and cisplatin, *Cancer* 55:1123, 1985.

173. Rosenberg B: *Cisplatin: its history and possible mechanisms of action*. In Prestayko AW, Crooke ST, Carter SK, editors: *Cisplatin: current status and new developments*, New York, 1980, Academic Press.

174. Rowinsky EK and others: Taxol: the first of the taxanes, an important new class of antitumor agents, *Semin Oncol* 19:646, 1992.

175. Sartorelli AC: Therapeutic attack of hypoxic cells of solid tumors, *Cancer Res* 48:775, 1988.

176. Sato Y and others: Combined surgery, radiotherapy, and regional chemotherapy in carcinoma of the paranasal sinuses, *Cancer* 25:571, 1967.

177. Scandolaro L, Bertoni F: Tolleranza cutanea e mucosa e risposte cliniche a breve termine nella associazione tra radioterapia e bleomicina per tumori del distretto cervico-cefalico, *Acta Otorhinol Ital* 2:213, 1982.

178. Schornagel JH and others: Randomized Phase III trial of edatrexate versus methotrexate in patients with metastatic and/or recurrent squamous cell carcinoma of the head and neck: a European organization for research and treatment of head and neck cancer cooperative group study, *J Clin Oncol* 13:1649, 1995.

179. Schramm VL, Strodes C, Myers EN: Cisplatin therapy for adenoid cystic carcinoma, *Arch Otolaryngol* 107:739, 1981.

180. Schuller DE and others: Preoperative chemotherapy in advanced resectable head and neck cancer: final report of the Southwest Oncology Group, *Laryngoscope* 98:1205, 1988.

181. Sessions RB and others: Intra-arterial cisplatin treatment of adenoid cystic carcinoma, *Arch Otolaryngol* 108:221, 1982.

182. Shah JP and others: Effects of retinoids on oral leukoplakia, *Am J Surg* 146:466, 1983.

183. Shanta Y, Krishnamurthi S: Combined bleomycin and radiotherapy in oral cancer, *Clin Radiol* 156:228, 1980.

184. Shanta V, Krishnamurthi S: Combined therapy of oral cancer bleomycin and radiation: a clinical trial, *Clin Radiol* 28:427, 1977.

185. Shantz SP and others: Immunologic determinants of head and neck cancer: response to induction chemotherapy, *J Clin Oncol* 7:857, 1989.

186. Shetty P and others: Controlled study in squamous cell carcinoma of base of tongue using conventional radiation, radiation with single drug, and radiation with multiple drug chemotherapy, *Proc Am Soc Clin Oncol* 4:152, 1985 (abstract).

187. Shibuya H and others: Reappraisal of trimodal combination therapy for maxillary sinus carcinoma, *Cancer* 50:2790, 1982.

188. Shigematsu Y, Sakai S, Fuchihata H: Recent trials in the treatment of maxillary sinus carcinoma with special reference to the chemical potentiation of radiation therapy, *Acta Otolaryngol* 71:63, 1971.

189. Shirinian MH and others: Laryngeal preservation by induction chemotherapy plus radiation therapy in locally advanced head and neck cancer: the MD Anderson Cancer Center experience, *Head Neck* 16: 39, 1994.

190. Simon RM: *Design and conduct of clinical trials*. In Devita VT Jr, Hellman S, Rosenberg SA, editors: *Cancer principles and practice of oncology*, ed 3, Philadelphia, 1989, JB Lippincott.

191. Slaughter DP, Southwick HW, Smejkal W: Field cancerization in oral stratified squamous epithelium, *Cancer* 6:193, 1953.

192. Snow GB and others: Prognostic factors of neck node metastasis, *Clin Otolaryngol* 7:185, 1982.

193. South-East Cooperative Oncology Group: A randomized trial of combined multidrug chemotherapy and radiotherapy in advanced squamous cell carcinoma of the head and neck, *Eur J Surg Oncol* 12:289, 1986.

194. Steel GG, Peckham MJ: Exploitable mechanisms in combined radiotherapy-chemotherapy: the concept of additivity, *Int J Radiat Oncol Biol Phys* 5:85, 1979.

195. Stefani S, Eells RW, Abbate J: Hydroxyurea and radiotherapy in head and neck cancer, *Radiology* 101:391, 1971.

196. Stell PM and others: Sequential chemotherapy and radiotherapy in advanced head and neck cancer, *Clin Radiol* 34:463, 1983.

197. Stich HF and others: Remission of oral leukoplakia and macronuclei in tobacco/betal quid chewers treated with beta-carotene and beta-carotene plus vitamin A, *Int J Cancer* 42:195, 1988.

198. Stich HF and others: Response of oral leukoplakias to the administration of vitamin A, *Cancer Lett* 40:93, 1988.

199. Strong MS, Incze J, Vaughan CW: Field cancerization in the digestive tract: its etiology, manifestation and significance, *J Otolaryngol* 13: 1, 1984.

200. Suen JY, Johns ME: Chemotherapy for salivary gland cancer, *Laryngoscope* 92:235, 1982.

201. Szpirglas H and others: Neo-adjuvant chemotherapy: a randomized trial before radiotherapy in oral and oro-pharyngeal carcinomas: end results. In *Proceedings of the 2nd International Head and Neck Oncology Research Conference*. Arlington, Va, September 10–12, 1987.

202. Tannock IF, Rotin D: Keynote address: mechanisms of interaction between radiation and drugs with potential for improvements in therapy, *NCI Monogr* 6:77, 1988.

203. Tannock IF, Sutherland DJ: Chemotherapy for adenocystic carcinoma, *Cancer* 46:452, 1980.

204. Tarpley JL and others: High-dose methotrexate as a preoperative adjuvant in the treatment of epidermoid carcinoma of the head and neck: a feasibility study and clinical trial, *Am J Surg* 130:481, 1975.

205. Taylor SG IV and others: Combined simultaneous cisplatin/fluorouracil chemotherapy and split course radiation in head and neck cancer, *J Clin Oncol* 7:846, 1989.

206. Taylor SG IV and others: Randomized comparison of neoadjuvant cisplatin and fluorouracil infusion followed by radiation versus concomitant treatment in advanced head and neck cancer, *J Clin Oncol* 12:385, 1994.

207. Testolin A and others: Vinorelbine in pretreated advanced head and neck squamous cell carcinoma. A phase II study, *Proc Am Soc Clin Oncol* 13:289, 1994.

208. Thornton D and others: A phase II trial of taxol in squamous cell carcinoma of the head and neck, *Proc Am Soc Clin Oncol* 13:288, 1994.

209. Toma and others: Beta-carotene in the treatment of oral leukoplakia, *Proc Am Soc Clin Oncol* 9:179, 1990 (abstract 695).

210. Toohill RJ and others: Cisplatin and fluorouracil as neoadjuvant therapy in head and neck cancer: a preliminary report, *Arch Otolaryngol Head Neck Surg* 113:758, 1987.

211. Troizzi PL and others: 5-Fluorouracil, cyclophosphamide, and vincristine for adenoid cystic carcinoma of the head and neck, *Cancer* 59: 887, 1987.

212. Truelson JM and others: DNA content and histologic growth pattern correlate with prognosis in patients with advanced squamous cell carcinoma of the larynx. The Department of Veterans Affairs Cooperative Laryngeal Cancer Study Group, *Cancer* 70:56, 1992.

213. Uen WC and others: A phase II study of piritrexim in patients with advanced squamous head and neck cancer, *Cancer* 69:1008, 1992.

214. Urba SG, Forastiere AA: Systemic therapy of head and neck cancer: most effective agents, areas of promise, *Oncology* 3:79, 1989.

215. Venook AP and others: Cisplatin, doxorubicin, and 5-fluorouracil chemotherapy for salivary gland malignancies: a pilot study of the Northern California Oncology Group, *J Clin Oncol* 5:951, 1987.

216. Vermeer RJ, Pinedo HM: Partial remission of advanced adenoid cystic carcinoma obtained with adriamycin, *Cancer* 43:1604, 1979.

217. Vermund H and others: Bleomycin and radiation therapy in squamous cell carcinoma of the upper aero-digestive tract: a phase III clinical trial, *Int J Radiat Oncol Biol Phys* 11:1877, 1985.

218. Veronesi A and others: High-dose versus low-dose cisplatin in advanced head and neck squamous cell cancer: a randomized study, *J Clin Oncol* 3:1105, 1985.

219. Verweij J, Alexiera-Figresch J, DeBoer MF: Ifosfamide in advanced head and neck cancer. A phase II study of the Rotterdam Cooperative Head and Neck Cancer Study Group, *Eur J Cancer Clin Oncol* 24: 795, 1988.

220. Verweij J, Clavel M, Chevalier B: Paclitaxel (taxol) and docetaxel (taxotere): not simply two of a kind, *Ann Oncol* 5:495, 1994.

221. Veterans Affairs Laryngeal Cancer Study Group: induction chemotherapy plus radiation in patients with advanced laryngeal cancer, *N Engl J Med* 324:1685, 1991.

222. Vogl SE and others: A randomized prospective comparison of methotrexate with a combination of methotrexate, bleomycin, and cisplatin in head and neck cancer, *Cancer* 56:432, 1985.

223. Vogler WR and others: Methotrexate therapy with or without citrovorum: factor in carcinoma of the head and neck, breast and colon, *Cancer Clin Trials* 2:227, 1979.

224. Vokes EE and others: Hydroxyurea, fluorouracil, and concomitant radiotherapy in poor prognosis head and neck cancer: a phase I-II study, *J Clin Oncol* 7:761, 1989.

225. Vokes EE and others: Induction chemotherapy with cisplatin, fluorouracil, and high-dose leucovorin for locally advanced head and neck cancer: a clinical and pharmacologic analysis, *J Clin Oncol* 8:241, 1990.

226. Vokes EE and others: A phase II study of piritrexim in combination

with methotrexate in recurrent and metastatic head and neck cancer, *Cancer* 67:2253, 1991.

227. Vokes EE and others: Induction chemotherapy followed by concomitant chemoradiotherapy for advanced head and neck cancer: impact on the natural history of the disease, *J Clin Oncol* 13:876, 1995.

228. Von Hoff DD, Rozencweig M, Piccart M: The cardiotoxicity of anticancer agents, *Semin Oncol* 9:23, 1982.

229. Wang SY, LaRosa GJ, Gudas LJ: Molecular cloning of gene sequences transcriptionally regulated by retinoic acid and dibutyrl AMP in cultured mouse teratocarcinoma cells, *Dev Biol* 107:75, 1985.

230. Weiss RB, Muggia FM: Cytotoxic drug-induced pulmonary disease: update 1980, *Am J Med* 68:259, 1980.

231. Weissberg JB and others: Randomized clinical trial of mitomycin C as an adjunct to radiotherapy in head and neck cancer, *Int J Radiat Oncol Biol Phys* 17:3, 1989.

232. Wendt TG and others: Cisplatin, fluorouracil with leucovorin calcium enhancement, and synchronous accelerated radiotherapy in the management of locally advanced head and neck cancer: a phase II study, *J Clin Oncol* 7:471, 1989.

233. Wheeler RH and others: High dose cisplatin and concomitant conventional fractionation radiation with or without prolonged infusion 5-fluorouracil in patients with unresectable stage III or IV squamous cell carcinoma of the head and neck. Presented at the Third International Head and Neck Oncology Research Conference, Las Vegas, Nev, Sept 26–28, 1990 (abstract 6.3).

234. Wheeler RH, Baker SR, Medvec BR: Single-agent and combination-drug regional chemotherapy for head and neck cancer using an implantable infusion pump, *Cancer* 54:1504, 1984.

235. Williams SD and others: Chemotherapy for head and neck cancer: comparison of cisplatin + vinblastine + bleomycin versus methotrexate, *Cancer* 57:18, 1986.

236. Wittes RE and others: cis-Dichlorodiammine platinum (II) in the treatment of epidermoid carcinoma of the head and neck, *Cancer Treat Rep* 61:359, 1977.

237. Wong DTW: Amplification of the C-erb B1 oncogene in chemically induced oral carcinomas, *Carcinogenesis* 8:1963, 1987.

238. Woods RL, Fox RM, Tattersall MHN: Methotrexate treatment of squamous cell head and neck cancers: dose response evaluation, *BMJ* 282:600, 1981.

239. Zatterstrom UK and others: Prognostic factors in head and neck cancer: histologic grading, DNA ploidy, and nodal status, *Head Neck* 13: 477, 1991.

240. Zielke-Temme BC and others: Combined intraarterial chemotherapy, radiation therapy and surgery for advanced squamous cell carcinoma of the head and neck, *Cancer* 45:1527, 1980.

Chapter 7

Head and Neck Cancer Staging

Ernest A. Weymuller, Jr.

Efforts to provide a classification system for cancer date back to the League of Nations Health Organization (1929), and subsequently to the International Commission on Stage Grouping and Presentation of Results of the International Congress of Radiology and the International Union Against Cancer (UICC, 1953).[4] The American Joint Committee on Cancer (AJCC) was organized in 1959 by multiple sponsoring organizations, including the American College of Surgeons, the American College of Radiology, the College of American Pathologists, the American College of Physicians, the American Cancer Society, and the National Cancer Institute. The AJCC orchestrated a sustained effort to provide unification of clinical cancer staging that resulted in the publication of the first edition of the *Manual for Staging of Cancer* in 1977. The fourth edition, published in 1992, is particularly important because it reflects the unified staging system now agreed on by the AJCC and the UICC.

BENEFITS OF A STAGING SYSTEM

The potential benefits of a staging system are numerous and include the following advantages: a staging system allows the physician to select an appropriate form of therapy for a given patient; it provides accurate prognostic information; it allows institutional assessment of therapeutic results; it allows collation of multiple institutional experiences; and it provides a foundation for the analysis of new forms of treatment.

Although these accomplishments are laudable and in many cases served by the existing system of staging, there is more to be done. This chapter includes a discussion of the current system's weaknesses and details some potential changes that could be made.

RULES OF THE AMERICAN JOINT COMMITTEE ON CANCER-INTERNATIONAL UNION AGAINST CANCER SYSTEM

Components of clinical classification

Tumor, node, metastasis (TNM) staging has evolved as a method to conveniently categorize the tumor burden of the patient. The assignment of specific criteria for these categories is a dynamic process related to evolving understanding of the prognostic significance of various aspects of tumor extent. The current system is anatomically based, with occasional recognition of the functional impact of tumor growth (for example, vocal cord fixation). Within the arena of head and neck cancer, the *Manual for Staging of Cancer* has specific classifications for the lip and oral cavity, the pharynx, the larynx, the maxillary sinus, the salivary glands, and the thyroid gland. The aerodigestive and maxillary sinus staging systems may be used for squamous cell carcinoma and malignancies of the minor salivary glands. The site-specific rules for head and neck do not include information gained during the surgical procedure as part of clinical staging. However, "all clinical and pathological data available before first definitive treatment may be used for clinical staging."[4] Thus physical examination, radiographic studies such as computed tomography (CT) scan and magnetic resonance imaging (MRI), endoscopy, and biopsy should be considered when determining the final clinical stage of a patient before treatment is initiated. When there is doubt regarding which stage to apply, it is recommended that the lower stage be selected. The intent of this recommendation is clear; the worst possible scenario would be to underestimate the necessary curative treatment modality for a given stage (Table 7-1).

Table 7-1. Current head and neck cancer staging

T stage	Mucosal squamous cell carcinoma
Lip and oral cavity	
T_X	Primary tumor cannot be assessed
T_0	No evidence of primary tumor
T_{is}	Carcinoma *in situ*
T_1	Tumor 2 cm or less in greatest dimension
T_2	Tumor more than 2 cm but not more than 4 cm in greatest dimension
T_3	Tumor more than 4 cm in greatest dimension
T_4	(lip) Tumor invades adjacent structures, e.g., through cortical bone, tongue, skin of neck
T_4	(oral cavity) Tumor invades adjacent structures, e.g., through cortical bone, into deep (extrinsic) muscle of tongue, maxillary sinus, skin
Pharynx (including base of tongue, soft palate, and uvula)	
Primary tumor (T)	
T_X	Primary tumor cannot be assessed
T_0	No evidence of primary tumor
T_{is}	Carcinoma *in situ*
Oropharynx	
T_1	Tumor 2 cm or less in greatest dimension
T_2	Tumor more than 2 cm but not more than 4 cm in greatest dimension
T_3	Tumor more than 4 cm in greatest dimension
T_4	Tumor invades adjacent structures, e.g., through cortical bone, soft tissue of neck, deep (extrinsic) muscle of tongue
Nasopharynx	
T_1	Tumor limited to one subsite of nasopharynx
T_2	Tumor invades more than one subsite of nasopharynx
T_3	Tumor invades nasal cavity or oropharynx
T_4	Tumor invades skull or cranial nerve(s)
Hypopharynx	
T_1	Tumor limited to one subsite of hypopharynx
T_2	Tumor invades more than one subsite of hypopharynx or an adjacent site, without fixation of hemilarynx
T_3	Tumor invades more than one subsite of hypopharynx or an adjacent site, with fixation of hemilarynx
T_4	Tumor invades adjacent structures, e.g., cartilage or soft tissues of neck
Larynx	
Primary tumor (T)	
T_X	Primary tumor cannot be assessed
T_0	No evidence of primary tumor
T_{is}	Carcinoma *in situ*
Supraglottis	
T_1	Tumor limited to one subsite of supraglottis with normal vocal cord mobility
T_2	Tumor invades more than one subsite of supraglottis or glottis, with normal vocal cord mobility
T_3	Tumor limited to larynx with vocal cord fixation or invades postcricoid area, medial wall of piriform sinus, or preepiglottic tissues
T_4	Tumor invades through thyroid cartilage or extends to other tissues beyond the larynx, e.g., to oropharynx, soft tissues of neck

From Beahrs OH and others, editors: *Manual for staging of cancer,* ed 4, Philadelpha, 1992, JB Lippincott.

Continued

Table 7-1. Current head and neck cancer staging—cont'd

T stage	Mucosal squamous cell carcinoma
Glottis	
T_1	Tumor limited to vocal cord(s) (may involve anterior or posterior commissures) with normal mobility
T_{1a}	Tumor limited to one vocal cord
T_{1b}	Tumor involves both vocal cords
T_2	Tumor extends to supraglottis or subglottis, or with impaired vocal cord mobility
T_3	Tumor limited to larynx with vocal cord fixation
T_4	Tumor invades through thyroid cartilage, or extends to other tissues beyond the larynx, e.g., oropharynx, soft tissues of neck
Subglottis	
T_1	Tumor limited to the subglottis
T_2	Tumor extends to vocal cord(s) with normal or impaired mobility
T_3	Tumor limited to larynx with vocal cord fixation
T_4	Tumor invades through cricoid or thyroid cartilage, or extends to other tissues beyond the larynx, e.g., oropharynx, soft tissues of neck

N & M stages	Mucosal squamous cell carcinoma
Maxillary sinus	
Primary tumor (T)	
T_X	Primary tumor cannot be assessed
T_0	No evidence of primary tumor
T_{is}	Carcinoma *in situ*
T_1	Tumor limited to the antral mucosa with no erosion or destruction of bone
T_2	Tumor with erosion or destruction of the infrastructure including the hard palate or the middle nasal meatus
T_3	Tumor invades any of the following: skin of cheek, posterior wall of the maxillary sinus, floor or medial wall of orbit, anterior ethmoid sinus
T_4	Tumor invades orbital contents or any of the following: cribriform plate, posterior ethmoid or sphenoid sinuses, nasopharynx, soft palate, pterygomaxillary or temporal fossae or base of skull
Lymph node (N)	
N_X	Regional lymph nodes cannot be assessed
N_0	No regional lymph node metastasis
N_1	Metastasis in a single ipsilateral lymph node, 3 cm or less in greatest dimension
N_2	Metastasis in a single ipsilateral lymph node, more than 3 cm but not more than 6 cm in greatest dimension, or multiple ipsilateral lymph nodes, none more than 6 cm in greatest dimension, or bilateral or contralateral lymph nodes, none more than 6 cm in greatest dimension
N_{2a}	Metastasis in a single ipsilateral lymph node, more than 3 cm but not more than 6 cm in greatest dimension
N_{2b}	Metastasis in multiple ipsilateral lymph nodes, none more than 6 cm in greatest dimension
N_{2c}	Metastasis in bilateral or contralateral lymph nodes, none more than 6 cm in greatest dimension
N_3	Metastasis in a lymph node more than 6 cm in greatest dimension
Distant metastasis (M)	
M_X	Presence of distant metastasis cannot be assessed
M_0	No distant metastasis
M_1	Distant metastasis

Salivary glands

This staging system is appropriate for all forms of carcinoma involving salivary glands. The histopathology grading system is the same as previously indicated.

From Beahrs OH and others, editors: *Manual for staging of cancer,* ed 4, Philadelphia, 1992, JB Lippincott.

Table 7-1. Current head and neck cancer staging—cont'd

N & M stages	

Primary tumor (T)

T_X	Primary tumor cannot be assessed
T_0	No evidence of primary tumor
T_1	Tumor 2 cm or less in greatest dimension
T_2	Tumor more than 2 cm but not more than 4 cm in greatest dimension
T_3	Tumor more than 4 cm but not more than 6 cm in greatest dimension
T_4	Tumor more than 6 cm in greatest dimension

Thyroid gland

The staging system for thyroid tumors in the TNM category includes all histopathologic types including anaplastic carcinoma, however the staging system suggests a separation of groupings so that papillary and follicular are reported separately from medullary and undifferentiated carcinomas.

Primary tumor (T)

All categories may be subdivided: (a) solitary; (b) multifocal—measure the largest for classification.

T_X	Primary tumor cannot be assessed
T_0	No evidence of primary tumor
T_1	Tumor 1 cm or less in greatest dimension limited to the thyroid
T_2	Tumor more than 1 cm but not more than 4 cm
T_3	Tumor more than 4 cm in greatest dimension limited to the thyroid
T_4	Tumor of any size extending beyond the thyroid capsule

Stage grouping

Separate stage groupings are recommended for papillary and follicular, medullary, and undifferentiated.

Papillary or follicular

Aged less than 45 years

Stage I	Any T, Any N, M_0
Stage II	Any T, Any N, M_1

Aged more than 45 years

Stage I	T_1, N_0, M_0
Stage II	T_2, N_0, M_0
	T_3, N_0, M_0
Stage III	T_4, N_0, M_0
	Any T, N_1, M_0
Stage IV	Any T, Any N, M_1

Medullary

Stage I	T_1	N_0	M_0
Stage II	T_2	N_0	M_0
	T_3	N_0	M_0
	T_4	N_0	M_0
Stage III	Any T	N_1	M_0
Stage IV	Any T	Any N	T_1

Undifferentiated

All cases are Stage IV

Stage IV	Any T	Any N	Any M

Other tumors, including skin tumors, melanoma, sarcoma, and lymphoma, have staging systems that are available for the interested reader but not included in this chapter.

Components of pathologic staging

AJCC pathologic staging (pTNM) uses the following designations to include information on the histopathologic type, or histologic grade, of cancer: G_x (cannot be assessed), G_1 (well differentiated), G_2 (moderately differentiated), G_3 (poorly differentiated), and G_4 (undifferentiated). Additional descriptors may include lymphatic invasion and venous invasion. Pathologic staging of lymph nodes is limited to the presence or absence of a tumor in the nodes.

Additional descriptors

The mTNM is used to indicate multiple primary tumors at a single site. When there are synchronous tumors at one site, the tumor with the higher stage should be selected for reporting. yTNM indicates that classification of the tumor was performed during or after multimodality therapy. rTNM indicates a recurrent tumor staged after a disease-free interval. This descriptor also allows for indication of the absence or presence of residual tumor after treatment. aTNM indicates that the tumor was first classified at autopsy.

STAGE GROUPING

The intent of clustering various combinations of TNM into stage groupings is to indicate a stratification of prognosis. The current AJCC stage groupings for squamous cell carcinoma are summarized in Table 7-2.

Whereas this system is accurate for the early stages (I and II), it is clear that even in the lower stages, multiple additional factors must be considered to refine the staging system. These issues are discussed in the second half of this chapter.

REPORTING OF RESULTS

Because one of the primary goals of a staging system is the reporting and comparison of results, a review of the nature of these reporting systems follows.

Essential data

The *Manual for Staging of Cancer* offers a full chapter that describes this information in greater detail. Ideally, each institution reporting its results would adhere to a predetermined format. Had this attitude been pervasive throughout the past two decades, much of the confusion regarding ideal forms of treatment might have been obviated. In the future, a major contribution to related literature would be a commitment to a uniform reporting format.[30] The essential components of such a system would include (1) demographic information regarding the age, race, and sex of a given patient; (2) a description of the disease that includes its histology, site, and stage; (3) precise treatment information (in this arena there is much work to be done regarding the accuracy of surgical information); (4) a definition of the start time of the first mode of therapy; and (5) the vital status of the patient (alive, dead, or unknown, and with or without tumor). "Completeness of the follow-up is crucial . . . even a small number of patients lost to follow-up may bias the data."[4]

Table 7-2. Stage grouping

Stage 0	T_{is}	N_0	M_0
Stage I	T_1	N_0	M_0
Stage II	T_2	N_0	M_0
Stage III	T_3	N_0	M_0
	T_1	N_1	M_0
	T_2	N_1	M_0
	T_3	N_1	M_0
Stage IV	T_4	N_0	M_0
	T_4	N_1	M_0
	Any T	N_2	M_0
	Any T	N_3	M_0
	Any T	Any N	M_1

From Beahrs OH and others, editors: *Manual for staging of cancer*, ed 4, Philadelphia, 1992, JB Lippincott.

A clear indication of the methodology for calculating the survival statistics of the study must also be included.

Options for calculating survival

There are numerous options for survival calculations. A broader description of these methods is included in Chapter 2 of the *Manual for Staging of Cancer.*

The direct method

The direct method system simply indicates the percentage of patients alive at the end of a designated interval, most commonly 5 years.

The actuarial or life table method

The actuarial or life table method allows the inclusion of patients who have been followed up for less than a specific interval such as 5 years; this provides "a means for using all follow-up information accumulated up to the closing date of the study."[4] It also "has the further advantage of providing information on the survival pattern . . . for example, do most patients die during the first year or is there a uniform death rate over 5 years?"[4]

The adjusted survival rate

The actuarial method includes death from all causes. Calculation of the adjusted survival rate requires accurate information on the cause of death. It "is the proportion of the initial patient group that escaped death due to cancer if all other causes of death were not operating . . . whenever reliable information on cause of death is available, an adjustment can be made for the deaths due to causes other than the disease under study."[4] This form of analysis "is particularly important in comparing patient groups that may differ with respect to factors such as sex, age, race, and socioeconomic status."[4]

The effect of using accurate cause-of-death information was highlighted by Brown,[5] who found "that there was a greater rate of noncancer deaths in cancer patients than in the population at large. . . . The excess of noncancer deaths in cancer patients occurred shortly after diagnosis, suggesting that *a large portion of the excess (of deaths) is attributable to treatment.*" The authors go on to indicate that "optimal medical treatment of a deadly disease may itself cause deaths. . . . The argument that we make is not that treatment-related deaths are either unexpected or evidence of poor treatment; rather it is that, in the assessment of outcome, deaths due to causes other than cancer cannot be ignored."[5]

The relative survival rate

When specific information regarding the cause of death cannot be obtained, an estimate called the relative survival rate can be accomplished by comparing "the ratio of the observed survival rate (of the group under study) to the expected rate for a group of people in the general population similar to the patient group with respect to race, sex, age and calendar period of observation."[4]

The Kaplan-Meier method

The details of the Kaplan-Meier method and multivariate analysis are beyond the intended scope of this chapter. It is important for the reader to note that the Kaplan-Meier method is similar to the actuarial (life table) method. However, depending on the data introduced, the Kaplan-Meier method can be used to calculate an adjusted survival rate or a relative survival rate.[4]

FUTURE OF STAGING

Strengths of the current system

The existing staging system has clearly provided a forum for the discussion of varying modes of therapy and has allowed an approach toward consistency in the prognoses that we can give to our patients. It is worthwhile to mention the report of the First Task Force of Laryngeal Cancer in 1961. Although it is compromised by the fact that it is retrospective, deals with a small number of patients (600), does not include information beyond pure 5-year survival figures (calculated by the direct method), and includes variable forms of therapy, this report comes to conclusions that are much the same as those that current attitudes reflect. Namely, "true cord (glottic tumors) have a much better prognosis;" "The most important factor in determining outcome of therapy . . . was the presence or absence of clinically palpable cervical lymph node metastases . . . survival dropped to 40% even when the local disease would allow a T_1 designation"; and "When the cancer extended beyond the larynx (T_4N_0), radiation was not effective."[26]

Likewise, the study of 1320 pharynx cancer cases reported by the AJCC in 1963 came to similar conclusions for carcinoma of the pharynx and added that "all sites demonstrated an increased survival in women."[27]

Confidence in the staging of laryngeal cancer is perhaps the most solid. This, no doubt, is influenced by the fact that there is a standardized surgical procedure for the management of advanced laryngeal cancer and for the salvage of postradiation recurrences. The Veterans Administration study CSP #268,[8] a comparison of surgery plus radiation versus induction chemotherapy plus radiation, is the only prospective multiinstitutional study in head and neck cancer that has addressed the problem of indistinct staging convincingly. Three important outcomes are the result of an entry population that was restricted to a tightly defined group of laryngeal cancer patients: (1) tumor staging in the larynx is more anatomically precise; (2) the surgical procedure is uniform (laryngectomy is a standardized operation); and (3) pathology margins are less often in question.

The specific criteria for the various T-stage categories continue to be debated and will undergo further refinement. However, because they are anatomically based and fairly well-tuned, emphasis in this area is probably misplaced. Far greater improvements will accrue if the other weaknesses in our staging system are addressed and resolved.

Weaknesses of the current system

As stated by Piccirillo and others,[21] "The dilemma of cancer staging occurs when multiple purposes are sought for a cancer staging system while only one type of prognostic variable is utilized." This statement encapsulates the challenge for the future. Because it has become clear that survival is dependent on multiple interactive biologic factors, we must develop a substantially more sophisticated system if we intend to ask for accurate answers regarding proper treatment and ultimate prognosis for a particular patient.

Stage groupings

The clustering of various subsets of TNM categories into four stages was undertaken in an attempt to stratify according to prognosis and to simplify communication. In many respects these goals were accomplished, but once again this clustering has resulted in a loss of accuracy. As indicated by the results of a poll of the membership of the American Society for Head and Neck Surgery:

The grouping together of the various T, N, and M combinations into stages was felt by many members to be inconsistent and biologically inaccurate. The original and current stage groupings were created based on *presumed* prognosis. No prospective, multi-variate analysis was performed to create the four stage groupings from the various combinations of T, N, and M.[21]

Impact of inadequate staging on multiinstitutional studies

The weaknesses in the current staging system are most apparent when it is applied to multiinstitutional studies, particularly those that include surgery as one of the treatment options. A recently published metaanalysis of adjuvant chemotherapy in head and neck cancer provides the following information: of 3977 patients available for analysis, the reduction in cancer mortality between patients treated in chemotherapy programs versus standard therapy programs is 2.8% (insignificant). In this detailed effort, Stell[28] provides clear evidence that there has been little progress in reducing overall cancer mortality through chemotherapy.

We are unable to document statistically significant improvement in survival through the use of single or multiagent chemotherapy; yet most clinicians are haunted by the obvious impact of chemotherapy on certain patients with head and neck cancer. The challenge is to identify those who will benefit from these toxic and expensive treatment regimens. The potential for a change in direction is implied in a presentation by Jacobs and Makuch[14] that evaluates a subset of patients treated in the Head and Neck Contracts program. They state:

One possible reason that efficacy of adjuvant chemotherapy has not been demonstrated is the heterogeneity of this disease with survival differences dependent on site and stage. There may be particular subgroups of patients who would benefit from adjuvant chemotherapy, but when combined in large trials, that improvement is obscured.

The article indicates that although there is a statistically significant improvement in "disease-free survival" rates in standard therapy over induction therapy or maintenance therapy, the overall or "absolute" survival rate is unchanged, regardless of the form of treatment. The authors ask, "Why have we failed to prove benefit from adjuvant chemotherapy for head and neck cancer? Perhaps the concept does not work." Further, they state that "improvement in disease free survival has not been translated into improved survival in these trials." It is imperative that we focus on the authors' statement that "the importance of proper stratification cannot be overemphasized." It is worth considering that the TNM system is inadequate for multiinstitutional trials and that until a better framework for the clinical staging of head and neck cancer is established, future efforts will continue to be frustrated by a failure to achieve significant results.[14]

As analysis of staging goes forward, there must be a concomitant improvement in the details regarding the specifics of surgical treatment. It is important to remain cognizant that what is done to treat the patient will have a bearing on the outcome and will influence the clinician's concepts of staging.[31]

Piccirillo[22] has further indicated that accounting for such variables as comorbidity, performance status, and nutritional and immune status, as well as therapeutic intent (palliative versus curative), will be important in more detailed analysis as the attempt is made to address questions that go beyond pure survival. We must be able to address more precisely the question of whether a single modality can offer an equal cure rate because that would obviously reduce the cost to the system and the cost to the patient in terms of time spent and side effects avoided.

This problem is not unique to head and neck cancer, as is indicated in the recent article by Gasparini and others,[12] which highlights the need for prospective multivariate analysis of prognostic and predictive indicators in node-negative breast cancer patients.

Of particular relevance to the assessment of treatment of head and neck cancer is the issue raised by Makuch and Johnson,[19] among others. Because there are relatively small numbers of patients each year who suffer from head and neck cancer and because there are multiple sites and multiple stages of cancer, the generation of sufficient numbers to achieve statistical relevance is a great problem.

The well-regarded adage of "garbage in, garbage out" applies fully to this situation. Multiinstitutional trials, as well as individual institutional studies, are fraught with the complexities of data stratification, and frequently promising single-institutional studies are not confirmed when reassessed in a multiinstitutional setting.[15] Head and neck surgeons must assert that until a well-established framework for study is constructed, further expenditures in multiinstitutional trials are inappropriate.

It is essential that improved stratification data related to tumor description and treatment, as well as multiple other variables, be included in prospective studies if there is any hope of determining which patients will benefit from treat-ment. This will require a concentrated effort that brings together the relevant treatment disciplines and the skills of biostatisticians to establish a mutually agreeable platform that could be applied to multiinstitutional and single-institutional trials.

POTENTIAL MODIFIERS OF STAGING

There is clearly no lack of contenders in the arena of potential modifiers of staging. The following section offers a brief commentary on two areas, imaging and biologic markers, that must be considered as refinements to the staging system.

As potentially significant prognostic markers evolve and are evaluated, it is particularly important that careful and well-defined statistical analysis be used. This issue was highlighted by Altman and others,[1] who demonstrated the risk involved in analyzing a continuous variable by selecting a single "optimal cut point" and including "the marker as a binary variable in a Cox multiple regression analysis." He recommended "that authors investigating the prognostic value of new markers use prespecified cut points, preferably three or four rather than just two."[1] It is clear that sophisticated statistical consultation will be critical to the analysis of each new prognostic marker as it is considered.

Imaging

CT and MRI are accepted as modifiers of clinical staging. They are particularly helpful in analyzing the extent of skull-base tumors, the degree of invasion of the mandible, and the assessment of metastases to the neck. A recent analysis of the accuracy of imaging, with respect to the evaluation of the N_0 neck, shows that CT scanning has a sensitivity of 93%, specificity of 83%, and accuracy of 89%, whereas MRI offers sensitivity of 90%, specificity of 89%, and accuracy of 87%. These are clearly superior to clinical palpation, which offers a sensitivity of 64%, specificity of 87%, and accuracy of 72%.[18] As a staging vehicle, ultrasound-guided fine-needle aspiration cytology may offer an appropriate supplement to CT and MRI scanning. As indicated by van den Brekel,[29] this type of cytology offers elimination of the false-positive study and may provide a sophisticated adjunct to other imaging studies.

Recently presented information regarding the applicability of positron emission tomography (PET) scanning to the staging of head and neck tumors provides an exciting window to the future of staging head and neck cancer. In particular, when a primary site cannot be identified, the application of PET scanning appears to provide information that may all but eliminate the T_x (primary not identified) category from the lexicon.[2]

Biologic markers

Host factors

There is a wide spectrum of potential biologic prognostic markers, Schantz[23] has suggested that these be divided along the lines of host and tumor factors. Immunologic factors, performance status, and genetic predisposition are included on the list of general host factors.

Immunologic factors. One of the earliest and yet still meaningful predictors of a poor prognosis is anergy to delayed hypersensitivity skin testing. More recently, the importance of natural killer (NK) cells has been identified for its association with prognosis.[23] Schantz[23] has also found that reduced NK cells are selectively important; this discovery has an increasingly significant impact on prognosis in poorly differentiated tumors. Another indicator of immunologic response capability, the ratio of $CD_4 : CD_8$ lymphocytes, was emphasized by Wolf as an effective prognostic tool.

Transfusion is suggested as an independent prognostic factor by multiple authors, although evidence to the contrary is offered by Schuller and others.[25] The interrelationship between transfusion and suppression of immune function has been recognized for many years.[10] Recently this phenomenon has been more completely characterized. Lenhard[17] identified two types of suppression *in vitro;* there was an early response to mitogenic and antigenic stimulation, felt to be monocyte-induced, and a late activation of T-suppressor cells observed up to 12 weeks after transfusion. Fischer and others[9] noted similar findings and added that repeated transfusion produced more pronounced and prolonged immunosuppression. Evaluating multiply transfused patients, Gascon and others[11] showed NK cell function to be severely depressed but demonstrated that $T_4 : T_8$ ratios did not significantly differ from normal. Kaplan,[16] studying similar population groups and using monoclonal antibodies for T_4 and T_8 subpopulations of lymphocytes, showed decreased $T_4 : T_8$ ratios and decreased NK cell captivity in transfused sickle cell and hemophiliac patients compared with healthy and nontransfused sickle cell patients. Using an animal model, Francis and Shenton[10] demonstrated that animals receiving allogeneic blood had significantly increased tumor growth and decreased lymphocyte responses compared with control animals receiving syngeneic blood or saline infusion.

Performance status. Nutritional status not only has a bearing on immediate posttreatment morbidity but also on long-term survival. Burns and others[6] found that there was a "dismal" survival rate for a group of patients with operable stage IV malignancies who had significant associated weight loss when they were diagnosed. Even in the face of nutritional rehabilitation and aggressive supportive care, only 2 of 14 patients survived longer than 6 months.[6] Likewise, Mick and others[20] identified weight loss as an important predictor of poor outcome in patients who are considered for multimodality regimens containing chemotherapy.

The presence of significant additional illness (comorbidity) has been defined as a predictor of poor survival by Piccirillo,[22] who found that "in each category of symptom stage, the survival rates were substantially lower when prognostic comorbidity was present." Piccirillo investigated symptoms that indicate the clinical severity of disease and found that there are specific severity indicators that sharpen

the "prognostic gradient" of the TNM system when it is applied to cancer of the larynx. His study points to an interesting new concept in fine-tuning the staging of head and neck cancer. However, it requires further analysis because the reported study made no account of the various forms of treatment, margin status, or pathologic indicators such as extracapsular spread.

An example of the impact of performance status on tumor control is provided by a study of the Radiation Therapy Oncology Group (RTOG) data of a large group of patients treated with definitive radiato therapy. A formula was derived for predicting tumor clearance at the 2-year level. Of particular note in this context is that the authors found three factors that had independent bearing on treatment outcome: primary tumor stage, N stage, and Karnofsky status. The Karnofsky performance correlated with a higher probability of ultimate control of the tumor.[13]

Genetic predisposition. The suggestion that genetic predisposition may play a role in susceptibility to head and neck cancer is included in the work of Saranough who has found, according to Schantz,[24] "that inheritable characteristics of the host (alleles of the 1-myc gene) govern phenotypic characteristics of their tumor." One of the challenges of the coming era will be to ascertain whether this genetic predisposition carries with it some modification of survival advantage or whether it contributes to the development of recurrence or second primary tumors.

Tumor factors. One of the most exciting and promising areas of further definition of the aggressiveness of head and neck cancer is the expanded understanding of cell biology.

Proliferation markers. Expression (or the lack of expression) of tumor antigens appears to have significant prognostic importance. For instance, the loss of expression of the major histocompatibility blood-group antigens is associated with a worsened prognosis, and increased expression of α_9 integrin is an independent predictor of tumor aggressiveness.[32]

Pathology. Other measures of tumor aggressiveness include analysis of deoxyribonucleic acid (DNA) content and flow cytometry. Wolf and others[33] demonstrated a higher metastatic rate in laryngeal cancers when the primary tumor had a high DNA index. Careful analysis of tumor depth has provided predictive information for early stage oral cavity and palate tumors.[3] Likewise, perineural invasion, angioinvasion, and extracapsular spread in lymph node disease clearly carry significant prognostic import that must be included in the refinement of the staging system.[7]

THE FUTURE

The current system of staging provides an effective framework for patient-care decisions but needs further definition and growth. The greatest challenge for the immediate future is to provide a foundation for the accumulation of large numbers of patient interactions. A common ground of data-gathering is necessary so that the refinements that promise to improve our understanding of the impact of treatment and comorbidity factors will help us deliver better care to future patients.

The National Cancer Institute and the National Institute for Deafness and Other Communicative Disorders co-sponsored a Strategic Planning Conference on Staging and Stratification for Multiinstitutional Trials in September of 1996. This meeting targeted the inadequacies of the TNM system for the purpose of statistical data-gathering in multiinstitutional trials. It should be reiterated that the TNM system provides a useful and well-accepted vehicle for communication among physicians. However, there are numerous weaknesses in the system. The conclusion of the participants in the Strategic Planning Conference was that an anatomically-based reporting system has the potential to provide a significant addition to current staging for multiinstitutional trials. It also was concluded that medical comorbidity will be an essential component of future staging systems.

REFERENCES

1. Altman DG and others: Dangers of using "optimal" cut points in the evaluation of prognostic factors, *J Natl Cancer Inst* 86:829, 1994.
2. Bailet JW and others: The use of positron emission tomography for the detection of unknown primary head and neck squamous cell malignancies, *Laryngoscope* 105:135, 1995.
3. Baredes S and others: Significance of tumor thickness in soft palate carcinoma, *Laryngoscope* 103:389, 1993.
4. Beahrs OH and others, editors: *Manual for staging of cancer*, ed 4, Philadelphia, 1992, JB Lippincott.
5. Brown BW: Noncancer deaths in white adult cancer patients, *J Natl Cancer Inst* 85:979, 1993.
6. Burns L, Chase D, Goodwin WJ: Treatment of patients with stage IV cancer: do the ends justify the means? *Otolaryngol Head Neck Surg* 97:8, 1987.
7. Close LG and others: Microvascular invasion in cancer of the oral cavity and oropharynx, *Arch Otolaryngol Head Neck Surg* 113:1191, 1987.
8. Department of Veterans Affairs Laryngeal Study Group: Induction chemotherapy plus radiation compared with surgery plus radiation in patients with advanced laryngeal cancer, *N Engl J Med* 324:1685, 1991.
9. Fischer E and others: Blood transfusion-induced suppression of cellular immunity in man, *Hum Immunol* 1:187, 1980.
10. Francis DMA, Shenton BK: Blood transfusion and tumor growth: evidence from laboratory animals, *Lancet* 2:871, 1981.
11. Gascon P, Zoumbos NC, Young NS: Immunologic abnormalities in patients receiving multiple blood transfusions, *Ann Intern Med* 100:173, 1984.
12. Gasparini G and others: Evaluating the potential usefulness of new prognostic and predictive indicators in node-negative breast cancer patients, *J Natl Cancer Inst* 85:1206, 1993.
13. Griffin TW and others: Predicting the response of head and neck cancers to radiation therapy with a multi-variate modeling system: an anal-
ysis of the RTOG head and neck registry, *Int J Radiat Oncol Biol Phys* 10:418, 1984.
14. Jacobs C, Makuch R: Efficacy of adjuvant chemotherapy for patients with resectable head and neck cancer: a subset analysis of the head and neck contracts program, *J Clin Oncol* 8:838, 1990.
15. Jacobs J, Adams GL: Current results and future directions of clinical trials in head and neck cancer, *Insights Otol* 3:1, 1988.
16. Kaplan J and others: Diminished helper/suppressor lymphocyte ratios and natural killer activity in recipients of repeated blood transfusions, *Blood* 64:308, 1984.
17. Lenhard V and others: Effect of blood transfusions on immunoregulatory mononuclear cells in prospective transplant recipients, *Transplant Proc* 15:1011, 1983.
18. Lenz M, Kersting-Sommerhoff B, Gross M: Diagnosis and treatment of the N0 neck in carcinomas of the upper aerodigestive tract: current status of diagnostic procedures, *Eur Arch Otorhinolaryngol* 250:432, 1993.
19. Makuch R, Johnson M: *Biostatistical considerations for head and neck cancer research.* In Wolf GT, editor: *Head and neck oncology*, Boston, 1984, M Nijhoff Pub.
20. Mick R and others: Prognostic factors in advanced head and neck cancer patients undergoing multimodality therapy, *Otolaryngol Head Neck Surg* 105:62, 1991.
21. Piccirillo JF: Purposes, problems, and proposals for progress in cancer staging, *Arch Otolaryngol* 121:145, 1995.
22. Piccirillo JF and others: New clinical severity staging system for cancer of the larynx: five-year survival rates, *Ann Otol Rhinol Laryngol* 103:83, 1994.
23. Schantz SP: Biologic markers, cellular differentiation, and metastatic head and neck cancer, *Eur Arch Otorhinolaryngol* 250:424, 1993.
24. Schantz SP, Goepfert H: Multimodality therapy and distant metastases, *Arch Otolaryngol Head Neck Surg* 113:1207, 1987.
25. Schuller DE and others: The effect of perioperative blood transfusion on survival in head and neck cancer, *Arch Otolaryngol Head Neck Surg* 120:711, 1994.
26. Smith RR and others: End results in 600 laryngeal cancers using the American Joint Committee's proposed method of stage classification and end results reporting, *Surg Gynecol Obstet* 113:435, 1961.
27. Smith RR and others: The American Joint Committee proposed method of stage classification and end result reporting applied to 1,320 pharynx cancers, *Cancer* 16:1505, 1963.
28. Stell PM: Adjuvant chemotherapy in head and neck cancer, *Semin Radiat Oncol* 2:195, 1992.
29. van den Brekel M: Assessment of lymph node metastases in the neck, doctoral thesis, Utrecht, 1992, Drukkerij Elinkwijk.
30. Weymuller EA: Uniformity of results reporting in head and neck cancer, *Head Neck* 275, 1991 (editorial).
31. Weymuller EA and others: Surgical reporting instrument designed to improve outcome data in head and neck cancer trials, *Ann Otol Rhinol Laryngol* 103:499, 1994.
32. Wolf GT, Carey TE: Tumor antigen phenotype, biologic staging, and prognosis in head and neck squamous carcinoma, *J Natl Cancer Inst Monogr* 13:67, 1992.
33. Wolf GT and others: DNA content and regional metastases in patients with advanced laryngeal squamous carcinoma, *Laryngoscope* 104:479, 1994.

Chapter 8

Skin Flap Physiology

George S. Goding, Jr.
Rick M. Odland

The creation of a flap applies specific stresses to healthy skin. These stresses include local tissue trauma and reduced neurovascular supply to the affected tissue. The extent to which skin can survive these injuries is a reflection of the anatomy and physiology of skin and of the cutaneous response to injury. Knowledge of these principles has led to improved skin flap survival rate by means of flap design and flap delay. Increasing cutaneous flap survival rate by minimizing the deleterious physiologic effects of flap transposition is an area of active research that has yet to produce techniques that have wide-spread clinical application.

ZONES OF PERFUSION

Maintenance of cell function and viability is the objective of the circulatory system at macrocirculatory, capillary, interstitial, and cellular levels. The importance of tissue vascularity is well recognized, but the complexity and diversity of tissue perfusion mechanisms require that the process be divided into components: each level of perfusion has different aspects, and optimal management is possible only if these differences are recognized. Johnson and Barker[118] described two levels of risk zones for flap failure, making a distinction between thrombosis at the arterial and capillary levels. By extension of this concept, four zones of the circulatory system can be considered for all hazards (Fig. 8-1). Proper function of each zone is crucial to tissue viability.

Zone I consists of the cardiopulmonary system, the conduits for blood flow (arteries and veins), neural control of those conduits, and the lymphatic system. Zone I has historically been recognized as essential for flap survival. The delay phenomenon is primarily a zone I affect. The development of the pedicled flap[13] underscores the importance of

zone I in extending flap survival time. Free microvascular tissue transfer also is a zone I manipulation.

Zone II comprises the capillary circulation. The importance of the capillary circulation is shown by the "no-reflow phenomenon," wherein a loss of nutritive blood flow occurs in the presence of an adequate vascular supply.[4]

Zone III is the interstitial space and its mechanisms of nutrient delivery. The capillary wall is included in zone III because capillary permeability is a main determinant of interstitial space properties. Failure of metabolites to enter and traverse the interstitial space can result in loss of cell viability, even though there is adequate zone I and even zone II function. Interstitial systems are an important link in skin flap survival rate.[203]

The cell and its membranes comprise zone IV. Maintaining viable cells is the ultimate determinant of flap survival. Prolongation of cell survival by selective changes in cell permeability and uptake is a potential future intervention that may improve flap survival rate.

ANATOMY AND PHYSIOLOGY OF SKIN

The skin serves as a sensory and as a protective organ. The thick epidermal layers are largely impermeable to gases and to most liquids. Because of this, many agents that could result in beneficial effects are ineffective when applied topically to intact skin.

The epidermis of the skin is derived from ectoderm in the early embryo. The glandular appendages of the skin (sebaceous glands, hair follicles) develop from tubes and solid cords that invaginate from the covering ectoderm.[184] The epidermis is a metabolically active, but avascular, stratified squamous epithelium. The average epidermal thickness for most of the body is 0.1 mm. The majority of cells undergo

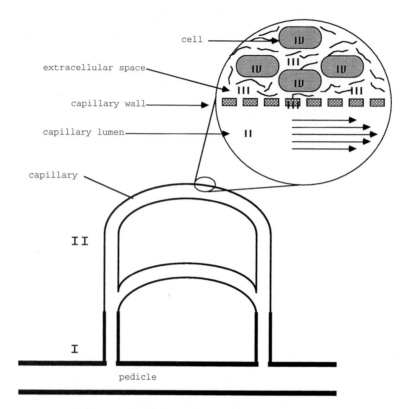

Fig. 8-1. Zones of perfusion. Zone I is the macrocirculatory system consisting of cardiopulmonary, neurovascular, and lymphatic function. Zone II is the capillary circulatory systems composed of arterioles, capillaries, venules, and arteriovenous shunts. The interstitial system is zone III and entails the capillary membranes and interstitial ground substance. The cell membrane, organelles, and intracellular space comprise zone IV, the cellular system.

keratinization and form the various epithelial layers.[116] The superficial keratinized cells of the skin are continuously replaced by cells originating from the mitotic activity in the basal layer of the epidermis. Melanocytes derived from neural crest cells also are found in the epithelium of skin and comprise a second cell type.

The dermis is derived from embryonic mesoderm and consists primarily of noncellular connective tissue. This relatively noncellular layer has metabolic requirements far less than those of the epidermis. Nerves, blood vessels, lymph vessels, and the base of the epidermal glandular appendages are found within the dermis.[116] The dermis is 15 to 40 times thicker than the epidermis, with a maximum width of 4 mm on the back.[120] The outer surface of the dermis has an uneven border contacting the epidermis and is known as the papillary layer. The papillary dermis is characterized by an abundant ground substance, irregularly arranged collagen bundles, and a highly developed microcirculation. The reticular dermis is composed of thick bundles of collagen and coarse elastic fibers. Fibrocytes and blood vessels are proportionally less numerous.

Deep to the reticular layer of the dermis, the anatomy of loose-skin and fixed-skin animals diverges. In fixed-skin animals (humans and swine), the subcutaneous layer consists of loose connective tissue and a varying amount of fat cells. It is a deeper continuation of the dermis and collagenous fibers continuous with those in the dermis. The density of the collagenous fibers is related to the degree of cutaneous mobility over the underlying structures. In the palms and soles, for example, these fibers are particularly numerous. The deep surface of the subcutaneous layer is attached to the superficial fascia of underlying muscle where it is present.

In loose-skin animals (rat, rabbit, dog), the panniculus carnosus muscle is firmly attached to the reticular dermis. The panniculus carnosus is separated from the superficial fascia of underlying muscles by a loose areolar tissue layer. This layer allows for increased mobility of the superficial cutaneous–panniculus carnosus complex relative to the underlying tissue. This mobility afforded by the loose areolar tissue layer creates a greater dependence on direct cutaneous arterial supply than is seen in humans.

Zone I: macrocirculatory system

Blood vessels travel by one of two main routes to terminate in the cutaneous circulation. Musculocutaneous arteries pass through the overlying muscle to which they provide

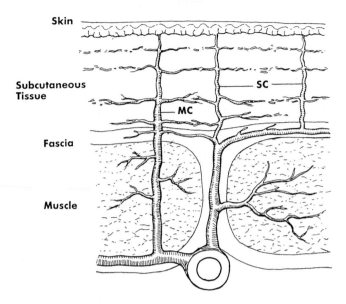

Fig. 8-2. Myocutaneous and septocutaneous arteries. Varying pathways to skin define musculocutaneous (*MC*) and septocutaneous (*SC*) arteries.

nutrition, whereas septocutaneous arteries[49] (also referred to as direct cutaneous arteries) travel through fascial septa that divide the muscular segments (Fig. 8-2).

The cutaneous portion of a septocutaneous artery typically runs parallel to the skin surface, providing nutrition to a large area of skin. Septocutaneous arteries typically have a pair of veins accompanying them and run above the superficial muscular fascia.[279] The more common musculocutaneous arteries leave the muscle and enter the subcutaneous tissue to supply a smaller region of skin.

Septocutaneous and musculocutaneous arteries empty into a diffuse interconnecting vascular network of dermal and subdermal plexi. This network provides a redundancy in the vascular supply to the skin. A collateral blood supply supports the vascular territory of each artery. Lymphatic vessels form a plexus running parallel and deep to the network of blood capillaries. The lymphatic capillaries end in blind sacs and conduct extracellular fluid back into the bloodstream. Lymphatic function is affected by inflammation and loss of blood vessel pulsations.[217]

The neural supply to the skin originates from sensory nerves and sympathetic nerves. The sensory nerves are distributed in segmental fashion, forming dermatomes, and participate in the skin's protective function. The postganglionic terminals of cutaneous sympathetic nerves contain the neurotransmitter, norepinephrine and are found in the area of cutaneous arterioles.[5,175]

Zone II: capillary system

The cutaneous capillary system serves two important functions: nutritional support and thermoregulation. Primarily because of its thermoregulatory function, the rate of blood flow through the skin is one of the most variable in the body. During ordinary skin temperatures, the amount of blood flowing through the skin (approximately 9 ml/min/100 g of tissue) is greater than the flow required for nutritional support.[286] Blood flow can increase to 20 times this value with maximal vasodilation. When the body is exposed to extreme cold, blood flow can be reduced to levels that are marginal for cutaneous nutrition.

Before entering the capillary bed, the arterioles branch into small vessels (terminal arterioles or metarterioles) surrounded by a discontinuous layer of smooth muscle. A simple ring of smooth muscle forms a sphincter at the point where the capillaries originate from the metarteriole. This sphincter can completely stop blood flow within the capillary. The capillary bed can be bypassed by arteriovenous shunts that allow the arterioles to empty directly into venules. During conditions of adequate systemic vascular pressure, preshunt and precapillary sphincters regulate the distribution of cutaneous blood flow.[86]

The preshunt sphincters are involved in regulating the changes in blood flow that affect thermoregulation and systemic blood pressure.[69,255] Release of norepinephrine by the postganglionic sympathetic fibers results in contraction of the preshunt sphincters. This diverts blood away from the skin surface wherein heat loss can occur. With increased body temperature, the sympathetic vasoconstrictor impulses decrease, allowing for increased blood flow to the skin. Local production of bradykinin may play a role in regulating skin blood flow by causing vasodilation.[90] The cutaneous circulation also is extremely sensitive to circulating norepinephrine and epinephrine. Even in areas of skin that have lost their sympathetic innervation, a mass discharge of the sympathetic system will still result in intense vasoconstriction in the skin.

The precapillary sphincter, which controls the amount of nutritive blood flow to the skin, responds to local hypoxemia and increased metabolic byproducts by dilation.[85,289] Capillary blood flow also is affected by elevated interstitial pressure, which can compress the capillary and decrease transcapillary flow. Conversely, as pressure decreases in the interstitium, the capillary expands, and flow increases.[237] Acute increases in systemic blood pressure cause an immediate increase in local blood flow followed by return of flow to near normal levels in less than 1 minute. This normalization of capillary blood flow is called *autoregulation*.[90] The metabolic theory for autoregulation proposes that an excess of oxygen and nutrients results in arteriolar constriction. This process is believed to be the primary functional mechanism of autoregulation. The myogenic theory suggests that stretching of the arteriolar muscle results in reflex contraction and may be a mechanism to protect capillaries from excessively high blood pressures. Reduction of blood flow also may occur as a result of increased interstitial pressure.

Zone III: interstitial system

The interstitial space is filled with proteoglycans and collagen.[237] In many tissues, hyaluronic acid filaments make up the interstitial ground substance. These filaments normally are woven through the interstitium, producing a medium that exhibits high resistance to fluid movement unless the tissue is well hydrated.[92] In tissues with excess edema, the filaments do not overlap, which will produce shear planes of free fluid within the interstitium.[89]

There are two processes by which substances can move across the interstitial space: diffusion and convection.[24] Diffusion is the process wherein a molecule passively moves to a lower concentration. Molecular movement by diffusion is affected by many factors. An important characteristic is lipid solubility. Lipid-soluble molecules tend to traverse cell membranes more easily and quickly than nonlipid soluble agents. Large molecules diffuse more slowly than small ones. As molecules diffuse away from the capillary, the concentration of that molecule decreases by the inverse square law. As edema occurs, diffusion distances increase.[104] The concentration of a molecule within the interstitium also varies from the arteriolar side to the venular side of a capillary.[174]

Convective flow, or bulk flow, is another way for molecules to move across the interstitium. Rather than a given agent diffusing to a lower concentration, the agent is swept along with the current of plasma that flows across the interstitial space in microchannels. The agents then diffuse the short distance from the microchannels to the cells.

The relative importance of diffusion and convective flow is controversial. Some authors believe diffusion is primarily responsible for cell nutrition. Convection becomes relatively more important for certain tissues, molecules, or pathologic states.

Convective flow of nutrient-laden plasma out of the capillaries and across the interstitial space is produced by a combination of hydrostatic and osmotic pressures as described by Starling in 1896. The formula[178] is:

$$Jv/A = Lp[(P_c - P_i) - \sigma(\pi_c - \pi_i)]$$

In descriptive terms, flow of plasma out of the capillary per unit area (Jv/A) is related to the product of the water permeability of the membrane (Lp) multiplied by the difference between hydrostatic pressure in the capillary (P_c) and interstitial space (P_i) minus the difference between osmotic pressure in the capillary (π_c) and the osmotic pressure in the interstitial space (π_i). The osmotic pressures are adjusted by the osmotic coefficient, σ, a measure of the "leakiness" of a semipermeable membrane.

In functional terms, over the length of the capillary, hydrostatic pressure decreases as fluid exits the capillary and hydraulic resistance is overcome. At the same time, oncotic pressure within the capillary increases as fluid exits the capillary and plasma proteins are retained. These changes in gradients favor return of fluid at the venular end of the capillary and in the immediately postcapillary venule. Pressure gradients also are responsible for bulk flow of fluid across the interstitial space in fluid microchannels.

A net change of 2 mOsm is sufficient to increase interstitial pressure beyond transmural capillary pressure,[148] thereby compressing the capillary. Increased venous pressure limits interstitial resorption of fluid and contributes to formation of an interstitial transudate.[237] Inflammation in a flap is probably a result of nociceptor pathway stimulation by handling of the flap. Even the relatively minor trauma of inserting a fine needle causes a "very large" increase in capillary permeability within minutes after insertion, as evidenced by rapid influx of proteins into the interstitium.[27] Ischemia also will produce inflammation. Capillary hyperpermeability has been found throughout ischemic flaps.[242]

The lymphatic system has two functions that affect zone III: to remove excess fluid, and to remove interstitial protein. There is some controversy in the physiology literature regarding the magnitude of the latter function.[95] If the lymphatic system is malfunctioning, interstitial fluid and interstitial protein will accumulate.[154]

Zone IV: cellular systems

The intracellular space is the endpoint for nutrient transport and the origin of metabolic waste. The cell wall is a fluid lipid bilayer, 7.5 to 10.0 nm thick. The lipid bilayer is a major barrier to movement of solutes across the membrane. The primary function of the cell membrane is to maintain or to vary in a controlled fashion the separation of the extracellular and intracellular environments. This separation is achieved by specific membrane proteins, which act as solute pumps and solute and solvent leaks. The osmotic pressure between the two environments also should be maintained to preserve normal cell volume. The sodium–potassium pump is important in maintaining osmotic equilibrium across the cell membrane and has a requirement for energy in the form of adenosine triphosphate (ATP).[150] A loss of energy substrate (oxygen and consequently ATP) produces an intracellular movement of sodium and an increase in intracellular osmotic pressure.[162] These changes occur quickly,[66,67,153,291] within 10 minutes after arterial occlusion.[112] Within seconds of hypoxia, levels of adenosine triphosphate begin to decrease, and cells begin to swell.[153] Relatively brief periods of ischemia result in a reversible swelling of the cell and organelles. If the ischemic insult is severe and prolonged, cell lysis and flap necrosis occur.

CLASSIFICATION OF FLAPS

The vascular supply to a flap is critical to its survival and is the basis of the most commonly used classification system of flaps (Fig. 8-3).[48,135]

Random cutaneous flaps

The blood supply to a random cutaneous flap is derived from musculocutaneous arteries near the base of the flap. Blood is delivered to the tip of the flap by the interconnecting subdermal plexus. The random cutaneous flap is commonly

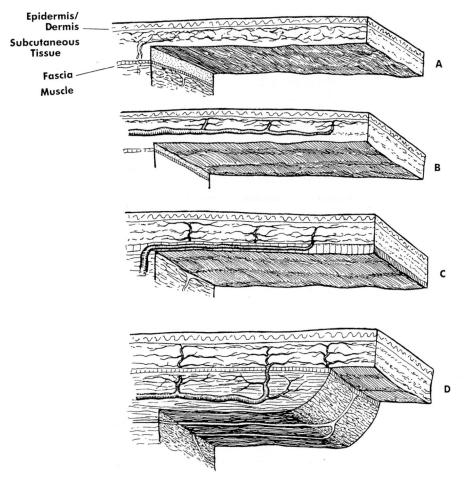

Fig. 8-3. Classification of flaps. Classification of skin flaps based on vascular supply. **A,** Random. **B,** Arterial cutaneous. **C,** Fasciocutaneous. **D,** Musculocutaneous.

used in local flap reconstruction and can be rotated, transposed, advanced, or tubed.

Length-to-width ratios of random cutaneous flaps have been recommended for various areas of the body. These differences reflect a regional variation of the neurovascular supply to the skin. Such a description can serve as a guide in designing random cutaneous flaps but should not imply that a wider flap would extend survival length.[36]

Arterial cutaneous flaps

Arterial cutaneous flaps (also called axial pattern flaps) typically have an improved survival length relative to random cutaneous flaps. This advantage results from the incorporation of a septocutaneous artery within its longitudinal axis. An island flap is an arterial flap with a pedicle consisting of nutrient vessels without the overlying skin. Island flaps can be useful to increase flexibility and decrease pedicle bulk in certain reconstructive procedures.

Use of arterial cutaneous flaps is limited by the availability of direct cutaneous arteries. Examples of arterial cutaneous flaps used in head and neck reconstruction are the deltopectoral flap, based on the anterior perforators of the internal mammary, and the midline forehead flap, based on the supratrochlear vessels.

The surviving length of an arterial flap is related to the length of the included septocutaneous artery. Survival beyond the arterial portion of the flap is based on the subdermal plexus and is essentially a random cutaneous extension of the flap. Flap necrosis resulting from ischemia can be said to occur only in the random portion of the flap (destruction of the arterial pedicle making the entire flap random).

Myocutaneous and fasciocutaneous flaps

Myocutaneous flaps represent an additional modification to improve flap survival. Myocutaneous flaps are based on distal segmental vessels leaving the local vasculature (perforators and cutaneous vessels) intact, which requires incorporation of muscle with the flap. Myocutaneous flaps are typically named for the donor muscle. Examples include the pectoralis myocutaneous flap, based on the pectoral branch of the thoracoacromial artery, and the latissimus dorsi myocutaneous flap, based on the thoracodorsal artery.

The increased blood flow and higher tissue oxygen tensions available with myocutaneous flaps[83] make this design superior in the management of contaminated or infected defects. Improved phagocytotic and bactericidal activity of leukocytes is seen in myocutaneous flaps relative to random pattern flaps in the canine model.[60] These physiologic benefits contribute to the ability of myocutaneous flaps to resist bacterial inoculation more effectively than random pattern flaps.

Like arterial flaps, it often is desirable to extend the surface area of the flap in clinical situations. A random portion of the flap can be incorporated based on the subdermal plexus. This random extension usually is the portion of the flap most at risk of ischemic necrosis.

Fasciocutaneous flaps use direct arterial (septocutaneous) vessels with the cutaneous branches at the level of the deep fascia forming a plexus, which supplies the subdermal plexus.[38] The appropriate size of fasciocutaneous flaps is less well-defined than axial pattern flaps with their obvious arterial supply. Fasciocutaneous flaps appear to rely more on potential skin vascular territories. Four types of fasciocutaneous flaps have been described based on the pattern of blood supply incorporated into the fascial component of the flap. Examples include the parascapular flap and the radial forearm flap.

Venous flaps

Flaps with only an intact venous supply show the minimal nutritional requirements needed for flap survival. Survival of venous flaps is most consistent when the vein is intact on entering and exiting the flap, providing a flow through the venous system.[78] Flaps with drainage from a single venous pedicle will survive, unlike flaps with an arterial pedicle alone, which necrose.[18] Surviving venous flaps show no evidence of arterial blood flow until the third postoperative day.[247] Venous injections show little uptake in venous flaps, arguing against a "to and fro" flow of nutrients from vein to capillary to vein.[282]

Rather than a capillary circulation, the venous drainage has been hypothesized to draw fluid and metabolites out of the flap, which are drawn into the capillaries from the interstitial space.[78] Oxygen and nutrients then diffuse into the flap from the recipient bed, allowing survival until revascularization occurs. Venous flaps were not found to have decreased lactate levels compared with composite grafts 6 hours after surgery[166] and, when compared with conventional arteriovenous flaps in a dog model, had decreased ATP but no increase in edema.[6] Revascularization occurs earlier in venous flaps compared with composite flaps, increasing another potential mechanism for flap survival. Venous flaps performed in humans have been most successful in the distal extremities, where there are multiple venous anastomoses and no valves.[32]

Free microvascular flaps

Free flaps are an increasingly popular form of reconstruction and hold several advantages over regional flaps. Tissue from a distant site can be harvested based on the characteristics of the donor site and the needs of the defect. Vascularity of the flap is maintained by microvascular anastomosis of the artery and vein. The flap can be harvested and customized to the defect in terms of absolute size and relative amounts of bone, muscle, skin, or nerve that is needed. Careful design of a free flap can eliminate a risk of partial necrosis caused by a random extension.

PHYSIOLOGY OF ACUTELY RAISED FLAPS

A number of changes detrimental to skin survival occur when a cutaneous flap is created. That flap survival occurs at all is a testimony to the minimal nutritional requirements of skin. The primary insult affecting flap survival is impaired vascular supply and the resultant ischemia. In the presence of adequate blood flow, complete flap survival occurs. Nerve section and inflammation influence flap survival primarily by affecting blood flow. Recovery from ischemia also can occur by the timely formation of new vascular channels between the transposed flap and the recipient bed.

Impairment of vascular supply

Partial interruption of the vascular supply (zone I) to the skin is the most obvious and critical change that occurs with elevation of a cutaneous flap. Myers[189] has emphasized that "fresh flaps are always both viable and ischemic." Flap survival depends on the degree of ischemia and the amount of time before recovery of nutrient blood flow. Flaps can tolerate an average of 13 hours of complete avascularity and survive.[130]

Limitation of the vascular supply results in a local decrease in perfusion pressure to the skin. In arterial or myocutaneous flaps, the blood supply to the skin overlying the vascular pedicle usually is adequate.[84] In random flaps or random extensions of flaps, the decrease in perfusion pressure becomes more pronounced with increasing distance from the base of the flap.[44,149] When perfusion is reduced in one area of a random flap, the adjacent vascular territories supplied by a separate perforating vessel can provide a low pressure blood supply through the subdermal plexus (Fig. 8-4). Because the nutritional requirements of skin are relatively low, a number of vascular territories can be compromised before necrosis will result.

The surviving length of the random portion of the flap depends on the physical properties of the supplying vessels (intravascular resistance) and the perfusion pressure.[48] When the perfusion pressure decreases below the pressure in the interstitial space, capillary blood flow ceases. The pressure at which there is no longer enough intravascular blood pressure to maintain capillary blood flow is called the *critical closing pressure*.

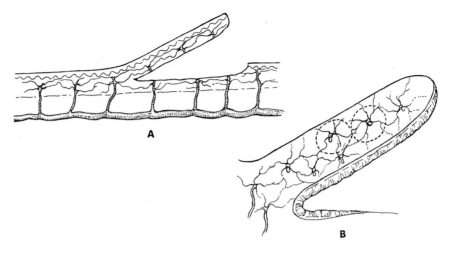

Fig. 8-4. A and **B**, Territories of flaps. Vascular territories in skin flap. Multiple perforating vessels exist and are interconnected at the periphery of their vascular territory. When some of these vessels are cut, blood supply can be replaced from nearby perforating vessels, and then tissue necrosis does not occur.

In the past, random cutaneous flaps often were designed relative to a desired length-to-width ratio—a wider base being needed to successfully transfer a longer flap. The wider random flap only includes additional vessels with the same perfusion pressure. The relationship between perfusion pressure and critical closing pressure is not altered, and no change in survival length occurs (Fig. 8-5).[179]

In free flaps, a secondary ischemia can occur when thrombus formation occurs at the anastomosis. Anastomosis failure is related to exposure of the vascular intima to platelets.[118,283] Platelet activation is caused by superficially exposed subendothelium or, with deeper vessel injury, exposure to collagen types I and III.[19] The geometry of the vascular arrangement often is a critical factor when experienced surgeons lose a free flap.

The venous outflow from the skin also is impaired with flap elevation. Venous flow can occur through the subdermal plexus or by venous channels that accompany the feeding artery in the pedicle. Complete venous occlusion in the early postelevation period may be more damaging to flap survival than inadequate arterial supply.[265] Fortunately, the subdermal plexus alone often is adequate to provide adequate venous outflow. Care should be taken to preserve venous outflow in flaps pedicled solely on the feeding vessels.

Impairment of lymphatic drainage with flap elevation also occurs. Reduction of the cutaneous lymphatic drainage results in an increase in interstitial fluid pressure that is compounded by increased leakage of intravascular protein associated with inflammation. The resulting edema leads to increased interstitial pressure, which decreases capillary perfusion by increasing the critical closing pressure (Fig. 8-6).[76,236] Alterations in the Starling's forces result in further ischemic swelling of cells and the interstitial space, setting a positive feedback cycle in motion.

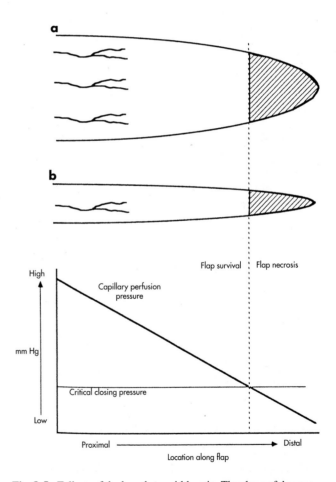

Fig. 8-5. Fallacy of the length-to-width ratio. The slope of decreasing perfusion pressure versus flap length does not change with incorporation of additional vessels (flap *a* versus flap *b*) with the same perfusion pressure. Flap necrosis occurs when perfusion pressure decreases below critical closing pressure of the capillary bed.

Microcirculatory changes

Necrosis in flaps is caused by prolonged loss of nutritional blood flow.[183,189,211] There are several proposed mechanisms for loss of nutritional flow, each of which may play a role. Erythrocyte sludging frequently has been noted in capillaries undergoing ischemia, often without thrombus formation.[242,264] Therefore, sludging is not necessarily caused by platelet activation unless there is a microvascular anastomosis or other vessel injury involved, such as tearing, stretching, laceration, or crushing of the vessel. Microemboli are commonly generated from a microvascular anastomosis.[19]

The reason for the erythrocyte sludging is multifactorial. Erythrocytes become turgid and lose the flaccid, biconcave disk in the acidic environment of ischemia. Narrowing of the capillaries,[245] presumably a result of external compression, also contributes to stacking of erythrocytes within the lumen of ischemic tissue capillaries. Sludging is seen less often if the hematocrit is kept below 30%.[20]

Capillary blood flow is further hindered by leukocyte adherence to the capillary wall.[245] The leukocytes probably are responding to cytokines released from the cells in response to initial injury. The leukocytes first roll along the capillary wall and then begin to stick. As time progresses, the leukocytes flatten onto the endothelial cell and eventually pass into the interstitium. Each step of the way has biochemical mediators. Carolina rinse solution will decrease sticking but not rolling.[231] Leukocyte depletion in patients undergoing heart transplantation prevents ultrastructural evidence of reperfusion injury.[219]

Ischemic cells of all tissues swell because of the loss of energy substrate needed to continue maintaining the osmotic gradient. Swelling of extravascular cells causes compression of the vascular lumen,[16] but endothelial cell swelling has a greater effect on capillary blood flow.[264] The effect of cell swelling is most dramatic in bone microcirculation, wherein a relatively small increase in cellular edema has a profound effect on vascular resistance.[185] A similar relationship between edema and increased vascular resistance has been shown in cardiac reperfusion studies.[2] Histologic evidence of edema can be used to grade the severity of free flap injury.[159] Nitric oxide synthase, an endothelial-derived vasodilator, has been studied for its effect in skin flaps.[144,146]

Neovascularization

In surviving flaps, blood flow gradually increases. If the flap is in a favorable recipient site, a fibrin layer forms within the first 2 days. Neovascularization of the flap begins 3 or 4 days after flap transposition.[77,273,276] Revascularization adequate for division of the flap pedicle has been shown as early as 7 days in animal models and humans.[40,142]

During revascularization, vascular endothelial cells play a major role in the formation of new vessels. Normally, endothelial cells are in a quiescent state, although when stimulated by angiogenic growth factors, these cells can dramatically proliferate. This normally occurs only during certain conditions, such as wound healing and ovulation.

Beginning with an angiogenic stimulus, the angiogenic process involves a number of discrete yet overlying steps (Fig. 8-7). Initially, the vessels become dilated and permeable with retraction of the endothelial cells and a decrease in endothelial junctions. The basement membrane then is dissolved by proteases, and the endothelial cells migrate from the vascular wall toward the angiogenic stimulus. Behind the leading front of migrating endothelial cells, endothelial cell replication begins forming a capillary sprout that elongates toward the angiogenic source. The nearby capil-

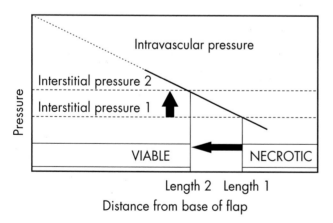

Fig. 8-6. The relationship between increased interstitial pressure and decreased surviving flap length. Intravascular perfusion pressure decreases along the length of the flap. At the distal end of the flap, intravascular perfusion pressure will become less than interstitial pressure, causing the capillaries to collapse (critical closing pressure). As edema is generated by ischemia and inflammation, interstitial pressure increases, which results in a decrease in surviving length from length 1 to length 2.

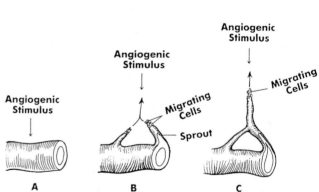

Fig. 8-7. Steps in angiogenesis. **A,** Initial stimulus with retraction of endothelial cells and thinning of basement membrane. **B,** Migration of endothelial cells and formation of capillary sprout. **C,** Formation of capillary loops, which become patent to form new blood vessels.

lary sprouts then anastomose to each other, forming capillary loops. As capillary loops and sprouts continue, the loops become patent, forming newly formed blood vessels. These blood vessels differentiate and lay down basement membrane consisting of type IV collagen, laminin, and proteoglycans. Pericytes and fibroblasts then migrate to the capillary loop sites.[75]

With the continued presence or absence of the angiogenic stimulus, substantial remodeling, regression, and rearrangement of the new capillaries occur.[75] Some capillaries join preexisting flap vessels (inosculation), but the majority of revascularization appears to involve direct ingrowth of recipient vessels into the flap (Fig. 8-8).[259] New capillaries can grow toward an angiogenic source at a mean rate of 0.2 mm/day. When the angiogenic stimulus is discontinued, the capillary vessels regress and eventually disappear over a period of weeks. Angiogenic growth factors can stimulate capillary growth over distances of 2 to 5 mm.[68]

To prevent an uncontrollable cascade of neovascularization, mechanisms to inhibit angiogenesis are believed to exist. Evidence suggests that pericytes can suppress endothelial growth by direct contact.[47] Thus, the physiologic response of angiogenesis may be analogous to the blood coagulation pathway that should be maintained at a constant steady state of control. In soft-tissue wound repair, macrophages, lymphocytes, mast cells, and platelets are involved in releasing various factors that modulate angiogenesis.[75] Tissues that are particularly high in angiogenic factors are bovine brain,[161] corpus luteum,[82] retina,[61] salivary glands,[111] and lymphatic tissues.[3] Benign and malignant tumors also can be sources of angiogenic growth factors.

Nerve section

Sensory and sympathetic nerves are severed in the process of flap elevation. Although loss of sensation may limit the usefulness of the flap after transfer, adrenergic denervation has implications for flap survival. When a sympathetic nerve is divided, catecholamines are released from the nerve terminal, and the mechanism for catecholamine reuptake is eliminated.[124,209,221] A local ''hyperadrenergic state'' exists, which produces vasoconstriction mediated by α-adrenergic receptors in the cutaneous vasculature.[209]

The vasoconstricting effect of sympathectomy further reduces the total flap blood flow[134,211] that has already been decreased by division of supplying vessels. This negatively affects the ratio of perfusion pressure to the critical closing pressure of the arterioles in the subdermal plexus. A greater proportion of the distal flap is excluded from the blood supply, and necrosis becomes more likely. The stored transmitter is depleted within 24 to 48 hours,[121,124] and blood flow increases as the concentration of norepinephrine declines.[211] In critical areas of the flap, the time to recovery of nutrient blood flow may be delayed sufficiently to produce additional necrosis.

Inflammation/prostaglandins

The surgical trauma and ischemia associated with an acutely raised flap result in an inflammatory response. Histamine, serotonin, and kinins are released into the extracellular compartment after flap elevation, increasing the permeability of the microcirculation. The result is an increase in the concentration of proteins and cells within the extracellular space. The presence of nonbacterial inflammation beginning a few days before flap elevation has been shown to improve flap survival.[156,160] This is presumably the result of an increase in local blood flow.

The inflammation created during flap elevation may have deleterious effects because of the resultant edema formation. In addition to compromising capillary blood flow and altering the relationships of the Starling equation, interstitial edema increases the diffusion distances between cells. The

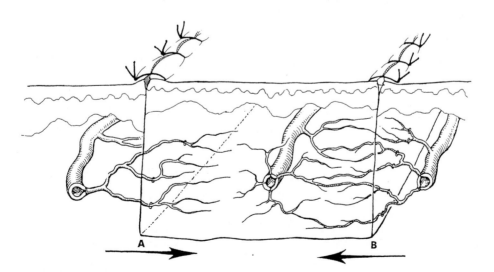

Fig. 8-8. Ingrowth of angiosomes. Cross-section of the flap, showing **A,** direct ingrowth versus **B,** inosculation.

effect is enhanced as a result of the inverse square law for diffusion. Edema also can constitute a direct barrier to diffusion.[102]

The action of the primary mediators of the inflammatory response (histamine, serotonin, and kinins) is short-lived. After kinin formation and in the presence of complement, prostaglandins are synthesized by injured cells. Prostaglandins play an important role in the later stages of the inflammatory reaction, while simultaneously initiating the early phases of injury repair.

Prostaglandins are derived from essential fatty acids that are incorporated in membrane phospholipids (Fig. 8-9). Activation of phospholipases results in the production of prostaglandin H_2 (PGH$_2$) by cyclooxygenase. Prostaglandin E_1 (PGE$_1$) and prostaglandin E_2 (PGE$_2$) can be synthesized from prostaglandin H_2 by isomerases in the vascular endothelium. PGE$_1$ and PGE$_2$ produce vasodilation. Prostaglandin D_2 (PGD$_2$) also is formed by an isomerase reaction and is the principal cyclooxygenase product of the mast cell. Its effects on the cutaneous microvasculature are similar to PGE$_1$. Prostacyclin (PGI$_2$) is a vasodilating agent and inhibitor of platelet aggregation that is derived from PGH$_2$ through the action of prostacyclin synthase. In the skin, PGI$_2$ is primarily produced in the endothelial cells of blood vessels.[96,125] Prostacyclin is metabolized to 6-keto-PGF$_{1a}$.

Thromboxane synthetase converts PGH$_2$ into thrombox-

ane A_2 (TxA$_2$) and is primarily located in the platelets. Its effects include vessel constriction and promotion of platelet aggregation.[127] TxA$_2$ is unstable and rapidly converted into thromboxane B_2 (TxB$_2$). Prostaglandin F_{2a} (PGF$_{2a}$) is derived from PGH$_2$ by a reductase reaction. A marked increase in resistance is seen in cutaneous arteries, arterioles, and venules in the presence of PGF$_{2a}$.[193]

The synthesis of prostaglandins and thromboxane can be altered by pharmacologic manipulation. The action of phospholipase A_2 can be inhibited by drugs that reduce the availability of Ca^{++}. Glucocorticoids also affect phospholipase A_2 activity by inducing the synthesis of a protein that inhibits the enzyme.[31] Aspirin and other nonsteroidal antiinflammatory drugs (NSAIDs) interfere with the cyclooxygenase enzyme inhibiting the synthesis of PGH$_2$.

Prostaglandins clearly play a role in the inflammatory response after flap surgery. Prostacyclin levels increase after flap elevation with a peak concentration around 7 days and then decrease to postoperative day 21.[96] PGE$_2$, PGF$_{2a}$, and TxB$_2$ also increase after the creation of a flap. The increase of PGE$_2$, PGF$_{2a}$, and TxB$_2$ can be blunted by creating a bipedicled flap. Conversion to a single pedicle flap (''delay'') results in decreased levels of thromboxane and an increased PGE$_2$, which remain at least to 7 days.[188] Whether these changes in prostaglandin levels represent a cause or a side effect of the observed phenomenon remains to be seen.

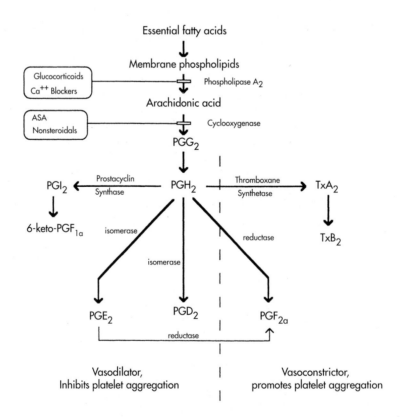

Fig. 8-9. Synthesis of prostaglandins and thromboxanes and their general effects in the cutaneous circulation.

Reperfusion injury

There is controversy and often confusion regarding the terms *no-reflow* and *reperfusion injury*. *No-reflow* is a term connoting the condition when zone I perfusion has been reestablished, but zone II or III failure prevails. *Reperfusion injury* describes the observation that tissues tolerate short periods of total ischemia fairly well but exhibit histologic injury after return of perfusion—thus injury apparently caused by reperfusion.[291] Both terms imply a period of ischemia, and both conditions result in microcirculatory failure.

All flaps experience some ischemia, and return of blood flow may result in microcirculatory impairment.[189,249] Free radicals form during reperfusion and result in tissue injury, but other causes such as hyperosmosis from lactic acid accumulation[265] have been implicated.[291]

Free radical formation

When oxygen becomes available with reperfusion, an additional menace to flap survival is produced—the free radical. This byproduct of reperfusion can cause damage at the cellular and subcellular levels,[133,262] contributing to postischemic tissue necrosis. The neutrophil appears to play a major role in the mediation of reperfusion injury.[155]

Free radicals are extremely reactive compounds because of an unpaired electron in their outer orbits. Oxygen free radicals are formed by the sequential univalent reduction of molecular oxygen. The superoxide anion radical (O_2-) is formed by the addition of a single electron to molecular oxygen. Superoxide is a by-product of ATP production in the mitochondria and other oxidation reduction reactions.[262] Polymorphonuclear cells are a second source of superoxide radicals that are released in response to bacterial inflammation.[17]

A major source of free radicals in ischemic tissue is the enzyme xanthine oxidase (Fig. 8-10).[172] With ischemia, high energy phosphate compounds are converted to hypoxanthine that accumulates in the tissues. When oxygen becomes available with reperfusion, xanthine oxidase catalyzes the conversion of hypoxanthine into uric acid, producing superoxide in the process. This reaction is believed to be an important mechanism in ischemic tissue injury in skin flaps.[171] The role of xanthine oxidase has been brought into question by the ability of some investigators to find xanthine oxidase activity in ischemic skin,[114,290] but others have not.[227] Xanthine oxidase activity has been found in normal rat skin and increases its activity after venous occlusion, reperfusion,[114] and flap elevation with the highest levels being present distally.[11] Tissue damage resulting from free radical production can occur from lipid peroxidation of the cellular membrane and denaturation of the intracellular matrix.[187,262] Delayed neovascularization has been proposed as another consequence of free radical damage affecting proliferating endothelial cells.[113]

Capillary obstruction (no-reflow)

Arterial and random flaps can tolerate several hours of total avascularity and remain viable.[130] When the critical ischemia time for a flap is exceeded, an ischemia-related obstruction to blood flow, known as the *no-reflow phenomenon*, develops. Even though large vessels (zone I) have adequate flow, there is no perfusion in zone II or III. The no-reflow phenomenon was described in skin flaps by May and others.[167] Swelling of the endothelial and parenchymal cells coupled with intravascular stasis and eventual thrombosis leads to loss of nutritive flow. Interactions between polymorphonuclear cells and endothelial cells appear to play a fundamental role in the generation of a reperfusion injury.[215,254] Both cell groups produce cytokine and proadhesive molecules that affect the inflammatory response.[229] Polymorphonuclear cells adhere to the vascular wall and generate pro-

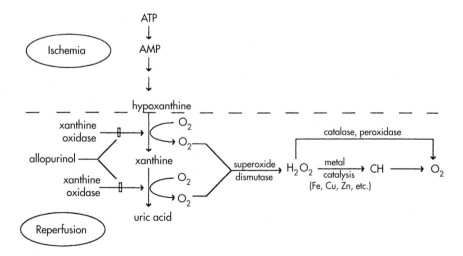

Fig. 8-10. Xanthine oxidase. Possible mechanism for formation of oxygen-free radicals during reperfusion after ischemia and the subsequent reduction of the superoxide radical.

teases and oxygen free radicals that injure the endothelial cells.[284]

A unique aspect of free flap physiology is microcirculatory failure related to showers of microemboli from the anastomosis.[19] These microemboli will flow through the microcirculation and sometimes will transiently occlude capillaries before finally clearing the microcirculation. Microemboli generated from the anastomosis have importance in management of microcirculatory failure and the no-reflow phenomenon as it applies to free flaps.[103]

RESEARCH METHODS

A large amount of literature is available on skin flap physiology. The results of several studies give conflicting results. Experimental results often are difficult to interpret because of variation in choice of animal model, timing of treatment, route of drug administration, method of data collection, and repeatability of the study.[131] Some standardization of flap research methods would help resolve some of these difficulties. Guidelines for pharmacologic investigation of skin flaps were suggested by Kerrigan and Daniel.[131] These recommendations include (1) postoperative treatment only, (2) control flaps on the same animal, (3) baseline fluorescein measurements, (4) double-blind experimental design, and (5) measurement of drug-induced changes in blood flow. No consensus has been reached regarding these or other guidelines.

Two basic experimental designs have been used to investigate the consequences of a vascular insult on a surgical flap. In one design, the blood supply to a flap is interrupted for varying amounts of time by occluding or otherwise interrupting flow through the vascular pedicle. The maximum amount of ischemic time the flap can survive in the experimental and control groups is determined. This design is useful to investigate the no-reflow phenomenon and ischemia tolerance. The second design involves flaps with a random extension in which the effect of an experimental manipulation on blood flow or flap survival is compared with a control. From this basic framework, a number of animal models and methods to assess blood flow and survival have been developed.

Animal models

The most common animals used in flap research are listed in Table 8-1. The most frequently used model for flap research is the rat. It is relatively inexpensive, and there is a large amount of reference data available. The rat is a loose-skinned animal and thus has a preponderance of skin supplied by direct cutaneous arteries, which is in contrast to humans. A pedicled abdominal or a random cutaneous dorsal flap can be created. The distal portion of a dorsal flap can survive as a free graft when in contact with the underlying bed. This "skin-graft effect" can be controlled by separating the flap from the underlying bed.[93] The variance seen in control animals often means that large numbers of animals are required to obtain meaningful results.

Pigs are another common animal model in flap research. Using pigs has a theoretic advantage in that they are fixed-skinned animals with numerous musculocutaneous arteries. The cutaneous blood supply is therefore closer to that of humans and also makes a good model for studying myocutaneous flaps. Flaps created from pig skin have been criticized for their use in research investigating changes in cutaneous surface area and thickness with tissue expansion.[22] The biomechanical properties of pig skin were found to be at variance with human skin.

Rabbits, like rats, are loose-skinned animals. Rabbits have been used as models in skin flap research when a larger skin area is desired in a random flap.[34] Myocutaneous flap studies in the rabbit may have little relevance to human myocutaneous flaps because of the paucity of musculocutaneous perforating arteries and their inability to support a cutaneous flap.[70,200]

The canine was the first animal model used in skin flap research.[54] The dog is a loose-skinned animal, and care should be used when investigating vascular changes in myocutaneous flaps. The biomechanical properties of canine skin have been found to be more like human skin than those seen in the pig model.[22] The expense and size of the model has limited its use when other models (rabbit, rat) can be substituted adequately.

Perfusion measurement

Direct observation of a flap is the most common method of assessing flap viability in clinical situations. Findings

Table 8-1. Animal models in skin flap research

Model	Cost	Skin type	Musculocutaneous vessels	Biomechanical properties*	Multiple flaps
Rat	Low	Loose	Few	Fair	No
Pig	Moderate	Fixed	Present	Poor	Yes
Rabbit	Low–moderate	Loose	Few	Fair	Few
Canine	Moderate–high	Loose	Few	Good	Yes

* Biomechanical similarity to human skin.

such as flap color, temperature, capillary refill, and bleeding at the distal edge give gross approximations of flap perfusion. Greater reliability is needed in clinical flaps with questionable viability and in the laboratory.

Perfusion measurements are used in research to (1) quantify the effect of a particular agent on the blood flow to a flap, (2) obtain a baseline measurement to assure that experimental and control flaps have an equivalent blood flow, and (3) predict the survival of a flap. Clinical uses of perfusion measurement have included monitoring the blood flow to a flap postoperatively and predicting flap viability at the time of surgery. Each technique has inherent advantages and disadvantages (Table 8-2) and inaccuracies (Fig. 8-11).

Microspheres

Microspheres are thought to be the most accurate means of estimating blood flow.[189] The technique depends on three

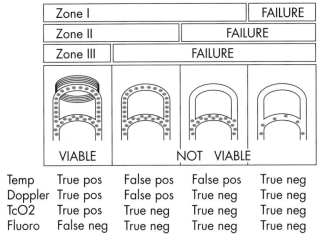

Zone I			FAILURE
Zone II		FAILURE	
Zone III		FAILURE	
VIABLE		NOT VIABLE	

Temp	True pos	False pos	False pos	True neg
Doppler	True pos	False pos	True neg	True neg
TcO2	True pos	True neg	True neg	True neg
Fluoro	False neg	True neg	True neg	True neg

Fig. 8-11. Perfusion types. Zones of circulatory impairment. The relationship of microcirculatory impairment and anomalous readings of common measurements of flap perfusion is shown. All zones should be functioning for cell viability, and zone III is the first to fail. Zone III failure is shown as a loss of interstitial flow, whereas capillary blood flow is potentially still present. Zone II failure occurs with loss of capillary blood flow. Arteriovenous shunt flow may still be present, but it is not nutritive. Finally, with zone I failure, the flap is ischemic. See text for a discussion of monitors of perfusion.

principles. First, the microspheres should be distributed to the tissues in direct proportion to their blood flow. For this to happen, the microspheres should be well mixed and rheologically similar to erythrocytes. Second, the microspheres should be trapped in the capillary bed in the first circulation. Finally, the systemic hemodynamics should not be affected by the embolization of the capillary beds.[213]

The microspheres are polystyrene beads of uniform size with isotopes placed inside. For measurement of capillary perfusion, the beads are typically 15 μm in size to allow trapping in the capillary beds but passage through A-V shunts. Larger microspheres (50 μm) can be used if trapping in the A-V shunts is desired. The microspheres are injected into the left ventricle, where they are mixed before being expelled with the blood and trapped in the tissue capillaries. The ratio of the blood flow in a specific tissue to the cardiac output equals the ratio of the number of microspheres trapped in that tissue to the total number of spheres injected. A blood sample is drawn at the time of microsphere injection to serve as a reference for calculating cardiac output and blood flow to the tissue being investigated.[213]

The microsphere technique was found to be linearly correlated with blood flow to the skin.[213] When skin blood flow was low (approximately 0.03 ml/min), the repeatability of the technique was hindered. This low blood flow is rarely seen in acute random flaps and occurs only when arterial spasm is at a maximum in the early postoperative period. By using different sets of microspheres, capillary blood flow can be measured simultaneously and consecutively to skin, muscle, and bone. A major disadvantage that prevents its clinical use is the need to sample the tissue at the end of the experiment. There are technical issues that should be considered when interpreting results of microsphere studies.[23,292]

Fluorescein

Sodium fluorescein dye ($C_{20}H_{10}Na_2O_5$; molecular weight, 376.3) is nontoxic at pharmacologic doses of 10 to 15 mg/kg.[212] The LD-50 is 1000 mg/kg in laboratory animals. When exposed to ultraviolet light (<510 nm), it will emit a yellow–green fluorescence. After intravenous injection, it moves quickly from the intravascular compartment to the extracellular space without penetrating the cell mem-

Table 8-2. Advantages and disadvantages of various perfusion measurements

Measurement	Clinical use	Advantage	Disadvantage
Microspheres	No	Most accurate	Requires biopsy, invasive, systemic injection
Fluorescein	Yes	Low toxicity, accurate at 24 hours	Single measurement or expensive, systemic injection
Laser Doppler	Yes	Noninvasive, qualitative reliability	$\pm$ Quantitative reliability, expensive
Temperature	Yes	Inexpensive, simple	Slow response
Clearance	No	Continuous monitoring	Radioactive systemic injection
Tissue oxygen	Yes	Continuous, noninvasive	Relative values

branes. Staining occurs in tissues with a nutrient blood flow. Fluorescence can be detected visually with a Wood's light, photographically with the appropriate filters, or with a dermofluorometer.

Visual and photographic detection require a relatively large dose of fluorescein (15 to 30 mg/kg). This dose can take 12 to 18 hours to clear, which limits the frequency with which the test can be performed. Lower doses of fluorescein (1.5 mg/kg) can be used with a fiberoptic dermofluorometer. For each estimation of blood flow with the dermofluorometer, the skin fluorescence before and after fluorescein injection is measured. The increase in fluorescence of the skin during investigation and a reference area is compared, and a dye fluorescence index (DFI) is calculated. By quantifying the fluorescence and decreasing the fluorescein dose, blood flow can be examined at more frequent intervals.

Areas in a skin flap with an increase in fluorescence that is approximately 30% of an area of normal skin (DFI = 30) would be expected to survive.[41,258,272] Arteriospasm[212] and interstitial acidosis[204] early after flap elevation will result in an underestimation of actual skin flap survival with fluorescein. At 18 to 24 hours after surgery, the prediction of flap survival was highly correlated with actual survival.[212,258] Measurement of fluorescein elimination with fiberoptic fluorometry can result in a method of continuous monitoring of tissue perfusion.[51]

Laser doppler

With the laser Doppler, a 2 mW helium–neon laser is used to produce a uniform light with a wavelength in air of 632.8 nm. A fiberoptic cable is used to carry the light to the skin surface and to transmit the backscattered light to a photodetector. Three different types of measurement can be obtained with a laser Doppler. A laser Doppler flow (LDF) signal is generated by measuring the movement of erythrocytes. The Doppler effect results in backscattered light from the surface of a stationary tissue plane having a different wavelength than light backscattered from a moving object (in this case, an erythrocyte). The number and average velocity of erythrocytes determine the LDF value. A second measurement is laser photometry (LP). This signal is generated by the total intensity of backscattered light. Because at this wavelength the light is mainly absorbed in the skin by the hemoglobin of the erythrocyte, the LP value is inversely proportional to the blood volume of the tissue studied. In newer versions of the laser Doppler, the velocity of the erythrocytes can be calculated.[226]

The laser Doppler can be used to differentiate arterial and venous occlusion while monitoring free flaps.[226,268] With arterial or venous occlusion, there was a dramatic decrease in flow through the tissue, but tissue engorgement was detected only with venous occlusion.

The quality of blood flow estimation with the laser Doppler has had mixed reviews,[65,101,157,165,258] so percentage change rather than absolute values often is followed when using the laser Doppler clinically. The laser Doppler has the advantages of being noninvasive and relatively simple to use. It is a viable option for continuous monitoring of revascularized tissue.[257]

Other methods

Metabolic monitoring

Monitoring the pH[52,277] or temperature[258] of a flap can provide a reliable measure of perfusion. Temperature monitoring is simple and has been used clinically but has a low response time.[277] Oxygen can be monitored by transcutaneous method[87] or by silastic tonometry.[105]

Clearance

The rate of removal of a particular substance can be used to estimate blood flow. Various isotopes have been used in this regard.[278,295] This technique was not believed to be useful in monitoring clinical flaps postoperatively. The use of fluorescein clearance is described previously.

Intravital microscopy

Barker and others[21] introduced the hairless mouse model using intravital microscopy to study microcirculatory changes and used the model to study drug effects[245] and hemodilution.[20] Skin flaps were created on the ears of hairless mice by microdissecting and occluding arterial vessels. The resultant changes in the microcirculation are observed directly with a computer-assisted microcirculatory analysis system (CAMAS), which has been able to show leukocyte adherence and erythrocyte sludging. Saetzler and others[66] used fluorescein isothiocyanate-labeled dextran as a marker. Barker and others have also used CAMAS in a free flap model using rat cremasteric muscle.[19] Although they note that microemboli frequently are seen downstream from a typical microvascular anastomosis, Barker and others use an ''intentionally thrombogenic arteriotomy/repair'' to produce consistent emboli. Intravital microscopy also was used in a dorsal flap in a hairless mouse model.[106]

ERRORS OF PERFUSION MONITORS

Methods to monitor perfusion focus on only one aspect of the zones of perfusion, so errors can occur. It is important to understand how a technique can be misleading (see Fig. 8-11).

Temperature probes are sensitive to nonnutritive shunt flow and will show the most false-positive results (i.e., indicating the tissue will survive when it will not). Laser Doppler reflects capillary blood flow but will still indicate adequate perfusion even though there is a zone III failure of interstitial nutrient flow. The transcutaneous oxygen monitor is more specific but may not be sensitive enough to distinguish zone III failure from zone II failure. Only fluorescein dye studies will produce a false-negative result in the first 24 hours, but clinically a false-negative result is a lessor error than a false-positive result. If the distal end of a flap stains with fluorescein dye, then the surgeon can be confident that the entire flap will survive. The error would be in excising tissue that did not stain because it may have survived. This is a lessor error than believing the tissue is viable when it will go on to necrosis.

ATTEMPTS TO ALTER SKIN FLAP VIABILITY

Increased blood supply

Skin flap failure can occur from extrinsic and intrinsic causes.[106] Extrinsic reasons for flap necrosis are those not resulting from the design of the raised flap. Examples include systemic hypotension, infection, and pedicle compression. These factors often can be overcome in the clinical situation. The primary intrinsic factor affecting flap survival is inadequate blood flow. Numerous experimental attempts have been made to influence flap microcirculation or decrease the deleterious effects of inadequate flap blood flow (Fig. 8-12). The most successful has been flap delay. Table

Table 8-3. Zones of perfusion affected by various interventions to increase flap survival

Intervention	Affected zones
Flap design	I
Delay	I, II
Vasodilators	II
Neovascularization	II
Rheology	II
Inflammation	II, III
Antioxidants	II, III, IV
Metabolic manipulation	II, IV
Increased oxygenation	IV

8-3 shows the affected zones of perfusion for various interventions to increase flap survival.

Delay

Four things are accepted about the delay phenomenon. First, it requires surgical trauma. Second, a large percentage of the neurovascular supply to the flap should be eliminated. Third, delay results in increased flap survival at the time of tissue transfer. Fourth, the beneficial effects can last up to 6 weeks in humans.[220] To explain this phenomenon, three theories regarding the mechanism of delay have been developed: (1) delay improves the blood flow, (2) delay conditions the tissue to ischemia,[173] and (3) delay closes arteriovenous shunts.[235] Most recent studies support a mechanism resulting in increased circulation to the flap. How this occurs remains to be proven.

The percentage of arteriovenous shunt flow to total blood flow is similar in delayed and acute flaps.[210] Delayed flaps simply have an increase in total blood flow. The addition of systemic norepinephrine decreases the blood flow in delayed flaps to the level seen in acute flaps. Thus, one effect of delay is a decrease in vasoconstriction in the distal portion of the flap.

Flaps delayed as few as 24 hours survive to a greater length[159] and can tolerate longer periods of ischemia.[7,280,281] Distal perfusion in the pig flank flap increases with a bipedicle flap delay up to 4 days. No further increase in perfusion occurs, extending delay up to 14 days.[211] Pang and others[211] theorized that after a delay, a reduced vasoactivity of the small arteries allows delivery of more blood to the distal portion of the flap. This modulation could occur by release of vasoconstrictive substances (norepinephrine, thromboxane, and serotonin) during elevation of the bipedicled flap. Degeneration release of norepinephrine oc-

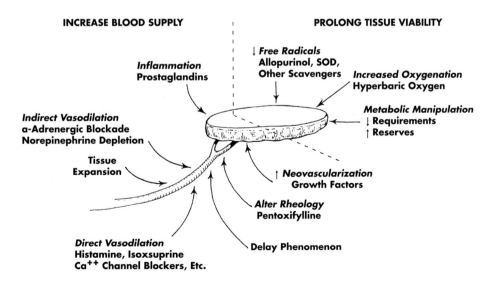

Fig. 8-12. Experimental attempts to affect flap survival.

curs soon after flap elevation with norepinephrine stores largely depleted in the first 24 to 48 hours.[121,124] In bipedicle flaps, Cutting and others[43] found the catecholamine level beginning to increase 4 days after flap construction, whereas others[121,124] have found the catecholamine levels to be depressed over a greater period. Necrosis is not seen with the first stage of delay because the bipedicled flap has an adequate blood supply. After depletion of the catecholamines, a relative state of sympathectomy develops. Because of the catecholamine depletion, conversion of the delayed flap to a single pedicle is not accompanied by the same degree of vasoconstriction.[210]

Early after elevation, the vasculature to the flap has an increased sensitivity to the effects of adrenergic drugs.[209] Intravenous norepinephrine will decrease blood flow to a myocutaneous flap even in the presence of increased blood flow to control skin.[183] This hypersensitivity to exogenous norepinephrine can be partially blocked by management with phenoxybenzamine, an α-adrenergic blocking agent. The period of hypersensitivity to norepinephrine lasts slightly less than 1 week[183] and correlates with the period of decreased tissue norepinephrine found after flap elevation.[43] Recovery from the hyperadrenergic state also appears to play a role in the delay phenomenon.

Reorientation of the major vascular channels is another mechanism to increase blood flow to the distal portion of the single pedicle flap.[42,88] The effect of delay is greater in narrow flaps than in wide flaps.[267] The longitudinal channeling is greater in narrow flaps because more of the transverse vessels are cut. Dilation of existing vessels is most evident in transitional areas between vascular territories of adjacent perforating arteries.[30] The effects of delay have been produced by inducing collateral blood flow by vessel occlusion in the laboratory setting[30,55,205,206] and clinically.[271] Longitudinal flow also is enhanced by vasodilating substances released by inflammation and mild ischemia.[267] Pang and others[210] believed that the depletion of vasoconstricting substances played a role in the early stage of delay, whereas locally released vasodilating substances were involved in the later stages.

Vasodilators

Indirect vasodilators. The intense vasoconstriction associated with release of norepinephrine after flap elevation should hinder flap survival. One of the benefits of flap delay seems to be depletion of norepinephrine before creation of the flap to be transferred. If this vasoconstriction could be blocked or reversed, the duration and severity of distal flap ischemia should be lessened. The result would be increased flap survival without the need for delay.

α-Adrenergic blocking agents are directed against the catecholamine-induced vasoconstriction seen after flap elevation. Using the rat model, phenoxybenzamine resulted in improving flap survival in some studies.[63,191,288] Phenoxybenzamine and phentolamine ointments applied topically

also were found to be effective in increasing flap survival in the rat model.[81] Other investigators have been unable to reproduce beneficial effects in the rabbit or pig.[131,190] Depletion of norepinephrine stores before flap elevation with reserpine[45,122,128,131] and guanethidine[1,62,94] also has met with mixed results and systemic toxicity.

Several anesthetic agents have vasoactive properties and may influence flap survival. Because general anesthetics often are used during the creation of larger flaps, any potential effects on flap survival are important. Isoflurane (a sympatholytic vasodilator) was found to significantly improve flap survival compared with nitrous oxide, which induces vasoconstriction.[53]

Direct vasodilators. Direct vasodilators such as histamine, hydralazine, and topical dimethylsulfoxide have showed a beneficial and no effect on skin flap survival.[131] Isoxsuprine is a phenylethylamine derivative of epinephrine having α-adrenergic receptor antagonistic and β-adrenergic receptor agonistic properties, resulting in relaxation of vascular smooth muscle. In high doses, it can decrease viscosity and inhibit platelet aggregation. Isoxsuprine was found to increase blood flow in the area of the dominant artery in porcine myocutaneous and arterial flaps. Unfortunately, no improvement in blood flow was seen in the distal random portion of the flaps or in flap survival.[134,196,214,293] The smaller vessels in the distal random portion of a flap were theorized to have a different sensitivity to vasodilator drugs than muscular or axial arteries. Manipulation of these distal vascular channels appears to be critical in increasing flap survival.

Calcitonin gene-related peptide (CGRP) is a bioactive neuropeptide found in primary sensory neurons. It is a potent vasodilator and is thought to stimulate smooth muscle relaxation by an endothelial-dependent mechanism. CGRP administration improves blood flow and survival in ischemic skin flaps[188] and delays the onset of the no-reflow phenomenon.[189] Pretreatment with capsaicin, which depletes neuropeptides from primary sensory neurons, results in a decreased flap survival.[140] These findings suggest a potential role for primary sensory neurons in cutaneous vascular control and flap survival.

Topical application of nitroglycerine was found to increase flap survival in some studies[232,241] but not in all.[199] Nitroglycerine acts as a vasodilator with more potent venodilator than arteriodilator effects. The action on the veins was believed to contribute to the increased flap survival. The ability to decrease platelet aggregation may be the main therapeutic benefit of nitroglycerine and other direct vasodilators that affect platelet function. Topical application of heparin, which has little vasodilatory effect, was found to have a survival benefit similar to PGE_1, a potent vasodilator that also decreases platelet aggregation.[251,252]

Neovascularization

Neovascularization can be accelerated with fibroblast growth factors. Application of fibroblast growth factors results in increased endothelial cell proliferation and vascular tube formation. Application of growth factor can generate functional blood vessels and nonsurgically anastomose divided vessels within 2 or 3 weeks.[28] The increased neovascularization also allows earlier ligation of the original vascular pedicle with complete tissue survival.[109,212] Growth factors have a short half-life and are more effective when delivered in a sustained release manner using a gelatin sponge.[110,263] The delay phenomenon does not work by an angiogenic mechanism, and attempts to increase survival of the random portion of a pedicled flap with fibroblast growth factors have had mixed results.[100,115,274] Growth factors may have their greatest clinical potential when a flap is transferred into an area of vascular compromise (e.g., irradiated soft tissue, diabetes, and steroid dependency).[109]

Rheology

In a homogeneous fluid that exhibits equal shear stress at different rates of shear, flow (Q) in a vessel can be approximated by Poiseuille's equation:

$$Q = \frac{\Delta P \cdot r^4 \cdot \pi}{1 \cdot 8 \cdot n}$$

where ΔP equals pressure gradient; r^4 equals the fourth power of the vessel radius; 1 equals vessel length; and n equals viscosity.[91] Although blood is a non-Newtonian fluid, the qualitative relationships in the equation remain. In larger vessels, the radius is a dominant factor, but in the capillary microcirculation, viscosity becomes more important. By decreasing the viscosity of blood, it may be possible to increase flow to the distal random portion of the acutely raised flap and beneficially affect flap survival. Viscosity is influenced by the hematocrit, serum proteins, temperature, erythrocyte deformability, aggregation, and other factors.[243] Each of these factors can be potentially manipulated with a resultant change in viscosity.

Hemodilution has been shown to decrease viscosity and have a beneficial effect on flap survival.[57,195,233] Reducing blood viscosity by protein depletion also results in increased flap survival in rats.[244]

Pentoxifylline and low viscosity whole blood substitutes (Fluosol-DA) will also lower viscosity. Pentoxifylline is a hemorrheologic agent that results in increased erythrocyte deformability[209] and decreased platelet aggregability.[243] When given 7 to 10 days before flap elevation, pentoxifylline improves flap survival.[243,294] Beneficial effects with limited preoperative dosing of pentoxifylline have not been uniform.[34,96,107,180,198] Fluosol-DA administration also has failed to consistently increase flap survival.[233,260]

Inflammation

The surgical trauma associated with an acutely raised or delayed flap results in an inflammatory response. This response results in a local increase in blood flow that could benefit flap survival. Improved flap blood flow and survival can occur with different methods of creating an inflammatory response before flap creation.[151,156] The beneficial effects of inflammation on flap survival also can be seen on a flap raised adjacent to a previously delayed flap.[119] Attempts to increase flap blood flow and survival with 5 days of low power laser burns have had mixed results.[126,260] These studies show that the inflammatory response has the potential to improve survival without sympathectomy or vascular division.

The mechanism by which inflammation produces a beneficial effect appears to involve the products of cyclooxygenase metabolism of arachidonic acid. Administration of PGI_2 results in dilation of the arterial pedicle and increased flap blood flow.[143] The result is increased flap survival.[59,238,248] Systemic administration of PGE_1 increases flap survival at low doses but can hinder flap survival at higher doses, causing hypotension.[266] Topical administration of PGE_1 also improves flap survival[252] but should be applied to the critical ischemic area to be effective.[253] Additional prostaglandin effects, such as increased erythrocyte deformity[152] and decreased platelet aggregation,[251] have been proposed as the mechanism of increased survival with prostaglandin administration.

Cyclooxygenase inhibitors such as indomethacin and ibuprofen have been shown to increase skin flap viability[240,248] and prolong tolerance of ischemia.[56] Glucocorticoids, which inhibit phospholipase activity, also have increased flap survival in some studies[147,176,177] but not in others.[194] Blocking TxA_2 synthesis has had mixed results.[127,208]

Tissue expansion

Tissue expansion has been shown to increase the size of the transferred flap in experimental animals and humans. Examination of expanded skin in the guinea pig has shown an increase in the thickness[14] and mitotic activity[73] of the epidermal layer, indicating epidermal proliferation. Blood flow in expanded tissue is greater than in skin overlying a noninflated expander 1 hour after creation of a pedicled flap.[164] The increase in blood flow to expanded skin seems to be short-lived.[80,239] Apart from the acute changes seen with expander manipulation, flap viability and blood flow in expanded skin appear to be similar to those seen in delayed flaps.[250]

Other

A number of drugs with multiple effects that should alter the blood flow to the flap have been tried with varying results. Ancrod, a defibrinogenating enzyme from the pit viper, has a selective affinity for fibrinogen and stimulates release of plasminogen activator with a resultant decrease in viscosity. The drug also causes increased endothelial generation of prostacyclin. When given postoperatively for 7 days, ancrod was unable to increase the viable surface area of porcine myocutaneous flaps.[182]

Chlorpromazine's effects include α-adrenergic blockade, stabilization of cell membranes, serotonin antagonism, metabolic depression, and cooling. All of these effects should be beneficial to the ischemic flap, but the results from experimental studies have been mixed.[12,25,108]

An interesting manipulation to increase survival of thin axial pattern skin flaps was proposed by Morrison and others.[186] In their study, the femoral artery and vein were implanted into the subdermal layer of skin in the rabbit model. After 8 to 12 weeks, sufficient neovascularization occurred to allow creation of a large skin flap based on the transferred pedicle. If confirmed in other laboratories, this technique may allow greater flexibility in the design of axial pattern flaps.

Prolonged viability

Protection against harmful agents

The formation of free radicals with reperfusion and the return of molecular oxygen to ischemic tissue places an increased burden on flap survival. Research has focused on decreasing the production of free radicals and using agents that remove free radicals (free radical scavengers) from the immediate environment.

Administration of allopurinol (a xanthine oxidase inhibitor) preoperatively prevents the increased xanthine oxidase activity seen with acute flap elevation.[290] Improved survival of dorsal rat flaps has been accomplished with allopurinol when given at high doses,[10,230] with lower doses having no effect.[228] The high doses required to obtain a beneficial effect have led to concern about the use of allopurinol to increase flap survival in the clinical setting.

A number of free radical scavengers are available to protect the tissues from destruction by free radicals. Superoxide dismutase (SOD), an intracellular free radical scavenger, catalyzes the conversion of superoxide to hydrogen peroxide (H_2O_2) and molecular oxygen. When given systemically, SOD is an effective scavenger of the superoxide radical regardless of its source.[171] SOD treatment has resulted in improved flap survival[74,182,298] and increased tolerance of flaps to ischemia.[169,246] Improved flap survival also has been shown with a number of other naturally occurring compounds with free radical scavenging properties. These include deferoxamine,[8] vitamin E, vitamin A, vitamin C, glutathione,[98] various amino acids,[216] and amino acid derivatives.[137]

The hydrogen peroxide formed by the dismutation of superoxide is not particularly harmful. In the presence of chelated metal complexes, hydrogen peroxide can be converted into a hydroxyl radical ($OH\cdot$).[50] The hydroxyl radical is much more reactive and may be responsible for much of the damage inflicted by oxygen free radicals.[97,262] The presence of a hematoma under a flap may decrease flap survival by increasing the available iron, which acts as a catalyst in the formation of free radicals.[9]

Hyperbaric oxygen

Improvement in flap survival with hyperbaric oxygen treatment has been documented,[129,222,225] but this has not been a consistent finding.[29] Hyperbaric oxygen treatment increases blood oxygen-carrying capacity by 20%.[129] This relative increase is greater with a low hematocrit because the additional oxygen is dissolved in the plasma rather than carried by hemoglobin. A greater effect of hyperbaric oxygen treatment may be increasing oxygen diffusion from surrounding perfused tissue to the ischemic portion of the flap.[46] Increased flap survival also occurs with treatments using hyperbaric air, showing that increased oxygen can be delivered with an increase in ambient pressure alone.[270]

The beneficial effect of hyperbaric oxygen in pedicled flaps includes decreased leukocyte adherence,[297] reduction of edema caused by vasoconstriction,[202] and neovascularization in irradiated tissue.[168] Animal studies have confirmed that it should be given early,[197] and one study suggested often.[222] There is little benefit from hyperbaric oxygen if the treatment is delayed by 24 hours or more after flap elevation.[123]

In a retrospective study of 65 patients with pedicled flaps that were determined by the surgeon to be in a high-risk group, hyperbaric oxygen was beneficial.[26] Although there is evidence that hyperbaric oxygen is effective for impaired flaps, it is not cost effective to treat every flap. Determining which flaps need treatment and which flaps will benefit is key. French investigators found that a hyperbaric oxygen challenge test (test dive) was predictive of successful outcome if the transcutaneous oxygen measurement rose 50 mm Hg or more. Still, the authors noted the need for further studies to determine indications for hyperbaric oxygen.[170]

Metabolic manipulation

Decreasing the metabolic requirements or increasing the metabolic reserves of skin are additional strategies for increasing flap survival. These approaches are based on the idea that flap necrosis occurs when tissue metabolic demand is greater than what the blood supply can deliver. Decreasing temperature is an effective way to reduce metabolic activity and delay necrotic changes, but improvement in flap survival is not seen.[79,136]

Administration of adenosine triphosphate-magnesium chloride complex was used to increase survival in the rat abdominal flap.[298] The metabolic support provided by this compound was believed to delay the onset of irreversible cell damage. Difluoromethylornithine (DFMO) was found to increase survival of abdominal flaps in rats.[224] DFMO appears to decrease metabolic demand by inhibiting the synthesis of polyamines, which are required for protein synthesis and cellular proliferation.

Increasing the individual cell's tolerance to ischemia also can be accomplished through stress conditioning. The production of heat-shock proteins can protect cells from a subsequent stress as long as an adequate recovery period (6 to 8 hours) from the initial stress occurs.[223] In an initial study, induction of heat-shock proteins resulted in improved flap survival.[145]

IMPAIRED FLAPS

In the majority of flaps, carefully designed and accomplished in healthy patients, flap survival is the rule, and methods improving survival or extensive monitoring or treatment of the flap are not warranted. The exceptions to the rule should be identified so extra efforts to ensure survival are reasonable and cost effective. Several risk factors place the patient in a higher risk category.

Smoking tobacco is associated with an increased chance of flap necrosis in facelift operations.[234] Exposure to tobacco smoke resulted in increased flap necrosis of dorsal flaps in rats[201] and hamsters.[39] The deleterious effects of nicotine appear to increase with prolonged exposure. The mechanism of tobacco or nicotine producing decreased flap survival is unknown but may involve direct endothelial damage, vasoconstriction caused by catecholamine release, or local concentrations of prostaglandins.[71] Long-term, low-dose nicotine (comparable with human smoking exposure) was used in a rat model[72] to document decreased capillary blood flow and survival—these effects could be avoided if the nicotine was withdrawn 2 weeks before raising the flap.

Radiation has been shown to be deleterious to flap survival in some studies[218,296] but not in others.[141,197,285] The reason for this discrepancy is probably because of differences in the radiation regimen administered (i.e., radiation dosage, fractionation, and surgical timing in respect to the radiation). Radiation treatment results in endarteritis obliterans and altered wound healing. Despite previous radiation, the delay phenomenon continues to improve flap survival.[64] Flap neovascularization is delayed but not eliminated after radiation. The use of angiogenic growth factors has the potential to increase the viability of irradiated skin flaps by means of accelerating revascularization.

The ischemia time occurring during the transfer of free flaps (called primary ischemia) appears to hinder the flap's ability to tolerate a second ischemic insult. The longer the period of perfusion after the microvascular anastomosis (called reperfusion period), the better a flap will tolerate secondary ischemia.[16] Porcine ventral arterial island flaps initially exposed to 2 hours of ischemia followed by 12 hours of blood flow had a 50% survival rate after a subsequent 7.2 hours of "secondary ischemia."[132] This is compared with 13 hours for the initial ischemic event needed to produce a 50% survival rate.[53]

Vascularity of the recipient bed is an important factor in free flaps. Experimentally, a pedicle can be divided at 6 days out,[35] and typically in clinical situations, the pedicle is no longer monitored after 1 week, although there are cases of late flap failure.[283] If the flap is placed into a bed with poor vascularity, dependence on the pedicle may be prolonged.

If there is late pedicle failure combined with a poor vascular bed in which neovascularization has not occurred, there could be an increased incidence of late complications.

Diabetes may be considered a risk factor because of the small vessel disease, although investigators did not find decreased flap survival in streptozotocin-induced diabetic rats. They did find slower endothelial growth at the anastomosis but concluded diabetes is not a contraindication to the use of a free flap.[37]

Ketamine and pentobarbital were found to decrease blood flow in the distal flap.[275] In a study on rats, older rats were found to have decreased tolerance to muscle ischemia than young rats, and this was assumed to be related to decreased mitochondrial function.[159] Fluid management also can have an impact on flap survival. Fluid overload will increase flap edema, and at the other extreme, intraoperative systemic hypotension has been shown to be detrimental.[256] Central venous pressure monitoring was not found to be helpful.[117] Other miscellaneous injuries documented in an isolated, perfused porcine flap include phototoxicity[181] and exposure to organic solvents.[138]

FLAP SALVAGE

Once a flap is identified as being at risk for necrosis, action can be taken to improve survival. Zone I manipulations are the most effective. In pedicled flaps, efforts to enhance zone I perfusion are limited to preoperative planning, flap execution and design, and surgical delay. If effectively executed, pedicled flap loss is a result of failure of zone II and III, which will develop slowly and involve the distal or random portion of the flap. Clinical efforts to improve zone II or III failure are limited to methods such as hyperbaric oxygen or leeching. Of the hundreds of pharmacologic agents that have been tested, none have gained widespread clinical use.

In contrast, the global ischemia of free flap failure often relates to a zone I failure—thrombosis or compression of the pedicle. This failure often is acute and relatively easy to detect and repair. If the zone I failure is not quickly resolved, the injury will progress to zone II and III.

Free flaps need intensive postoperative monitoring. There are several different methods of monitoring free flaps, but none are foolproof, and frequent observation by experienced personnel is still the gold standard. Pedicle failure can be determined early, and the flap can be salvaged by exploring the anastomosis and clearing the thrombus in many cases.

Because of the accessibility of the vessels and a short period of nonperfusion (primary ischemia), the question was raised whether washing out flap vessels could potentially improve survival in the event of secondary ischemia,[242] analogous to organ transplantation. University of Wisconsin solution has been used to effectively decrease perivascular swelling in the microvasculature of organ systems.[192] The solution has been used as a washout solution to improve survival in free flaps by Babajanian and others.[15,16]

An intriguing application of perfusion washout technology is extracorporeal circulation,[163] which investigators theorize could be used if there were no suitable donor site vessels. Extracorporeal circulation was studied in a flow-through venous free flap. Only a plasma solution was able to maintain viability over 3 days of extracorporeal infusion, although three other test perfusates caused massive edema and total obstruction to perfusion.

Perfusion washout also has been studied for its ability to improve survival after the thrombosis is cleared from the anastomotic site. University of Wisconsin solution caused greater improvement when used during secondary ischemia than during primary ischemia, indicating that it may be better for flap salvage than prophylaxis.[15] Urokinase has been used for the antithrombotic effects at the anastomosis and, because of microemboli, at the capillaries (zone II).[103] Intravascular heparin was not useful after thrombus formation.[158]

Medicinal leeches have been used clinically.[99] The leeches are thought to relieve microcirculatory congestion during active feeding and for several hours afterwards because of the antithrombotic effect of the leeches' salivary fluid. There is a risk of aeromonas infection. The "chemical leech"[283] and mechanical leeches have been described.[261] Relief of vascular congestion and edema also may be possible with microdialysis techniques, which have been used to reduce skin flap edema in a rat model.[207]

Hyperbaric oxygen has been used for free flap salvage. In a study of a rat epigastric free flap after 8 hours of global ischemia, hyperbaric oxygen increased survival and increased distal blood flow by laser Doppler.[297] In a similar model, hyperbaric oxygen inhibited the xanthine oxidase system and improved free flap survival after 18 hours of nonperfused storage.[269] Hyperbaric oxygen therapy will not be effective treatment unless the thrombosis has been cleared, but it may prolong viability and increase neovascularization.

SUMMARY

The blood flow required for nutritional support of the skin is dramatically less than what is available to carry out its thermoregulatory function, which allows skin to survive a compromise of its blood supply during creation of local flaps. The surviving length of a particular flap depends on the relationship between the proximal perfusion pressure (zone I) and the critical closing pressure of the arterioles, capillaries, and venules in the subdermal and subpapillary plexi (zone II). The interstitial space (zone III) is a critical link in this process. Cell viability (zone IV) is the ultimate determinate of flap survival. Appropriate flap design is the most critical factor in maintaining an adequate relationship between the zones of the circulatory system and avoiding tissue necrosis.

During the first 48 hours after raising a flap, the transferred tissue must survive a number of hazards. After the initial ischemia that all flaps undergo, reperfusion injury occurs by the formation of free radicals and other factors that can further damage tissue. An inflammatory response begins the process of wound healing but also may impair perfusion in zones II and III. Beyond the first few days, neovascularization and wound healing lessen the surviving flap's dependence on the pedicle.

Attempts to improve flap survival have involved improving flap design, altering the early physiologic impairment of blood flow, and increasing tissue resistance to ischemia. The most effective efforts to improve survival have been focused on zone I—surgical delay to decrease distal ischemia in pedicled flaps, and revision of a microvascular anastomosis to avoid global ischemia in free flaps. Treatment of zones II to IV includes pharmacologic manipulations designed to improve blood flow or increase tissue tolerance of ischemia—these treatments have not achieved sufficient and reproducible results required for incorporation into common clinical usage.

REFERENCES

1. Aarts HF: Regional intravascular sympathetic blockade for better results in flap surgery: an experimental study of free flaps, island flaps and pedicle flaps in the rabbit ear, *Plast Reconstr Surg* 66:690, 1980.
2. Acar C and others: Studies of controlled reperfusion after ischemia XIX: reperfusate composition: benefits of blood cardioplegia over Fluosol DA cardioplegia during regional reperfusion—importance of including blood components in the initial reperfusate, *J Thorac Surg* 101:248, 1991.
3. Amerbuch R, Kuban L, Sidley Y: Angiogenesis induction by tumors, embryonic tissues and lymphocytes, *Cancer Res* 36:3435, 1976.
4. Ames A and others: Cerebral ischemia. II: the no-reflow phenomenon, *Am J Pathol* 52:437, 1968.
5. Anden N, Carlsson A, Haggendal J: Adrenergic mechanisms, *Ann Rev Pharmacol* 9:119, 1969.
6. Angel MF and others: Biochemical analysis of the venous flap in the dog, *J Surg Res* 53:24, 1992.
7. Angel MF and others: A biochemical study of acute ischemia in rodent skin free flaps with and without prior elevation, *Ann Plast Surg* 26:419, 1991.
8. Angel M and others: Deferoxamine increases skin flap survival: additional evidence of free radical involvement in ischaemic flap surgery, *Br J Plast Surg* 39:469, 1986.
9. Angel M and others: The etiologic role of free radicals in hematoma-induced flap necrosis, *Plast Reconstr Surg* 77:795, 1986.
10. Angel M and others: Augmentation of skin flap survival with allopurinol, *Ann Plast Surg* 18:494, 1987.
11. Angel M and others: The critical relationship between free radicals and degrees of ischemia: evidence for tissue intolerance of marginal perfusion, *Plast Reconstr Surg* 81:233, 1988.
12. Angel MF and others: The beneficial effect of chlorpromazine on dorsal skin flap survival, *Ann Plast Surg* 23:492, 1989.
13. Ariyan S: The pectoralis major myocutaneous flap. A versatile flap for reconstruction in the head and neck area, *Plast Reconstr Surg* 63:73, 1979.
14. Austad E and others: Histomorphic evaluation of guinea pig skin and soft tissue after controlled tissue expansion, *Plast Reconstr Surg* 70:704, 1982.
15. Babajanian M and others: Prolongation of secondary critical ischemia time of experimental skin flaps using UW solution as a normothermic perfusate, *Otolaryngol Head Neck Surg* 108:149, 1993.
16. Babajanian M and others: Temporal factors affecting the secondary

critical ischemia of normothermic experimental skin flaps, *Arch Otolaryngol Head Neck Surg* 117:1360, 1991.

17. Babior B, Kipnes R, Curnutte J: Biological defense mechanisms: the production by leukocytes of superoxide, a potential bactericidal agent, *J Clin Invest* 52:741, 1973.

18. Baek S and others: Experimental studies in the survival of tenuous island flaps without arterial inflow, *Plast Reconstr Surg* 75:88, 1985.

19. Barker JH and others: Microcirculatory disturbances following the passage of emboli in an experimental free-flap model, *Plast Reconstr Surg* 90:95, 1992.

20. Barker JH and others: Direct monitoring of capillary perfusion following normovolemic hemodilution in an experimental skin-flap model, *Plast Reconstr Surg* 86:946, 1990.

21. Barker JH and others: Direct monitoring of nutritive blood flow in a failing skin flap: the hairless mouse ear skin-flap model, *Plast Reconstr Surg* 84:303, 1989.

22. Bartell TH, Mustoe TA: Animal models of human tissue expansion, *Plast Reconstr Surg* 83:681, 1989.

23. Bassingthwaighte JB: Discussion of Hjortdal VE, Hansen ES and others: The microcirculation of myocutaneous island flaps in pigs studied with radioactive blood volume tracers and microspheres of different sizes, *Plast Reconstr Surg* 89:116, 1992.

24. Bert JL, Pearce RH: The interstitium and microvascular exchange. In *Handbook of physiology*, 4, part 1, Bethesda, Md, 1984, American Physiologic Society.

25. Bibi R, Ferder M, Strauch B: Prevention of flap necrosis by chlorpromazine, *Plast Reconstr Surg* 77:954, 1986.

26. Bowersox J, Strauss MB, Hart GB: Clinical experience with hyperbaric oxygen therapy in the salvage of ischemic flaps and grafts, *J Hyperbar Med* 1:141, 1986.

27. Brace RA: Progress toward resolving the controversy of positive vs. negative interstitial fluid pressure, *Circ Res* 49(2):281, 1981.

28. Brown DM and others: Platelet-derived growth factor BB induces functional vascular anastomoses in vivo, *Proc Natl Acad Sci U S A* 92:5920, 1995.

29. Caffe H, Gallagher T: Experiments on the effects of hyperbaric oxygen on flap survival in the pig, *Plast Reconstr Surg* 81:954, 1988.

30. Callegari PR and others: An anatomic review of the delay phenomenon: I. experimental studies, *Plast Reconstr Surg* 89:397, 1992.

31. Campbell WB: *Lipid-derived autacoids: eicosanoids and platelet-activating factor*. In Gilman AG and others, editors: *Goodman and Gilman's the pharmacologic basis of therapeutics*, New York, 1990, Pergamon Press.

32. Chavoin J and others: Island flaps with an exclusively venous pedicle. A report of eleven cases and a preliminary haemodynamic study, *Br J Plast Surg* 40:149, 1987.

33. Chowdary R and others: Fluorocarbon enhancement of skin flap survival in rats, *Plast Reconstr Surg* 79:98, 1987.

34. Chu B, Deshmukh N: The lack of effect of pentoxifylline on random skin flap survival, *Plast Reconstr Surg* 83:315, 1989.

35. Clarke H, Chen G: Peripheral neovascularization of muscle and musculocutaneous flaps in the pig, *Plast Reconstr Surg* 89:109, 1992.

36. Cook TA: *Reconstruction of facial defects*. In Cummings CW, editor: *Otolaryngology—head and neck surgery*, St Louis, 1986, Mosby.

37. Cooley BC and others: The influence of diabetes on free flap transfer: I. flap survival and microvascular healing, *Ann Plast Surg* 29:58, 1992.

38. Cormack GC, Lamberty GH: A classification of fascio-cutaneous flaps according to their patterns of vascularization, *Br J Plast Surg* 37:80, 1984.

39. Craig S, Rees T: The effects of smoking on experimental skin flaps in hamsters, *Plast Reconstr Surg* 75:842, 1985.

40. Cummings C, Trachy R: Measurement of alternative blood flow in the porcine panniculus carnosus myocutaneous flap, *Arch Otolaryngol* 111:598, 1985.

41. Cummings C and others: Prognostication of myocutaneous flap viabil-

ity using laser doppler velocimetry and fluorescein microfluorometry, *Otolaryngol Head Neck Surg* 92:559, 1984.

42. Cutting C, Bardach J, Tinseth F: Haemodynamics of the delayed skin flap: a total blood flow study, *Br J Plast Surg* 34:133, 1981.

43. Cutting C and others: Changes in quantitative norepinephrine levels in delayed pig flank flaps, *Plast Reconstr Surg* 69:652, 1982.

44. Cutting CA: Critical closing and perfusion pressures in flap survival, *Ann Plast Surg* 9:524, 1982.

45. Cutting C, Robson M, Koss N: Denervation supersensitivity and the delay phenomenon, *Plast Reconstr Surg* 61:881, 1978.

46. Cutting C: *Skin flap physiology*. In Cummings CW, editor: *Otolaryngology—head and neck surgery*, St Louis, 1986, Mosby.

47. D'Amore PA: *The role of growth factors and cell-cell communication in the control of angiogenesis*. In Cederholm-Williams SA, Ryan TJ, Lydon MJ, editors: *Fibrinolysis and angiogenesis in wound healing*, Princeton, NJ, 1987, Excerpta Medica.

48. Daniel RK: *The anatomy and hemodynamics of the cutaneous circulation and their influence on skin flap design*. In Grabb WC, Myers MB, editors: *Skin flaps*, Boston, 1975, Little, Brown.

49. Daniel RK, Kerrigan CL: *Principles and physiology of skin flap surgery*. In McCarthy JG, editor: *Plastic surgery*, vol 1, Philadelphia, 1990, WB Saunders.

50. Del Mastro R: An approach to free radicals in medicine and biology, *Acta Physiol Scand Suppl* 492:153, 1980.

51. Denneny J and others: Flourescein elimination as a measure of island flap perfusion, *Otolaryngol Head Neck Surg* 95:200, 1986.

52. Dickson M, Sharpe D: Continuous subcutaneous tissue pH measurement as a monitor of blood flow in skin flaps: an experimental study, *Br J Plast Surg* 38:39, 1985.

53. Dohar J, Goding G, Azarshin K: The effects of inhalation anesthetic agents on survival in a pig random skin flap model, *Arch Otolaryngol* 118:37, 1992.

54. Donovan WE: *Experimental models in skin flap research*. In Grabb WC, Myers MB, editors: *Skin flaps*, Boston, 1975, Little, Brown.

55. Dorion D, Boyd J: Augmentation of transmidline skin perfusion and viability in transverse rectus abdominis myocutaneous (TRAM) flaps in the pig, *Plast Reconstr Surg* 88:642, 1991.

56. Douglas B and others: Beneficial effects of ibuprofen on experimental microvascular free flaps: pharmacologic alteration of the no-reflow phenomenon, *Plast Reconstr Surg* 79:366, 1987.

57. Earle A, Fratianne R, Nunez F: The relationship of hematocrit levels to skin flap survival in the dog, *Plast Reconstr Surg* 54:341, 1974.

58. Ehrly A: Improvement of the flow properties of blood: a new therapeutic approach in occlusive arterial disease, *Angiology* 27:188, 1976.

59. Emerson D, Sykes P: The effect of prostacyclin on the experimental random skin flap in the rat, *Br J Plast Surg* 34:264, 1981.

60. Eshima I, Mathes SJ, Paty P: Comparison of the intracellular bacterial killing activity of leukocytes in musculocutaneous and random-pattern flaps, *Plast Reconstr Surg* 86:541, 1990.

61. Federman JL and others: Experimental ocular angiogenesis, *Am J Ophthalmol* 89:231, 1980.

62. Finseth F, Adelberg MG: Prevention of skin flap necrosis by a course of treatment with vasodilator drugs, *Plast Reconstr Surg* 61:738, 1978.

63. Finseth F, Zimmerman J: Prevention of necrosis in island myocutaneous flaps in the pig by treatment with isoxsuprine, *Plast Reconstr Surg* 64:536, 1979.

64. Fisher J and others: The effect of delay on flap survival in an irradiated field, *Plast Reconstr Surg* 73:99, 1984.

65. Fischer J, Parker P, Shaw W: Laser doppler flowmeter measurements of skin perfusion changes associated with arterial and venous compromise in the cutaneous island flap, *Microsurgery* 6:238, 1985.

66. Fishman RA: Brain edema, *N Engl J Med* 292:706, 1975.

67. Flores J and others: The role of cell swelling in ischemic renal damage and the protective effect of hypertonic solute, *J Clin Invest* 51:118, 1972.

68. Folkman J: How is blood vessel growth regulated in normal and neoplastic tissue? *Cancer Res* 46:467, 1986.

69. Folkow B: Role of the nervous system in the control of vascular tone, *Circulation* 21:760, 1960.

70. Forrest C, Pang C: Latissimus dorsi musculocutaneous flap model in the rabbit: a hemodynamic and anatomical study, *Ann Plast Surg* 21:335, 1988.

71. Forrest C, Pang C, Lindsay W: Dose and time effects of nicotine treatment on the capillary blood flow and viability of random pattern skin flaps in the rat, *Br J Plast Surg* 40:295, 1987.

72. Forrest CR and others: Pathogenesis of ischemic necrosis in random-pattern skin flaps induced by long-term nicotine treatment in the rat, *Plast Reconstr Surg* 87:518, 1991.

73. Francis A, Marks R: Skin stretching and epidermopoiesis, *Br J Exp Pathol* 58:35, 1977.

74. Freeman TJ and others: Inhibition of endogenous superoxide dismutase with diethyldithiocarbamate in acute island skin flaps, *Otolaryngol Head Neck Surg* 103:938, 1990.

75. Furcht LT: Critical factors controlling angiogenesis: cell products, cell matrix, and growth factors, *Lab Invest* 55:505, 1986.

76. Gaskell P, Krisman AM: Critical closing pressure of vessels supplying the capillary loops of the nail fold, *Circ Res* 7:461, 1958.

77. Gatti J and others: Assessment of neovascularization and timing of flap division, *Plast Reconstr Surg* 73:396, 1984.

78. Gencosmanoglu R and others: Mechanisms of viability in rabbit flank venous flaps, *Ann Plast Surg* 30:60, 1993.

79. Goding G, Cummings C, Bright D: *Effects of local hypothermia on the porcine myocutaneous flap.* In Stucker FJ, editor: *Plastic and reconstructive surgery of the head and neck, proceedings of the fifth international symposium,* Philadelphia, 1991, BC Decker.

80. Goding G, Cummings C, Trachy R: Tissue expansion and cutaneous blood flow, *Laryngoscope* 98:1, 1988.

81. Goshen J, Wexler M, Peled I: The use of two alpha blocking agents, phenoxybenzamine and phentolamine, in ointment and injection form to improve skin flap survival in rats, *Ann Plast Surg* 15:431, 1985.

82. Gospodarowicz D, Thakoral KK: Production of a corpus luteum angiogenic factor responsible for the proliferation of capillaries and revascularization of the corpus luteum, *Proc Natl Acad Sci U S A* 75:874, 1978.

83. Gottrup F and others: The dynamic properties of tissue oxygen tension in healing flaps, *Surgery* 95:527, 1983.

84. Gottrup F and others: A comparative study of skin blood flow in musculocutaneous and random-pattern flaps, *J Surg Res* 37:443, 1984.

85. Grange H, Goodman A, Grange N: Role of resistance and exchange vessels in local microvascular control of skeletal muscle oxygenation in the dog, *Circ Res* 38:379, 1976.

86. Greene N: Physiology of sympathetic denervation, *Ann Rev Med* 13:87, 1962.

87. Gross JE. Friedman JD: Monitoring, *Orthop Clin North Am* 24(3):531, 1993.

88. Guba A: Study of the delay phenomenon in axial pattern flaps in pigs, *Plast Reconstr Surg* 63:550, 1979.

89. Guyton A, Hall J: *The body fluid compartments: extracellular and intracellular fluids: interstitial fluid and edema.* In *Textbook of medical physiology,* ed 9, Philadelphia, 1996, WB Saunders.

90. Guyton A, Hall J: *Local control of blood flow by the tissues, and humoral regulation.* In *Textbook of medical physiology,* ed 9, Philadelphia, 1996, WB Saunders.

91. Guyton A, Hall J: *Overview of the circulation: medical physics of pressure, flow, and resistance.* In *Textbook of medical physiology,* ed 9, Philadelphia, 1996, WB Saunders.

92. Guyton AC, Schell K, Murphres D: Interstitial fluid pressure: III. its effect on resistance to tissue fluid mobility, *Circ Res* 19:412, 1966.

93. Hammond DC and others: The dorsal skin-flap model in the rat: factors influencing survival, *Plast Reconstr Surg* 91:316, 1993.

94. Hannington-Kiff J: Intravenous regional sympathetic block with guanethidine, *Lancet* 1:1019, 1974.

95. Hargens AR: *Introduction and historical perspectives.* In Hargens AR, editor: *Tissue fluid pressure and composition,* Baltimore, 1971, Williams & Wilkins.

96. Hauben D, Aijlstra F: Prostacyclin formation in delayed pig flank flaps, *Ann Plast Surg* 13:304, 1984.

97. Hayden R and others: The effect of hydroxyl radical scavenging on acute axial-random skin flap survival, *Laryngoscope* 98:106, 1988.

98. Hayden R and others: The effect of glutathione and vitamins A, C, and E on acute skin flap survival, *Laryngoscope* 97:1176, 1987.

99. Hayden RE, Pillips JG, McLear PW: Leeches. Objective monitoring of altered perfusion in congested flaps, *Arch Otolarynol Head Neck Surg* 114:1395, 1988.

100. Hayward PG and others: Local infiltration of an angiogenic growth factor does not stimulate the delay phenomenon, *Br J Plast Surg* 44:526, 1991.

101. Heden P, Jurell G, Arnander C: Prediction of skin flap necrosis: a comparative study between laser doppler flowmetry and fluorescein test in a rat model, *Ann Plast Surg* 17:485, 1986.

102. Henrich DE and others: The influence of arterial insufficiency and venous congestion on composite graft survival, *Laryngoscope* 105:565, 1995.

103. Hirigoyen MB and others: Improved efficacy of urokinase further prolongs ischemic skin-flap survival, *J Reconstr Microsurg* 11:151, 1995.

104. Hjortdal VE and others: Differential release of endothelin in myocutaneous island flaps in response to gradually insetting venous stasis or arterial ischemia, *Metabolism* 43:1201, 1994.

105. Hjortdal VE and others: Tissue oxygen tension in myocutaneous flaps, *Eur J Surg* 157:307, 1991.

106. Hochberg J and others: Development and evaluation of an in vivo mouse model for studying myocutaneous flap microcirculation and viability before and after suturing or stapling, *Int J Microcirc* 14:67, 1994.

107. Hodgson R, Brummett R, Cook T: Effects of pentoxifylline on experimental skin flap survival, *Arch Otolaryngol Head Neck Surg* 113:950, 1987.

108. Hoft HD and others: Can chlorpromazine prevent flap necrosis? *Br J Plast Surg* 43:587, 1990.

109. Hom D, Assefa G: Effects of endothelial cell growth factor on vascular compromised skin flaps, *Arch Otolaryngol Head Neck Surg* 118:624, 1992.

110. Hom D and others: Utilizing angiogenic agents to expedite the neovascularization process in skin flaps, *Laryngoscope* 98:521, 1988.

111. Huffman H and others: An endothelial growth stimulating factor from salivary glands, *Exp Cell Res* L02:269, 1976.

112. IIannotti Y, Crowell RM, Klato I: Brain tissue in focal cerebral ischemia, *J Neurosurg* 62:83, 1975.

113. Im MJ and others: Effects of sympathetic denervation and oxygen free radicals on neovascularization in skin flaps, *Plast Reconstr Surg* 92:736, 1993.

114. Im M and others: Effect of allopurinol on the survival of hyperemic island skin flaps, *Plast Reconstr Surg* 73:276, 1984.

115. Ishiguro N and others: Basic fibroblast growth factor has a beneficial effect on the viability of random skin flaps in rats, *Ann Plast Surg* 32:356, 1994.

116. Jakubovic HR, Ackerman AB: *Structure and function of skin.* In Moschella SL, Hurley HJ, editors: *Dermatology,* Philadelphia, 1992, WB Saunders.

117. Jensen NF and others: The efficacy of routine central venous monitoring in major head and neck surgery: a retrospective review, *J Clin Anesth* 7:119, 1995.

118. Johnson P, Barker J: Thrombosis and antithrombotic therapy in microvascular surgery, *Clin Plast Surg* 19:799, 1992.

119. Jonsson K and others: Tissue oxygen measurements in delayed skin

flaps: a reconsideration of the mechanisms of the delay phenomenon, *Plast Reconstr Surg* 82:328, 1988.

120. Junqueira LC, Carneiro J, Kelley RO: *Basic histology*, ed 8, Norwalk, Conn, 1995, Appleton & Lange.

121. Jurell G: Adrenergic nerves and the delay phenomenon, *Ann Plast Surg* 17:497, 1986.

122. Jurell G, Jonsson CE: Increased survival of experimental skin flaps in rats following treatment with antiadrenergic drugs, *Scand J Plast Reconstr Surg* 10:169, 1976.

123. Jurell G, Kaijser L: The influence of varying pressure and duration of treatment with hyperbaric oxygen on the survival of skin flaps: an experimental study, *Scand J Plast Reconstr Surg* 7:25, 1973.

124. Jurell G, Norberg K, Palmer B: Surgical denervation of the cutaneous blood vessels, *Acta Physiol Scand* 74:511, 1968.

125. Kaley G and others: *Role of prostaglandins in microcirculatory function*. In Neri GG and others, editors: *Advances in prostaglandin, thromboxane, and leukotriene research*, New York, 1985, Raven Press.

126. Kami T and others: Effects of low-power diode lasers on flap survival, *Ann Plast Surg* 14:278, 1985.

127. Kay S, Green C: The effect of a novel thromboxane synthetase inhibitor dazegrel (UK38485) on random pattern skin flaps in the rat, *Br J Plast Surg* 39:361, 1986.

128. Kennedy TJ, Pistone G, Miller SH: The effect of reserpine on microcirculatory flow in rat flaps, *Plast Reconstr Surg* 63:101, 1979.

129. Kernahan D, Zingg W, Kay C: The effects of hyperbaric oxygen on the survival of experimental skin flaps, *Plast Reconstr Surg* 36:19, 1965.

130. Kerrigan C, Daniel R: Critical ischemia time and the failing skin flap, *Plast Reconstr Surg* 69:986, 1982.

131. Kerrigan C, Daniel R: Pharmacologic treatment of the failing skin flap, *Plast Reconstr Surg* 70:541, 1982.

132. Kerrigan C, Daniel R: Skin flap research: a candid view, *Plast Reconstr Surg* 13:383, 1984.

133. Kerrigan CL: Skin flap failure: pathophysiology, *Plast Reconstr Surg* 72:766, 1983.

134. Kerrigan C, Zelt R, Daniel R: Secondary critical ischemia time of experimental skin flaps, *Plast Reconstr Surg* 74:522, 1984.

135. Kerrigan C and others: The pig as an experimental animal in plastic surgery research for the study of skin flaps, myocutaneous flaps and fasciocutaneous flaps, *Lab Animal Sci* 36:408, 1986.

136. Kiehn C, Desprez J: Effects of local hypothermia on pedicle flap tissue, *Plast Reconstr Surg* 25:349, 1960.

137. Kim YS, Im MJ, Hoopes JE: The effect of a free-radical scavenger, N-2-mercaptopropionylglycine, on the survival of skin flaps, *Ann Plast Surg* 25:18, 1990.

138. King JR, Monteiro-Riviere NA: Effects of organic solvent vehicles on the viability and morphology of isolated perfused porcine skin, *Toxicology* 69:11, 1994.

139. Kjartansson J, Dalsgaard C: Calcitonin gene related peptide increases survival of a musculocutaneous critical flap in the rat, *Eur J Pharmacol* 142:355, 1987.

140. Kjartansson J, Dalsgaard C, Jonsson C: Decreased survival of experimental critical flaps in rats after sensory denervation with capsaicin, *Plast Reconstr Surg* 79:218, 1987.

141. Kleiman LA and others: The effects of carbocisplatin and radiation on skin flap survival, *Arch Otolaryngol Head Neck Surg* 118:68, 1992.

142. Klingenstrom P, Nylen B: Timing of transfer of tubed pedicles and cross flaps, *Plast Reconstr Surg* 37:1, 1966.

143. Knight K and others: Pharmacologic modification of blood flow in the rabbit microvasculature with prostacyclin and related drugs, *Plast Reconstr Surg* 75:692, 1985.

144. Knox LK and others: Nitric oxide synthase inhibitors improve skin flap survival in the rat, *Microsurgery* 15:708, 1994.

145. Koenig WJ and others: Improving acute skin-flap survival through stress conditioning using heat shock and recovery, *Plast Reconstr Surg* 90:659, 1992.

146. Kreidstein ML and others: Evidence of endothelium-dependent and endothelium-independent vasodilation in human skin flaps, *Can J Physiol Pharmacol* 70:1208, 1992.

147. Kristensen J, Wadskov S, Henriksen O: Dose-dependent effect of topical corticosteroids on blood flow in human cutaneous tissue, *Acta Derm Venereol* 58:145, 1978.

148. Kutchai HC: Cellular membranes and transmembrane transport of solutes and water. In Berne RM, Levy MN, editors: *Physiology*, St Louis, 1988, Mosby.

149. Landis E: Microinjection studies of capillary permeability, *Am J Physiol* 82:217, 1927.

150. Lasiter W, Gottschalk C: *Volume and composition of the body fluids*. In Mountcastle VB, editor: *Medical physiology*, St Louis, 1980, CV Mosby.

151. Lawrence W and others: Prostanoid derivatives in experimental flap delay with formic acid, *Br J Plast Surg* 37:602, 1984.

152. Layton CT and others: Pharmacologic enhancement of random skin flap survival by prostaglandin E2, *Arch Otolaryngol Head Neck Surg* 120:56, 1994.

153. Leaf A: Cell swelling: a factor in ischemic tissue injury, *Circulation* 47:455, 1973.

154. Leak LV, Burke JF: *Early events of tissue injury and the role of the lymphatic system in early inflammation*. In Zweifach, Grant, McCluskey, editors: *The inflammatory process*, ed 2, New York, 1974, Academic Press.

155. Lee C, Kerrigan CL, Picard-Ami LA: Cyclophosphamide-induced neutropenia: effect on postischemic skin-flap survival, *Plast Reconstr Surg* 89:1092, 1992.

156. Liston S: Nonbacterial inflammation as a means of enhancing skin flap survival, *Laryngoscope* 94:1075, 1984.

157. Liu A, Cummings C, Trachy R: Venous outflow obstruct in myocutaneous flaps: changes in microcirculation detected by the perfusion fluorometer and laser doppler, *Otolaryngol Head Neck Surg* 94:164, 1986.

158. Li X and others: Intravascular heparin protects muscle flaps from ischemia/reperfusion injury, *Microsurgery* 16:90, 1995.

159. Lu X and others: Effect of age upon ischemia/reperfusion injury in rat muscle free flaps, *J Surg Res* 55:193, 1993.

160. Macht S, Frazier W: The role of endogenous bacterial flora in skin flap survival, *Plast Reconstr Surg* 65:50, 1980.

161. Maciag T and others: An endothelial cell growth factor, *Proc Natl Acad Sci* 76:5674, 1979.

162. Macknight ADC: *Cellular response to injury*. In Staub NC, Taylor AE, editors: *Edema*, New York, 1984, Raven Press.

163. Maeda M and others: Extracorporeal circulation for tissue transplantation (in the case of venous flaps), *Plast Reconstr Surg* 91:113, 1993.

164. Marks M and others: Enhanced capillary blood flow in rapidly expanded random pattern flaps, *J Trauma* 26:913, 1986.

165. Marks N, Trachy R, Cummings C: Dynamic variation in blood flow as measured by laser doppler velocimetry: a study in rat skin flaps, *Plast Reconstr Surg* 73:804, 1984.

166. Matsushita K and others: Blood flow and tissue survival in the rabbit venous flap, *Plast Reconstr Surg* 91:127, 1993.

167. May JW Jr, Chait LA, O'Brien BM: The no-reflow phenomenon in experimental free flaps, *Plast Reconstr Surg* 61:256, 1978.

168. Marx RE: A new concept in the treatment of osteoradionecrosis, *J Oral Maxilliofac Surg* 41:351, 1983.

169. Marzella L and others: Functional and structural evaluation of the vasculature of skin flaps after ischemia and reperfusion, *Plast Reconstr Surg* 81:742, 1988.

170. Mathieu DR and others: Pedicle musculocutaneous flap transplantation: prediction of final outcome by transcutaneous oxygen measurements in hyperbaric oxygen, *Plast Reconstr Surg* 91:329, 1993.

171. McCord J: Improved survival of island flaps after prolonged ischemia

by perfusion with superoxide dismutase, discussion, *Plast Reconstr Surg* 77:643, 1986.

172. McCord J: Oxygen-derived free radicals in postischemic tissue injury, *N Engl J Med* 312:159, 1985.

173. McFarlane RM, DeYoung G, Henry RA: The design of a pedicle flap in the rat to study necrosis and its prevention, *Plast Reconstr Surg* 35:177, 1965.

174. Meldon JH, Garby L: The blood oxygen transport system, *Acta Med Can Suppl* 19:19, 1975.

175. Mellander S, Johansson B: Control of resistance, exchange, and capacitance functions in the peripheral circulation, *Pharmacol Rev* 20:117, 1968.

176. Mendelson B, Woods J: Effect of corticosteroids on the surviving length of skin flaps in pigs, *Br J Plast Surg* 31:293, 1978.

177. Mes L: Improving flap survival by sustained cell metabolism within ischemic cells: a study using rabbits, *Plast Reconstr Surg* 65:56, 1980.

178. Michel CC: *Fluid movements through capillary walls*. In *Handbook of physiology*, part 1 Bethesda, Md, 1984, American Physiologic Society.

179. Milton S: Fallacy of the length-width ratio, *Br J Plast Surg* 57:502, 1971.

180. Monteiro D, Santamore W, Nemir P: The influence of pentoxifylline on skin-flap survival, *Plast Reconstr Surg* 77:277, 1986.

181. Monteiro-Riviere NA and others: Development and characterization of a novel skin model for cutaneous phototoxicology, *Photodermal Photoimmunal Photomed* 10:235, 1994.

182. Moore G, Cummings C: The effect of ancrod on perfusion of myocutaneous flaps, *Arch Otolaryngol Head Neck Surg* 114:1175, 1988.

183. Moore GK, Trachy RE, Cummings CW: The effect of alpha-adrenergic stimulation and blockade on perfusion of myocutaneous flaps, *Otolaryngol Head Neck Surg* 94:489, 1986.

184. Moore KL, Persaud TVN: *The developing human*, Philadelphia, 1993, WB Saunders.

185. Moran CG and others: Preservation of bone graft vascularity with the University of Wisconsin cold storage solution, *J Orthop Res* 11:840, 1993.

186. Morrison WA and others: Prefabrication of thin transferable axial-pattern skin flaps: an experimental study in rabbits, *Br J Plast Surg* 43:645, 1990.

187. Mulliken J, Im M: The etiologic role of free radicals in hematoma-induced flap necrosis—discussion, *Plast Reconstr Surg* 77:802, 1986.

188. Murphy R and others: Surgical delay and arachidonic acid metabolites: evidence for an inflammatory mechanism: an experimental study in rats, *Br J Plast Surg* 38:272, 1985.

189. Myers B: Understanding flap necrosis, *Plast Reconstr Surg* 78:813, 1986 (editorial).

190. Myers MB: *Attempts to augment survival in skin flaps—mechanism of the delay phenomenon*. In Grabb WC, Myers MB, editors: *Skin flaps*, Boston, 1975, Little, Brown.

191. Myers MB, Cherry G: Enhancement of survival in devascularized pedicles by the use of phenoxybenzamine, *Plast Reconstr Surg* 41:254, 1968.

192. Naka Y and others: Canine heart-lung transplantation after twenty-four-hour hypothermic preservation with Belzer-UW solution, *J Heart Lung Transplant* 10:296, 1991.

193. Nakano J: *General pharmacology of prostaglandins*. In Cuthbert MF, editor: *The prostaglandins*, Philadelphia, 1973, JB Lippincott.

194. Nakatsuka T and others: Effect of glucocorticoid treatment on skin capillary blood flow and viability in cutaneous and myocutaneous flaps in the pig, *Plast Reconstr Surg* 76:374, 1985.

195. Neilsen R, Parkin J: Skin flap survival: influence of infection, anemia and tubing, *Arch Otolaryngol* 102:727, 1976.

196. Neligan P and others: Pharmacologic action of isoxsuprine in cutaneous and myocutaneous flaps, *Plast Reconstr Surg* 75:363, 1985.

197. Nemiroff P and others: Effects of hyperbaric oxygen and irradiation on experimental skin flaps in rats, *Otolaryngol Head Neck Surg* 93:485, 1985.

198. Nemiroff P: Synergistic effects of Pentoxifylline and hyperbaric oxygen on skin flaps, *Arch Otolaryngol Head Neck Surg* 114:977, 1988.

199. Nichter L, Sobieski M, Edgerton M: Efficacy of topical nitroglycerin for random-pattern skin-flap salvage, *Plast Reconstr Surg* 75:847, 1985.

200. Nieto C and others: Survival of myocutaneous flaps, *Arch Otolaryngol* 111:43, 1985.

201. Nolan J and others: The acute effects of cigarette smoke exposure on experimental skin flaps, *Plast Reconstr Surg* 75:544, 1985.

202. Nylander G and others: Reduction of postischemic edema with hyperbaric oxygen, *Plast Reconstr Surg* 76:596, 1985.

203. Odland RM, Cohen JI: Measurement of interstitial tissue compliance in skin flaps, *Arch Otolaryngol Head Neck Surg* 114:1276, 1988.

204. Odland R and others: Fluorescein and acidosis: implications for flap perfusion studies, *Arch Otolaryngol Head Neck Surg* 110:712, 1992.

205. Odland R, Rice R: A comparison of tunable dye and KTP lasers in nonsurgical delay in cutaneous flaps, *Otolaryngol Head Neck Surg* 113:92, 1995.

206. Odland R and others: Use of the tunable dye laser to delay McFarlane skin flaps, *Arch Otolaryngol Head Neck Surg* 121:1158, 1995.

207. Odland R and others: Reduction of tissue edema by microdialysis, *Arch Otolaryngol Head Neck Surg* 121:662, 1995.

208. Ono I and others: A study on the effectiveness of a thromboxane synthetase inhibitor (OKY-046) in increasing survival length of skin flaps, *Plast Reconstr Surg* 86:1164, 1990.

209. Palmer B: Sympathetic denervation and reinnervation of cutaneous blood vessels following surgery, *Scand J Plast Reconstr Surg* 4:93, 1970.

210. Pang C and others: Augmentation of blood flow in delayed random skin flaps in the pig: effect of length of delay period and angiogenesis, *Plast Reconstr Surg* 78:68, 1986.

211. Pang CY and others: Hemodynamics and vascular sensitivity to circulating norepinephrine in normal skin and delayed and acute random skin flaps in the pig, *Plast Reconstr Surg* 78:75, 1986.

212. Pang C and others: Assessment of the fluorescein dye test for prediction of skin flap viability in pigs, *J Surg Res* 41:173, 1986.

213. Pang C, Neligan P, Nakatsuka T: Assessment of microsphere technique for measurement of capillary blood flow in random skin flaps in pigs, *Plast Reconstr Surg* 74:513, 1984.

214. Pang C and others: Pharmacologic manipulation of the microcirculation in cutaneous and myocutaneous flaps in pigs, *Clin Plast Surg* 12:173, 1985.

215. Pang CY: Ischemia-induced reperfusion injury in muscle flaps: pathogenesis and major source of free radicals, *Reconstr Microsurg* 6:77, 1990.

216. Paniello R, Hayden R, Bello S: Improved survival of acute skin flaps with amino acids as free radical scavengers, *Arch Otolaryngol Head Neck Surg* 114:1400, 1988.

217. Parsons RJ, McMaster PD: The effect of the pulse upon the formation and flow of lymph, *J Exp Med* 68:353, 1938.

218. Patterson T and others: *The effect of radiation in survival of experimental skin flaps*. In Grabb WC, Myers MB, editors: *Skin flaps*, Boston, 1975, Little, Brown.

219. Pearl JM and others: Leukocyte-depleted reperfusion of transplanted human hearts prevents ultrastructural evidence of reperfusion injury, *J Surg Res* 52:298, 1992.

220. Pearl R: The delay phenomenon—why the fuss, *Ann Plast Surg* 13:307, 1984.

221. Pearl R: A unifying theory of the delay phenomenon—recovery from the hyperadrenergic state, *Ann Plast Surg* 7:102, 1981.

222. Pellitteri PK, Kennedy TL, Youn BA: The influence of intensive hyperbaric oxygen therapy on skin flap survival in a swine model, *Arch Otolaryngol Head Neck Surg* 118:1050, 1992.

223. Perdrizet GA and others: Stress conditioning, a novel approach to organ preservation, *Curr Surg* 46:23, 1989.

224. Perona BP and others: Acute diflurоromethylornithine treatment increases skin flap survival in rats, *Ann Plast Surg* 25:26, 1990.

225. Perrins D: *The effect of hyperbaric oxygen on ischemic skin flaps.* In Grabb W, Myers MB, editors: *Skin flaps,* Boston, 1975, Little, Brown.

226. Phillips J, Hayden R, McLear P: Real time multivariable laser doppler analysis of arterial and venous compromise, *Am J Otolaryngol* 10: 26, 1989.

227. Picard-Ami LA, Kerrigan CL: Pathophysiology of ischemic skin flaps: difference in xanthineoxidase levels between rat, pig and man, *Plast Reconstr Surg* 87:750, 1991.

228. Picard-Ami LA, MacKay A, Kerrigan CL: Effect of allopurinol on the survival of experimental pig flaps, *Plast Reconstr Surg* 89:1098, 1992.

229. Pober JS, Cotran RS: The role of endothelial cells in inflammation, *Transplantation* 50:537, 1990.

230. Pokorny A, Bright D, Cummings C: The effects of allopurinol and superoxide dismutase in a rat model of skin flap necrosis, *Arch Otolaryngol Head Neck Surg* 115:207, 1989.

231. Post S and others: Effects of Carolina rinse and adenosine rinse on microvascular perfusion and intrahepatic leukocyte-endothelium interaction after liver transplantation in the rat, *Transplantation* 55:972, 1993.

232. Price MA, Pearl RM: Multiagent pharmacotherapy to enhance skin flap survival: lack of additive effect of nitroglycerin and allopurinol, *Ann Plast Surg* 33:52, 1994.

233. Ramasastry S and others: Effect of fluosol-DA (20%) on skin flap survival in rats, *Ann Plast Surg* 15:436, 1985.

234. Rees T, Liverett D, Guy C: The effect of cigarette smoking on skin flap survival in the face lift patient, *Plast Reconstr Surg* 73:911, 1984.

235. Reinisch JF: The pathophysiology of skin flap circulation: the delay phenomenon, *Plast Reconstr Surg* 54:585, 1974.

236. Reneman RS and others: Muscle blood flow disturbances produced by simultaneously elevated venous pressure and total muscle pressure, *Microvasc Res* 20:307, 1980.

237. Renkin EM: *Control of microcirculation and blood-tissue exchange.* In *Handbook of physiology,* part 2, Bethesda, Md, 1984, American Physiologic Society.

238. Reus W and others: Effect of intraarterial prostacyclin on survival of skin flaps in the pig: biphasic response, *Ann Plast Surg* 13:29, 1984.

239. Ricciardeli E and others: Acute blood flow changes in rapidly expanded and adjacent skin, *Arch Otolaryngol Head Neck Surg* 115: 182, 1989.

240. Robson M, DelBeccaro E, Heggers J: The effects of prostaglandins on the dermal microcirculation after burning and the inhibition of the effect by specific pharmacological agents, *Plast Reconstr Surg* 63: 781, 1979.

241. Rohrich R, Cherry G, Spira M: Enhancement of skin-flap survival using nitroglycerin ointment, *Plast Reconstr Surg* 73:943, 1984.

242. Rosen HM, Slivjak BS, McBrearty FX: Preischemic flap washout and its effect on the no-reflow phenomenon, *Plast Reconstr Surg* 76:737, 1985.

243. Roth A and others: Augmentation of skin flap survival by parenteral pentoxifylline, *Br J Plast Surg* 41:515, 1988.

244. Ruberg RL, Falcone RE: Effect of protein depletion the surviving length in experimental skin flaps, *Plast Reconstr Surg* 61:581, 1978.

245. Saetzler R and others: Visualization of nutritive perfusion following tourniquet ischemia in arterial pattern skin flaps: effect of vasoactive medication, *Plast Reconstr Surg* 94:652, 1994.

246. Sagi A and others: Improved survival of island flaps after prolonged ischemia by perfusion with superoxide dismutase, *Plast Reconstr Surg* 77:639, 1986.

247. Sasa M and others: Survival and blood flow evaluation of canine venous flaps, *Plast Reconstr Surg* 82:319, 1988.

248. Sasaki G, Pang C: Experimental evidence for involvement of prosta-

glandins in viability of acute skin flaps: effects on viability and mode of action, *Plast Reconstr Surg* 67:335, 1981.

249. Sasaki G, Pang C: Hemodynamics and viability of acute neurovascular island skin flaps in rats, *Plast Reconstr Surg* 65:152, 1980.

250. Sasaki G, Pang C: Pathophysiology of skin flaps raised on expanded pig skin, *Plast Reconstr Surg* 74:59, 1984.

251. Sawada Y, Hatayama I, Sone K: The effect of continuous topical application of heparin on flap survival, *Br J Plast Surg* 45:515, 1992.

252. Sawada Y and others: A study of topical and systemic prostaglandin E1 and survival of experimental skin flaps, *Br J Plast Surg* 46:670, 1993.

253. Sawada Y and others: The relationship between prostaglandin E1 applied area and flap survival rate, *Br J Plast Surg* 45:465, 1992.

254. Schmie-Schonbein GW: Capillary plugging by granulocytes and the no-reflow phenomenon in the microcirculation, *Fed Proc* 46:2397, 1987.

255. Sherman J: Normal arteriovenous anastomoses, *Medicine* 42:247, 1963.

256. Sigurdsson GH: Perioperative fluid management in microvascular surgery, *J Reconstr Microsurg* 11:57, 1995.

257. Silverman D and others: Comparative assessment of blood flow to canine island flaps, *Arch Otolaryngol Head Neck Surg* 111:677, 1985.

258. Sloan G, Sasaki G: Noninvasive monitoring of tissue viability, *Clin Plast Surg* 12:185, 1985.

259. Smahel J: *The healing of skin grafts.* In Montandon D, editor: *Clinics in plastic surgery,* Philadelphia, 1977, WB Saunders.

260. Smith RJ and others: The effect of low-energy laser on skin-flap survival in the rat and porcine animal models, *Plast Reconstr Surg* 89:306, 1992.

261. Smoot EC and others: Mechanical leech therapy to relieve venous congestion, *J Reconstr Microsurg* 11:51, 1995.

262. Southorn P, Powis D: Free radicals in medicine. I. Chemical nature and biologic reactions, *Mayo Clin Proc* 63:381, 1988.

263. Stepnick DW and others: Effects of tumor necrosis factor alpha and vascular permeability factor on neovascularization of the rabbit ear flap, *Arch Otolaryngol Head Neck Surg* 121:667, 1995.

264. Strock PE, Majno G: Microvascular changes in acutely ischemic rat muscle, *Surg Gynecol Obstet* 1213, 1969.

265. Su CT and others: Tissue glucose and lactate following vascular occlusion in island skin flaps, *Plast Reconstr Surg* 70:202, 1982.

266. Suzuki S and others: Effect of intravenous prostaglandin E1 on experimental flaps, *Ann Plast Surg* 19:49, 1987.

267. Suzuki S and others: Experimental study on "delay" phenomenon in relation to flap width and ischemia, *Br J Plast Surg* 41:389, 1988.

268. Svensson H and others: Detecting changes of arterial and venous blood flow in flaps, *Ann Plast Surg* 15:35, 1985.

269. Tai YJ and others: The use of hyperbaric oxygen for preservation of free flaps, *Ann Plast Surg* 28:284, 1992.

270. Tan C and others: Effect of hyperbaric oxygen and hyperbaric air on survival of island skin flaps, *Plast Reconstr Surg* 73:27, 1984.

271. Taylor G and others: An anatomic review of the delay phenomenon: II. Clinical applications, *Plast Reconstr Surg* 89:408, 1992.

272. Thomson J, Kerrigan C: Dermofluorometry: thresholds for predicting flap survival, *Plast Reconstr Surg* 83:859, 1989.

273. Tsur H, Daniller A, Strauch B: Neovascularization of skin flaps: route and timing, *Plast Reconstr Surg* 66:85, 1980.

274. Uhl E and others: Improvement of skin perfusion by subdermal injection of recombinant human basic fibroblast growth factor, *Ann Plastic Surg* 32:361, 1994.

275. Uhl E and others: Influence of ketamine and pentobarbital on microvascular perfusion in normal skin and skin flaps, *Int J Microcirc* 14: 308, 1994.

276. Verlander E: Vascular changes in a tubed pedicle. 5: an experimental study, *Acta Chir Scand Suppl* 322:1, 1964.

277. Warner K and others: Comparative response of muscle and subcutane-

ous tissue pH during arterial and venous occlusion in musculocutaneous flaps, *Ann Plast Surg* 22:108, 1989.

278. Waterhouse N and others: Observations on dermal blood flow as reflected by technetium-99m pertechnetate clearance, *Br J Plast Surg* 39:312, 1986.

279. Webster JP: Thoraco-epigastric tubed pedicles, *Surg Clin North Am* 17:145, 1937.

280. Weinberg H, Song Y, Douglas B: Enhancement of blood flow in experimental microvascular free flaps, *Microsurg* 6:121, 1985.

281. Weinberg H and others: Vascular island skin-flap tolerance to warm ischaemia: an analysis by perfusion fluorometry, *Plast Reconstr Surg* 73:949, 1984.

282. Weinberg H: Survival and blood flow evaluation of canine venous flaps—discussion, *Plast Reconstr Surg* 82:326, 1988.

283. Weinzweig N, Gonzalez M: Free tissue failure is not an all-or-none phenomenon, *Plast Reconstr Surg* 96:648, 1995.

284. Weis SJ: Tissue destruction by neutrophils, *N Engl J Med* 320:365, 1989.

285. Weisman R and others: Fluorometric assessment of skin flap viability in the rat: effect of radiation therapy, *Otolaryngol Head Neck Surg* 91:151, 1983.

286. West JB: *Best and Taylor's physiological basis of medical practice*, ed 12, Baltimore, 1991, Williams & Wilkins.

287. Westin M, Heden P: Calcitonin gene-related peptide delays the no-reflow phenomenon in the rat island flap, *Ann Plast Surg* 21:329, 1988.

288. Wexler MR and others: The effect of phenoxybenzamine, phentol-amine, and 6-hydroxydopamine on skin flap survival in rats, *J Surg Res* 19:83, 1975.

289. Wideman M, Tuma R, Mayorvitz H: Defining the precapillary sphincter, *Microvasc Res* 12:71, 1976.

290. Wilkins EG and others: Identification of xanthine oxidase activity following reperfusion in human tissue, *Ann Plast Surg* 31:60, 1993.

291. Willms-Kretschmer K, Manjo G: Ischemia of the skin, *Am J Pathol* 54:327, 1969.

292. Wood MB: Discussion of Clarke H, Chen G: peripheral neovascularization of muscle and musculocutaneous flaps in the pig, *Plast Reconstr Surg* 89:109, 1992.

293. Wray R, Young V: Drug treatment and flap survival, *Plast Reconstr Surg* 73:939, 1984.

294. Yessenow R, Maves M: The effects of pentoxifylline on random skin flap survival, *Arch Otolaryngol Head Neck Surg* 115:179, 1989.

295. Young C, Hopewell W: The evaluation of an isotope clearance technique in the dermis of pig skin: a correlation of functional and morphological parameters, *Microvasc Res* 20:182, 1980.

296. Young CMA, Hopewell JW: The effects of preoperative x-irradiation on the survival and blood flow of pedicle skin flaps in the pig, *Int J Radiation Oncology Biol Phys* 9:865, 1983.

297. Zamboni WA and others: The effect of hyperbaric oxygen on reperfusion of ischemic axial skin flaps: a laser doppler analysis, *Ann Plast Surg* 23:339, 1992.

298. Zimmerman T, Sasaki G, Khattab S: Improved ischemic island skin flap survival with continuous intraarterial infusion of adenosine triphosphate-magnesium chloride and SOD: a rat model, *Ann Plast Surg* 18:218, 1987.

Chapter 9

Free Tissue Transfer

Bruce H. Haughey
Ewain P. Wilson

Free tissue transfer is a technique whereby tissue units, either homogenous or composite, are completely separated from their blood supply and transported from one part of the body to another for reconstruction. Restoration of blood supply by vascular anastomosis at the recipient site is performed with magnification (usually a microscope), may have an associated nerve anastomosis, and has been performed on most parts of the body, i.e., cranium and scalp, head and neck, trunk, extremities, and within the thoracic, abdominal, and pelvic cavities. The technique has been applied extensively to reconstruction of head and neck defects, resulting from elective neoplastic surgical resections and from congenital, traumatic, inflammatory, thermal, and radiation-related tissue loss.

The unique advantages of this technique include immediate delivery of well-vascularized tissue to the recipient site in a single stage, with the potential for rapid wound healing, sealing of critical compartments, such as the subarachnoid space or aerodigestive tract, and efficient restoration of functions, such as mastication and swallowing. Reconstruction of contour and external tissue endows major cosmetic restoration.

This chapter will cover general aspects of the technique as it relates to reconstruction of the head, neck, face, and upper aerodigestive tract.

HISTORY

In 1907, Carrel[15] reported experimental free transfer of bowel for reconstruction of an esophageal defect in dogs, preceded by orthotopic replantation experiments. Seidenberg and others in 1959[106] reported replacement of a cervical esophageal defect with a free jejunal segment using small vessel anastomosis in a canine series and a human case. Hiebert and Cummings[46] reported transfer of a gastric antrum segment for pharyngoesophageal reconstruction in 1961. Thus the concept of autotransplantation with restoration of blood supply by anastomosis of small vessels had become a clinical reality, but until magnification with an operating microscope[90] had been applied to small vessels,[51] the technique was hampered by inaccurate anastomosis. Development of small-scale, atraumatic needles and a knowledge of the vascular territories of the body also were needed.

Credit for the first clinical transfer of skin flaps is difficult to assign because it depends on whether precedence is given to actual surgery dates or publication dates, but it has been contended by Liu and Kumar[73] that the first such successful operation was a flap transferred by Antia and Buch in 1966, reported in 1971.[5] This was a free abdominal dermofat groin flap based on the superficial epigastric artery and the saphenous vein. Other early transfer reported were those by McLean and Buncke in 1972[81] (free omentum transfer to scalp) and by Daniel and Taylor in 1973,[21] in which a free groin flap based on the superficial inferior epigastric was transferred to the leg. Kaplan and others[54] also reported on a free groin flap used for oral cavity reconstruction in 1973, and Harii and others[39] described distant transfer of free deltopectoral flaps in 1974. Panje and others[93] from the University of Iowa were the first otolaryngologists to publish a study on free tissue transfer for oral cavity reconstruction.

The next phase saw a rapid escalation in anatomic studies, especially those using cadaver dissection, injection, or radiography to define independent vascular territories, which could be used as donor sites. This was accompanied by a more refined demonstration of how musculocutaneous blood is supplied to the body surface, with axial vessels underlying major muscles being shown to send musculocutaneous perforators through the muscle for supply of the overlying skin and subcutaneous tissue. Soon after, fasciocutaneous units, especially those on the limbs, also were clearly defined. An important anatomic concept, espoused by Taylor,[125] was the presence of 40 angiosomes and corresponding venosomes, which, when adjacent, may have anastomotic connections between intramuscular vascular networks (Fig. 9-1). An angiosome is that anatomic territory that relies on blood supply from a segmental vessel and spans the superficial to deep plane between skin and underlying bone. The thickness of encompassed tissue is variable, and the anastomotic connec-

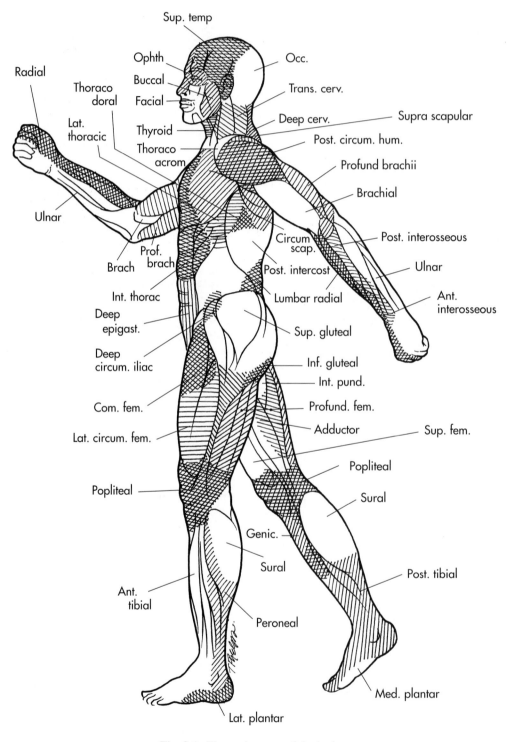

Fig. 9-1. The angiosomes of the body.

tions between adjacent angiosomes may either be true dissectable anastomoses or reduced caliber, retiform anastomoses ("choke" connections). Importantly, it was this knowledge that allowed a unit of vascularized soft tissue, bone, nerve, and tendon to be reliably transferred on a specific vascular pedicle. All or part of the tissue in the adjacent angiosome also can usually be incorporated in the flap, vascularized by retiform anastomoses.[125] Bone transfer was found to be particularly germane in the management of segmental mandibular defects because healing at the osteosynthesis sites was rapid and secure, contouring osteotomies were feasible, and the bone tolerated plating, screwing, and osseointegrated implant insertion with or without postoperative radiation. This has led to near-ideal conditions for reconstruction of the mandible, even in patients with bone defects that communicate with the mouth, facial skin, or both.

Clinical practice of free tissue transfer is now a routine part of the head and neck surgery program in modern medical centers. However, the technique remains a major logistical undertaking, and because each of the many steps contributes to a successful outcome, intense concentration on details is critical.

INDICATIONS FOR FREE TISSUE TRANSFER

The indications for free tissue transfer are derived from a balanced assessment of the advantages (Box 9-1) and disadvantages of the technique. The latter include lengthy operations, donor site morbidity, and relatively high cost. These factors are weighed against other reconstructive alternatives for managing a particular head and neck defect. Such alternatives include no reconstruction, primary closures, skin grafts, local flaps, regional and pedicle flaps from the trunk, or prosthetic appliances. There are currently reconstructive situations where the free flap is the procedure of choice, and the use of, for example, a pedicled flap for a major defect is controversial. Table 9-1 lists defects in the head and neck wherein free tissue transfer is a highly appropriate method of reconstruction, along with possible donor sites.

Box 9-1. Relative advantages of free flaps compared with pedicled flaps in head and neck reconstruction

Portability
Simultaneous harvest option
Donor sites abundant, although often hidden
Composite tissue abundant
Bulk adjustment, matched with recipient site
Vascularity in a radiated or scarred recipient site
Pliability and maneuverability for accurate inset
Motor and sensory innervation options
Functional recovery potential, e.g., mastication

Although in many patients free tissue transfer offers an improvement over formerly used techniques, this modality has not solved all the problems of reconstruction. Free flaps share some of the disadvantages of pedicled flaps because both techniques involve the repair of a defect with tissue that by definition is different from the original. Donor site morbidity also is an intrinsic disadvantage of both techniques. No currently used flap is absolutely ideal, but the desirable characteristics of a free flap are listed in Box 9-2. Different authorities may have varying preferences for reconstructing individual defects and may have valid reasons for disagreeing with the choices of these authors.

Among the general, logistic indications for free flaps are the availability of hospital facilities with appropriate personnel, equipment, and space for intraoperative and postopera-

Table 9-1. Defects suitable for reconstruction with free flaps and appropriate choices of donor sites

Defect	Donor site
Pharyngoesophagus with or without neck skin	Radial forearm fasciocutaneous Lateral thigh cutaneous Jejunum
Mandible	Fibula Iliac crest Scapula Radius
Oromandibular composite (bone, mucosa, and/or skin)	Fibular osteocutaneous Scapular osteocutaneous Iliac crest osseomyocutaneous Radial forearm osteofasciocutaneous
Tongue with motile component remaining	Radial forearm (sensory) innervated Lateral arm innervated Ulnar forearm innervated
Tongue, total	Latissimus dorsi motor innervated Tensor fascia lata motor and sensory innervated Rectus abdominus (noninnervated) Lateral thigh
Lip or cheek full thickness, total	Radial forearm, 180° folded with tendon
Skull base, dura exposed or grafted	Rectus abdominis Radial forearm fascial
Temporal bone or lateral skull	Rectus abdominis myocutaneous Latissimus dorsi myocutaneous Radial forearm
Scalp or skull vertex	Rectus abdominis myocutaneous Latissimus dorsi myocutaneous Omentum
Midface, palate composite	Radial forearm osteofasciocutaneous Serratus anterior rib osseomyocutaneous Scapular osteocutaneous Rectus abdominis myocutaneous
Nose, total	Radius osteocutaneous
Skin defect, large	Latissimus dorsi, perforator based Rectus abdominis, perforator based Radial forearm fasciocutaneous Lateral arm fasciocutaneous

---

> **Box 9-2.** Characteristics of "ideal" free flaps for head and neck reconstruction
>
> Donor site previously unviolated
> Bulk and color matched to defect
> Composition of tissue similar to defect
> Harvest expeditious, dry, simultaneous
> Supine position of patient maintained intraoperatively
> Length and caliber of vessels adequate
> Innervation with sensory or motor nerves feasible
> Functional recovery of resected structure(s) facilitated
> Cosmetic potential excellent
> Donor site morbidity minimal

---

tive phases. In addition, trained rehabilitation experts who have an understanding of the specific techniques and pertinent problems associated with free tissue transfer are necessary.

PATIENT SELECTION

General patient factors that affect selection of candidates for free tissue transfer include comorbidity, performance status, social habits and circumstances, and the patient's preferences.

Comorbid disease conditions have the potential for complicating any or all phases of management, but they are especially relevant in assessing candidacy for a prolonged anesthetic. If correctable conditions are noted preoperatively, management can be instituted or intensified to minimize their effects. Patients with renal insufficiency, cardiac failure or ischemic heart disease, and hepatic insufficiency need to be appropriately evaluated for anesthesia risk. Close liaison needs to be maintained with anesthesia staff and the internal medical services to determine the risks and benefits of undergoing major surgery, especially considering perioperative fluid management.

Advanced age

Several studies suggest that age *per se* does not constitute a contraindication to free tissue transfer.[4,16,109] However, elderly patients are somewhat more likely to have comorbidities, thereby increasing the risks.

Diabetes

Diabetic patients in general can be expected to have a higher incidence of postsurgical infection, as well as to have a greater degree of pedicle and recipient vessel atherosclerosis. These issues are not serious enough to exclude diabetic patients from free tissue transfer,[18] but diabetic patients need to be monitored closely for neck wound infection, which would threaten the microvascular pedicle.

Arterial factors

Atherosclerosis

Atherosclerotic vessels may be narrowed or occluded and contain plaques that add to the technical difficulty of anastomosis. For example, the peroneal artery is commonly diseased near its origin, whereas the circumflex scapular and subscapular vessels are seldom affected. These problems should be anticipated in patients with known hypertension and diabetes.

Arteritis

The presence of a collagen vascular disease may be a relative contraindication to microvascular procedures.[120] The authors have performed successful procedures on patients with such a condition, but patients and surgeons should be aware of the higher potential for complications related to the arteritis and a history of steroid use.

Hypertension

Arteries in patients with long-standing hypertension are more likely to undergo vasospasm, thickening of the media, or perianastomic rupture. It is important that hypertension be controlled perioperatively, in case weak areas (created by dissection or clumping) rupture the arterial pedicle.

Hematologic disorders

Sickle cell sufferers are known to be hyperthrombotic, and this condition is a relative contraindication to free flap surgery.[101] Hemophilia and polycythemia vera also are relative contraindications to microvascular procedures.[4]

Smoking

Studies have confirmed the vasoconstrictive effects of nicotine and the adverse effects of smoking on wound healing.[100,127] Everything possible should be done to dissuade patients from smoking or from using other nicotine-containing products before surgery.

Medications

Patients on steroids can be expected to have delayed wound healing.[4] Caution also should be exercised when operating on patients taking aspirin or coumadin because therapeutic levels of anticoagulation predispose to hematoma accumulation in the early postoperative period.

Previous irradiation

Recipient vessels that have been radiated may be thickened by endarteritis obliterans, making the microvascular anastomosis technically more difficult. In addition, the intima is frequently roughened, irregular, and replete with pedunculated fragments, which float into the lumen. These findings are not necessarily associated with an increased risk of morbidity or thrombosis.[37] Baker[7] has nevertheless suggested that previous irradiation, when taken with other adverse factors and because of irreversible vascular fibrosis and intimal proliferation,[8] may tip the balance toward failure of the flap. Radiation also will delay wound healing at the periphery of the flap as a result of recipient bed fibrosis.

SURGICAL PLANNING AND ANESTHESIA MANAGEMENT

The usual principles of good anesthesia management apply to free flap surgery as they do to other types of surgery. There are certain unique factors that need to be considered. The surgery is typically lengthy, and the anesthesiologist will have difficulty achieving access to the patient once the procedure is underway. Keeping a patient warm is a problem, especially during surgical prepping and securing intravenous lines and monitoring cables. Changes in the position of the patient are sometimes necessary during the procedure, and the anesthesiologist should be able to accommodate this safely. Intubation and the securing of the airway require careful attention, with special care during tracheotomy to avoid exposing or damaging the anterior jugular venous system. Central hemodynamic monitoring is important, with, at the least, measurement of the central venous pressure being advocated.[128] Patients with a history of cardiorespiratory instability should be considered for placement of a Swan-Ganz catheter. Finally, placement of pneumatic hose is important, although it may not be possible to do this bilaterally because of the need for access to the donor site.

The following physiologic parameters have been emphasized by several authors.[50,74,104,111,128]

Cardiac output and perfusion pressure

No absolute pulse pressure values for optimal free tissue transfer have been proven, but empirically, a systolic arterial pressure of 100 mm Hg or more should be maintained.[74] This is to maintain blood flow in the flap according to the Pouseille-Hagen law. Achievement of this goal involves limitation of the use of myocardial depressants, maintenance of hydration, judicious use of cardiac afterload reduction, and avoidance of histamine-releasing agents.[111] Pressors should be avoided unless they are absolutely necessary for life-threatening hypotension because many of them cause intense peripheral vasoconstriction. Denervated flaps also are thought to be hypersensitive to circulating catecholamines.

Hemodilution

Hemodilution improves blood flow to the flap by viscosity reduction, and oxygen delivery to the tissues is increased down to a hematocrit of 30% through a compensatory increase in the cardiac output.[83] It is considered preferable by some to achieve this through slight overhydration and to maintain the central venous pressure at about 2 mm Hg above baseline.[74,111]

Normothermia

Decreased body temperature results in peripheral vasoconstriction.[38] It is therefore important to warm the patient,

use warm infused fluids, and maintain the temperature in the operating room at around 24° to 25° C.

Normocapnia

Overventilation should be avoided because hypocapnia is known to result in peripheral vasoconstriction.[128] The use of a carbon dioxide monitor is essential.

Fluid balance

Sigurdsson[111] has asserted, "The present state of knowledge favors the use of colloids rather than large volumes of isotonic crystalloids for plasma substitution." Apart from the systemic risks of overhydration, flap and recipient site edema should be avoided because they will create difficulties in insetting and have the potential for compromising perfusion. Crystalloids should be used for the correction of preoperative dehydration and for the replacement of insensible losses.[36,65] Colloids should be used to restore volume to the point where the hematocrit indicates that the administration of packed erythrocytes is necessary.

There is debate as to the best colloid to use. Synthetic preparations may be preferable because of their lower expense and the lower risk of disease transmission.[9] Low molecular weight dextran has several desirable characteristics, including antithrombotic properties, but it may cause anaphylaxis, and because of the potential for bleeding, the daily dosage of dextran should be limited to 1.5 g/kg.[83] Hetastarch also may result in allergic reactions and may have effects on hemostasis.[118] The medium molecular weight agent, pentastarch, may have several advantages, including fewer adverse reactions, desirable blood flow characteristics by inhibition of rouleaux formation,[74] and effective volume expansion.[111,118]

Once blood loss and hemodilution have resulted in a hematocrit below 25%, transfusion with packed erythrocytes should be considered.

The ideal inhalational combination will result in modest vasodilation without marked reduction of cardiac output.[111] The drugs of choice presently are isoflurane and nitrous oxide.[26] Fentanyl is a good choice of analgesic, and vecuronium currently is considered the best nondepolarizing muscle relaxant by Sigurdsson[111] because of its minimal histamine-releasing and sympatholytic effects.

DONOR SITE CHOICE AND FLAP HARVEST

The variety of donor sites offering different tissue components for head and neck reconstruction has afforded surgeons the luxury of choosing a flap that is well tailored to meet the needs of the recipient site. Flaps and their available tissue components commonly used in head and neck reconstruction are listed in Table 9-2. It is not only the presence of specific donor tissue or a structure that determines choice but also the quality and quantity of that tissue. For example, if an innervated skin flap with minimal bulk is required for pharyngeal wall reconstruction, the radial forearm flap may be

Table 9-2. Tissue components available for commonly used donor sites in head and neck reconstruction

Flap	Skin	Bone	Muscle	Fascia	Sensory nerve	Motor nerve	Tendon	Mucosa
Radial forearm	+ +	+	+	+	+ (LABCN, MABCN)		+	
Fibula	+ +	+ +	+		+			
Rectus abdominis	+ +		+ +	+				
Iliac crest	+	+	+					
Lateral arm	+ +	+			+			
Lateral thigh	+ +		+	+	+ (LCNT)			
Latissimus dorsi	+ +	+ (Rib)	+ +			+		
Gracilis	+		+			+		
Scapula	+ +	+						
Serratus	+	+ (Rib)	+ +			+		
Jejunum								+
Gastroomentum								+
Colon								+

+ + Denotes large amount available.

ideal. If less bulk is available on that patient's forearm than is required for sensate tongue base reconstruction, the lateral thigh or lateral arm may be preferable. There are tissue variations from patient to patient on the same donor site, necessitating careful review of the patient and his or her potential sites. Quality and quantity of bone for osteotomies and implants may be a determining factor in choice of donor site for mandibular reconstruction.[33]

Intraoperative factors in donor site choice should include potential for blood loss and ease of access for simultaneous harvest and resection. Flaps harvested from the limbs, e.g., fibula, usually can be obtained during tourniquet control, thus minimizing hemorrhage. The iliac crest, by contrast, creates a relatively sanguineous harvest.

Simultaneous harvest of the flap with the head and neck resection can save considerable time, although it requires an accurate knowledge of the likely size, shape, and missing components of the defect to be reconstructed. If surgery is two-teamed, combined preoperative planning and precise communication about the proposed resection is optimal. For example, in the authors' hands, the decision to use a sensate, folded radial forearm flap versus a motor-innervated latissimus dorsi flap for tongue reconstruction is determined by the presence or absence, after the glossectomy, of a viable, motor-innervated, contracting tongue remnant. If the latter is present and confirmed by nerve stimulation, the authors usually will choose the sensate forearm flap option. If absent, the motor-innervated latissimus musculocutaneous flap may endow a superior functional result. Such a decision is a watershed in preoperative judgment and intraoperative case management because the forearm flap is harvested simultaneously with the patient in the supine position, whereas the latissimus necessitates a shoulder up or even lateral decubitus position.

Another critical factor in choice of donor site is the potential for morbidity. Although rare and unlikely, immediate morbidity may result, such as peritoneal or gastrointestinal tract perforations, when harvesting rectus or iliac crest flaps, or peripheral nerve injuries, when harvesting flaps from the limbs. Intermediate and late effects, such as speed of resumption of walking after harvest of fibular versus iliac flaps may be determinant. Donor site morbidity tends to be downplayed by surgeons and, to some extent, by patients in the context of major head and neck malignancies, trauma, or deformities. Symptoms usually can be elicited if sought, but in a survey of 20 of the authors' patients after free flap reconstruction, they noticed that the impact of those symptoms on quality of life had usually become minimal 6 to 12 months after surgery.

RECIPIENT SITE PREPARATION

Recipient site preparation is a vital phase of head and neck free tissue transfer. It seeks to provide appropriate placement of skin incisions, suitable surfaces for coaptation and healing to the donor tissue, a high quality set of recipient vessels, and a layout that avoids kinking, twisting, or compression of the pedicle.

In simultaneous, combined ablative and reconstructive procedures, conditions set by the oncologic resection create the initial operative defect to be reconstructed. The ablative team therefore should have a clear knowledge of factors that are critical for the reconstructive effort. Placement of neck incisions, for example, should avoid three point junctions or vertical limbs running along the course of the great vessels or external jugular vein. Postoperative breakdown of skin at these sites, especially in previously radiated necks, may leave the pedicle, especially the venous component, exposed. If pedicles must lie beneath neck incisions, it is best to have the axis of the incision perpendicular to the axis of the pedicle or to cover the pedicle with vascularized soft tissue. If a neck dissection is performed, the ablative team should use gentle handling of potential recipient arteries and veins, be willing to use microvascular clamps rather than the hemostat "crush and tie" technique, adopt simple pledget pressure for venotomies and arteriotomies on small vessels (rather than attempting to hand tie or cauterize), and know to avoid monopolar electrocautery. Monopolar electrical stimulation of vessels causes depolarization of the existing charge across the vessel wall, and mechanical vessel injury during ablation also contributes to excessive platelet–fibrin clot accumulation, endangering any anastomosis performed on the injured vessel.

When the resection field is available for assessment, the reconstructive team evaluates the dimensions, location, and missing structures of the defect; ensures that cancer margins are clear by frozen section analysis; trims mucosal or skin margins with cold steel instruments to optimize healing; and evaluates the potential recipient arteries, veins, and nerves. The harvest is hopefully sufficiently advanced at this stage to have measurements of the donor vessel diameters and an idea of flap pedicle length available. Recipient vessels are chosen with the latter variables in mind, aiming for a good match of vessel diameters, wall thickness, and wound contour, which will allow a favorable lie for the pedicle. Another common point of judgment is whether, after a modified neck dissection, there is a stump on the internal jugular vein that is long enough to clamp and anastomose versus an end-to-side jugular anastomosis.

The authors next perform sufficient, naked-eye dissection and mobilization of arteries and veins to allow them to lie without tension on a clean, moist sponge for subsequent microdissection. The operating microscope then is brought to the field for vessel trimming, dilation, heparin flushing, and adventitial stripping in preparation for the anastomosis. The reader is referred to a manual of microvascular surgery[2] for a description of the relevant techniques.

MICROVASCULAR AND MICRONEURAL TECHNIQUE

Exhaustive detail of microsurgical technique is beyond the scope of this chapter, but the standard texts are available.[2,7,122] In this section, the tools and skills necessary for the microsurgical aspects of free tissue transfer will be reviewed and the basic procedure will be outlined.

Laboratory

Accurate microsurgical technique requires practice and patience, and the appropriate place to acquire the initial technical skills is in the microvascular laboratory. The rat model for such training has been well described.[2]

Equipment

The operating microscope is used by most surgeons for microsurgery. It offers magnification of ×10 to ×40 and has opposing binocular assemblies for simultaneous use by the surgeon and the assistant. The use of loupes is reviewed later in this chapter.

Instruments are of critical importance in microvascular surgery, and it is essential that they be gently used and well maintained. The minimum instrumentation required for good microsurgical practice includes jeweler's forceps, microbipolar cautery forceps, a microneedle holder, straight and curved microscissors, a vessel dilator, and atraumatic microvascular clamps. Sliding, cleated approximator clamps mounted on a tying frame also are useful and are routinely used by the authors. Nonabsorbable monofilament suture on an atraumatic needle is the standard, with a needle of 75 to 100 μm being appropriate for head and neck microvascular work. Suture sizes of 9-0 or 10-0 are typically used for vessel anastomoses, and 8-0 to 9-0 for neural anastomoses (epineural technique).

Preoperative planning

The details of the surgical procedure need to be delineated well in advance, with the individual steps being communicated to the medical, nursing, and anesthesia personnel involved. Care should be taken to ascertain that the appropriate equipment is available and in working order. The surgeon selects and prepares an alternative donor site in case the primary choice is not feasible. In addition, a surgical site for a pedicled flap, such as the pectoralis major, should be included in the draping of the patient in case microvascular techniques cannot be used. A centrous venous sheath for invasive hemodynamic monitoring may be placed the night before surgery to save operating room time. Preoperative hydration is helpful to avoid the blood pressure swings characteristic of general anesthesia in dehydrated patients. The need for blood transfusion should be expected in most patients, particularly when the resection is done at the same session.

Informed consent is of paramount importance, as with all surgical procedures. Explaining the multiplicity of surgical sites, each with their attendant possible complications, to patients requires time on the part of the surgical team.

Microvascular technique

Gentle, accurate microsurgical technique is extremely important. Essential to a successful anastomosis are the avoidance of tension at the anastomotic site and the minimization of twisting and kinking of the vessels. Once the anastomosis has been done, it is important to check for kinking of the vessels by turning the head to the neutral position.

A physiologic irrigating solution, such as balanced salt solution or Ringers lactate, should be mixed with heparin, at a ratio of 10:20 units/ml, which is then used to clean thrombus from within the lumen of the vessels. Vessel spasm, more of a potential problem in arterial repairs than in venous repairs because of the paucity of muscle in the vein wall, may be ameliorated by the use of lidocaine in concentrations of up to 20 mg%.[114] Papaverine also may be used.[114] Mechanical dilation with a vessel dilator is the most effective strategy to overcome spasm, but it is only applicable before anastomosis.

The most commonly performed and simplest type of anastomosis is the end-to-end technique. On occasion, this is not possible, and an end-to-side anastomosis should be performed. Everything possible should be done to harvest the flap with a pedicle that is long enough to reach the recipient vessels in the neck. On the rare occasions when this is not possible, either venous interposition grafts (to either or the artery and the vein) will be necessary or the proximal cephalic vein should be dissected out and turned over into the neck if the primary problem is insufficient venous length.

Arterial anastomosis

The adventitia of the donor and recipient vessels are trimmed under the microscope with curved scissors. This can be accomplished by dissection of the adventitia or by the ''circumcision'' technique, in which the adventitial sleeve is gently pulled over the end of the vessel and amputated with straight scissors. In most patients, it is advisable to trim the adventitia of the recipient vessel to its point of origin from its parent vessel because this minimizes twisting, facilitates draping, and, as is the case in irradiated fields, alleviates constriction. The edges of the donor and recipient vessels also are checked to make sure the cuts are clean and revised, if necessary, under the microscope. Copious irrigation is used to clear away blood clots, and the vessel ends are gently dilated. It is imperative to check for blood flow through the recipient vessels by releasing the arterial clamp before commencing anastomosis. If something less than a strong pulsatile flow from the end of the vessel is obtained, the artery should be dilated or resected a short distance, and the flow should be checked again. The two ends of the vessels to be anastomosed are then placed in an approximating frame, such as the Acland double-approximating frame. The vessel ends are approximated so that the repair is accomplished under no tension. A blue background is used, and it is helpful to surround the field with clean, moist sponges.

A variety of anastomotic techniques have been described. The classic technique and that most advisable for the beginning surgeon is the triangulation technique as described by Acland.[2] Two stay sutures are placed in the superficial wall of the vessels 120° apart and applied to the opposing cleats during straight tension. The anterior wall is then repaired, while the tension allows the deep wall to fall away from the needle and minimize the possibility of ''through'' stitching. The tips of the jeweler's forceps are gently introduced into the lumen of the first vessel to be penetrated by the needle to evert the vessel edge. The needle should be introduced perpendicularly and it is important to keep the needle tip in sight at all times. The whole vessel wall should not be grasped by the forceps, and direct contact with the endothelium should be minimized. The needle should penetrate the vessel wall approximately 1.5 to 2.0 needle diameters from the edge of the vessel, and three half knots should be thrown, taking care to make them square. Once the superficial wall is repaired, the frame is turned over. Another stay suture is placed through the opposite wall, 120° from each of the previously placed stay sutures, and left long enough to reach both cleats. This stitch is cleated, and the second row of sutures is placed. The stay suture is removed from the cleat and taken across to the opposing cleat, whereby the final segment of vessel wall is presented for suturing. After completion of the anastomosis, the approximating frame is removed, but the proximal arterial clamps are left in place. An alternative technique of arterial anastomosis is to use a continuous technique, which is better suited to vessels that do not have a major size mismatch, and has the advantage of being quicker. This technique is less forgiving than the interrupted technique and is best reserved for the more advanced surgeon, especially in venous anastomosis. The lumen is narrowed slightly, so this technique also is best reserved for those whose vessels are greater than 1 mm in diameter. The surgeon is now ready to complete the venous anastomosis.

The end-to-side technique is useful to have in the surgeon's armamentarium, although it is not necessary in the majority of head and neck cases. It is needed when there are no suitable side branches from the external carotid system, when the only venous recipient vessel is a large caliber vein such as the internal jugular, or when there is a size mismatch between vessels of more than approximately 3 to 1.[126] After the vessel has been clamped, the adventitia is trimmed as usual around the proposed anastomotic site, and an arteriotomy is made. The arteriotomy is made very slightly larger than the caliber of the flap vessel, and it is useful to place a stay suture through the wall of the recipient vessel at the site of the arteriotomy to assist with stabilization. It also is important to angle the entry of the flap vessel into the recipient vessel to minimize turbulence.[123]

Venous anastomosis

Venous anastomosis is more difficult than arterial anastomosis because the vein walls are thinner, resulting in collapse and infolding of the walls after the vessel has been transected. The low-flow state of the blood also makes it more likely to thrombose. Adventitial trimming should be conservative and done with great care because the potential for inadvertent venotomy is high. The principles of anastomosis are the same for the venous repair as for the arterial repair, but the dangers of including the back wall of the vessel in a suture are higher, as is the possibility of suturing a fold in the vessel wall rather than the end of the vessel and misidentifying adventitia as the vessel media. It is helpful to place the initial stay sutures under irrigating fluid because this allows the vessel walls to float apart, opening the lumen. The suture interval required may be larger than in arterial repairs because of the low pressure venous blood, but because the vein caliber usually is larger, typically the same number of sutures, around 10, is required.

Several mechanical ring anastomotic devices, such as the Nakayama ring pin system and the 3M Precise system, have been described[70] based on the original concept described by Payr in 1904.[95] In these authors' hands, this method has been consistently successful for selected venous anastomoses, with considerable time saved.

The need for a vein graft has been shown to be associated with a significantly higher rate of complication in a large series.[110] This complication rate may be kept to a minimum by anticipating and planning for the possibility of the graft. Because of the need for extra anastomoses, there is a slightly higher risk of thrombosis, and alternative methods are superior, such as using flaps with longer pedicles or using recipient vessels on the contralateral side of the neck.

After the vessel clamps are released, it is necessary to test for vessel patency. Signs of vessel patency include bright red bleeding from the edges of the flap and expansile arterial pulsation.[3] Alternatively, the "strip" test can be used. In this test, the vessel is emptied by sliding compression between two forceps and then is allowed to refill, although this is traumatic to the endothelium.[96] A test for distal venous outflows away from the flap is to gently compress the recipient vein where it is accessible closest to the heart, assess the intraluminal pressure proximally by finger palpation, and then release the distal compression to confirm a proximal pressure reduction. Observation of the flap after completion of the anastomosis and during inset provides an important opportunity to detect correctable problems.

Microneural anastomosis

Trimmed epineurium of the nerve is coapted with nonabsorbable suture, usually size 8-0. Six to eight sutures usually are sufficient to eliminate gaps. It is important to avoid suture line tension.

FLAP INSET

The flap inset phase of a free tissue transfer procedure may be performed before or after the microvascular anastomosis, depending on the type of reconstruction, the tissue conditions, and the surgeon's preference.

The advantages of preanastomosis flap inset are predetermined pedicle positioning in the wound, an accurate judgment of required pedicle length, and minimal postanastomotic manipulation of the vessels. The advantages of postanastomosis inset are decreased ischemia time and maximal physical access for execution of the microvascular anastomosis. Such access can be difficult, for example, when reconstructing the mandible with a vascularized bone flap. Recipient vessels located superiorly on the carotid artery can be substantially concealed by the bone if it is inset before the anastomosis. In general, if the surgeon elects to anastomose before flap inset, he or she should have an accurate idea of how the donor tissue will lie in the wound and whether

wound closure, such as mandibulotomy repair, will cause excessive compression of the flap. A trial of simulated closure, with judicious trimming of excess tissue bulk, should precede the final wound closure. These authors have left one osteosynthesis site in a mandibular reconstruction unscrewed until edema has settled 6 or 7 days later to avoid acute pedicle or soft-tissue compression.

Another critical factor in flap inset technique is tissue manipulation to simulate the resected structure. An obvious example is the need for contouring osteotomies for fibular reconstruction of curved segments of the mandible. Also, sutures and folds that are introduced into soft-tissue flaps, enabling them to sit well and resemble a resected structure such as the tongue, may be important in the patient's final functional performance. Conversely, if a flap is used to close a defect without shaping and sculpting, mediocre function may result. For example, the authors have found that articulation seems to be correlated with the degree to which their patients' tongue reconstructions can be made to oppose the hard palate and lips. A series of folds used for radial forearm flaps was introduced[42] to optimize this result.

The timing of neurorrhaphy also is planned to coordinate with the rest of the procedure. Assuming postanastomotic flap inset, a convenient interval for this step is during the perfusion period immediately after vascular anastomosis when the microscope is still in the field. Access to the "donor" nerve usually is still available, whereas gross manipulation of the flap is undesirable during this platelet–fibrin clot "wash-out" phase.

COMPLICATIONS, MONITORING, AND SALVAGE

Roberts and Bailey[102] have comprehensively described the complications that may occur after the completion of a free flap. The systemic complications common to all types of surgery pertain equally to free flap surgery, and some, such as deep venous thrombosis, may be potentially more problematic because of the length of the procedures. These general systemic complications will not be described in this chapter. Local complications occur at the donor and recipient sites.

Donor site complications include hemorrhage, wound breakdown, nerve damage, scarring, functional deficits, and cosmetic deformities.

Recipient site complications occur in the immediate, early, and late stages. Immediate problems include anastomotic leak, anastomotic failure, and flap compression, whereas early complications include anastomotic occlusion, vascular thrombosis, edema of the flap, secondary hemorrhage, and infection. Late complications include infection, dehiscence, fistula, poor cosmesis, and loss of function. Hemorrhage, fistula, and infection should be aggressively managed, surgically if necessary, because the presence of saliva, pus, or an expanding hematoma in the vicinity of the pedicle may compromise the flap.

The viability of a free tissue graft depends on the maintenance of sufficient arterial and venous blood flow. In general, factors that could be expected to reduce the blood flow can be considered as those external to the vessel wall, in the vessel wall, and within the lumen. Factors extrinsic to the vessel wall include mechanical compression from neighboring anatomic structures, from tight skin flaps, from edema, or hematoma. Vessel spasm is an intrinsic vessel wall factor that can limit blood flow to the point of thrombosis, whereas mechanical disruption of the wall and release of thromboplastins invites platelet–fibrin clot formation. Stasis of blood flow will result in thrombosis, which, if not corrected promptly, will result in the loss of the flap.

Endothelium is critical in preventing thrombosis in the vascular system. Among its numerous other functions, vascular endothelium synthesizes and expresses antithrombotic factors, such as antithrombin III, and fibrinolytic factors, such as plasminogen activator.[129] When the endothelium is breached or damaged, such as at the site of anastomosis, the coagulation cascade may be triggered. The events intrinsic to this sequence are platelet deposition, degranulation, and the clotting cascade.[115] Platelets adhere to exposed collagen in the subepithelial layer, form a platelet clot, transform, and degranulate. Degranulation releases factors that activate the traditional clotting cascade, in particular the intrinsic system. The endpoint of the cascade is the deposition of fibrin, which converts the platelet plug into an entity that is more tenacious, less prone to embolize, and more difficult to lyse.[63] Once thrombin is formed on the vessel endothelial surface, the effect of heparin is attenuated.[52] It is thought that intact endothelium may be functionally damaged and may lose its antithrombotic effect.[117] In their comprehensive review of thrombosis and antithrombotic therapy in microvascular surgery, Johnson and Barker[52] suggest that the causes of thrombosis in some patients may be more complex, and simple technical anastomotic issues may not be the sole cause of flap failure. In an animal model, Hjortdal and others[47] have shown that a "poor" arterial anastomosis is not significantly more thrombogenic than an arterial clamping technique and that the accumulation of platelets and fibrinogen seen in the distal microcirculation of the failing flap is less a result of emboli from the anastomotic site than a result of adhesion to an ischemia-damaged endothelium. They also found an increase in platelet and fibrinogen accumulation in venous ischemic flaps with major tissue edema, which, in contrast with arterial ischemic flaps, is aggravated by the reestablishment of blood flow.[48]

Concerning the role of flow in thrombosis, blood flow through a nonlaminar system follows the Pouseille/Hagan law, which states that flow is proportional to the perfusion pressure and the fourth power of the radius of the vessel and is inversely proportional to the viscosity and the length of the vessel.[129] Below a critical rate of blood flow, the erythrocytes form a rouleaux pattern, and flow is more likely to become stagnant. This effect increases with increasing viscosity. Above a critical rate of flow, the flow becomes laminar with a faster rate of flow in the central lumen. In this state, the viscosity is at its lowest level.[34,55] It is thought that a critical closing pressure exists whereby below a certain threshold of perfusion pressure, the peripheral arterioles and capillaries are not supplied with blood.[20]

Skin blood supply is well described in standard physiology textbooks,[11,38] and a detailed analysis of its characteristics is beyond the scope of this chapter. In brief, the skin has different types of vessels, consisting of a resistance system of capillaries and arterioles that provide the nutritive blood supply to the skin and a capacitance system of arteriovenous anastomoses and subdermal venous plexus. Precapillary sphincters, predominantly under the control of circulating metabolites and hormones, regulate flow into the nutritive bed, whereas the capacitance vessels are largely under the control of the neural system. The skin is predominantly concerned with temperature regulation, and vessels constrict in response to cold and dilate in response to heating. Constriction of these skin vessels also occurs in response to decreasing of blood pressure as flow is shunted away from the integument to more vital organs.

In a review of the factors thought to contribute to failure of free flaps, Khouri[61] describes preoperative, operative, and postoperative causes. Once the surgeon has achieved a level of technical proficiency allowing him or her to successfully complete the microvascular anastomosis, failure of a given free flap is likely to result from the accumulation of several perioperative factors, including poor patient selection, unmanaged or undiagnosed comorbidity, inappropriate selection of recipient vessels, inappropriate selection of donor flap, and poor execution of the procedure.

Operative factors contributing to free flap failure include lack of surgical precision, small vessel size, inadequate exposure, and poor hemostasis. Rough handling of recipient vessels and anastomotic errors, such as a stitch through the back wall or adventitia trapped in the lumen, also will contribute to failure of a flap and may result from surgeon discomfort and fatigue. Avoidance of kinking is critical, and it is imperative to identify and to act on potential problems intraoperatively.[80]

Other detrimental factors include one versus two venous anastomosis, vein grafts, intraoperative thrombosis of the pedicle, or major general deviation from a surgeon's set practices. Postoperatively, care should be taken to avoid hypovolemia, hypotension, hypothermia, interstitial edema, and mechanical compression of the pedicle by wound closure or hematoma.

Animal studies have suggested that the free flap may be viable independent of its pedicle after as few as 8 days,[12] after which time the collateral blood supply maintains perfusion. Typically, survival of the flap is not to be relied on for less than 2 to 3 weeks in nonirradiated fields and perhaps double that time in irradiated fields. This is the critical interval before neovascularization at the periphery of the flap renders it independent of pedicle's axial blood supply.

After 12 hours of complete ischemia, it is unlikely that the flap tissue is salvageable, even if a patent anastomosis is restored. This has been termed the *no-reflow phenomenon.*[77] This length of time that a flap may be ischemic and survive has been termed the *critical ischemia time,*[56] and in animal experiments, this was found to be about 13 hours. The time varies for different tissues, with muscle being less resistant to ischemia than skin, which is less resistant than bone. Some degree of necrosis may be expected after 6 hours of ischemia, and there is a risk after this time that the whole flap may be lost.[7] It is thought that a flap that has suffered one period of ischemia may be less able to tolerate subsequent episodes of ischemia, with the secondary critical ischemia time being half as long as the primary critical ischemia time in animal experiments.[59] During the first 72 postoperative hours, it is essential that a prompt diagnosis of ischemia be made and that blood flow be immediately reestablished. Paradoxically, the resumption of blood flow may result in the so-called reperfusion-ischemia injury described in detail elsewhere.[58,82,92] Oxygen-derived free radicals, including the superoxide anion and hydroxyl radicals and hydrogen peroxide, are formed after an ischemic flap is reperfused, resulting in peroxidation of cellular membranes and cell death. Various other molecular mediators of inflammation, such as thromboxane A_2 and leukotriene B_4 are thought to cause leukocyte-endotheral adhesion, an associated event in reperfusion injury.

The clinical features of a compromised flap are different for arterial and venous insufficiency. Arterial insufficiency signs are a cool, pale, flaccid flap with capillary refill prolonged beyond approximately 4 seconds, and no bleeding from cuts or punctures made into the flap.[40] Evidence of venous compromise is blue or purple, turgid, congested-looking flaps, with rapid refill of less than approximately 1 second and dark blood oozing from the suture line or into the wound from cut surfaces. Failure of the venous side of the pedicle is more common as an initial event than arterial failure,[7] but eventually a compromised flap will have arterial and venous insufficiency. Clinical monitoring as described previously is difficult when the flaps are buried or when there is combined arterial and venous insufficiency. Even with the best clinical judgment, once there is evidence of venous arterial compromise, the underlying thrombotic process may be far advanced in the microcirculation.

For this reason, more sophisticated electronic monitoring methods, either invasive or noninvasive, have been introduced and are under evaluation. The two different types are those that monitor blood flow through the pedicle and those that evaluate tissue perfusion at the arteriolar or capillary level. Numerous methods have been described.[29,32,53,76,88] These techniques include radioisotope bone scanning, temperature probes, Doppler ultrasound, colorflow Doppler, impedance plethysmography, oxygen tension measurement, and laser Doppler velocimetry. Many of the techniques' common disadvantages are excessive cost, artifact, and mo-

tion sensitivity. The laser Doppler probe seems to be the most promising of the current technologies. The rationale for hourly monitoring during the first 72 hours is to provide an opportunity for immediate salvage intervention when problems are noted.[69] Monitoring less frequently, e.g., every 2 to 4 hours, should probably continue for an additional 2 to 3 days, but successful salvage is rarely necessary or achievable during this phase. The need for continued monitoring also can be balanced against the flaps' ''job description.'' If the reconstruction is sealing the subarachnoid space, protecting the carotid from salivary contamination, monitoring should probably continue for 7 days. A skin coverage flap is less critical.

Numerous pharmacologic strategies have been explored for increasing the chances of flap survival maneuvers. Broadly, they may be divided into methods that decrease the likelihood of thrombosis, those that increase blood flow, and those that protect the flap against the metabolic effects of ischemia.

Antithrombotic pharmacologic agents

Pharmacologic prophylaxis against thrombosis is a controversial subject, and therefore, practices vary.[22] Agents that are commonly but not universally used are heparin, aspirin, and rheologic agents.

Heparin

Heparin binds to antithrombin III, inactivated thrombin, and several other esterases of the clotting cascade.[52] It is thought to increase the electronegative potential of the endothelium and thereby decrease platelet adhesiveness.[122] It appears that high local concentrations of heparin are necessary to achieve this beneficial effect.[112] Dosing systemically to achieve the same concentration may result in excessive operative bleeding.[60] A retrospective review of heparin use in a large series of patients was recently published.[66] Although not statistically significant, their findings suggest that the use of a low-dose intraoperative bolus of intravenous heparin followed by a 20 to 30-unit/hour infusion of heparin for 5 to 7 days reduced flap loss without resulting in a higher rate of hematoma formation. The routine use of heparin in topical irrigating solutions is recommended.[7,52,122]

Aspirin

Aspirin exerts its effect by inhibiting the action of cyclooxygenase and interferes with the synthesis of prostaglandin H2.[34] This inhibits the degranulation of platelets, but the benefit of aspirin on microvascular patency rates has not been conclusively proven. A 650-mg daily dose of aspirin started by suppository at the time of anastomosis is used by some[122] and has a positive effect in some clinical series on flap survival.

Dextran

A loading dose of low molecular weight dextran given immediately before the microvascular clamps are released and continued for 5 days postoperatively has been proposed[60] because of the supposed antithrombin and antifibrin effect of dextran.

Goding[34] has examined the means by which the free flap may be manipulated to improve local blood flow. These techniques include surgical delay and the use of vasodilators, such as calcium channel blockers. The routine use of thymoxamine has been advocated by some.[94] The use of antiinflammatories, rheologic agents such as pentoxyphylline, and growth factors also has been described experimentally.[34]

Increased resistance to ischemia is another approach to improving flap viability. The use of hyperbaric oxygen has been described,[132] and of current interest is the use of free radical scavengers such as allopurinol and superoxide dismutase.[57,58]

Once the diagnosis of vascular compromise has been made, the primary management in the first 3 to 5 days is surgical. The mainstay of flap salvage is immediate surgical exploration. Depending on findings, one or both existing anastomoses may need revision, or alternative recipient vessels may need to be used. Thrombus commonly found propagating throughout the pedicle is gently evacuated once the vessels are opened. The rate of flap failure through ischemia ranges from 5% to 10% in modern series, with a salvage rate of approximately 40%.[7,58,62]

Adjuvant use of pharmacologic agents for flap salvage is advisable. Liberal topical and intravascular heparin irrigation should be used, and systemic heparin commenced[52] to keep partial thromboplastin time at twice normal. Salvage of a failing flap by the continuous infusion of intraarterial heparin also has been described.[78] An alternative is heparin infusion by microcatheterization of a side branch of the arterial pedicle with 50 units of heparin per hour postsalvage. Streptokinase, which activates plasminogen by binding with the plasminogen molecule to lyse thrombus, is infused through the flap by injection of 75,000 units into the flap artery. This distributes the drug throughout the flap and usually results in a rapid increase in the venous outflow. The latter is collected on sponges and discarded to avoid systemic distribution of streptokinase. After approximately 30 minutes of sustained perfusion, the recipient artery is clamped while one venous anastomosis is performed. All clamps are released again for full perfusion. The use of systemic streptokinase is not advised postoperatively because of the risk of generalized bleeding, but the successful use of local infusions of streptokinase has been described.[35,72] It has been asserted in the cardiology literature that the use of fibrinolytic needs to be followed by the use of heparin or aspirin to prevent rethrombosis.[116] The addition of aspirin should be considered whether fibrinolytics are used. Free radical scavenger use has not become established despite considerable experimental interest.

The management of a congested flap may be assisted with the use of the medicinal leech.[23,130] The leech is indicated when a flap has venous congestion, but arterial flow is still established. It may be used in a mildly congested flap for 4 to 5 days or postoperatively after flap salvage. The leech manufactures hementin, a local anesthetic, and hirudin, which inhibits the conversion of fibrinogen to fibrin. The gut of the leech harbors a gram-negative β lactamase-producing commensal, aeromonas hydrophile,[113] which may cause extensive necrotic soft-tissue infection of the flap in 10% to 15% of patients. The patient needs to be covered with gram-negative parenteral β lactamase-resistant antibiotic coverage, such as ciprofloxin or a third generation cephalosporin. Another hazard of prolonged leeching is significant blood loss requiring transfusion.

Once it is obvious that the flap has died, it needs to be resected in a timely, but nonemergent fashion because of the risk of infection and disseminated intravascular coagulation. The loss of a free flap is a major complication and may result in life-threatening sequelae. In most patients, the situation will need to be salvaged by the use of a pedicled flap, such as the pectoralis major myocutaneous flap or another free flap.

OUTCOMES

The current appropriate focus on outcomes measurement of treatment intervention in medicine has resulted in a modicum of data being available on free tissue transfer in the head and neck. In general, the categories into which these outcomes divide are morbidity, mortality, functional measures, quality of life, and cost. Some studies include data that incorporate outcomes related to the defect and the reconstructive process.

Mortality and morbidity rates in free tissue transfer to the head and neck have been considered low enough to offer this method of reconstruction routinely. Perioperative mortality rates have been approximately 2% in most series,[98] and morbidity, at least as measured by flap series survival rates of approximately 94% to 97%, also has been low.[110] Other causes of morbidity, such as hematomas, fistulae, delayed healing, and infections, vary from series to series, but are not beyond what is expected for major head and neck surgery even without free tissue transfer.[17,66,99,126]

Donor site morbidity has been studied in detail for flaps such as the fibula. Although the majority of patients ultimately do well, ankle instability can be problematic. This is because of the fibula's small, but measurable, contribution to weight-bearing and deepening of the ankle mortise. Loss of the interosseous membrane and disruption of muscles also has an effect.[6] In a questionnaire study recently performed in the authors' clinic, approximately 75% of patients with a variety of flaps admitted to donor site symptoms, but none ultimately rated the impact of those symptoms on their ability to function as worse than mild. A study of donor site problems for the radial forearm also indicated insignificant morbidity.[14]

Functional measures after free tissue transfer, either ''objective'' tools, which can be administered and quantified by the medical or paramedical professions, or "subjective" patient questionnaires may be generally categorized as follows:

- Appearance[27,45]
- Facial movement analysis[86,87]
- Mastication[13]
- Speech or intelligibility[43]
- Swallowing[89]
- Voice[25]

These can be supplemented by objective physical tests that may or may not correlate with the previous measures, e.g., sizing of chewed food particles,[85] intraoral pressure measurement,[75,103] simultaneous manometry and video images,[79] oropharyngeal swallow efficiency (percent bolus swallowed/transit time),[97] or voice.[91]

Quality of life instruments may be general in nature (e.g., general health measures MOSF-36) or specific,[41] but they will require further refinement before a more precise measure can be given for free flap patients. The clinical application of "measured" quality of life requires considerable further investigation and refinement. Interpretation of such outcomes should be tempered by the knowledge that surgeons strive to select cases to optimize the outcome of their technical efforts. The cost of free tissue transfer surgery also has been assessed and found to be comparable with pedicled reconstruction.[67,68]

FUTURE DEVELOPMENT OF FREE TISSUE TRANSFER

Refinement of techniques and instrumentation for free tissue transfer continues to allow translation of laboratory experiments into useful clinical advances.

Magnification

At a technical level, methods of magnification and imaging continue to develop. Loupe magnification was advocated by Shenaq and others[108] after their report of a 251-case series in which 5.5 × loupes were used for a 97.2% flap and replant success rate. There was an 8.3% intraoperative revision rate in the 199 free flap cases, although it was concluded that in practiced hands, loupes provided cost-effectiveness, portability, efficiency, and operator freedom, except in those patients with vessels 1.0 mm or less in diameter or in children. Serletti and others[107] were similarly impressed with their success rate of 99% in a series of 119 free flaps performed with 3.5 × loupes. They stressed the need to revert to microscopes when dealing with patients with vessels 1.5 mm or less in diameter or with children, but they were pleased with the access that use of loupes created for surgeon and assistants and the success of their procedures in community hospitals wherein microscopes were not available.

Another system of magnification and image presentation is the three-dimensional on-screen microsurgical system (TOMS). Franken and others[31] reported laboratory and clini-

cal use of this equipment, in which the two eye pieces on a microscope are replaced by cameras, and the image is relayed to a monitor that is viewed directly by the surgeon wearing polarizing glasses to enhance depth perception. Surgeons responded favorably to the comfort and operation of the equipment and its educational potential.[31]

Anastomosis methods

Novel anastomosis methods and connector systems also have been investigated. Lasers with wavelengths from 10,600 nm (CO_2) to 514 to 488 nm (argon) have achieved acceptable patency rates with much reduced operating time. Pseudoaneurysm formation has been consistently observed. More recently, the 830-nm diode laser used in a contact method with fiberoptic "wand" transmission[71] or with a noncontact beam[124] also has been shown to be reliable but without microaneurysm formation. Clinical series of laser anastomoses have been reported, with the major advantage being much reduced anastomotic time.

Mechanical devices such as the 3M ring pin system also are excellent time savers, although the authors found these are best reserved for venous anastomosis. Microstapled anastomosis technology may prove suitable for arterial anastomosis in the future.

Endoscopic flap harvest

Early reports of clinical endoscopic harvest techniques have been made by Fine and Eaves.[28,30] Both reports describe harvest of latissimus dorsi muscle flaps using endoscopic assistance, delivering the muscle through shortened donor site incisions, but prolonging harvest time by up to 4 hours. Rectus abdominus muscle harvest techniques have been reported in cadavers.[10] Laparoscopic jejunum and omentum harvest has been reported in clinical cases and investigated in animals.[84,105] The future of endoscopic harvest techniques will undoubtedly hinge on the technique being proved to reduce scarring and donor site morbidity, whereas operating times, cost, flap survival, and complication rates need to become comparable with conventional harvest techniques.

Prefabrication

Prefabrication of flaps custom-prepared for the recipient site is a potential area for future development in free tissue transfer. Vessel pedicles can be inserted into randomly vascularized soft tissue, bone, or both, converting the recipient areas into vessel pedicle–based transferable units.[131] Pretransfer expansion, lamination, and grafting of tissue also customizes flaps for use in the recipient site.[1,19,64] Further, alloplastic materials can be incorporated into free flaps before transfer so that a sculpted composite unit is ready for transfer to the nose or auricle.[19] Bioengineered tissue now is being developed in which biodegradable polymer scaffolds and growth factor-enriched media are seeded with progenitor cells. Production of a structure of predetermined size and shape around a vascular pedicle *in vitro* may allow vascularized attachment of complex prefabricated organs such as nose, ear, and facial skeletal structures.

Allotransplantation

Transfer of cadaver-derived flap allografts holds potential for precise reconstruction of functionally complex organs, such as the larynx,[119] tongue,[44] trachea,[24] or mandible.[49] In all previously described cases, feasibility of animal allotransplantation during immunosuppression with agents such as cyclosporine and FK506 has been demonstrated, in some experimental situations with return of neuromuscular function.[43] Clinical allotransplantation of whole organs will hinge on further experimental proof that recovery of function in the transplanted organs is adequate, and especially that cancer patients who receive such transplantation will not be harmed by immunosuppression.

REFERENCES

1. Abbase EA and others: Prefabricated flaps: experimental and clinical review, *Plast Reconstr Surg* 96:1218, 1995.
2. Acland RD: *Microsurgery practice manual,* St Louis, 1980, Mosby.
3. Acland RD: Signs of patency in small vessel anastomosis surgery, *Surgery* 72:744, 1972.
4. Al Qattan MM, Bowen V: Effect of pre-existing health conditions on the results of reconstructive microvascular surgery, *Microsurgery* 14: 152, 1993.
5. Antia NH, Buch VI: Transfer of an abdominal dermofat graft by direct anastomosis of blood vessels, *Br J Plast Surg* 24:15, 1971.
6. Babhulkar SS, Ketan CP, Babhulkar S: Ankle instability after fibular resection, *J Bone Joint Surg* 77:258, 1995.
7. Baker SR: *Complications of microvascular surgery.* In Baker SR, editor: *Microsurgical reconstruction of the head and neck,* New York, 1989, Churchill Livingstone.
8. Baker SR, Krause CJ, Panje WR: Radiation effects on microvascular anastomosis, *Arch Otolaryngol Head Neck Surg* 104:103, 1978.
9. Baron JF and others: How molecular weight hydroxyethyl starch 6% compared to albumin 4% during intentional hemodilution, *Intensive Care Med* 17:141, 1991.
10. Bass LS and others: Endoscopic harvests of the rectus abdominis free flap: balloon dissection in the fascial plane, *Ann Plast Surg* 34(3): 274, 1995.
11. Berne RM, Levy MN: *Principles of physiology,* St Louis, 1990, Mosby.
12. Black MJM and others: How soon may the axial vessels of a surviving free flap be safely ligated: a study in pigs, *Br J Plast Surg* 31:295, 1978.
13. Boretti G, Bickel M, Seeing AH: A review of masticatory ability and efficiency, *J Prosthet Dent* 74:400, 1995.
14. Brown MT and others: Assessment of functional morbidity in the radial forearm free flap donor site, *Arch Otolaryngol Head Neck Surg* 122:991, 1996.
15. Carrel A: The surgery of blood vessels, etc, *Bull Johns Hopkins Hosp* 18:18, 1907.
16. Chick LR and others: Free flaps in the elderly, *Plast Reconstr Surg* 90:87, 1992.
17. Clayman GL and others: Outcome and complications of extended cranial-base resection requiring microvascular free-tissue transfer, *Arch Otolaryngol Head Neck Surg* 121:1253, 1995.
18. Cooley BC and others: The influence of diabetes on free flap transfer: I. flap survival and microvascular healing, *Ann Plast Surg* 29:58, 1992.
19. Costa H and others: Prefabricated flaps for the head and neck: a preliminary report, *Br J Plast Surg* 46:223, 1993.
20. Cutting C and others: Critical closing pressure, local perfusion pressure, and the failing skin flap, *Ann Plast Surg* 8:504, 1982.
21. Daniel RK, Taylor GI: Distant transfer of an island flap by microvascular anastomosis, *Plast Reconstr Surg* 12:111, 1973.
22. Davies DM: A world survey of anticoagulation practice in clinical microvascular surgery, *Br J Plast Surg* 35:96, 1982.
23. de Chalain TMB: Exploring the use of the medicinal leech: a clinical risk–benefit analysis, *J Reconstr Microsurg* 12:165, 1996.
24. Delaere PR and others: Experimental tracheal allograft revascularization and transplantation, *J Thorac Cardiovasc Surg* 110(3):728, 1995.
25. Deschler DG and others: Tracheoesophageal voice following tubed free radial forearm flap reconstruction of the neopharynx, *Ann Otol Rhinol Laryngol* 103(12):929, 1994.
26. Dohar JE, Goding GS, Maisel RH: The effects of the inhalational anesthetic agent combination, isoflurane-nitrous oxide, on survival in a pig random skin flap model, *Arch Otolaryngol Head Neck Surg* 120:74, 1994.
27. Dropkin M and others: Scaling of disfigurement and dysfunction in post operative head and neck patients, *Head Neck Surg* 6(1):559, 1983.
28. Eaves FF and others: Invited discussion: endoscopic-assisted muscle flap, *Ann Plast Surg* 33(5):469, 1994.
29. Fernando B, Young VL, Logan SE: Miniature implantable laser doppler probe monitoring of free tissue transfer, *Ann Plast Surg* 20(5): 434, 1988.
30. Fine NA, Orgill DP, Pribaz JJ: Early clinical experience in endoscopic-assisted muscle flap harvest, *Ann Plast Surg* 33(5):465, 1994.
31. Franken RJPM and others: Microsurgery without a microscope: laboratory evaluation of a three-dimensional on-screen microsurgery system, *Microsurgery* 16:746, 1995.
32. Furnas H, Rosen JM: Monitoring in microvascular surgery, *Ann Plast Surg* 26:265, 1991.
33. Genden E, Haughey BH: Mandibular reconstruction by vascularized free tissue transfer, *Am J Otolaryngol* 17(4):219, 1996.
34. Goding GS, Hom DB: *Skin flap physiology.* In Baker SR, Swanson NA, editors: *Local flaps in facial reconstruction,* St Louis, 1995, Mosby.
35. Goldberg JA, Pedeom WC, Barwick WJ: Salvage of free tissue transfers using thrombolytic agents, *J Reconstr Microsurg* 5:351, 1989.
36. Gruber UF, Messimer K: Colloids for blood volume support, *Prog Surg* 15:49, 1977.
37. Guelinckx PJ and others: Scanning electron microscopy of irradiated recipient blood vessels in head and neck free flaps, *Plast Reconstr Surg* 74(2):217, 1984.
38. Guyton AC: *Human physiology and mechanisms of disease,* Philadelphia, 1987, WB Saunders.
39. Harii K, Ohmori K, Ohmori S: Free deltopectoral skin flaps, *Br J Plast Surg* 24:231, 1974.
40. Harrison DH, Girling M, Mott G: Experience in monitoring the circulation in free-flap transfers, *Plast Reconstr Surg* 68(4):543, 1981.
41. Hassan SJ, Weymuller EA Jr: Assessment of quality of life in head and neck cancer patients, *Head Neck* 15(6):485, 1993.
42. Haughey BH: *Specialized reconstruction of the oral cavity and oropharynx.* In Robbins KT, editor: *Head and neck cancer: function, treatment, rehabilitation and reconstruction,* 1997, Singular Publishing.
43. Haughey BH, Beggs JC, Bong JP: Allotransplantation of the canine tongue. Abstracts of the 11th Annual Meeting American Society for Reconstructive Microsurgery, Tuscon, Ariz, January, 1996.
44. Haughey BH, Beggs JC, Bong JP: Microneurovascular allotransplantation of the canine hemitongue. Abstracts of the American Society for Head and Neck Surgery, Palm Desert, Calif, April, 1995.

45. Hay GC, Heather BB: Changes in psychometric test results following cosmetic nasal operations, *Br J Psychiatry* 122:89, 1973.

46. Hiebert CA, Cumings GO: Successful replacement of the cervical esophagus by transplantation and revascularization of a free graft of gastric antrum, *Ann Surg* 154:103, 1961.

47. Hjortdal VE and others: Venous ischemia in skin flaps: microcirculatory intravascular thrombosis, *Plast Reconstr Surg* 93:366, 1994.

48. Hjortdal VE and others: Arterial insufficiency in skin flaps: microcirculatory intravascular thrombosis, *Plast Reconstr Surg* 93:375, 1994.

49. Hoehnke C and others: Vascularized composite tissue mandibular transplantation in dogs long-term survival under FK 506 immunosuppression. Abstracts of the American Society for Reconstructive Microsurgery. 11th Annual Meeting, p. 169, Tuscon, Ariz, January, 1996.

50. Inghs MS and others: The anesthetic management of patients undergoing free flap reconstruction surgery following resection of head and neck neoplasms—a review of 64 patients, *Ann R Coll Surg Engl* 70: 235, 1988.

51. Jacobsen JH, Suarez EL: Microsurgery in anastomosis of small vessels, *Surg Forum* 11:243, 1960.

52. Johnson PC, Barker JH: Thrombosis and antithrombotic therapy in microvascular surgery, *Clin Plast Surg* 19(4):799, 1992.

53. Jones NF: Intraoperative and postoperative monitoring of microsurgical free tissue transfers, *Clin Plast Surg* 19(4):783, 1992.

54. Kaplan EN, Buncke HJ, Murray DE: Distant transfer of cutaneous island flaps in humans by microvascular anastomosis, *Plast Reconstr Surg* 52:301, 1973.

55. Kerrigan CL: Skin flap failure: pathophysiology, *Plast Reconstr Surg* 72(6):766, 1983.

56. Kerrigan CL, Daniel RK: Critical ischemia time and the failing skin flap, *Plast Reconstr Surg* 69:986, 1982.

57. Kerrigan CL, Daniel RK: Pharmacologic treatment of the failing skin flap, *Plast Reconstr Surg* 70:641, 1982.

58. Kerrigan CL, Stotland MA: Ischemia reperfusion injury: a review, *Microsurgery* 14:165, 1993.

59. Kerrigan CL, Zelt RG, Daniel RK: Secondary critical ischemia time of experimental skin flaps, *Plast Reconstr Surg* 74:522, 1984.

60. Ketchum LD: Pharmacological alterations in the clotting mechanisms: use in microvascular surgery, *J Hand Surg Am* 3(5):407, 1978.

61. Khouri RK: Avoiding free flap failure, *Clin Plast Surg* 19:773, 1992.

62. Khouri RK: Free flap surgery: the second decade, *Clin Plast Surg* 19:757, 1992.

63. Khouri RK and others: Thrombosis of microvascular anastomosis in traumatized vessels: fibrin versus platelets, *Plast Reconstr Surg* 86:110, 1990.

64. Khouri RK and others: Facial reconstruction with prefabricated induced expanded (PIE) supraclavicular skin flaps, *Plast Reconstr Surg* 95(6):1007, 1995.

65. Kramer GC, Wallfisch HK: Recent trends in fluid therapy, *Curr Opin Anesthesiol* 5:272, 1992.

66. Kroll SS and others: Anticoagulants and hematomas in free flap surgery, *Plast Reconstr Surg* 96(3):643, 1995.

67. Kroll SS and others: Comparison of the rectus abdominis free flap with the pectoralis major myocutaneous flap for reconstructions in the head and neck, *Am J Surg* 164(6):615, 1992.

68. Kroll S, Schusterman MA, Reece GP: Costs and complications in mandibular reconstruction, *Ann Plast Surg* 29(4):341, 1992.

69. Reference deleted in pages.

70. Lee S and others: A review of vascular anastomosis with mechanical aids and non-suture techniques, *Head Neck Surg* 3:58, 1980.

71. Lewis WJ, Uribe A: Contact diode laser microvascular anastomosis, *Laryngoscope* 103:850, 1993.

72. Lipton HA, Jupiter JB: Streptokinase salvage of a free tissue transfer: case report and review of the literature, *Plast Reconstr Surg* 79:977, 1987.

73. Liu J, Kumar VP: The unrecognized giants, *Plast Reconstr Surg* 97(2):486, 1996.

74. Macdonald DJF: Anaesthesia for microvascular surgery: a physiological approach, *Br J Anaesth* 57(9):904, 1985.

75. Mahmood WA and others: Use of image analysis in determining masticatory efficiency in patients presenting for immediate dentures, *Int J Prosthedont* 5(4):359, 1992.

76. Manktelow RT, Ahm DS: Monitoring free muscle transfer, *Microsurgery* 12:367, 1991.

77. May JW and others: The no-reflow phenomenon in experimental free flap, *Plast Reconstr Surg* 61:256, 1978.

78. May JW, Rothkopf DM: Salvage of a failing microvascular free muscle flap by direct continuous intravascular infusion of heparin: a case report, *Plast Reconstr Surg* 83:1045, 1989.

79. McConnel FM, Mendelsohn MS, Logemann JA: Examination of swallowing after total laryngectomy using manofluorography, *Head Neck Surg* 9(1):3, 1986.

80. McKee NH: Operative complications and the management of intraoperative flow failure, *Microsurgery* 14:158, 1993.

81. McLean DH, Buncke HJ: Autotransplant of omentum to a large scalp defect with microsurgical revascularization, *Plast Reconstr Surg* 49(3):268, 1972.

82. Mellow CG and others: The biochemical basis of secondary ischemia, *J Surg Res* 52:226, 1992.

83. Messmer KF: The use of plasma substitutes with special attention to their side effects, *World J Surg* 11(1):69, 1987.

84. Miller MJ: Minimally invasive techniques of tissue harvest in ear and neck reconstruction, *Clin Plast Surg* 21:149, 1994.

85. Montana F, Heath MR, Auger D: Automated optical scanning for rapid sizing of chewed food particles in masticating tests, *J Oral Rehabil* 22(2):153, 1995.

86. Neely JG and others: Quantitive assessment of the variation within grades of facial paralysis, *Laryngoscope* 106:438, 1996.

87. Neely JG and others: Computerized quantitative dynamic analysis of facial motion in the paralyzed and synkinetic face, *Am J Otol* 13(2):97, 1992.

88. Neligan PC: Monitoring techniques for the detection of flow failure in the postoperative period, *Microsurgery* 14:162, 1993.

89. Newton HB and others: Swallowing assessment in primary brain tumor patients with dysphagia, *Neurology* 44(10):1927, 1994.

90. Nylen CO: The microscope in aural surgery: its first use and later development, *Acta Otolaryngol Suppl* 116:226, 1954.

91. Painter C: Semi-automated voice evaluation, *Am J Otolaryngol* 12:329, 1991.

92. Pang CY, Forrest CR, Morissey R: Pharmacologic intervention in ischemia induced reperfusion injury in the skeletal muscle, *Microsurgery* 14:176, 1993.

93. Panje WR, Bardach J, Krause CJ: Reconstruction of the oral cavity with a free flap, *Plast Reconstr Surg* 58(4):415, 1976.

94. Patel C, Marsili A, Sykes PJ: Augmentation of flap survival by thymoxamine, *Br J Plast Surg* 35(1):88, 1982.

95. Payr E: Zur Frage der circularen Vereinigung von Blutegafassen mit resorbirbaren Prothesen, *Arch Klinische Chirurgie* 72:32, 1904.

96. Petry JJ, French TS, Worthan KA: The effect of the "patency-test" on arterial endothelial surface, *Plast Reconstr Surg* 77:960, 1986.

97. Rademaker AW and others: Oropharyngeal swallow efficiency as a representative measure of swallowing function, *J Speech Hear Res* 37(2):314, 1994.

98. Reece GP and others: Morbidity and functional outcome of free jejunal transfer reconstruction for circumferential defects of the pharynx and cervical esophagus, *Plast Reconstr Surg* 96(6):1307, 1995.

99. Reece GP and others: Morbidity associated with free-tissue transfer after radiotherapy and chemotherapy in elderly cancer patients, *J Reconstr Microsurg* 10(6):375, 1994.

100. Reus WF, Colen LB, Straker DJ: Tobacco smoking and complications in elective microsurgery, *Plast Reconstr Surg* 89:490, 1992.

101. Richards RS, Bowen CVA, Glynn MFX: Microsurgical free tissue transfer in sickle cell disease, *Ann Plast Surg* 29:278, 1992.

102. Roberts J, Bailey B: *The management of post-operative problems.* In Soutar DS, editor: *Microvascular surgery and free tissue transfer,* Boston, 1993, Little, Brown.

103. Robin DA, Somodi LB, Luschei E: *Measurement of tongue strength and endurance in normal and articulation disordered subjects.* In Moore C, Yorkston K, Beukelman DR, editors: *Dysarthria and apraxia of speech: perspectives on management,* Baltimore, 1991, Paul H. Brookes.

104. Robins DW: The anaesthetic management of patients undergoing free flap transfer, *Br J Plast Surg* 36:231, 1983.

105. Saltz R and others: Laparoscopically harvested omental free flap to cover a large soft tissue defect, *Ann Surg* 217:542, 1993.

106. Seidenberg B and others: Immediate reconstruction of the cervical esophagus by a revascularized isolated jejunal segment, *Ann Surg* 149:162, 1959.

107. Serletti JM and others: Comparison of the operating microscope and loupes for free microvascular tissue transfer, *Plast Reconstr Surg* 95(2):270, 1995.

108. Shenaq SM, Klebuc MAJ, Vargo D: Free-tissue transfer with the aid of loupe magnification: experience with 251 procedures, *Plast Reconstr Surg* 95(2):261, 1995.

109. Shestak KC and others: Effect of advanced age and medical disease on the outcome of microvascular reconstruction for head and neck defects, *Head Neck* 14:14, 1992.

110. Schusterman MA and others: A single center's experience with 308 free flaps for repair of head and neck cancer defects, *Plast Reconstr Surg* 93:472, 1994.

111. Sigurdsson GH, Thomson D: Anaesthesia and microvascular surgery: clinical practice and research, *Eur J Anaesthesiol* 12:101, 1995.

112. Sinclair S: The importance of topical heparin in microvascular anastomosis: a study in the rat, *Br J Plast Surg* 33:422, 1980.

113. Snower DP and others: Aeromonas hydrophila infection associated with the use of medicinal leeches, *J Clin Microbiol* 27:1421, 1989.

114. Sonnenfeld T, Cronenstrand R: Pharmacological vasodilation during reconstructive vascular surgery, *Acta Chir Scand* 141:9, 1980.

115. Steed DL: *Basic science review for surgeons.* In Simmons RL, Steed DL, editors: *Basic science review for surgeons,* Philadelphia, 1992, WB Saunders.

116. Stein B, Fuster V: Antithrombotic therapy in acute myocardial infarction: prevention of venous, left ventricular and coronary artery thrombo embolism, *Am J Cardiol* 64:338, 1989.

117. Stern DM and others: Self regulation of procoagulant events on the endothelial cell surface, *J Exp Med* 162(4):1223, 1985.

118. Strauss RG and others: Pentastarch may cause fewer effects on coagulation than hetastarch, *Transfusion* 28:257, 1988.

119. Strome M, Strome S: Laryngeal transplantation: a program for investigating new parameters, *J Voice* 8(1):92, 1994.

120. Sullivan M, Baker S: *Microsurgical reconstruction of the head and neck.* In Baker SR, editor: *Microsurgical reconstruction of the head and neck,* New York, 1989, Churchill Livingstone.

121. Sullivan M, Baker S: *Microvascular surgical technique.* In Baker SR, editor: Microsurgical reconstruction of the head and neck, New York, 1989, Churchill Livingstone.

122. Swartz WM, Banis JC: *Head and neck microsurgery,* Baltimore, 1992, Williams & Wilkins.

123. Szilagyi DE and others: The laws of fluid flow and arterial grafting, *Surgery* 47:55, 1960.

124. Tang J and others: Microarterial anastomosis using a noncontact diode laser versus a control study, *Lasers Surg Med* 14:229, 1994.

125. Taylor GI, Razaboni RM: *Michel Salmon's anatomical studies. Book 1: Arteries of the muscles of the extremities and the trunk,* St Louis, 1994, Quality Medical Publishing.

126. Urken ML and others: Microvascular free flaps in head and neck reconstruction: report of 200 cases and review of complications, *Arch Otolaryngol Head Neck Surg* 120(6):633, 1994.

127. Van Adrichem LN and others: The effect of cigarette smoking on the survival of free vascularized and pedicled epigastric flaps in the rat, *Plast Reconstr Surg* 97:86, 1996.

128. Vance JP, Soutar D: *General anaesthesia for microvascular surgery.* In Soutar DS, editor: *Microvascular surgery and free tissue transfer,* Boston, 1993, Little, Brown.

129. Webster MW, Ramadan F: *Vascular physiology.* In Simmons RL, Steed DL, editors: *Basic science review for surgeons,* Philadelphia, 1992, WB Saunders.

130. Wells MD and others: The medicinal leech: an old treatment revisited, *Microsurgery* 14:183, 1993.

131. Yao ST: Microvascular transplantation of a prefabricated free thigh flap, *Plast Reconstr Surg* 69:568, 1982.

132. Zamboni WA and others: The effect of hyperbaric oxygen on reperfusion of ischemic axial skin flaps: a laser doppler analysis, *Ann Plast Surg* 28(4):339, 1992.

Chapter 10

Wound Healing

Mark T. Brown

Wound healing is a complex, multistep process. It relies on the integration and coordination of many cellular and humoral elements. Many endogenous and exogenous influences, such as radiation, infection, nutrition, systemic factors, and surgical technique, affect this process, and a basic understanding is incumbent on any practicing surgeon.

This chapter focuses on the mechanisms of cutaneous wound healing. Future directions for wound healing research, including growth factor applications, are explored.

MECHANISMS OF WOUND HEALING

Primary injury

The first priority after wounding is the formation of a hemostatic plug composed of platelets and fibrin. Injury to capillary endothelium exposes basement membrane adhesive proteins, collagen, fibronectin, and von Willebrand factor to the flow of blood. These structures stimulate platelets to aggregate.[28] Activated platelets, tissue factor (a membrane protein found on the surface of fibroblasts and macrophages), and other perivascular proteins initiate the clotting cascade.[114] Activated plasma coagulation factors, normally quiescent in the serum, catalyze a sequence of reactions, which ultimately result in fibrin production. These fibrin molecules are polymerized by thrombin on the surface of the aggregated platelets to crosslink and stabilize the hemostatic plug.[28] This coagulum also is the initial framework for wound healing. Early migration of fibroblasts, macrophages, endothelial cells, and epithelial cells depends on the presence of fibrin polymers.[70,114]

Activated platelets in the hemostatic plug release chemotactic factors and arachadonic acid metabolites (e.g., leukotrienes, thromboxanes, and prostaglandins), which attract an inflammatory infiltrate into the wound.[69] The arachadonic acid metabolites also serve as vasoconstrictors to assist with hemostasis.

Platelets also produce growth factors.[24] When released from stores in α granules, these factors have chemotactic properties and modulate the inflammatory infiltrate, which is critical to the first phase of wound healing.

Inflammatory phase

Polymorphonuclear leukocytes (PMN) predominate the population of inflammatory cells initially recruited to the wound. PMNs phagocytose devitalized tissue and bacteria.[70] After 48 hours, the PMN's influence on the wound declines with the influx of monocytes. Circulating monocytes are drawn to the wound by chemotactic factors elaborated by PMNs, platelets, and the clotting cascade. The monocytes, now called *macrophages*, enter the injured tissue and continue débridement of the wound.[69]

Lymphocytes also are present in the inflammatory infiltrate. Although their specific role in the wound healing process is not completely clear,[37] it is known that lymphocytes release macrophage migration inhibition factor and macrophage activating factor.[69] These soluble mediators stimulate macrophages and maintain their presence in the wound.

The inflammatory phase persists for 72 to 96 hours. Eventually, all devitalized debris is removed in preparation for definitive repair of the injury.

Proliferative phase

Shortly after the initial injury, epithelial cells at the wound margin, fibroblasts, and capillary endothelial cells activate metabolically to cover and fill the wound.[69,70] This migration is predicated on the presence of a scaffolding on which the cells can move. The framework, initially made of fibrin polymers, is replaced during the inflammatory and proliferative phases with collagen, hyaluronic acid, fibronectin, and chondroitin sulfate.[25] This lattice, called the *extracellular matrix* (ECM), is derived primarily from fibroblasts.[32,70] Its function goes beyond providing a pathway for cellular migration. The ECM influences chemotaxis of leukocytes, neoangiogenesis, and collagen deposition.[25] In normal, unwounded skin it helps organize the geometry of the tissues.[1]

Macrophages are the central directors of the healing sequence. Because of their ability to tolerate the low tissue oxygen tensions present in the wound dead space, macrophages are able to lead the advancing front of neovascularization and fibroblast proliferation. They elaborate growth factors and coordinate migrations of other cells. Fibroblasts respond with migration and collagen production.[69] The presence of macrophages has a direct effect on neoangeogenesis.[24] Epithelial cells also are stimulated to cover the wound.[69] Granulation tissue is formed as the fibroblasts, capillary endothelial cells, and macrophages migrate together across the wound.[24,70]

These granulation fibroblasts have contractile properties and are termed *myofibroblasts*. They have the functional capacity of smooth muscle as seen by their reaction to histamine, serotonin, bradykinin, epinephrine, norepinephrine, and prostaglandins *in vitro*. By electron microscopy, myofibroblasts and smooth muscle share the presence of contractile proteins.[76] As the wound fills with granulation, myofibroblasts pull the wound edges together, a phenomenon seen clinically as contracture.[33]

Oxygen tension in the wound increases as new blood vessels form and improve circulation. This inhibits fibroblast proliferation but stimulates the production of extracellular collagen.[69,70] During the next 7 to 10 days, the wound fills with collagen and is covered by epithelial cells. The long process of scar maturation then begins.

Maturation phrase

The maturing of a wound is a dynamic process, which can continue for up to 2 years. Over time, macrophage influence decreases as does the vascularity of the healing wound. Myofibroblasts disappear from the wound.[32] Eventually, a relatively avascular collection of extracellular collagen interspersed with fibroblasts remains.

Secreted collagen is a macromolecule that consists of a triple helix of α chains with unique amino acid residues. Glycine represents every third amino acid molecule. There are major extracellular modifications. Proline and lysine residues are enzymatically hydroxylated, which is important for glycosylization reactions, stable crosslinking, and maintenance of the triple helix structure.[71] Initially, immature extracellular collagen (type III) and ground substance (proteoglycans and glycosaminoglycans) dominate the wound. As the maturation proceeds, macrophages release proteases and collagenases, which degrade the immature collagen at the same rate at which it is replaced.[69] Ground substance

decreases, and the wound fills with type I collagen, which characterizes the mature scar. This new collagen is aligned and crosslinked such that strength is maximized (typically 80% that of normal skin).

The overproduction of collagen characterizes hypertrophic scars and keloids.[102] Persistent hypervascularity and inflammation are associated with abnormal arrangements and the accumulation of type III (immature) collagen.[59] Activity of lysyl hydroxylase is increased as compared with normal scars.[71] Clinically, abnormal scar tissue manifests itself in two ways. Hypertrophic scars are large, erythematous, and resolve with steroid injection and time. In contrast, keloids tend to grow beyond the bounds of the wound and are progressive.[59] Their response to steroid and other therapies is variable.[102]

Growth factors

The complex sequence described previously is coordinated to a great extent by growth factors. These soluble polypeptides are elaborated by the inflammatory, mesenchymal, and hematogenous cells involved in the healing process.[57] The term *growth factors* is misleading. These substances, along with the extracellular matrix, control the wound healing process through stimulatory or inhibitory influences, depending on the concentrations and ratios of the factors present.

Cells susceptible to the effects of growth factors have surface receptors specific for these or other homologous substances. The binding of the growth factor to its receptor results in the phosphorylation of intracellular proteins.[29,37] These proteins carry a message to the nucleus by a mechanism, which is not yet elucidated.[29,121] The effect on the genome is to produce a target protein, stimulate cellular proliferation, or both.[121]

The following describes the groups of growth factors that are known to impact on the healing process. Under each major heading are several different substances. The discussion will focus on the properties that generally characterize each group.

Transforming growth factor beta

Transforming growth factor β (TGF-β) is found in all phases of wound healing as a controlling agent for cell differentiation and growth.[30] Platelets contain this factor in α granules, which are released at adhesion and activation during hemostasis. At this stage, TGF-β is chemotactic to macrophages and stimulates their production and elaboration of other growth factors.[26] During the proliferative phase, TGF-β controls and coordinates neovascularization and mesenchymal cell proliferation.[58] Fibroblasts are stimulated to produce ECM and collagen.[26] Myofibroblasts produce α smooth muscle actin.[31] Neoangiogenesis is enhanced.[26] Finally, epidermal cells are stimulated to migrate but not to replicate.[70] Thus, TGF-β is central to many aspects of the wound healing process.

Epidermal growth factors

Epidermal growth factors (EGFs) are found in platelets and macrophages.[26] They have chemotactic properties and stimulate proliferation of keratinocytes.[58] In epithelial cell culture[70] and in a skin explant model,[11] topical application enhances epidermal growth and metabolism. There also is activity in the stimulation of fibroplasia, neovascularization, and granulation tissue formation.[25,26]

Fibroblast growth factors

Fibroblast growth factors (FGF) have wide-ranging activity in the healing wound. Basic FGF is primarily produced by activated macrophages.[25] It also is stored in the ECM and released on injury.[58] Despite the name, it is one of the most potent angiogenesis stimulators. In response to FGF, endothelial cells release digestive enzymes and migrate through the ECM.

Another member of this family, keratinocyte growth factor (KGF) has a specific effect on epidermal cells. Produced by fibroblasts lacking receptors for KGF, it stimulates keratinocytes to divide.[129] When applied experimentally to partial and full-thickness wounds, epidermal coverage is quicker as compared with controls.[119]

Platelet-derived growth factors

Platelets, macrophages, fibroblasts, and endothelial cells produce platelet-derived growth factors (PDGF),[121] which are active during the inflammatory phase, stimulating leukocyte degranulation and phagocytosis. In the proliferative phase, PDGF stimulates fibroblasts to divide, migrate, and produce collagen. Epithelial and endothelial cells also are activated by this factor.[26] Finally, wound contraction is enhanced by stimulation of myofibroblasts.[25] Thus, PDGF has wide-ranging effects on the healing process.

Insulin-like growth factors

Insulin-like growth factors (IGF) are unique relative to the other growth factors mentioned because significant levels of IGFs circulate in the plasma. Binding proteins, with which the IGFs are associated, enhance the activity of the IGFs systemically[27] and locally in wound healing.[68,74] Activated platelet granules release IGF into the wound. Endothelial cells, for which the IGFs are mitogenic,[58] and fibroblasts[122] also produce IGF locally.[124] There is some evidence that these peptides potentiate the activity of PDGFs.[120]

Interleukins

The interleukins (IL) are a group of peptides that were originally described as modulators of the immune system. Evidence now exists that ILs play an active role in acute inflammation.[26] Macrophages produce IL-1,[69] which enhances fibroblast deposition of ECM deposition in the proliferative phase and collagen production and remodeling in the maturation phase.[26] IL-6 is thought to moderate epithelial migration.[90]

Thus, growth factors are a diverse and varied group of substances, which impact on the healing process. As more is learned about the mechanisms of action and interactions of these peptides, the intricacies of the healing process and how it can be manipulated will be uncovered.

INTRINSIC FACTORS AFFECTING WOUND HEALING

Nutrition

The association between good nutrition and successful wound healing is well established.[47] Unfortunately, in the head and neck cancer patient population, some degree of malnutrition is common.[18] Many of these patients have dysphagia and odynophagia, which precludes adequate oral intake. This deficit is compounded by the cachexia often associated with malignancy. Evidence suggests that patients with malignancy have altered metabolism[78] and even malabsorption.[47] Therefore, it is imperative that the surgeon be cognizant of this issue and attempt to correct nutritional deficits.

Assessment of the patient's metabolic status is easily accomplished using serum indicators. Albumin, transferrin, and hemoglobin are easily obtainable and are consistently decreased in patients with nutritional deficits. Elevated red cell volumes are reliable indicators of folate or B_{12} deficiencies. Finally, the total lymphocyte count is a sensitive indicator of protein malnutrition.[93] More elaborate tests of body mass and adipose content are available[47] but less convenient for most clinicians.

Several major nutritional components are required for wound healing. Adequate protein, lipids, carbohydrates, vitamin C, and vitamin A are necessary for the healing sequence to proceed appropriately. The use of supplemental zinc and other trace metals to enhance wound healing in well-nourished patients is controversial.

Protein undernutrition is common in alcoholic patients as a result of poor diet. These patients have limited availability of amino acid building blocks for angiogenesis, collagen production, and wound contraction.[93] Additionally, protein-calorie malnutrition increases complications in hospitalized patients.[81]

Carbohydrate and lipid deficiencies are less common than protein malnutrition. Thus, severe energy deficiency associated with clinical starvation is rare, although tumors clearly act as ''glucose drains.'' Study of glucose use and insulin levels show that glucose consumption occurs at a greater rate than would be predicted based on metabolic state in cancer patients.[21]

Vitamin C is necessary for the hydroxylation of proline residues in collagen synthesis.[93] Ascorbic acid deficiency decreases production of collagen and results in poor wound healing.[130] This is quickly reversed with supplementation.

Vitamin A plays a major role in the synthesis of glycoproteins. As these molecules are found in every cell, the importance of adequate dietary supplementation is obvious.[130] Hypovitaminosis A impairs collagen synthesis, increases wound infections, and delays epithelialization.[93]

Zinc is a trace element that acts as a cellular and organelle membrane stabilizer and is widely distributed throughout the body.[19] Zinc is particularly important to tissues with high cellular turnover.[38] As a result, deficiency is associated with healing difficulties, dermatitis, and alopecia.[123] Dietary supplementation is needed for deficient patients only.[19] Topical application of zinc oxide may be useful. Experimental studies show that zinc oxide induces insulin-like growth factor-1 messenger ribonucleic acid (mRNA), which supports the healing process.[123]

Nutrition supplementation to improve wound healing in the postoperative or trauma patient enjoys scientific support. Experimentally, parenteral and enteral nutrition after surgical intervention improves wound breaking strength and decreases postoperative weight loss.[61,133] Prospective human studies in trauma patients support this notion. Immediate institution of enteral feeding improves nitrogen balance and decreases infectious complications.[86]

Adequate nutrition is vital to any patient with a healing wound. In patients undergoing head and neck surgery, the prevalence of malnutrition requires the clinician to maintain a high index of suspicion and supplement the patient aggressively. This strategy will reduce the incidence of complications.

Diabetes mellitus

Increased serum glucose has a major impact on wound healing. This is likely a multifactorial process because hyperglycemia causes many deleterious effects on molecular and cellular physiology.

Although traditional teaching is that the etiology of diabetic complications is microvascular occlusive disease, recent research does not support this.[36] Several defects that may influence the healing process are now known. Sorbitol, a toxic by-product of glucose metabolism, accumulates in tissues and is implicated in many of the renal, ocular, and vascular complications associated with diabetes.[42] Increased dermal vascular permeability results in pericapillary albumin deposition, which impairs the diffusion of oxygen and nutrients.[37] Hyperglycemia-associated nonenzymatic glycosylation inhibits the function of structural and enzymatic proteins.[92] Additionally, glycosylated collagen is resistant to enzymatic degradation and less soluble than the normal protein product.[42]

Experimental studies of diabetic animal models and wound healing show decreased granulation, decreased collagen in granulation tissue, and defects in collagen maturation.[132] Human studies of healing in diabetic patients parallel these findings, showing slow wound maturation and decreased numbers of dermal fibroblasts.[92]

Growth factor abnormalities also are shown in recent studies. Wounds in diabetic rats have decreased amounts of acidic and basic FGF and KGF.[128] The application of FGFs[84]

and PDGFs[3] to wounds in diabetic animal models has shown promise, although human trials have not produced consistently good results.[101]

Clinically, the diabetic patient requires special attention. Perioperatively, it is critical to meticulously control blood glucose levels.[106] Currently, this is the only tool that the surgeon has to impact on the wound healing process in these patients. As further research defines the specific healing deficits, growth factor manipulation may offer improved outcomes for these patients.

Genetic disease

Heritable disorders of collagen tissue impair wound healing. Ehlers-Danlos and Menkes' kinky hair syndromes represent this type of genetic defect. Cutis laxa and osteogenesis imperfecta also may be categorized in this group.[59,97]

There are multiple genotypes of the Ehlers-Danlos syndrome. Some forms are a result of mutations in type I or type III procollagen genes. Others are the result of defects in the copper enzyme lysyl hydroxylase.[97] The type of inheritance also is broad; autosomal dominant, autosomal recessive, and X-linked recessive patterns are seen.[59] Ultrastructural study of dermal fibroblasts from a patient with Ehlers-Danlos reveals decreased amounts of endoplasmic reticulum and ribosomes.[113] This indicates a lack of protein production capacity. Clinically, the skin is fragile, hyperextendable, and scars poorly. Some subtypes are prone to hemorrhage as a result of friable perivascular connective tissue.[7,50]

Menke's kinky hair syndrome is similar phenotypically to the Elhers-Danlos syndrome. The metabolic defect is localized to the inability to properly metabolize copper. The functional deficiency of this essential trace element results in dysfunctional lysyl hydroxylase and in poor stability of crosslinked collagen.[2,71,111]

Recognition of these patients preoperatively is vital. Preparation for intraoperative bleeding and generally poor cosmetic results should be made before any surgical intervention.

Hypothyroidism

The incidence of hypothyroidism in head and neck cancer patients after treatment is high because of the effects of radiation and surgery on the gland itself. Experimental data and anecdotal series support delayed wound healing in the head and neck.[4,41] Rats pharmacologically rendered hypothyroid have decreased collagen production as measured by extractable soluble hydroxyproline levels.[73] Hypothyroidism also significantly decreases wound tensile strength in rats.[77] Irradiation of hypothyroid pigs results in poor healing.[22] These studies indicate the deleterious effect of inadequate thyroid hormone levels on fibroblast function and subsequent wound strength. Compounding these local effects are the systemic complications (i.e., higher risk of heart failure, intraoperative hypotension risk, neuropsychiatric disturbances, lack of postoperative fever) for which the postoperative hypothyroid patient is at risk.[75] Thus, vigilance in seeking out thyroid deficiency is important to ensure against inadequate healing and systemic complications. This is particularly true in patients who have previously undergone treatment for head and neck malignancies.

Age

It is well accepted that aging patients have higher rates of complications and mortality than do younger persons undergoing major head and neck surgery.[82] It also is widely accepted that the elderly population heals more slowly than younger patients.[45,126] This information should be balanced with the fact that older patients generally have more comorbidities than younger patients. Coronary artery disease, peripheral vascular disease, diabetes, and pulmonary compromise are more common with aging and may affect the healing process independent of age.

Experimental studies show that the inflammatory and proliferative phases are less efficient in older animals, particularly compared with very young subjects.[126] Longitudinal study of hamster fibroblast cultures over the span of the animal's life show progressively decreasing proliferative capacity over time.[17] Studies of healthy human volunteers do not completely support these findings. Skin graft donor sites have slower reepithelialization rates in older persons, although the deposition of dermal collagen is equivalent between young and older, otherwise healthy, volunteers. The fact that proteins other than collagen are less abundant in older subjects' wounds may indicate age-related differences in the production of the extracellular matrix.[55] In another clinical study, wound transudate collected from occlusive dressings over skin graft donor sites from patients aged more than 55 years have significantly decreased concentrations of TGF-α and IL-1.[94] However, cultured human fibroblasts subjected to the cytokines (EGF, tumor necrosis factor-α, PDGF, fetal bovine serum) respond with equivalent mitogenic response and collagen synthesis regardless of patient age. These findings suggest that the defect in age-related wound healing is related to abnormal initiation of healing as a result of insufficient presence of growth factors.[43] Future research aimed at identifying the imbalance and normalizing the growth factor profile may dramatically improve our ability to improve our surgical care of older patients.

EXTRINSIC FACTORS AFFECTING WOUND HEALING

Infection

It is intuitive that infection is disruptive to the healing process. Bacteria use oxygen and nutrients and lower tissue pH through anaerobic metabolism. The cellular inflammatory response is prolonged, especially because of complement activation. Increased local tissue destruction results. Additionally, bacteria release toxins that directly injure the

cells, thus inhibiting their function and prolonging the healing process.[99] Thus, the avoidance of postoperative infection is critical. Perioperative antibiotic therapy to prevent infection in those undergoing head and neck surgery is successful,[110] although the appropriate agents, dosages, and length of use are still subject to debate.

Head and neck oncologic surgeries that require skin and mucosal incisions are considered to be clean contaminated. In this setting, the use of antibiotics against oral flora is appropriate.[66] Some authors suggest the use of topical rinses to reduce oral bacterial flora and to potentially decrease the inevitable contamination of the neck intraoperatively.[98] However, this effect can be accomplished either topically[98] or systemically.[48]

The recommended length of antibiotic prophylaxis is 24 hours, as determined by prospective randomized trials. With appropriate antibiotic selection, 1-day coverage is as effective as 2-[39] or 5-[64,65] day coverage. This is not universally practiced. Some maintain antibiotic coverage until all drains are removed[46] with similar infection rates.

Smoking

Clinically, the association between smoking and wound healing difficulties is clear. Cigarette smoke contains thousands of toxic substances, some of which directly impact on delayed wound closure. Nicotine is an addictive and vasoconstrictive substance that decreases proliferation of erythrocytes, macrophages, and fibroblasts. Hydrogen cyanide is inhibitory to oxidative metabolism enzymes. Carbon monoxide decreases the oxygen-carrying capacity of hemoglobin by competitively inhibiting oxygen binding.[117] These are shown in a study of human volunteers whose subcutaneous Po_2 decreased significantly after 10 minutes of cigarette smoking. The effect lasted almost 1 hour.[63] Taken together, this triad has obvious implications for the reduction of the cellular response and efficiency of the healing process.

This effect is shown clearly in clinic reports. The healing of oral wounds after bone grafting is suboptimal in patients who smoke.[67] Smoking affects the cosmetic appearance of wounds,[116] which has serious ramifications for the smoker who desires facial cosmetic surgery. Abstinence from smoking should be observed for at least 48 hours preoperatively.[106]

Corticosteroids

Antiinflammatory steroid medications globally inhibit cell growth and production.[96] They also are well known to have widespread negative effects on the wound healing process. This is seen clinically and experimentally.

A decreased inflammatory infiltrate is the most obvious impact of steroids.[122] The macrophage response to chemotactic factors is inhibited. Effective phagocytosis by PMNs and macrophages also is decreased as a result of the stabilizing effect of steroids on lysosomes.[34] Because of the lack of an appropriate initial inflammatory response, these cells do not produce the typical growth factor profile.[13] This has been shown experimentally. Insulin-like growth factor-1 is decreased in a rat model of steroid-inhibited wound healing, although application of exogenous IGF-1 locally on the wound reverses the effect.[122]

Glucocorticoids also inhibit epithelial regeneration. KGF levels decrease in corticosteroid-treated mice as a result of a direct effect on the mesenchymal cells, which produce KGF.[13] The application of hydrocortisone to epidermal cultures decreases cell proliferation. Use of topical TGF-α decreases this effect.[23]

Steroids have a direct inhibitory effect on the fibroblast genome, which is shown in cell culture.[13,96] Ultrastructurally, corticosteroid-treated rat fibroblasts have minimal endoplasmic reticulum, indicating a low-secretory state.[6] Without the appropriate deposition and maturation of collagen, wound strength is less, and wound dehiscence is likely. Vitamin A supplementation reverses steroid disruption of normal wound healing.[106]

Surgery on steroid-treated patients should be approached with caution. Complications in these patients should be anticipated and managed expectantly.

Ionizing radiation and chemotherapy

Many procedures in otolaryngology—head and neck surgery are performed on previously radiated tissue. Although it is obvious to most practitioners that radiation slows healing, the specific mechanisms of this inhibition are still being explored.

Ionizing radiation either directly damages the genome or it injures the DNA through the production of free radicals.[35] This effect has short- and long-term consequences for radiated tissue.

In patients with acute radiation injury, the skin becomes erythematous and edematous. Histologically, dilation of fine blood vessels, endothelial edema, and lymphatic obliteration are seen. As the acute response abates, thrombosis and fibrinoid necrosis of capillaries occur.[9] In this setting, although perfusion of radiation-damaged skin is seen with fluorescein injection,[106] effective tissue oxygenation is inadequate. Blood vessel appearance is varied: thick-walled, telangectatic, or thrombosed. The deposition of dense, hyalinized collagen characterizes radiated dermis. The endpoint of chronic radiation damage is the nonhealing ulcer. Obvious necrotic tissue is seen, and there is loss of epithelial coverage.[105,107] Electron microscopy of human radiation ulcers reveals varying degrees of vascular injury and few myofibroblasts.[105]

The mechanisms of radiation damage and inhibited wound healing are currently being studied. Experimentally, healing immediately after irradiation is hampered by slowed fibroblast proliferation, migration, and contraction.[127,131] Impairment of the acute inflammatory response and granulation formation also occurs.[9,127] The production of mRNA coding for collagen is delayed up to 2 weeks.[8] Clinically, few surgeries are performed on patients with acutely radiated tissues. The greater concern lies with the patient who has chronic radiation damage.

Cultures of fibroblasts from radiation ulcers proliferate at a slower rate compared with those cells from nearby unirradiated tissue.[108] Effects vary between patients. Each person has a differing sensitivity to radiation injury. Human fibroblasts cultured from patients with severe radiation reactions have poor survival rates relative to those from patients who have a less severe injury.[118] Thus, fibroblast defects have emerged as a central problem in the inhibited healing of chronic radiation injury.

Cellular mechanisms of phagocytosis and bacteriocidal metabolic functions in PMNs harvested from tissue with chronic radiation damage also are impaired. The effect increases as time passes after therapy, which cannot be a result of a direct effect of radiation on the neutrophils because their life span is too short. The local wound environment is the locus of the problem. Irradiated tissue may not ''prime'' the neutrophils with the appropriate cytokines and growth factors needed for activation,[44] which has a major impact on the incidence of postoperative infection in previously irradiated patients.

The association between radiation damage and postoperative complications is debated. In retrospective studies, patients undergoing surgery after failing primary radiotherapy for early staged tumors do not show an increase in severity of complications or length of hospital stay.[79,80] One prospective trial comparing antibiotic regimens did not show any increase in wound infection rate in radiated patients,[65] although other investigators have shown increased rates of postoperative infections[5] and major wound complications.[46]

With the advent of more aggressive radiation regimens, concern regarding increased operative complications has surfaced. Twice-a-day hyperfractionation protocols versus once-a-day radiation do not seem to increase the surgical morbidity.[85]

Chemotherapy now is included in many ''organ-preservation'' protocols in an attempt to cure patients with head and neck cancer without disfiguring or functionally devastating surgery. If given perioperatively, the resultant bone marrow suppression inhibits the formation of an adequate inflammatory response needed for the initiation of the healing process.[35] Experimental studies show the inhibition of fibroblast collagen production[53] and a decreased ability to fight off wound infection[5] with the application of antineoplastic agents. These effects appear to be transient as opposed to the progressive nature of radiation damage. The combination of radiation and chemotherapy increases the risk of serious postoperative complications.[95] This risk appears to decrease if surgery is delayed for more than 1 year.[112]

Surgery for patients with previous radiotherapy should be approached cautiously. Nutritional status and thyroid functions are important parameters to maximize preoperatively. Careful surgical planning and avoidance of tight closures are paramount. However, in patients with wound healing problems (i.e., pharyngocutaneous fistula, open granulating wound), the use of postoperative radiotherapy is not contraindicated. Healing proceeds despite the radiation effects.[62] Experimental studies in the use of exogenously applied growth factor (namely TGF-β) have shown improved wound tensile strength and collagen deposition in acute[30] and chronic[88] radiation models.

Surgical technique and wound care

The influence of the physician on the healing of a surgical wound begins preoperatively. It is imperative to identify all conditions potentially detrimental to the healing process. Correction of metabolic abnormalities (i.e., diabetes, hypothyroidism, malnutrition) and curbing alcohol intake and smoking are critical to improving healing and to avoiding local and systemic complications. Intraoperatively, the appropriate use of prophylactic antibiotics decreases the incidence of infection. Preparing the skin with a disinfectant is effective.[15]

Gentle handling of tissues and dissection techniques that do not devitalize tissue improve the healing outcome. Once the procedure is completed, there are a large number of suture materials available for wound closure. The choice of a nonreactive suture that is quickly removed or degraded results in the least inflammation and disruption of the healing progression. A discussion of this topic is beyond the scope of this chapter. A detailed review is listed in the reference list.[100]

The avoidance of tension in suturing of the wound is critical to cosmetic result. Increased closing tension is associated with depressed and hypertrophic scars,[106] although increased tension results in improved tensile strength experimentally. As the closing tension increases, the strength and width of the wound increase dramatically.[87]

There are many dressings and topical preparations used to protect the wound and to enhance the healing environment after closure. Experimentally, topical antibiotics are capable of improving the rate of healing. Mupirocin, bacitracin, and neosporin are associated with enhanced reepithelialization and granulation formation.[15] The effectiveness of most cleaning and dressing agents is associated with side effects, and they should be used with care.[99]

Finally, hyperbaric oxygen has found use in patients with healing difficulties related to poor oxygen delivery. Experimentally, normal and ischemic tissues have improved wound healing under 100% oxygen applied at two atmospheres.[125] Clinically, nonhealing ulcers close at a faster rate with oxygen supplied at an increased pressure versus air delivered the same way.[51] Hyperbaric oxygen also increases osseointegration of titanium implants for bone-anchored prostheses in previously radiated patients.[49]

The use of hyperbaric oxygen in cancer patients increases the concern of potentiation of residual tumor by management. This effect is not yet consistently shown in experimen-

tal models. One study shows the inhibition of tumor induction, but tumor growth stimulation occurs once the cancer is established.[83] Another study of xenograft tumor implantation fails to show any effect by the hyperbaric oxygen on tumor growth.[52] Thus, hyperbaric oxygen should be used with caution, and there should be a heightened suspicion for recurrence until further information is available.

THE FUTURE OF WOUND HEALING

Fetal wound healing

As research in prenatal surgery has progressed, interest in the phenomenon of scarless fetal wound healing has grown. Although confirmation of the "scarless" part of this process is still questioned by some,[60] the evidence continues to accumulate regarding the differences between pre- and postnatal healing.

In the fetal sheep model, wounding the animal *in utero* results in a different response to injury as compared with the adult animal. There is almost no inflammatory response if the injury occurs early enough in gestation.[1] Collagen deposition is highly organized and resembles normal dermis. Neovascularization and endothelial proliferation are absent, and epithelialization is rapid. The regenerated epidermis has a structure that is identical to uninjured skin.[14]

There is intense interest in unraveling the differences between adult and fetal healing mechanisms. The ECM, collagen deposition, growth factor profile, and the responses of immature fibroblasts are implicated as playing some part in the phenomenon.[1,40] The balance of growth factors is different in the prenatal injury versus in the adult. In particular, TGF-β and PDGF, both of which induce adult scarring patterns in the fetal model, are mostly absent in the fetal wound.[14] In support of this observation is the report of decreased scar formation in adult rats with the application of anti-TGF-β antibodies.[115]

Human clinical trials of growth factor application

The importance of growth factors to the healing process is apparent. The availability of these substances in therapeutic quantities allows the design of clinical randomized, prospective, blinded trials. Most of the current studies are conducted in industry, although those trials presented in the scientific literature show promise.

The rate of healing of split-thickness skin graft donor sites improved by 1.5 days with the application of topical epidermal growth factor. Punch biopsies from the healing wounds show increased thickness and maturity of the epithelium versus controls.[16] Application of a preparation of autologously harvested platelet preparation containing at least five different platelet-derived growth factors increases the rate of healing of chronic ulcerations on lower extremities.[72] However, topical basic FGF alone has not shown improvement in healing diabetic ulcers.[101] Finally, placental angiogenic and growth factors applied to venous stasis ulcers speed the appearance of granulation after wound care in preparation for skin grafting.[20] Although promising, all of these trials are small and await validation.

The improvement of cosmetic scars in those undergoing facial plastic surgery is a focus of the development of growth factor applications. The daunting problem of healing the radiated patient may provide fertile ground for the use of these technologies. However, appropriate fears exist regarding the possible potentiation of microscopic tumor residue by the application of growth factors.[54]

REFERENCES

1. Adzick NS, Lorenz HP: Cells, matrix, growth factors, and the surgeon, *Ann Surg* 220:10, 1994.
2. Al-Qattan MM, Thomson HG: Menkes' syndrome: wound healing in a long-term survivor, *Ann Plast Surg* 32:550, 1993.
3. Albertson S and others: PDGF and FGF reverse the healing impairment in protein-malnourished diabetic mice, *Surgery* 114:368, 1993.
4. Alexander MV, Zajtchuk JT, Henderson RL: Hypothyroidism and wound healing, *Arch Otolaryngol* 108:289, 1982.
5. Ariyan S, Kraft RL, Goldberg NH: An experimental model to determine the effects of adjuvant therapy on the incidence of postoperative wound infection: II. Evaluating preoperative chemotherapy, *Plast Reconst Surg* 65:338, 1980.
6. Beck LS and others: One systemic administration of transforming growth factor-β1 reverses age- or glucocorticoid-impaired wound healing, *J Clin Invest* 92:2841, 1993.
7. Beighton P, Horan FT: Surgical aspects of the Ehlers-Danlos syndrome, *Br J Surg* 56:255, 1969.
8. Bernstein EF and others: Healing impairment of open wounds by skin irradiation, *J Dermatol Surg Oncol* 20:757, 1994.
9. Bernstein EF and others: Collagen gene expression and wound strength in normal and radiation-impaired wound healing, *J Dermatol Surg Oncol* 19:564, 1993.
10. Reference deleted in pages.
11. Bhora FY and others: Effect of growth factors on cell proliferation and epithelialization in human skin, *J Surg Res* 59:236, 1995.
12. Reference deleted in pages.
13. Brauchle M, Fassler R, Werner S: Suppression of keratinocyte growth factor expression by glucocorticoids in vitro and during wound healing, *J Invest Dermatol* 105:579, 1995.
14. Broker BJ, Reiter D: Fetal wound healing, *Otolaryngol Head Neck Surg* 110:547, 1994.
15. Brown CD, Zitelli JA: A review of topical agents for wounds and methods of wounding, *J Dermatol Surg Oncol* 19:732, 1993.
16. Brown GL and others: Enhancement of wound healing by topical treatment with epidermal growth factor, *N Engl J Med* 321:76, 1989.
17. Bruce SA, Deamond SF: Longitudinal study of in vivo wound repair and in vitro cellular senescence of dermal fibroblasts, *Exp Gerontol* 26:17, 1991.
18. Bumpous JM, Johnson JT: The infected wound and its management, *Otolaryngol Clin North Am* 28:987, 1995.
19. Burch RE, Sullivan JF: Clinical and nutritional aspects of zinc deficiency and excess, *Med Clin North Am* 60:675, 1976.
20. Reference deleted in pages.
21. Byerley LO and others: Insulin action and metabolism in patient with head and neck cancer, *Cancer* 67:2900, 1991.
22. Cannon CR: Hypothyroidism in head and neck cancer patients: experimental and clinical observations, *Laryngoscope* 104:1, 1994.
23. Chernoff EAG, Robertson S: Epidermal growth factor and the onset of epithelial epidermal wound healing, *Tissue Cell* 22:123, 1990.
24. Clark RAF: Basics of cutaneous wound repair, *J Dermatol Surg Oncol* 19:693, 1993.
25. Clark RAF: Biology of dermal wound repair, *Derm Clin* 11:647, 1993.
26. Cohen IK, Bettinger D: Pharmacologic enhancement of chronic wounds, *Adv Plast Reconstr Surg* 11:151, 1995.
27. Cohick WS, Clemmons DR: The insulin-like growth factors, *Annu Rev Physiol* 55:131, 1993.
28. Coleman RW and others: *Plasma coagulation factors*. In Coleman RW and others, editors: *Hemostasis and thrombosis*, ed 3, Philadelphia, 1994, JB Lippincott.
29. Cox DA: Transforming growth factor-beta 3, *Cell Biol Int* 19:357, 1995.
30. Cromack DT and others: Acceleration of tissue repair by transforming growth factor β_1: identification of in vivo mechanism of action with radiotherapy-induced specific healing deficits, *Surgery* 113:36, 1993.
31. Desmouliere A, Gabbiani G: Modulation of fibroblastic cytoskeletal features during pathological situations: the role of extracellular matrix and cytokines, *Cell Motility Cytoskeleton* 29:129, 1994.
32. Desmouliere A: Factors influencing myofibroblast differentiation during wound healing and fibrosis, *Cell Biol Int* 19:471, 1996.
33. Diwan R and others: Secondary intention healing, *Arch Otolaryngol Head Neck Surg* 115:1248, 1989.
34. Dostal GH, Gambrell RL: The differential effect of corticosteroids on wound disruption strength in mice, *Arch Surg* 125:636, 1990.
35. Drake DB, Oishi SN: Wound healing considerations in chemotherapy and radiation therapy, *Clin Plast Surg* 22:31, 1995.
36. Falanga V: Chronic wounds: pathophysiologic and experimental considerations, *J Invest Dermatol* 100:721, 1993.
37. Falanga V: Growth factors and wound healing, *Derm Clin* 11:667, 1993.
38. Falchuk KH: *Disturbances in trace element metabolism*. In Isselbacher KJ and others, editors: *Harrison's principles of internal medicine*, New York, 1994, McGraw-Hill.
39. Fee WE and others: One day vs. two days of prophylactic antibiotics in patients undergoing major head and neck surgery, *Laryngoscope* 94:612, 1984.
40. Ferguson MWJ and others: Scar formation: the spectral natural of fetal and adult wound repair, *Plast Reconst Surg* 97:854, 1996.
41. Finkelstein Y, Talmi YP, Zohar Y: Pharyngeal fistulas in postoperative hypothyroid patients, *Ann Otol Rhinol Laryngol* 98:267, 1989.
42. Foster DW: *Diabetes mellitus*. In Isselbacher KJ and others, editors: *Harrison's principles of internal medicine*, New York, 1994, McGraw-Hill.
43. Freedland M and others: Fibroblast responses to cytokines are maintained during aging, *Ann Plast Surg* 35:290, 1995.
44. Gabka CJ and others: An experimental model to determine the effect of irradiated tissue on neutrophil function, *Plast Reconstr Surg* 96:1676, 1995.
45. Gerstein AD and others: Wound healing and aging, *Dermatol Clin* 11:749, 1993.
46. Girod DA and others: Risk factors for complications in clean-contaminated head and neck surgical procedures, *Head Neck* 17:7, 1995.
47. Goodwin WJ, Byers PM: Nutritional management of the head and neck cancer patient, *Med Clin North Am* 77:597, 1993.
48. Grandis JR and others: Efficacy of topical amoxicillin plus clavulanate/ticarcillin plus clavulanate and clindamycin in contaminated head and neck surgery: effect antibiotic spectra and duration of therapy, *J Infect Dis* 170:729, 1994.
49. Granstrom G and others: Bone-anchored reconstruction of the irradiated head and neck cancer patient, *Otolaryngol Head Neck Surg* 108:334, 1993.
50. Guerrerosantos J, Dicksheet S: Cervicofacial rhytidoplasty in Ehler-Danlos syndrome: hazards on healing, *Plast Reconst Surg* 75:100, 1985.
51. Hammarluned C, Sundberg T: Hyperbaric oxygen reduced size of chronic leg ulcers: a randomized double-blind study, *Plast Reconst Surg* 93:829, 1994.
52. Headley DB and others: The effect of hyperbaric oxygen on growth of

human squamous cell carcinoma xenografts, *Arch Otolaryngol Head Neck Surg* 117:1269, 1991.

53. Hendriks T and others: Inhibition of basal and TGFβ-induced fibroblast collagen synthesis by antineoplastic agents, implications for wound healing, *Br J Cancer* 67:545, 1993.

54. Herndon DN and others: Growth hormones and factors in surgical patients, *Adv Surg* 25:65, 1992.

55. Holt DR and others: Effect of age on wound healing in healthy human beings, *Surgery* 112:293, 1992.

56. Reference deleted in pages.

57. Hom DB: Growth factors and wound healing in otolaryngology, *Otolaryngol Head Neck Surg* 110:560, 1994.

58. Hom DB: Growth factors in wound healing, *Otolaryngol Clin North Am* 28:933, 1995.

59. Hunt TK: Disorders of wound healing, *World J Surg* 4:271, 1980.

60. Hurley JV: Inflammation and repair in the mammalian fetus: a reappraisal, *Microsurgery* 15:811, 1994.

61. Irvin TT: Effects of malnutrition and hyperalimentation of wound healing, *Surg Gynecol Obstet* 146:33, 1978.

62. Issacs JH and others: Postoperative radiation of open head and neck wounds, *Laryngoscope* 97:267, 1987.

63. Jensen JA, Goodson WH, Hunt TK: Cigarette smoking decreases tissue oxygen, *Arch Surg* 126:1131, 1991.

64. Johnson JT and others: Antimicrobial prophylaxis for contaminated head and neck surgery, *Laryngoscope* 94:46, 1984.

65. Johnson JT and others: Antibiotic prophylaxis in high-risk head and neck surgery: one-day vs. five-day therapy, *Otolaryngol Head Neck Surg* 95:554, 1986.

66. Johnson JT and others: Prophylactic antibiotics for head and neck surgery with flap reconstruction, *Arch Otolaryngol Head Neck Surg* 118:488, 1992.

67. Jones JK, Triplett RG: The relationship of cigarette smoking to impaired intraoral wound healing, *J Oral Maxillofac Surg* 50:237, 1992.

68. Jyung RW and others: Increased wound-breaking strength induced by insulin-like growth factor I in combination with insulin-like growth factor binding protein-1, *Surgery* 115:233, 1994.

69. Kanzler MH, Gorsulowsky DC, Swanson NA: Basic mechanisms in the healing cutaneous wound, *J Dermatol Surg Oncol* 12:1156, 1986.

70. Kirsner RS, Eaglstein WH: The wound healing process, *Derm Clin* 11:629, 1993.

71. Kivirikko KI, Risteli L: Biosynthesis of collagen and its alterations in pathological states, *Med Biol* 54:159, 1976.

72. Knighton DR and others: Stimulation of repair in chronic, nonhealing, cutaneous ulcers using platelet-derived wound healing formula, *Surg Gynecol Obstet* 170:56, 1990.

73. Kowalewski K, Young S: Hydroxyproline in healing dermal wounds of normal and hypothyroid rats, *Acta Endocrinol* 54:1, 1967.

74. Kratz G, Lake M, Kratz G: Insulin like growth factor-1 and -2 and their role in the reepithelialization of wounds: interactions with insulin like growth factor binding protein type 1, *Scand J Plast Reconstr Hand Surg* 28:107, 1994.

75. Ladenson PW and others: Complications of surgery in hypothyroid patients, *Am J Med* 77:261, 1984.

76. Larrabee WF, Bolen JW, Sutton D: Myofibroblasts in head and neck surgery, an experimental and clinical study, *Arch Otolaryngol Head Neck Surg* 114:982, 1988.

77. Lennox J, Johnston ID: The effect of thyroid status on nitrogen balance and the rate of wound healing after injury in rats, *Br J Surg* 60:309, 1973.

78. Linn BS, Robinson DS, Klimas NG: Effects of age and nutritional status on surgical outcomes in head and neck cancer, *Ann Surg* 207:267, 1988.

79. Marcial VA and others: Does preoperative irradiation increase the rate of surgical complications in carcinoma of the head and neck? *Cancer* 49:1297, 1982.

80. Marcial VA and others: Tolerance of surgery after radical radiotherapy of carcinoma of the oropharynx, *Cancer* 46:1910, 1980.

81. Mason JB, Rosenberg IH: *Protein-energy malnutrition.* In Isselbacher KJ and others, editors: *Harrison's principles of internal medicine*, New York, 1994, McGraw-Hill.

82. McGuirt WF and others: The risks of major head and neck surgery in the aged population, *Laryngoscope* 87:1378, 1977.

83. McMillan T and others: The effect of hyperbaric oxygen therapy of oral mucosal carcinoma, *Laryngoscope* 99:241, 1989.

84. Mellin TN and others: Acidic fibroblast growth factor accelerates dermal wound healing in diabetic mice, *J Invest Dermatol* 104:850, 1995.

85. Metson R, Freehling DJ, Wang CC: Surgical complications following twice-a-day versus once-a-day radiation therapy, *Laryngoscope* 98:30, 1988.

86. Moore EE, Jones TN: Benefits of immediate jejunostomy feeding after major abdominal trauma—a prospective, randomized study, *J Trauma* 26:874, 1986.

87. Morrin G and others: Wound healing: relationship of closing tension to tensile strength in rats, *Laryngoscope* 99:783, 1989.

88. Nall AV and others: Transforming growth factor β_1 improves wound healing and random flap survival in normal and irradiated rats, *Arch Otolaryngol Head Neck Surg* 122:171, 1996.

89. Reference deleted in pages.

90. Nishida T and others: Interleukin 6 promotes epithelial migration by a fibronectin-dependent mechanism, *J Cell Physiol* 153:1, 1992.

91. Nowak R: Moving developmental research into the clinic, *Science* 266:567, 1994.

92. Reference deleted in pages.

93. Ondrey FG, Hom DB: Effects of nutrition on wound healing, *Otolaryngol Head Neck Surg* 110:557, 1994.

94. Ono I and others: Evaluation of cytokines in donor site wound fluids, *Scand J Plast Reconstr Hand Surg* 28:269, 1994.

95. Panje WR and others: Surgical management of the head and neck cancer patient following concomitant multimodality therapy, *Laryngoscope* 105:97, 1995.

96. Pratt WB: The mechanism of glucocorticoid effects in fibroblasts, *J Invest Dermatol* 71:24, 1978.

97. Prockop DJ, Kivirikko KI: Heritable disease of collagen, *N Engl J Med* 311:376, 1984.

98. Redleaf MI, Bauer CA: Topical antiseptic mouthwash in oncological surgery of the oral cavity and oropharynx, *J Laryngol Otol* 108:973, 1994.

99. Reed BR, Clark RAF: Cutaneous tissue repair: practical implications of current knowledge. II, *J Am Acad Dermatol* 13:919, 1985.

100. Reiter D: Methods and materials for wound management, *Otolaryngol Head Neck Surg* 110:550, 1994.

101. Richard J and others: Effect of topical basic fibroblast growth factor on the healing of chronic diabetic neuropathic ulcer of the foot, *Diabetes Care* 18:64, 1995.

102. Rockwell WB and others: Keloids and hypertrophic scars: a comprehensive review, *Plast Reconstr Surg* 84:827, 1989.

103. Reference deleted in pages.

104. Reference deleted in pages.

105. Rudolph R, Arganese T, Woodward M: The ultrastructure and etiology of chronic radiotherapy damage in human skin, *Ann Plast Surg* 9:282, 1982.

106. Rudolph R, Hunt TK: *Healing in compromised tissues.* In Rudolph R, editor: *Problems in aesthetic surgery: biological causes and clinical solutions*, St Louis, 1986, Mosby.

107. Rudolph R and others: The ultrastructure of chronic radiation damage in rat skin, *Surg Gynecol Obstet* 152:171, 1981.

108. Rudolph R and others: Slowed growth of cultured fibroblasts from human relation wounds, *Plast Reconst Surg* 82:669, 1988.

109. Reference deleted in pages.

110. Saginur R, Odell PF, Poliquin JF: Antibiotic prophylaxis in head and neck cancer surgery, *J Otolaryngol* 17:78, 1988.

111. Sander C, Niederhoff H, Horn N: Life-span and Menkes kinky hair syndrome: report of a 13 year course of this disease, *Clin Genet* 33: 228, 1988.

112. Sassler AM, Esclamado RM, Wolf GT: Surgery after organ preservation therapy, *Arch Otolaryngol Head Neck Surg* 121:162, 1995.

113. Scarpelli DG, Goodman RM: Observations on the fine structure of the fibroblast from a case of Ehlers-Danlos syndrome with the Marfan syndrome, *J Invest Dermatol* 50:214, 1968.

114. Schafer AI: *Coagulation cascade: an overview.* In Loscalzo J, Schafer AI, editors: *Thrombosis and hemorrhage*, Boston, 1994, Blackwell Scientific Publications.

115. Shah M, Foreman DM, Ferguson MWJ: Control of scarring in adult wounds by neutralising antibody to transforming growth factor β, *Lancet* 339:213, 1992.

116. Siana JE, Rex S, Gottrup F: The effect of cigarette smoking on wound healing, *Scand J Plast Reconstr Surg* 23:207, 1989.

117. Silverstein P: Smoking and wound healing, *Am J Med* 93:22S, 1992.

118. Smith KC and others: Radiosensitivity *in vitro* of human fibroblasts derived from patients with a severe skin reaction to radiation therapy, *Int J Radiation Oncol Biol Phys* 6:1573, 1980.

119. Staiano-Coico L and others: Human keratinocyte growth factor effects in a porcine model of epidermal wound healing, *J Exp Med* 178:865, 1993.

120. Steenfos HH, Jansson JO: Growth hormone stimulates granulation tissue formation and insulin-like growth factor-I gene expression in wound chambers in the rat, *J Endocrinol* 132:293, 1992.

121. Steenfos HH: Growth factors and wound healing, *Scand J Plast Reconstr Hand Surg* 28:995, 1994.

122. Suh DK, Hunt TK, Spencer EM: Insulin-like growth factor-I reverses the impairment of wound healing induced by corticosteroids in rats, *Endocrinol* 131:2399, 1992.

123. Tarnow P and others: Topical zinc oxide treatment increases endogenous gene expression of insulin-like growth factor-I in granulation tissue from porcine wounds, *Scand J Plast Reconstr Hand Surg* 28: 255, 1994.

124. Taylor WR, Alexander RW: Autocrine control of wound repair by insulin-like growth factor I in cultured endothelial cells, *Am J Physiol* 265:C801, 1993.

125. Uhl E and others: Hyperbaric oxygen improves wound healing in normal and ischemic skin tissue, *Plast Reconst Surg* 93:835, 1994.

126. Van De Kerkhof PCM and others: Age-related changes in wound healing, *Clin Exp Dermatol* 19:369, 1994.

127. Wang Q and others: Electron irradiation slows down wound repair in rat skin: a morphological investigation, *Br J Dermatol* 130:551, 1994.

128. Werner S and others: Induction of keratinocyte growth factor expression is reduced and delayed during wound healing in the genetically diabetic mouse, *J Invest Dermatol* 103:469, 1994.

129. Werner S and others: Large induction of keratinocyte growth factor expression in the dermis during wound healing, *Proc Natl Acad Sci U S A* 89:6896, 1992.

130. Wilson JD: *Vitamin deficiency and excess.* In Isselbacher KJ and others, editors: *Harrison's principles of internal medicine*, New York, 1994, McGraw-Hill.

131. Yanase A and others: Irradiation effects on wound contraction using a connective tissue model, *Ann Plast Surg* 30:435, 1993.

132. Yue DK and others: Effects of experimental diabetes, uremia, and malnutrition on wound healing, *Diabetes* 36:295, 1987.

133. Zaloga GP and others: Immediate postoperative enteral feeding decreases weight loss and improves wound healing after abdominal surgery in rats, *Crit Care Med* 20:115, 1992.

Chapter 11

Laser Surgery: Basic Principles and Safety Considerations

Robert H. Ossoff
Lou Reinisch
C. Gaelyn Garrett

Laser light is the brightest monochromatic (single color) light existing today. In addition to being a standard tool in the research laboratory, the laser is currently used in communications, surveying, manufacturing, diagnostic medicine, and surgery. Supermarket bar code scanners, lecture pointers, and compact disc players have even moved lasers into everyday life. The addition of lasers and the development of new lasers to the surgical armamentarium in otolaryngology offers new and exciting possibilities to improve conventional techniques and to expand the scope of this specialty.

This chapter reviews the principles, applications, and safety considerations associated with the use of lasers in the upper aerodigestive tract. The material presented provides a foundation for the otolaryngologist to begin to apply this exciting technology in daily practice.

LASER PHYSICS

Laser is an acronym for *l*ight *a*mplification by the *s*timulated *e*mission of *r*adiation. Einstein[30] postulated the theoretical foundation of laser action, stimulated emission of radiation, in 1917. In his classic publication "Zur Quantem Theorie der Strahlung" ("The Quantum Theory of Radiation"), he discussed the interaction of atoms, ions, and molecules with electromagnetic radiation. He specifically addressed absorption and spontaneous emission of energy and proposed a third process of interaction: stimulated emission. Einstein postulated that the spontaneous emission of electromagnetic radiation from an atomic transition has an en-hanced rate in the presence of similar electromagnetic radiation. This "negative absorption" is the basis of laser energy.

Many attempts were made in the following years to produce stimulated emission of electromagnetic energy, but it was not until 1954 that this was successfully accomplished. In that year, Gordon and others[41a] reported their experiences with stimulated emission of radiation in the microwave range of the electromagnetic spectrum. This represented the first maser (*m*icrowave *a*mplification by the *s*timulated *e*mission of *r*adiation) and paved the way for the development of the first laser.

In 1958, Schawlow and Townes[105] published "Infrared and Optical Masers," in which they discussed stimulated emission in the microwave range of the spectrum and described the desirability and principles of extending stimulated emission techniques to the infrared and optical ranges of the spectrum. Maiman[68] expanded on these theoretical writings and built the first laser in 1960. With synthetic ruby crystals, this laser produced electromagnetic radiation at a wavelength of 0.69 μm in the visible range of the spectrum. Although the laser energy produced by Maiman's ruby laser lasted less than 1 ms, it paved the way for explosive development and widespread application of this technology.

Commercial lasers were being sold for laboratory use within 1 year of being invented. Partially reacting to the recently discovered dangers of x-rays, scientists were concerned about the safety of lasers and how laser light might damage living tissue.

This concern over the safety of laser light prompted much

of the early transition of the laser from the scientific laboratory to the medical clinic. In 1962, Zaret and others[138] published one of the first reports of laser light interacting with tissue. They measured the damage caused by lasers incident on rabbit retina and iris. Goldman and others[40,41] consulted with Zaret to study the occupational hazards of the laser. Similarly, Zweng and others[139] were using ruby lasers on patients for eye care. In 1964, the argon (Ar) and neodymium: yttrium-aluminum-garnet (Nd:YAG) lasers were developed.[39] Excited by the ophthalmologists' progress in using the laser as a therapeutic tool, Goldman used his medical laser laboratory to look at the hazards of the laser and to consider the potential uses of the laser in medicine.

Two important advances allowed the laser to be useful in otolaryngology: in 1965, the carbon dioxide (CO_2) laser was developed, in 1968, Polanyi[101] developed the articulated arm to deliver the infrared radiation from the CO_2 laser to remote targets. He combined his talents with Jako and used the articulated arm and the CO_2 laser in laryngeal surgery. Simpson and Polanyi[114] described the series of experiments and new instrumentation that made this work possible.

A laser is an electrooptical device that emits organized light (rather than the random-pattern light emitted from a light bulb) in a very narrow intense beam by a process of optical feedback and amplification. Because the explanation for this organized light involves stimulated emission, a brief review of quantum physics is necessary.

In the semiclassical picture of the atom, each proton is balanced by an electron that orbits the nucleus of the atom in one of several discrete shells or orbits. Shells correspond to specific energy levels, which are characteristic of each different atom or molecule. The smaller shells, where the electron is closer to the nucleus, have a lower energy level than the larger shells, where the electron is farther from the nucleus. Electrons of a particular atom can only orbit the nucleus at these shells or levels. Radiation of energy does not occur while the electrons remain in any of these shells.

Electrons can change their orbits, thereby changing the energy state of the atom. During excitation, an electron can make the transition from a low-energy level to a higher energy level. Excitation that comes from the electron interacting with light (a photon) is termed *absorption*. The atom always seeks its lowest energy level (i.e., the ground state). Therefore, the electron will spontaneously drop from the high-energy level back to the lowest energy level in a very short time (typically 10^{-8} sec). As the electron spontaneously drops from the higher energy level to the lower energy level, the atom must give up the energy difference. The atom emits the extra energy as a photon of light in a process termed the *spontaneous emission of radiation* (Fig. 11-1).

Einstein[30] postulated that an atom in a high-energy level could be induced to make the transition to a lower energy state even faster than the spontaneous process if it interacted with a photon of the correct energy. This process can be imagined as a photon colliding with an excited atom, resulting in two identical photons (one incident and one produced by the decay) that leave the collision. The two photons have the same frequency and energy and travel in the same direction in spatial and temporal phase. This process, which Einstein called *stimulated emission of radiation*, is the underlying principle of laser physics (Fig. 11-1).

All laser devices have an optical resonating chamber (cavity) with two mirrors; the space between these mirrors is filled with an active medium, such as argon (Ar), Nd:YAG, or CO_2. An external energy source (e.g., an electric current) excites the active medium within the optical cavity. This excitation causes many atoms of the active medium to be raised to a higher energy state. A population inversion occurs when more than half of the atoms in the resonating chamber have reached a particular excited state. Spontaneous emission is taking place in all directions; light (photons) emitted in the direction of the long axis of the laser is retained within the optical cavity by multiple reflections off of the precisely aligned mirrors. One mirror is completely reflective, and the other is partially transmissive (Fig. 11-2). Stimulated emission occurs when a photon interacts with an excited atom in the optical cavity, yielding pairs of identical photons that are of equal wavelength, frequency, and energy and are in phase with each other. This process occurs at an increasing rate with each passage of the photons through the active medium; the mirrors serve as a positive feedback mechanism for the stimulated emission of radiation by reflecting the photons back and forth. The partially transmissive mirror emits some of the radiant energy as laser light. The radiation leaving the optical cavity through the partially transmissive mirror quickly reaches an equilibrium with the pumping mechanism's rate of replenishing the population of high-energy state atoms. (In the preceding discussion, the term *atom* refers to the active material. In reality, the active material can consist of molecules, ions, atoms, semiconductors, or even free electrons in an accelerator. These other systems do not require the bound electron to be excited but may instead use different forms of excitation, including molecular vibrational excitation or the kinetic energy of an accelerated electron.)

The radiant energy emitted from the optical cavity is of the same wavelength (monochromatic), is extremely intense and unidirectional (collimated), and is temporally and spatially coherent. The term *temporal coherence* refers to the waves of light oscillating in phase over a given time, whereas *spatial coherence* means that the photons are equal and parallel across the wave front. These properties of monochromaticity, intensity, collimation, and coherence distinguish the organized radiant energy of a laser light source from the disorganized radiant energy of a light bulb or other light source (Fig. 11-3).[87]

After the laser energy exits the optical cavity through the partially transmissive mirror, the radiant energy typically passes through a lens that focuses the laser beam to a very

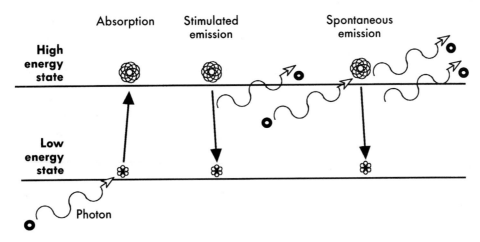

Fig. 11-1. The interaction of light (a photon) with an atom. Three processes are shown: the absorption of a photon by an atom in a low-energy state, the spontaneous emission of a photon from an atom in an excited state, and the stimulated emission of a photon by a second photon of the same wavelength from an excited-state atom.

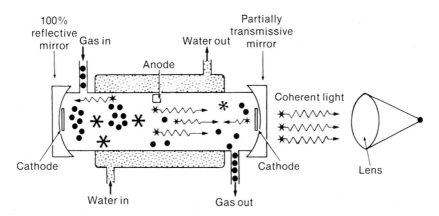

Fig. 11-2. The optical resonating chamber of a carbon dioxide laser. The gas molecules are excited by an electric current. The gas is cooled by a water jacket. The two mirrors provide the optical feedback for the amplification. The emitted light is coherent, monochromatic, and collimated. The light can be focused to a small point with an external lens.

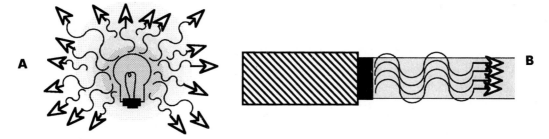

Fig. 11-3. A, Light emitted from a conventional lamp. The light travels in all directions, is composed of many wavelengths, and is not coherent. **B,** Light emitted from a laser. The light travels in the same direction, it is a single wavelength, and all of the waves are in phase (the light is coherent).

small diameter, or spot size, ranging from 0.1 to 2.0 mm. When necessary, the lens system is constructed to allow the visible helium-neon aiming laser beam and the invisible CO_2 or Nd:YAG laser beam to be focused in a coplanar manner. The optical properties of each focusing lens determine the focal length or distance from the lens to the intended target tissue for focused use.

CONTROL OF THE SURGICAL LASER

With most surgical lasers, the physician can control three variables: (1) power (measured in watts), (2) spot size (measured in millimeters), and (3) exposure time (measured in seconds).

Power

Of power, spot size, and exposure time, power is the least useful variable and may be kept constant with widely varying effects, depending on the spot size and the duration of exposure. For example, the relationship between power and depth of tissue injury becomes logarithmic when the power and exposure time are kept constant and the spot size is varied.[87]

Irradiance is a more useful measure of the intensity of the beam at the focal spot than power is because it considers the surface area of the focal spot. Specifically, irradiance is expressed (in W/cm^2) as: Irradiance = Power in the focal spot/Area of the focal spot.

Spot size

Power and spot size are considered together, and a combination is selected to produce the appropriate irradiance. If the exposure time is kept constant, the relationship between irradiance and depth of injury is linear as the spot size is varied. Irradiance is the most important operating parameter of a surgical laser at a given wavelength. Therefore, surgeons should calculate the appropriate irradiance for each procedure to be performed; these calculations allow the surgeon to control, in a predictable manner, the tissue effects when changing from one focal length to another (e.g., from 400 mm for microlaryngeal surgery to 125 mm for hand-held surgery). Irradiance varies directly with power and inversely with surface area. This relationship of surface area to beam diameter is important when evaluating the power density. The larger the surface area, the lower the irradiance; conversely, the smaller the surface area, the higher the irradiance. Surface area (A) is expressed as:

$$A = \pi r^2 \text{ or } A = \pi d^2/4$$

where r is the beam radius and d is the beam diameter (d = 2r). Surface area and irradiance vary with the square of the beam diameter.[87] Doubling the beam diameter (e.g., from d to 2d) increases the surface area by four times and reduces irradiance to one fourth; halving the beam diameter (e.g., from d to d/2) yields only one fourth of the area and increases irradiance by a factor of four.

Current CO_2 lasers emit radiant energy with a characteris-

tic beam intensity pattern. This beam pattern ultimately determines the depth of tissue injury and vaporization across the focal spot; therefore, the surgeon should be aware of the characteristic beam pattern of the laser. Transverse electromagnetic mode (TEM) refers to the distribution of energy across the focal spot and determines the shape of the laser's spot. The most fundamental mode is TEM_{00}, which appears circular on cross section; the power density of the beam follows a gaussian distribution. The greatest amount of energy is at the center of the beam and diminishes progressively toward the periphery. TEM_{01} and TEM_{11} are less fundamental modes that have a more complex distribution of energy across their focal spot, causing predictable variations in tissue vaporization depth. Additionally, their beams cannot be focused to as small a spot size as TEM_{00} lasers at the same working distance.[37]

Although simple ray diagrams normally show parallel light focused to a point, the actual situation is a bit more complicated. A lens focuses a gaussian beam to a beam waist or a finite size. This beam waist is the minimum spot diameter (d) and can be expressed as:

$$d \sim 2f\lambda/D$$

where f is the focal length of the lens, λ is the wavelength of light, and D is the diameter of the laser beam incident on the lens (Fig. 11-4). The beam waist occurs over a range of distances, termed the *depth of focus*, which can be expressed as:

$$\text{Depth of focus} \sim \pi d^2/2\lambda$$

Depth of focus is realized when a camera is focused. With a camera, a range of objects is in focus, which can be set without carefully measuring the distance between the object and the lens. The above equations show that a long focal length lens leads to a large beam waist, which also translates as a large depth of focus.

The size of the laser beam on the tissue (spot size) can therefore be varied in two ways: (1) because the minimum

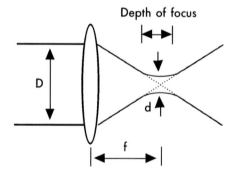

Fig. 11-4. The beam waist of parallel light focused by a lens. The focal length of the lens is f and the incident beam is transverse electromagnetic mode (TEM $_{00}$) and has a diameter incident on the lens of D The beam waist has a diameter of d.

beam diameter of the focal spot increases directly with increasing the focal length of the laser focusing lens, the surgeon can change the focal length of the lens to obtain a particular beam diameter. As the focal length decreases, a corresponding decrease occurs in the size of the focal spot; also, the smaller the spot size is for any given power output, the greater the corresponding power density. (2) The surgeon can also vary the spot size by working in or out of focus. The minimum beam diameter and highest power concentration occur at the focal plane, where much of the precise cutting and vaporization is carried out (Fig. 11-5, *A*). As the distance from the focal plane increases, the laser beam diverges or becomes unfocused (Fig. 11-5, *B*). The cross-sectional area of the spot increases and thus lowers the power density for a given output. The size of the focal spot depends on the focal length of the laser lens and whether the surgeon is working in or out of focus. Figure 11-6 shows these concepts using arbitrary ratios accurate for a current model TEM_{00} CO_2 laser. The laser lens setting (focal length) and working distance (focus/unfocus) combinations determine the size of the focal spot. The height of the various cylinders represents the amount of tissue (depth and width) vaporized after a 1-sec exposure at the three focal lengths.

Exposure time

The surgeon can vary the amount of energy delivered to the target tissue by varying the exposure time. Fluence refers to the amount of time (measured in seconds) that a laser beam irradiates a unit area of tissue at a constant irradiance. Fluence is a measure, then, of the total amount of laser energy per unit area of exposed target tissue and is expressed (in J/cm^2) as:

$$\text{Fluence} = \text{Power density} \times \text{Time}$$

Fluence varies directly with the length of the exposure time, which can be varied by working in the pulsed mode (duration, 0.05 to 0.5 sec) or in the continuous mode.

TISSUE EFFECTS

When electromagnetic energy (incident radiation) interacts with tissue, the tissue reflects, absorbs, and transmits and scatters portions of the light. The surgical interaction of this radiant energy with tissue is caused only by that portion of light that is absorbed (i.e., the incident radiation minus the sum of the reflected and transmitted portions).[9]

The actual tissue effects produced by the radiant energy of a laser vary with the laser's wavelength. Each type of laser exhibits different characteristic biologic effects on tissue and is therefore useful for different applications. However, certain similarities exist regarding the nature of interaction of all laser light with biologic tissue. The lasers used in medicine and surgery today can be ultraviolet, in which the interactions are a complex mixture of heating and photodissociation of chemical bonds. The more commonly used lasers emit light in the visible or the infrared region of the electromagnetic spectrum, and their primary form of interaction with biologic tissue leads to heating. Therefore, if the radiant energy of a laser is to exert its effect on the target tissue, it must be absorbed by the target tissue and converted to heat (Fig. 11-7). Scattering tends to spread the laser energy over a larger surface area of tissue, but it limits the penetration depth (Fig. 11-8). The shorter the wavelength of light, the more it is scattered by the tissue. If the radiant energy is reflected from or transmitted through the tissue (Figs. 11-9

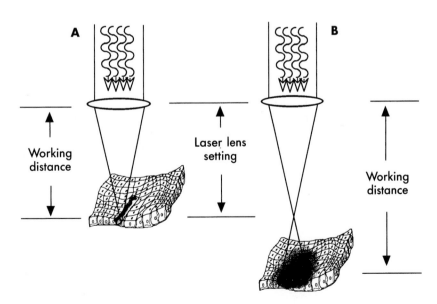

Fig. 11-5. A, Laser-tissue interaction when the tissue is the focal distance away from the lens. Note the minimum beam diameter in the focal plane. **B,** Laser-tissue interaction when the tissue is not in the focal plane of the lens. The laser covers a much larger area on the tissue surface.

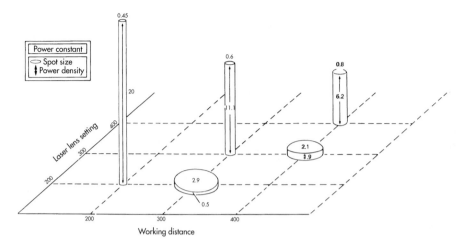

Fig. 11-6. Power density versus spot size. The ratios are arbitrary for a current model carbon dioxide laser. The cylinder height represents the amount of tissue vaporized after a 1-sec exposure at the three designated focal lengths.

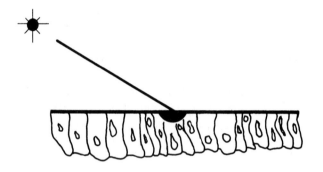

Fig. 11-7. Absorption.

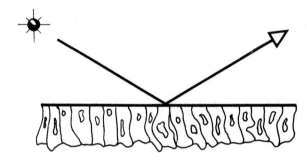

Fig. 11-9. Reflection.

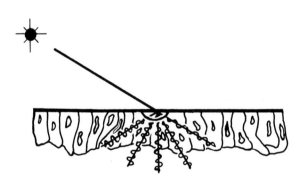

Fig. 11-8. Scattering.

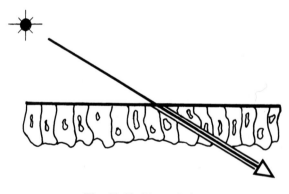

Fig. 11-10. Transmission.

and 11-10), no effect will occur. To select the most appropriate laser system for a particular application, the surgeon should thoroughly understand these characteristics regarding the interaction of laser light with biologic tissue.[36]

The CO_2 laser creates a characteristic wound (Fig. 11-11). When the target absorbs a specific amount of radiant energy to increase its temperature to between 60° C and 65° C,

protein denaturation occurs. Blanching of the tissue surface is readily visible, and the deep structural integrity of the tissue is disturbed. When the absorbed laser light heats the tissue to approximately 100° C, vaporization of intracellular water occurs, causing vacuole formation, craters, and tissue shrinkage. Carbonization, disintegration, smoke, and gas generation with destruction of the laser-radiated tissue oc-

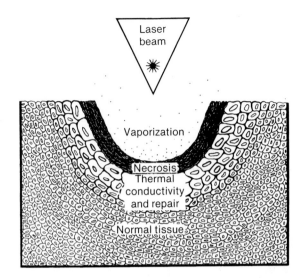

Fig. 11-11. The wound created by the carbon dioxide laser, showing the representative zones of injury.

curs at several hundred degrees centigrade. In the center of the wound is an area of tissue vaporization, where just a few flakes of carbon debris are noted. Immediately adjacent to this area is a zone of thermal necrosis (about 100 μm wide). Next is an area of thermal conductivity and repair (usually 300 to 500 μm wide). Small vessels, nerves, and lymphatics are sealed in the zone of thermal necrosis; the minimal operative trauma combined with the vascular seal probably account for the absence of postoperative edema characteristic of laser wounds.[77]

Comparison animal studies have been performed on the histologic properties of healing and the tensile strength of the healing wound after laser- and scalpel-produced incisions. Several studies noted impaired wound healing with the CO_2 laser incision when compared with the scalpel-produced incision.* Other studies of the healing properties of laser-induced incisions concluded that laser incisions have equivalent or better healing results than surgical knife wounds.[32,81,104,126] Buell and Schuller[13] compared the rate of tissue repair after CO_2 laser and scalpel incisions on hogs. In this study, the tensile strength of the laser incisions was less than that of similar scalpel incisions during the first 3 weeks after surgery; after this time, the tensile strength of both wounds rapidly increased at a similar rate.

Regardless of which studies accurately depict the effects of the CO_2 laser on wound healing, the incidental, collateral thermal damage is indisputable. To minimize lateral thermal damage from thermal diffusion, the tissue should be ablated with a short laser pulse.

To understand how a pulsed laser reduces thermal diffusion, consider the analogy of filling a large bucket with a hole in the bottom. If a narrow stream of water is used to

fill the bucket, the filling process will take a long time and a considerable amount of water will leak out of the hole during the filling process. Instead, if the bucket is filled in one quick dump from an even larger bucket, the water will have little time to leak out of the hole during the filling process.

This analogy can also be used to understand the ablation process. In ablation, the water represents laser energy and the filled bucket represents sufficient energy deposited in the tissue to cause ablation. The hole in the bottom of the bucket represents the thermal diffusion of heat away from the ablation site while the energy is being deposited. A low-intensity, continuous laser beam is similar to the narrow stream of water. The short-pulsed, high-peak power laser is similar to the larger bucket in that it dumps energy into the ablation site.

LASER TYPES AND APPLICATIONS

Six types of lasers are commonly used in otolargyngology: the Ar laser, Ar tunable dye laser, Nd:YAG laser, potassium-titanyl–phosphate (KTP) laser, flash lamp pumped dye laser, and CO_2 laser. Many more types are in various stages of development. The potential clinical applications of these surgical lasers are determined by wavelength and the specific tissue-absorptive characteristics. Therefore, the surgeon should consider the properties of each wavelength when choosing a particular laser to achieve the surgical objective with minimal morbidity and maximal efficiency (Table 11-1).

Argon laser

Ar lasers produce blue-green light in the visible range of the electromagnetic spectrum with primary wavelengths of 0.488 and 0.514 μm. The radiant energy of an Ar laser may be strongly absorbed, scattered, or reflected depending on the specific biologic tissues with which it interacts. Its extinction length (i.e., the thickness of water necessary to absorb 90% of the incident radiation) in pure water is about 80 m. Therefore, the radiant energy from an Ar laser is readily transmitted through clear aqueous tissues (e.g., cornea, lens, and vitreous humor) and is absorbed and reflected to varying degrees by tissues white in color (e.g., skin, fat, and bone). Light from an Ar laser is absorbed by hemoglobin and pigmented tissues; a localized thermal reaction occurs within the target tissue, causing protein coagulation. The clinician uses this selective absorption of light from an Ar laser to photocoagulate pigmented lesions, such as port-wine stains, hemangiomas, and telangiectasis.[4,98] The heat produced destroys the epidermis and upper dermis. Therefore, the surgeon should minimize the amount of laser energy delivered to the vascular cutaneous lesion to decrease the tendency of scarring in the overlying skin. The technique, called *minimal treatment/retreatment*, seems ideally suited to limit the scarring in the overlying skin.[56,97] The method uses the lowest power setting and exposure time necessary to blanch the

* Refs. 16, 28, 33, 43, 45, 66, 67.

Table 11-1. Laser choices for various lesions

Laser	Second-choice laser	Anatomic site	Lesion	Reason
Argon		Ear	Lysis of middle ear adhesions	Optical fiber delivery, hemaglobin absorption
Argon pumped dye laser			Photodynamic therapy	Can tune the laser to maximum absorption of photosensitizer
CO_2		Glottis	Nodules	Microspot, precision
CO_2		Glottis	Polyps	Microspot, precision
CO_2		Glottis	Reinke's edema	Microspot, precision, microflap technique
CO_2		Glottis	T1 midcordal squamous cell carcinoma with no anterior commissure involvement	Excisional biopsy
CO_2	KTP	Larynx	Laryngoceles, cysts, granulomas	Coagulation, hands-off technique
CO_2		Larynx	Laryngomalacia	Aryepiglottic fold division, precision, coagulation
CO_2		Larynx	Stenoses (glottic, posterior, and subglottic)	Micro–trap door techniques
CO_2		Lingual tonsils	Recurrent tonsillitis, hypertrophy	Minimal edema with complete vaporization
CO_2		Oral cavity	Carcinoma (verrucous, superficial T1)	Less pain and edema, covers a large area
CO_2		Oral cavity	Premalignant (leukoplakia, erythroplakia)	Vaporization, excision, can cover a large area
CO_2	KTP	Glottis	Bilateral vocal cord paralysis	Laser arytenoidectomy, coagulation
CO_2	KTP	Larynx	Recurrent respiratory papilloma	Hands-off technique, less scarring, precision (although KTP may be faster)
CO_2	KTP	Larynx	Suprahyoid supraglottic T1 squamous cell carcinoma	Excision with frozen section control
CO_2	KTP	Oral cavity	Tongue T1 and limited T2 cancer	Less pain and edema, precision, coagulation
CO_2	KTP or Argon	Ear	Stapedotomy	Minimal trauma
CO_2	KTP or Nd:YAG	Oral cavity	Lymphangioma	Minimal edema, coagulation
CO_2	KTP or Nd:YAG	Oropharynx	T1 and T2 squamous cell carcinoma	Precision, coagulation, less edema, contact tip with Nd:YAG
CO_2	Nd:YAG	Nose	Turbinate hypertrophy	Coagulation, less scabbing and scarring
CO_2	Nd:YAG	Subglottis	Hemangioma	Defocused beam, shrinkage, coagulation
Flash lamp pumped dye laser			Port-wine stains	Selective photothermolysis
KTP		Nose	Polyps, concha bullosa	Debulking for visualization, coagulation
KTP	CO_2	Larynx	Obstructing squamous cell carcinoma	Debulking airway, staging, coagulation
KTP	CO_2	Oropharynx	Sleep apnea (uvulopalatopharyngoplasty)	Coagulation
KTP	CO_2	Palatine tonsils	Recurrent tonsillitis, obstructive apnea	Coagulation ? less postoperative pain
KTP	Nd:YAG	Nose	Epistaxis	Fiber delivery, coagulation, hands-off technique
Nd:YAG	KTP	Nose	Hereditary hemorrhagic telangiectasias	Coagulation, hands-off technique
Nd:YAG	KTP or CO_2	Trachea	Obstructing malignant lesions	Debulking, coagulation, fiber delivery

CO_2—Carbon dioxide; KTP—Potassium-titanyl–phosphate; Nd:YAG—neodymium:yttrium-aluminum-garnet.

vascular cutaneous lesion. The Ar laser energy is delivered with a 1-mm spot size in an overlapping beading pattern.

When the beam of the Ar laser is focused to a small focal spot, its power density increases sufficiently to vaporize the target tissue. This characteristic allows otologists to perform stapedotomy in patients with otosclerosis.[99,123] Bone, being a white tissue, reflects most of the incident radiation from an Ar laser. Therefore, to perform an Ar laser stapedotomy,

it is necessary to place a drop of blood on the stapes to initiate absorption. Other applications of this laser in the middle ear include lysis of middle ear adhesions[20] and spot welding of grafts in tympanoplasty surgery.[31,44]

Argon tunable dye laser

The Ar tunable dye laser works on the principle of the Ar laser; it makes a high-intensity beam that is focused on dye that is continuously circulating in a second laser optically coupled with the Ar laser. The Ar laser beam energizes the dye, causing it to emit laser energy at a longer wavelength than the pump beam. By varying the type of dye and using a tuning system, different wavelengths can be obtained. The laser energy from this dye laser can be transmitted through flexible fiberoptics and delivered through endoscopic systems or inserted directly into tumors. The major clinical use of this laser is with selective photodynamic therapy (PDT) for malignant tumors after the intravenous injection of the photosensitizer, hematoporphyrin derivative.[25]

After intravenous injection, the hematoporphyrin derivative disseminates to all of the cells of the body, rapidly moving out of normal tissue but remaining longer in neoplastic tissue. After a few days, a differential in concentration exists between the tumor cells and the normal cells. When the tumor is exposed to red light (630 nm), the dye absorbs the light, causing a photochemical reaction. Toxic oxygen radicals such as singlet oxygen are produced within the exposed cells, causing selective tissue destruction and cell death. Because healthy tissues contain less photosensitizer, a much less severe reaction or no reaction occurs. Long-term tumor control has been achieved using PDT for recurrent nasopharyngeal cancer.[65] The main technical problem is getting enough light to the target area. The Ar tunable dye laser has helped to solve this problem.[46] Additional research to increase the laser intensity and simplify the sometimes cumbersome setup is being conducted with gold vapor lasers and Ar pumped titanium sapphire lasers.[100]

Many investigators in the United States have shown that the premise of treating selected neoplasms with hematoporphyrin derivative followed by activation with red light is valid.[17,24,42,137] The overall potential and the place of maximum value of this form of management remain to be established. Areas that appear very promising include carcinoma of the urinary bladder,[131] endobronchial lesions of the lung,[47] selected carcinomas of the upper aerodigestive tract,[136] skin cancers,[69] and metastatic dermal breast cancers.[23] Trials are being conducted in certain specialties on intraoperative PDT in conjunction with conventional surgery and on PDT as the sole modality for selected superficial mucosal carcinomas.[8] The potential for this compound to serve as a tumor marker in sites where multicentric tumors are common (e.g., mucosal surfaces lining the upper aerodigestive tract) has been discussed.[83] The use of a krypton laser with an image intensifier system to facilitate endoscopic detection of hematoporphyrin derivative fluorescence looks promising in the tracheobronchial tree.[22]

Neodymium: yttrium-aluminum-garnet laser

Nd:YAG lasers produce light with a wavelength of 1.064 μm in the near infrared (invisible) range of the electromagnetic spectrum. Pure water weakly absorbs the radiant energy of the Nd:YAG laser. The extinction length is about 40 mm. Therefore, its radiant energy can be transmitted through

clear liquids, facilitating its use in the eye or other water-filled cavities (e.g., the urinary bladder). Absorption of light from this laser is slightly color dependent, with increased absorption in darkly pigmented tissues and charred debris. In biologic tissue, strong scattering, both forward and backward, determines the effective extinction length, which is usually 2 to 4 mm. Backward scattering can account for up to 40% of the total amount of scattering. The zone of damage produced by the incident beam of a Nd:YAG laser produces a homogeneous zone of thermal coagulation and necrosis that may extend up to 4 mm deep and lateral from the surface, making precise control impossible.

The primary applications for the Nd:YAG laser in otolaryngology include palliation of obstructing tracheobronchial lesions,[10,26,109,130] palliation of obstructing esophageal lesions,[34] photocoagulation of vascular lesions of the head and neck,[102,108] and photocoagulation of lymphatic malformations.[5] The contact Nd:YAG laser is reportedly useful in the removal of malignant tumors in the oral cavity and oropharynx, where it is difficult to maintain a generous safety margin.[79] The Nd:YAG laser has several distinct advantages in the management of obstructing lesions of the tracheobronchial tree. Hemorrhage is the most frequent and dangerous complication associated with laser bronchoscopy, and its control is extremely important. Control of hemorrhage is more secure with this laser because of its deep penetration in tissue.

Nd:YAG laser application through an open, rigid bronchoscope allows for multiple distal suction capabilities simultaneous with laser application and rapid removal of tumor fragments and debris to prevent hypoxemia. Patients for Nd:YAG laser bronchoscopy should be selected after flexible fiberoptic bronchoscopic examination of the tracheobronchial tree and tracheal polytomography or computed tomography; patients in whom extrinsic compression of the airway can be shown should be excluded. The radiant energy from the Nd:YAG laser can be transmitted through flexible fiberoptic delivery systems, allowing its use with flexible endoscopes. In the management of patients with obstructing neoplasms of the tracheobronchial tree, it is considered safer to use a rigid ventilating bronchoscope rather than a flexible fiberoptic bronchoscope.[27] With this approach, the laser fiber is passed down the lumen of the rigid bronchoscope with a rod lens telescope and suction catheter.[26]

Other advantages of the use of this laser with a rigid bronchoscope include ventilatory control of the compromised airway, palpation of the tumor/cartilage interface, use of the bronchoscope tip as a "cookie cutter," and use of the bronchoscope tip to compress a bleeding tumor bed for temporary hemostasis. The flexible fiberoptic bronchoscope is often used through the open rigid scope to provide pulmonary toilet and more distal laser application after the major airway is secure.

This laser is an excellent surgical instrument for tissue coagulation; vaporization and incision also can be performed with the Nd:YAG laser. When this laser is used for these functions, however, precision is lacking and tissue damage is widespread. The major disadvantage of the Nd:YAG laser is its comparatively less predictable depth of tissue penetration. This laser is used primarily to rapidly photocoagulate tumor masses in the upper and lower aerodigestive tract at 40- to 50-W, using 0.5- to 1-second exposures. Whenever possible, the laser beam is applied parallel to the wall of the tracheobronchial tree. The rigid tip of the bronchoscope is used mechanically to separate the devascularized tumor mass from the wall of the tracheobronchial tree.

Otolaryngologists may use this laser with the CO_2 laser when performing bronchoscopic laser surgery. The effective coagulating properties of the Nd:YAG laser should augment the predictable vaporizing properties of the CO_2 laser when treating patients with obstructive tracheal and proximal endobronchial cancers, especially if an ulcerative or actively bleeding tumor is present.[95]

Carbon dioxide laser

CO_2 lasers produce light with a wavelength of 10.6 μm in the infrared (invisible) range of the electromagnetic spectrum. A second, built-in, coaxial helium neon laser is necessary because its red light indicates the site where the invisible CO_2 laser beam will impact the target tissue. Thus, this laser acts as an aiming beam for the invisible CO_2 laser beam. The radiant energy produced by the CO_2 laser is strongly absorbed by pure, homogeneous water and by all biologic tissues high in water content. The extinction length of this wavelength is about 0.03 mm in water and in soft tissue; reflection and scattering are negligible. Because absorption of the radiant energy produced by the CO_2 laser is independent of tissue color and because the thermal effects produced by this wavelength on adjacent nontarget tissues are minimal, the CO_2 laser has become extremely versatile in otolaryngology. With current technology, light from this laser cannot be transmitted through existing flexible fiberoptic endoscopes, although research and development of a suitable flexible fiber for transmission of this wavelength is being carried out internationally. At present, the radiant energy of this laser is transmitted from the optical resonating chamber to the target tissue via a series of mirrors through an articulating arm to the target tissue.[87] This laser can be used free-hand for macroscopic surgery, attached to the operating microscope for microscopic surgery, and adapted to an endoscopic coupler for bronchoscopic surgery;[89,94] this latter application requires rigid nonfiberoptic bronchoscopes.[84]

The CO_2 laser is indispensable in laryngology, bronchology, neurootology, and pediatric otolaryngology. Many upper aerodigestive tract procedures that previously required prolonged hospitalization and tracheotomy can now be performed without the need for tracheotomy[50] and often as an outpatient procedure. In the field of neurootology and neurosurgery, reports have shown that the length of stay and perioperative morbidity associated with laser removal of acoustic neuromas is reduced when compared with those associated with conventional techniques.[15]

In the oral cavity, benign tumors can be excised with the laser.[71] A one-stage tongue release can be performed for patients requiring rehabilitation of speech after composite resection with tongue flap reconstruction.[64] Multiple areas of leukoplakia can be precisely excised; often, a graft is not necessary to resurface the operative field. Selected superficial carcinomas can be precisely excised with the use of the laser, and large, recurrent, or inoperable tumors can be debulked for palliation.[122]

The laser has also been used in the management of nasal and paranasal sinus disease. Choanal atresia,[49] hypertrophic inferior turbinates,[78] squamous papilloma, and hereditary hemorrhagic telangiectasia have been managed with the CO_2 laser,[116] although the Ar laser is more efficacious for the management of hereditary hemorrhagic telangiectasia.

In the field of facial plastic surgery, the CO_2 laser has shown promise in the excision of rhinophyma,[112] the excision of benign and malignant skin tumors,[57] and the vaporization and excision of nevi and tattoos.[61]

The CO_2 laser is best used in otolaryngology in the microscopic surgical management of benign and malignant diseases of the larynx. Surgery for recurrent respiratory papillomatosis has advanced with the use of the laser. The increased ability to preserve normal laryngeal structures while maintaining the translaryngeal airway more than offsets the initial disappointment associated with the laser's inability to cure the disease.[115] In a published survey, the CO_2 laser was preferred for the management of recurrent respiratory papillomatosis by 92% of the respondents.[19] In pediatric patients, surgery for webs, subglottic stenosis, capillary hemangiomas, and other space-occupying airway lesions has been significantly improved by the precision, preservation of normal tissue, and predictably minimal amount of postoperative edema associated with the judicious use of the CO_2 laser.[73]

In adults, surgery for polyps, nodules, leukoplakia, papillomas, cysts, granulomas, and other benign laryngeal conditions can be performed effectively with the laser.[132] A new era of conservation surgery or phonosurgery for benign laryngeal disease has been created by the laser. In the past, microlaryngeal surgery for benign disease has been mucosal stripping with healing by regrowth of the mucosal layer. Now, normal mucosal tissue can be preserved by elevating and advancing mucosal flaps with endoscopic laser techniques.[54] The addition of the microspot micromanipulator has furthered these techniques.[90,111]

Management of laryngotracheal stenosis is a difficult problem for the otolaryngologist. Retrospective analysis has determined that stenotic lesions appropriate for endoscopic management have three features in common:[114] (1) All lesions treated with endoscopic techniques must retain intact external cartilaginous support. (2) Lesions appropriate for endoscopic management are usually less than 1 cm in vertical length, yet favorable results have been reported for lesions up to 3 cm in length when endoscopic incision is combined with prolonged stenting.[110,135] (3) Total cervical tracheal or subglottic stenosis does not usually respond well to endoscopic management. Again, however, successful cases have been reported for when endoscopic management is combined with prolonged stenting of the stenotic area.[110]

The micro–trap door flap technique uses the CO_2 laser to make a horizontal incision in the mucosa overlying the stenosis. The laser is then used to vaporize the underlying scar tissue. The micro–trap door flap has been used in a sequential, staged manner on circumferential stenosis with fair to good results.[11,134]

The addition of the CO_2 laser to endoscopic arytenoidectomy allows the surgeon to precisely vaporize the mucosa and underlying arytenoid cartilage layer by layer in a dry field.[92] The precision associated with the laser facilitates performance of this operation, even by surgeons who have difficulty mastering the conventional techniques of endoscopic arytenoidectomy.[128]

The transoral management of squamous cell carcinoma of the larynx using the CO_2 laser is an obvious extension of the application of this surgical instrument. The advantages of precision, increased hemostasis, and decreased intraoperative edema allow the surgeon to perform exquisitely accurate and relatively bloodless endoscopic surgery of the larynx. Determinate cure rates with this method of management are reported to be equivalent to those of radiotherapy.[12,58]

Bronchoscopic indications for CO_2 laser surgery include management of recurrent respiratory papillomatosis or granulation tissue within the tracheobronchial tree, excision of selected subglottic or tracheal strictures, excision of bronchial adenomas, and re-establishment of the airway in patients with obstructing tracheal or endobronchial cancers. In this latter indication, palliation or reduction of the patient's symptoms of airway obstruction or hemoptysis is the desired goal.[95]

The laser-assisted uvulopalatoplasty was developed by Kamami[53] in the late 1980s. The procedure was introduced to the United States in 1992, where it has continued to grow in popularity. The procedure is designed to correct snoring caused by airway obstruction and soft-tissue vibration at the level of the soft palate by reducing the amount of tissue in the velum and uvula. At present, the procedure is being looked at very closely by several institutions to determine its place in the management of obstructive sleep apnea.[76]

Potassium-titanyl–phosphate laser

The KTP laser has also been used in surgery. It emits at 532 nm and is therefore comparable with the Ar laser. The scattering and absorption by skin pigments are nearly the same as the Ar laser. Yet the KTP laser light is more strongly absorbed by hemoglobin.

The KTP laser has shown success in stapedotomies.[9] It has also been shown to enhance safety and efficacy of the revision stapedectomy.[72] Thedinger[127] has promoted the

KTP laser for chronic ear surgery, specifically for removing hyperplastic infected mucosa, disarticulating mobile stapes suprastructure in a complete cholesteatoma removal, and removing previously inserted middle ear implants. Hand-held probes also facilitate use of the KTP laser for functional endoscopic sinus surgery and other intranasal applications[62] and for microlaryngeal applications.[6] The optical fiber delivery of the 532-nm laser light can be manipulated through a rigid pediatric bronchoscope as small as 3 mm, facilitating lower tracheal and endobronchial lesion treatment in infants and neonates.[133] Other examples of hand-held KTP laser applications include tonsillectomy[52,59,60,63,124] and excision of benign and malignant laryngeal lesions.[7] The KTP laser can also be used an automatic scanning device to manage pigmented dermal lesions, such as port-wine stains.[70]

The KTP crystal actually doubles the frequency (halves the wavelength) of a Nd:YAG laser. Therefore, with this laser, the output between the 532-nm KTP light and the 1064-nm Nd:YAG light can usually be switched.

Flash lamp pumped dye laser

The management of hemangiomas and port-wine stains with lasers has benefited from the application of the flash lamp pumped dye laser. The dye was initially selected for maximum absorption by the oxyhemoglobin at 577 nm. Tan and others[125] showed that at 585 nm, hemoglobin absorption is maximal with minimal scattering and absorption by melanin and other pigments. The light pulse is about 400 μsec long to minimize thermal diffusion in the tissue. Although dark skin types show little or no selective vascular photothermolysis with the laser, lighter skin types show significant results. At a threshold dose, specific vascular injury is observed without disruption of the adjacent tissue in lightly pigmented skin.[125]

The flash lamp pumped dye laser has also been effective in the management of uncomplicated and recalcitrant warts,[55] with response rates as high as 99% for body, limb, and anogenital warts. The laser effectively destroys the warts without damaging the surrounding skin.

Other lasers

In an effort to have a more controlled laser effect with less damage to adjacent tissue, several lasers in the near to mid infrared region have been investigated, including the erbium:YAG (Er:YAG) and the holmium:YAG (Ho:YAG). The Er:YAG emits at the infrared peak of water absorption at 2.94 μm. The extinction length in water is less than 2 μm. The laser produces very clean incisions with a minimal amount of thermal damage to the adjacent tissue. The negative aspects include: (1) The wavelength is too long to be transmitted through normal optical fibers. This gives a distinct advantage to lasers that produce light that can be transmitted through fibers. (2) More importantly, the thermal propagation is so short there is practically no tissue coagulation and no hemostasis. This laser is therefore unsuitable for use in highly vascular tissue.

The Ho:YAG laser operates at 2.1 μm. This wavelength can be effectively transmitted through fibers. The extinction length in water is about 0.4 mm, which suggests that this laser light should interact with tissue very similar to the CO_2 laser. The Ho:YAG has been combined with fiberoptic endoscopy for sinus surgery.[106] The hemostasis is good, and the soft bone ablation is readily controlled. Adjacent thermal damage zones varied from 130 to 220 μm in a study by Stein and others.[120] The laser is as effective in sinus surgery as conventional surgical techniques with less blood loss but increased postoperative edema.[74]

Other materials that operate in the near infrared region of the spectrum are also being evaluated, e.g., the cobalt: magnesium fluoride laser (tunable from 1.8 to 2.14 μm), alexandrite lasers (750 nm), and titanium sapphire lasers (tunable from 0.6 to 1.0 μm). Ultimately, many parameters (e.g., cost, reliability, size, and tissue response) influence choice of lasers in medicine.

PULSE STRUCTURE

As mentioned, the surgeon has three parameters to select when using a particular laser. The intensity of the laser is the least useful. The exposure time is important in that it controls the total amount of light incident on the tissue (i.e., the radiant exposure). The pulse structure of the laser light within the given exposure time is also crucial. The pulse structure is a characteristic of the active medium and the cavity configuration. It is often fixed and cannot be changed or modified by the surgeon.

Continuous wave lasers

Many lasers operate in a continuous wave mode. In this mode, the laser is always on. The instantaneous intensity and the average laser intensity are essentially the same. A shutter, external to the laser cavity, usually controls the exposure time, allowing the laser to operate independent of the exposure time or the frequency of exposures. This gives the most stable operation. A surgical CO_2 or Nd:YAG laser will operate in continuous wave mode at intensities of a few watts to more than 50 W.

Flash lamp pulsed lasers

Certain lasers operate in a pulsed mode. Flash lamp pumped lasers can pulse from about 0.5 μsec to several 100 ms. The first ruby laser operated in a pulsed mode. The flash lamp used to pump the ruby crystal had about a 1-ms pulse duration. The laser output of this first laser clearly was irregular and unstable. When observed with a fast detector and oscilloscope, the output intensity was found not to be a 1-ms long laser pulse but a series of irregular spikes. Each spike is a few microseconds long with several microseconds between the spikes. The stimulated emission in the ruby is so efficient that it quickly depletes the population inversion

and the operation stops, after which the flash lamp can reestablish the population inversion and operation can resume. This process repeats until the flash lamp stops. Most of the long-pulsed lasers operate in a spiking mode.

Q-switched laser

The spiking of the laser output can be controlled to produce a single very short laser pulse, much shorter than the flash lamp lifetime. One technique to produce the short pulses is Q-switching, in which the laser pumping process (usually a flash lamp) builds up a large population inversion inside the laser cavity. Blocking or removing one of the mirrors prevents the laser from emitting. After a large population inversion has developed, the feedback is restored and a short intense burst of laser light depletes the accumulated population inversion, typically in 10 to 50 ns. Q-switching can be accomplished by several different methods. The most direct and earliest method is rotating the end mirror so that the light amplification by stimulated emission can occur during the short interval when the mirror is correctly aligned. Waring blender motors were often used as fast, stable motors. However, uncertain timing, lack of reliability, and vibration (not to mention the noise) led to many problems, particularly with the alignment. Electrooptic polarization rotators and acoustooptic beam deflectors are now commonly used for Q-switching.

Cavity dumped lasers

Cavity dumping produces slightly shorter pulses of light. In this technique, the laser is pumped and allowed to operate between completely reflecting mirrors. The light energy is trapped in the cavity until it reaches a maximum. Then one of the mirrors is "removed" from the cavity and allows all the light to leave the cavity. The laser pulse has a physical length of twice the cavity length. Thus, the duration of the laser pulse is $2\lambda/c$ where λ is the length of cavity and c is the speed of light (c is about 3×10^{10} cm/sec or 1 foot/ns).

Mode locked lasers

Mode locking produces pulses of light as short as a few picoseconds. A Q-switched laser operates in several longitudinal modes (or slightly shifted frequencies). A fast saturable dye brings all these modes into phase. The nanosecond macropulse of light is actually a train of micropulses, each of which is several picoseconds long and repeats at about 100 MHz. These pulses can be further compressed by various techniques. The shortest laser light pulses achieved in the laboratory are less than four wave oscillations long (about 6 fs or 6×10^{-15} sec).

The pulsed laser dramatically changes the interaction of the light with tissue. The intensity of the laser during the pulse is extremely high (approaching 10^9 W). The high intensity and short pulse duration enable the laser light efficiently to ablate tissue before the thermal energy spreads by thermal diffusion. The pulse should be significantly shorter than the thermal diffusion time to prevent thermal diffusion from spreading damage. Typically, a tissue under laser irradiation reaches thermal equilibrium within a few milliseconds. The heat will spread over several micrometers in less than 10 μsec.[103] Also, the transverse mode structure of the laser beam must be preserved in the short pulses to yield the small focal spot size.

SAFETY CONSIDERATIONS

Education

The laser is a precise but potentially dangerous surgical instrument that must be used with caution. Although distinct advantages are associated with the use of laser surgery in the management of certain benign and malignant diseases of the upper aerodigestive tract, these advantages must be weighed against the risks of complications. Because of these risks, the surgeon must first determine if the laser offers an advantage over conventional surgical techniques. For the surgeon to use good judgment in the selection and use of lasers in practice, prior experience in laser surgery is necessary. Therefore, some type of formal laser education program should be a prerequisite to using this technology. Many hospitals now require evidence of participation in a laser use and safety course prior to granting laser privileges. The surgeon who has not received training in laser surgery as a resident should attend one of the many excellent hands-on training courses in laser surgery given in the United States. Such a course should include laser biophysics, tissue interactions, safety precautions, and supervised hands-on training with laboratory animals. After completing such a course, the surgeon should practice laser surgery on cadaver or animal specimens before progressing to the more simple procedures on patients.

Hospitals that offer laser surgery should appoint a laser safety officer and set up a laser safety committee consisting of the laser safety officer, two or three physicians using the laser, one or two operating room nurses, a hospital administrator, and a biomedical engineer. The purpose of this committee is to develop policies and procedures for the safe use of lasers within the hospital. The safety protocols established by this committee will vary with each specialty and use of the laser. In addition, the laser safety committee should (1) make recommendations regarding the appropriate credential-certifying mechanisms required for physicians and nurses to become involved with each laser, (2) develop educational policies for surgeons, anesthesiologists, and nurses working with the laser, (3) accumulate laser patient data in cases where an investigational device was used, and (4) conduct a periodic review of all laser-related complications.

Aside from a few minor eye injuries from a laser beam exposure, most serious accidental injuries related to laser use can be traced to the ignition of surgical drapes and airway tubes.[117] Because the anesthesiologist is also concerned with the airway and because potent oxidizing gases pass through the airway in close approximation to the path of the laser beam, it is necessary to develop a team approach to the anesthetic management of the patient undergoing laser surgery of the upper aerodigestive tract. It is recommended that anesthesiologists involved with laser surgery cases attend a didactic session devoted to this subject. Finally, the operating room staff must be educated with regard to laser surgery. Attendance at an inservice workshop with exposure to clinical laser biophysics and the basic workings of the laser as well as hands-on orientation should be the minimal requirement for nurses to participate in laser surgery.[119]

Safety protocol

Development of an effective laser safety protocol that stresses compliance and meticulous attention to detail by the operating room personnel (laser surgery team) is probably the most important reason this potentially dangerous surgical instrument can be used safely in treating patients with diseases of the upper aerodigestive tract.[96] Such a laser safety protocol is usually general enough to list all the major and most minor precautions necessary when laser surgery is being performed within the specialty of otolaryngology. General considerations concern provisions for protection of the eyes and skin of patients and operating room personnel, and for adequate laser plume (smoke) evacuation from the operative field. Additional precautions concern the choice of anesthetic technique, the choice and protection of endotracheal tubes, and the selection of proper instruments, including bronchoscopes.

Eye protection

Several structures of the eye are at risk; the area of injury usually depends on which structure absorbs the most radiant energy per volume of tissue. Depending on the wavelength, corneal or retinal burns, or both, are possible from acute exposure to the laser beam. The possibility for corneal or lenticular opacities (cataracts) or retinal injury exists after chronic exposure to excessive levels of laser radiation. Retinal effects occur when the laser emission wavelength occurs in the visible and near-infrared range of the electromagnetic spectrum (0.4 to 1.4 μm). When viewed directly or secondary to reflection from a specular (mirrorlike) instrument surface, laser radiation within this wavelength range would be focused to an extremely small spot on the retina, causing serious injury. This occurs because of the focusing effects of the cornea and lens. Laser radiation in the ultraviolet (<0.4 μm) or in the infrared range of the spectrum (>1.4 μm) produces effects primarily at the cornea, although certain wavelengths also may reach the lens.[3]

To reduce the risk of ocular damage during cases involving the laser, certain precautions should be followed. Protecting the eyes of the patient, surgeon, and other operating room personnel must be addressed; the actual protective device will vary according to the wavelength of the laser used. A sign should be placed outside the operating room door warning all persons entering the room to wear protective glasses

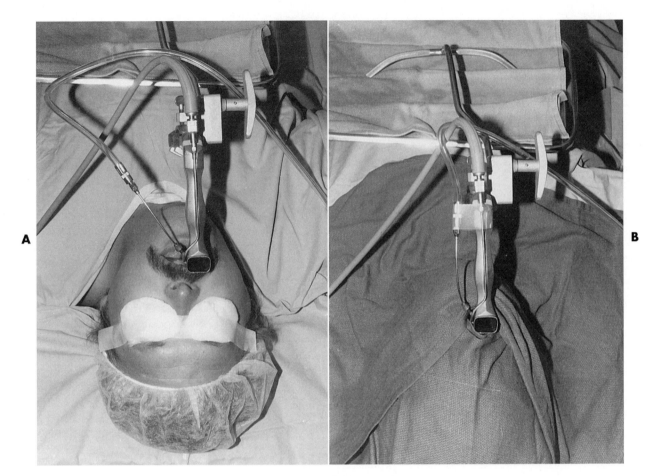

Fig. 11-12. Patient undergoing carbon dioxide laser microlaryngoscopy with jet ventilation. **A,** Saline-moistened eye pads are secured with silk tape. The eyes are first taped closed with silk tape to prevent corneal abrasions from the eye pads. **B,** Saline-moistened towels are placed around the patient's head to cover all skin surfaces.

because the laser is in use. In addition, extra glasses for the specific wavelength in use should be placed on a table immediately outside the room. The doors to the operating room should remain closed during laser surgery with the CO_2 laser and locked during laser surgery with the Nd:YAG or Ar laser.

Patients undergoing CO_2 laser surgery of the upper aerodigestive tract should have a double layer of saline-moistened eye pads placed over the eyes (Fig. 11-12 *A, B*). All operating room personnel should wear protective glasses with side protectors. Regular eyeglasses or contact lenses protect only the areas covered by the lens and do not provide protection from possible entry of the laser beam from the side. When working with the operating microscope and the CO_2 laser, the surgeon need not wear protective glasses; the optics of the microscope provide the necessary protection (Fig. 11-13).[93] When working with the Nd:YAG laser, all operating room personnel (and the patient) must wear wavelength-specific protective glasses that are usually blue-green. Although the beam direction and point of impact may appear to be confined

within the endoscope, inadvertent deflection of the beam may occur because of a faulty contact, a break in the fiber, or accidental disconnection between the fiber and endoscope. Special wavelength-specific filters are available for flexible and rigid bronchoscopes; when these filters are in place, the surgeon need not wear protective glasses.[42]

When working with the Ar, KTP, or dye lasers, all personnel in the operating room, including the patient, should again wear wavelength-specific protective glasses that are usually amber. When undergoing photocoagulation for selected cutaneous vascular lesions of the face, the patient usually wears protective metal eye shields rather than protective glasses.[21] Similar precautions are necessary for the visible and near-infrared wavelength lasers. The major difference is the type of eye protection that is worn.

Skin protection

The patient's exposed skin and mucous membranes outside the surgical field should be protected by a double layer of saline-saturated surgical towels, surgical sponges, or lap

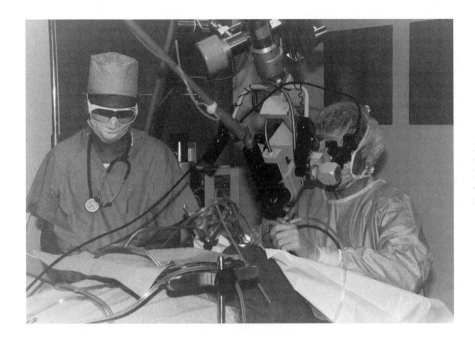

Fig. 11-13. Protective eyewear is worn by the anesthesiologist during carbon dioxide laser microlaryngoscopy. The surgeon's eyes are protected by the optics of the operating microscope.

pads. When microlaryngeal laser surgery is being performed, the beam might partially reflect off the proximal rim of the laryngoscope rather than go down it. Thus, saline-saturated surgical towels completely drape the patient's face; only the proximal lumen of the laryngoscope is exposed. Great care must be exercised to keep the wet draping from drying out; it should occasionally be moistened during the procedure. Teeth in the operative field also need to be protected; saline-saturated Telfa, surgical sponges, or specially constructed metal dental impression trays can be used. Meticulous attention is paid to the protective draping procedures at the beginning of the surgery; the same attention should be paid to the continued protection of the skin and teeth during the surgical procedure.[93]

Smoke evacuation

Two separate suction setups should be available for all laser cases in the upper aerodigestive tract; one provides for adequate smoke and steam evacuation from the operative field, whereas the second is connected to the surgical suction tip for the aspiration of blood and mucus from the operative wound.[119] When performing laser surgery with a closed anesthetic system, the surgeon should use constant suctioning to remove laser-induced smoke from the operating room; this helps to prevent inhalation by the patient, surgeon, or operating room personnel. When the anesthetic system is open or has jet ventilation systems, suctioning should be intermittent to maintain the forced inspiratory oxygen at a safe level. Laryngoscopes, bronchoscopes, operating platforms, mirrors, and anterior commissure and ventricle retractors with built-in smoke-evacuating channels facilitate the evacuation of smoke from the operative field.[86] One report suggested that the smoke created by the interaction of the

CO_2 laser with tissue may be mutagenic.[129] Filters in the suction lines should be used to prevent clogging by the black carbonaceous smoke debris created by the laser.[80] Although papillomavirus and other viral particles have been detected in the laser plume, no cases of clinical transmission of diseases are documented.[1,38]

Anesthetic considerations

Optimal anesthetic management of the patient undergoing laser surgery of the upper aerodigestive tract must include attention to the safety of the patient, the requirements of the surgeon, and the hazards of the equipment. Most patients undergo general anesthesia for upper airway endoscopy. Some laser procedures in the oral cavity and oropharynx may be performed under local anesthesia, with or without intravenous sedation. Most patients undergoing upper airway laser endoscopy, however, require general anesthesia. Any nonflammable general anesthetic is suitable; halothane and enflurane are most often used. Because of the risk of fire associated with general endotracheal anesthesia, the inspired concentration of oxygen, a potent oxidizing gas, is important. Mixtures of helium, nitrogen, or air plus oxygen are commonly used to maintain the forced inspiratory oxygen around but not greater than 40% and to ensure that the patient is adequately oxygenated. Nitrous oxide is also a potent oxidizing gas and should not be used in the anesthetic mixture to cut the oxygen concentration. When performing laser surgery in the tracheobronchial tree through the rigid, ventilating bronchoscope, the surgeon may use 100% oxygen. In either case, intravenous supplementation with small doses of narcotics or tranquilizers is often used to shorten the emergence period after anesthesia. Muscle relaxation is required to prevent movement of the vocal cords during surgery in the larynx. Jet ventilation techniques during laser surgery are effective for selected patients, such as those with subglottic stenosis.[29] Successful use of this ventilation technique requires that the anesthesiologist be experienced in this technique.

At present, a nonflammable, universally accepted endotracheal tube for laser surgery of the upper aerodigestive tract does not exist. The traditional polyvinyl endotracheal tube should not be used, either wrapped or unwrapped. It offers the least resistance to penetration by the laser beam of all the endotracheal tubes that have been tested, fire-breakdown products are toxic, and tissue destruction associated with combustion of this tube is the most severe. The Ruysch red rubber tube offers some resistance to penetration by the laser beam and causes mild to moderate damage to the tracheobronchial tree if a fire occurs. The silicone tube offers more resistance to penetration than the red rubber tube; however, silica ash can be seen in the airway after fires with these tubes and raises the possibility of future problems with silicosis.[91] Although the Norton metal tube[82] is nonflammable, rigidity problems, inner-to-outer diameter ratios, gas leakage, and lack of a cuff have prevented it from becoming the universally accepted tube of choice for CO_2 laser surgery. Endotracheal tubes for laser surgery (wavelength specific) are now available from several manufacturers.

Protection of the endotracheal tube from direct or reflected laser beam irradiation is of primary importance. If the laser beam strikes an unprotected endotracheal tube carrying oxygen, ignition of the tube could result in a catastrophic, intraluminal, blowtorch-type endotracheal tube fire.[107] Use of red rubber endotracheal tubes wrapped circumferentially from the cuff to the top with reflective metallic tape reduces the risk of intraluminal fire when a special laser-protective endotracheal tube cannot be used. Metallic tape covered with Merocel is another acceptable alternative. Mylar tape offers no protection from the laser and should not be used.[88] Ventilation tubes made of fluoroplastic were preferred when compared with silastic, red rubber, and polyvinyl chloride tubes under maximum power irradiation from CO_2, Nd:YAG, and KTP lasers.[51]

Protection should also be provided for the cuff of the endotracheal tube. Methylene blue–colored saline should be used to inflate the cuff.[91] Saline-saturated cottonoids are then placed above the cuff in the subglottic larynx to further protect the cuff. These cottonoids require frequent moistening during the procedure. If the cuff deflates from an errant hit by the laser beam, the already saturated cottonoids turn blue to warn the surgeon of impending danger. The tube should then be removed and replaced with a new one. Use of the microlaryngeal operating platform is strongly recommended as further protection against potential danger. Inserted into the subglottic larynx above the level of the packed cottonoids, this unique instrument serves as a back stop to protect the cottonoids, endotracheal tube, and cuff from any direct or reflected laser beam irradiation.[85]

The Nd:YAG laser has a different interaction with endotracheal tubes than the CO_2 laser. *In vitro* testing of various endotracheal tubes with the Nd:YAG laser has shown that the safest tube to use is a colorless or white polyvinyl endotracheal tube or a silicone endotracheal tube without any dark-colored lettering on the tube itself. Also, the tube should not have any lead-lined marking. The Ruysch red rubber tube with or without metallic tape does not protect against ignition with the Nd:YAG laser.[113]

Instrument selection

The surface characteristics of instruments used in laser surgery should provide for low specular or direct reflectance and large diffuse or scattered reflectance of the laser beam, if the beam inadvertently strikes the instrument. Plastic instruments should be avoided because they can melt with the laser irradiation. Use of instruments with these surface characteristics will help minimize tissue injury or endotracheal tube ignition from direct or reflected laser beam irradiation.

Rigid instrumentation is the preferred method of laser bronchoscopy with the CO_2 or Nd:YAG laser; if active bleeding occurs during bronchoscopy, it would be extremely difficult or impossible to successfully control the airway and evacuate the blood with flexible instrumentation. Additionally, rigid instrumentation allows the surgeon to pass one, two, or three suction cannulas through the bronchoscope to facilitate blood evacuation and airway control. This point must be emphasized because of the proliferation of Nd:YAG laser surgery and the ability of this laser light to be delivered through flexible fiberoptic and rigid endoscopes. Bronchoscopic couplers for CO_2 laser surgery must have an optical system that allows the visible helium-neon–aiming laser beam to be passed coaxially with the invisible CO_2 laser beam. In addition, the surgeon should be able to center the beam within the lumen of the bronchoscope to avoid the hazards of the beam reflecting off the inside wall of the bronchoscope, with subsequent loss of power and possible heating of the bronchoscope itself. Burns of the trachea, larynx, pharynx, and oral cavity have occurred as a direct result of such an event.[88]

Effectiveness of a safety protocol

Strong and Jako[121] and later Snow and others[118] warned of the possible complications associated with laser surgery of the upper aerodigestive tract, including the risks of endotracheal tube fires and tissue damage from reflection of the laser beam. After these early warnings, complications uniquely attributable to use of the CO_2 laser were reported in the literature.[2,14,18,75] In a survey of laser-related complications by Fried,[35] 49 of 152 otolaryngologists who used the laser reported 81 complications, including 28 incidents of endotracheal tube fires. An analysis of complications unique to the use of the laser that occurred under a rigid safety protocol at Northwestern University Medical School and affiliated hospitals revealed a 1.7% incidence of complications; no fires were reported in this group.[91] Healy and others[48] reported a 0.2% complication rate in 4416 cases of CO_2 laser surgery in the upper aerodigestive tract. Ossoff[96] published an extensive view of laser-related complications experienced by 218 past registrants of hands-on laser surgery training courses that he directed. Seven surgeons experienced eight complications and no endotracheal tube fires. The complication rate was 0.1% in more than 7200 laser surgical procedures. These papers have similar conclusions: (1) certain precautions are necessary when performing laser surgery of the upper aerodigestive tract, and (2) adherence to a rigid safety protocol allows laser surgery of the airway to be performed safely and with an extremely small risk of serious complications.

REFERENCES

1. Abramson AL and others: Is papillomavirus detectable in the plume of laser-treated laryngeal papilloma? *Arch Otolaryngol Head Neck Surg* 116:604, 1990.
2. Alberti PW: The complications of CO_2 laser surgery in otolaryngology, *Acta Otolaryngol (Stockh)* 91:375, 1981.
3. American National Standards Institute: *American national standard for the safe use of lasers, Z136. 1*, New York, 1981, American National Standards Institute.
4. Apfelberg DB and others: The argon laser for cutaneous lesions, *JAMA* 245:2073, 1981.
5. April MM and others: Laser therapy for lymphatic malformations of the upper aerodigestive tract: an evolving experience, *Arch Otolaryngol Head Neck Surg* 118:205, 1992.
6. Atiyah RA, Friedman CD, Sisson GA: The KTP/532 laser in glossal surgery: KTP/532 clinical update, *Laserscope* 22:1, 1988.
7. Atiyah RA: The KTP/532 laser in laryngeal surgery KTP/532 clinical update, *Laserscope* 21:1, 1988.
8. Balchum OJ, Dorion DR, Huth GC: Photoradiation therapy of endobronchial lung cancers employing the photodynamic action of hematoporphyrin derivative, *Lasers Surg Med* 4:13, 1984.
9. Bartels LJ: KTP laser stapedotomy: is it safe? *Otolaryngol Head Neck Surg* 103:685, 1990.
10. Bemis JF Jr and others: Endoscopic laser therapy for obstructing tracheobronchial lesions, *Ann Otol Rhinol Laryngol* 100:413, 1991.
11. Beste DJ, Toohill RJ: Microtrapdoor flap repair of laryngeal and tracheal stenosis, *Ann Otol Rhinol Laryngol* 100:420, 1991.
12. Blakeslee D and others: Excisional biopsy in the selective management of T1 glottic cancer: a three-year follow-up study, *Laryngoscope* 94:488, 1984.
13. Buell BR, Schuller DE: Comparison of tensile strength in CO_2 laser and scalpel skin incisions, *Arch Otolaryngol Head Neck Surg* 109:465, 1983.
14. Burgess GE, LeJeune FE: Endotracheal tube ignition during laser surgery of the larynx, *Arch Otolaryngol Head Neck Surg* 105:561, 1979.
15. Cerullo LJ, Mkrdichian E: Acoustic nerve tumor surgery before and since the laser: comparison of results, *Laser Surg Med* 7:224, 1987.
16. Cochrane JPS and others: Wound healing after laser surgery: experimental study, *Br J Surg* 67:740, 1980.
17. Cortese DA, Kinsey JH: Hematoporphyrin-derivative phototherapy for local treatment of cancer of the tracheobronchial tree, *Ann Otol Rhinol Laryngol* 91:652, 1982.
18. Cozine K and others: Laser-induced endotracheal tube fire, *Anesthesiology* 55:583, 1981.
19. Derkay CS: Task force on recurrent respiratory papillomas: a preliminary report, *Arch Otolaryngol Head Neck Surg* 121:1386, 1995.
20. DiBartolomeo JR, Ellis M: The argon laser in otology, *Laryngoscope* 90:1786, 1980.
21. DiBartolomeo JR: The argon and CO_2 lasers in otolaryngology: which one, when and why? *Laryngoscope* 91(suppl 26):1, 1981.
22. Dorion DR and others: Fluorescence bronchoscopy for detection of lung cancer, *Chest* 76:27, 1984.
23. Dougherty TJ and others: Photoradiation in the treatment of recurrent breast carcinoma, *J Natl Cancer Inst* 62:231, 1979.
24. Dougherty TJ and others: Photoradiation therapy for the treatment of malignant tumors, *Cancer Res* 38:2628, 1978.
25. Dougherty TJ and others: Photoradiation therapy II: cure of animal tumors with hematoporphyrin and light, *J Natl Cancer Inst* 55:115, 1975.
26. Dumon JF and others: Treatment of tracheobronchial lesions by laser photoresection, *Chest* 81:278, 1982.
27. Dumon JF: Principles for safety in application of neodymium-YAG laser in bronchology, *Chest* 86:163, 1984.
28. Durkin GE and others: Wound healing of the true vocal cord squamous epithelium after CO_2 laser ablation and cup forceps stripping, *Otolaryngol Head Neck Surg* 95:273, 1986.
29. Edelist G, Alberti PW: Anesthesia for CO_2 laser surgery of the larynx, *J Otolaryngol* 11:107, 1982.
30. Einstein A: Zur Quantem Theorie der Strahlung, *Phys Zeit* 18:121, 1917.
31. Escudero L and others: Argon laser in human tympanoplasty, *Arch Otolaryngol Head Neck Surg* 105:252, 1979.
32. Finsterbush A and others: Healing and tensile strength of CO_2 laser incisions and scalpel wounds in rabbits, *Plast Reconstr Surg* 70:360, 1982.
33. Fisher SE and others: Comparative histological study of wound healing following CO_2 laser and conventional surgical excision of canine buccal mucosa, *Arch Oral Biol* 28:287, 1983.
34. Fleischer D: Endoscopic laser therapy for gastrointestinal neoplasms, *Otolaryngol Clin North Am* 64:947, 1984.
35. Fried MP: A survey of the complications of laser laryngoscopy, *Arch Otolaryngol Head Neck Surg* 110:31, 1984.
36. Fuller TA: The characteristics of operation of surgical lasers, *Surg Clin North Am* 64:843, 1984.
37. Fuller TA: The physics of surgical lasers, *Lasers Surg Med* 1:5, 1980.
38. Garden JM and others: Papillomavirus in the vapor of carbon dioxide laser-treated verrucae, *JAMA* 259:1199, 1988.
39. Geusic JE, Marcos HM, Van Uitert LG: Neodymium doped yttrium-aluminum-garnet laser material, *Appl Phys Letters* 4:182, 1964.
40. Goldman L and others: Effect of the laser beam on the skin, *J Invest Dermatol* 40:121, 1963.
41. Goldman L and others: Pathology of the effect of the laser beam on the skin, *Nature* 197:912, 1963.
41a. Gordon JP, Zeiger HZ, Townes CH: Microwave amplification by stimulated emission, *Phys Rev* 95:282, 1954.
42. Laser Institute of America: *Guide for the selection of laser eye protection*, Toledo, Ohio, 1984, Laser Institute of America.
43. Hall RR: The healing of tissues incised by carbon dioxide laser, *Br J Surg* 58:222, 1971.
44. Hanna E and others: Laser welding of fascial grafts and its potential application in tympanoplasty: an animal model, *Otolaryngol Head Neck Surg* 108:356, 1993.
45. Hashimoto K and others: Laser wound healing compared with other surgical modalities, *Burns* 1:13, 1971.
46. Hayata Y and others: Hematoporphyrin derivative and laser photoradiation in the treatment of lung cancer, *Chest* 81:269, 1982.
47. Hayata Y and others: Photoradiation therapy with hematoporphyrin derivative in early and stage 1 lung cancer, *Chest* 86:169, 1984.
48. Healy GB and others: Complications of CO_2 laser surgery of the aerodigestive tract: experience of 4416 cases, *Otolaryngol Head Neck Surg* 92:13, 1984.

49. Healy GB and others: Management of choanal atresia with the carbon dioxide laser, *Ann Otol Rhinol Laryngol* 87:658, 1978.

50. Holinger LD: Treatment of severe subglottic stenosis without tracheotomy: a preliminary report, *Ann Otol Rhinol Laryngol* 91:407, 1982.

51. Hunsaker DH: Anesthesia for microlaryngeal surgery: the case for subglottic jet ventilation, *Laryngoscope* 104(suppl 65):1, 1944.

52. Joseph M, Reardon E, Goodman M: Lingual tonsillectomy: a treatment for inflammatory lesions of the lingual tonsil, *Laryngoscope* 94:179, 1984.

53. Kamami Y-V: Laser CO_2 for snoring: preliminary results, *Acta Otorhinolaryngol Belg* 44:451, 1990.

54. Karlan MS, Ossoff RH: Laser surgery for benign laryngeal disease: conservation and ergonomics, *Surg Clin North Am* 64:981, 1984.

55. Kauvar AN, McDaniel DH, Geronemus RG: Pulsed dye laser treatment of warts, *Arch Fam Med* 4:1035, 1995.

56. Keller GS, Doiron D, Weingarten C: Advances in laser skin surgery for vascular lesions, *Otolaryngol* 111:437, 1985.

57. Kirschner RA: Cutaneous plastic surgery with the CO_2 laser, *Surg Clin North Am* 64:871, 1984.

58. Koufman JA: The endoscopic management of early squamous carcinoma of the vocal cord with the carbon dioxide surgical laser: clinical experience and a proposed subclassification, *Otolaryngol Head Neck Surg* 95:531, 1986.

59. Krespi YP and others: Laser laryngeal tonsillectomy, *Laryngoscope* 99:131, 1989.

60. Kuhn F: The KTP/532 laser in tonsillectomy: KTP/532 clinical update, *Laserscope* 6:1, 1988.

61. Levine H, Balin P: Carbon dioxide laser treatment of cutaneous hemangiomas and tattoos, *Arch Otolaryngol Head Neck Surg* 108:236, 1982.

62. Levine HL: Endoscopy and the KTP/532 laser for nasal sinus disease, *Ann Otol Rhinol Laryngol* 98:46, 1989.

63. Linden BE and others: Morbidity in pediatric tonsillectomy, *Laryngoscope* 100:120, 1990.

64. Liston SL, Giordano A: Tongue release using the CO_2 laser, *Laryngoscope* 91:1010, 1981.

65. Lofgren LA and others: Photodynamic therapy for recurrent nasopharyngeal cancer, *Arch Otolaryngol Head Neck Surg* 121:997, 1995.

66. Luomanen M, Meurman JH, Lehto VP: Extracellular matrix in healing CO_2 laser incision wound, *J Oral Pathol* 16:322, 1987.

67. Madden JE and others: Studies in the management of the contaminated wound: resistance to infection of surgical wounds made by knife, electrosurgery and laser, *Am J Surg* 119:222, 1970.

68. Maiman TH: Stimulated optical radiation in ruby, *Nature* 187:493, 1960.

69. McCaughan JS Jr and others: Hematoporphyrin-derivative and photoradiation therapy of malignant tumors, *Lasers Surg Med* 3:199, 1983.

70. McDaniel DH, Mordon S: Hexascan: a new robotized scanning laser handpiece, *Cutis* 45:300, 1990.

71. McDonald GA, Simpson GT: Transoral resection of lesions of the oral cavity with the carbon dioxide laser, *Otolaryngol Clin North Am* 16:839, 1983.

72. McGee TM, Diaz-Ordaz EA, Kartush JM: The role of KTP laser in revision stapedectomy, *Otolaryngol Head Neck Surg* 109:839, 1993.

73. McGill TJI, Friedman EM, Healy GB: Laser surgery in the pediatric airway, *Otolaryngol Clin North Am* 16:865, 1983.

74. Metson R: Holmium:YAG laser endoscopic sinus surgery: a randomized, controlled study, *Laryngoscope* 106:1, 1996.

75. Meyers A: Complications of CO_2 laser surgery of the larynx, *Ann Otol Rhinol Laryngol* 90:132, 1981.

76. Mickelson SA: Laser-assisted uvulopalatoplasty for obstructive sleep apnea, *Laryngoscope* 106:10, 1996.

77. Mihashi S and others: Laser surgery in otolaryngology: interaction of the CO_2 laser in soft tissue, *Ann N Y Acad Sci* 267:263, 1976.

78. Mittelman H: CO_2 laser turbinectomies for chronic obstructive rhinitis, *Lasers Surg Med* 2:29, 1982.

79. Miyaguchi M, Sakai S: The contact Nd-YAG laser for oral and oropharyngeal malignant tumors, *Auris Nasus Larynx* 21:226, 1994.

80. Mohr RM and others: Safety considerations and safety protocol for laser surgery, *Surg Clin North Am* 64:851, 1984.

81. Norris CW, Mullarry MB: Experimental skin incision made with the carbon dioxide laser, *Laryngoscope* 92:416, 1982.

82. Norton ML, DeVos P: New endotracheal tube for laser surgery of the larynx, *Ann Otol Rhinol Laryngol* 87:554, 1978.

83. Ossoff RH and others: Potential applications of photoradiation therapy in head and neck surgery, *Arch Otolaryngol Head Neck Surg* 110:728, 1984.

84. Ossoff RH, Karlan MS: A set of bronchoscopes for carbon dioxide laser surgery, *Otolaryngol Head Neck Surg* 91:336, 1983.

85. Ossoff RH, Karlan MS: Instrumentation for CO_2 laser surgery of the larynx and tracheobronchial tree, *Surg Clin North Am* 64:973, 1984.

86. Ossoff RH, Karlan MS: Instrumentation for micro-laryngeal laser surgery, *Otolaryngol Head Neck Surg* 91:456, 1983.

87. Ossoff RH, Karlan MS: *Laser surgery in otolaryngology*. In Ballenger JJ, editor: *Diseases of the nose, throat, ear, head and neck*, Philadelphia, 1985, Lea & Febiger.

88. Ossoff RH, Karlan MS: Safe instrumentation in laser surgery, *Otolaryngol Head Neck Surg* 92:664, 1984.

89. Ossoff RH, Karlan MS: Universal endoscopic coupler for carbon dioxide laser surgery, *Ann Otol Rhinol Laryngol* 91:608, 1982.

90. Ossoff RH and others: Advanced microspot microslad for the CO_2 laser, *Otolaryngol Head Neck Surg* 105:411, 1991.

91. Ossoff RH and others: Comparison of tracheal damage from laser-ignited endotracheal tube fires, *Ann Otol Rhinol Laryngol* 92:333, 1983.

92. Ossoff RH and others: Endoscopic laser arytenoidectomy for the treatment of bilateral vocal cord paralysis, *Laryngoscope* 94:1293, 1984.

93. Ossoff RH and others: The CO_2 laser in otolaryngology—head and neck surgery: a retrospective analysis of complications, *Laryngoscope* 93:1287, 1983.

94. Ossoff RH and others: The universal endoscopic coupler for bronchoscopic carbon dioxide laser surgery: a multi-institutional clinical trial, *Otolaryngol Head Neck Surg* 93:824, 1985.

95. Ossoff RH: Bronchoscopic laser surgery: which laser when and why? *Otolaryngol Head Neck Surg* 94:378, 1986.

96. Ossoff RH: Laser safety in otolaryngology—head and neck surgery: anesthetic and educational considerations for laryngeal surgery, *Laryngoscope* 99:1, 1989.

97. Parkin JL, Dixon JA: Argon laser treatment of head and neck vascular lesions, *Otolaryngol Head Neck Surg* 93:211, 1985.

98. Parkin JL, Dixon JA: Laser phototherapy in hereditary hemorrhagic telangiectasia, *Otolaryngol Head Neck Surg* 89:204, 1981.

99. Perkins RC: Laser stapedotomy for otosclerosis, *Laryngoscope* 90:228, 1980.

100. Petrucco OM and others: Ablation of endometriotic implants in rabbits by hematoporphyrin derivative photoradiation therapy using the gold vapor laser, *Lasers Surg Med* 10:344, 1990.

101. Polanyi TG: Laser physics, *Otolaryngol Clin North Am* 16:753, 1983.

102. Rebeiz E and others: Nd-YAG laser treatment of venous malformations of the head and neck: an update, *Otolaryngol Head Neck Surg* 105:655, 1991.

103. Reinisch L: Laser induced heating and thermal propagation: a model of tissue interaction with light, *Proc Conf Lasers Elect Optics* 11:TuR4, 1989.

104. Robinson JK and others: Wound healing in porcine skin following low-output carbon dioxide laser irradiation of the incision, *Ann Plast Surg* 18:499, 1987.

105. Schawlow AL, Townes CH: Infrared and optical masers, *Physiol Rev* 112:1940, 1958.

106. Schlenk E and others: Laser assisted fixation of ear prostheses after stapedectomy, *Lasers Surg Med* 10:444, 1990.

107. Schramm VL, Mattox DE, Stool SE: Acute management of laser-ignited intratracheal explosion, *Laryngoscope* 91:1417, 1981.

108. Shapshay SM, Oliver P: Treatment of hereditary hemorrhagic telangiectasia by Nd-YAG laser photocoagulation, *Laryngoscope* 94:1554, 1984.

109. Shapshay SM, Simpson GT: Lasers in bronchology, *Otolaryngol Clin North Am* 16:879, 1983.

110. Shapshay SM, Beamis JF Jr, Dumon JF: Total cervical tracheal stenosis: treatment by laser, dilation, and stenting, *Ann Otol Rhinol Laryngol* 98:890, 1989.

111. Shapshay SM and others: New microspot micromanipulator for carbon dioxide laser surgery in otolaryngology, *Arch Otolaryngol Head Neck Surg* 114:1012, 1988.

112. Shapshay SM and others: Removal of rhinophyma with the carbon dioxide laser, *Arch Otolaryngol Head Neck Surg* 106:257, 1980.

113. Shapshay SM: Personal communication, 1983.

114. Simpson GT, Polanyi TG: History of the carbon dioxide laser in otolaryngologic surgery, *Otolaryngol Clin North Am* 16:739, 1983.

115. Simpson GT, Strong MS: Recurrent respiratory papillomatosis: the role of the carbon dioxide laser, *Otolaryngol Clin North Am* 16:887, 1983.

116. Simpson GT and others: Rhinologic surgery with the carbon dioxide laser, *Laryngoscope* 92:412, 1982.

117. Sliney DH: Laser safety, *Lasers Surg Med* 16:215, 1995.

118. Snow JC, Norton ML, Saluja TS: Fire hazard during CO_2 laser microsurgery on the larynx and trachea, *Anesth Analg* 55:146, 1976.

119. Spilman LS: Nursing precautions for CO_2 laser surgery, *Symposium Proceedings, The Laser Institute of America* 37:63, 1983.

120. Stein E and others: Acute and chronic effects of bone ablation with a pulsed holmium laser, *Lasers Surg Med* 10:384, 1990.

121. Strong MS, Jako GJ: Laser surgery in the larynx, *Ann Otol Rhinol Larynol* 81:791, 1972.

122. Strong MS and others: Transoral resection of cancer of the oral cavity: the role of the CO_2 laser, *Otolaryngol Clin North Am* 12:207, 1979.

123. Strunk CL Jr, Quinn FB Jr: Stapedectomy surgery in residency: KTP-532 laser versus argon laser, *Am J Otol* 14:113, 1993.

124. Strunk CL, Nichols ML: A comparison of the KTP/532-laser tonsillectomy vs. traditional dissection/snare tonsillectomy, *Otolaryngol Head Neck Surg* 103:966, 1990.

125. Tan OT and others: Histologic comparison of the pulsed dye laser and copper vapor laser effects on pig skin, *Lasers Surg Med* 10:551, 1990.

126. Tauber C and others: Healing of CO_2 laser incision in the skin and fascia, *Harefuah* 98:1, 1980.

127. Thedinger BS: Applications of the KTP laser in chronic ear surgery, *Am J Otol* 11:79, 1990.

128. Thornell WC: Intralaryngeal approach for arytenoidectomy in bilateral abductor vocal cord paralysis, *Arch Otolaryngol Head Neck Surg* 47:505, 1984.

129. Tomita Y, Mihashi S, Nagata K: Mutagenicity of smoke condensates induced by CO_2 laser irradiation and electrocauterization, *Mutat Res* 89:145, 1981.

130. Toty A and others: Bronchoscopic management of tracheal lesions using the Nd:YAG laser, *Thorax* 36:175, 1981.

131. Tsuchiya A and others: Hematoporphyrin derivative and laser photoradiation in the diagnosis and treatment of bladder cancer, *J Urol* 130:79, 1983.

132. Vaughan CW: Use of the carbon dioxide laser in the endoscopic management of organic laryngeal disease, *Otolaryngol Clin North Am* 16:849, 1983.

133. Ward RF: Treatment of tracheal and endobronchial lesions with the potassium titanyl phosphate laser, *Ann Otol Rhinol Laryngol* 101:205, 1992.

134. Werkhaven JA, Weed DT, Ossoff RH: Carbon dioxide laser serial microtrapdoor flap excision of subglottic stenosis, *Arch Otolaryngol Head Neck Surg* 119:676, 1993.

135. Whitehead E, Salam MA: Use of the carbon dioxide laser with the Montgomery T-tube in the management of extensive subglottic stenosis, *J Laryngol Otol* 106:829, 1992.

136. Wile AG and others: Laser photoradiation therapy of cancer: an update of the experience at the University of California, Irvine, *Lasers Surg Med* 4:5, 1984.

137. Wile AG, Novotny J, Mason GR: Photoradiation therapy of head and neck cancer, *Am J Clin Oncol* 6:39, 1984.

138. Zaret M and others: Biomedical experimentation with optical masers, *J Opt Soc Am* 52:607, 1962.

139. Zweng HC and others: Experimental laser photocoagulation, *Am J Ophthalmol* 58:353, 1964.

Chapter 12

Anesthesia and Management of the Difficult Airway

Allan C.D. Brown

Anesthesiology is the art and science of rendering a patient insensible to pain while maintaining physiologic functions. Anesthesiologists most commonly practice within the environs of an operating room, but the past several decades have seen their increasing involvement in intensive care units, pain clinics, respiratory therapy units, and obstetric labor units.

HISTORY

Development of general anesthesia

The beginnings of surgical anesthesia are usually dated from "ether day"—October 16, 1846—when William Thomas Green Morton of Worcester County, Massachusetts, publicly exhibited the use of diethyl ether for the first time at the Massachusetts General Hospital. The operation was for the excision of a tumor from the jaw of Gilbert Abbot by a noted surgeon of the day, Dr. John C. Warren.[7] Unbeknownst to the rest of the medical community, Dr. Crawford Williamson Long of Georgia had already successfully used ether for surgery—on March 30, 1842.[38] However, as Sir Francis Darwin stated in 1914, "In science, the credit goes to the man who convinces the world, not the man to whom the idea first occurs."

The time was ripe for the introduction of anesthesia. The discipline of chemistry was developing apace. Henry Hickman's work in England on the anesthetic effects of carbon dioxide had preceded Morton's demonstration, and in 1845, Horace Wells had tried unsuccessfully to demonstrate in public the use of nitrous oxide for surgical anesthesia. After Morton's demonstration, in 1847 James Young Simpson introduced chloroform into clinical use in Scotland.[59]

The need for a general term to describe this new state of insensibility for surgery was evidenced by the number of synonyms in use by 1847. Learned articles on the use of chloroform were referring to its effects with the term *etherization*. The word *anesthesia* was first suggested by Oliver Wendell Holmes. Holmes appears to have thought that he invented the word itself,[70] but Plato's previous use of the word in the sense of "lack of philosophic perception" had preempted his claim. The early development of anesthesia in the United States took a decisively different turn from its development in Britain and Europe. This was associated with the well-publicized controversy that surrounded the preeminence of claims to its discovery, and the fact that Morton, a dentist, tried to patent the use of ether under the name of "Letheon." Physicians on the other side of the Atlantic not only recognized the importance of the discovery, but also considered it an appropriate discipline for medical practice and investigation. The medical profession in anesthesia's country of origin, in the face of the early scandals, was more circumspect in accepting its part in medical practice. This situation was not to be rectified until early in the twentieth century and only after the administration of anesthetics by nonphysicians had become established.

Thus it was European physicians who accomplished much of the initial development of anesthetic equipment and techniques. Britain was fortunate to have Dr. John Snow (1813-1858), a physician of established reputation who was interested in respiratory physiology; he took an immediate interest in anesthesia and devoted his remaining professional life to its practice. His early, careful observations established the groundwork for clinical anesthesia, but the infrastructure for the widespread application of that knowledge did not exist. Britain at that time was approaching the height of its industrial power and was in a position to create the means for routine anesthetic administration. The principles for the controlled vaporization of agents were incorporated into the inhalers of Snow and Clover. In 1862, Thomas Skinner, an obstetrician, invented a wire mask for the administration of chloroform, later improved by Karl Schimmelbusch. However, the introduction of the first practical anesthesia machine by Sir Frederick Hewitt in 1887 had to await the development of compressed gas cylinders in 1868 by the Medical Pneumatic Appliance Company in London. In 1880, Macewen introduced oral endotracheal intubation, and Kirstein described the first direct-vision laryngoscope in 1895.

Boothby and Cotton introduced a sight-feed nitrous oxide and oxygen flowmeter in 1912, and in 1920 Guedel's first paper on the signs of anesthesia was published, which refined Snow's original signs.[36] At this time, Magill and Rowbotham were refining the techniques of endotracheal anesthesia, and in 1923 Ralph Waters, in Wisconsin, first used carbon dioxide absorption on a human. It was also Waters who became professor and chair of the first academic department of anesthesiology in the United States at the University of Wisconsin in Madison and trained many of the first generation of academic anesthesiologists in the United States.

The ideal general anesthetic

It was fortunate that diethyl ether inaugurated painless surgery because this drug was physiologically safe and had a high therapeutic index. Its two major drawbacks were its flammability and its unpleasant after-effects for patients and attendants. These shortcomings explained the sustained popularity of chloroform, which was much more pleasant to inhale and allowed a more dignified emergence because of the lower incidence of nausea and emesis. However, the toxic effects of chloroform on the heart and liver spurred the search for an ideal inhalational anesthetic agent, which has continued to this day. The ideal inhalational anesthetic should allow a pleasant, rapid induction and emergence. It should be chemically stable when stored and should not decompose on contact with the materials used in anesthetic circuits. It should neither be flammable nor support combustion. It should be nontoxic and biochemically stable, undergoing no biotransformation in the body and being excreted unchanged through the lungs. It should be sufficiently potent to allow high oxygen concentrations to be delivered. It should exhibit neither chemical nor physiologic interactions with other drugs. If the target organs are not exclusively the brain and nervous system, the anesthetic should at least depress other organ activity to a lesser extent for a given dose of the drug. At this time, such a drug has not been found.

A triad of properties are desirable in all inhalational anesthetics—narcosis, relaxation, and analgesia. The original choice of the word *analgesia* was probably a misnomer because absence of pain implies the blocking of a sensation, which can only be perceived when a person is conscious. Because patients are not conscious during general anesthesia, the third desirable property of the triad is more correctly described as *reflex suppression*. The term *analgesia* is probably better confined to conduction block and infiltration anesthetic techniques. Fortunately, the dose of diethyl ether required to achieve unconsciousness also achieved sufficient muscular relaxation and reflex suppression for operations on most parts of the body, without dangerous depression of brainstem vital functions. Ether's drawbacks remained, but as each new agent was introduced and investigated, it was found that although some were more acceptable in terms of flammability and patient comfort, none had the basic triad of properties in the same balance as ether. Over the years, many inhalation agents were introduced to clinical practice and enjoyed popularity among anesthesiologists for varying periods of time. This work was somewhat random in approach, relying on the investigation of newly identified compounds for anesthetic and toxic properties in the hope of discovering a clinically useful drug. In 1951, C. W. Suckling, armed with the knowledge and techniques of modern organic chemistry, brought a new approach to fruition with the synthesis of halothane (Fluothane) in the laboratories of Imperial Chemical Industries, near Manchester, England.[63] In response to the request from anesthesiologists for an ideal agent with a predefined list of desirable properties, he succeeded in building the halothane molecule from the "atom up." This new agent was studied pharmacologically by Raventos[51] and introduced to clinical practice by Johnstone.[29] Halothane heralded a new era in anesthesia; this drug is four or five times more potent than diethyl ether and twice as potent as chloroform. Its vapor is pleasant to inhale and is not an irritant, but most important, it is nonflammable and nonexplosive when mixed with oxygen in any concentration. Here was a drug similar to ether in terms of its triad of properties, but with high patient acceptability, and it held out to the surgeon the promise of the unrestricted use of electrocautery and diathermy. That these were significant advantages was evidenced by the rapid spread of the use of halothane throughout anesthetic practice around the world. However, amid the initial euphoria, it became evident that halothane was still not the perfect agent. Its potency demanded skill and the redesigning of equipment for its safe use. Its poor analgesic properties were a relative drawback. Of interest is its propensity to sensitize the myocardium to catecholamines[2,45] and the rare occurrence of liver failure[66] in association with its use. Therefore the search for the ideal agent continued.

Variations on the halogenated aliphatic compound theme (Fig. 12-1) have been introduced to clinical practice over the past two decades to overcome the problems identified with halothane. The major thrust of the work has been to develop agents less likely to be metabolized in the body, thereby minimizing the chances of hepatic- and nephrotoxi-

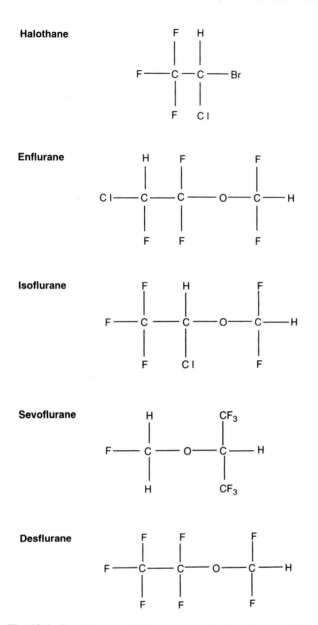

Fig. 12-1. The halogenated inhalation anesthetic agents available in the United States (halothane, enflurane, its isomer isoflurane, sevoflurane, and desflurane).

popularity, and with experience, its use has largely replaced that of halothane, except in pediatric practice. The most common concerns associated with isoflurane involve the cardiovascular system and represent the spectrum of its pharmacologic properties rather than any specific toxicity. Hypotension, similar to that seen with the other potent vapors, is especially evident in the absence of significant surgical stimulation. Tachycardia and the remote possibility of coronary blood flow "steal" may be of importance in patients who have coronary artery disease. The relative absence of hepatic complications is a major advantage. Overall, isoflurane is remarkable for its lack of serious complications, and this accounts for its current popularity among the inhalation anesthetics. However, it has been found to be somewhat irritating to the airway in conscious patients, thus halothane is still preferred when an inhalation induction is required, e.g., with the management of the difficult airway and for pediatric inductions. More recently, two new agents have been approved for clinical use in the United States, sevoflurane and desflurane. Both agents approach the ideal in some ways and fall short in others. Both agents have low blood–gas and blood–tissue partition coefficients that allow rapid induction and emergence. Desflurane is difficult to handle because of its physical properties and requires specially designed heated vaporizers and may possibly be limited to closed-circuit use because of its cost; sevoflurane resembles isoflurane in physical properties. Desflurane is almost inert under normal conditions and has less metabolic breakdown than isoflurane; sevoflurane is unstable in alkali (i.e., carbon dioxide absorbers) and can be metabolized, including the production of fluoride, which may reach nephrotoxic levels during long operations. If these new agents find a permanent place in clinical practice, it will most likely be associated with short outpatient procedures.

Development of local anesthesia

Carl Koller (1858-1944) graduated from the University of Vienna in 1882 and went on to specialize in ophthalmic surgery. He soon became dissatisfied with the operating conditions and patient problems created by the general anesthetic techniques of the time, which prompted him to search for better methods of pain relief in ophthalmology. Koller had been interested in the properties of cocaine since medical school. After animal experiments, Koller tried topical use of cocaine on his patients with great success and reported his findings to the German Ophthalmological Congress in 1884.[32] In the same year, the noted American surgeon William Steward Halsted (1852-1922) performed the first successful nerve block—a block of the mandibular nerve with cocaine.

In 1891, Quincke in Germany and Essex Wynter in England demonstrated lumbar puncture to be a practical clinical procedure. In 1898, August Bier (1861-1949) gave the first deliberate spinal anesthetic.[5] In addition to his many surgical achievements, he also developed the intravenous use of pro-

city. The first widely accepted agent was enflurane. Major complications unique to enflurane occur infrequently. Reasons for its declining popularity today may involve the narrow margin between adequate anesthesia and unacceptable hypotension more than any specific toxicity of the drug. It can induce a distinctive seizure activity, but it is rare, self-limited, and without apparent consequences. Hepatic dysfunction also is rare, but biotransformation of enflurane can lead to the release of free fluoride, especially when anesthesia is prolonged or when renal dysfunction is present. However, the usual levels of fluoride required to produce nephrotoxicity (40 to 50 μmol) are rarely exceeded except during long operations. Isoflurane was the next agent to achieve caine to induce anesthesia.[6] Tropococaine, isolated by Giesel in 1891, was the first alternative to cocaine, but a local anesthetic drug with relatively low toxicity was not found until 1904, when Alfred Einhorn synthesized procaine. In 1890, Redard of Geneva introduced the ethyl chloride spray for topical analgesia, and in 1892, Karl Ludwig Schleich (1859-1922) introduced infiltration analgesia.

The scene was now set for Heinrich Friedrich Braun (1862-1934), the "father of local analgesia." His interest in local analgesia was developed while he was director of the Deaconess Hospital in Leipzig. In 1902, he added epinephrine to cocaine solutions to prolong analgesic action,[8] and in 1905 he pioneered the use of the new drug procaine.[9] The year 1905 also saw the publication of his classic textbook *Local Anesthesia*. It was Braun who first coined the term *conduction anesthesia*. A pupil of Braun, Arthur Lawen (1876-1958), went on to describe paravertebral conduction anesthesia and in 1910 demonstrated that extradural analgesia was a safe and practical technique for pain relief.

Fortunately for the development of local anesthesia, its successful clinical application did not have to generate its own equipment. The hypodermic syringe and hollow needle had been developed concurrently but independently. The principle of injection had been demonstrated as early as 1657, when Sir Christopher Wren and Robert Boyle, using a bladder attached to a sharpened quill, had injected tincture of opium intravenously into a dog. In 1827, von Neuner described one of the first practical hypodermic devices, which was used for veterinary ophthalmology. Zophar Jayne of Illinois patented an early device for human use in 1841.[42] In 1853, Pravaz of Lyons (1791-1853) invented the syringe made of glass, and in the same year, Alexander Wood of Edinburgh (1817-1874) introduced the hypodermic syringe and hollow needle as we know them today.

As might be expected, the development of local anesthetic drugs did not occur without problems. Natives of the Andean foothills had chewed the leaves of the coca shrub for their mood-elevating effect since time immemorial. Scientific expeditions to South America brought the shrub back to Europe, where chemists endeavored to separate the active principle. In 1855, Gaedicke isolated the alkaloid erythroxylin, but it was not until 1860 that Albert Niemann succeeded in isolating cocaine from the erythroxylin extract, remarking that the crystals numbed his tongue. Eight years elapsed before a monograph appeared, in 1868, by a Peruvian army surgeon, Thomas Moreno y Maiz, describing experiments with cocaine. This probably was the first publication suggesting cocaine's potential as a local anesthetic and coincidentally the first description of cocaine-induced seizures,[67] preceding Koller's definitive work by 16 years.

Although cocaine's benefits were beyond doubt, so were the toxic and addictive properties of the drug. These problems prompted the search for better drugs. Willstatter in 1895 succeeded in defining the chemical structure of cocaine, identifying it as the benzoic acid ester of ecgonine.

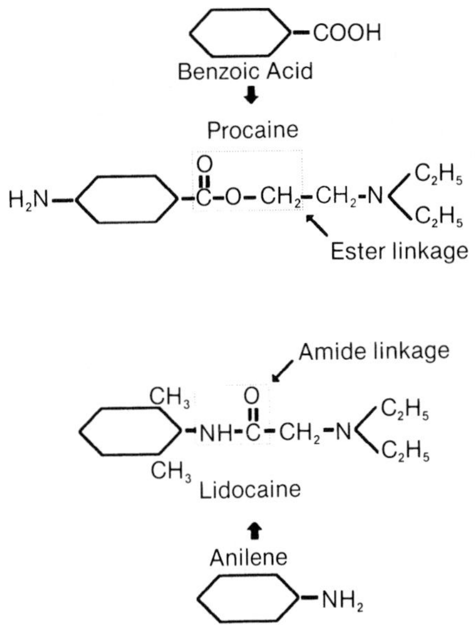

Fig. 12-2. The two major groups of local anesthetic agents—the ester group, derived from benzoic acid, and the amide group, derived from aniline.

Further investigation of the benzoic acid esters resulted in the introduction of tropococaine by Giesel and stovaine by Fourneau. However, both these drugs were toxic and irritant and did not supplant cocaine in practice. Not until the introduction of procaine did a benzoic acid ester of low toxicity become available to clinicians. Modifications of procaine's structure have since yielded many new agents, current examples being tetracaine and chloroprocaine.

Procaine and its derivatives held sway in clinical practice until 1948, when the Swedish chemist Lofgren discovered lidocaine during his investigations of aniline derivatives.[37] The discovery of lidocaine was as important to local anesthesia as the discovery of halothane was to be to general anesthesia. Lidocaine is a potent, stable drug with relatively low toxicity and high tissue penetration but without cocaine's habituating properties. It was the progenitor of many new "amide" local anesthetics, including prilocaine and bupivacaine (Fig. 12-2).

THE ANESTHETIC STATE

The anesthetic state has three component properties: narcosis, relaxation, and reflex suppression. In the case of general anesthetic agents, all three components can be achieved with the use of single drug, primarily by the central depression of brain activity. *General anesthesia* may be defined as a progressive, reversible depression of nervous tissue, leading to the controlled production of unconsciousness.

Theories of general anesthesia

The mechanism by which general anesthetics cause loss of consciousness is unknown. A number of theories have been advanced; each is based on either the physicochemical properties of the drug or the localization of a site of action. Many compounds, with widely differing chemical structures, are capable of producing anesthesia, making a strictly structural theory untenable. The purely physical theories, based on the intermolecular forces exerted between the drug molecules themselves and evidenced by proposed correlations between boiling points, vapor pressure, van der Waals constants, and so on, are not informative relative to the interaction between the drug and its site of action. Thus, recent thought has concentrated on two main areas, solubility and sites of actions.

Solubility theories

Work on the physicochemical theories of general anesthesia has revolved around differentiating between their behavior in aqueous media and their behavior in nonaqueous media. The aqueous theories are based on the apparent relationship between the anesthetic partial pressure and the decomposition pressure of the gas hydrates (clathrates) formed by the anesthetics. The postulate is that anesthetic action occurs in the aqueous or hydrophilic areas of the central nervous system, where clathrates are stabilized with charged protein sidechains, impeding neural impulse conduction, while the ordering effect on adjacent water molecules interferes with neural membrane transport.[45,49] The aqueous theories are no longer tenable because they fail to correlate the potency of the fluorocarbons and do not predict the additive effects of anesthetic potencies observed in clinical practice; in addition, some volatile agents do not form clathrates under the proposed conditions.

The nonaqueous theories have developed out of the Meyer-Overton fat solubility hypothesis,[43,47] which relates the onset of narcosis to the attainment of a certain molar concentration of the agent in the lipids of the cell, the effective concentration depending on the nature of the cell rather than on the agent. This theory accounts for the strong relationship between the anesthetic pressure of a compound and its lipid solubility. The correlation appears to hold true over a range of anesthetic agent potencies.[21,26] However, alkaloids do not fit the theory, and many fat-soluble substances have no anesthetic action. This approach does not address the mechanism of anesthetic action in the area of the nonaqueous medium.

Site-of-action theories

The surface tension theory of anesthesia holds that the adsorption of anesthetic agents by cell surfaces alters permeability and the dielectric constant, interfering with metabolic process and neural transmission.[13] The cell permeability theory states that anesthetic agents stabilize cell membranes, thereby interfering with sodium transport mechanisms. The biochemical theories endeavor to explain the anesthetic state in terms of interference with subcellular enzyme systems. The decreased oxygen consumption observed with clinical concentrations of inhalation agents[16] and barbiturates[10] sug-

gests decreased enzyme activity, but whether this is a cause or an effect of anesthesia is moot. The same question of cause versus effect can be leveled at all the site-of-action theories.

Mechanisms of local anesthesia

Local anesthetics are drugs that reversibly block the initiation and propagation of nerve action potentials distal to the point of application. This is achieved by a combination of mechanisms. By hydrophobic bonding, the drug base is adsorbed by the cell membrane, thereby hindering sodium access. By virtue of lipid solubility, the drug base dissolves in the phospholipids of the cell membrane, causing swelling, which tends to obstruct the ion channels through the membrane. The base that penetrates to the axoplasm dissociates to the degree dictated by the particular drug's pK_a, and the cation, held in place by electrostatic forces, closes the inner mouth of the sodium channels.[54] The cation from dissociated drug on the exterior membrane also binds to the dipolemolecular coat on the exterior surface of the membrane, where its charge tends to repel sodium ions. Local anesthetic block is a nondepolarizing type of block.[61] The resting potential of the axon is unchanged, as are its metabolic activity and the resting membrane permeability. These mechanisms apply equally to the saltatory conduction in myelinated axons, but because the exposure of the membrane at the nodes of Ranvier is small, a higher concentration of drug is required to block conduction in myelinated nerves than in nonmyelinated nerves. Also, because of the skipping of the impulse over one or more blocked nodes,[64] it is necessary to expose several adjacent nodes to the agent to ensure a block.

Stages of general anesthesia

In 1920, Arthur Guedel published a systemized description of the signs of anesthesia. This description was based on observations of the use of diethyl ether as a single anesthetic agent. Ether is so soluble in blood that its uptake from the lungs to a sufficient dose to achieve and deepen anesthesia is slow. Guedel was, therefore, able to describe four stages of anesthesia, each of which is characterized by a distinct combination of signs:

1. Analgesic stage—from the beginning of induction to loss of consciousness; characterized by a varying degree of true surgical analgesia and the patient's ability to respond to commands.
2. Excitement stage—from loss of consciousness to the onset of automatic respiration; characterized by increased skeletal muscle tone and irregular breathing. Excitement and involuntary activity may be absent or marked. Hypertension, tachycardia, breath holding, laryngospasm, swallowing, and vomiting may occur.
3. Surgical anesthesia stage—from the onset of automatic respiration to respiratory paralysis; character-

ized by loss of skeletal muscle tone and eyelid and conjunctival reflexes.

4. Overdose stage—from respiratory paralysis to death. All reflex activity is lost, and pupils are widely dilated.

Guedel originally described four progressive planes within stage 3 (surgical anesthesia), which were based on the progressive suppression of ocular signs and respiratory activity, but these may be condensed into three functional planes of surgical anesthesia.

1. Light anesthesia—until eye movement disappears
2. Medium anesthesia—increasing intercostal paralysis
3. Deep anesthesia—diaphragmatic respiration

In otolaryngology, these stages may still be seen because of the occasional need for the inhalation induction of anesthesia in the presence of airway problems. In anesthesia for most other branches of surgery, however, the original concept of anesthetic depth is outmoded because combinations of drugs are used in balanced techniques. Newer agents do not follow such an orderly sequence. Thiobarbiturates may induce surgical anesthesia without stages 1 and 2 being evident. The muscle relaxants simulate most of the signs of anesthesia without rendering the patient anesthetic at all. However, the need to assess the patient's conscious state and degree of reflex suppression remains, and the orthodox stages have been restated in modern terms.[35] When the surgeon commences surgical preparation and positioning, the patient sometimes moves (much to the mortification of the anesthesiologist). Movement does not necessarily mean that the patient is awake. The usual explanation is that the surgeon is stimulating the patient while he or she is still in stage 2, either because the intravenous induction agent's effects are wearing off before the inhalation agent's have had sufficient time to replace them or because injected muscle relaxants have not yet achieved full effect. The surgeon should always wait for the anesthesiologist to give the word to proceed. This precaution is even more important if an inhalation induction is being undertaken because any stimulation of the patient, including auditory, may unleash the full excitation of stage 2, with vomiting and laryngospasm and their associated serious sequelae. It should be remembered that the stages of anesthesia are traversed on emergence and on induction. Thus patients in the anesthesia recovery room should be allowed to awaken with as little stimulation as possible. In this context, mentioning the small problem associated with estimated surgical closing time also is worthwhile. The anesthesiologist usually asks for an estimate to gauge when to start to reverse anesthesia so as not to waste unnecessary time at the end of the operation. The surgeon who estimates 10 minutes and in fact requires 20 minutes may find that the patient tends to make the final skin closure and dressings difficult.

ASSESSMENT OF THE PATIENT FOR ANESTHESIA

The purpose of this section is not to provide a comprehensive review of the basic clinical skills of eliciting a history or conducting a thorough physical examination, but rather to emphasize those areas in the preoperative assessment of the patient that are important to the conduct of anesthesia. All anesthetic agents are cellular poisons, some with a low therapeutic index, that give rise to potentially adverse physiologic changes even in healthy patients. There is such a thing as minor surgery, but there is no such thing as a minor anesthetic; the patient's life always is at risk when he or she is under the influence of anesthetic drugs.

Physical status assessment

The American Society of Anesthesiologists (ASA) has sponsored several attempts to develop a classification of anesthetic risk according to the preexisting diseases and conditions of the patient and the operation to be undertaken. These efforts have met with only partial success because a positive correlation between these factors is not evident.[31] What has developed from this work is the ASA physical status classification system, which may not directly reflect the anesthetic risk:

ASA 1—a normal healthy patient
ASA 2—a patient with a mild systemic disease
ASA 3—a patient with a severe disease that limits activity but is not incapacitating
ASA 4—a patient with an incapacitating systemic disease that is a constant threat to life
ASA 5—a moribund patient not expected to survive 24 hours with or without operation

Each of the classes may be modified with the letter *E*, denoting an emergency presentation and all that implies for the patient's preoperative preparation. The problems associated with the preoperative assessment of risk are evident if one considers the case of a young healthy adult with a minor deformity of the second branchial arch structures, which, although not being apparent in everyday life, poses major anatomic problems for safe endotracheal intubation. Similarly, a young healthy patient with a family history of malignant hyperthermia, although at considerable risk from anesthesia, could still be classed as an ASA 1 patient. Thus the preoperative anesthetic assessment is aimed not only toward the assessment of the general physical status of the patient, which at best is an indicator of the general state of the patient's integrated physiologic systems, but also toward detecting specific problems posed by coexisting disease, the requirements of the operation, and any significant medication being taken, as well as problems and points in the history suggesting a true anesthetic risk. Of particular importance is a history of previous problems with anesthesia or a difficult intubation.

Physical status assessment requires that two major questions be answered: (1) What is the patient's general physiologic ability to respond to stress (anesthetic and surgical)? (2) What currently existing disease conditions might modify or limit that response? The history of the patient's response to the level of physical activity undertaken in everyday living usually is the best guide to the patient's probable response to the iatrogenic stresses of the operating room. However, some individuals appear to lead perfectly satisfying lives without exposing themselves to a stress sufficient to gauge the appropriateness of the response from the history. Asking the patient to accompany the interviewer up some stairs is usually sufficient to form a valid clinical impression.[25] The heart rate and rhythm, blood pressure (BP), respiratory pattern, and general state of distress may certainly suggest the need for quantitative laboratory investigation. Preexisting systemic disease would modify one's enthusiasm and the number of stairs, but in general the approach to physical assessment is the same. It is the patient's integrated response to stress that is being assessed, even if it is modified by disease, rather than any specific problems of management posed by the disease itself.

The presence of systemic disease necessitates the answering of a number of specific questions:

1. Is the disease process under the best medical control possible, or in the case of an emergency situation, has everything reasonable been attempted to stabilize the patient's condition?
2. What drugs are being used to control the disease, and do any of them interact with anesthetic drugs?
3. Does the disease process impose any limits on what may be undertaken surgically and anesthetically in terms of positioning, technique, and duration of the procedure?
4. Who will manage the disease during the perioperative period?
5. Have the expected gains of the surgical intervention been appropriately weighed against the estimated risks of anesthesia associated with the systemic disease under this degree of control?
6. Does this disease process pose any specific perioperative problems for surgical or anesthetic management?
7. Does the anesthetic technique pose any problems for the perioperative management of the disease?

A patient with a poor physical status because of disease generally has impaired homeostatic control and is particularly vulnerable to the depressant effects of an inhalational anesthetic drug given as the sole anesthetic agent. This tends to necessitate the use of balanced anesthetic techniques with muscle relaxant drugs. In some operations, the possible necessity of using a nerve stimulator might persuade the surgeon to delay elective surgery until the patient's physical status is improved. Should the anesthesiologist, in consultation with the patient and the surgeon, elect to proceed with conduction anesthesia or infiltration anesthesia with the anesthesiologist standing by, a new set of problems and limitations emerges. Will the patient's condition permit correct positioning for surgery? Can the patient breathe while lying flat? Can the patient tolerate lying on the operating table for sufficient time to complete the proposed procedure?

These alternatives are not particularly promising in those with serious pulmonary, cardiac, or arthritic conditions. It is worth emphasizing that if a patient for elective surgery with a major systemic disease is not considered to be in the best possible medical condition, stand-by local anesthesia is not an appropriate choice to ''get away with surgery'' on an improperly prepared patient. Long operations during local infiltration anesthesia frequently require local anesthetic drug dosages approaching or exceeding safe levels. Even then, general anesthesia still may be required if the patient cannot tolerate the duration of the procedure, thereby subjecting the patient to two sets of risks that could have been avoided. No anesthesiologist should allow this situation to occur because of misplaced concern for either patient or surgical convenience.

The anesthesiologist should be concerned not only about the effects of systemic disease on the conduct of anesthesia but also about the impact of the anesthetic on the subsequent course and management of the disease. A respiratory cripple imprudently paralyzed and ventilated for surgery may not be able to be weaned from the ventilator postoperatively. An association exists between the stress of surgery and anesthesia and exacerbation of multiple sclerosis. Anesthetic management may create major problems in reestablishing the myasthenic or diabetic patient on stable medication postoperatively. Is the withdrawal of long-term medication to permit the safe use of one anesthetic technique really in the patient's interest when another, perhaps less ideal, technique would permit continuation of the medication? These are all necessarily matters of judgement, only to be decided after consultation between the anesthesiologist, the surgeon, the appropriate internist, and the patient. Systemic medication should always be reviewed at the preoperative visit, with particular attention being paid to possible interactions with anesthetic drugs. It also is important to remember that some patients will not volunteer information concerning over-the-counter drugs; because these drugs were not prescribed by a physician, some patients do not consider them ''real'' drugs. Similarly, a patient admitted for surgery with a serious systemic disease may neglect to mention drugs being taken for an unrelated, older chronic condition.

Examples encountered in practice include elderly patients whose mild hypertension has been managed successfully for many years with reserpine and patients who may be taking long-acting anticholinesterases such as echothiophate for glaucoma. Both drugs have serious interactions with drugs used in anesthetic practice. Reserpine blocks peripheral adrenergic neurons by depleting synaptic norepinephrine stores; this is associated with supersensitivity to direct-acting and insensitivity to indirect-acting sympathomimetic amines, which may be used to counteract hypotension during anesthesia.[14,24] Echothiophate iodide, a long-acting anticholinesterase, interferes with the hydrolysis of the depolarizing muscle relaxant succinylcholine by pseudocholinesterase, thereby prolonging its clinical action dramatically.

As a general rule, if a patient is sufficiently ill to require systemic medication while awake, the same medication is required during anesthesia. The anesthesiologist's preoperative assessment should allow modifications to a proposed anesthetic technique to consider the actions and interactions expected from these systemic drugs. This is particularly true for most antihypertensive drugs and drugs used to control cardiac and pulmonary disease. A few drugs have potential interactions so devastating that their withdrawal before anesthesia should be considered.[60] However, some medications, although posing additional risks to the patient requiring anesthesia, are an essential part of the treatment of the patient's presenting condition and cannot be withdrawn for anesthetic considerations. An example of this situation is the antibiotic chemotherapeutic agents such as the anthracyclines. Anthracyclines are used to manage lymphomas and solid tumors such as breast, lung, and thyroid. Chronic cardiotoxicity associated with anthracycline administration is a dose-dependent cardiomyopathy that leads to congestive heart failure in 2% to 10% of patients. Adriamycin-induced myocardial injury appears to be the result of oxygen free radical formation.[30] Cardiac tissue is low in catalase, the enzyme that detoxifies free radicals. It is thought that dilation of the sarcoplasmic reticulum and a buildup of calcium deposits in cardiac myocytes results from free radical-induced injury, which ultimately results in cardiac failure. Another one of the group, bleomycin is a chemotherapeutic agent that is primarily dose-limited by pulmonary toxicity, occurring in 5% to 10% of patients treated. The antitumor effects of bleomycin and its toxicity are the result of its binding to cellular deoxyribonucleic acid (DNA). When bleomycin binds to DNA, a ferrous ion on the bleomycin molecule undergoes oxidation to the ferric state, liberating electrons. The electrons are accepted by oxygen and form superoxide and oxygen free radicals.[58] The lungs are the primary target for bleomycin toxicity because they have a high concentration of oxygen, and the lung is low in the enzyme bleomycin hydrolase, a metabolic inactivator of the drug. The actual mechanism of pulmonary damage is controversial. When these agents are encountered in practice, it is important that their implications for anesthetic technique be recognized and the management of the potential adverse effects of any cardiac and pulmonary toxicity be anticipated in an appropriate anesthetic plan.

Another factor to be considered is the possible effect of chronic systemic medication on the usual biologic clearance mechanisms of anesthetic drugs. Saturation of the normal enzyme detoxification pathways' capacity in the liver is thought to lead to detoxification of anesthetic drug metabolites by alternative pathways. Alternative degradation pathways are thought to be one of the possible mechanisms leading to "halothane hepatitis."[52] Enzyme induction in the liver from chronic medication may also decrease the anticipated effects of anesthetic drugs given in normal dosage. Similarly, many drugs, such as the aminoglycoside antibiotics, are nephrotoxic and will impair renal clearance sufficiently to prolong the action of anesthetic drugs relying on that route for excretion.

Airway assessment

The airway and the general anatomy require particularly careful assessment at the preoperative visit because these two factors are likely to impose limitations on surgical positioning and on the choice of technique for anesthetic induction and maintenance. A morbidly obese patient not only may pose problems of access for the surgeon but also may cause difficulty for the anesthesiologist in intubation and choice of technique to minimize well-recognized postoperative sequelae of the condition.[50] The elderly patient with limitation of movement or with joint deformity requires careful attention to positioning and the protection of pressure points. When the temporomandibular joints are involved, access to the airway may be a problem. Of concern in the elderly patient with systemic vascular disease is the presence of carotid plaques with or without bruit. If the operation requires exaggerated rotation of the head, as for posterior auricular approaches, it is important to check preoperatively to see that the patient can rotate his or her head without fainting, in the hope of preventing a potentially fatal maneuver during anesthesia. Airway compromise usually is evident from the general history and examination. However, to detect occult impending airway compromise requires detailed examination of the airway. Congenital anomalies of the airway may involve any part of the respiratory tract, but the most commonly underestimated ones occur in structures originating from the first and second branchial arch structures. The classic syndromes—Treacher Collins, Hallermann-Streiff, and so on—are obvious, but similar deformities of a lesser degree are not. These may occur in otherwise healthy patients who compensate for their deformities with muscular effort. Premedication or induction of anesthesia modifies or abolishes this compensatory effort, leading to airway obstruction.

Anatomic variations also contribute to technical difficulties with laryngoscopy and intubation. A larynx easily visualized with indirect or fiberoptic laryngoscopy may not be visualized as easily with direct laryngoscopy. Of particular interest in anticipating such problems is the presence of micrognathia, microstomia, macroglossia or relative macroglossia; unusual angulation of the larynx; a short, thick neck; or combinations of these conditions. In the clinical examination of the upper airway, attention should be paid to the patency and size of the nasal passages in regard to the potential use of nasal endotracheal tubes. The full facial view should be examined for symmetry, and a full lateral view should be examined for the size and position of the mandible relative to the maxilla. The state and presentation of dentition should be noted, as should the presence of a narrow, high-arched hard palate. A high-arched palate in association with closely spaced, parallel upper alveolar ridges can make the simultaneous manipulation of laryngoscope and endotracheal tube impossible (Fig. 12-3). The position of the larynx relative to the mandible should be identified. If the distance between the prominence of the thyroid cartilage and the lower border of the mandible admits one and one half finger breadths (3 cm) or more (Fig. 12-4), a high larynx tucked under the base of the tongue will probably not be encountered. The mobility of the larynx should be observed by asking the patient to swallow, and the presence of induration or scarring in the base of the tongue and hypopharynx should be sought by palpation of the soft tissues beneath the mandible. Palpation of the neck will confirm the midline position of the trachea and identify the possibility of an awkward laryngeal presentation resulting from edema or scarring, together with the presence of any tumors impinging on the trachea, which might make the passage of an endotracheal tube difficult. Finally, the full and free movement of the cervical spine and the atlantooccipital joints should be confirmed, as well as the patient's ability to open the mouth without limitation.

If the inability to intubate or ventilate the patient is encountered unexpectedly at anesthetic induction, the presence of a short, thick neck makes a safe rapid tracheostomy more difficult, thereby placing the patient's life in immediate jeopardy. The need for a thorough preoperative examination of the patient's airway cannot be overemphasized. However, none of the many clinical indicators of difficulty that have been advocated have been found to be particularly reliable or consistent when used alone.[15] Each has considerable inter- and intraobserver variation with low sensitivity, therefore diagnosis depends more on an "index of suspicion," which becomes greater as more and more abnormal findings and variations are uncovered. If for any reason the patient is suspected by the surgeon of having a difficult airway, preoperative notification of the anesthesiologist concerned is in the patient's best interest.

Laboratory testing

The use of the laboratory to document the obvious and the irrelevant in the preoperative patient has increased, is increasing, and should be decreased. A few tests can be justified as "routine," and any test ordered to pander to the attending physician's insecurities rather than further the patient's interest is to be condemned. A review of the cost-effectiveness of "routine" preoperative testing has been presented elsewhere.[55] It will suffice here to discuss a reasonable approach to the use of the laboratory for anesthetic purposes.

The first question to be asked before ordering a laboratory test is: "Will the result, anticipated or unanticipated, be

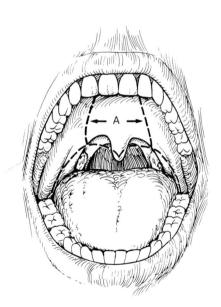

Fig. 12-3. Examination of the mouth may reveal a high-arched palate where the upper teeth lie more parallel *(A)* than usual, restricting laryngoscopy maneuvers. An upwardly bulging tongue may indicate macroglossia or displacement resulting from a small mandible.

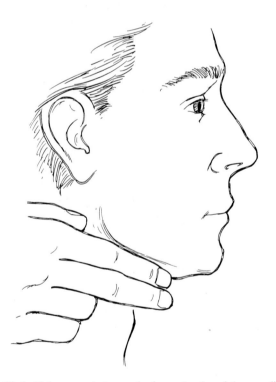

Fig. 12-4. If the space between the lower border of the mandible and the prominence of the thyroid cartilage admits more than one and one half finger breadths (3 cm), a high larynx with difficult visualization is unlikely.

likely to lead the anesthesiologist to change the anesthetic plan suggested by his or her clinical assessment?'' If not, the test will serve no useful preoperative purpose and is therefore superfluous. This is not to suggest that the degree of impairment of physiologic functions resulting from a patient's preexisting medical conditions should not be quantified if, in the clinical judgment of the anesthesiologist, the anesthetic itself might be expected to cause a deterioration in the patient's condition intraoperatively or postoperatively. However, it does preclude the routine preoperative chest radiograph in the absence of clinical indications, as well as an electrocardiogram for most younger patients coming to operation. The prime purpose of anesthetic preoperative laboratory tests is to define the limits of anesthetic maneuvering intraoperatively. Because the anesthesiologist has two principal duties—to render the patient insensitive to pain and to maintain an adequate supply of oxygen to the tissues—preoperative testing should be aimed at ensuring the basis for these two functions in all patients.

The ability to render the patient insensitive to pain depends on the choice of anesthetic technique—local anesthesia, conduction blockade, or general anesthesia. Local anesthesia does not require preoperative testing to confirm patient suitability in the absence of a history of specific agent sensitivity. Conduction blockade poses more potential problems than local anesthesia, even in some ASA 1 patients. For example, the technical difficulties posed by serious kyphoscoliosis in an otherwise apparently healthy patient would certainly justify radiographic studies to define the extent of the anatomic problem and lung volume studies before one proceeds with a spinal anesthetic. Any situation in which abnormal coagulation might be expected, or in which the patient has been taking over-the-counter proprietary preparations containing aspirin, would justify preoperative coagulation studies to ascertain the likelihood of hemorrhage into the nerve trunk after the block. The major problem with general anesthetic techniques is introducing sufficient doses of anesthetic agents into the patient's circulation while still maintaining an adequate circulation. The decrease in BP resulting from a combination of decreased peripheral vascular resistance and decreased cardiac output in the presence of anesthetic agents is usually exaggerated by a preexisting reduction in circulating volume. Reduced circulating volumes may be anticipated, for example, in the previously undiagnosed mild hypertensive, the relatively malnourished elderly patient living alone, the young child with a fever who is starved overnight for surgery, and the fit young woman misguidedly trying to control her weight with diuretic preparations. Such presentations justify electrolyte and hematocrit studies, which in the case of diuretic use may uncover a clinically unacceptable hypokalemia. An intravenous infusion of crystalloid solution can be started earlier than usual to preload such patients, or an alternative anesthetic technique can be chosen if appropriate.

The preoperative measurement of hemoglobin concentration and hematocrit can be more easily justified as routine in all patients because these have a direct bearing on the oxygen supply to tissues. The term *available oxygen* refers to the quantity of oxygen passing through the root of the aorta each minute; this quantity can be determined from the oxygen transport equation:

$$\text{Available oxygen} = \text{Cardiac output} \times \text{Arterial saturation}$$
$$\times \text{Hemoglobin concentration} \times 1.34$$

$$1000 \text{ ml/min} = 5250 \text{ ml/min} \times \frac{95}{100} \times \frac{15 \text{ g/ml}}{100} \times 1.34 \text{ ml/g}$$

In the normal patient who does not smoke, the oxygen-hemoglobin combining power 1.34 is a constant. The other three factors are variables; if any one is reduced while the other two remain constant, the available oxygen is reduced proportionately. However, if two of the variables are reduced simultaneously while the third remains constant, the effect on available oxygen will be the product of the individual changes. Thus, if cardiac output and hemoglobin saturation are reduced by half, oxygen availability decreases to a quarter of the normal value, which in the case of the above example is approximately 250 ml/min, which may not be compatible with safety in some patients.

It is evident that the only variable usually amenable to preoperative intervention is the hemoglobin concentration. A decrease in cardiac output occurs to some extent in all patients as a normal concomitant of anesthetic induction. Transient decreases in excess of 30% of normal are not unusual. If any difficulty occurs in maintaining the airway and normal ventilation, the hemoglobin oxygen saturation will also decrease, so the patient is always at risk during induction of anesthesia, regardless of ASA status. Should preexisting pathology cause the values for any of the variables to be below normal, the risk is increased. This is the physiologic basis for the long-standing 10 g/100 ml rule, which can be such a bone of contention between anesthesiologists and surgeons. Although anesthesiologists have become more liberal in their application of the rule to elective surgery over the years, it still rests on sound principles. It is known that patients with chronic anemia are better able to withstand the insult of anesthetic induction than those with acute anemia. The risks and questionable ethics of a rapid preoperative blood transfusion to increase the hemoglobin concentration above the 10 g/100 ml limit have become better defined. It remains imprudent, however, to perform elective surgery on a patient who is anemic, unless there is a well-defined medical reason to proceed other than convenience, and 10 g/100 ml still constitutes a reasonable reference point against which medical judgments can be made. On this basis, the routine measurement of hemoglobin and hematocrit can be justified.

Of more recent interest is the thorny question of the use of volatile halogenated agents in the presence of liver dysfunction. ''Halothane hepatitis,'' not unique to halothane, is a diagnosis made by exclusion of other possible causes. No direct causal relationship between halothane exposure and halothane hepatitis can be proved, nor is there a unique pathologic picture that can be considered pathognomonic of the condition. However, there is sufficient circumstantial evidence to make the prudent anesthesiologist hesitant in repeatedly exposing the same patient to halothane over a short period of time, and a history of jaundice after halothane exposure in the past suggests its avoidance altogether in the future. The real problem is whether to give halogenated agents in the face of active liver disease. There does not appear to be an increased risk to a patient who has made a complete recovery from infectious hepatitis in the past, but common prudence would suggest avoidance during active hepatitis. Some studies have shown that a surprising number of patients presenting for elective surgery are incubating hepatitis, and it is tempting to postulate that it is exposure to metabolites under these circumstances that could explain the occurrence of halothane hepatitis. Whatever the final answer may be, it would appear reasonable to screen a patient's liver function, perhaps with nothing more than an estimation of serum glutamic pyruvate transaminase (SGPT), and avoid halogenated agents when the level is significantly increased.

Informed consent

A California court has stated:

"A physician violates his duty to his patient and subjects himself to liability if he withholds any facts which are necessary to form the basis of an intelligent consent by the patient to the proposed treatment. Likewise the physician may not minimize the known dangers of a procedure or operation in order to induce his patient's consent."[28]

The opinion then goes on to recognize the dilemma that sometimes full disclosure may not promote the patient's welfare because it may further alarm a patient who is already apprehensive. This dilemma has led to the existence of two competing rules—the "professional standard of consent," which holds that the amount of information disclosed is a matter of reasonable professional judgment, and the "lay standard of reasonableness," which holds that the crux of the matter is not what the physician thinks the patient should know, but what the patient should know to make an informed decision.

Anesthesiology has not had a high public profile in the past, and today patients still have only a vague idea of what anesthesia entails. The last thing that most patients consider is the possibility of being maimed or killed by the anesthetic process when they come to the hospital for surgery. There is something particularly poignant about an anesthetic catastrophe in a patient admitted for an operation that in retrospect he or she could have done perfectly well without. Because anesthesia cures little or nothing, it should not injure. Unfortunately it does. Thus the anesthesiologist has a particular duty to inform the patient of serious adverse effects, even

if the incidence is low. Because most of the serious adverse sequelae of anesthesia are rare, the physician seeking consent should be sufficiently conversant with the anesthetic literature to be aware of their existence and significance in the light of the condition of the patient. It is unwise, therefore, for the surgeon to seek consent for anesthesia at the same time as that for operation and certainly foolhardy to anticipate the choice of anesthetic technique unless he or she is willing to proceed with infiltration anesthesia alone. Informed consent can be obtained only by the physician who is responsible for administering the anesthetic. This is a potential liability problem for surgeons working with nurse anesthetists without the aid of anesthesiologists.

PREPARATION OF THE PATIENT FOR ANESTHESIA

Preparations on the ward

The preparation of the patient for anesthesia begins with the anesthesiologist's preoperative visit and evaluation. The anesthesiologist has to try to establish rapport quickly with the previously unknown patient. Informed consent has to be obtained. Frequently any lingering questions and doubts concerning the proposed operation have to be addressed without contradicting or undermining what the surgeon has already told the patient. This is accomplished the evening before surgery, but with the developing practice of "day-of-surgery admission," care must be taken not to detract from the thoroughness of the preoperative visit.

Apart from becoming familiar with the patient's medical problems and devising the appropriate anesthetic plan, the anesthesiologist may have a number of objectives to be achieved through preoperative medication:

1. The prime objective is always the relief of the patient's anxiety when it is judged to be significant. Methods used may range from reassurance with "light" anxiolytic medication, to time-consuming hypnotic suggestion, to "heavy" premedication with sedatives or narcotics. Some studies have suggested that the relief of anxiety before surgery depends more on the rapport the anesthesiologist establishes with the patient than on the choice of drugs for premedication.
2. When preoperative pain is present, it is important to prescribe analgesics in sufficient dosage to minimize exacerbation from the movements involved in transporting the patient from the bed to the operating table.
3. When a light, balanced anesthetic technique is contemplated, an amnesic drug should form part of premedication to protect the patient's psyche from the trauma of awareness.
4. The inclusion of an antisialogogue is frequently required for head and neck surgery and endoscopy because the patient's airway is not accessible for manual suctioning by the anesthesiologist. The reduction in volume of secretions also will facilitate endoscopy.

5. When the suppression of cardiovascular reflexes is considered important for induction of anesthesia or the surgical procedure, sedation and vagolytic agents are indicated.
6. Depressant premedicant drugs also can facilitate the anesthetic technique itself by smoothing inhalation inductions and reducing the requirement for intraoperative agents.
7. Premedicant drugs also can be used to reduce the incidence of postoperative nausea and vomiting, although to achieve effective antiemesis for operations of the inner ear, premedicant effects usually should be reinforced with drugs such as droperidol just before the patient emerges from anesthesia.

The patient must eat nothing for at least 6 to 8 hours before anesthesia, although in any patient this period does not guarantee an empty stomach. Even when "empty," the stomach contains approximately 200 ml of strong hydrochloric acid, which poses the ever-present risk of acid-aspiration pneumonitis at induction. This fact has led some anesthesiologists routinely to prescribe an H_2-histamine blocker (such as ranitidine). When hiatus hernia with acid reflux is suspected, the addition of an antacid by mouth on the morning of surgery has been recommended. The question of whether a patient should be subjected to an absolute fast (nothing by mouth [NPO] after midnight), thereby depriving the patient of a significant fluid intake during the fast period, is now being questioned for adults and small children undergoing elective surgery.[62] However, any relaxation of fasting rules should be approached with care as, despite claims to the contrary, some patients become confused if offered even reasonable choices, and compliance with instructions decreases.

Preparation in the operating room

Before the patient is brought to the operating room, the anesthesiologist's first task, and probably the most important one of the day, is to prepare the drugs and check the equipment that are to be used. In this area the practice of anesthesia differs drastically from that of surgery. Whereas the surgeon relies on the operating room nurse to assemble instruments and perhaps draw up any local anesthetic that the surgeon is to use, the anesthesiologist has a duty to check everything personally. An anesthetic drug drawn up in the wrong syringe and then in error injected intravenously cannot be retrieved, and malfunctioning equipment may lead to a rapid hypoxic disaster for the patient. The checking process must be obsessively thorough, and the anesthesiologist must not be distracted while it is going on.

When the patient arrives in the operating room, his or her identity is confirmed together with the site of operation. Then he or she is made comfortable on the operating table. An intravenous cannula is inserted during intradermal local anesthesia to provide a drug injection route. An intravenous

infusion may be started if intraoperative hydration or blood replacement is anticipated. The appropriate clinical measuring instruments are applied according to the patient's condition, but a minimum standard of care now dictates the use of at least the following with every patient:

1. Indirect blood pressure measurement
2. Electrocardiogram
3. Temperature
4. Oxygen analysis, at least on the circuit supply line
5. Expired carbon dioxide analysis
6. Pulse oximetry

While the final preparations are made for induction, the patient is "preoxygenated" by mask with 100% oxygen to create an oxygen reserve in the patient's functional residual capacity (FRC) and thus increase the time available for maneuver in the event of a difficult induction. When all is prepared, the surgeon should be summoned before induction begins, if he or she is not already present.

The surgical outpatient

Persons having outpatient surgery require special mention, not because their preoperative evaluation differs dramatically from that of the surgical inpatient, but because certain additional requirements must be considered. Because there is insufficient time for the full evaluation of major systemic disease on the day of surgery, the surgeon must ensure that this is done thoroughly during the patient's outpatient clinic visit and that appropriate medical consultations are obtained at that time.

As outpatient surgery has developed in the United States, the emphasis has been on ASA 1 patients to minimize the supposed difficulties associated with postoperative management. This approach has been overly conservative. Modern anesthetic techniques, appropriately selected, permit rapid recovery and pose few problems for the patient discharged home. It is now feasible to include ASA 2 patients and carefully selected ASA 3 patients, as long as admission to hospital after surgery is available if anything untoward develops. As a general rule, the following factors would militate against outpatient surgery:

1. The need for extensive medical preparation, rather than just "tuning up" the medical control of chronic disease
2. The need for postoperative intravenous therapy of any sort
3. The need for invasive monitoring during operation
4. A nonconducive home situation for the patient; for instance, an elderly patient living alone or a patient living at great distance from the hospital, with difficult access to emergency care
5. Procedures that are expected to produce serious postoperative pain, which may not be amenable to management with oral analgesics

6. Conditions for which extensive postoperative medical management is required
7. The patient's lack of ability to comprehend and follow postoperative instructions

It is the surgeon's responsibility to ensure that the patient has fasted since the previous evening and is accompanied by a competent adult into whose care and protection the patient will be discharged. Premedication, if any, is usually given by the anesthesiologist intravenously after the patient has been evaluated and informed consent has been obtained. Before discharge, each patient must be given written and oral instructions cautioning him or her against undertaking any activities that may pose a hazard to him- or herself or others as a result of the "hangover" effect of anesthetic drugs still being cleared from the body over the next 24 to 48 hours, which can affect the patient's judgment and reflexes. Such warning should encompass driving, operating machinery, nursing infants, the hazards of the domestic kitchen, and signing any legal documents.

As its cost advantages become more widely appreciated, outpatient surgery is becoming more common. However, it should be understood that the usual inpatient ratios of patient preparation space to operating rooms and staffing levels are not adequate for a safe, efficient outpatient program. Outpatient surgery is space- and labor-intensive, particularly in terms of the requirements for patient preparation, recovery, and discharge.

CONDUCT OF ANESTHESIA

Operating room setup

The anesthetic setup for otolaryngology surgery is dictated by the competition for the airway between the anesthesiologist and the surgeon. In ophthalmic surgery and neurosurgery, the anesthesiologist usually has some restricted access to the oral endotracheal tube. In otolaryngologic surgery, even if the surgeon is not working in the aerodigestive tract itself, the patient's head is usually draped completely (Fig. 12-5).

The clustering of the surgeons, the scrub nurse, and the instrument tables about the patient's head usually means that the anesthesiologist and his or her equipment are forced toward the foot of the table. This situation dictates a meticulous setup after induction, with a well-secured airway and close monitoring of the anesthetic circuit's integrity throughout the operation. The situation demands close cooperation from the surgeon. Any changes in the surgical field, such as increased oozing, dark blood, or surgical manipulation around the carotid bodies, must be communicated to the anesthesiologist immediately. If the anesthesiologist in turn has any concern about the patient's condition, the surgeon should be informed and the matter resolved with good grace, by undraping the patient if necessary. There are no "points" to be scored between professionals in operating rooms.

Anesthetic induction is always undertaken with the anesthesiologist at the head of the patient. If a tracheostomy is to be undertaken, the anesthesiologist remains at the patient's head, where he or she has control of the endotracheal tube and can assist the surgeon. When the trachea is exposed, the tube cuff is deflated, and the tube is advanced into the right mainstem bronchus. This prevents the cuff from being incised with the trachea and enables the anesthesiologist to seal the airway if the surgeon encounters bleeding problems. Once the window in the trachea has been made without incident, the anesthesiologist withdraws the tube until the surgeon informs him or her that the tip is level with the upper border of the window. The tube is never withdrawn from the larynx completely until after the surgeon has inserted, secured, and tested the correct position of the tracheostomy tube.

If the surgical intention is to undertake endoscopy or microsurgery of the larynx, the operating table is rotated 90°,

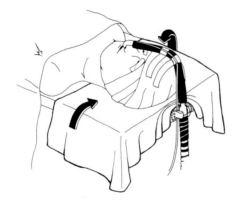
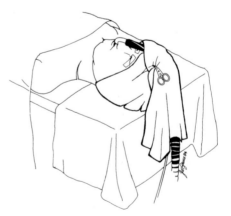

Fig. 12-5. The nasal endotracheal tube offers great security for otolaryngologic surgery because the tube itself is surrounded by bone. The stability of circuit connections is further enhanced by the use of a wrap-around head drape.

and the anesthesiologist remains near but below the left side of the patient's head. This position allows the anesthesiologist to make and secure various ventilatory attachments to whatever endoscopes may be used or permits him or her to ensure manually that the endotracheal tube is not inadvertently dragged from the larynx by the surgeon during endoscopic manipulation.

For most other procedures the anesthesiologist is to the side of the operating table and near the foot or actually at the foot. The advantage of being off to one side is that this position permits the use of a standard circle circuit without modification, and some anesthesiologists feel more comfortable if the airway is at least within reach, if not immediately

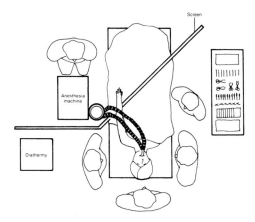

Fig. 12-6. The anesthesiologist at the side of the operating table and using a standard circle circuit with carbon dioxide absorber.

accessible (Fig. 12-6). The disadvantage of the position is the crowding and potential interference with anesthetic equipment and the circuit inherent if more than one surgeon is involved in the procedure. If the anesthesiologist sits at the foot of the table, this latter problem is overcome, but special circuits must then be used (Fig. 12-7). A "long" circle circuit may be used, but the increased volume of the circuit introduces additional compression and distension errors in ventilator settings, and although these may be compensated for in normal patients, in those with reduced chest compliance, ventilation management may become difficult. These problems are largely circumvented by the use of coaxial circuits, such as the Bain high-flow circuit (Fig. 12-8). The single tube is light and easy to secure; although because the avoidance of expired carbon dioxide rebreathing is achieved by using high gas flows,[4] the use of this coaxial circuit consumes more anesthetic agent than does the circle circuit. Conservation of heat and water with soda lime adsorption also is lost unless an artificial "nose" is interposed between the endotracheal tube and the circuit. An additional advantage of the Bain circuit is that the metal "head" containing the expiratory valve and various hose attachments can be clamped to the operating table itself, further minimizing the chance of circuit disconnection resulting from any changes in table position requested by the surgeon during the procedure (Fig. 12-9). Coaxial circle circuits are now available for use with soda lime, which help conserve heat and moisture and the volume of anesthetic gases used. They are long enough for this setup when used with extension tubes. The foot position affords a better, more symmetric

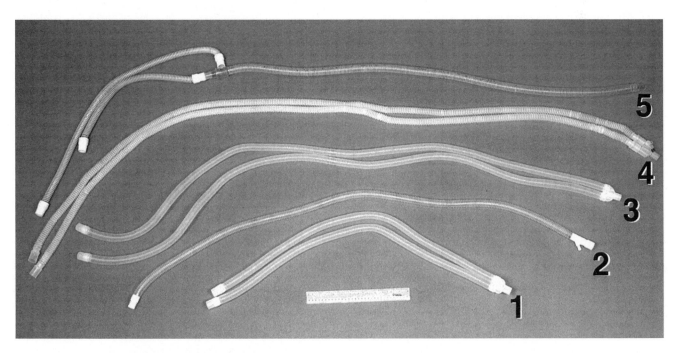

Fig. 12-7. The various circuits available for head and neck surgery: (*1*) A standard short circle. (*2*) The coaxial high-flow Bain circuit. (*3*) A standard long circle. (*4*) An adjustable long circle. (*5*) The coaxial low-flow circle with extension tubes. A 1-foot ruler is included for reference.

view of chest wall movement during anesthesia and gives the anesthesiologist access to both sides of the table.

Anesthetic techniques

Five main groups of anesthetic techniques are available to the otolaryngologic patient.

Infiltration anesthesia

Infiltration anesthesia, with or without standby for monitoring, sedation, or resuscitation by the anesthesiologist, is most commonly used for minor, superficial operations or operations in the middle ear. The surgeon is solely responsible for the use and dosage of whatever local anesthetic agent is selected and should ensure that the safe total dose with or without epinephrine is not exceeded. The surgeon should exercise care when selecting patients, so that the procedure planned can be completed in the time made available by the technique and the patient can tolerate the experience. The safety of the technique depends on not exceeding safe drug dosages and on frequent aspiration during injection with a constantly moving needle to minimize the risk of inadvertent intravenous injection. This is not a "second-best" technique to "get away" with surgery on inadequately prepared patients already rejected for general anesthesia.

Topical anesthesia

Topical anesthesia is used primarily for diagnostic or therapeutic endoscopy—particularly when patient cooperation is required, as with Teflon injection of the vocal cords. Again, attention to total drug dosage and the careful selection of those patients who will tolerate the experience are important. The secret of consistent success is to take sufficient time at each step to allow full analgesia to develop. The lip and gums are "painted" first and then tongue, epiglottis,

and larynx in turn under direct or indirect vision. Rather than spraying the larynx, some may prefer to achieve laryngeal anesthesia by applying cotton pledgets soaked in local anesthetic to the piriform fossae using Krause forceps or by percutaneous injection through the neck. At the conclusion of paintup, a small amount of viscous lidocaine is given to the patient to gargle and swallow.

Conduction anesthesia

Conduction anesthesia is the technique whereby a local anesthetic agent is introduced through a needle to the immediate proximity of a specific nerve, series of nerves, or nerve trunk to produce analgesia over the sensory distribution. Anesthesiologists use the technique for head and neck surgery infrequently. The common technique of spinal anesthesia theoretically can be used for analgesia of the head and neck, and has been used in the past.[33] However, achieving a sensory block high enough to be of use to the surgeon results in a simultaneous motor block of the muscles of respiration. This requires control of the patient's respiration, necessitating general anesthesia, which somewhat defeats the purpose of conduction blockade in the first place. Blockade of the cervical nerves is a more viable technique, which creates a favorable operating field—one that can be used to advantage for thyroid surgery or lymph node dissections. However, the two fundamental disadvantages of conduction blockade are encountered. The duration of surgical analgesia depends on the accuracy of initial injection and the properties of the drug injected. Therefore if the surgical procedure takes longer than anticipated and if the block wears off, general anesthesia with its concomitant risks has to be superimposed. The other major drawback is the time required for the block to be executed and for analgesia to develop. It is because of the induction time and the inflexibility of a "one shot" technique that these blocks are not used more frequently. Despite these considerations, conduction blockade still has two well-established roles in head and neck surgery: blockade for surgery on the teeth, supporting structures, and oral mucous membrane[41] and the control of the chronic pain syndromes.[12]

Monitored anesthesia care

Monitored anesthesia care (MAC) refers to the situation wherein an anesthesiologist is present to supervise and monitor patient sedation during a local anesthetic technique. Sedation is desirable for a patient who is concerned about recall of intraoperative events and to minimize the systemic stresses associated with the experience. This may be required with any form of local technique whether it be topical, infiltration, or conduction blockade. It is sometimes desirable for procedures where no local anesthetic drugs are used and it is the patient's medical condition that is the only concern. It should be emphasized that the anesthesiologist must ensure that the operation is not performed during an inadequate local anesthetic, resulting in progressive depression of the

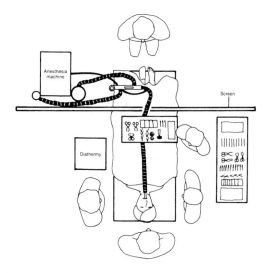

Fig. 12-8. The anesthesiologist at the foot of the operating table and using a coaxial circuit with high fresh gas flow to prevent rebreathing.

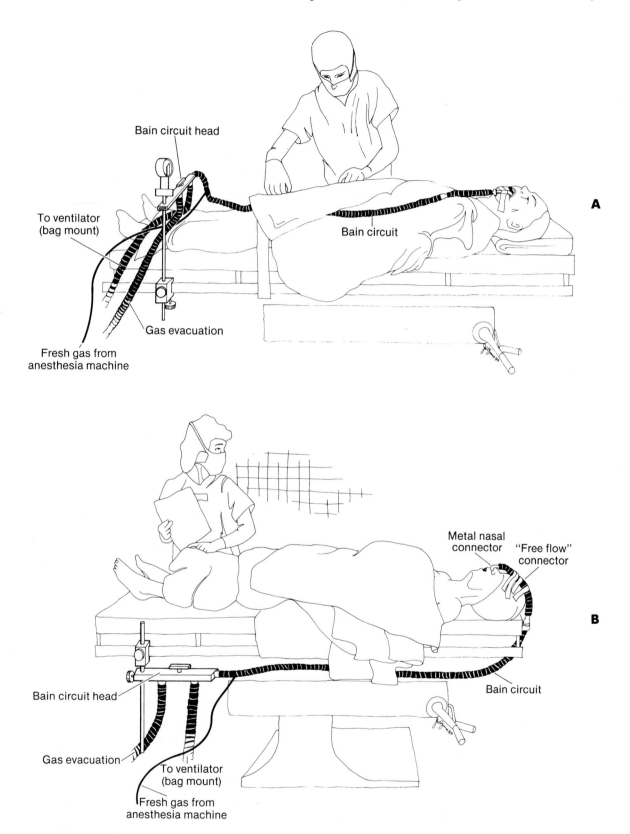

Bain circuit head

To ventilator
(bag mount)

Bain circuit

A

Gas evacuation

Fresh gas from
anesthesia machine

Metal nasal
connector

"Free flow"
connector

B

Bain circuit

Bain circuit head

Bain circuit

Gas evacuation

To ventilator
(bag mount)

Fresh gas from
anesthesia machine

Fig. 12-9. The use of the coaxial anesthetic circuit (Bain). **A,** Setup for oral endotracheal tube. **B,** Setup for nasal endotracheal tube.

patient's cerebrum and brainstem with increasing doses of intravenous drugs. Such a situation demands either abandonment of the procedure or conversion to a formal general anesthetic, which in turn implies that the patient has undergone preoperative evaluation and preparation with this eventuality in mind.

The term *MAC* has been defined and approved by the ASA,[1] but other terms are still in use, such as *local standby anesthesia, intravenous amnesia, conscious sedation*, and *monitored anesthesia and pharmacologic support*. The term *MAC* should not be confused with the same term used in two other contexts by anesthesiologists: (1) Mac is also the slang abbreviation for the curved anesthetic laryngoscope blade first described by Sir Robert Macintosh and is still in common use; (2) MAC is also the acronym for the minimum alveolar concentration in stable state of an anesthetic gas or vapor that blocks reflex response in 50% of a group of animals to a standardized noxious stimulus. Although the concept is used with respect to patients by anesthesiologists, it was originally developed as a standardized laboratory measure to compare the potencies of different anesthetic agents.

MAC implies that an anesthesiologist is providing specific anesthesia services to a patient undergoing a planned surgical procedure and is in control of his or her nonsurgical medical care, including being available to perform immediate resuscitation, administering additional anesthetics, or providing other medical care as appropriate. The ASA specifically includes MAC in the Standard for Basic Intraoperative Monitoring, thereby requiring the same level of care for MAC as is required for all other anesthetic procedures. Therefore, the term should be limited to the practice of anesthesiologists observing the standards of care promulgated by their specialist society. The American Dental Association also has adopted definitions and standards related to "conscious sedation" in dental practice. Over the years dentists have become particularly aware of their vulnerability in the face of patient disaster when a single dentist has tried to act as operator and monitoring anesthetist simultaneously. Thus, when a patient requires anything greater than the lightest level of sedation and in the absence of an anesthesiologist, a second dentist should be in attendance to monitor the patient's condition during continuing sedation. Unfortunately this is not the case with many medical specialties where patients are still occasionally oversedated for invasive and diagnostic procedures by physicians acting as operator/anesthetists. These physicians sometimes miss the signs of impending central nervous system depression because they are concentrating on the procedure in hand. However, the realities and demands of daily practice also must be acknowledged. There is an insufficient supply of anesthesiologists and nurse anesthetists to staff the many minor operative and diagnostic procedures that require some level of sedation in the many outpatient clinics and office practices across the country. Fortunately few of the patients undergoing procedures in such environments come to any harm. Therefore,

to avoid the occasional disaster and while keeping within the bounds of reasonable cost, it is suggested that certain precautions be considered when the surgeon uses sedation outside the operating room environment.

1. Prepare for the unexpected patient collapse by keeping within reach an office resuscitation box, including the means for high-volume suction, artificial ventilation, supplementary oxygen, and drugs suitable for managing hypotension, cardiac dysrhythmias, anaphylactic reactions, bronchospasm, and local anesthetic seizures. Several companies produce such ready-stocked cases at a reasonable cost. Ensure that the contents are checked regularly.

2. Train office or clinic staff in advance concerning their duties in an emergency. Ensure that the appropriate telephone numbers for use in an emergency are known, posted, and updated.

3. Select patients carefully to exclude those with severe obesity and those with major pulmonary or cardiac function impairment or severe hypertensive disease, and also other patients who do not have a responsible adult to accompany them to and from the office. Even with these exclusions, patients remaining will fall into ASA classes 1 through 3.

4. Monitoring of the patients selected is predicated on the rigor of the exclusion criteria adopted in any practice. The more physiologic modalities to be monitored, the more the need for an independent observer such as a trained nurse. The maximum intensity of monitoring in a nonoperating room environment should encompass no more than four indirect modalities. The most informative are probably end-tidal carbon dioxide, pulse oximetry (PO), BP, and single-channel electrocardiogram (ECG), in descending order of importance. Capnography, although the most useful early warning monitor of apnea, requires practice to obtain a usable trace in conscious patients who are not intubated. Nasal oxygen prongs attached to the sampling tube and secured with tape to the patient's nose or lower lip usually are effective, but sometimes a small sampling catheter passed a little way into the nostril is required. It must be determined whether the patient breathes primarily through the mouth or nose. If the surgeon is alone, these monitors should be automated with easily visible and interpreted displays together with audible limit alarms that have distinctive sounds and an audible beat-to-beat monitor on the pulse oximeter. Any patient who requires more than this should be cared for in a hospital operating room during formal MAC. Such automated monitors are not cheap, but their costs are dwarfed by the costs of chronic dependency after a patient accident. The purpose of these monitors is to detect the occurrence of one of the four common clinical scenarios that may result from patient sedation:

1. The onset of apnea (end-tidal carbon dioxide first; PO later)
2. Hypoventilation leading to hypoxia (PO first—end-tidal carbon dioxide may not trigger its apnea alarm)
3. Hypotension or cardiovascular collapse (BP first ± ECG and PO)
4. Dysrhythmia (ECG ± PO)

In each situation, if the PO alarm sounds, it is a late warning because desaturation is already occurring, requiring an immediate response. The types of monitors used in operating rooms are robust but bulky and may not be ideal for the more limited space in clinics and offices. However, recently, miniaturized compact "compound" monitors designed for transporting patients in hospitals have become available; these may prove far more suited to the office environment (Fig. 12-10).

5. Technique and the choice of sedatives and analgesics to be used is very much a question of personal preference and experience. It is probably far more important to be intimately familiar with the scope and limitations of the pharmacology of a few drugs rather than to have a variety of less well-understood techniques available.

The object of the procedure is to establish good analgesia with whatever local anesthetic technique has been chosen and then to sedate the patient to a satisfactory level. Although sedation may be established first, it is then very difficult to judge whether satisfactory local anesthesia has been achieved. But what is satisfactory sedation? The reader will appreciate that any agent capable of achieving satisfactory

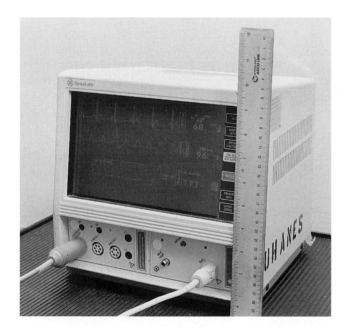

Fig. 12-10. An example of a multichannel transport monitor, which may be best suited for office procedures. A 1-foot ruler is included for reference.

sedation also is capable of achieving general anesthesia if given in sufficient quantity. Therefore the final point lies somewhere on the continuum between normal consciousness and stage 4 general anesthesia. Because stages 2 through 4 are inimical to patient safety outside the hospital environment, stage 1 or lighter anesthesia should be the objective for office procedures. The patient should be conscious, able to respond to commands, with some degree of amnesia and systemic analgesia. The onset of snoring, irregular breathing, the loss of swallowing, and the ability to handle secretions, confusion, and increasing reflex activity all suggest that the patient is becoming too sedated. Therefore the surgeon should establish a satisfactory local anesthetic and then pause to induce and confirm an appropriately stable level of sedation before proceeding further. If, during the procedure, further sedation appears to be required, it should first be established that the local block is still effective. It is the administration of supplemental doses of sedatives and narcotics during the procedure, when the surgeon's attention is concentrated elsewhere, that most often leads to overdose. The surgeon also should guard against the patient who appears to be properly sedated during a stimulating procedure but lapses into a dangerous state of sedation during recovery when the stimulus is removed. The elderly patient is particularly at risk, and it increases the need for monitoring into the recovery period.

In one cross-over study of the use of sedation in outpatients,[39] 85% of patients preferred sedation with local anesthesia over local anesthesia alone. Patient satisfaction is reported to be higher with more profound sedation irrespective of the route of administration.[40] However, increasing sedation leads to increasing ventilatory depression and risk for the patient; therefore the use of supplemental oxygen through nasal prongs should be considered as a routine. Of patients in one study who did not receive supplemental oxygen during local anesthesia with sedation, 40% showed clinically significant oxygen desaturation[69]; hypoxia also occurred in some patients receiving only local anesthesia. Information concerning the relative safety of different techniques is scarce, although one large review of outpatient procedures[23] involving more than 83,000 cases reported the following general incidence of postoperative complications:

Local anesthesia only	1/268
Local anesthesia with sedation	1/106
General anesthesia	1/120
Regional block	1/277

Many drugs and drug combinations are being used for the sedation of surgical patients. The most popular techniques are probably those involving the use of combinations of benzodiazepines (e.g., diazepam, midazolam, lorazepam) and opioid analgesics (e.g., alfentanyl, fentanyl, sufentanyl). Certainly among anesthesiologists involved in performing MAC, the midazolam/fentanyl combination has achieved considerable popularity. But even with an anesthesiologist in attendance and one who is free to concentrate on achieving a safe level of patient sedation, a recent study[3] has sounded a note of caution.

More than 80 deaths in the United States have been reported to the Department of Health and Human Resources[19] associated with the use of midazolam in sedating patients during various diagnostic or therapeutic medical and surgical procedures. Most of the deaths occurred in patients who were breathing spontaneously, usually without supplemental oxygen. In many cases, opioids also had been administered. However, similar accidents may be expected with any combination of depressant drugs injudiciously used, whether opioids with the older barbiturate sedatives or the newer ultra–short-acting combinations such as propofol and alfentanil. The latter combination, although effective and gaining widespread acceptance among anesthesiologists for MAC, should under no circumstances be used by the surgeon working alone. The combination is administered most effectively as a continuous intravenous drip or with an infusion pump, which requires continuous informed attention because complete general anesthesia may be achieved with ease and speed.

In conclusion, surgeons working alone should limit themselves to a few drugs with which they are familiar, should supply supplemental oxygen for all patients undergoing sedation, and should insist on appropriate monitoring. If a trained nurse is available to watch the patient during the procedure, so much the better. It is prudent to select procedures that require only one episode of sedation so that surgeons can be certain that appropriate levels of sedation have not been exceeded before they concentrate on surgical manipulations. Where the length or nature of a planned procedure is such that continuing adjustment of sedation is likely to be required, it probably is wiser to schedule such a patient for formal MAC with the assistance of an anesthesiologist.

General anesthesia

Despite the availability of a rapidly increasing variety and number of anesthetic drugs, general anesthetic techniques can still be divided into two broad categories: single-agent techniques and balanced techniques. The fundamental difference between the two categories lies in the use of muscle relaxants to decrease or abolish skeletal muscle tone.

A single agent can achieve all three properties of the anesthetic triad, but profound degrees of skeletal muscle relaxation are achieved only by a relative overdose of the agent compared with that required for narcosis and reflex suppression. This means that maintenance of the circulation becomes more difficult with greater degrees of muscle relaxation. The problem is overcome with muscle relaxant drugs. These drugs, however, mandate the full control of the patient's ventilation with an endotracheal tube and, by definition, convert the normal negative intrathoracic pressure to positive with the associated implication for venous pressure

and surgical field oozing. With single-agent anesthesia, spontaneous respiration through a mask or endotracheal tube can be maintained, albeit with some intermittent support of ventilation for the longer surgical procedures to minimize peripheral lung gas absorption collapse. Even with spontaneous respiration, the problem of oozing in the surgical wound is not completely overcome because the anesthetized respiratory center requires a higher driving tension of carbon dioxide than normal (45 to 55 mm Hg as opposed to 38 to 42 mm Hg), and hypercapnia itself can lead to increased oozing. Because otolaryngology always requires a secure airway, an endotracheal tube is indicated for most procedures, no matter which type of technique is being used. Thus the choice of preferred technique for surgery, in the absence of specific patient medical problems, is reduced to a consideration of a few general advantages and disadvantages in different surgical situations.

Single-agent technique	Balanced technique
1. Simple: reduces number of potential adverse reactions to drugs	Complex: more drugs, more potential adverse reactions
2. Control of circulation more difficult; patient usually requires fluid ''loading''	Can be tailored to maintain circulation more easily
3. Cardiac dysrhythmia with exogenous catecholamines more common	Can be tailored to minimize catecholamine dysrhythmias
4. Nerve stimulator use unaffected	Response to nerve stimulator abolished or diminished
5. With stable state, patient immobility can be nearly guaranteed	Even with blockade monitoring, patient immobility cannot be guaranteed without excessive paralysis
6. Muscle relaxant reversal not required	Muscle relaxant reversal required; may be incomplete and ''recurarization'' can occur postoperatively
7. Anesthetic effects completely reversible as long as patient is breathing with a clear airway	Excretion of intravenous drugs depends primarily on liver and renal excretion, which may be impaired
8. Awareness during anesthesia extremely rare	Awareness occurs
9. Spontaneous respiration an option with or without a mask	Controlled respiration; use of mask ill advised
10. Particularly suited to initial management of difficult airway	Contraindicated for initial management of difficult airway
11. Involves use of halogenated hydrocarbon agents	Volatile agents can be excluded with hepatitis risk
12. Increases cerebral blood flow and intracranial pressure	Can be used to decrease intracranial pressure
13. Associated risk of malignant hyperthermia	Can be tailored to avoid known triggers of malignant hyperthermia

These are the major considerations that influence the selection of technique. The list is not exhaustive because specific diseases may favor choice of the technique opposite to that which might be chosen for a healthy patient undergoing the same surgical procedure. A knowledge of the general approach that anesthesiologists use in choosing anesthetic technique should assist the surgeon in anticipating problems in patients during the initial outpatient visit. This should in turn permit the surgeon to consult with the anesthesiologist earlier than the preoperative visit to avoid any last-minute cancellations and delays which, in the minds of patients, always decrease the reputations of those physicians involved.

Discussing the pharmacology of each anesthetic drug is not possible in a general chapter such as this, therefore the reader is referred to a standard anesthetic pharmacology textbook for the answers to questions of detail concerning individual drug dosage, precautions, and usage.[65]

SPECIAL ANESTHETIC TECHNIQUES

Microsurgery of the ear

When using an operating microscope, the otologist requires a patient who remains still and a relatively bloodless field, and he or she should consider the possible effects of nitrous oxide in the anesthetic carrier gas mixture. The operating microscope magnifies everything it sees. The slightest patient movement becomes an earthquake; blood oozing into the field looks like a flood. Therefore the anesthesiologist should pay particular attention to providing an adequate depth of anesthesia, in the case of a single-agent technique, or an appropriate level of muscle blockade, in the case of a balanced technique, to ensure that the patient does not move.

To prevent major oozing into the wound, meticulous attention to the airway is required to avoid an inadvertent positive end-expiratory pressure. Airway pressure should equal atmospheric pressure during the end-expiratory pause, whether the patient is breathing spontaneously or being ventilated, to avoid an increased venous pressure. Venous drainage from the area can be facilitated by a slight head-up tilt of the patient, but this increases the risk of occasional air embolism from the wound. If this position is adopted, the standard precautions of a chest Doppler and a central venous line for aspiration are suggested. Expired carbon dioxide and nitrogen analysis also will give warning of the condition. With any technique, allowing the blood pressure to decrease somewhat from normal values is useful when this is deemed safe for the patient. Some surgeons and anesthesiologists believe that formal controlled hypotensive techniques have much to offer in improving the operative field. In the shorter operations on the middle ear—such as tympanoplasty, in which oozing may lift a technically successful graft—the shorter-acting agents such as sodium nitroprusside or trimethaphan, given by intravenous infusion, are indicated. When a longer operation on the structures of the inner ear

and neural canals is contemplated, better conditions can be maintained with the older, longer-acting ganglionic blockers such as pentolinium.

Where sensory-evoked potentials are being used to facilitate cochlear implants, muscle relaxants may be required to eliminate background electrical ''noise'' from muscle activity. If this is required, the anesthesiologist should be informed of the need well in advance.

Air under pressure in the closed middle ear cavity is usually vented passively through the normal eustachian tube. Nitrous oxide in the anesthetic carrier gas mixture, although relatively insoluble in blood, is still much more soluble than nitrogen, the major constituent of air. Therefore, more nitrous oxide molecules will present themselves in the walls of the cavity and slide down the diffusion gradient into the contained gas than can be compensated for by the removal of nitrogen molecules down their own diffusion gradient by the same blood. For every molecule of nitrogen leaving the cavity, 10 molecules of nitrous oxide are available. With time, this net increase in molecules leads to increasing intracavity pressure. If for any reason normal passive venting is impaired, pressure can increase rapidly to levels that can rupture the normal tympanum and disrupt tympanic grafts. Because nitrous oxide is a relatively insoluble gas, its uptake and washout from the blood is rapid. Turning the gas off approximately 30 minutes before a tympanic graft is placed is usually sufficient to avoid the problem.

Also, the rapid diffusion of nitrous oxide out of the middle ear cavity may cause subatmospheric pressures and retraction of the tympanum or graft. Occasional cases of irreversible sensorineural hearing loss in patients who have undergone previous stapedectomies with prosthesis insertion have been attributed to the pressure effects of nitrous oxide.[48] Of more recent interest are the possible beneficial effects of the agent in evacuating fluid from the middle ear and elevating retracted membranes preparatory to ventilation tube insertion.

Microsurgery of the larynx

When a laryngologist has declined to operate on a conscious patient, several methods are available for the management of general anesthesia. The major problem is the difficulty of securing the airway against contamination because of the close proximity of surgical activity. If a small, standard cuffed endotracheal tube is used, normal inhalation techniques are feasible. However, the surgeon's access to the structures of the larynx is restricted, which may be unacceptable if work is to be done on the posterior vocal folds, where the tube comes to lie naturally. If laryngeal polyps or papillomata are the reason for surgery, difficulty in working around the tube may be insurmountable, and some consider the risk of passing the tube through such a glottis in the first place unacceptable.

An alternative is the use of venturi jet ventilation as part of a balanced technique. Jet ventilation may be achieved by using a rigid injector above or protruding below the larynx and attached to the laryngoscope or by using the cuffed Carden tube (Fig. 12-11) placed below the larynx and independent of the laryngoscope. Each is attached to a high-pressure gas source, either oxygen or a nitrous oxide–oxygen mixture from a high-pressure blender, and intermittent pulses of gas are used to inflate the patient's lungs by means of a manual or automatic pneumatic switch. The high-pressure gas stream in theory entrains room air from the pharynx. In prac-

tice, entrainment is slight if the injector orifice is below the cords, and when a nitrous oxide–oxygen mixture is used, anesthetic tensions can be achieved. The patient should be fully paralyzed to facilitate ventilation, and the surgeon should ensure a clear expiratory pathway at all times to prevent pressure injury to the lungs. Intravenous adjuvants are used to ensure an adequate depth of anesthesia. The rigid jet (Fig. 12-12) used in modifications of the Toronto ventilating laryngoscope improves access compared with a standard

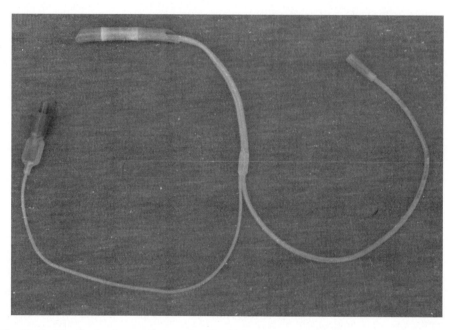

Fig. 12-11. The Carden jet-ventilation tube. The high-pressure connection tube is to the *right*; the cuff inflation tube to the *left* (should not be used for laser applications).

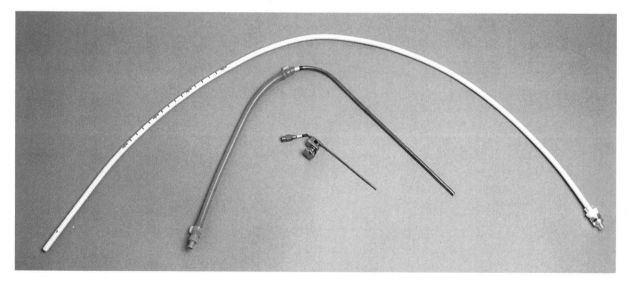

Fig. 12-12. Various high pressure injectors available for jet ventilation techniques. (1) A Cook exchange catheter rigged with a Luer lock. (2) A homemade injector fashioned for use with a Jako suspension laryngoscope. (3) The classic Sanders' jet ventilation attachment with several applications, including rigid laryngoscopy and rigid bronchoscopy.

tube but is still inflexible. The advantage of the Carden tube is that only the small cuff inflation tube and the jet tube protrude above the larynx, and because both are made of soft flexible material, the surgeon can lift them out of the way if necessary. With venturi jet techniques, when the injector orifice is above the cords, the surgeon should remember the risks of blowing blood and particulate matter into the unprotected tracheobronchial tree.

Laser surgery

The laser (the word is an acronym for "light amplification by stimulated emission of radiation") is finding an increasing number of applications as a tool for surgery. The lasers of particular interest in otolaryngologic surgery are the carbon dioxide laser, the argon laser, and the neodymium/yttrium-aluminum-garnet (Nd:YAG) laser. Although each differs from the others in its physical properties and applications, the requirements for anesthetic management are similar:

1. Complete patient immobility to ensure that normal tissue is not hit accidentally
2. Unencumbered surgical access to and visibility of the target area
3. Protection of the patient from stray laser radiation or reflection

When the use of a laser in the airway is contemplated, further precautions are needed:

1. Protection of the airway against blood and the products of vaporization
2. Removal of smoke and debris
3. Prevention of airway fires

Although the use of lasers for stapedectomy, extirpation of base-of-skull tumors, and operations on the nose has been described, these applications should be considered under development, if not still experimental. Applications in the airway, however, have already established the laser as an important treatment modality.

The need for absolute immobility demands the use of muscle relaxants and hence general anesthesia. The choice of the method of ventilation and the choice of the method for maintaining the airway depend on the site of the target lesion. The carbon dioxide laser is used with the microscope for susceptible lesions in the larynx. Here access for the surgeon is difficult, and two methods of ventilation are available: use of a small cuffed endotracheal laser tube or, if that restricts access to the lesion, venturi ventilation with the orifice of the injector attached to the laryngoscope sited below the cords (Fig. 12-13). The positioning of the injector

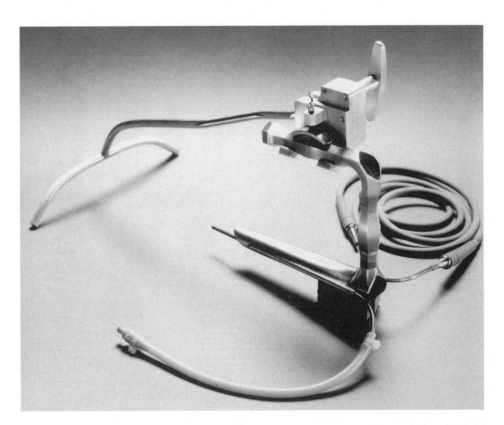

Fig. 12-13. Suspension laryngoscopy setup for use with jet ventilation. Originally designed to hold two fiberoptic light guides, the guide on the left of the Jako has been replaced with a homemade metal injector, which may be adjusted by the surgeon so that the orifice is sited above or below the vocal folds.

below the target minimizes the risk of blowing blood into the lungs, and the expired gases are effective in removing smoke. However, the relaxed vocal cords balloon with ventilation, necessitating synchronization of surgical activity on the cords with the ventilatory cycle so as not to have to hit a moving target.

The use of an endotracheal tube introduces the risk of intratracheal fires. Initial efforts to minimize this risk involved wrapping standard tubes with dampened muslin or metallic tape to disperse or reflect the aberrant laser strike. This approach was not particularly successful because tubes still ignited. Energy would be transferred from the laser beam to the tube in the form of heat, and once the "flash point" for the material constituting the tube was reached, ignition occurred. The subsequent fire was fed by the anesthetic carrier gases, creating a reasonable facsimile of a blowtorch within the trachea. Different tube materials and coatings have been tried to minimize this risk, but it now seems clear that the all-metal tube or the silicone-coated metal tube (Fig. 12-14) is the instrument of choice for ventilation.[46] Even these tubes are not without problems. With rough handling of the all-metal tubes, metal burrs are created that can lead to direct trauma with placement, and the tube can still heat up with laser impacts and cause contact tissue burns. For control of the airway, a latex cuff has to be added, which apart from causing allergic responses in some patients also can ignite. This risk is minimized by inflation with 1% aqueous lidocaine rather than air, so that if the cuff ignites and ruptures, the escaping liquid will tend to quench the fire and minimize any local tissue burn reaction. The metal spiral is designed to leak gases, which some consider a major disadvantage. The silicone-coated metal tubes are gas tight but have a small lumen relative to external diameter, which can lead to ventilation problems and limits the choice of methods for placement with a difficult airway.

For palliative procedures to relieve neoplastic obstruction of the trachea, when getting below the laser target is not possible, venturi ventilation through an uncuffed metal tube is indicated. For endobronchial procedures using an Nd: YAG laser through a fiberoptic bronchoscope, the airway may be maintained by using an old rigid ventilating bronchoscope with a Sanders' venturi ventilation attachment.[56] If the patient already has a tracheostomy, the tube should be exchanged for a metal tracheostomy tube that has been suitably protected.

Additional general precautions are required for the conduct of laser surgery. Care should be exercised to ensure that the patient is electrically grounded. The patient's eyes should be protected with wet eye patches secured with canvas tape (plastic tapes should be avoided because they can melt onto the skin). The immediate area surrounding the operative site should be draped with wet linen towels. All personnel in the operating room should wear protective eye glasses appropriate to the laser, with side guards.

If despite precautions taken, a laser fire still occurs, the flow of anesthetic gases should be cut off and the laser discontinued immediately. If the endotracheal tube is involved, it should be quickly removed and the patient immediately re-intubated with a standard tube before edema can develop. The fire should be quenched with water held in readiness

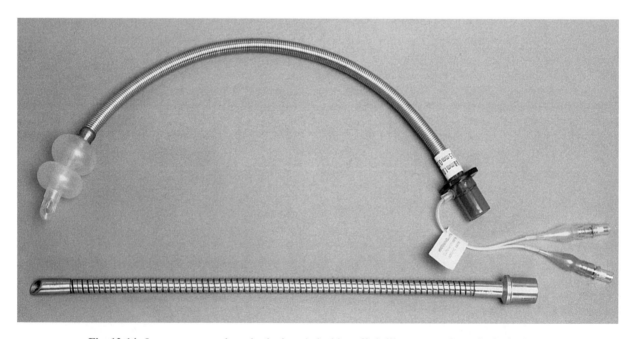

Fig. 12-14. Laser surgery endotracheal tubes. A double-cuffed silicone-coated metal tube is above. The proximal cuff is inflated first with saline or lidocaine solution. The distal cuff is held in reserve in case of rupture of the proximal cuff. The all-metal Norton tube is pictured below.

on the instrument table for such an eventuality. The standard therapeutic and respiratory support measures for severe airway burns should then be instituted.[57]

General endoscopy

The ''paint-up'' technique discussed previously for intubating the larynx in the awake patient is equally suited to laryngoscopy and bronchoscopy—although less so for esophagoscopy because of patient discomfort. Therefore it only remains to add here a few points that can facilitate the technique. When the procedure is to be undertaken electively, starving the patient is wise because his or her reflexes will be obtunded, and a light premedication with a benzodiazepine or barbiturate will facilitate the paintup if they are not contraindicated by an airway already compromised by disease. When the surgeon's practice requires large planned endoscopy clinics, the services of an anesthesiologist in preparing the second and subsequent patients while the surgeon is working speed matters considerably. When the use of a topical technique is inappropriate, the following methods of management during general anesthesia are available:

1. *Laryngoscopy,* as far as the anesthesiologist is concerned, involves two types of surgical technique—suspension and manual. When the laryngoscope is suspended and manipulation kept to a minimum, venturi ventilation with or without a Carden tube is indicated because it gives the surgeon the best possible access. The patient should be fully paralyzed, and maximum inflation pressures should be monitored with care. The surgeon should ensure a clear expiratory pathway at all times to avoid barotrauma to the lungs. Anesthesia is induced with a thiobarbiturate depolarizing relaxant sequence in the usual way, but the anesthesia is maintained with intravenous agents, because standard vaporizers cannot be used in high-pressure systems.

Should a ''manual'' laryngoscopic technique be used for diagnostic work, particularly when the surgeon is exploring the hypopharyngeal area, venturi ventilation should not be used because intermittent interruption of the expiratory pathway occurs too frequently. If biopsies are being taken when the larynx is not in view continuously, the additional risk of blood contaminating the tracheobronchial tree has to be recognized. Therefore in this situation, a small cuffed endotracheal tube is the best choice for securing the airway, with anesthesia being maintained by means of inhaled vapors.

2. *Bronchoscopy* allows four main variations in technique:
   a. The rigid ventilating bronchoscope allows maintenance of anesthesia with a standard anesthetic vapor through a side arm with a 15-mm connector, which permits attachment to standard anesthetic circuits. Surgeons derive some protection from anesthetic gases by using glass eyepieces, but these should be firmly attached during positive-pressure ventilation, otherwise they can blow off into the eyes. An alternative is to use a Sanders' venturi attachment and proceed with a balanced intravenous technique.
   b. Fiberoptic bronchoscopy permits the passage of the instrument through the lumen of a standard endotracheal tube, which allows the airway to be secured against aspiration at all times while permitting standard anesthetic maintenance techniques. The connection between the circuit and tube is made with a right-angled swivel connector with a perforated rubber diaphragm that permits access for the bundle while maintaining a gas-tight seal. The limitation of the approach is the resistance to expiration, which is determined by the cross-sectional area of the instrument relative to the area of the lumen of the tube. Anatomy dictates the size of the tube lumen, but the size of the bundle is a matter of technology. The ability to manufacture ever-smaller fiberoptic bundles with satisfactory optical properties is improving rapidly, and now the technique may be considered even in small children.
   c. Apneic oxygenation uses the principle of oxygenation by diffusion in a fully paralyzed patient. Intravenous drugs are used to maintain anesthesia. Once anesthesia is induced, profound hypocapnia is achieved with hyperventilation by mask. A small-gauge catheter is passed through the larynx to the carina under direct vision. A 1- to 3-l min/flow of oxygen is attached to the catheter, and the patient is turned over to the surgeon. The duration of uninterrupted access is limited only by the rate of increase of endogenous carbon dioxide to significant levels, as long as the patient remains fully paralyzed. The technique works well in patients without major pulmonary disease, but the surgeon should be sparing and careful in the use of suction through the bronchoscope.
   d. Deep inhalation anesthesia is another established technique; it is particularly helpful in small children. Anesthesia is induced, and the patient is allowed to breathe an anesthetic vapor in oxygen spontaneously. Any of the standard agents is suitable, but the most prolonged uninterrupted access to the airway is achieved with the highly blood-soluble, potent analgesic vapor of methoxyflurane. Anesthesia is taken to the deepest safe level. When the mask is removed, the surgeon proceeds while the patient lightens slowly, still breathing spontaneously. (Techniques *c* and *d* are equally suited to flexible or rigid bronchoscopy.)
3. *Esophagoscopy* requires full control of the airway when the procedure is performed during general anes-

thesia. With a large, rigid esophagoscope, some difficulty may be experienced in passing the instrument past the posterior tracheal bulge of the tube cuff. Therefore the anesthesiologist should be ready to deflate the cuff transiently to assist the surgeon. As the instrument passes the arch of the aorta, an occasional patient will develop profound reflex bradycardia requiring intervention, although the major risk is perforation of the esophagus, so the patient should remain immobile. Some surgeons maintain that if the patient is breathing spontaneously, the residual muscle tone, particularly in the inferior pharyngeal constrictor, permits them to judge more accurately the amount of force they are using to pass the instrument.

The mentally retarded patient

Otolaryngology is one of the specialties that involves frequent contact with mentally retarded patients. Mental retardation often is associated with congenital abnormalities resulting in multiple otolaryngologic problems, particularly with hearing.

Anesthetic evaluation of these patients is frequently difficult. The history obtained is often sketchy and unreliable, and a disproportionate reliance must be placed on the opinions of available lay observers. Rapport may be impossible to establish, and the physical examination can bear more resemblance to a wrestling match than a dignified medical procedure. Nonetheless, associated congenital deformities of the cardiovascular system, airway, and skeletal system must be identified, if present, to formulate an anesthetic plan. It is particularly important in institutionalized patients to remember their high exposure to infectious hepatitis, necessitating liver function studies preoperatively.

The anesthesiologist should develop a healthy skepticism concerning the adequacy of the standard preoperative safety precautions in these patients. The mentally retarded patient's stomach is never assumed to be empty, even when he or she has been starved. Some patients manage to thwart the efforts of even the most dedicated ward nurse, and an interesting variety of objects, other than food, have been retrieved from their stomachs during the course of anesthesia.

Premedication also poses problems. Some form of sedation is usually indicated, but persuading the patient to take it is another matter. The severely mentally retarded, similar to children, do not take kindly to needles, which should be reserved for use in the operating room. Many of these patients are already taking behavior-modifying medication, and enzyme induction is to be expected, with unpredictable implications for the effects of standard premedicant drug dosages. The standard drug mixtures may or may not work. The author has come to rely increasingly on an orally administered combination of a butyrophenone (haloperidol) and a benzodiazepine (diazepam) mixed with a small amount of fruit preserve, if necessary, on the basis of trial and error only.

If the patient is tranquil on arrival in the operating room, the choice of anesthetic technique may be made in the usual way. However, if the patient is not cooperative, the problem of how to prepare the patient for anesthesia has to be faced. Reasoning with the patient is rarely an effective option. The surreptitious intramuscular use of ketamine (4 mg/kg), injected into whichever limb muscle may conveniently present itself for a few seconds, is suggested. The niceties of removing clothing and of skin preparation before injection may have to be dispensed with in the face of patient counterattack. The assistance of able-bodied operating room staff is invaluable. Once the drug has taken effect, monitors and an intravenous infusion can be set up and a modified anesthetic induction begun. Because of the possibility of a full stomach, cricoid pressure should be used with all such inductions.

Some mentally retarded patients frequently swallow foreign objects and, consequently, make frequent visits to the hospital. The anesthesiologist experiences brief glory if he or she is able to retrieve a foreign object from the hypopharynx at induction without surgical assistance. The anesthesiologist should be aware of the possibility of hypopharyngeal location to avoid pushing the object into a less favorable position. Multiple visits of this nature should not lead the patient's attendants to relax the normal standards of care. These patients are rarely legally competent, so time should be taken to ensure that the person signing the consent is the legal guardian and not merely the patient's custodian.

Cancer surgery

Several factors justify the separate consideration of anesthesia for cancer surgery of the head and neck including the propensity for large blood loss and the requirement for fine dissection around nerves and vessels. These factors necessitate an increased capacity for intravenous infusion and the more direct measurement of BP; in addition, the use of controlled hypotension may be considered to limit blood loss and provide a drier surgical field. The use of controlled hypotension is still a matter of controversy even after 60 years of experience.[22]

Many techniques have been described for the deliberate lowering of BP during anesthesia,[34] but only a few are suitable for use in head and neck surgery. The advantages claimed for the technique may be summarized as follows:

1. Reduced bleeding leads to better visualization of the field for fine dissection, especially with the shallow depth of focus of an operating microscope. This statement has two implications:
   a. Better visualization decreases the risk of accidental damage to important structures (e.g., facial nerve in parotidectomy).
   b. Better visualization encourages more definitive dissection, thereby improving the chances of success in cancer surgery.
2. Reduced bleeding reduces the need for blood transfusion, with its associated risks. This claim has been

clearly substantiated for selected operations (e.g., the commando procedure).

3. For some operations, reduced bleeding makes the ''impossible'' possible (e.g., resection of a juvenile angiofibroma).

4. It also is claimed that reduced bleeding results in less of the surgeon's time being spent in securing hemostasis. This has a number of advantages. There is less necrotic tissue in the wound from diathermy use, less foreign material in the form of hemostatic ligatures, and less tissue handling in the first place. These factors are said to result in less wound infection and breakdown and to lead to better wound scars. It is further claimed that the reduced time spent on hemostatis maneuvers results in shorter surgical procedures, but on this point the literature is equivocal.

5. The continuation of BP control into the postoperative period is said to reduce the incidence of rebound hypertension and wound hematomas.

Before deciding to use controlled hypotension, one should set these advantages against the supposed risks for the patient. Those who have experience in the technique cite various contraindications, but one fact has been clear from the technique's inception: institutions that use controlled hypotension frequently have a far lower complication rate attributable to the technique itself than those that use it only occasionally. The complications associated with the improper use of the technique are serious, and it should not be undertaken lightly.[27] For the details of the various drugs and methods available, refer to the extensive literature on the topic. The remarks that follow will be confined to the general standard of care applicable to the use of the technique in head and neck surgery.

All patients require a large-volume line for fluid infusion and transfusion if necessary. A second, low dead-space line is required for the administration of the potent hypotensive agents. The recent advances and general availability of sophisticated monitoring equipment now mandate the direct measurement of arterial pressure and electrocardiography. Arterial blood samples should be taken at frequent intervals for blood gas analysis and hematocrit and hemoglobin–oxygen saturation determinations to confirm pulse oximetry. Core temperature should be monitored in all patients, although no measures should be taken to warm the patient actively because of the risk of thermal burns over pressure points as skin circulation pressure decreases. Particular care should be taken in older patients with atrophic skin because mere body weight on pressure points will produce damage more quickly with controlled hypotension; placing a synthetic sheepskin under the patient is a suitable precaution.

Recent advances in the understanding of the changes that occur in ventilation–perfusion ratios in the lungs at low pulmonary perfusion pressures mandate the full control of ventilation with a cuffed endotracheal tube and intermittent positive-pressure ventilation by machine. To avoid excessive cerebral vasoconstriction, care must be exercised to maintain $Paco_2$ at close to normal levels. This frequently requires an artificial dead space between the tube and the anesthesia circuit. Patients at the extremes of age are ''vagal dominant,'' but those in between tend to respond to attempts to lower their blood pressure with a compensatory tachycardia. This may prove troublesome if it is allowed to become established, so β-adrenergic blocking drugs are indicated early in the case. The availability of a fully staffed recovery room with nurses trained in the specific condition of the patient is a *sine qua non* of safe practice. The remaining points of technique are still a matter of opinion based on the anesthesiologist's personal experience.

From the point of view of the surgeon, it is suggested that the procedures most likely to benefit from controlled hypotension are the major cancer dissections of the head and neck, the fine dissection required with operations on the parotid gland, and a few ear procedures, such as tympanoplasty. The classic indication is the intranasal juvenile angiofibroma. All these operations require a reduced BP held stable for an extended period of time. This requirement is best met with the longer-acting ganglionic blockers and with a slight degree of head-up tilt on the operating table.

The surgeon should be cautioned that arteries still bleed profusely when cut and that tissues are more susceptible to injury from careless handling. In particular, the surgeon should guard against ''retractor ischemia'' when nerves or vessels are retracted. The technique has much to offer the competent surgeon but will not improve pedestrian efforts.

Of more recent interest is the introduction of free-flap techniques for the closure of the more extensive cancer resections of the head and neck. This surgical technique is responsible for the growing rarity of controlled deliberate hypotension in head and neck surgery as low perfusion pressures are inimical to the survival of free-flaps. In the past, thermal homeostasis for the patient undergoing head and neck resections has not been a particular problem because most of the patient's body was outside the surgical field and could be effectively ''cocooned'' to minimize heat loss and active warming was contraindicated when deliberate hypotension was used. With the introduction of free-flap techniques, body temperature control has become an issue. With the improved ability to close a wound, resections have become more extensive, and the flap attachment phase has prolonged the operation. This has had the expected result of greater fluid requirements for third-spacing, but one problem that was not anticipated was the large body surface area required for surgical preparation. The standard operating table underbody warming pad has not proved adequate for the new conditions, and only a small upper surface area is available for additional active warming of the patient. Because operation time is extended over many hours, relying on a sustained increase in operating room ambient tempera-

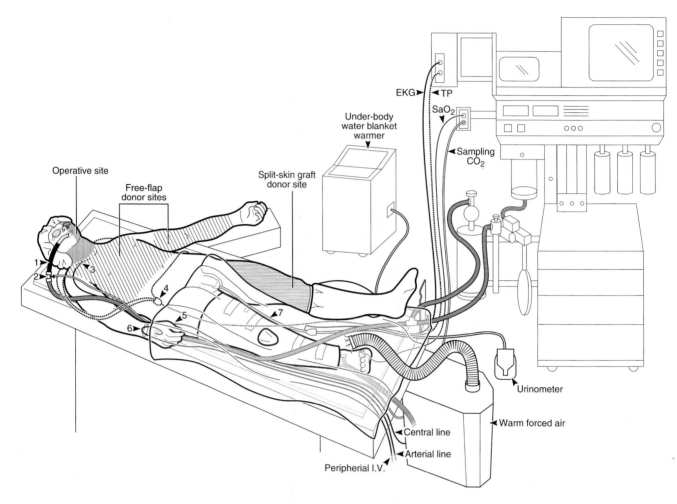

Fig. 12-15. Operating room setup for radical resections with free-flap closure. Note that the various preparation areas leave a large surface open to evaporative heat and water loss. The donor sites are preferably on the nondominant side of the patient's body but that means that most of the anesthetic lines have to be inserted on the dominant side. The forced air warming blanket is placed over the dominant side of the lower body with the nondominant leg on top. The anesthesia circuit and fluid lines are led up from the feet under the blanket to aid in heat conservation.

1. Flexible free-flow connector from endotracheal tube (ETT) to circuit to permit changes in head position without circuit disruption. If a full face operative site is required, a nasal ETT can be substituted.

2. Carbon dioxide monitor sampling T-piece mounted at the distal end of the coaxial circle with extensions.

3. The central line monitor (CVP or Swann-Ganz) is inserted in the subclavian vein on the dominant side. However, if the extent of surgery prevents this a central line may be passed up the median antecubital or the femoral veins.

4. The electrocardiogram contact leads are secured out of the surgical preparation areas.

5. A cannula is inserted into the dominant side radial artery for continuous blood pressure monitoring.

6. A large bore intravenous infusion is also started on the dominant arm.

7. A temperature-sensing Foley catheter is placed and attached to a urinometer.

ture did not seem a reasonable solution if operating room staff comfort and efficiency were to be maintained. The setup illustrated in Figure 12-15 using a forced air lower body warming blanket in conjunction with a circle circuit under the blanket has been found particularly effective in addressing these problems. A coaxial circle makes secure positioning even easier.

Difficult airway

Attorneys tell us that the anesthesiologist is the hospital's expert in the management of the airway. Unfortunately, nothing is so humbling for our expert than finding that, having induced anesthesia, he or she is unable either to ventilate the patient by mask or secure the airway with an endotracheal tube. Luckily the truly difficult airway is rare, but because death or serious morbidity may result from mismanagement, the anesthesiologist is obliged to master the several techniques that may be used to avert disaster. Anesthesiologists working in otolaryngology have more than their fair share of difficult airways to contend with, but at least they are working with surgeons who are skilled in tracheotomy. It is useful to divide patients with airway problems into three distinct groups to discuss their management:

1. Patients in extremis with severe airway obstruction and hypoxia. These patients will have accompanying hypercapnia, delirium, or unconsciousness. The situation is an emergency, and cardiac arrest will occur if the airway is not cleared immediately.
2. Patients with respiratory distress. These patients represent the largest group requiring anesthesia. They may exhibit stridor, tracheal tug, intercostal retraction, labored breathing, and agitation. Although increasingly fatigued, they are able to compensate sufficiently to maintain adequate oxygenation and remain alert and cooperative.
3. Patients with occult impending obstruction. Such patients volunteer little information in their history to suggest difficulties, and a cursory physical examination reveals little to warn of the management problems that are to follow the induction of anesthesia.

The management of the first group is self-evident. Oxygenation should be reestablished immediately. If the patient is unconscious and relaxed, it is worthwhile to use a few seconds to attempt rapid laryngoscopy and intubation, but no time should be wasted. If intubation is obviously not going to be easy, the surgeon or anesthesiologist should perform an immediate cricothyroidotomy to reestablish the airway before moving the patient to the operating room for formal tracheotomy. (It is exceedingly rare that a so-called emergency tracheotomy is done under unfavorable conditions by an inexperienced surgeon in the hospital environment.) If the patient is still moving some air into his or her lungs, laryngoscopy should be omitted because this could lead to total obstruction. The patient should have his or her airway supported and be transferred to the operating room breathing 100% oxygen by mask. A cricothyroidotomy is indicated should the patient's condition deteriorate in transit, therefore the equipment should accompany the patient.[68]

An alternative to cricothyroidotomy is transtracheal jet ventilation.[17] This technique requires access to a line with 100% oxygen at 50 psi and a Luer-lock connector. The airway is controlled by puncturing the trachea or cricothyroid membrane with a 16-gauge plastic-sheathed needle. The needle is withdrawn, leaving the sheath in the trachea; the sheath is then attached to the high-pressure line through a pressure regulator control, and ventilation is accomplished using a manual interruptor switch. As with any technique for emergency airway management, it should be practiced in a controlled setting, and the equipment should be available. This technique has proved valuable in the management of infectious and neoplastic sudden obstruction of the upper airway and can be relied on to support ventilation for as long as 30 to 60 minutes while arrangements for more formal airway management are being undertaken, but the risk of barotrauma with the technique always should be remembered. The other two groups of patients permit the anesthesiologist and the surgeon the luxury of planning airway management in advance. A word of caution is in order for those patients in respiratory distress. The worst possible place in which to manage an airway crisis is the radiology department, especially at night. The absolute need for formal radiologic examination, particularly if the patient is obviously tiring, should be carefully considered. Most needed information about the airway can be obtained in the operating suite with a C-arm image intensifier with all the equipment necessary to handle a crisis immediately to hand.

The purpose of the management plan is to achieve full control of the airway to guarantee oxygenation while sealing it against contamination. The ideal method is to achieve control from above the larynx by inserting an oral endotracheal tube, under direct vision, into a relaxed anesthetized patient. This is assumed to cause the least trauma to the patient's anatomy and psyche. This of course is the normal configuration for the majority of general anesthetics, although when pathology intervenes, the patient's best interests may be served by deviations from the ideal; the choices to be made are represented by the ''decision tree'' in Figure 12-16.

If the problems involved are severe, the surgeon may elect to do a tracheotomy during local anesthesia without an endotracheal tube. This is less desirable than doing a tracheotomy after the protection afforded by an endotracheal tube cuff is in place, even in an awake patient. Similarly, visualized manipulations always are preferable to blind, and oral approaches are preferable to nasal, with their increased risk of damage to the structures of the nasal cavity and the posterior pharyngeal wall and associated bleeding. The height of folly is to undertake surgery during general anesthesia with a totally uncontrolled airway, but even this has been tried with the use of ketamine as the all-purpose single-agent anesthetic and is the not uncommon result of the poorly conducted local anesthesia ''stand-by'' case. In the second group of patients—those with respiratory distress—it is the technical skill of the anesthesiologist that determines the airway control plan and its success. In patients with occult impending obstruction, the anesthesiologist's diagnostic abilities in detecting that a problem is present in the first place are paramount.

Most occult problems result from subtle congenital anatomic abnormalities for which the patient compensates with muscular effort. The only clue to the condition may be a history of obstructive sleep apnea. However, under direct questioning, the patient may admit only to early waking, and the true sequence of events is frequently obtained only from

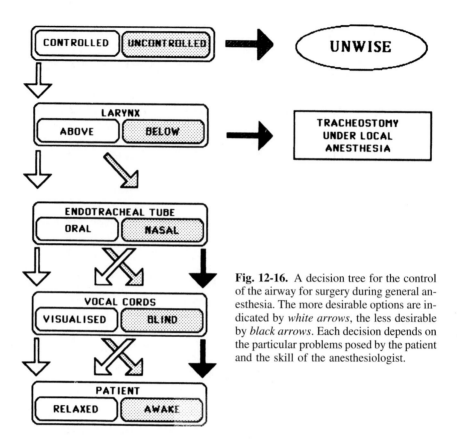

Fig. 12-16. A decision tree for the control of the airway for surgery during general anesthesia. The more desirable options are indicated by *white arrows*, the less desirable by *black arrows*. Each decision depends on the particular problems posed by the patient and the skill of the anesthesiologist.

the patient's bedmate, who is awakened by heavy snoring and then hears the onset of obstruction or "choking," followed by the patient's awakening. The normal anesthetic induction abolishes all muscle tone and promptly precipitates complete obstruction, which, because of the anatomic abnormalities involved, usually is not amenable to the normal methods of reestablishing the airway. In addition, the use of relaxant drugs in the induction sequence for any difficult airway will not only abolish the airway but also prolong the interval during which the patient cannot breathe spontaneously. If the patient cannot be actively ventilated and if the period of apnea exceeds the oxygen reserves in the patient's body, disaster is certain. Thus exists the need to maintain spontaneous ventilation and to increase the oxygen reserve in the FRC by preoxygenation. Premedication alone may be sufficient to precipitate a crisis. Besides congenital conditions, some patients with morbid obesity or carcinomas of the base of tongue behave in this manner, as do those with epiglottitis.

Having assessed the patient, the anesthesiologist should consider the means of achieving airway control. If the desirable condition is oral intubation during general anesthesia, alternatives have to be decided by a process of exclusion. Ludwig's angina, with its large upwardly swelling tongue, precludes the use of an oral tube, but passage of a nasal tube with fiberoptic visualization may be feasible. However, the leukemic coagulopathy resulting in a large tongue also would render any nasal intubation attempt unwise. Similarly, although micrognathia might preclude the desirable oral visualization of the larynx and the passage of an oral tube, blind nasal intubation may be easily achieved. Any friable hemorrhagic tumor above the larynx or a large pointing abscess in the pharynx would be an absolute contraindication to any blind technique and could dissuade most from visualized techniques. This would leave local anesthesia for awake tracheotomy as the only viable alternative.

Regardless of the approach chosen, certain precautions should be observed. Patients with airway compromise should receive no depressant premedicant drugs without most careful consideration. The neck is prepared for tracheotomy before any intubation procedures are started. The patient is fully preoxygenated. The surgeon, fully scrubbed, remains in the operating room until the airway is secured by whatever means. If general anesthesia is to be induced, an inhalation technique is elected so that in the event of the development of difficulties in the maintainance of airway patency, the induction process may be reversed and the patient awakened. Once given, intravenous drugs cannot be retrieved in the face of developing obstruction. Sudden obstruction can still occur, and if a pharyngeal airway or rapid laryngoscopy does not resolve the problem, the use of a laryngeal mask or a Combitube may save the situation; if not, immediate cricothyrotomy or tracheotomy is indicated.

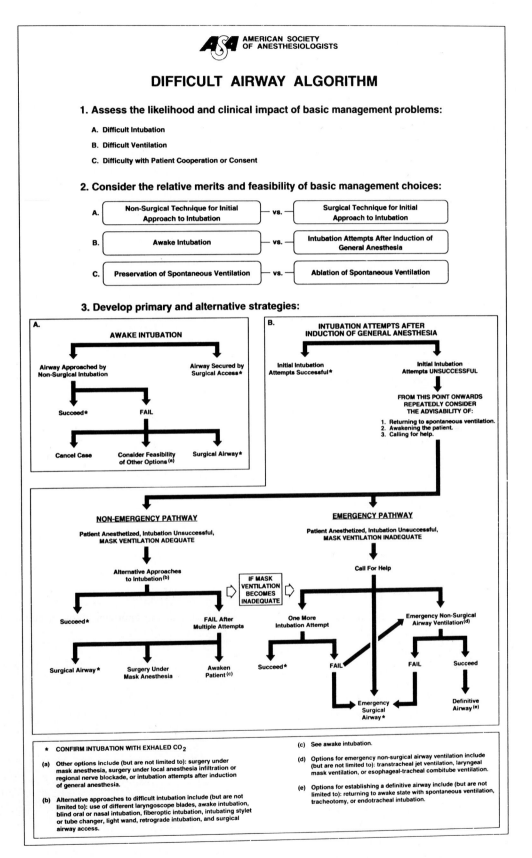

Fig. 12-17. The American Society of Anesthesiologists Difficult Airway Algorithm. (Reproduced with permission.)

If the induction is successful, numerous methods are available to persuade tubes to pass into the trachea in various situations; these have been described elsewhere.[11] One point should be emphasized with regards to choice of intubation technique. If fiberoptic intubation is considered an appropriate alternative choice for intubation, it should be used first because previous attempts with other methods may cause bleeding in the airway and make the subsequent use of fiberoptic instruments impossible. The prerequisites of consistent success in the management of the difficult airway are thorough preoperative assessment, good planning with viable first, second, and third alternative techniques, and full cooperation between the anesthesiologist and the surgeon. An algorithmn for guidance in selecting from the various approaches to the difficult airway has been promulgated recently by the ASA (Fig. 12-17). Finally, never persist too long in the face of a failed plan because of the risk of laryngospasm and iatrogenic edema of the airway. Back out and reconsider.

POSTOPERATIVE RECOVERY

Patients recovering from general anesthesia traverse the stages of anesthesia in reverse and should be watched closely throughout the process. If the patient is still in the third stage, without an endotracheal tube, laryngeal mask, or tracheostomy, continued airway support is needed. As stage 2 is traversed, muscle tone progressively returns, and the patient becomes irritable and salivates, which can lead to coughing and swallowing. External stimulation should be kept to a minimum to avoid the risk of laryngospasm or vomiting (which are not mutually exclusive). In stage 1, the patient is rousable but in a state of analgesia. However, some time may elapse before normal mental faculties and spatial and temporal orientation are regained. It is during this period that the perception of postoperative pain first intrudes. All forms of anesthesia potentially reduce cardiac output and peripheral vascular resistance. This leads to increased ventilation–perfusion mismatch in the lungs and a reduced Pao_2. Therefore, all postoperative patients should be supported with supplemental oxygen administered by mask (nasal prongs are not reliable without Pao_2 determination), giving an inspired oxygen concentration of at least 30% to 35%. This is equally true for patients who are still intubated and being ventilated. All patients benefit from humidification of the inspired gas, particularly those with an irritable airway.

If a difficult intubation has been encountered at induction of anesthesia, it is usual to transfer the patient from the operating room with the endotracheal tube in place. The patient is allowed to awaken fully before any consideration is given to removing the tube. If the patient fights the tube during second stage emergence, it should not be removed but rather the patient sedated and his or her vital signs controlled as appropriate. Once the patient is fully conscious and oriented and the anesthesiologist is satisfied with the adequacy of the patient's spontaneous ventilation, a standard protocol for extubation should be followed:

1. Prepare equipment for reintubation including an endotracheal tube one full size smaller.
2. If reintubation is required and fails, what is the plan?
3. Instill 4 ml of 2% lidocaine down the endotracheal tube into the patient's trachea.
4. Suction tracheal and pharyngeal secretions if necessary and preoxygenate the patient.
5. The anesthesiologist then deflates the tube cuff and stops the tube (obstructs the lumen with his or her thumb) to see if the patient can breathe around the tube. If he or she can:
6. Pass a tube guide (e.g., teflon guide, Cook catheter, or gumelastic bougie) through the tube into the trachea.
7. Withdraw the tube over the guide leaving the guide in place.
8. Secure the guide through an oxygen mask and observe the patient for developing obstruction.

Patients will tolerate the presence of a guide for extended periods and can talk around it (Fig. 12-18). If there is no evidence of developing obstruction, it usually is safe to remove it after 30 minutes. However, if there is any suggestion of deterioration in the function of the patient's airway, the guide is used to immediately "railroad" a new tube of similar size or smaller back into the trachea. If the patient cannot breathe around the original tube when "stopped," obstruction after extubation is more likely so the patient's surgeon should be consulted before proceeding further. The surgeon may wish to be present during extubation attempts or may decide to return the patient to the operating room for an elective tracheotomy with

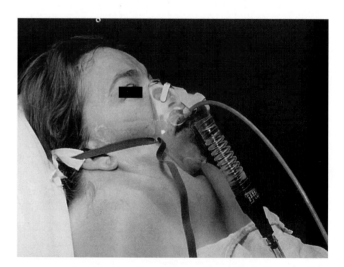

Fig. 12-18. Extubation of the difficult airway patient over a tube-guide. Several different types of guides are available; in this case, a gumelastic bougie was used. Patients tolerate the procedure well and are able to talk around the guide.

the existing endotracheal tube in place. These precautions are no protection against the occasional late airway obstruction that does occur. Therefore if the patient is difficult to intubate this should be communicated to the postoperative ward and clearly noted.

The effects of anesthetics on the circulation at the end of an operation may be masked by the release of endogenous catecholamines in response to the final surgical maneuvers. By the time the patient reaches the recovery room, the catecholamine response usually has subsided, exposing the true degree of anesthetic depression or inadequate fluid replacement. Both conditions can usually be managed with a fluid load rather than with vasopressors; it should always be remembered that blood pressure, even with adequate circulating volume, will not return to normal preoperative values until the initial phases of anesthetic recovery are complete.

Depression of respiration also continues into the recovery phase. Patients who have received a single volatile agent may be relied on to progressively return to normal as long as spontaneous respiration with a clear airway is maintained. This is not so true for patients undergoing a balanced technique, in which the timing of the last dose of muscle relaxant or narcotic drug is important. All nondepolarizing relaxants should be reversed with a mixture of anticholinesterase, such as neostigmine, and an anticholine drug, such as atropine, to block the undesirable muscarinic effects of the former. The reversal is affected by overriding the competitive inhibition of neuromuscular transmission. The degree of override is governed by the law of mass action, and the final balance in patients is unpredictable, although the nerve stimulator gives a useful indication. However, the reversed state is itself reversible, and changes in body temperature or pH can cause bound inactive relaxant drug molecules to ionize and become active again, leading to recurarization.

The surgeon also should be aware of the risk associated with the use of some of the antibiotics he or she may prescribe postoperatively. Most of the ''mycin'' antibiotics are weak muscle blockers in their own right and can act in synergy with residual anesthetic relaxants to a degree that poses a serious risk to the patient. If this situation should develop, rather than attempting reversal of the block with additional anticholinesterases, thereby incurring the risk of a mixed block, the anesthesiologist should reintubate the patient and ventilate him or her until normal excretion takes care of the problem.

The narcotics pose parallel difficulties in terms of circulatory and central respiratory depression, and the injudicious use of additional postoperative analgesics can lead to profound depression. Therefore, the need for additional narcotics should be carefully evaluated, with small intravenous doses being given until the patient's overall clinical condition is better defined. If major narcotic depression is suspected, narcotic antagonists such as naloxone may be used, but it should be remembered that the duration of action of the narcotic usually exceeds the duration of action of the antagonist, so late renarcotization can occur. Once these potential ''normal'' emergence problems have been overcome, the patient's continued presence in the recovery unit is not justified. The following criteria are of use in determining patients' readiness for discharge to general care:

System	Observation	Score
Respiration	Patient is able to breathe freely	2
	Respiratory effort limited (splinting or dyspnea)	1
	Absence of spontaneous respiration	0
Blood pressure	Systolic pressure ±20% of preoperative level	2
	Systolic pressure ±20% to 50% of preoperative level	1
	Systolic pressure ±50% of preoperative level	0
Consciousness	Fully alert and oriented	2
	Only rousable when called by name	1
	Auditory stimulus fails to produce response	0
Color	Normal ''pink'' mucous membranes and nail beds	2
	Discoloration—anything but pink or blue	1
	Frank cyanosis	0
Activity	Able to move all four limbs on command	2
	Able to move only two limbs	1
	Unable to move extremities	0

Modified from Aldrete JA, Kronlik D: A post-anesthetic recovery score, *Anesth Analg Curr Res* 49:924, 1970.

The score for each section is added, and patients having a total score in the range of 8 to 10 are considered ready for discharge to general care. It is unlikely that a patient can achieve a top score in four sections and a zero in the fifth; the one exception is the patient with chronic respiratory paralysis, in which case continued ventilatory support would require admission to intensive care rather than general care for initial convalescence.

Several additional factors should be considered in the discharge of outpatients. The patient should not only be stable, but also ''street ready.'' Activity assessment should include the return of the postural reflexes required for standing and walking safely. Postoperative pain should be under good control. The patient should demonstrate the ability to micturate before discharge. Immediate postoperative surgical problems should be excluded, and significant nausea and vomiting should be controlled. Last but not least, the outpatient may be discharged only into the care of a competent adult for transport home and should remain under supervision at home for the first 24 hours after anesthesia.

ANESTHETIC COMPLICATIONS AND MORTALITY

A recent survey of the English-language literature on anesthesia safety concludes that the risk of death attributable to anesthesia has dropped from 1 in 2680 to about 1 in 10,000 over the past 30 years.[18] Those who have studied the subject believe that all Western nations experience similar mortality rates. If this rate is applied to the approximately 20 million patients to whom anesthetics are administered annually in the United States, at least 2000 deaths may be anticipated. Put another way, the average practicing anesthesiologist will lose two or three patients to causes directly attributable to anesthesia during his or her practice lifetime. Some authorities have suggested, with the benefit of hindsight, that between 50% and 90% of these deaths could be prevented.

Studies of individual cases suggest that the causes of death may be attributed to three broad categories of factors: human factors, patient factors, and technology-related factors.

Of the three, human factors, such as failure to detect disconnection of the anesthetic circuit, are thought to play the decisive part in approximately 70% of the incidents reported. This belief has stimulated the rapid development of "smart," microprocessor-controlled monitoring and measuring devices to supplement the vigilance of the anesthesiologist. Patient factors, such as malignant hyperthermia and anaphylactic anesthetic drug reactions, are much rarer. Technology-related factors are involved in the incidents related to the quality of design and manufacture of anesthesia equipment. One by one, specific problems with anesthesia equipment have been identified and corrected until the equipment manufactured today is much safer than that used even 10 years ago, but vigilance is still required because the more complex a machine is, the more prone it is to malfunction.

Serious complications of anesthesia by which the patient is not killed are rare but devastating because most involve variable degrees of hypoxic brain damage and the high medical costs of chronic dependency. The problem is not limited to short periods of anoxia associated with an acute airway or circuit accident but also includes prolonged "suboxygenation," which may occur in several ways in patients of poor physical status undergoing major surgery. The line between adequate and inadequate tissue oxygenation may be fine, and the situation is not easily measured or monitored.

Despite this depressing cataloging of serious problems, the average patient still has less chance of sustaining a serious injury from anesthesia than of being killed or seriously injured in a traffic accident.

Of more interest to the patient are the chances of experiencing the minor unpleasant complications of anesthesia. More work remains to be done to quantify the true incidence of these complications. Existing studies show a range of variation in incidence.[53] This fact results in part from different patient populations undergoing different operations with varying anesthetic techniques, but also it appears to be related to differences in elapsed time between the end of anesthesia and the patient interview. For example, the reported incidence of postanesthetic nausea varies from 27% of pa-

tients interviewed within 24 hours of anesthesia to 70% of patients interviewed after 3 days.

The common side effects of general anesthesia that the patient should be warned of are as follows:

Complication	Reported incidence
Headache	2% to 60%
Sore throat	6% to 38%
Muscle pains (following suxamethonium)	0% to 100% (muscled males susceptible)
Nausea and vomiting	27% to 70%
Venous complications (following intravenous drugs)	1% to 11%

In addition, minor complications associated with specific techniques or surgical procedures should be remembered. These complications can result from poor positioning and poor protection measures of the patient during anesthesia. Nerve compression (e.g., ulnar) and stretching (e.g., brachial plexus in the abducted arm) can result from poor positioning, but even with apparently appropriate precautions there appears to be an underlying incidence of these problems. Corneal abrasions from lack of adequate eye protection and careless mask technique, and jaw and neck pain from overforceful laryngoscopy and head extension, have been reported. A recurring source of patient complaint is minor damage to the teeth and lips associated with laryngoscopy. Most of these incidents can be prevented with care, but the patient should still be warned of their possible occurrence in advance.

The surgeon should be particularly aware of the delayed complications that may develop after the patient has returned to his or her care. Manipulation of the airway, whether by surgeon or anesthesiologist, is the commonest cause of laryngospasm and acute airway obstruction in the recovery room. Recurarization and renarcotization, leading to hypoxia, always should be considered in the restless patient. Restlessness is usually a result of pain, hypovolemia, or hypoxia, in that order of frequency, *but it should be assumed to be due to hypoxia until proved otherwise.* The persistence of nerve compression paresthesia, hypotension, urinary retention, or altered mental status into the postoperative period always should be taken seriously. A careful watch should be kept for the appearance of postoperative pulmonary complications and the development of jaundice. Such occurrences always warrant the courtesy of consultation with the anesthesiologist concerned when they are first recognized.

As we grow older

The population of the Western world, and of the United States in particular, is aging. Increasing numbers of elderly patients submit themselves for minor and major surgery each year. As life expectancy increases, so does the need for pharmacologic "servicing" of the chronic controllable medical conditions acquired along the way. Many elderly patients no longer die of a disease but rather of total physiologic systems failure in the face of one pathologic, or therapeutic, stress too many. When that stress is likely to be surgical in nature, it usually is the anesthesiologist who is expected to get the patient off the table alive.

The walking pharmacologic "minefields" who constitute an increasing proportion of our patients, are effecting a subtle change in the practice of anesthesia. In the past, the anesthesiologist, having satisfied himself or herself as to the patient's safety, would then concentrate on creating good operating conditions and generally facilitating the rapid and efficient conduct of the procedure in the operating room. Today, the increasing complexity of coexisting medical conditions and associated therapeutic agents is restricting the anesthesiologist's ability to comply with some of the surgeon's requirements. Surgeons are finding that anesthesiologists appear less accommodating about accepting patients who are not as well prepared medically as they might be.

This reluctance should not be attributed to the assertiveness of a young specialty; the smaller margins for error in the patients we now care for should be considered. For some reason, it appears to be difficult for surgeons to grasp why setting up the monitors and completing the anesthetic induction process required for an octogenarian with serious multiple-system disease sometimes takes longer than performing the operation itself.

As patients present more and more complex anesthetic management problems, the practice of surgery will become less efficient and more costly in terms of operations completed per unit of time. This is the new reality, and to minimize its effects, every surgical specialty should make an increasing commitment to achieving the optimum medical preparation of its patients to avoid cancellations and delays of planned operations.

The elderly patient population presents another problem: how to care for the patient when surgery can offer no more. Already the careful management of acute, time-limited postoperative pain can succumb to the pressures of a busy schedule and exaggerated fears of narcotic addiction. The patient with chronic terminal pain may fare even worse. The surgeon should endeavor to enlist the aid of a pain clinic before the patient acquires the reputation of a troublesome surgical failure.

These examples of the increasing requirements for complex medical–surgical management and time for patient clinical care are occurring against the background of the tighter regulation of the permissible costs and scope of medical practice. To ensure the maintenance of minimally acceptable medical standards in the future care of our patients will require a renewed commitment to the traditionally close cooperation between the otolaryngologist and the anesthesiologist.

REFERENCES

1. American Society of Anesthesiologists: *Position on monitored anesthesia care*, Park Ridge, Ill, 1986, The Society.
2. Andersen N, Johansen SH: Incidence of catecholamine-induced arrhythmias during halothane anesthesia, *Anesthesiology* 24:51, 1963.
3. Bailey PL: Frequent hypoxemia and apnea after sedation with midazolam and fentanyl, *Anesthesiology* 73:826, 1990.
4. Bain JA, Spoerel MD: A streamlined anesthetic system, *Can Anaesth Soc J* 19:426, 1972.
5. Bier A: Versuche über Cocainisirung des Ruchenmarkes, *Dtsch Z Chir* 51:361, 1899.
6. Bier A: Uber einen neuen Weg Lokalanasthesie und den Gliedmassen zu erzeugen, *Verh Dtsch Ges Chir* 37:204, 1908.
7. Bigelow HJ: Insensibility during surgical operation produced by inhalation, *Boston Med Surg J* 35:309, 1846.
8. Braun H: Uber den Einfluss der Vitalitat der Gewebe auf die ortlichen und allgemeinen Giftwirkungen localanaesthesirender Mittel und über die Bedeutung des Adrenalins fur die Localanaesthesis, *Arch Klin Chir* 69:541, 1902.
9. Braun H: Uber einige neue ortliche Anaesthetica, *Dtsch Med Wochenschr* 31:1667, 1905.
10. Brody TM, Bain JH: Barbiturates and oxidative phosphorylation, *J Pharmacol Exp Ther* 110:148, 1954.
11. Brown ACD: *Anesthetic management*. In Norton ML, Brown ACD, editors: *Atlas of the difficult airway*, St Louis, 1991, Mosby.
12. Carron H: Control of pain in the head and neck, *Otolaryngol Clin North Am* 14:631, 1981.
13. Clements JA, Wilson KM: The affinity of narcotic agents for interfacial films, *Proc Natl Acad Sci U S A* 48:1008, 1962.
14. Coakley CS, Alpert S, Boling JS: Circulatory responses during anesthesia of patients on *Rauwolfia* therapy, *JAMA* 161:1143, 1956.
15. Cobley M, Vaughan RS: Recognition and management of difficult airway problems, *Br J Anaesth* 68:90, 1992.
16. Cohen PJ: Effects of anesthetics of mitochondrial function, *Anesthesiology* 39:153, 1973.
17. Cummings CW and others: *Atlas of laryngeal surgery*, St Louis, 1984, Mosby.
18. Davies JM, Strunin L: Anesthesia in 1984: how safe is it? *Can Med Assoc J* 131:437, 1984.
19. Department of Health and Human Resources Office of Epidemiology and Biostatistics, Center for Drug Evaluation and Research, Data Retrieval Unit HFD-737, June 27, 1989.
20. Reference deleted in pages.
21. Eger EI and others: Anesthetic potencies of sulfur hexafluoride, carbon tetrafluoride, chloroform and Ethrane in dogs, *Anesthesiology* 30:129, 1969.
22. Enderby GEH, editor: Special issue on controlled hypotension, *Br J Anaesth* 47:743, 1975.
23. Federated Ambulatory Surgery Association: Special Study I, no 520, Alexandria, Va, 1986.
24. Gelder MG, Vane JR: Interaction of the effects of tyramine, amphetamine and reserpine in man, *Psychopharmacology* 3:231, 1962.
25. Greene NM: Evaluation of perioperative risk, *Anesth Analg* 60:623, 1981.
26. Halsey MJ: *Molecular mechanisms in general anaesthesia*. In *Structure activity relationships of general anaesthetics, Glax. Symposia*, New York, 1974, Longman.
27. Hampton LJ, Little DM: Complications associated with the use of controlled hypotension in anesthesia, *Arch Surg* 67:549, 1953.
28. Informed consent: *Salgo v Leland Stanford Jr Univ Bd of trustees*, 154 Cal App 2d560, 317 P.2d170, 1957.
29. Johnstone M: The human cardiovascular response to fluothane anesthesia, *Br J Anaesth* 28:392, 1956.
30. Jones SE, Ewy GA, Grove BM: Electrocardiographic detection of adriamycin heart disease, *Proc Am Soc Clin Oncol* 16:228, 1975.
31. Keats AS: The ASA classification of physical status—a recapitulation, *Anesthesiology* 49:233, 1978.
32. Koller C: Uber die Verwendung des Cocain zur Anaesthesirung am Auge, *Wien Med Bull* 7:1352, 1884.
33. Koster H: Spinal anesthesia with special reference to its use in surgery of head and neck and thorax, *Am J Surg* 5:554, 1928.

34. Larson AG: Deliberate hypotension, *Anesthesiology* 25:682, 1964 (review).

35. Laycock JD: Signs and stages of anesthesia—a restatement, *Anaesthesia* 8:15, 1953.

36. Little DM: Classical file, *Surv Anesth* 10:514, 1966.

37. Lofgren N: *Xylocaine: a new synthetic drug.* In *Studies on local anesthetics*, Stockholm, 1948, Hoeggstroms.

38. Long CW: An account of the first use of sulphuric ether by inhalation as an anesthetic in surgical operations, *South Med Surg J* 5:705, 1849.

39. Lundgren S, Rosenquist JB: Amnesia, pain experience, and patient satisfaction with intravenous diazepam, *J Oral Maxillofac Surg* 41:99, 1983.

40. Lundgren S, Rosenquist JB: Comparison of sedation, amnesia and patient comfort produced by intravenous and rectal diazepam, *J Oral Maxillofac Surg* 42:646, 1984.

41. Martof AB: Anesthesia of the teeth, supporting structures and oral mucous membrane, *Otolaryngol Clin North Am* 14:653, 1981.

42. McAuley JE: The early development of local anesthesia, *Br Dent J* 121:139, 1966.

43. Meyer HH: Zur Theorie der Alkoholnarcose, I. Mit welche Eigenschaft der Anasthetika bedingt ihre narkotische Wiring? *Arch Exp Path Pharmak* 42:109, 1899.

44. Millar RA, Gilbert RGB, Brindle GF: Ventricular tachycardia during halothane anesthesia, *Anaesthesia* 13:164, 1958.

45. Millar SL: A theory of gaseous anesthetics, *Proc Natl Acad Sci U S A* 47:1515, 1961.

46. Norton ML, deVos P: A new endotracheal tube for laser surgery of the larynx, *Ann Otol Rhinol Laryngol* 87:554, 1978.

47. Overton E: *Studien über die Narkose Zugleich ein Beitrag zur allgemeinen Pharmakologie*, Jena, 1901, G Fischer.

48. Patterson ME, Bartlett PC: Hearing impairment caused by intratympanic pressure changes during general anesthesia, *Laryngoscope* 86:399, 1976.

49. Pauling L: A molecular theory of general anesthesia, *Science* 134:15, 1961.

50. Putnam L and others: Anesthesia in the morbidly obese patient, *South Med J* 67:1411, 1974.

51. Raventos J: The action of fluothane—a new volatile anaesthetic, *Br J Pharmacol* 11:394, 1956.

52. Ray DC, Drummond GB: Halothane hepatitis, *Br J Anaesth* 67:84, 1991 (review).

53. Riding JE: Minor complications of general anesthesia, *Br J Anaesth* 47:91, 1975.

54. Ritchie JM: Mechanism of action of local anesthetic agents and biotoxins, *Br J Anaesth* 47:191, 1975.

55. Roizen MF: *Routine preoperative evaluation.* In Miller RD, editor: *Anesthesia*, Edinburg, 1981, Churchill Livingstone.

56. Sanders RD: Two ventilating attachments for bronchoscopy, *Del Med J* 39:170, 1967.

57. Schramm VL, Mattox DE, Stool SE: Acute management of laser ignited intratracheal explosion, *Laryngoscope* 91:1417, 1981.

58. Sikic BI: Biochemical and cellular determinants of bleomycin cytotoxicity, *Cancer Surv* 5:81, 1986.

59. Simpson JY: On a new anaesthetic agent more efficient than sulphuric ether, *Lancet* II:549, 1847.

60. Smith RB: Drug interaction and drug reactions, *Otolaryngol Clin North Am* 14:615, 1981.

61. Strichartz G: Molecular mechanisms of nerve blocks by local anesthetics, *Anesthesiology* 45:421, 1976.

62. Strumin L: How long should patients fast before surgery? Time for new guidelines, *Br J Anaesth* 70:1, 1993.

63. Suckling JCW: Some chemical and physical factors in the development of fluothane, *Br J Anaesth* 29:466, 1957.

64. Tasaki I: *Nervous transmission*, Springfield, Ill, 1953, Charles C Thomas.

65. Vickers MD, Morgan M, Spencer PSJ, editors: *Drugs in anaesthetic practice*, Boston, 1991, Butterworth-Heinemann.

66. Virtue RW, Payne KW: Postoperative death after fluothane, *Anesthesiology* 19:562, 1958.

67. von Oettingen WF: The earliest suggestion of the use of cocaine for local anesthesia, *Ann M Hist* 5:275, 1933.

68. Weis S: A new emergency cricothyroidotomy instrument, *J Trauma* 23:155, 1983.

69. White CS and others: Incidence of oxygen desaturation during oral surgery outpatient procedures, *J Oral Maxillofac Surg* 47:167, 1989.

70. Willet E: The origin of the term anaesthetics, *BMJ* 2:898, 1894.

Chapter 13

Allergy and Immunology of the Upper Airway

Fuad M. Baroody
Robert M. Naclerio

The importance of the immune system in health and disease has long been recognized. Not only does the immune system distinguish self from nonself, it also mounts an inflammatory response to defend the body against foreign invaders. This chapter reviews the immune system and its various components and discusses the pathophysiology of immunoglobulin E (IgE)-mediated allergic rhinitis.

SELF AND NONSELF

The essence of specific immunity is the ability to discriminate at the molecular level between self and nonself. This ability allows the immune system to attack and destroy potentially harmful microorganisms without simultaneously destroying the person infected by these agents. This crucial function is mediated by the molecules determined by the human leukocyte antigen (HLA) complex. Initial study of the HLA system focused on the role of these antigens in determining the success of organ and tissue transplantation. The HLA complex and its homologues in other species were thus termed the *major histocompatibility complex* (MHC). In humans, the MHC occupies about 4000 KD of DNA on the short arm of chromosome 6 and contains many genes that encode molecules for various functions. Among these molecules, a group of glycoproteins belonging to the immunoglobulin supergene family are present on the cell surface and play a major role in allowing the immune system to distinguish between self and nonself. These are MHC class I molecules (HLA-A, -B, and -C) and class II molecules (HLA-DR, -DQ, and -DP).

MHC class I molecules are present on the surface of most nucleated somatic cells. They are responsible for presenting endogenous antigen to cytotoxic T cells, allowing the recognition and elimination of virus-infected cells and cells containing autoantibodies. A class I molecule and an antigenic (e.g., viral) peptide are recognized as a complex by the T-cell receptor (TCR). When cytotoxic T-lymphocyte precursors recognize the combination of a particular foreign peptide and a particular class I molecule on a sensitizing cell, they proliferate and differentiate to become mature cytotoxic T-lymphocytes (CD8$^+$). These mature lymphocytes recognize and kill only target cells that bear the same class I molecule and the same viral peptide as were present on the sensitizing cells. Cytotoxic T-lymphocyte killing is peptide-specific (lymphocytes will not lyse a target cell bearing the same class I molecule infected with a different virus) and class I restricted (lymphocytes will not lyse a cell bearing a different class I molecule infected with the same virus).

In contrast to class I molecules, MHC class II molecules are expressed primarily on immunocompetent antigen-presenting cells (APC), including macrophages, monocytes, dendritic cells, B lymphocytes, and activated T lymphocytes; they can be upregulated by interferon (IFN)-γ on a several cell types (macrophages, monocytes, endocrine and endothelial cells) in states of inflammation. Class II molecules allow binding of peptides of 10 to 25 amino acids, and the bound peptide and the class II molecule constitute the ligand for the receptor on a CD4$^+$ T lymphocyte (T-helper cell). Thus, just as class I molecules restrict the recognition of peptides by CD8$^+$ T cells, class II molecules restrict the recognition of peptides by CD4$^+$ T cells. Therefore, class II molecules are necessary for the presentation of exogenous antigen to T-helper cells.

INNATE AND ACQUIRED IMMUNITY

Innate immunity

The immune system has two functional divisions: the innate (or nonspecific) and acquired (or specific). Innate immune responses are independent of the function of B and T lymphocytes. This form of immunity is available rapidly on encounter with a pathogen, does not require immunization, and does not exhibit memory for previous encounters with the same pathogen. The components of the innate immune system include physical barriers to pathogen invasion (skin, mucous membranes, cilia, mucus) and many cellular and serum factors that can be activated by secreted or cell-surface products of the pathogen. Among these factors are activated phagocytes (including neutrophils, monocytes, and macrophages) and secreted inflammatory cytokines and chemokines, including interleukin (IL)-1, tumor necrosis factor (TNF)-α, IL-6, and arachidonic acid metabolites.[20] All of these products lead to an acute inflammatory response, which is accompanied by the production (primarily by hepatocytes) of the acute phase reactants that promote phagocytosis and killing of microorganisms by multiple mechanisms (e.g., C-reactive protein).[160]

The skin is the most effective first line of defense of the innate immune system. Most infectious organisms cannot penetrate intact skin. Mucosal surfaces of the upper airway, gut, lungs, and genitourinary tract, on the other hand, are less resistant than the skin and are thus more frequent portals for offending pathogens. The innate immune system reduces that vulnerability by the presence of various physical and biochemical factors. A good example is the enzyme lysozyme, which is distributed widely in secretions and can split the cell walls of most bacteria. Other protective substances are the mucus and cilia that cover the upper and lower airway mucosa, spermine in semen, acid in the stomach, sebaceous gland secretions, and the normal flora of the gut and the vagina. If an offending organism penetrates this first line of defense, bone marrow–derived phagocytic cells engulf and destroy it. These cells are located in fixed sites, such as liver sinusoids (Kupffer's cells), or travel through the blood (neutrophils and monocytes) and are ready to enter tissues in response to invasion by a foreign organism.

Other components of the innate system include acute phase proteins, complement, and IFN. Acute phase proteins increase in the serum in response to infection. For example, C-reactive protein binds the C protein of pneumococci, promotes binding of complement, and thus facilitates the uptake of these bacteria by phagocytes (opsonization). The complement system consists of serum proteins, which increase in concentration during infections. The components of this system interact with each other and with other components of the innate and adaptive immune systems through two pathways of activation: classical and alternative. IFNs constitute a group of proteins that are produced early during viral infections. They can be released by the virally infected cells or by activated T lymphocytes to induce a state of viral resistance in uninfected cells. They also modulate the response of lymphocytes and natural killer (NK) cells.

Acquired immunity

If the defense of the innate immune system is penetrated, the acquired immune system, controlled by lymphocytes, mounts a specific response to the pathogen in an attempt to eradicate it. The acquired system remembers prior pathogens, and thus future responses occur more rapidly. Lymphocytes are the major effector cells in acquired immunity. Although each lymphocyte recognizes antigen, the entire immune system with its many lymphocytes recognizes thousands. When an antigen penetrates the barriers of innate immunity, it binds and activates the lymphocytes with the best fitting receptors, a process called *clonal selection*. Because different antigens may have similar antigenic determinants between which lymphocytes cannot distinguish, cross-reactions between tissues can develop. Harmful side effects may ensue, such as rheumatic heart disease after streptococcal infection.

The innate and acquired immune systems act in concert to rid the body of foreign invaders. When T lymphocytes are stimulated, they stimulate the production of antibodies by B cells, which in turn help phagocytes recognize their targets. T lymphocytes also produce lymphokines, which stimulate phagocytes directly to destroy infectious agents more effectively. Macrophages, which are components of the innate immune system, help lymphocytes by presenting antigens and releasing cytokines.

DEVELOPMENT OF THE IMMUNE SYSTEM

The human immune system consists of a dispersed organ system (spleen, thymus, lymph nodes) and of cells capable of moving from the bone marrow to the blood and the lymphatic system. The pluripotent stem cells, which are derived from the yolk sac and ultimately reside in the bone marrow, are the progenitor cells from which all cells of the immune system are derived (Fig. 13-1). These pluripotent stem cells give rise to a lymphoid stem cell and a myeloid stem cell. The lymphoid stem cell differentiates into the T lymphocyte, the B lymphocyte, and the non-T, non-B large granular lymphocyte. Lymphocytes represent about 25% of leukocytes in the peripheral blood. The relative contribution of each subtype to this percentage is as follows: T lymphocytes, 80%; B lymphocytes, 10%; non-T, non-B large granular lymphocytes, 10%. The myeloid stem cell gives rise to mast cells, basophils, neutrophils, eosinophils, monocytes, macrophages, megakaryocytes, and erythrocytes. Differentiation of the myeloid stem cell occurs in the bone marrow, as does the development of B lymphocytes and non-T, non-B lymphocytes. In contrast, T-cell progenitors leave the bone mar-

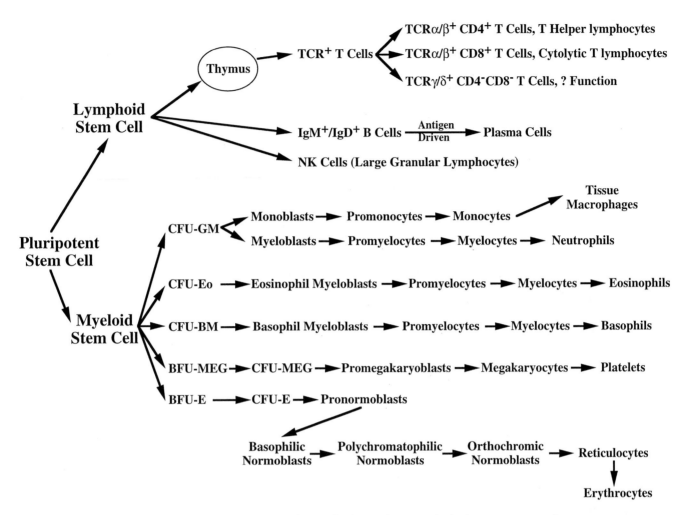

Fig. 13-1. The development of the various cells that are important in the immune response from their pluripotent stem cell origin to their final stages of maturation.

row and migrate to the thymus, where they differentiate into T lymphocytes.

Differentiation of lymphoid and myeloid stem cells is dependent on their interaction through their surface receptors with soluble ligands (cytokines) or surface ligands (cell interaction molecules). Therefore, proliferation and differentiation along one of the myeloid or lymphoid lineages are controlled (1) through the spatially and temporally regulated exposure of these stem cells to different ligands or factors and (2) through the differential expression of receptors on the stem cells. Cytokines have pleiotropic effects on the development of lymphoid and myeloid cells, affecting growth and maintenance of pluripotent stem cells and development and differentiation of specific lineages. Stromal cells within the bone marrow and thymus also regulate cell growth and differentiation by releasing cytokines, such as IL-4, IL-6, IL-7, IL-11, granulocyte-macrophage colony-stimulating factor (GM-CSF), and others.[49] They also participate in cell-cell interactions with progenitors through engagement of cell-surface molecules that provide additional regulatory stimuli

and participate in the development of the intercellular matrix (e.g., collagen, fibronectin).[49,187]

T cells

Lymphoid stem cells leave the bone marrow and reach the thymus gland via the bloodstream. At this stage of development, these cells lack surface antigens that comprise the TCR complex and mature T-cell markers (e.g., CD4, CD8) associated with specific effector functions. These progenitor cells develop into descendant cells with α and β or γ and δ genes of the TCR, resulting in immature T cells that are now TCR+. Cell-surface expression of the TCR depends on coexpression of the CD3 molecule, which with the TCR forms the TCR complex.[94] Maturation continues within the thymus under the control of specialized thymic cortical cells, either by cell-to-cell contact or by the elaboration of cytokines. Mature T cells can distinguish between self and nonself antigens presented in the context of MHC molecules. Cytokines that are important in the maturation of T lymphocytes in the thymus include IL-1, produced by thymic epithelial cells, which promotes the differentiation of T-cell precursors into CD3[42] IL-2 and IL-4 seem capable of promoting the development of $\alpha \beta$ and $\gamma \delta$ thymocytes and of antagonizing their development;[12] IL-6 acts as co-stimulator of IL-1– or IL-2–induced proliferation of CD4$^-$ CD8$^-$ thymocytes.

At the end of the maturation process, two types of cells leave the thymus and begin to circulate in the peripheral blood, lymphatic system, and tissues: TCR-α/β^+ CD4$^+$ T cells and TCR-α/β^+ CD8$^+$ T cells. Less than 10% of mature T cells leave the thymus as TCR-γ/δ^+ T cells, which are predominantly CD4$^-$ CD8$^-$ and have an unknown physiologic role. All peripheral T cells bear the TCR complex, and thus CD3 serves as a pan T-cell marker. The two major subpopulations of T cells, CD4$^+$ and CD8$^+$, were originally characterized by expression of the respective antigen and by their functional ability. Human CD4$^+$ cells provided help for antibody synthesis and were thus referred to as *T-helper cells*, and cells expressing CD8 developed into cytotoxic cells and were thus referred to as *T-suppressor cells*. More recently, these cell types have been classified according to the antigen-presenting molecule used for TCR interaction: CD4$^+$ cells recognize antigen in the context of MHC class II molecules, whereas CD8$^+$ cells recognize antigen presented by class I molecules.

B cells

B cells mature in the bone marrow and are characterized by expression of cell membrane immunoglobulin (Ig), with most expressing IgM and IgD.[8] This stage of the development process is antigen independent. Subsequent steps in the differentiation of the IgM$^+$, IgD$^+$ B cells; the activation of mature B cells into Ig-secreting B cells or long-lived memory cells; and final differentiation into plasma cells are antigen driven. Upon activation and cross-linking of surface Ig by specific antigen, B cells proliferate and differentiate to produce plasma cells that are nondividing, specialized cells that function only to secrete Ig. Switching to production of a specific Ig (isotype switching) involves rearrangement of Ig heavy-chain genes and DNA splicing and is a process that is under T-cell control. This switching mechanism involves T- and B-cell contact and secretion of IL molecules that make accessible the 5′ switch regions of the heavy-chain DNA sequence so that the γ, α, or ϵ gene can be transcribed, leading to the production of IgG, IgA, or IgE, respectively. As in T-cell development, multiple cytokines are thought to affect the maturation and differentiation of B lymphocytes. IL-1 and IL-2 promote B-cell activation and growth; IL-4 induces switching to the IgE isotype[64]; IL-13, which is closely related to IL-4, has many similar effects on B cell[141]; IL-5 enhances B-cell growth and terminal differentiation; IL-6 increases the rate of secretion of Ig by B cells; and IL-7 promotes proliferation of pre-B cells. B-cell proliferation and differentiation occurs in the germinal centers of lymph nodes.

Large granular lymphocytes

Large granular lymphocytes are the third major subtype of lymphocytes and are referred to as *natural killer (NK) cells*. These cells are usually larger than typical lymphocytes and display less nuclear material and more cytoplasm. They possess electron-dense, peroxidase-negative granules and a well-developed Golgi apparatus. These cells lack rearranged Ig or TCR genes and therefore do not express surface Ig or the TCR complex. NK cells provide nonspecific cytotoxic activity toward virally infected cells and tumor cells. They can also mediate antibody-dependent cellular cytotoxicity (ADCC) by activation through their IgG Fc receptors and the subsequent production of cytokines such as IFN-γ, which can affect the proliferation and differentiation of other cell types. Resting NK cells can be induced to proliferate and can be activated by IL-2 derived from antigen-activated T cells.[71]

Monocytes and macrophages

Monocytes and macrophages arise from colony-forming unit–granulocyte-macrophage (CFU-GM) progenitors, which differentiate into monoblasts, promonocytes, and monocytes. Mature monocytes leave the bone marrow and circulate in the bloodstream until they enter tissues, where they develop into tissue macrophages (e.g., alveolar macrophages, Kupffer's cells, microglial cells). Monocytes account for about 10% of circulating leukocytes. Several cytokines, including stem cell factor (SCF), IL-3, IL-6, IL-11, and GM-CSF, promote the development of myeloid-lineage cells from CD34$^+$ stem cells, predominantly in the early stages of differentiation. Macrophage colony-stimulating factor (MCSF) acts at the later stages of development and induces maturation of macrophages.[76]

Neutrophils

Neutrophils arise from CFU-GM progenitor cells that give rise to myeloblasts, which differentiate into promyelocytes, myelocytes, and finally, mature neutrophils. After maturation in the bone marrow, neutrophils circulate in the peripheral blood, where they account for 60% to 65% of leukocytes. As for monocytes, SCF, IL-3, IL-6, IL-11, and GM-CSF promote the growth and development of neutrophil precursors. Other cytokines that exhibit more specific effects on neutrophils include granulocyte colony-stimulating factor (G-CSF), which induces maturation of neutrophil precursors into neutrophils.[112] IL-4 also enhances neutrophil differentiation induced by G-CSF.

Eosinophils

Eosinophils are derived from colony-forming unit–eosinophil (CFU-Eo), a progenitor that differentiates into an eosinophilic myeloblast, promyelocyte, myelocyte, and finally a mature eosinophil. Eosinophils comprise 2% to 5% of circulating leukocytes. GM-CSF and IL-3 promote eosinophil growth and differentiation.[181] IL-5 maintains the viability of eosinophils through inhibition of apoptosis[161] and enhances the differentiation and functional activation of eosinophils.[106]

Basophils and mast cells

Basophils mature from a progenitor colony-forming unit–basophil mast cell (CFU-BM) into basophilic myeloblasts, promyelocytes, myelocytes, and then mature basophils. Mast cells are thought to develop from the same progenitor, but less is known about their specific stages of development. IL-3 and SCF induce the most consistent effects on human basophil and mast cell growth and differentiation. These cytokines act synergistically to induce basophil and mast cell development from CD34$^+$ progenitor cells.[88] SCF induces functional maturation of human mast cells. Nerve growth factor and GM-CSF[170] affect basophil growth, and IL-5 enhances basophil differentiation.[47]

Platelets and erythrocytes

Platelets and erythrocytes are derived from stem cell progenitors, which in turn differentiate into burst-forming units–megakaryocytes (BFU-MEG) in the case of platelets and into burst-forming units–erythroid (BFU-E) in the case of erythrocytes. BFU-MEG then differentiate into CFU-MEG, promegakaryoblasts, megakaryocytes, and platelets. IL-1, IL-3, GM-CSF, IL-6, and IL-11 affect the growth and differentiation of platelets.[123,159,164] The erythrocyte precursor BFU-E differentiates into colony-forming unit–erythroid (CFU-E), pronormoblasts, basophilic normoblasts, polychromatophilic normoblasts, orthochromic normoblasts, reticulocytes, and erythrocytes. Cytokines important in the various stages of erythrocyte differentiation and development include GM-CSF, SCF, IL-9, and erythropoeitin.[58]

LYMPHOID ORGANS

The primary lymphoid organs, sites where lymphocytes differentiate and mature from stem cells into effector cells, include the thymus and bone marrow. The secondary lymphoid organs are sites where mature lymphocytes reside and immune responses are generated. These organs are divided into the systemic immune system, which includes the spleen and lymph nodes, and the mucosal immune system, which includes the tonsils, Peyer's patches, scattered lymphoid follicles, intraepithelial lymphocytes, and the lamina propria of mucosal tissues. The spleen protects the body from antigens in the bloodstream, whereas lymph nodes respond to antigens delivered through lymphatics draining the skin and deeper tissues. The secondary lymphoid organs, specifically lymph nodes and the mucosal immune system, are of particular interest to otolaryngologists because they are located in the head and neck.

Lymph nodes

Lymph nodes occur as chains or groups. They are oval structures with a hilus—where blood vessels enter and leave the node—and a surrounding fibrous capsule. After entering the node, blood vessels and nerves branch within the fibrous trabeculae that traverse the node to its various parts. Beneath the lymph node capsule, a sinus receives afferent lymphatic vessels from the structures that drain into the lymph nodes. These vessels carry antigen-processing cells and foreign antigens that are subsequently transported into the substance of the lymph node.

Lymph nodes are divided into two major regions, the cortex and the medulla. The cortex contains numerous primary and secondary lymphoid follicles in which B cells predominate. Primary follicles, consisting of a mantle zone without germinal centers, contain resting B cells expressing surface IgM or IgD and CD23. In addition to an outer mantle zone, secondary follicles contain inner germinal centers, which form in response to antigen stimulation. Immunoglobulin class switch, affinity maturation through somatic mutation, and development of memory B cells occur within germinal centers. CD4$^+$ T cells are also found in these centers and play a key role in the above-mentioned B-cell responses through interactions between CD40 (expressed on the B cell) and the ligand for CD40 (CD, present on activated CD4$^+$ cells). The paracortical region of the lymph node cortex surrounds the lymphoid follicles and contains mostly T cells (both CD4$^+$ and CD8$^+$) and some macrophages, dendritic cells, and B cells (accessory cells). The accessory cells present peptide antigens in association with MHC molecules to the TCR on T cells, resulting in their activation. The medulla, the region at the center of the lymph node, is divided into medullary cords surrounded by medullary sinuses that drain into the hilus. Medullary cords contain B cells, T cells, macrophages, and many plasma cells. These cells are joined by B and T cells that migrate from the cortex to the medulla. Efferent lymphatic vessels leave the hilus carrying antibodies and mature B and T cells that migrate to other tissues and act as memory cells during subsequent immune exposure. The lymphatic system eventually drains into the thoracic duct and into the circulation, therefore allowing lymphocytes to circulate throughout the body.

Mucosal immune system

Mucosal surfaces and skin encounter the environment and possess an immune system capable of responding to pathogens and foreign antigens. The mucosal immune system is composed of the organized mucosal immune system (including tonsils, Peyer's patches, and isolated lymphoid follicles) and the diffuse mucosal immune system (including intraepithelial lymphocytes and lamina propria).

Tonsils

Three lymphoid structures surround the entrance to the throat: the adenoids, the palatine tonsils, and the lingual tonsils. These structures reach full development in childhood and begin to involute around puberty. The palatine tonsils are surrounded by a poorly organized capsule, except at the pharyngeal surface, which is covered with stratified squamous epithelium. Trabeculae extend from the capsule and divide the tonsils into lobules. Blood vessels and nerves enter through the capsule and extend within the trabeculae. The tonsillar surface is covered by pits, which open into crypts that branch down within the tissue of the tonsil, maximizing the surface area exposed to the pharynx. Each lobule contains numerous lymphoid follicles with germinal centers that contain predominantly B cells,[63] whereas the lymphoid tissue that surrounds the follicles contains T cells, macrophages, dendritic cells, and some B cells. These structures are strategically located at sites of entry of airborne particles through the nose (adenoids) and mouth (tonsils) and at sites of food particle entry (tonsils); the structures filter unwanted organisms and antigens and function as a mucosal immune barrier.

Peyer's patches and lymphoid follicles

Peyer's patches are aggregates of lymphoid follicles within the mucosa of the jejunum and ileum, with the most in the terminal ileum. The full development of this component of the mucosal immune system, including the formation of follicles containing germinal centers, occurs several weeks after birth, and their number increases until puberty and then decreases. Lymphoid follicles, another component of the mucosal immune system with structures similar to follicles of a Peyer's patch, are scattered throughout the gastrointestinal, respiratory, and genitourinary tract mucosa. These lymphoid organs facilitate antigen presentation from the intestinal lumen to T and B cells. Unlike the epithelium of the gastrointestinal tract, the epithelium overlying Peyer's patches and isolated lymphoid follicles lacks villi and contains very few goblet cells. Antigen uptake occurs in this epithelium through specialized epithelial cells (M cells) through pinocytosis. The epithelium also expresses MHC class II antigens (with the exception of M cells) but not the immunoglobulin receptor required for secretion of IgA. The subepithelial region contains many T cells (including CD4+ cells); beneath this region is the dome, which contains many T cells, macrophages, dendritic cells, and some B cells. Antigens, pinocytosed by M cells, are transported to the dome region, where they are presented to T cells by macrophages and dendritic cells. Follicles lie beneath the dome region and contain mantle zones with predominantly resting B cells, most of which express IgM and IgD on their surface. Most Peyer's patch follicles have germinal centers containing activated B cells, dendritic cells, CD4+ T cells, and macrophages. An interfollicular region contains many CD4+ and CD8+ T cells, dendritic cells, macrophages, and some B cells.

Intraepithelial lymphocytes

Intraepithelial lymphocytes are found at the basal surface of the epithelium and are interdigitated with epithelial cells. Initially, they were considered to be lamina propria cells that invaded the epithelial layer. However, it is now clear that they are phenotypically and probably functionally distinct from lamina propria T cells. Most are T cells (CD8+ or CD4− CD8−), and although most express the TCR-α/β, some express the TCR-γ/δ, further setting them apart from other lymphoid sites. The function of intraepithelial lymphocytes is not well understood, but studies have shown their capacity to generate cytotoxic activity.[68,101]

Lamina propria

The lamina propria, located beneath the epithelium, is a loosely structured tissue populated by various groups of cells. One of the key functions of this tissue is the secretion of IgA antibody from the many IgA plasma cells.[81] IgA is transported from the lamina propria to the epithelium and is then secreted into the lumen. The lamina propria also contains many CD4+ and CD8+ T lymphocytes in a ratio of about 2:1. In contrast to intraepithelial lymphocytes, most lamina propria T cells express the TCR-α/β. Other effector cells of the lamina propria include IgG B cells, macrophages, dendritic cells, eosinophils, mast cells, and a few neutrophils.

ANTIGEN PRESENTATION

Antigen presentation is carried out by specialized cells referred to as antigen-presenting cells (APC), which include a diverse group of leukocytes, such as monocytes, macrophages, dendritic cells, and B cells. These cells are found primarily in the solid lymphoid organs and the skin. Follicular dendritic cells are specialized APC in the B-cell areas of lymph nodes and the spleen and are important in the generation and maintenance of memory B cells by trapping antigen-antibody complexes. Peripheral tissue dendritic cells engulf and process antigen and then leave the tissues and home to T-cell areas in draining lymph nodes or the spleen. The predominant APC of the skin are Langerhans' cells, which are found in the epidermis and deliver antigens entering the skin to the effector cells of the lymph nodes. In the lymph nodes, these APC can directly present processed antigens to resting T cells to induce their proliferation and differentiation. Monocytes-macrophages exist as monocytes in blood and as macrophages (a more differentiated form) in various tissues, such as the lungs, liver, and brain. In addition to phagocytic and cytotoxic functions, these cells have receptors for various cytokines (IL-4, IFN-γ), which can regulate their function. Activated macrophages are also a major source of several cytokines (IFN, IL-1, TNF), complement proteins, and prostaglandins.[145] All APC have MHC class II surface molecules.

Foreign or self proteins undergo hydrolytic cleavage within the APC and become oligopeptides, which are then loaded onto antigen-binding grooves of MHC molecules before expression at the cell surface (Fig. 13-2). Class I molecules usually bind peptides that are 8 to 10 amino acids long and are derived from proteins synthesized intracellularly (e.g., tumor antigens, viruses), whereas class II molecules bind peptides that are 14 to 22 amino acids long and are

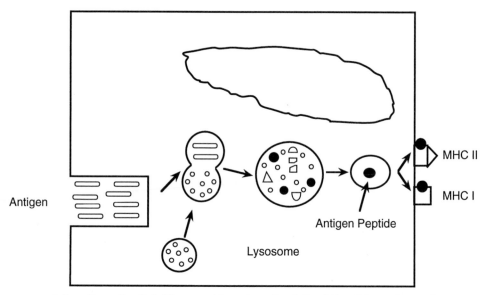

Antigen-Presenting Cell: (Monocyte, Macrophage, B cell, Dendritic cell, Langerhans cell)

Fig. 13-2. Antigen processing and presentation. Antigen undergoes hydrolytic cleavage within antigen-presenting cells, and the resultant oligopeptides are loaded on antigen-binding grooves of major histocompatibility complex molecules and expressed at the cell surface.

derived from proteins synthesized extracellularly (e.g., non-replicating vaccines, extracellular bacteria).

In addition to the mechanism of presentation of oligopeptide antigens to lymphocytes via MHC molecules, T cells can recognize haptens, which are covalently or noncovalently complexed with peptides residing in the MHC-binding groove. Another exception is the presentation of superantigens, which are about 30 kD proteins produced by a broad spectrum of microbes ranging from retroviruses to bacteria. These antigens do not undergo processing to oligopeptides but bind intact to class II MHC molecules and the TCR outside the antigen-binding grooves. They can activate more T cells than conventional peptide antigens can.

CELL-MEDIATED IMMUNE RESPONSES

Initial lymphocyte activation is a two-step event; the first activation signal is provided by antigen. As mentioned, the antigens that stimulate T cells are limited to oligopeptides (or haptens attached to peptides) that reside within the antigen-binding groove of a self MHC molecule. TCRs do not bind antigen in solution. B cells, on the other hand, can be stimulated by antigens in solution or fixed to a solid matrix. The second signal necessary for T-cell activation is provided by accessory molecules expressed on the surface of the APC for stimulation of T cells or on the surface of a T-helper cell for activation of B lymphocytes. The growth and differentiation of T cells and B cells also require stimulation with one or more cytokines, which are secreted by activated T cells and APC.

T lymphocytes expressing the TCR-α/β are divided into two major subpopulations based on the class of the MHC

molecule that their TCR recognizes. T cells expressing CD4, or T helper (TH) cells, recognize antigen bound to class II MHC molecules, whereas T cells expressing CD8, or T-suppressor cells, recognize antigen bound to MHC class I molecules. CD8$^+$ T cells are commonly cytotoxic T-lymphocytes (CTL) and are important effectors of the cell-mediated immune response. The ratio of CD4 to CD8 cells in peripheral blood is usually 2:1, but may vary considerably.

CD4$^+$ T cells

After recognizing antigens presented by MHC class II molecules, CD4$^+$ cells become activated to secrete IL-2, partly in response to monocyte-derived IL-1 and partly in response to autocrine stimulation by IL-2 as part of a positive feedback loop (Fig. 13-3). Activated CD4$^+$ cells interact with other CD4$^+$ or CD8$^+$ cells by secreting IL-2 and with B cells by secreting B-cell growth and differentiation factors (IL-2, IL-4, IL-6). Thus, CD4$^+$ cells augment immune responses by stimulating B cells sensitized by antigen and by stimulating CD8$^+$ cells sensitized by binding of antigen in the context of MHC class I molecules. The activities of these CD4$^+$ cells are thus largely mediated via the secretion of cytokines, which are small protein hormones that control the growth and differentiation of cells in the microenvironment. The pattern of cytokine secretion of TH cells allows further subdivision into TH-1 and TH-2 cells.[118] TH-1 cells elaborate inflammatory cytokines involved in effector functions of cell-mediated immunity, such as IL-2 and IFN-γ, whereas TH-2 cells elaborate cytokines such as IL-4 and IL-13, which control and regulate antibody responses. Some CD4$^+$ cells, capable of secreting both TH1 and TH2 cytokines, are desig-

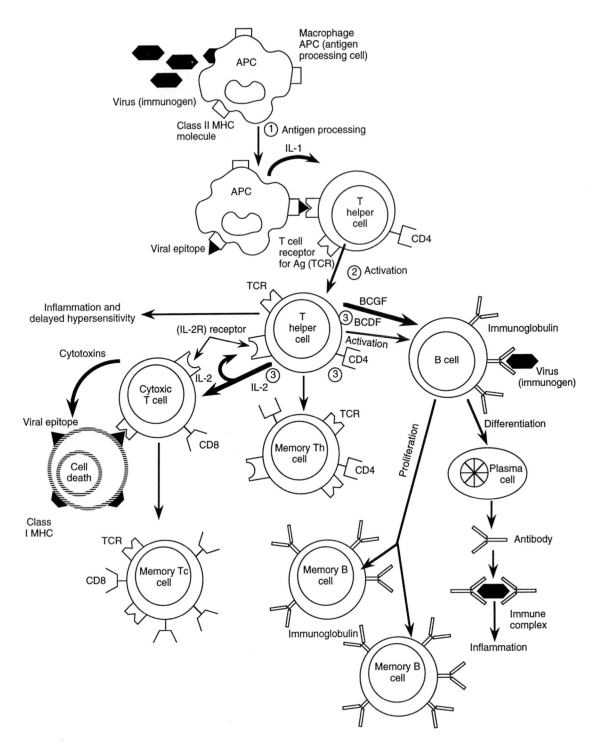

Fig. 13-3. Summary of the cell-mediated immune response showing the events that follow exposure to an immunogen and the role of the T-helper cell in orchestrating these events. (From Stites DP, Terr AI, editors: *Basic and clinical immunology*, ed 7, Norwalk, Conn, 1991, Appleton & Lange.)

nated TH-0 cells and may be the precursors of fully differentiated TH-1 and TH-2 cells. Differentiation into TH-1 versus TH-2 cells is regulated by positive feedback loops promoted primarily by IL-12 and IL-4, respectively.[154] In addition to their central role in initiating and regulating immune re-

sponses, CD4+ T lymphocytes are important effectors of cell-mediated immunity by virtue of the cytokines that they elaborate. These cytokines, particularly IFN-γ, are essential contributors to the generation of chronic inflammatory responses characterized by mononuclear cellular infiltration and activated macrophages. Furthermore, CD4$^+$ cells can contribute to the cellular immune response by functioning as cytotoxic effectors, directly as CTL or by secreting cytotoxic cytokines such as TNF-β.

In addition to orchestrating the immune response by secreting various cytokines and contributing to T-lymphocyte cytotoxic activities, the characteristic inflammatory reaction induced by CD4$^+$ T lymphocytes is delayed-type hypersensitivity (DTH). DTH is elicited by challenge with antigen in immune, sensitized persons. The typical example is the cutaneous reaction to challenge with the purified protein derivative (PPD) of *Mycobacterium tuberculosis* in previously infected, or vaccinated, persons. Clinically, DTH is manifested by local erythema and induration 24 to 48 hours after challenge. Microscopically, the lesion shows perivascular accumulations of leukocytes (initially neutrophils, later lymphocytes and activated macrophages), edema, and fibrin deposition. Chronic DTH reactions result in the formation of granulomas (nodular collections of macrophages and lymphocytes) and possibly fibrosis as a result of the cytokines produced by macrophages, which stimulate fibroblast proliferation and collagen synthesis. DTH involves reactions by various immune system components. A sensitized person has activated and memory T lymphocytes specific for the immunizing antigen. A subsequent antigen challenge induces local inflammation and the release of cytokines that stimulate the expression of intercellular adhesion molecule (ICAM)-1 and vascular cell adhesion molecule (VCAM)-1 on vascular endothelium. These molecules bind activated and memory T lymphocytes, which express a high level of ligands that interact with ICAM-1 (lymphocyte function antigen ([LFA-1]) and VCAM-1 (very late antigen [VLA-4]). These interactions lead to tissue accumulation of T lymphocytes, which are presented with the antigen by APC in the context of MHC molecules (in the case of a PPD-DTH reaction, the T lymphocytes are CD4$^+$ and the MHC molecules are class II). Recognition of antigen by the T lymphocytes leads to an increase in the affinity of T-cell LFA-1 and VLA-4 for their specific ligands. For example, VLA-4 binds to fibronectin in the extracellular matrix and therefore promotes the retention of antigen-stimulated T cells in the extravascular tissue. Activated T cells also secrete cytokines. The most important cytokines in DTH are IFN-γ (a potent activator of macrophages) and TNF, which increases the expression of leukocyte adhesion molecules on endothelium and initiates recruitment of leukocytes (neutrophils and monocytes) to the site. IL-2 is also secreted by activated T cells and stimulates the proliferation of T cells. As mentioned, these cytokines are produced by the T helper-1 cells. The recruited inflammatory leukocytes and the resident activated tissue macrophages then phagocytose the antigen and secrete various substances with microbicidal activity (reactive oxygen intermediates, lysosomal enzymes), which also contribute to tissue injury. DTH is seen in various clinical situations, such as in the skin lesions of contact sensitivity to chemicals,

in infections with certain microbes (*M. tuberculosis*), in some fungal and parasitic infections,[87] and in certain autoimmune diseases.[37,186]

Another type of inflammation that occurs in some T-cell–mediated immune responses is characterized by the accumulation of eosinophils and is caused by the activation of T helper-2 cells. These secrete IL-4 and IL-5, which promote the recruitment and survival of eosinophils in tissue sites of inflammation. Allergic reactions are a good example of this process; the pathophysiology of allergic rhinitis is discussed later in this chapter.

CD8$^+$ T cells and cytotoxicity

The best understood function of CD8$^+$ cells is that of cytotoxic effectors. Their function as suppressors of the immune response is more controversial, and the mechanism of this activity is not very well understood and, in some instances, is thought to be mediated by the production of nonspecific inhibitory cytokines. Although CD4$^+$ and CD8$^+$ lymphocytes can act as cytotoxic effectors, the CD8$^+$ population has a higher frequency of cytotoxic effectors than does the CD4$^+$ population.

The initial event in the destruction of target cells by cytotoxic effectors involves contact with the target cell membrane components. When the cytotoxic effector is a CD8$^+$ cell (as is most often the case), the foreign peptide is recognized by a class I MHC molecule on the target cell. Transmembrane signaling then occurs; the adhesion between the two cells is strengthened, and conjugation takes place. This nonspecific adhesion between the two cells is achieved by the binding of LFA-1 on the cytotoxic effectors to ICAM-1 on the target cells, when available, and CD2 on the cytotoxic effectors to LFA-3 on the target cells. A lethal hit is then delivered by the cytotoxic effector to the target cell by exocytosis of cytotoxic effectors granules into the junctional region between effector and target. These granules contain perforins, which are proteins that create pores within the target cell membrane, making it permeable. Granzymes and other proteases and granule mediators released from the cytotoxic effector can then enter the target cell and effect internal disintegration. After delivering a lethal hit to a target cell, the cytotoxic effector still contains additional granules and can immediately recycle to engage and lyse additional target cells. Because of an unidentified property of their plasma membranes, cytotoxic effectors are resistant to lysis by their own exocytosed granules.

Another pathway for cytotoxic cell function involves the cell-surface molecule Fas, which is a member of the TNF receptor–nerve growth factor receptor–CD40 superfamily and mediates apoptosis.[82] Binding of the cell-surface Fas molecule on a target cell to the Fas ligand on the cytotoxic effector leads to apoptosis of the target cell. Fas-mediated cytotoxicity is thought to play a role in the negative selection process in T-cell development; however, the role of this pathway for cytolysis in various infectious diseases has not been defined. Another mechanism for the induction of cytotoxicity, which is thought to play a key role in many inflammatory processes, involves the secretion of cytolytic cytokines by cytotoxic effectors (e.g., TNF).

CTL exert cell contact–dependent cytotoxic functions through the mechanisms mentioned. The perforin-dependent pathway of cytotoxicity is largely responsible for cell-mediated clearance of infectious viruses (e.g., cytomegalovirus, Epstein-Barr virus, hepatitis B and C, human immunodeficiency virus–1, influenza A and B, measles, mumps, respiratory syncytial virus, rubella, vaccinia,) and certain intracellular bacterial infections and for the rejection of allogenic tissue grafts and tumors. The Fas antigen/ligand pathway of cytotoxicity appears to be important in the elimination of T cells during differentiation and tolerance induction.

Natural killer cell cytotoxicity

The ability of $CD4^+$ and $CD8^+$ T cells to recognize only peptides presented by self MHC molecules is termed *MHC restriction*, and cytolytic activity mediated by these cells is known as *MHC-restricted cytotoxicity*. In contrast to these two cell types, NK cells (large granular lymphocytes), are capable of cytotoxic activity that is not restricted to recognition of target cells that display MHC molecules; this process is termed *unrestricted toxicity*.

NK cells are distinct from T cells or B cells and can manufacture and release various cytokines, including IFN-γ, TNF-α, and GM-CSF. These cells express a unique pattern of surface molecules not usually expressed on other lymphocytes, including CD16 (FcγRIII), a receptor for the Fc portion of immunoglobulin, and CD56, an adhesion molecule that is also expressed on neural cells.[98,121,136,168] In addition, they express CD2, which is also expressed on T cells.[121] These cells are present in the peripheral circulation and in the spleen, lungs, and liver.[31,180] They are not found in lymph nodes and do not recirculate through the thoracic duct lymph. The cytotoxic mechanisms of NK cells appear to be similar to those of CTL, including perforin-mediated destruction of cells, receptor-induced apoptosis, and release of cytokines such as TNF-β. The structures that are recognized by NK cells and that lead to NK cell activation have not been well defined, but a clear specificity to target recognition exists. At least a part of this specificity is the result of an inhibitory effect of MHC class I molecules, such that natural killing is inhibited when target cells express class I MHC antigens.[86,161]

NK cells can lyse susceptible tumor cells *in vivo* and *in vitro*. When tumor cells are injected into NK cell–depleted animals, tumor growth and spread are facilitated.[153] Such studies support a role for NK cells in host defense against malignancy, particularly against tumor metastasis. There is good evidence that NK cells play a role in host defense against viruses, particularly herpesvirus infections.[184] NK cells also have a role in host defense against intracellular bacterial pathogens, such as *Listeria monocytogenes*, which activates macrophages to produce TNF-α and IL-12, both of which lead to IFN-γ production by NK cells, an important response in host defense.[9] A similar sequence of events occurs after infection with certain intracellular parasites and is also important in host defense. Another important function of NK cells is the regulation of other lymphocytes. Because NK cells produce IFN-γ, they may help govern the path of TH cell activation, leading to the preferential proliferation of TH-1 cells, which predominantly produce IL-2 and IFN-γ.

HUMORAL IMMUNE RESPONSE

T-cell dependent and T-cell independent B-cell responses

Humoral immunity consists of responses that are T-cell dependent (TD) and T-cell independent. T-cell independent B-cell responses occur with large antigens that have repeating antigenic determinants, such as carbohydrates, which constitute the capsule and cell wall components of bacteria. This T-cell response represents a major protective role against bacterial pathogens such as *Streptococcus pneumoniae*. These pathogens bridge immunoglobulins on the B-cell surface, causing activation and the subsequent secretion of antibodies, primarily of the IgM class. Antibodies to *S. pneumoniae* mediate the opsonization of bacteria by binding to the bacterial cell surface, thereby targeting them for destruction by Fc receptor–bearing macrophages. Young children and the elderly, who generally respond poorly to T-cell independent antigens, are at increased risk for these bacterial infections. Protective immunity against *Haemophilus influenzae* and meningococcal infections is also mediated by T-cell independent B-cell responses.

The sequence of events in TD B-cell responses starts by the processing of antigen by B cells, which, as mentioned, are capable of antigen processing and presentation. Membrane IgM and membrane IgD are capable of capturing antigen and mediating presentation. A special advantage of B-cell antigen presentation is that very low concentrations of antigen can be captured by membrane immunoglobulins bearing the appropriate specificity and targeted within the cell for presentation to TH cells.[99] The membrane Ig move antigen into the B cell; their primary function on resting B cells seems to be capturing antigen and mediating its presentation. This finding is supported by the observation that targeting of antigen to membrane Ig is more effective than targeting of antigen to other cell-surface proteins, such as MHC class I molecules.[169]

In the B cell, antigen is proteolytically degraded and associated with class II MHC molecules on the cell surface. This activity is followed by the formation of conjugates between the antigen-presenting B cells and antigen-specific T cells. Stabilization of these conjugates is facilitated by the interaction of antigen presented by the B cell with the TCR, CD4 molecules on T cells and the class II MHC molecules on B cells and by the interaction between LFA-1 on T cells and ICAM-1 on B cells. Once activated by the antigen-presenting B cells, TH cells express gp39,[125] the ligand for CD40, a membrane protein expressed on all mature B cells and a potent mitogenic receptor for B cells. This membrane protein is transiently expressed on activated TH cells and, on binding to CD40, triggers B cells to enter the cell cycle. Antimurine gp39 inhibits primary and secondary humoral immune responses *in vivo*,[60] supporting the essential role of this membrane protein in humoral immunity. An additional interaction between B and T cells occurs next, namely, the cross-linking of CD28, a costimulatory molecule on the T-helper cell surface, to its counterreceptor on the B cell, B7/BB1 (CD80). This interaction results in enhanced T-cell proliferation and lymphokine production.[104]

Multiple lymphokines are therefore produced by TH cells and encounter B cells that have been rendered responsive to the growth and differentiating effects of these lymphokines via the actions of CD40. Among these cytokines, IL-4 and IL-10 are important growth factors, especially for CD40-triggered B cells. IL-4 also mediates the production of IgE and IgG4 from CD40-activated B cells,[83] and IL-10 is an important factor regulating the production of IgG and IgA.[44] TGF-β induces the switching of B cells to IgA production, and multiple other cytokines (IL-1, IL-2, IL-3, IL-6, IFN-γ, TNF-α) have modulating roles in the magnitude of B-cell responses.[43]

Antibody-dependent cellular cytotoxicity

Antibody-dependent cellular cytotoxicity (ADCC) can lead to the destruction of invading foreign organisms (bacteria, helminths), virus-infected cells, or tumor cells. In the process of destruction of invading organisms, ADCC involves the targeting of effector cells to these organisms by antibodies. The antibody's variable regions provide specificity for the organism, whereas the antibody's constant region focuses effector cells to the site via various Fc receptors. In ADCC directed against altered self cells, the process involves the reaction of antibodies with cell-surface receptors producing antibody-coated target cells for reaction with NK cells that secondarily destroy these altered self cells. The process occurs via binding of the antibody to FcγRIII receptor (CD16) on NK cells.

An example of such an antibody-mediated cytotoxic reaction is the accumulating *in vitro* evidence of involvement of IgE ADCC in host defense against helminths. Macrophages, eosinophils, and platelets have been implicated in this process. A finding that supports this mechanism is that macrophages and platelets can mediate damage to schistosomula only when IgE antibodies are present, and depletion of IgE from immune sera inhibits the killing reaction of these cells.[173] Eosinophils may contribute to this cytotoxic reaction, probably by virtue of their recently discovered low-affinity IgE receptor, FcγRII. When eosinophils interact via this receptor with large, antibody-coated surfaces that do not

undergo phagocytosis (e.g., worms), they release the contents of their granules onto these surfaces. Antigen-specific IgA antibodies can also opsonize antigen-bearing particles and facilitate ADCC reactions, via their FcαR receptor, leading to activation and mediator release by phagocytes.[69]

Immunoglobulins

The antibodies (immunoglobulins) secreted by activated B cells are glycoproteins composed of polypeptide (82% to 96%) and carbohydrate (4% to 18%). They account for approximately 20% of the total plasma proteins and, on serum electrophoresis, migrate to the γ-globulin and β-globulin zones. Immunoglobulin molecules consist of four polypeptide chains divided into two light (L) and two heavy (H) chains linked by disulfide bonds (Fig. 13-4). Each polypeptide chain consists of domains formed between intrachain disulfide bonds. The amino (N)-terminal domain (the variable region, V) of each chain shows greater variation in amino acid sequence than the carboxy (C)-terminal end (the constant region, C). The N-terminal of these chains is referred to as the *Fab,* or *antigen-binding, fragment.* The antigen-binding site of the antibody molecule represents few amino acids in the V regions of the H and L chains. The C-terminal end of immunoglobulin molecules consists only of H chains and is referred to as the *Fc fragment.* This fragment is responsible for conferring biologic activity to immunoglobulins, such as placental transfer, complement fixation, and cell binding.

The isotype of a heavy or light chain is defined by the constant region antigenic determinants that are defined by the particular constant region gene of that isotype. All isotypes are present in a healthy person. Because there are nine known separate heavy-chain, constant region genes, there are nine heavy-chain isotypes that define the class and subclass of the antibody molecule. These are designated γ1, γ2, γ3, γ4, μ, α1, α2, δ, and ϵ, and the corresponding immunoglobulin isotypes (class or subclass) are IgG1, IgG2, IgG3, IgG4, IgM, IgA1, IgA2, IgD, and IgE. Light-chain isotypes are known as types (κ and λ) and subtypes. Monomers consist of a single immunoglobulin molecule (e.g., IgG), whereas polymers have multiple basic units (e.g., IgM has five basic units, dimeric IgA has two units). The polymerization of these immunoglobulins is facilitated by the presence of a small glycopeptide with an unusually high content of aspartic acid, known as the J chain.

Immunoglobulin G

IgG constitutes approximately 75% of the total serum immunoglobulins and consists of four subclasses (IgG1, IgG2, IgG3, IgG4). It is a monomer with a molecular weight of 150,000 D. IgG1, IgG3, and to a lesser extent, IgG2 can bind and fix complement. Specific Fc receptors for IgG are present on monocytes, macrophages, and neutrophils, and IgG is usually bound to the Fc receptor before binding with antigen. Because of these interactions with antigen and phag-

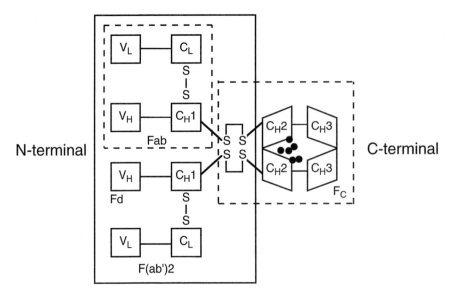

Fig. 13-4. Immunoglobulin structure. Human Immunoglobulin G1 is a representative example of immunoglobulin structure. H—heavy chains, L—light chains, V—variable regions, C—constant regions. *Dark circles* represent carbohydrate residues between the C_H^2 domains. (From Wright A, Shin SU, Morrison SL: *Crit Rev Immunol* 12:125, 1992, Copyright CRC Press).

ocytic cells, IgG functions as an opsonin that facilitates phagocytosis. The Fc receptors for IgG include $Fc\gamma RI$ on monocytes and macrophages, $Fc\gamma RII$ on most hematopoeitic cells except erythrocytes, and $Fc\gamma RIII$ on NK cells, eosinophils, neutrophils, and macrophages. Interaction of IgG with NK cells can generate ADCC, which is one mechanism of lymphocyte-mediated killing of bacteria, virus-infected cells, and tumor cells. In general, the IgG antibody response to soluble protein antigens involves the IgG1 and IgG3 subclasses, whereas polysaccharide antigens elicit primarily IgG2 antibodies. IgG is the immunoglobulin primarily involved in secondary or recall immune responses and is the only immunoglobulin that can cross the placenta and protect the neonate. IgG can fix complement, leading to neutralization, opsonization, bacteriolysis, agglutination, and hemolysis.

Immunoglobulin M

IgM constitutes approximately 10% of serum immunoglobulins. IgM normally exists as a pentamer of five IgM subunits linked by disulfide bonds and J chains with a molecular weight of 900,000 D. It is the major immunoglobulin (along with IgD) expressed on the surface of B cells. Membrane IgM functions as the earliest antigen receptor on B cells. Antigen binding results in B-cell activation and differentiation, leading to pentameric IgM secretion. Because pentameric IgM contains 10 antibody-binding sites, binding avidity is greatly enhanced. IgM predominates in the early humoral response, and levels then decline rapidly and are replaced by IgG of the same specificity. IgM is the most efficient complement fixing antibody, which, similar to IgG, increases its array of biologic activities.

Immunoglobulin A

IgA constitutes 15% of the total serum immunoglobulins and exists in both monomeric and polymeric forms (the IgA dimer is a single J chain joined to two IgA monomeric subunits). Each immunoglobulin molecule has a molecular weight of 160,000 D. Humans produce more IgA than any other immunoglobulin class, and the major role of this immunoglobulin is mucosal immunity. Monomeric IgA is synthesized by plasma cells located in the interstitial space of exocrine glands. These monomers combine with the J chain, which is also synthesized by IgA plasma cells, to form IgA2-J dimers. These dimers are too large to cross the tight junctions of the exocrine gland epithelium. They are therefore transported across the epithelium by an active secretory component–dependent mechanism.[95] The secretory component is synthesized by epithelial cells and is located at the basolateral surface of epithelial cells, which are exposed to locally produced IgA dimers. The secretory component specifically binds to the J chain of IgA dimers, and the resultant, noncovalently associated secretory component–IgA dimer complex is endocytosed into intracellular vesicles and transported across epithelial cells to the apical plasma membrane. During transport, IgA dimer covalently links to the secretory component by a disulfide bond, and the newly formed complex of IgA dimer and secretory component is referred to as *secretory IgA*. Finally, secretory IgA cleaves from the membrane-anchoring domain of the membrane secretory component and is subsequently released into exocrine secretions by exocytosis. Secretory IgA appears to be derived from locally produced IgA, not intravascular IgA.[45] IgA is the predominant immunoglobulin in external secretions; because of its abundance in saliva, tears, bronchial secretions, nasal mucosa, prostatic fluid, vaginal secretions, and small intestinal mucous secretions, IgA provides the primary defense mechanism against local mucosal infections. The main function of IgA is to neutralize foreign substances and prevent their systemic access.

Immunoglobulin E

IgE comprises only 0.004% of the total serum immunoglobulins and normally exists as a monomer with a molecular weight of 200,000 D. IgE-specific Fc receptors exist on mast cells and basophils, neutrophils, eosinophils, macrophages, and platelets. Cross-bridging of IgE molecules on the surface of mast cells and basophils by antigen triggers mediator release from mast cells and basophils. These mediators, the most notable being histamine, are responsible for allergic reactions. In addition to mediating immediate hypersensitivity reactions, IgE can mediate antibody-mediated cellular cytotoxicity.

Immunoglobulin D

IgD constitutes 0.2% of the total serum immunoglobulins and exists as a monomer with a molecular weight of 180,000 D. The primary function of IgD appears to be that of a membrane-bound antigen receptor on the B-cell surface.

THE COMPLEMENT SYSTEM

The complement system consists of approximately 20 plasma proteins that are sequentially activated and can interact with each other, with antibodies, and with cell membranes. These interactions mediate functions such as immune adherence, phagocytosis, chemotaxis, and cytolysis. Complement system proteins comprise about 15% of the globulin fraction of plasma and circulate as inactive molecules. Complement activation centers around cleavage of C3, which can be achieved by classical or alternative pathways (Fig. 13-5).

The classical pathway comprises C1, C4, and C2. C1, in turn, consists of C1q, C1r, and C1s. Antigen-antibody complexes (containing IgG1, IgG2, IgG3, or IgM) activate C1 into C1′, which cleaves C2 and C4 with the subsequent formation of C4b,2. The C4b,2 complex then cleaves C3 into C3a and C3b. From this point on, the classical and alternative pathways merge.

The alternative pathway can be activated in the absence of specific antigen-antibody complexes, thus providing host protection before the initiation of a humoral immune response. Insulin, zymosan, bacterial polysaccharides, IgG4, IgA, IgE, and aggregated immunoglobulins can activate this pathway. The proteins in this pathway consist of properdin, C3, and factors B and D. C3b, which is generated continu-

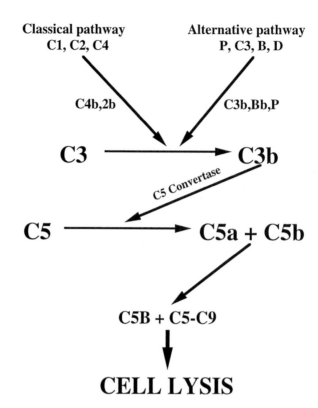

Fig. 13-5. Complement system. Classical and alternative pathways produce C3b, which in turn continues the complement cascade that ultimately results in cell lysis. (From Baroody FM, Naclerio RM: An overview of immunology, *Otolaryngol Clin North Am* 26:571, 1993.)

ously in small amounts, reacts with factors B and D to generate C3bBb, the alternative pathway C3 convertase which cleaves C3 into C3a and C3b. The newly generated C3b enters into a positive feedback loop to combine with factors B and D, forming more C3bBb. Properdin stabilizes the C3 convertase, forming C3bBbP.

After cleavage of C3, the classical and alternative pathways of complement activation converge to initiate the terminal sequence, which culminates in the formation of the membrane attack complex. C3b interacts with other complement components and forms C5 convertase, which cleaves C5 into C5a and C5b. C6, C7, and C5b then bind successively to form the C5b,6,7 complex. Formation of membrane-bound C5b,6,7 permits binding of C8 to the C5 fragment to cause a partial membrane lesion, which results in slow cell lysis. By binding with C9, the cytolytic reaction is accelerated.

In addition to cell lysis, breakdown products of this cascade serve other biologic functions that result in better defense against foreign substances. C3a and C5a are anaphylatoxins, and they stimulate chemotaxis of neutrophils. They also have powerful effects on blood vessel walls, leading to an increase in vascular permeability. Bound C3 and C4 fragments act as opsonins, enhancing phagocytosis and stimulating the exocytosis of granules that contain powerful proteolytic enzymes and free radicals from neutrophils, monocytes, and macrophages.

CYTOKINES

Cytokines are a diverse group of small, secreted protein mediators that are an important means of interaction between the different effector cells of the human immune response. Each cytokine may have multiple activities on different cell types, and several cytokines often have related functions. They can also have synergistic or antagonistic activities and can inhibit or induce the synthesis of other cytokines. The different cytokines, their principal cell sources, and their main effects in humans are summarized in Table 13-1.

PHAGOCYTES

The phagocytic system consists of circulating and fixed cells. Monocytes and granulocytes circulate, whereas Kupffer's cells, macrophages, and brain microglial cells remain fixed. Migration of phagocytic cells can occur randomly or in response to a directed signal, a process known as *chemotaxis*. Substances with chemotactic properties include complement and bacterial products. Once attracted to a particular site, phagocytes engulf foreign material. Phagocytosis is facilitated by opsonization, which coats foreign material with antibodies. After phagocytosis, an intracellular vacuole forms around the foreign material and lysosomal enzymes released into the vacuole destroy the foreign invader.

Monocytes originate in the bone marrow from progenitors common to monocytic and granulocytic cells. Once re-

Table 13-1. Cell sources and predominant effects of cytokines

Cytokine	Cell sources	Predominant effects
IL-1	Macrophages	Hematopoietic and proinflammatory effects, B-cell activation
IL-2	T lymphocytes	T-lymphocyte, B-lymphocyte, and natural killer cell proliferation
IL-3	T lymphocytes	Myeloid progenitor cell, eosinophil, mast cell, and basophil growth
IL-4	T lymphocytes	B and T cell growth, IgE switch
IL-5	T lymphocytes	Eosinophil proliferation and differentiation
IL-6	Macrophages, fibroblasts	T-cell proliferation, B-cell antibody production
IL-7	Stromal cells	pre–B-cell and pre–T-cell growth
IL-8, gro (CXC chemokines)	Macrophages, fibroblasts, platelets	Neutrophil chemotaxis and activation
RANTES, MIP1α,β (CC chemokines)	T cells, fibroblasts, macrophages	Monocyte chemotaxis and activation, potent eosinophil chemoattractant effects (RANTES)
IL-9	T lymphocytes	Erythroid progenitor maturation, T-cell tumor growth
IL-10	T and B lymphocytes	Inhibited cytotoxic or inflammatory responses, enhanced antibody responses
IL-11	Fibroblasts	Hematopoietic growth factor for megakaryocyte precursors
IL-12	Macrophages, B cells	Enhanced cell-mediated and cytotoxic responses, enhanced differentiation of precursors into TH1 cells
IL-13	T lymphocytes	B-cell growth, IgE switch
GM-CSF	T lymphocytes, keratinocytes, stromal cells	Proliferation and differentiation of hematopoietic progenitor of granulocytes and macrophages
Interferon-γ	T lymphocytes, natural killer cells	Macrophages and natural killer cells activation, antiviral effects, antagonizes interleukin-4 effects, enhanced differentiation of precursors into TH1 cells
Tumor necrosis factor-α or lymphotoxin	Macrophages, T lymphocytes, natural killer cells, keratinocytes	Monocyte and neutrophil activation, vascular leakage induction, septic shock mediation, infected or malignant cell destruction
Transforming growth factor-β1, -β2, or -β3	Macrophages, chondrocytes, megakaryocytes	Wound healing and remodeling, B-cell switch to IgA production, inhibition of T- and B-cell proliferation and B-cell antibody secretion
Stem cell factor	Stromal cell, fibroblasts	Functions as a cofactor for proliferation of early hematopoietic progenitors
Leukemia inhibitory factor	T lymphocytes, fibroblasts, monocytes	Hematopoietic progenitor proliferation

IL—Interleukin; RANTES—Regulated on activation; normal T cell expressed and secreted; MIP—Macrophage inflammatory protein; GM-CSF—Granulocyte-macrophage colony-stimulating factor; INF—Interferon; TNF—Tumor necrosis factor.

leased into the peripheral blood, they circulate until migration into various organs occurs. In tissues, mitogens, such as colony-stimulating factor (CSF), produced by fibroblasts, lymphocytes, and monocytes, induce the maturation of circulating monocytes into macrophages. Circulating monocytes possess a well-developed Golgi apparatus and many intracytoplasmic lysosomes, which contribute to the intracellular killing of organisms. Monocytes and macrophages bind to foreign organisms through specialized receptors for carbohydrates, IgG, and complement on the surface of organisms. They also have receptors for lymphokines. In addition, monocytes produce complement components, prostaglandins, IFN, and cytokines such as IL-1 and TNF.

Granulocytes released into the circulation are short-lived (2 to 3 days) compared with monocytes and macrophages (months and years). Granulocytes include neutrophils, eosinophils, and basophils. From the circulation, these cells migrate to sites of acute inflammation and, together with antibodies and complement, protect primarily against microorganisms.

Neutrophils represent more than 90% of circulating granulocytes. They possess azurophilic cytoplasmic granules, which contain acid hydrolases, myeloperoxidase, and lysozyme, and secondary granules, which contain lactoferrin and lysozyme. Besides their ability to phagocytize foreign organisms, neutrophils can release their cytotoxic substances extracellularly in response to appropriate stimuli, such as immune complexes. Neutrophils are expert phagocytes by virtue of their expression of several specialized receptors. The opsonic attachment of microorganisms to neutrophils occurs via Fcγ receptors and through receptors for the complement-derived opsonin C3b. After an opsonized microbe attaches to the neutrophil membrane via these receptors, the cell surrounds it, forming a phagosome; the microbe becomes susceptible to the highly concentrated nonoxidative and oxidative products that the neutrophil spills into the phagosome as it develops into a phagolysosome.

Eosinophils comprise 2% to 5% of blood granulocytes in healthy persons. Produced in the bone marrow from distinct progenitors, eosinophils enter and leave the circulation rapidly. Their half-life in blood is 3 to 8 hours, whereas it is several days in tissues. Although they possess phagocytic activity, eosinophils are much less efficient in this process than are neutrophils. Eosinophils possess several surface markers and receptors involved in differentiation, recruitment into tissues, activation, and synthesis and release of their multiple mediators. Receptors that are constitutively expressed on normal blood eosinophils or induced during priming or activation include receptors for the eosinophil-active cytokines and chemokines, such as IL-1, IL-5, GM-CSF, IFN-γ, IL-8, RANTES (regulated on activation, normal T cell expressed and secreted), and macrophage inflammatory protein-1α. Eosinophils also possess the low-affinity IgG receptor (FcγRII) and an FcαR, which makes secretory IgA a potent secretagogue for stimulation of eosinophil de-

granulation and mediator release.[1] Complement receptors for anaphylatoxins, such as C5a, are expressed on eosinophils; C5a is a potent eosinophil chemoattractant *in vitro*. To facilitate eosinophil recruitment into sites of tissue inflammation, eosinophils possess several members of the $\beta2$ integrin family of adhesion proteins that allow them to bind to various adhesion molecules. These include CD11a (LFA-1), CD11b (Mac-1, CR3), and CD11c (p150,95), in association with the shared CD18 β chain. These proteins are also expressed on neutrophils and on monocytes and macrophages, unlike VLA-4, which is expressed only on eosinophils. This adhesion protein on eosinophils is responsible for the specific adherence of this cell type to VCAM-1 on IL-1-[29] or IL-4-[150] activated endothelial cells and is probably responsible, at least in part, for selective recruitment of eosinophils into tissues. Inducible surface markers identified primarily on activated eosinophils *in vivo* or *in vitro* include the T-cell–associated markers CD4, HLA-DR, Mac-2, and FcϵRII (CD23). CD4 expression may be functionally relevant because eosinophils undergo chemotaxis *in vitro* to various CD4-binding ligands,[142] and HLA-DR may be functionally relevant to the potential of eosinophils to serve as MHC class II–restricted APC *in vitro*.[73]

The eosinophil's cationic granule proteins have been studied extensively; they include major basic protein (MBP), eosinophil peroxidase (EPO), eosinophil cationic protein (ECP), and eosinophil-derived neurotoxin (EDN). Another prominent protein of the eosinophil is the Charcot-Leyden crystal (CLC) protein, which constitutes an estimated 7% to 10% of total cellular protein, possesses lysophospholipase activity, and forms the distinctive hexagonal bipyramidal crystals that are the hallmark of eosinophil-associated inflammation. MBP is present in eosinophils and basophils (at much lower concentrations than in eosinophils), and mast cells may acquire MBP by endocytosis and vesicular uptake. MBP is a potent cytotoxin and helminthotoxin *in vitro*. It can kill bacteria and many types of normal and neoplastic mammalian cells, stimulate histamine release from basophils and mast cells, activate neutrophils and platelets, and augment superoxide generation by alveolar macrophages. It can also induce bronchoconstriction and transient airway hyperreactivity when instilled into the monkey trachea.[2] As with MBP and ECP, EPO is highly cationic and exerts some cytotoxic effects on parasites and mammalian cells in the absence of hydrogen peroxide. However, it is highly effective in combination with hydrogen peroxide and a halide cofactor (iodide, bromide, or chloride) from which EPO catalyzes the production of the toxic hypohalous acid. In the presence of these compounds, EPO is highly toxic to various unicellular, multicellular, and other targets, including viruses, mycoplasma, bacteria, fungi, and parasites. ECP, similar to MBP, has marked toxicity for helminth parasites, blood hemoflagellates, bacteria, and mammalian cells and tissues. Purified ECP has been used in several studies in which respiratory epithelial damage (epithelial stripping, mucus plugging), similar to that in severe asthmatics, has been reproduced. EDN induces a syndrome of muscle rigidity, ataxia, eventual paralysis, widespread loss of Purkinje's cells, and spongiform degeneration of the white matter of the cerebellum, brainstem, and spinal cord when injected intrathecally or intracerebrally into experimental rabbits or guinea pigs. Unlike the other eosinophil granule cationic proteins, EDN is a poor cationic toxin, with only limited toxicity for helminths and mammalian cells at very high concentrations. In allergic conditions, eosinophils may play a dual role. They can suppress the local tissue response to inflammatory mediators involved in IgE-mediated hypersensitivity reactions by inactivating histamine, platelet-activating factor, and heparin. On the other hand, eosinophils can augment the destruction by the toxic effects of the products they release on degranulation. The balance between these two seemingly contradictory functions of eosinophils in IgE-mediated reactions is still under investigation.

Basophils are very sparse in the circulation and are characterized by deep blue granules that can be identified by alcian blue staining. Basophils, similar to mast cells, have high-affinity Fc receptors for the IgE antibody. They participate in allergic reactions by releasing several inflammatory mediators, such as histamine and leukotriene C_4, and they produce IL-4.[152]

IMMUNOPATHOLOGY

As described, the two major effector arms of the specific immune response are humoral and cellular. In the defense against infections, antibodies are operative against bacteria or bacterial products, whereas cell-mediated immunity operates primarily against viral, fungal, and mycotic infections. With few exceptions, antibody-mediated immune mechanisms work best when directed to extracellular infections, whereas cell-mediated immunity is effective against intracellular infections. The killing effects of immune reactions are extremely efficient and, when specifically directed to a given infection, can eliminate many organisms in a short time. However, these same immune mechanisms may cause host tissue destruction and therefore lead to disease states. This destructive effect of immune reactions is termed *allergy* or *hypersensitivity* and is considered an immunopathologic reaction.

For several years, these reactions were divided into four types according to the Gell and Coombs classification proposed in 1963:[66] type I, immediate hypersensitivity (IgE mediated); type II, cytotoxic reactions (IgG, IgM mediated); type III, immune complex reactions (IgG, IgM complex mediated); and type IV, delayed hypersensitivity reactions (T-cell mediated). The division of these immune reactions into neat categories, although easy to comprehend, is oversimplified. For example, allergic reactions are classified as IgE-mediated, type I immunopathologic responses but involve all components of the immune system.

Type I mast cell–mediated reactions

Possibly as a remnant of host defense mechanisms to parasites,[155,183] the immediate hypersensitivity reaction uses the release of mast cell or basophil mediators to create immediate and delayed (4 to 8 hours) responses to sensitizing allergens. These reactions can be IgE-dependent (anaphylactic), requiring allergen-specific IgE antibody to attach to IgE receptors on mast cells or basophils to initiate a clinical reaction, such as anaphylaxis to penicillins or allergic rhinitis to ragweed pollen. Type I reactions can also be IgE-independent (anaphylactoid) and can be caused by IgE-independent mechanisms of mast cell or basophil degranulation, such as sensitivity to iodide contrast media.

Type II antibody–mediated reactions

Type II antibody (non-IgE)–mediated immune reactions involve IgG and IgM antibodies binding to antigens on the surface of target cells (e.g., erythrocytes, neutrophils, platelets, and epithelial cells of glandular or mucosal surfaces) or to antigens on tissues such as basement membranes. The sensitizing antigens in these cases can be natural cell-surface antigens, modified cell-surface antigens, or haptens attached to cell surfaces. This interaction between IgG and IgM antibodies and cell-surface antigens leads to destruction of these cells by one of three mechanisms: opsonization, complement activation, and cell lysis and ADCC. These mechanisms afford protection against infections and eradication of malignant cells but can also damage self antigens in various tissues.

One example of such a reaction includes the phagocytic cell destruction of antibody-coated platelets (opsonization), leading to thrombocytopenia. Another example occurs when penicillin binds to the surfaces of erythrocytes, creating a nonself antigen composed of penicillin-modified erythrocyte cell surfaces.[138] Antipenicilloyl antibodies, initially IgM and later IgG, fix to these surfaces and concomitantly activate complement, leading to the lysis of the cell by penetration of the terminal hydrophobic complement components, C7 to C9. Clinically, this condition is known as penicillin-induced autoimmune hemolytic anemia. Similar reactions are quinidine-induced autoimmune thrombocytopenia and methyldopa-induced autoimmune hemolytic anemia. In these reactions, activated complement components generated from a few target cells under immune attack by antibody can damage target cells and non–antibody-bound target cells. Another example of a type II reaction is binding of eosinophils via Fc γRII receptors to IgG-bound helminths and release of cytolytic major basic protein, resulting in destruction of the parasite via ADCC.

Type III immune complex–mediated reactions

Type III reactions are similar to type II reactions in that they involve antibody-mediated inflammation. However, in type III reactions the antibody and its antigen form low-solubility immune complexes, which are deposited in normal tissues and precipitate an immune response. These immune complexes are usually deposited around the basement membranes of vessels with a high plasma outflow. They activate complement and set off an inflammatory response characterized primarily by neutrophil influx, which inflicts tissue injury. Knowledge of this immunologic disease became widespread in the early 1900s, when physicians began using immune animal sera, usually equine sera, to treat bacterial infections, which led to serious illness and even death of the treated subjects.[91] Immune complexes of antibody (IgM or IgG) and antigen, activated complement components, and neutrophil chemotaxis are important participants in this hypersensitivity reaction, which is better known as *serum sickness*. Immune complex vasculitis in the skin can also occur in a series of clinical conditions, such as systemic lupus erythematosus, rheumatoid arthritis, drug reactions, and infections.

Type IV cell–mediated reactions

This category of the classical hypersensitivity reactions is caused by antibody-independent mechanisms involving T cells or NK cells. These reactions are the pathologic variants of a normal T-cell–mediated immune response in which the T-cell response to an environmental antigen becomes exaggerated. The typical type IV immune response is the delayed hypersensitivity reaction caused by sensitized T cells, in particular the CD4+ (helper) cell population. A clinical example of such a reaction is the cutaneous reaction to challenge with the PPD of *M. tuberculosis* in previously infected or vaccinated patients.

Although the focus is on delayed hypersensitivity reactions involving the skin and sensitizing antigens, other reactions involving other organ systems and target antigens are known. Examples of such reactions are the T-cell infiltration of tumor beds and the T-cell infiltration of blood vessels and alveoli in chronic asthma. Some type IV hypersensitivity responses are also mediated by CD8+ T cells and NK cells. In contrast to the neutrophilic infiltration of the tissues in type III reactions, the cell infiltrate in type IV reactions is dominated by lymphocytes, monocytes, and macrophages.

PATHOPHYSIOLOGY OF ALLERGIC RHINITIS

Allergic rhinitis, a chronic disease defined as a clinical hypersensitivity of the nasal mucosa to foreign substances mediated through IgE antibodies, affects millions of Americans and is encountered frequently by the otolaryngologist in the clinical setting. This IgE-dependent disease is an example of more than a mast cell–mediated reaction. The pathophysiologic events involved in allergic rhinitis illustrate the interactions of multiple components of the immune response.

Sensitization and immunoglobulin E production

During the initial stage of the natural history of the disease, low-dose exposure leads to the production of specific IgE antibodies, a primary humoral response. During subsequent exposure, a secondary humoral response occurs in conjunction with an inflammatory response. Antigen that is deposited on the nasal mucosa is engulfed by APC (macrophages, dendritic cells, Langerhans' cells) and is partially degraded within their phagolysosomes. Portions of the antigen are then exteriorized on the surfaces of APC and are recognized by T-helper cells and class II MHC molecules. IL-1–activated T-helper cells then secrete cytokines, which promote the growth and differentiation of other cells involved in the immune response.

TH-2 CD4+ cells are thought to be an important contributor to allergic reactions because they secrete the cytokines IL-4 and IL-5. IL-4 promotes B-cell isotype switching to the production of IgE.[46] Increased production of IL-4 by peripheral blood mononuclear cells has been associated with high serum IgE levels,[65] whereas IFN-γ (secreted by TH-1 cells) has the opposite effect.[134] The importance of TH-2 cells and IL-4 is further supported by the preferential release of TH-2 cytokines from allergen-specific T-cell clones of atopic donors.[133] Durham and others,[51] using *in situ* hybridization, found message for IL-4 in nasal biopsy specimens of patients with allergic rhinitis 24 hours after provocation with allergen. Antigen-specific IgE then attaches to high-affinity receptors on mast cells and basophils and to low-affinity receptors on other cells, thereby sensitizing the nasal mucosa. On subsequent exposure to the offending allergen, the IgE antibodies on the surface of these cells serve as receptors for the antigen molecules. Cross-linking of adjacent IgE molecules on mast cells leads to the release of inflammatory mediators that stimulate nerves, glands, and blood vessels to cause the clinical manifestations of the disease, namely sneezing, pruritus, rhinorrhea, and nasal obstruction. These events are known as the early or immediate allergic response. Secondary rises in specific IgE occur in response to nasal challenge and seasonal exposure. The role of this secondary response is unknown.

The early response to antigen

Within minutes after exposure of an allergic patient to antigen, an inflammatory response occurs. After antigen provocation, the patient first senses tingling and pruritus, followed by sneezing, rhinorrhea, and lastly, nasal congestion. These subjective feelings correlate with physiologic changes that are measured after antigen provocation, such as increases in nasal secretions and nasal airway resistance (NAR).[13] In addition to these physiologic changes, increases are noted in the levels of histamine,[120] kinins, albumin,[22] plasma and glandular kallikrein,[21,23] mast cell tryptase,[38] prostaglandin D_2 (PGD_2),[22] leukotriene C_4 (LTC_4),[41] leukotriene B_4 (LTB_4),[61] MBP,[19] platelet-activating factor (PAF),[113] and total protein and lactoferrin in recovered nasal lavage specimens.[144] These increases in mediators and biologic markers do not occur in allergic patients challenged with diluent or nonallergic controls. Histamine and tryptase are found in mast cell granules, and their detection in nasal secretions after antigen provocation provides support for mast cell degranulation during the nasal allergic reaction. PGD$_2$, a newly synthesized mediator of the cyclooxygenase pathway, is also secreted by mast cells. Direct evidence for the role of nasal mast cells in the immediate allergic reaction was provided by Gomez and others,[67] who biopsied the nasal mucosa in allergic patients 20 minutes after provocation with either antigen or saline. Mast cells in the nasal mucosa were significantly more degranulated after allergen provocation than after saline or antigen challenge of nonallergic controls.

Neuronal contribution

Sneezing and itching during the early response to allergen provocation involve the nervous system. Konno and Togawa[93] and others[16,143] showed the importance of neural reflexes in patients with allergic rhinitis when stimulation of one nasal cavity with histamine led to bilateral nasal secretions. Unilateral intranasal challenge with antigen in patients with allergic rhinitis led to an increase in sneezes, rhinorrhea, nasal secretions, histamine, NAR,[15] and PGD$_2$[144,176] on the side of challenge. Contralateral to the challenge, rhinorrhea, secretion weights, and PGD$_2$ increased significantly.[176] The contralateral secretory response was rich in the glandular markers lactoferrin and lysozyme[144] and was inhibited by atropine, an anticholinergic,[16] suggesting that the efferent limb was cholinergically mediated. The muscarinic receptors that mediate the actions of acetylcholine in the nasal mucosa have been characterized pharmacologically in human inferior turbinates by use of receptor-binding assays, localized by autoradiography, and examined functionally *in vitro* by assays of mucus secretion from cultured nasal mucosal explants.[128] These studies showed the presence of muscarinic (M$_1$) and M$_3$ receptor subtypes in the human nasal mucosa, with 45% of the total receptors being M$_1$. High densities of M$_1$ and M$_3$ receptors coexisted in submucosal glands, M$_3$ receptors predominated in vessels, and M$_2$ receptors were not found. M$_1$ and M$_3$ receptors were implicated in methacholine-induced respiratory glycoconjugates and lactoferrin glandular secretion, but M$_2$ receptors did not appear to be involved.

Immunohistochemical studies have established the presence of several neuropeptides in addition to sympathetic and parasympathetic nerves and their transmitters in the nasal mucosa. These neuropeptides are secreted by unmyelinated nociceptive C fibers (tachykinins, calcitonin gene-related peptide [CGRP], neurokinin [NKA], gastrin-releasing peptide), parasympathetic nerve endings (vasoactive intestinal peptide [VIP], peptide histidine methionine), and sympathetic nerve endings (neuropeptide Y). Substance P (SP), a member of the tachykinin family, is often found as a cotransmitter with NKA and CGRP and has been found in high density in arterial vessels and, to some extent, in veins, gland acini, and epithelium of the nasal mucosa.[10] In addition to the identification of these neuropeptides in the nasal mucosa, several studies support the concept that neuronal mecha-

nisms mediated by these peptides amplify the inflammatory allergic reaction. Nasal provocation with neuropeptide Y, a 36–amino acid peptide co-localized with norepinephrine in sympathetic fibers, increases the expression of ICAM-1.[163] Nasal challenge with SP induces few changes in healthy patients, but leads to a modest increase in vascular permeability, NAR, and eosinophil and neutrophil chemotaxis in rhinitics.[35] In an *in vitro* study, Okamoto and others[127] incubated nasal biopsy specimens of patients with perennial rhinitis and nonallergic rhinitis with SP or mite allergena, they then tested for messenger ribonucleic acid (mRNA) of different cytokines by using semiquantitative analysis by reverse transcription polymerase chain reaction (RT-PCR).[127] SP and allergen challenge resulted in significant increases in mRNA for IL-1β, IL-2, IL-3, IL-4, IL-5, IL-6, TNF-α, and IFN-γ in nasal biopsy specimens of allergic patients; these increases were blocked by an SP antagonist. Such upregulation was not observed in biopsy samples of nonallergic patients. Because these cytokines are important in allergic reactions, this study supports the importance of SP as a proinflammatory neuropeptide. Schierhorn and others[149] provided further evidence for the importance of SP in allergic reactions when they showed that SP stimulation of human nasal mucosal biopsy specimens in culture resulted in significant elevation of histamine content, decreased density of mast cells, and increased percentage of degranulated mast cells. VIP stimulates serous cell secretion,[11] dilates nasal vessels,[107] and regulates mucociliary clearance in dogs.[122]

To implicate these neuropeptides further in allergic reactions, Mosimann and others[117] challenged allergic rhinitic patients with histamine and antigen and measured levels of neuropeptides in recovered nasal washes. Only VIP increased above baseline after histamine challenge, whereas levels of SP, CGRP, and VIP increased significantly immediately after antigen challenge and returned to baseline within 2 hours. In patients who experienced a late reaction, only SP increased slightly, but it increased significantly at the peak of the reaction. SP and CGRP were not significantly increased in atopic patients or nonatopic controls challenged with irrelevant antigen.

In similar experiments, Nieber and others[124] detected significantly higher levels of SP–like immunoreactivity at baseline in nasal lavages of patients with allergic rhinitis compared with nonallergic volunteers.[124] They also showed a significant increase of SP–like immunoreactivity in the allergic patients but not in healthy subjects 10 minutes after allergen challenge. These experiments suggest that neuropeptides are released *in vivo* in humans after allergen challenge and might be partly responsible for symptoms of the allergic reaction. Furthermore, the recovery of VIP after histamine challenge suggests that histamine-induced cholinergic reflexes induce the release of VIP.

Repetitive application of capsaicin, the essence of chili peppers, depletes sensory nerves of their content of SP and

CGRP and initiates both central and axonal reflexes.[79] Capsaicin causes a burning sensation and profuse bilateral rhinorrhea when applied to one side of the nasal cavity, and repeated administration causes tachykinin depletion and tachyphylaxis.[18,137] Unlike its effects in rodents, the capsaicin-induced nasal secretory response in humans is glandular and not caused by increased vascular permeability.[140] To investigate possible proinflammatory effects of capsaicin, Philip and others[139] challenged patients with allergic rhinitis and healthy subjects using intranasal capsaicin and examined subsequent cellular influx into nasal secretions, as sampled by lavage. Capsaicin challenge caused significant increases in leukocyte counts from the prechallenge baseline at 10 minutes, 30 minutes, and 4 hours after challenge, with no difference between rhinitic and healthy subjects. The rise in the number of inflammatory cells represented significant increases in neutrophils, eosinophils, and mononuclear cells, supporting a nonspecific inflammatory effect of sensory nerve activation.

The neuropeptide-depleting property of capsaicin decreased symptoms of nonallergic chronic rhinitis.[96] Lacroix and others[76] showed also that the decrease in symptoms of these patients correlated with a significant decrease in CGRP in the nasal mucosa. Furthermore, capsaicin desensitization reduces sneezing in response to antigen and histamine challenges.[92] Therefore, several experimental findings point to the importance of neurogenic control of the allergic response, including the presence of nasonasal reflexes after nasal antigen provocation, the presence of neuropeptides in nasal tissues and their recovery in nasal secretions after antigen challenge, the ability of these peptides to produce symptoms and inflammatory responses similar to those obtained after exposure to antigen, and finally, the clinical efficacy of capsaicin, which depletes the stores of these substances. More specific delineation of the role of each of these substances awaits the development of specific antagonists.

The early reaction to allergen challenge with the release of mast cell mediators results in increased symptoms. However, these changes are measured in minutes, in contrast to clinical disease in which symptoms last for hours after exposure to allergen. Furthermore, other discrepancies exist between the early reaction and clinical disease, such as the chronic inflammation and hyperresponsiveness seen in allergic patients during the allergy season and the lack of inhibition of the early response by systemic corticosteroids that are effective in the treatment of allergic rhinitis. Therefore, the early response does not mimic all aspects of clinical disease, and investigations should evaluate the events that occur hours after antigen exposure.

The late response to antigen

Hours after antigen challenge, some patients experience a recurrence of their earlier symptoms, most notably nasal congestion. This is termed the *late-phase reaction*. Several investigators have documented elevations in NAR that occur 4 to 10 hours after antigen challenge, with a peak around 6 hours and resolution by 24 hours.[53,135] The production of mediators during the late reaction was documented by challenging allergic patients with allergen and collection of nasal secretions hourly for up to 12 hours after provocation.[119] The early rise in mediators as part of the early reaction was followed by a recurrence of symptoms and increases in the levels of histamine, tosyl-L-arginine methyl ester (TAME)-esterase, and kinins, but not PGD_2. Other mediators, including eosinophil products, have also been detected.[19] The peak of mediator production during the late phase varied among patients, and some had multiphasic responses, but these changes were unique to allergic patients after challenge and did not occur in allergic patients after diluent challenge or in nonallergic controls after antigen challenge.

Recently, levels of nitric oxide (NO) have been detected in exhaled air during nasal and oral breathing in patients with seasonal allergic rhinitis and in healthy subjects.[110] Concentrations of nasally exhaled NO were significantly higher in the allergic patients than in the healthy subjects, suggesting a role for this mediator in the pathophysiology of allergic rhinitis. Nitric oxide is synthesized from L-arginine in various cell types by the action of NO synthases, including the constitutive forms of nitric oxide synthase in vascular endothelial cells (type III nitric oxide synthase) and neurons (type I nitric oxide synthase) and the inducible form (type II nitric oxide synthase) induced by cytokines in macrophages, neutrophils, mast cells, smooth muscle cells, and fibroblasts. NO has vasodilatory properties, and its increased production in the nose could contribute to nasal obstruction and plasma protein extravasation in allergic disease.

Furukawa and others[62] investigated the presence and localization of type III and II nitric oxide synthase in the inferior nasal turbinates of patients with turbinate hypertrophy and septal deviation by using immunohistochemistry and *in situ* hybridization. Type III nitric oxide synthase immunoreactivity and mRNA were observed in endothelial cells, surface epithelium, and submucosal glands, whereas type II nitric oxide synthase immunoreactivity was less intense and was observed in surface epithelium, vascular endothelial and smooth muscle cells, submucosal glands, and inflammatory cells, and mRNA for type II nitric oxide synthase was localized mainly to inflammatory cells. Type II nitric oxide synthase immunoreactivity was more intense in the specimens with more severe inflammatory changes and correlated with the extent of inflammation. Bacci and others[6] reported on the presence of neuronal nitric oxide synthase immunoreactivity in mast cell granules in biopsy specimens of normal nasal mucosa from four patients undergoing rhinoplasties. These studies support the presence of nitric oxide synthase in the nasal mucosa and suggest a possible role for NO in the pathophysiology of nasal diseases, including allergic rhinitis.

To investigate the role of the neuronal contribution to

the late nasal allergic reaction, levels of histamine in nasal secretions were measured hourly, for 10 hours, after allergen or control provocations from the site of challenge and from the contralateral nostril.[175] As previously shown, histamine release occured at the site of challenge during the early response and hours after allergen provocation but not after control challenge. On the contralateral side of challenge histamine production showed no significant increase during the early phase but significant increase in histamine (compared with challenge in healthy subjects) during the late phase. In another group of subjects, an influx of basophils to the contralateral nasal cavity occurred 24 hours after provocation with allergen but not after control challenge. These studies suggest a neuronal contribution to the late inflammatory response.

Cellular events

Along with the physiologic changes and inflammatory mediator production that occur hours after antigen provocation, inflammatory cellular influx occurs in the nasal mucosa and in recovered nasal secretions after experimental provocation and in seasonally exposed patients. A slight initial increase in eosinophils in nasal secretions occurred within 1 to 2 hours of challenge and was followed by a peak 6 to 8 hours later.[17] MBP, a mediator secreted by eosinophils, was also recovered in nasal lavages hours after antigen provocation, and its levels correlated with the number of eosinophils, suggesting that these cells influx into nasal secretions and release inflammatory mediators.[19] Juliusson and others[84] examined nasal inflammatory cellular influx by lavaging the nasal cavities and obtaining brush samples from the nasal mucosa hours after antigen challenge. They observed a rapid and significant increase in the number of eosinophils in allergic patients as early as 2 hours after challenge in the lavage specimens and 4 hours after challenge in the brush samples. The percentage of activated eosinophils (as assessed by cytoplasmic vacuolization) in brush samples increased and reached a peak 8 hours after provocation, and the basal values of eosinophils correlated significantly with symptoms of congestion, sneezing, and rhinorrhea observed after challenge.[84] To examine changes in eosinophil numbers and activation status during natural exposure, Bentley and others[25] performed nasal biopsies in allergic patients during the pollen season and reported significant seasonal increases in total MBP and activated (EG2+) eosinophils in the submucosa of these patients compared with preseasonal eosinophil numbers or from nonallergic subjects.

To compare cellular influx into nasal secretions with that into the nasal mucosa, Lim and others[102] obtained nasal lavages and inferior turbinate biopsy specimens before and 24 hours after challenging allergic patients with allergen. Similar to findings reported by other investigators, the number of eosinophils and polymorphonuclear cells in nasal lavages and the number of eosinophils and mononuclear cells in the nasal mucosa were significantly increased. The predominant cell types in nasal secretions were polymorphonuclear cells and eosinophils, whereas mononuclear cells predominated in the nasal mucosa, suggesting that nasal secretions and the nasal mucosa are two separate compartments with different inflammatory cellular predominance during allergic inflammation.

Cells that stained positive with alcian blue were also recovered in nasal lavages in small, but significantly increased numbers during the late-phase response.[17] They constituted 1% of the recovered cells, and 68% were classified as basophils on light microscopy. Furthermore, their number correlated significantly with levels of histamine recovered in nasal secretions during the late-phase response (r = 0.72, $P < 0.0001$), suggesting that these cells are the source of the late rise in histamine. Juliusson and others[84] observed significant increases in metachromatic cells 8 to 10 hours after allergen provocation in brush samples and 8 to 12 hours after provocation in lavages of the nasal mucosa, with more metachromatic cells obtained by the brush technique. Light microscopic morphology and ultrastructural observations indicated that these cells were mast cells rather than blood basophils. Cell pellet histamine levels were also measured, and allergen challenge led to lower histamine: metachromatic cell quotients, suggesting that the mast cells were activated and secreting histamine. Furthermore, the basal number of metachromatic cells in the nasal mucosa correlated significantly with symptoms of congestion and sneezes after antigen provocation, suggesting that the baseline metachromatic cell content of the nasal mucosa was a predictor of the extent of clinical symptoms after antigen provocation.

Similar changes have been observed during seasonal exposure of allergic patients, lending credibility to the observations after experimental allergen challenge. In separately conducted studies, Bryan and Bryan[36] and Okuda and Ohtsuka[130] observed basophilic cells in nasal secretions during seasonal exposure of allergic patients to pollen. Ultrastructural and light microscopic studies of these cells suggested that most are identical to blood basophils.[74,129,131] In contrast to nasal secretions, which represent the most superficial compartment of the nasal mucosa, examination of nasal mucosal scrapings[126,131] or biopsy specimens,[57,131] which sample deeper layers, showed that most metachromatic cells in these compartments were mast cells. The mast cells were divided into two subpopulations, one located in the epithelium and the other located deeper, in the lamina propria.[132] Unlike allergic patients during seasonal exposure, nonallergic individuals had fewer basophilic cells in nasal secretions and few mast cells in the mucosa.[74,131] Enerback and others,[57] using biopsies and cytologic imprints to examine the cellular content of the nasal mucosa during the birch pollen season in Sweden, showed a seasonal increase in mast cells on the surface of the nasal epithelium after 4 or 5 days of exposure to pollen. Because the overall number of mast cells in the nasal mucosa remained unchanged, they suggested that seasonal exposure led to migration of mast cells from the deeper layers of the lamina propria to the epithelium. Bentley and others[25] reported a similar significant increase in intraepithelial tryptase-positive mast cells in nasal biopsy specimens of allergic patients during the pollen season compared with preseasonal biopsy specimens and samples from nonallergic controls. The consensus of most authors is that basophils predominate in nasal secretions, whereas mast cells are more abundant in the epithelium and lamina propria of allergic patients exposed to antigen either experimentally or naturally.

Eosinophils and mast cells, which are most frequently associated with allergic reactions, occur in the nasal submucosa, but most cells in this location are mononuclear cells (lymphocytes and monocytes). To examine the different types of mononuclear cells in the nasal mucosa after antigen provocation, Varney and others[172] used immunohistochemical staining to analyze nasal biopsy specimens obtained from allergic patients 24 hours after challenge with diluent or the relevant antigen. The numbers of CD4[+] (T helper) lymphocytes and CD25[+] (IL-2 receptor–bearing) cells were significantly increased after antigen challenge compared with challenge with the diluent. Eosinophils (MBP[+]) and neutrophils (neutrophil elastase positive) were also significantly increased. The number of IL2-receptor–bearing cells (CD25[+]) correlated positively with the numbers of CD3[+] and CD4[+] cells, suggesting that CD25[+] cells were activated lymphocytes. To support these observations, Hamid and others[72] used double immunofluorescent staining to show that 60% to 100% of CD25[+] cells identified in the nasal mucosa 24 hours after antigen challenge were also CD3[+]. Unlike changes after antigen provocation, there were no significant increases in CD45[+], CD3[+], CD4[+], CD8[+], CD25[+], CD68[+] cells, or neutrophils in the nasal submucosa during the season.[25] This might be related to the lower dose of antigen to which allergic patients are exposed during the season compared with the amount during experimental provocation or related to the site of the nasal biopsy and the placement of allergen.

Another important cell type detected in the nasal mucosa of allergic patients are Langerhans' cells, which are large mononuclear dendritic cells that are important in antigen presentation. Fokkens and others[59] examined nasal biopsy specimens of allergic patients before, during, and after the grass pollen allergy season and compared them with nasal biopsy specimens from healthy subjects. They used immunohistochemistry with CD1 monoclonal antibody, which identifies Langerhans' cells. The numbers of intraepithelial CD1[+] cells in healthy subjects and grass-allergic patients before and after the pollen season were not different, the numbers of intraepithelial CD1[+] cells were significantly increased during the allergy season compared with the other time points and with nonallergic subjects. In another study involving patients with perennial allergic rhinitis, the same investigators showed a significant decrease in Langerhans'

cells in the epithelium after 3 months of treatment with fluticasone propionate.[78] These studies support the importance of Langerhans' cells in the allergic reaction, specifically as antigen presenters, and suggest that they are not constitutively more numerous in patients with allergic rhinitis but are more likely to be upregulated upon exposure to allergen.

Detection of cytokines in nasal secretions and cells after allergen provocation

In addition to the different preformed and newly generated inflammatory mediators secreted by mast cells and other inflammatory cells during the allergic reaction, cytokines have recently been identified in the nasal mucosa and in nasal secretions of allergic patients during natural exposure and allergen provocation. Several approaches have been used to detect these cytokines, including measurement of the protein in nasal secretions, immunohistochemical staining for the protein in nasal biopsy specimens using monoclonal antibodies, and the use of *in situ* hybridization to identify mRNA.

Sim and others[156] challenged allergic patients with diluent, followed by increasing doses of allergen, until a symptomatic response was obtained. They collected nasal secretions by applying filter paper strips to the nasal mucosa after the challenges and then hourly for 10 hours during the late-phase response. Compared with the diluent challenges, there were significant increases in the levels of IL-1β during the early- and late-phase responses, and of GM-CSF and IL-6 during the late-phase response in all patients. In five of eight patients studied, there were significant elevations of IL-5 during the early- and late-phase responses. Levels of IL-2 or IL-4 were not detectable after challenge. Levels of IL-1β correlated with symptom scores during the early and late reactions, and levels of GM-CSF and IL-6 correlated with symptoms during the late response, suggesting that these cytokines had a role in the clinical manifestations of allergic rhinitis. In a similar study, the same investigators measured levels of cytokines and chemokines in nasal lavages after allergen provocation and studied the effect of premedication with intranasal corticosteroids.[157] In addition to duplicating their findings with IL-1β and GM-CSF, they showed significant increases in levels of macrophage inflammatory protein-1α during the early and late responses and IL-8 and RANTES during the late response when the patients were receiving placebo. Pretreatment with intranasal corticosteroids significantly inhibited the rise in the levels of all the cytokines and chemokines measured. Furthermore, as in the previous studies, the levels of these cytokines correlated with nasal symptoms. Using nasal lavage to sample nasal secretions after allergen challenge, Gosset and others[70] detected significant elevations in levels of IL-1α and IL-6 in patients with dual early and late responses. Levels were elevated during the early and late responses, with higher levels in the late hours after allergen challenge. Bachert and others[7] also measured significant increases in levels of IL-1β and TNF within 2 hours after challenge in nasal lavage specimens and increases in levels of IL-6 and IL-8, 6 to 8 hours after challenge. They detected significantly elevated baseline levels of IL-1β, IL-6, and IL-8 in patients with seasonal allergic rhinitis compared with those of healthy subjects. Finally, similar increases in levels of IL-1β and GM-CSF were detected by Linden and others[103] in nasal lavage specimens from allergic patients shortly after challenge with antigen.

In an attempt to identify cytokines in nasal tissues, Bradding and others[33,34] used immunocytochemistry with monoclonal antibodies against human IL-4, IL-5, IL-6, and IL-8 to stain nasal biopsy specimens from patients with perennial allergic rhinitis and from nonatopic healthy subjects. They detected significantly more IL-4$^+$ cells in the nasal mucosa of perennial rhinitis patients compared with healthy subjects and no positive signal when using an irrelevant antibody. Using staining of 2-μm adjacent sections with antibodies against mast cell tryptase, CD3, and eosinophil cationic protein, the investigators showed that 78% to 100% of the IL-4$^+$ cells contained mast cell tryptase. In one rhinitic patient, IL-4 antibody co-localized to cells staining positively for ECP, i.e., eosinophils. Immunoreactivity for IL-5, IL-6, and IL-8 was present in most biopsy specimens from perennial rhinitic patients and healthy subjects, and there were no significant differences between the two populations in the number of cytokine-positive cells. Consecutive-section staining showed that most IL5$^+$ cells were mast cells, with some eosinophils. Most IL-6$^+$ cells were mast cells, and IL-8 was localized to the cytoplasm of epithelial cells.[33] No cytokine reactivity was localized to CD3$^+$ or CD4$^+$ cells. These data suggest that IL-4, IL-5, and IL-6 are localized to mast cells in the nasal mucosa of patients with perennial allergic rhinitis, but the data do not prove that mast cells are responsible for the secretion of these cytokines, because they could simply be storing them. The investigators attribute the lack of localization of any of the cytokines to T lymphocytes to the fact that cytokines generated by activated T cells are rapidly transported from the cell and do not accumulate in sufficient concentrations to be detected by their technique. They hypothesize that mast cells provide the initial burst of IL-4, which enhances other cells (e.g., T lymphocytes) to continue secreting this and other cytokines, thus perpetuating the inflammatory allergic reaction. The same investigators used similar techniques to study the effect of pretreatment with fluticasone propionate on inflammatory cells in the nasal mucosa of allergic patients during the grass pollen season.[32] Treatment with intranasal corticosteroids suppressed the seasonal increases in epithelial eosinophils, submucosal eosinophils, and epithelial mast cells and also led to a significant suppression of IL-4$^+$ cells in the nasal submucosa, without significant effects on the number of IL-5 and IL-6 immunoreactive cells.

In another approach to investigating the importance of cytokines and their relationship to eosinophil influx in allergic rhinitis, Durham and others[51] performed nasal biopsies on 10 allergic patients 24 hours after local nasal provocation with allergen or diluent.[51] The tissues were processed for *in situ* hybridization with RNA probes for IL-2, IL-3, IL-4, IL-5, GM-CSF, and IFN-γ and for immunohistochemistry with a monoclonal antibody against EG2 to identify activated eosinophils. When the biopsy samples after allergen challenge were compared with those after site diluent challenge, there were significant increases in cells bearing mRNA for IL-3, IL-4, IL-5, and GM-CSF, but not for IL-2 or IFN-γ. Activated eosinophils (EG2$^+$) increased significantly after allergen challenge and correlated positively with mRNA expression for IL-5, IL-4, GM-CSF, IL-3, and IL-2 but not for IFN-γ; the strongest correlation was with IL-5 (r = 0.9, P < 0.0001), and the weakest correlations were with IL-3 (r = 0.63, P = 0.05) and IL-2 (r = 0.65, P = 0.04). To identify the cells bearing mRNA for IL-5, Ying and others[185] developed a method of simultaneous immunocytochemistry and nonradiolabeled *in situ* hybridization and used it to stain nasal biopsy samples of allergic patients obtained 24 hours after antigen challenge. Most IL-5 mRNA$^+$ cells were also CD3$^+$ (83%), and the rest were positive for tryptase (16.4%). This suggests that T lymphocytes are a major contributor to IL-5 in nasal allergic reactions. The same investigators also studied the effects of therapeutic intervention with intranasal corticosteroids and immunotherapy on the expression of mRNA for the different cytokines in the nasal mucosa. Pretreatment with fluticasone propionate before allergen challenge and subsequent biopsy resulted in significant inhibition of nasal symptoms and inhibition of an allergen-induced increase in cells expressing mRNA for IL-4 but not for IL-5.[111] Pretreatment with intranasal corticosteroids also significantly inhibited allergen-induced increases in submucosal IL-2 receptor–bearing cells (CD25$^+$) and activated eosinophils (EG2$^+$). Immunotherapy, in addition to inhibiting cellular influx into the nasal mucosa, also induced a TH-1 cell response, with a significant increase in cells expressing mRNA for IFN-γ.[52]

The various techniques of cytokine detection all support the importance of these proteins in the allergic reaction *in vivo*. Difficulty measuring some cytokines in nasal secretions, most notably IL-4 and IL-5, might be related to the lack of sensitivity of available assays. The techniques of immunohistochemistry and *in situ* hybridization have been helpful in detecting cells bearing the protein itself or mRNA for the protein. The cytokine profile observed after allergen provocation in the *in situ* studies supports the involvement of TH-2 cells in the allergic reaction. Because IL-5 promotes the differentiation,[39] vascular adhesion,[179] and *in vitro* survival[106] of eosinophils and enhances histamine release from basophils,[77] and because IL-4 is a mast cell growth factor[147] and promotes the switching of B cells to the production of IgE,[134] TH-2-like T cells are thought to be particularly important in allergic disease. Bradding and others[33,34] support the importance of IL-4 and IL-5 in the pathophysiology of perennial allergic rhinitis and raise the interesting possibility that mast cells are, at least in part, responsible for the production of these crucial cytokines.

Adhesion molecules and cellular recruitment

Cellular trafficking is integral to human immune response because it allows cells to be selectively recruited from the bloodstream into sites of tissue inflammation. Cellular recruitment into sites of allergic reactions is an example of such trafficking. As detailed, numerous inflammatory cells are present in the nasal mucosa and in nasal secretions of allergic patients during allergen exposure but not in healthy subjects. Mechanisms should therefore exist for the migration and accumulation of these effector cells during allergic inflammation. Recruitment of cells such as eosinophils and activated T lymphocytes are mediated, in part, by interactions between adhesion molecules on the cells themselves and those on vascular endothelial cells, with cytokines playing various regulating roles in these interactions.

The molecules responsible for adhesion on leukocytes belong to different families, such as the integrin family, which consists of molecules with three α chains (CD11a, b, or c) and a common $\beta2$ chain (CD18, $\beta2$ integrin), which can combine noncovalently to form LFA-1, Mac-1, and p150,95, respectively.[4] Another set of adhesion proteins present on leukocytes possesses a different common β subunit, $\beta1$ (CD29), and at least seven α chains and comprises the VLA antigen family.[75] Another leukocyte adhesion protein, L-selectin, belongs to the selectin adhesion molecule family and allows attachment to endothelium under conditions of shear stress caused by blood flow.[27] Adhesion molecules on the vascular endothelial cell surface include ICAM-1 (CD54),

ICAM-2, E-selectin (formerly endothelial-leukocyte adhesion molecule-1), P-selectin (GMP-140, CD62), and VCAM-1.[158] Receptor-counterreceptor pairs for adhesion molecules include LFA-1 with ICAM-1 and ICAM-2, Mac-1 with ICAM-1, VLA-4 with VCAM-1, the carbohydrate structure sialyl-Lewis X with E-selectin and P-selectin, and the recently identified structure GlyCAM-1 for L-selectin.[4,27]

It is currently thought that a series of events occurs during the migration of circulating leukocytes into tissues (Fig. 13-6). The cells initially undergo reversible margination and can be seen rolling along the endothelial surface on intravital microscopy.[158] These changes are mediated by interactions between carbohydrates and selectins. Leukocyte activation occurs next, presumably as a result of exposure to chemoattractants or other activating factors released by endothelial cells or by nearby tissue-dwelling cells; it is associated with changes in affinity and expression of adhesion molecules on the leukocyte surface. Leukocytes also may be activated directly by their interaction with adhesion molecules on activated endothelial cells.[105] Activated leukocytes then attach to endothelial cells and migrate across the endothelium into the extravascular space. These events are mediated by one or more members of the integrin, selectin, and immunoglobulin families of adhesion molecules. Furthermore, it is likely that the preferential recruitment of leukocytes involves multiple steps, such as leukocyte activation, vascular endothelial cell expression of adhesion molecules, adhesion of leukocytes to vascular endothelium, transendothelial migration, chemotaxis, and localized survival within the tissues. Multiple cytokines and other factors are important in upregulating adhesion molecules on circulating leukocytes and vascular

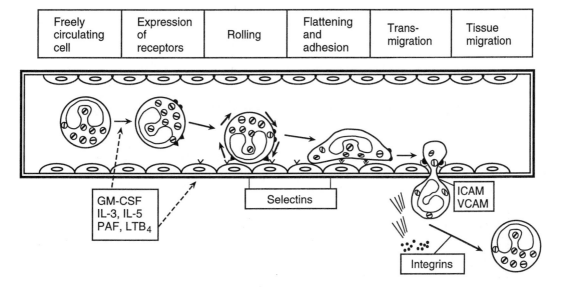

Fig. 13-6. Cellular adhesion and recruitment. An eosinophil is seen from the early stage of free circulation, on to rolling, adhesion to the vascular endothelium, transendothelial migration, and, finally, tissue migration. In the case of the eosinophil, these events are regulated and mediated by multiple cytokines and adhesion molecules. (From Mygind N and others, editors: *Essential allergy*, ed 2, Oxford, 1996, Blackwell Scientific Publications.)

endothelium and are crucial in chemotaxis and leukocyte survival within the tissues.

Because the eosinophil consistently increases in tissues and in secretions of patients with allergic rhinitis, *in vitro* and *in vivo* evidence helps elucidate the mechanism of selective eosinophil recruitment into inflammatory sites. Several investigators have used a nonrotational, static adhesion assay to show that exposure of endothelial cells to IL-1 or TNF induces endothelial expression of ICAM-1, E-selectin, and VCAM-1 and enhances adhesion of eosinophils, basophils, and neutrophils.[26,28,97,151] Blocking antibodies to VCAM-1 were extremely effective in inhibiting eosinophil adherence and, to a lesser degree, basophil adherence but had no effect on neutrophil adherence, suggesting that eosinophils and basophils, in contrast to neutrophils, recognize VCAM-1.[29] Consistent with these observations were the findings that neutrophils did not express VLA-4, the counterligand for VCAM-1, whereas eosinophils and basophils did[29,48,178,182] and the antibodies to VLA-4 inhibited eosinophil but not neutrophil adhesion.[48,178] These studies show that the VLA-4 and VCAM-1 interaction may be important in eosinophil recruitment, and they raise the possibility that conditions leading to selective VCAM-1 expression on endothelial cells result in the preferential adherence of eosinophils. The cytokine IL-4 induces VCAM-1 expression selectively in endothelial cells,[167] and incubation of endothelial cells with IL-4 induced eosinophil and basophil adherence with no effect on the adherence of neutrophils.[150] Much of this adherence was inhibited by addition of anti–VCAM-1 or anti–VLA-4 blocking antibodies.[150] These findings were consistent with the observations *in vivo* that mice transgenic for IL-4 developed eosinophilic inflammatory lesions[165] and that mice injected with a tumor cell line producing IL-4 form an intense eosinophilic infiltrate at the site of the tumor.[166] Therefore, IL-4–induced VCAM-1 expression is probably important in inflammatory responses; however, its interaction with VLA-4 cannot, by itself, explain selective eosinophil recruitment because VLA-4 is also expressed on other cell types, including lymphocytes and monocytes.

After adhering to vascular endothelial cells, eosinophils leave the circulation and enter local inflammatory sites by migrating across the endothelium. In a study of this phenomenon *in vitro*, endothelial cells were cultured to confluence on plastic supports, leukocytes were added, and the cells that migrated were recovered beneath the monolayer and counted. Similar to the findings with adhesion to endothelial cells, managing endothelial monolayers with IL-1 or TNF induced the expression of E-selectin, ICAM-1, and VCAM-1 and increased transendothelial migration of neutrophils[108,115] and eosinophils.[56,116] For eosinophils, transendothelial migration through IL-1–activated endothelium was inhibited almost completely by antibodies to CD18 (β2 integrin), whereas CD29 (β1 integrin, one of the chains of VLA antigens) antibody had essentially no effect.[56] A combination of antibodies against ICAM-1, E-selectin, and VCAM-1 was more effective than anti–ICAM-1 alone in inhibiting eosinophil transmigration.[55] These data suggest that transendothelial migration of eosinophils is mediated by adhesion molecules on the eosinophils and the vascular endothelium, and that the mechanisms of adhesion may be different from those of transmigration.

In addition to cytokines and chemoattractants that can affect the function and expression of leukocyte and endothelial adhesion molecules, another family of mediators, the chemokines, has recently been described. One of these mediators, IL-8, is released by epithelial cells and appears to be necessary for transendothelial migration of neutrophils.[80] Another member of this family, RANTES, selectively promotes chemotaxis of memory T lymphocytes, monocytes,[148] and eosinophils.[3,54,85,146] In the transendothelial migration assay, RANTES stimulates eosinophil migration but has no effect on neutrophils.[175] In contrast to previous studies in which anti-β2 integrin antibody almost completely inhibited eosinophil transendothelial migration, a combination of anti-β2 and anti–VLA-4 antibodies was required for complete inhibition of RANTES-induced transmigration across activated endothelium.[54] Corroborating the importance of these chemokines in allergic reactions is the fact that RANTES, macrophage inflammatory protein-1α, and IL-8 have been detected in nasal lavages after allergen provocation.[157] IL-8 protein has also been localized to the nasal mucosa of patients with perennial allergic rhinitis and healthy subjects.[33] Finally, RANTES has been detected in nasal polyp tissues obtained at the time of sinus surgery and was localized mainly to the sinus epithelium.[24]

There is clear evidence that endothelial activation occurs during allergic rhinitis *in vivo*. Montefort and others[114] compared the expression of endothelial cell adhesion molecules in nasal biopsy specimens from patients with perennial allergic rhinitis and healthy subjects.[114] They found enhanced expression of ICAM-1 and VCAM-1, but not E-selectin, in the mucosa of allergic patients. Lee and others[100] obtained biopsy specimens from the nasal mucosa of allergic patients 24 hours after antigen challenge and compared them with biopsy samples from the same allergic patients without challenge and from nonallergic subjects.[100] They found significant upregulation in the expression of VCAM-1 in the biopsy specimens of allergic patients obtained 24 hours after antigen challenge compared with that in the other groups. Concomitantly, the number of eosinophils significantly increased 24 hours after allergen challenge in the allergic patients compared with those in the other groups. These studies of adhesion molecules *in vivo* suggest that these molecules, along with their counterligands on circulating leukocytes, have an important role in cellular recruitment to allergic inflammatory sites. Further studies are needed for better definition of the role of these adhesion mechanisms in allergic rhinitis and for determination of whether interfering with the process of adhesion will modify the course and severity of the disease.

Hyperresponsiveness

One of the hallmarks of allergic rhinitis is the hyperresponsiveness of allergic patients to specific stimuli, such as antigen (a phenomenon known as *priming*), and to nonspecific stimuli, such as environmental strong odors during the allergen season. Priming has been investigated in the context of allergen provocation and seasonal exposure.

Specific hyperresponsiveness

Many allergic patients report worsening symptoms as the allergy season progresses, despite unchanged or decreased pollen counts. This phenomenon is probably caused by a shift in the threshold of responsiveness. Connell[40] investigated this phenomenon by performing daily antigen challenges in allergic patients and found that the dose of pollen necessary to create symptoms decreased more than fivefold by the fourth day. To examine changes in inflammatory mediators and cells in nasal lavages during priming, Wachs and others[174] challenged asymptomatic allergic patients with increasing doses of antigen on consecutive days.[174] When the patients were challenged 24 hours after prior exposure, they had significantly more sneezes in response to provocation, and the threshold for the initiation of sneezes decreased. The dose necessary to initiate sneezing during the priming response was reduced to about 100 grains of ragweed extract, a dose easily inhaled over a brief period during the pollen season, compared with 10,000 grains needed to initiate sneezing during a regular challenge. Concomitant with the priming response observed for sneezes, there were significantly higher levels of histamine, TAME-esterase activity, and kinins in nasal lavage samples compared with the levels in the initial challenge. There was also an increase in the number of total cells, neutrophils, eosinophils, and basophils in nasal lavages on the days when priming occurred than on the initial challenge day. These observations suggest that mechanisms of priming involve cellular infiltration, increased mediator production and possible increased end organ responsiveness. Influxing inflammatory cells are hypothesized to alter the mucosal penetration of antigen and to provide additional targets for antigen stimulation and increased generation of inflammatory mediators, which would, in turn, encounter more responsive end organs, thus leading to the exaggerated response noted after repeated antigen exposure.

Nonspecific hyperresponsiveness

Increased reactivity to irritant stimuli is often reported by allergic patients. This phenomenon has been studied by observation of the nasal response to nonantigenic nasal secretagogues, such as histamine and the cholinergic agonist methacholine. Walden and others[177] challenged allergic patients with increasing doses of histamine and showed a dose-dependent increase in sneezes and in the levels of albumin and TAME-esterase, indices of vascular permeability, in re-

covered nasal lavage specimens.[177] The patients were then challenged with antigen, and 24 hours later, a histamine challenge was repeated. Increased sensitivity to histamine was observed, compared with the baseline challenge. This increased responsiveness to histamine plateaud and was reversible. Other investigators confirmed the increased responsiveness to histamine 24 hours after antigen challenge and inhibited this phenomenon by pretreatment with topical corticosteroids.[5,14] The number of eosinophils 24 hours after antigen challenge correlated with the magnitude of reactivity to histamine, as assessed by levels of TAME-esterase activity in recovered nasal lavage samples ($r = 0.67$, $P = 0.03$); inhibition by topical corticosteroids was accompanied by an inhibition of the increase of eosinophils in nasal secretions.[14]

To examine the effect of seasonal exposure on nasal responsiveness to histamine, Majchel and others[109] challenged allergic patients with histamine before, at the peak of, near the end of, and 2 weeks after the ragweed pollen season and monitored the response by symptoms and markers of vascular permeability in recovered nasal lavage specimens.[109] They observed a significant increase in all monitored parameters at the peak of the pollen season; these returned to baseline with the disappearance of pollen. However, the increase above baseline at the peak of the season was not significant for any of the parameters measured, suggesting that increased reactivity to histamine with seasonal exposure represents a change in baseline rather than an increased sensitivity to histamine itself. This change in baseline reactivity was inhibited in patients undergoing immunotherapy.

Similar studies show nasal hyperresponsiveness to the cholinomimetic agonist methacholine. Druce and others[50] compared the responsiveness of atopic and nonatopic patients to intranasal administration of methacholine by measuring levels of total proteins in recovered nasal washes. They showed significantly more responsiveness in atopic versus nonatopic patients.[50] Measuring the volume of generated nasal secretions in response to increasing doses of methacholine, Borum[30] showed that patients with perennial rhinitis had a significantly more pronounced secretory response than did healthy subjects.[30] Klementsson and others[89] also measured the secretory response to methacholine before and after antigen challenge of allergic patients out of season and observed significant increases over baseline in methacholine-induced secretions at 2, 4, 6, 8, 10, and 24 hours after antigen challenge. Although the numbers of eosinophils in nasal secretions increased significantly after antigen challenge, their numbers did not correlate with the increase in nonspecific hyperresponsiveness to methacholine. The same investigators also showed increased responsiveness to methacholine and a significant increase in eosinophils in nasal brushings during a weak pollen season; both were inhibited significantly by pretreatment with budesonide.[90] Again, number of eosinophils did not correlate with the degree of secretory responsiveness. These observations suggest that the allergen-induced increase in nonspecific responsiveness to methacholine is a complex phenomenon that is not solely dependent on eosinophil influx into the nasal mucosa.

In allergic patients during the allergy season, the hyperresponsiveness caused by nonspecific irritants probably reflects complex interactions among inflammatory cellular influx, epithelial injury, and increased end organ responsiveness caused by exposure to antigen.

The pathophysiologic mechanisms in allergic rhinitis can be synthesized in the following scenario (Fig. 13-7): sensitization of the nasal mucosa to a certain allergen entails multiple interactions among APC cells, T lymphocytes, and B cells that lead to the production of antigen-specific IgE antibodies, which then localize to mast cells and basophils. Subsequent exposure leads to cross-linking of specific IgE receptors on mast cells and their resultant degranulation, with the release of a host of inflammatory mediators that are, in large part, responsible for allergic nasal symptoms. Other proinflammatory substances are also generated after antigen exposure, most prominent is eosinophil products and cytokines. Cytokines are thought to be generated, in part, by lymphocytes, which are abundant in resting and stimulated nasal mucosa. Recent evidence also points to an important

role for mast cells in the storage and probable production and secretion of cytokines. Cytokines will upregulate adhesion molecules on the vascular endothelium, and possibly on marginating leukocytes, and lead to the migration of these inflammatory cells into the site of tissue inflammation. Various cytokines will also promote the chemotaxis and survival of these recruited inflammatory cells and lead to a secondary immune response by virtue of their capability to promote IgE synthesis by B cells. Also important is the nervous system, which amplifies the allergic reaction by central and peripheral reflexes that result in changes at sites distant from those of antigen deposition. These changes lower the threshold of mucosal responsiveness to various specific and nonspecific stimuli, making allergic patients more responsive to stimuli to which they are exposed every day.

This overview of the immune system examines its different components, which include cell-mediated and humoral immunity, the complement system, and the various phagocytic cells functioning in concert to protect the body from foreign invaders. When the immune system behaves in a misdirected fashion, however, disease states develop from the injurious effects of this powerful system. The pathophysiology of one such disease process frequently

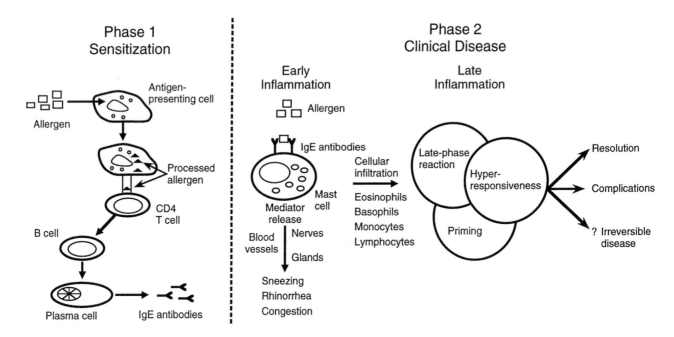

Fig. 13-7. Pathophysiology of allergic rhinitis. The first stage of development of allergic rhinitis involves antigen processing and the production of specific immunoglobulin E (IgE) antibodies, which attach to mast cells, basophils, and other inflammatory cells. On subsequent exposure to the same allergen, IgE receptors on the surface of mast cells are cross-linked, leading to the degranulation of these cells and the release of preformed and newly synthesized mediators that are responsible for symptoms of the disease. There is also recruitment of inflammatory cells to the nasal mucosa and a resultant state of chronic inflammation with a heightened state of reactivity to specific and nonspecific stimuli, a hallmark of allergic nasal disease. In addition to the early and late inflammatory responses, exposure to allergen leads to a secondary immune response with increased production of specific IgE and a perpetuation of the state of susceptibility to allergen. (From Naclerio RM: Allergic rhinitis, *N Engl J Med* 325:860, 1991.)

encountered by otolaryngologists, allergic rhinitis, is discussed in detail.

REFERENCES

1. Abu-Ghazaleh RI and others: IgA-induced eosinophil degranulation, *J Immunol* 42:2393, 1989.
2. Ackerman SJ: *Eosinophils: biologic and clinical aspects in allergy and inflammation.* In Rich RR and others, editors: *Clinical immunology: principles and practice,* vol 1, St Louis, 1996, Mosby–Year Book.
3. Alam R and others: RANTES is a chemotactic and activating factor for human eosinophils, *J Immunol* 150:3442, 1993.
4. Albelda SM, Buck CA: Integrins and other cell adhesion molecules, *FASEB J* 4:2868, 1990.
5. Andersson M, Andersson P, Pipkorn U: Allergen-induced specific and non-specific nasal reactions: reciprocal relationship and inhibition by topical glucocortico-steroids, *Acta Otolaryngol (Stockh)* 107:270, 1989.
6. Bacci S and others: Localization of nitric oxide synthase immunoreactivity in mast cells of human nasal mucosa, *Histochemistry* 102:89, 1994.
7. Bachert C, Wagenmann M, Hauser U: Proinflammatory cytokines: measurement in nasal secretion and induction of adhesion receptor expression, *Int Arch Allergy Immunol* 107:106, 1995.
8. Bancereau J, Rousset F: Human B lymphocytes: phenotype, proliferation, and differentiation, *Adv Immunol* 52:125, 1992.
9. Bancroft GJ, Schreiber RD, Unanue ER: Natural immunity: a T cell-independent pathway of macrophage activation, defined in the scid mouse, *Immunol Rev* 124:5, 1991.
10. Baraniuk JN and others: Substance P and neurokinin A in human nasal mucosa, *Am J Respir Cell Mol Biol* 4:228, 1991.
11. Baraniuk JN and others: Vasoactive intestinal peptide (VIP) in human nasal mucosa, *J Clin Invest* 86:825, 1990.
12. Barcena A and others: Interplay between IL-2 and IL-4 in human thymocyte differentiation: antagonism or agonism, *Int Immunol* 3:419, 1991.
13. Baroody FM and others: Histamine (HIS) release and physiologic changes during the early reaction to antigen, *J Allergy Clin Immunol* 89:303, 1992 (abstract).
14. Baroody FM and others: Intranasal beclomethasone inhibits antigen-induced nasal hyperresponsiveness to histamine, *J Allergy Clin Immunol* 90:373, 1992.
15. Baroody FM and others: Physiologic responses and histamine release after nasal antigen challenge: effect of atropine, *Am J Respir Crit Care Med* 149:1457, 1994.
16. Baroody FM, Wagenmann M, Naclerio RM: A comparison of the secretory response of the nasal mucosa to histamine and methacholine, *J Appl Physiol* 74:2661, 1993.
17. Bascom R and others: Basophil influx occurs after nasal antigen challenge: effects of topical corticosteroid pretreatment, *J Allergy Clin Immunol* 81:580, 1988.
18. Bascom R, Kagey-Sobotka A, Proud D: Effect of intranasal capsaicin on symptoms and mediator release, *J Pharmacol Exp Ther* 259:1323, 1991.
19. Bascom R and others: Major basic protein and eosinophil-derived neurotoxin concentrations in nasal lavage fluid after antigen challenge: effect of systemic corticosteroids and relationship to eosinophil influx, *J Allergy Clin Immunol* 84:338, 1989.
20. Baumann H, Gauldie J: The acute phase response, *Immunol Today* 15:74, 1994.
21. Baumgarten CR and others: Concentration of glandular kallikrein in human nasal secretions increases during experimentally induced allergic rhinitis, *J Immunol* 137:1323, 1986.
22. Baumgarten CR and others: Influx of kininogens into nasal secretions following antigen challenge of allergic individuals, *J Clin Invest* 76:191, 1985.
23. Baumgarten CR and others: Plasma kallikrein during experimentally induced allergic rhinitis: role in kinin formation and contribution of TAME-esterase activity, *J Immunol* 137:977, 1986.
24. Beck LA and others: Detection of the chemokine RANTES and endothelial adhesion molecules in nasal polyps, *J Allergy Clin Immunol* 98:766, 1996.
25. Bentley AM and others: Immunohistology of the nasal mucosa in seasonal allergic rhinitis: increase in activated eosinophils and epithelial mast cells, *J Allergy Clin Immunol* 89:877, 1992.
26. Bevilacqua MP and others: Interleukin 1 acts on cultured human vascular endothelium to increase the adhesion of polymorphonuclear leukocytes, monocytes and related leukocytic cell lines, *J Clin Invest* 76:2003, 1985.
27. Bevilacqua MP, Nelson RM: Selectins, *J Clin Invest* 91:379, 1993.
28. Bochner BS and others: Adherence of human basophils to cultured umbilical vein vascular endothelial cells, *J Clin Invest* 81:1355, 1988.
29. Bochner BS and others: Adhesion of human basophils, eosinophils, and neutrophils to interleukin 1-activated human vascular endothelial cells: contribution of endothelial cell adhesion molecules, *J Exp Med* 173:1553, 1991.
30. Borum P: Nasal methacholine challenge: a test for the measurement of nasal reactivity, *J Allergy Clin Immunol* 63:253, 1979.
31. Bouwens L, Wisse E: Pit cells in the liver, *Liver* 12:3, 1992.
32. Bradding P and others: Cytokine immunoreactivity in seasonal rhinitis: regulation by a topical corticosteroid, *Am J Respir Crit Care Med* 151:1900, 1995.
33. Bradding P and others: Immunolocalization of cytokines in the nasal mucosa of normal and perennial rhinitic subjects: the mast cell as a source of IL-4, IL-5, and IL-6 in human allergic mucosal inflammation, *J Immunol* 151:3853, 1993.
34. Bradding P and others: Interleukin 4 is localized to and released by human mast cells, *J Exp Med* 176:1381, 1992.
35. Braunstein G and others: Clinical and inflammatory responses to exogenous tachykinins in allergic rhinitis, *Am Rev Respir Dis* 144:630, 1991.
36. Bryan WTK, Bryan MP: Significance of mast cells in nasal secretions, *Trans Am Acad Ophthalmol Otolaryngol* 63:613, 1959.
37. Castano L, Eisenbarth GS: Type-I diabetes: a chronic autoimmune disease of human, mouse, and rat, *Annu Rev Immunol* 8:647, 1990.
38. Castells M, Schwartz LB: Tryptase levels in nasal lavage fluid as an indicator of the early allergic reaction, *J Allergy Clin Immunol* 82:348, 1988.
39. Clutterbuck EJ, Hirst EMA, Sanderson CJ: Human interleukin-5 (IL-5) regulates the production of eosinophils in human bone marrow cultures: comparison and interaction with IL-1, IL-3, IL-6 and GM-CSF, *Blood* 73:1504, 1989.
40. Connell JT: Quantitative intranasal pollen challenge: III. The priming effect in allergic rhinitis, *J Allergy* 43:33, 1969.
41. Creticos PS and others: Peptide leukotriene release after antigen challenge in patients sensitive to ragweed, *N Engl J Med* 310:1626, 1984.
42. Dalloul AH and others: Thymic epithelial cell-derived supernatants sustain the maturation of human prothymocytes: involvement of interleukin 1 and CD23, *Eur J Immunol* 21:2633, 1991.
43. DeFrance T, Banchereau J: *Role of cytokines in the ontogeny, activation and proliferation of B lymphocytes,* London, 1990, Academic Press.
44. DeFrance T and others: Interleukin 10 and transforming growth factor beta cooperate to induce anti-CD40-activated naive human B cells to secrete immunoglobulin A, *J Exp Med* 175:671, 1992.
45. Delacroix DL and others: Selective transport of polymeric immunoglobulin A in bile, *J Clin Invest* 70:230, 1982.
46. Del Prete G and others: IL-4 is an essential co-factor for the IgE synthesis induced in vitro by human T cell clones and their supernatants, *J Immunol* 140:4193, 1988.

47. Denburg JA, Silver JE, Abrams JS: Interleukin-5 is a human baso-philopoietin: induction of histamine content and basophilic differentiation of HL-60 cells and of peripheral blood basophil-eosinophil progenitors, *Blood* 77:1462, 1991.

48. Dobrina A and others: Mechanisms of eosinophil adherence to cultured vascular endothelial cells: eosinophils bind to the cytokine-induced endothelial ligand vascular cell adhesion molecule-1 via the very late activation antigen-4 integrin receptor, *J Clin Invest* 88:20, 1991.

49. Dorshkind K: Regulation of hemopoiesis by bone marrow stromal cells and their products, *Annu Rev Immunol* 8:111, 1990.

50. Druce HM and others: Cholinergic nasal hyperreactivity in atopic subjects, *J Allergy Clin Immunol* 76:445, 1985.

51. Durham SR and others: Cytokine messenger RNA expression for IL-3, IL-4, IL-5, and granulocyte/macrophage-colony-stimulating factor in the nasal mucosa after local allergen provocation: relationship to tissue eosinophilia, *J Immunol* 148:2390, 1992.

52. Durham SR, Kay AB, Hamid Q: Changes in allergic inflammation associated with successful immunotherapy, *Int Arch Allergy Immunol* 107:282, 1995.

53. Dvoracek JE and others: Induction of nasal late-phase reactions by insufflation of ragweed-pollen extract, *J Allergy Clin Immunol* 73:363, 1984.

54. Ebisawa M and others: Eosinophil transendothelial migration induced by cytokines: III. Effect of the chemokine RANTES, *J Immunol* 153:2153, 1994.

55. Ebisawa M and others: Eosinophil transendothelial migration induced by cytokines: II. Potentiation of eosinophil transendothelial migration by eosinophil-active cytokines, *J Immunol* 152:4590, 1994.

56. Ebisawa M and others: Eosinophil transendothelial migration induced by cytokines: I. Role of endothelial and eosinophil adhesion molecules in IL-1 β-induced transendothelial migration, *J Immunol* 149:4021, 1992.

57. Enerback L, Pipkorn U, Granerus G: Intraepithelial migration of nasal mucosal mast cells in hay fever, *Int Arch Allergy Appl Immunol* 80:44, 1986.

58. Erickson N, Quesenberry PJ: Regulation of erythropoiesis: the role of growth factors, *Med Clin North Am* 76:745, 1992.

59. Fokkens WJ and others: Fluctuation of the number of CD-1 (T6)-positive dendritic cells, presumably Langerhans cells, in the nasal mucosa of patients with an isolated grass-pollen allergy before, during, and after the grass-pollen season, *J Allergy Clin Immunol* 84:39, 1989.

60. Foy TM and others: *In vivo* CD40-gp39 interactions are essential for thymus-dependent immunity: II. Prolonged in vivo suppression of primary and secondary humoral immune responses by an antibody targeted to the CD40 ligand, gp39, *J Exp Med* 178:1567, 1993.

61. Freeland H and others: Leukotriene B$_4$ as a mediator of early and late reactions to antigen in humans: the effect of systemic glucocorticoid treatment in vivo, *J Allergy Clin Immunol* 83:634, 1989.

62. Furukawa K and others: Expression of nitric oxide synthase in the human nasal mucosa, *Am J Respir Crit Care Med* 153:847, 1996.

63. Gadol N, Peacock MA, Ault KA: Antigenic phenotype and functional characterization of human tonsil B cells, *Blood* 71:1048, 1988.

64. Gascan H and others: Human B cell clones can be induced to proliferate and to switch to IgE and IgG4 synthesis by interleukin 4 and a signal provided by activated CD4$^+$ T cell clones, *J Exp Med* 173:747, 1991.

65. Gascan H and others: Regulation of human IgE synthesis, *Clin Exp Allergy* 21:162, 1991.

66. Gell PGH, Coombs RRA: *Clinical aspects of immunology,* Oxford, 1963, Blackwell.

67. Gomez E and others: Direct *in vivo* evidence for mast cell degranulation during allergen-induced reactions in man, *J Allergy Clin Immunol* 78:637, 1986.

68. Goodman T, Lefrancois L: Intraepithelial lymphocytes: anatomical

69. Gorter A and others: IgA- and secretory IgA-opsonized *S. aureus* induce a respiratory burst and phagocytosis by polymorphonuclear leucocytes, *Immunology* 61:303, 1987.

70. Gosset P and others: Interleukin-6 and interleukin-1 alpha production is associated with antigen-induced late nasal response, *J Allergy Clin Immunol* 92:878, 1993.

71. Gray JD, Horwitz DA: Lymphocytes expressing type 3 receptors proliferate in response to interleukin 2 and are the precursors of lymphokine-activated killer cells, *J Clin Invest* 81:1247, 1988.

72. Hamid Q and others: Co-expression of CD25 and CD3 in atopic allergy and asthma, *Immunology* 75:659, 1992.

73. Hansel TT and others: Induction and function of eosinophil intercellular adhesion molecule-1 and HLA-DR, *J Immunol* 149:2130, 1992.

74. Hastie R, Heroy JH, Levy DA: Basophil leukocytes and mast cells in human nasal secretions and scrapings studied by light microscopy, *Lab Invest* 40:554, 1979.

75. Hemler ME: VLA proteins in the integrin family: structures, functions, and their role on leukocytes, *Annu Rev Immunol* 8:365, 1990.

76. Heyworth CM and others: Stem cell factor directly stimulates the development of enriched granulocyte-macrophage colony-forming cells and promotes the effects of other colony stimulating factors, *Blood* 80:2230, 1992.

77. Hirai K and others: Enhancement of human basophil histamine release by interleukin 5, *J Exp Med* 172:1525, 1990.

78. Holm AF and others: Effect of 3 months' nasal steroid therapy on nasal T cells and Langerhans cells in patients suffering from allergic rhinitis, *Allergy* 50:204, 1995.

79. Holzer P: Capsaicin: cellular targets, mechanisms of action, and selectivity for thin sensory neurons, *Pharmacol Rev* 43:143, 1991.

80. Huber AR and others: Regulation of transendothelial neutrophil migration by endogenous interleukin-8, *Science* 254:99, 1991.

81. Husband AJ, Gowans JL: The origin and antigen-dependent distribution of IgA-containing cells in the intestine, *J Exp Med* 148:1146, 1978.

82. Itoh N and others: The polypeptide encoded by the cDNA for human cell surface antigen Fas can mediate apoptosis, *Cell* 66:233, 1991.

83. Jabra HJ and others: CD40 and IgE: synergism between anti-CD40 monoclonal antibody and interleukin 4 in the induction of IgE synthesis by highly purified human B cells, *J Exp Med* 172:1861, 1990.

84. Juliusson S and others: Mast cells and eosinophils in the allergic mucosal response to allergen challenge: changes in distribution and signs of activation in relation to symptoms, *J Allergy Clin Immunol* 90:898, 1992.

85. Kameyoshi Y and others: Cytokine RANTES released by thrombin-stimulated platelets is a potent attractant for human eosinophils, *J Exp Med* 176:587, 1992.

86. Karre K and others: Selective rejection of H-2 deficient lymphoma variants suggests alternative immune defense strategy, *Nature* 319:675, 1986.

87. Kaufmann SHE: Immunity to intracellular bacteria, *Annu Rev Immunol* 11:129, 1993.

88. Kirshenbaum AS and others: Effect of IL-3 and stem cell factor on the appearance of human basophils and mast cells from CD34$^+$ pluripotent progenitor cells, *J Immunol* 148:772, 1992.

89. Klementsson H and others: Changes in non-specific nasal reactivity and eosinophil influx and activation after allergen challenge, *Clin Exp Allergy* 20:539, 1990.

90. Klementsson H and others: Eosinophils, secretory responsiveness and glucocorticoid-induced effects on the nasal mucosa during a weak pollen season, *Clin Exp Allergy* 21:705, 1991.

91. Kojis FG: Serum sickness and anaphylaxis: analysis of 6,211 patients treated with horse serum for various infections, *Am J Dis Child* 64:93, 1942.

92. Kokumai S and others: Effect of capsaicin as a neuropeptide-releasing

substance on sneezing reflex in a type 1 allergic animal model, *Int Arch Allergy Immunol* 98:256, 1992.

93. Konno A, Togawa K: Role of the vidian nerve in nasal allergy, *Ann Otol Rhinol Laryngol* 88:258, 1979.

94. Krensky AM and others: T-lymphocyte-antigen interactions in transplant rejection, *N Engl J Med* 322:510, 1990.

95. Kuhn LC, Kraehenbuhl JP: Role of secretory component, a secreted glycoprotein, in the specific uptake of IgA dimer by epithelial cells, *J Biol Chem* 254:11072, 1979.

96. Lacroix JS and others: Improvement of symptoms of non-allergic chronic rhinitis by local treatment with capsaicin, *Clin Exp Allergy* 21:595, 1991.

97. Lamas AM, Mulroney CR, Schleimer RP: Studies on the adhesive interaction between human eosinophils and cultured vascular endothelial cells, *J Immunol* 140:1500, 1988.

98. Lanier LL and others: The relationship of CD16 (Leu-11) and Leu-19 (NKH-1) antigen expression on human peripheral blood NK cells and cytotoxic T lymphocytes, *J Immunol* 136:4480, 1986.

99. Lanzavecchia A: Antigen-specific interaction between T and B cells, *Nature* 314:537, 1985.

100. Lee BJ and others: Upregulation of vascular cell adhesion molecule-1 (VCAM-1) after nasal allergen (Ag) challenge, *J Allergy Clin Immunol* 94:1006, 1994.

101. Lefrancois L, Goodman T: In vivo modulation of cytolytic activity and Thy-1 expression in TCR $\gamma\delta$ intraepithelial lymphocytes, *Science* 243:1716, 1989.

102. Lim MC, Taylor RM, Naclerio RM: The histology of allergic rhinitis and its comparison to nasal lavage, *Am J Respir Crit Care Med* 151:136, 1995.

103. Linden M and others: Nasal cytokines in common cold and allergic rhinitis, *Clin Exp Allergy* 25:166, 1995.

104. Linsley PS and others: Binding of the B cell activation antigen B7 to CD28 costimulates T cell proliferation and interleukin 2 mRNA accumulation, *J Exp Med* 173:721, 1991.

105. Lo SK and others: Endothelial-leukocyte adhesion molecule-1 stimulates the adhesive activity of leukocyte integrin CR3 (CD11b/CD18, Mac-1, $\alpha_m\beta_2$) on human neutrophils, *J Exp Med* 173:1493, 1991.

106. Lopez AF and others: Recombinant human interleukin 5 is a selective activator of human eosinophil function, *J Exp Med* 167:219, 1988.

107. Lung MA, Widdicombe JG: Lung reflexes and nasal vascular resistance in the anaesthetized dog, *J Physiol* 386:465, 1987.

108. Luscinskas FW and others: Cytokine-activated human endothelial monolayers support enhanced neutrophil transmigration via a mechanism involving both endothelial-leukocyte adhesion molecule-1 and intracellular adhesion molecule-1, *J Immunol* 146:1617, 1991.

109. Majchel AM and others: The nasal response to histamine challenge: effect of the pollen season and immunotherapy, *J Allergy Clin Immunol* 90:85, 1992.

110. Martin U and others: Increased levels of exhaled nitric oxide during nasal and oral breathing in subjects with seasonal rhinitis, *J Allergy Clin Immunol* 97:768, 1996.

111. Masuyama K and others: Topical glucocorticosteroid (fluticasone propionate) inhibits cells expressing cytokine mRNA for interleukin-4 in the nasal mucosa in allergen-induced rhinitis, *Immunology* 82:192, 1994.

112. Mendoza JF and others: Evidence that G-CSF is a fibroblast growth factor that induces granulocytes to increase phagocytosis and to present a mature morphology, and that macrophages secrete 45-kd molecules with these activities as well as with G-CSF like activity, *Exp Hematol* 18:903, 1990.

113. Miadonna MA and others: Evidence of PAF-acether metabolic pathway activation in antigen challenge of upper respiratory airways, *Am Rev Respir Dis* 140:142, 1989.

114. Montefort S and others: The expression of leukocyte-endothelial adhesion molecules is increased in perennial allergic rhinitis, *Am J Respir Cell Mol Biol* 7:393, 1992.

115. Moser R and others: Interleukin 1 and tumor necrosis factor stimulate

116. Moser R and others: Migration of primed human eosinophils across cytokine-activated endothelial cell monolayers, *Blood* 79:2937, 1992.

117. Mosimann BL and others: Substance P, calcitonin gene-related peptide, and vasoactive intestinal peptide increase in nasal secretions after allergen challenge in atopic patients, *J Allergy Clin Immunol* 92:95, 1993.

118. Mosmamn TR, Coffman RL: THI and TH2 cells: different patterns of lymphokine secretion lead to different functional properties, *Annu Rev Immunol* 7:145, 1989.

119. Naclerio RM and others: Inflammatory mediators in late antigen-induced rhinitis, *N Engl J Med* 313:65, 1985.

120. Naclerio RM and others: Mediator release after airway challenge with antigen, *Am Rev Respir Dis* 128:597, 1983.

121. Nagler A and others: Comparative studies of human FcRIII-positive and negative natural killer cells, *J Immunol* 143:3183, 1989.

122. Nathanson I, Widdicombe JG, Barnes PJ: Effect of vasoactive intestinal peptide on ion transport across dog tracheal epithelium, *J Appl Physiol* 55:1844, 1983.

123. Neben TY and others: Recombinant human interleukin-11 stimulates megakaryocytopoiesis and increases peripheral platelets in normal and splenectomized mice, *Blood* 81:901, 1993.

124. Nieber K and others: Substance P and b-endorphin-like immunoreactivity in lavage fluids of subjects with and without allergic asthma, *J Allergy Clin Immunol* 90:646, 1992.

125. Noelle RJ, Ledbetter JA, Aruffo A: CD40 and its ligand, an essential ligand-receptor pair for thymus-dependent B cell activation, *Immunol Today* 13:431, 1992.

126. Ohtsuka H and others: Heterogeneity of metachromatic cells in the human nose: significance of mucosal mast cells, *J Allergy Clin Immunol* 76:695, 1985.

127. Okamoto Y and others: Cytokine expression after the topical administration of substance P to human nasal mucosa: the role of substance P in nasal allergy, *J Immunol* 151:4391, 1993.

128. Okayama M and others: Muscarinic receptor subtypes in human nasal mucosa: characterization, autoradiographic localization, and function in vitro, *Am J Respir Cell Mol Biol* 8:176, 1993.

129. Okuda M, Kawabori S, Otsaka H: Electron microscope study of basophilic cells in allergic nasal secretions, *Arch Otorhinolaryngol* 221:215, 1978.

130. Okuda M, Ohtsuka M: Basophilic cells in allergic nasal secretions, *Arch Otorhinolaryngol* 214:283, 1977.

131. Okuda M, Ohtsuka H, Kawabori S: Basophil leukocytes and mast cells in the nose, *Eur J Respir Dis* 64(suppl 128):7, 1983.

132. Okuda M and others: Ultrastructural heterogeneity of the basophilic cells in the allergic nasal mucosa, *Ann Allergy* 154:152, 1985.

133. Parronchi P and others: Allergen and bacterial antigen-specific T cell clones established from atopic donors show a different profile of cytokine production, *Proc Natl Acad Sci U S A* 88:4538, 1991.

134. Parronchi P and others: IL-4 and IFN (alpha and gamma) exert opposite regulatory effects on the development of cytolytic potential by T_{H1} or T_{H2} human T cell clones, *J Immunol* 149:2977, 1992.

135. Pelikan Z: Late and delayed responses of the nasal mucosa to allergen challenge, *Ann Allergy* 41:37, 1978.

136. Perussia B, London L, Trinchieri G: Phenotypic characteristics of human natural killer cells, *Biomed Pharmacother* 39:13, 1985.

137. Petersson G and others: Capsaicin evokes secretion of nasal fluid and depletes substance P and calcitonin-gene related peptide from the nasal mucosa in the rat, *Br J Pharmacol* 98:930, 1989.

138. Petz LD, Branch DR: *Drug induced immune hemolytic anemia.* In Chaplin H, editor: *Methods in hematology,* vol 12, New York, 1985, Churchill Livingstone.

139. Philip G, Sanico AM, Togias A: Inflammatory cellular influx follows capsaicin nasal challenge, *Am J Respir Crit Care Med* 153:1222, 1996.

140. Philip G and others: The human nasal response to capsaicin, *J Allergy Clin Immunol* 94:1035, 1994.

141. Punnonen J and others: Interleukin 13 induces interleukin 4-independent IgG4 and IgE synthesis and CD23 expression by human B cells, *Proc Natl Acad Sci U S A* 90:3730, 1993.

142. Rand TH and others: CD4-mediated stimulation of human eosinophils: lymphocyte chemoattractant factor and other CD4-binding ligands elicit eosinophil migration, *J Exp Med* 173:1521, 1991.

143. Raphael GD and others: Pathophysiology of rhinitis: II. Assessment of the sources of protein in histamine-induced nasal secretions, *Am Rev Respir Dis* 139:791, 1989.

144. Raphael GD and others: The pathophysiology of rhinitis: V. Sources of protein in allergen-induced nasal secretions, *J Allergy Clin Immunol* 88:33, 1991.

145. Rappolee DA, Werb A: *Macrophage-derived growth factors.* In Russell SW, Gordon S, editors: *Macrophage biology and activation,* Berlin, 1992, Springer-Verlag.

146. Rot A and others: RANTES and macrophage inflammatory protein 1 alpha induce the migration and activation of normal human eosinophil granulocytes, *J Exp Med* 176:1489, 1992.

147. Saito H and others: Selective differentiation and proliferation of hematopoietic cells induced by recombinant human interleukins, *Proc Natl Acad Sci U S A* 85:2288, 1988.

148. Schall TJ and others: Selective attraction of monocytes and T lymphocytes of the memory phenotype by cytokine RANTES, *Nature* 347:669, 1990.

149. Schierhorn K and others: Substance-P-induced histamine release from human nasal mucosa in vitro, *Int Arch Allergy Immunol* 107:109, 1995.

150. Schleimer RP and others: IL-4 induces adherence of human eosinophils and basophils but not neutrophils to endothelium: association with expression of VCAM-1, *J Immunol* 148:1086, 1992.

151. Schleimer RP, Rutledge BK: Cultured human vascular endothelial cells acquire adhesiveness for leukocytes following stimulation with interleukin-1, endotoxin, and tumor promoting phorbol esters, *J Immunol* 136:649, 1986.

152. Schroeder JT and others: IgE-dependent IL-4 secretion by human basophils: the relationship between cytokine production and histamine release in mixed leukocyte cultures, *J Immunol* 153:1808, 1994.

153. Seaman WE and others: Depletion of natural killer cells in mice by monoclonal antibody to NK-1.1: reduction in host defense against malignancy without loss of cellular or humoral immunity, *J Immunol* 138:4539, 1987.

154. Seder RA, Paul WE: Acquisition of lymphokine-producing phenotype by CD4+ T cells, *Annu Rev Immunol* 12:635, 1994.

155. Sher A, Ottesen E: *Immunoparasitology.* In Samter M and others, editors: *Immunological diseases,* ed 4, Boston, 1988, Little, Brown.

156. Sim TC and others: Proinflammatory cytokines in nasal secretions of allergic subjects after antigen challenge, *Am J Respir Crit Care Med* 149:339, 1994.

157. Sim TC and others: Secretion of chemokines and other cytokines in allergen-induced nasal responses: inhibition by topical steroid treatment, *Am J Respir Crit Care Med* 152:927, 1995.

158. Springer TA: Adhesion receptors of the immune system, *Nature* 346:425, 1990.

159. Stahl CP and others: Differential effects of sequential, simultaneous, and single agent interleukin-3 and granulocyte-macrophage colony-stimulating factor on megakaryocyte maturation and platelet response in primates, *Blood* 80:2479, 1992.

160. Steel D, Whitehead AS: The major acute phase reactants: C-reactive protein, serum amyloid P component and serum amyloid A protein, *Immunol Today* 15:81, 1994.

161. Stern M and others: Apoptosis in human eosinophils: programmed cell death in the eosinophil leads to phagocytosis by macrophages and is modulated by IL-5, *J Immunol* 148:3543, 1992.

162. Storkus WJ and others: Reversal of natural killing susceptibility in target cells expressing transfected class I HLA genes, *Proc Natl Acad Sci U S A* 86:2361, 1989.

163. Sung CP, Arleth AJ, Feverstein GZ: Neuropeptide Y upregulates the adhesiveness of human endothelial cells for leukocytes, *Clin Res* 68:314, 1991.

164. Takahashi T and others: Megakaryocyte potentiating activity of IL-1, IL-6 and GM-CSF as evaluated by their action on in vitro human megakaryocytic colonies, *Br J Haematol* 78:480, 1991.

165. Tepper RI and others: IL-4 induces allergic-like inflammatory disease and alters T cell development in transgenic mice, *Cell* 62:457, 1990.

166. Tepper RI, Pattengale PK, Leder P: Murine interleukin-4 displays potent anti-tumor activity in vivo, *Cell* 57:503, 1989.

167. Thornhill MH, Kyan-Aung U, Haskard DO: IL-4 increases human endothelial cell adhesiveness for T cells but not for neutrophils, *J Immunol* 144:3060, 1990.

168. Timonen T, Ortaldo JR, Herberman RB: Characteristics of human large granular lymphocytes and relationship to natural killer and NK cells, *J Exp Med* 153:569, 1981.

169. Tony H, Phillips NE, Parker DC: Role of membrane immunoglobulin (Ig) crosslinking in membrane Ig-mediated, major histocompatibility complex-restricted T cell-B cooperation, *J Exp Med* 162:1695, 1985.

170. Tsuda T and others: Synergistic effects of nerve growth factor and granulocyte-macrophage colony-stimulating factor on human basophilic cell differentiation, *Blood* 77:971, 1991.

171. Underdown BJ, Schiff JM: Immunoglobulin A: strategic defense initiated at the mucosal surface, *Annu Rev Immunol* 4:389, 1986.

172. Varney VA and others: Immunohistology of the nasal mucosa following allergen-induced rhinitis, *Am Rev Respir Dis* 146:170, 1992.

173. Verwaerde C and others: Functional properties of a rat monoclonal IgE antibody specific for Schistosoma mansoni, *J Immunol* 138:4441, 1987.

174. Wachs M and others: Observations on the pathogenesis of nasal priming, *J Allergy Clin Immunol* 84:492, 1989.

175. Wagenmann M and others: Bilateral increases in histamine after unilateral nasal allergen challenge, *Am J Respir Crit Care Med* 155:426, 1997.

176. Wagenmann M and others: Unilateral nasal allergen challenge leads to bilateral release of prostaglandin D$_2$, *Clin Exp Allergy* 26:371, 1996.

177. Walden SM and others: Antigen-provoked increase in histamine reactivity: observations on mechanisms, *Am Rev Respir Dis* 143:642, 1991.

178. Walsh GM and others: Human eosinophil, but not neutrophil, adherence to IL-1 stimulated human umbilical vascular endothelial cells is a 4β1 (very late antigen-4) dependent, *J Immunol* 146:3419, 1991.

179. Walsh GM and others: IL-5 enhances the in vitro adhesion of human eosinophils, but not neutrophils, in a leukocyte integrin (CD11/18)-dependent manner, *Immunology* 71:258, 1990.

180. Weissler JC and others: Natural killer cell function in human lung is compartmentalized, *Am Rev Respir Dis* 135:941, 1987.

181. Weller PF: Cytokine regulation of eosinophil function, *Clin Immunol Immunopathol* 62:S55, 1992.

182. Weller PF and others: Human eosinophil adherence to vascular endothelium mediated by binding to vascular cell adhesion molecule-1 and endothelial leukocyte adhesion molecule-1, *Proc Natl Acad Sci U S A* 88:7430, 1991.

183. Weller PF: The immunobiology of eosinophils, *N Engl J Med* 324:1110, 1991.

184. Welsh RM, Vargas-Cortes C: *Natural killer cells in viral infection.* In Lewis CE, McGee JO'D, editors: *The natural killer cell,* Oxford, 1992, Oxford University Press.

185. Ying S and others: Phenotype of cells expressing interleukin-5 mRNA in the nasal mucosa after local allergen provocation, *J Allergy Clin Immunol* 91:252, 1993 (abstract).

186. Zamvil SS, Steinman L: The T lymphocyte in experimental allergic encephalomyelitis, *Annu Rev Immunol* 8:579, 1990.

187. Zuckemman KS, Prince CW, Gay S: *The hemopoietic extracellular matrix.* In Tavassoli M, editor: *Handbook of the hemopoietic microenvironment,* Clifton, NJ, 1989, Humana Press.

Chapter 14

Head and Neck Manifestations of Human Immunodeficiency Virus Infection

Howard W. Francis

HUMAN IMMUNODEFICIENCY VIRUS INFECTION

The human immunodeficiency virus (HIV) attacks the immune system, producing progressive immunocompromise that culminates in the acquired immunodeficiency syndrome (AIDS). The patient becomes increasingly susceptible to an ever widening spectrum of pathologic conditions, including the life-threatening opportunistic infections and neoplasms associated with AIDS.

Cases of idiopathic immune deficiency and unusual infections in homosexual men that were anecdotally reported in the early 1980s have given way to one of the most deadly epidemics in recent history. AIDS remains a major medical challenge as we enter the new millenium, despite unprecedented research efforts by medical, public health, and basic science communities and despite the rapid growth of knowledge about the virology and pathophysiology of HIV infection. The World Health Organization estimates that by the year 2000, HIV will infect 30 million adults and 10 million children.[80] In the United States, more than 15,000 new cases of non-AIDS HIV infection and more than 85,000 new AIDS cases were reported in the year ending June 1994.[32] Approximately 400,000 cases of AIDS have been diagnosed since the beginning of the epidemic.

HIV infection results when body fluids from an infected person inoculate the blood stream of another through a breach in the skin or mucosa or through intravenous infusion. Viral transmission most commonly occurs through homosexual and heterosexual intercourse, the sharing of needles by intravenous drug users (IVDU), the transfusion of contaminated blood products, perinatal transmission from mother to child, and rarely, by accidental puncture wounds in health care workers. In North America, Western Europe, and Australia, HIV transmission by male homosexual intercourse accounts for 60% of cases, whereas transmission through the sharing of needles by IVDUs accounts for 22% of cases.[80] Heterosexual transmission is the fastest growing means of HIV transmission in the United States; the rate of increase of male homosexual and bisexual transmission has slowed.

Biology

HIV is a retrovirus of the lentivirus subfamily, which has an affinity for cells with the CD4$^+$ cell surface marker (e.g., T-helper lymphocytes, macrophages). The primary reservoir of HIV and the epicenter of a deteriorating immune system is the T-helper lymphocyte (CD4$^+$ cell), which coordinates many limbs of the immunologic response to infection.[53,70,159,167] After HIV infects these cells, viral RNA undergoes reverse transcription to deoxyribonucleic acid (DNA), which is then integrated into the host genome. After a dormant period of variable duration, these lymphocytes are activated, resulting in replication of the viral genome and shedding of viral progeny, which infect other cells.[144] The clinical course and manifestations of HIV infection and AIDS are diverse, because of viral heterogeneity and poorly understood host

Table 14-1. Immune dysfunction in human immunodeficiency virus

Components of immune system	Effects of HIV infection
T-helper lymphocytes	Decreased
Macrophages	Impaired antigen presentation, phagocytosis, and chemotaxis
Neutrophils	Dysfunctional or decreased
B lymphocytes	Decreased antigen-specific immunoglobulin production
Complement activation	Defective

factors, which are the cause of much frustration in vaccine development. Frequent transcription errors and the selection over time of the least immunogenic and most pathogenic strains lead to a gradual increase in the virulence of HIV within the same host.[70,159]

As T-helper cells become increasingly dysfunctional and fewer in number, cell-mediated and humoral immunity are adversely affected, resulting in increased vulnerability to infection and neoplasia (Table 14-1).[53] HIV infection is also associated with abnormal immune regulation, resulting in increased atopy and autoimmune disease (e.g., demyelinating neuropathy).

The dysfunction of macrophages, neutrophils, and B lymphocytes in HIV infection compound CD4$^+$ cell deficits, increasing host susceptibility to opportunistic diseases.[70,159] HIV infection impairs the antigen-presenting function of macrophages to the detriment of CD4$^+$ cell response to various organisms. Furthermore, impaired macrophage chemotaxis and phagocytosis and defective intra- and extracellular killing render the patient vulnerable to opportunistic infections (e.g., candidiasis, toxoplasmosis). The production of immunoglobulins by B lymphocytes in response to infection and immunization is blunted, increasing the patient's vulnerability to encapsulated organisms and other bacteria.[29,53,70,119,198] Susceptibility to bacterial and fungal organisms is further increased by neutropenia and neutrophil dysfunction.[51,134] Iatrogenic neutropenia may result from agents used by the HIV-infected patient, such as zidovudine, ganciclovir, and antineoplastic chemotherapy.[46] Concurrent infection with cytomegalovirus (CMV) may also impair neutrophil function.[76,214]

Natural history

Most sequelae of HIV infection in the head and neck region result from its detrimental effects on host immunity. Subtle changes in different arms of the immune system eventually give way to profound immunocompromise and AIDS, rendering the patient increasingly vulnerable to infections and neoplasms. Morbidity may also result from the neurotropism of HIV and its ability to cause neurologic and neurotologic dysfunction.[107]

Approximately 50% of HIV-infected homosexual men are estimated to progress to AIDS within about 9 years from the date of seroconversion.[122,132] The rate of progression may vary with the route of transmission and patient age, shorter latencies occur in congenital and tranfusion-acquired infections.[121] The 5-year mortality rate from the time of diagnosis of AIDS is approximately 80%.[32] The cause of death in most cases is overwhelming infection or disseminated neoplasm.

The differential diagnosis of any lesion in the HIV-infected patient depends on the immune status as indicated by laboratory and clinical data. An especially strong correlation exists between the progression to AIDS and the fall in the absolute number of T-helper lymphocytes or CD4$^+$ cells in the blood. This correlation has led to the use of the CD4$^+$ count in diagnosis, prognosis, and classification of HIV infection. Measurements of quantitative HIV burden using plasma HIV RNA assays are widely used as a guideline for initiating antiretroviral therapy, for monitoring therapy, and for assessing prognosis.[112] Although HIV RNA assays are more predictive of prognosis, the CD4$^+$ count best indicates the likelihood of developing specific HIV-related complications. The otolaryngologist must therefore evaluate each case in the context of the patient's evolving immune status, including the CD4$^+$ count. A knowledge of the Centers for Disease Control (CDC) classification of HIV infection is helpful in this regard.

Diagnosis and classification

HIV infection can be diagnosed when anti-HIV antibodies are detected in the serum by enzyme-linked immunosorbent assay (ELISA) and Western blot. Persistent antibodies against HIV appear within 3 months of infection.

The CDC classification system for HIV infection is based on the history of clinical manifestations and the CD4$^+$ count.[30,52,132] This scheme helps to estimate the level of immunocompromise and associated risks of life-threatening opportunistic diseases in adults and helps to direct prophylactic and antiretroviral therapy. The three clinical categories are (A) asymptomatic HIV infection, persistent generalized lymphadenopathy (PGL), or acute HIV infection (a mononucleosis-like syndrome); (B) symptomatic conditions that are attributed to HIV infection and associated defects in cell-mediated immunity but that are not in categories (A) or (C), e.g., fever and diarrhea of 1 month's duration or more, oral thrush, oral hairy leukoplakia, and fungal sinusitis; and (C) AIDS (Box 14-1).

Patients in each category are further stratified according to their CD4$^+$ counts: (1) 500 cells/μl or more, (2) 200 to 499 cells/μl, and (3) less than 200 cells/μl. The lowest accurate CD4$^+$ count, not the most recent one, is used for classification purposes. AIDS is diagnosed for any patient in category C or 3.

Box 14-1. Conditions that define acquired
immunodeficiency syndrome

Candidiasis, pulmonary or esophageal
Cervical cancer, invasive
Coccidioidomycosis, disseminated or extrapulmonary
Cryptococcosis, extrapulmonary
Cryptosporidiosis, chronic intestinal (> 1 month)
Cytomegalovirus disease (liver, spleen, and nodes excluded)
Cytomegalovirus retinitis
Encephalopathy, human immunodeficiency virus–related
Herpes simplex, chronic ulcers (> 1 month), pulmonary or esophageal
Histoplasmosis, disseminated or extrapulmonary
Isosporiasis, chronic intestinal (> 1 month)
Kaposi's sarcoma
Non-Hodgkin's lymphoma
Mycobacterium avium complex, *Mycobacterium kansasii*, or other species, disseminated or extrapulmonary
Mycobacterium tuberculosis, any site
Pneumocystis carinii pneumonia
Pneumonia, recurrent
Progressive multifocal leukoencephalopathy
Salmonella septicemia, recurrent
Toxoplasmosis of brain
Wasting syndrome caused by human immunodeficiency virus
CD4$^+$ T-helper lymphocyte count less than 200 cells/μl

Taken from Centers for Disease Control: 1993 Revised classification system for HIV infection and expanded surveillance case definition for AIDS among adolescents and adults, *MMWR Morb Mortal Wkly Rep* 41:1, 1992.

Box 14-2. Differential diagnosis of
lymphadenopathy in human
immunodeficiency virus infection

Infectious

Mycobacterial lymphadenitis: tuberculous* and atypical organisms†
Pneumocystis lymphadenitis*
Pneumocystis thyroiditis*
Viral lymphadenitis: cytomegalovirus, Epstein-Barr virus
Toxoplasma lymphadenitis
Bacterial lymphadenitis or abscess secondary to oropharyngeal infection
Cat-scratch disease

Neoplastic

Lymphoma
  Non-Hodgkin's†
  Hodgkin's disease
Metastatic Kaposi's sarcoma†
Metastatic carcinoma
Metastatic melanoma
Salivary gland tumors
Thyroid tumors

Idiopathic

Persistent generalized lymphadenopathy*
Lymphoepithelial cysts of the parotid gland*

* Incidence is significantly increased in human immunodeficiency virus infection.
† Incidence is significantly increased in acquired immunodeficiency syndrome.

CERVICAL DISEASE

The otolaryngologist is often consulted to evaluate cervical adenopathy in the HIV-infected patient. Ideopathic follicular hyperplasia is the most common cause of cervical adenopathy in this patient population and is clinically evident in 12% to 45% of patients.[18,82] However, in this background of hyperplastic adenopathy, cases of infectious and neoplastic etiology exist, including Mycobacterium tuberculosis, Pneumocystis carinii, lymphoma, and Kaposi's sarcoma (KS), and other processes that also occur in the general population (Box 14-2).[100]

Persistent generalized lymphadenopathy

PGL is a common early symptom of HIV infection and a common cause of cervical adenopathy. PGL is defined as lymphadenopathy without an identifiable infectious or neoplastic etiology, which involves two or more extra-inguinal sites for at least 3 months, in a patient at risk for or confirmed to be HIV infected.[9,25,44]

The neck is the third most common site of PGL after the axillary and inguinal regions. In decreasing order, cervical adenopathy occurs in the posterior triangle (85%), the pre- and postauricular regions (51%, 47%), the submandibular triangle (37%), and the occipital region (30%).[2] Enlarged nodes are usually asymptomatic, but when bulky they sometimes elicit pain in the postauricular and axillary regions.[2]

Associated lymphoid hyperplasia in the pharynx may be present, resulting in middle ear effusions secondary to eustachian tube obstruction.

Three histologic patterns occur in PGL lymph nodes: (1) In follicular hyperplasia, follicles increase in number and size and the mantle zones are either irregular (fragmented) or intact (non-fragmented); (2) in follicular involution, follicles are small and mantle zones are absent, whereas germinal centers are either inactive or scarred; (3) in lymphoid depletion, the node is infiltrated by immunoblasts and plasma cells, follicles are absent, and microvascular proliferation is significant.[9,25,44]

As HIV infection approaches end-stage AIDS, the lymph node architecture degenerates from one histologic type to another. Of patients with follicular hyperplasia, 77% progress to follicular involution and lymphoid depletion.[34] It has been proposed that lymph node architecture is of prognostic value in HIV infection because the incidence of constitutional symptoms and opportunistic infections is increased and the life expectancy for patients who progress through these histologic stages is decreased.[9,25,34,44] Proposed mechanisms for this histologic progression include a direct cytopathic effects of HIV or similar effects by other viruses, including Epstein-Barr virus (EBV), CMV, or herpesviruses.

Diagnostic approaches to cervical lymphadenopathy

In an HIV-infected patient, cervical lymphadenopathy due to pathologic processes that pose a health risk to the patient, such as tuberculosis (TB), lymphoma, and metastatic carcinoma, must be differentiated from PGL.

The diagnostic workup of cervical lymphadenopathy (Fig. 14-1) starts with a thorough history and physical examination. All patients with cervical adenopathy of uncertain etiology should be questioned about risk factors for HIV infection and should be tested for the presence of antibodies to HIV. The clinician should question the patient about risk factors for infectious causes of cervical adenopathy, including contact with cats and dogs and exposure to TB, and risk factors for head and neck malignancy, including tobacco and alcohol use. An enlarged lymph node is more likely to be pathologic when certain local and constitutional features are found on history and physical examination.

Bacterial lymphadenitis or lymphomas are suspicious when constitutional symptoms are present in association with enlarged neck nodes. Cervical lymphadenopathy caused by granulomatous disease and lymphoma in HIV infection is associated with weight loss in 33%, night sweats in 50% and fever in 67% of cases.[1,104] However, PGL is also associated with a relatively high incidence of weight loss (24%), night sweats (35%), and fever (47%) caused by other HIV-related processes. Therefore constitutional symptoms by themselves are not very sensitive indicators of infection or malignancy as the cause of cervical lymphadenopathy in an HIV-infected patient.

A thorough head and neck examination should search for possible primary sites of infection or malignancy. The clinician should note the distribution of lymphadenopathy in the neck. The size and mobility of the nodes and the presence of tenderness should also be noted.

Cervical lymphadenopathy that is greater than 2 cm, unilateral, localized, or asymmetric is suspicious for pathology, especially granulomatous disease and lymphomas.[1,175] Pathologic cervical lymphadenopathy should also be suspected in a patient with a moderately to severely depressed CD4+ count who did not have lymphadenopathy at higher cell counts but who now presents with new and rapid-onset adenopathy. Tender adenopathy is more likely to be secondary to bacterial infections, including TB, whereas nontender enlarging neck nodes may result from malignancy.[26] The abdomen should be evaluated for hepatosplenomegaly by percussion and palpation because this finding suggests lym-

phoma. The presence of adenopathy in the axilla and inguinal regions suggests PGL. Laboratory tests and chest radiograph will help narrow the differential diagnosis of cervical lymphadenopathy.

The differential diagnosis of cervical adenopathy is influenced by the immune status as indicated by the history of opportunistic infections and the CD4+ count. For example, lymphoma or mycobacterial infection are more likely to be present when the CD4+ count is less than 100 cells/μl or a history of AIDS is present, whereas PGL is more likely when the CD4+ count is more than 500 cells/μl. Mediastinal adenopathy and pulmonary lesions on chest radiograph may represent lymphoma, TB, fungal infection, or carcinoma related to disease in the neck. The purified protein derivative (PPD) or tuberculin skin test may facilitate the diagnosis of mycobacterial lymphadenitis, but the sensitivity is low, especially in patients with advanced HIV infection, because of the anergy resulting from cellular immunodeficiency. The criterion for a positive result in an HIV-infected patient is a skin reaction greater than 5 mm in diameter, rather than 10 mm as in the general population. The tendency for multiple pathologic processes to co-exist in the HIV-infected patient and the poor sensitivity of many clinical findings and tests often make it necessary to perform microbiologic and histologic evaluations of lymph node tissue.

The high prevalence of PGL in HIV-infected patients makes open biopsy of all suspicious nodes an expensive and unnecessary policy; only 5% to 15% of biopsies would significantly influence therapy if all enlarged cervical nodes were biopsied.[1,104] In some cases, the need for tissue sampling is eliminated by a favorable clinical response to empiric antibiotic therapy. Fine-needle aspiration (FNA) should be the initial method of tissue sampling in most cases of suspicious cervical lymphadenopathy in the HIV-infected patient. Material obtained by FNA should undergo microbacterial and cytologic studies. If lymphoma is diagnosed on FNA, the histologic type should be confirmed by open biopsy before definitive management is rendered.

The diagnostic yield of FNA is increased with multiple passes of the needle while suction is applied to the plunger. The presence of a cytopathologist or a technician is beneficial for two reasons: preparation of the specimen for cytology can be properly and judiciously carried out, and the adequacy of the aspirate for diagnosis can be determined and FNA repeated if necessary. Ultrasound guidance increases the diagnostic yield, especially in nodes that are difficult to palpate. False-negative results can be caused by sampling errors, improper preparation of cytopathology slides, and misinterpretation of the cytologic features.

An FNA diagnosis of follicular hyperplasia should therefore be based on the clinical picture and should not by itself absolve the clinician's suspicion of lymphoma. The false-negative rate for diagnosis of lymphoma by FNA is as high as 40%.[21] Sampling error is the likely cause, especially for Hodgkin's disease (HD), in which diagnosis is based on

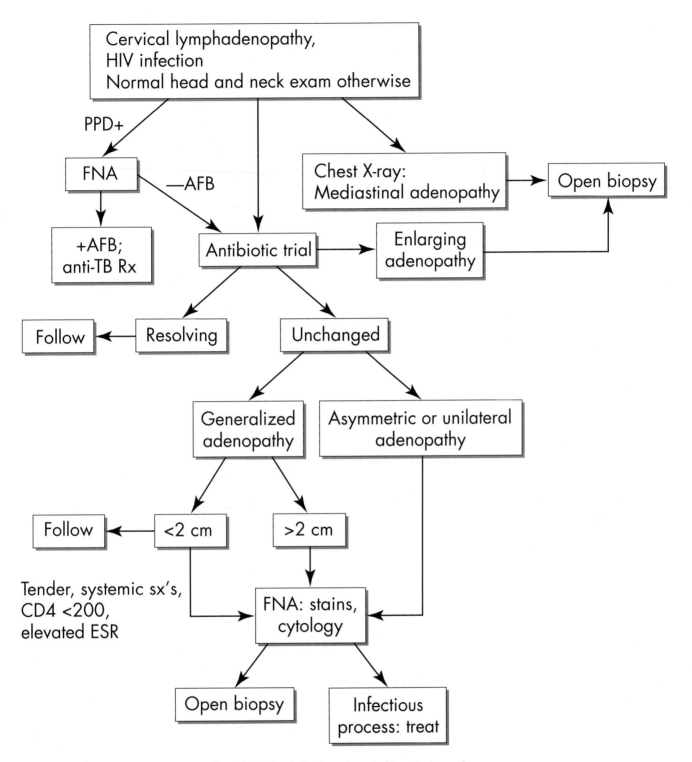

Fig. 14-1. The evaluation of cervical lymphadenopathy.

Box 14-3. Indications for open biopsy of cervical lymphadenopathy in human immunodeficiency virus

Infection

Fine-needle aspiration cytology suggestive of malignancy
Fine-needle aspiration cytology negative and any of the following:
    Enlarging node
    Asymmetric, localized or unilateral adenopathy
    Nodes larger than 2 cm
    Low CD4+ count and new lymphadenopathy
    Fever, night sweats, weight loss
    Significant mediastinal or abdominal adenopathy

---

the presence of Reed-Sternberg cells in the aspirate. Close follow-up and serial examinations of the neck are recommended. Open biopsy should be performed if lymphadenopathy becomes larger or if constitutional symptoms occur.

The decision to perform a diagnostic open biopsy should be driven by a suspicion of malignancy or infection in the setting of a negative or inconclusive FNA (Box 14-3).[43] Nodal tissue should be sampled if nodes are greater than 2 cm and growing; if onset is associated with a low CD4+ count; if lymphadenopathy is asymmetric, unilateral, or localized; and if constitutional symptoms of unknown origin are present. Open biopsy to rule out lymphoma should be performed in a patient with severe immunocompromise or AIDS, mediastinal adenopathy, or hepatosplenomegaly. In the less immunocompromised patient with an otherwise normal physical examination, FNA should be performed first; based on culture, stain, and serology, empiric therapy should be instituted. Open biopsy can follow if FNA is nondiagnostic or if cervical lymphadenopathy becomes larger despite antibiotic therapy. Open biopsy of suspected metastatic carcinoma should be avoided and if possible, the diagnosis made by FNA. When metastatic carcinoma is diagnosed, a thorough examination of the upper aerodigestive tract should be performed under general anesthesia in search of a primary tumor.

Fresh biopsy specimens should be sent directly to the pathologist, who should be informed of the possibility of lymphoma. Tissue should also be sent for culture and stains for mycobacteria and fungi.

HUMAN IMMUNODEFICIENCY VIRUS–ASSOCIATED CYSTIC LYMPHOEPITHELIAL DISEASE OF THE PAROTID GLAND

The major salivary glands and their contained lymph nodes are potential locations of benign and malignant disease. The incidence of primary parotid tumors does not appear to differ between HIV-infected and general populations.

However, the HIV-infected patient is at increased risk for parotid enlargement resulting from benign and malignant lymphoproliferative processes[172] and metastatic disease occurring in intraglandular lymph nodes. For example, lymphoid hyperplasia similar to PGL is an intraglandular nodal response to HIV infection.[147]

Of children with HIV infection, 30% have bilateral parotid enlargement resulting from lymphocytic infiltration of gland parenchyma, which is often associated with pulmonary lymphoid hyperplasia.[163,211] In the severely immunocompromised adult, parotid enlargement may result from an opportunistic malignancy, such as non-Hodgkin's lymphoma (NHL) or metastatic KS.[154] However, in most instances, parotid swelling in adults results from a benign cystic lymphoproliferative process that is associated with ductal metaplasia, known as *benign lymphoepithelial lesion* (BLL).

Parotid cystic lymphoepithelial disease occurs in the earlier stages of HIV infection, almost always in association with PGL.[183,191,197] Parotid swelling is often the only symptom of HIV infection, providing the otolaryngologist the opportunity to make an early diagnosis.[190]

Cystic lymphoepithelial disease produces persistent but nonprogressive and nontender enlargement of the parotid gland with varying proportions of solid and cystic components.[164,191] Parotid disease may be only clinically evident unilaterally, but cystic changes are almost always seen bilaterally on computed tomography (CT) or magnetic resonance imaging (MRI).[188] The histology of BLL is similar to that of Sjogren's syndrome.[196] An exuberant lymphoid hyperplasia almost replaces the parotid parenchyma. Germinal centers, epimyoepithelial islands representing metaplasia of ductal epithelium, and cystic dilation of ducts differentiate this lesion from a lymphoma (Fig. 14-2).[141,183]

HIV-related cystic lymphoepithelial disease of the parotid gland is thought to arise in intraglandular lymph nodes as part of a continuum of lymphoid responses to HIV or associated viral infections.[183] The occurrence of xerophthalmia and xerostomia in a subset of patients and the histologic similarities of BLL in HIV-related parotid swelling and Sjogren's disease suggest that an autoimmune process may be responsible for some cases of parotid enlargement in HIV infection.[188]

The differential diagnosis of parotid enlargement in any patient should include cystic lymphoepithelial disease associated with HIV infection (Box 14-4). A thorough history should include the time of onset; the rate of growth of the mass; the presence of any associated symptoms, such as pain consistent with bacterial sialadenitis, and weight loss, fever, and night sweats consistent with lymphoma or TB. On physical examination, signs of malignancy should be sought, such as induration, fixation, and facial nerve dysfunction. The demonstration of unilateral or bilateral cystic parotid enlargement and PGL on physical examination or radiographic imaging is highly suggestive of cystic lymphoepithelial disease. A chest radiograph should be examined for any associ-

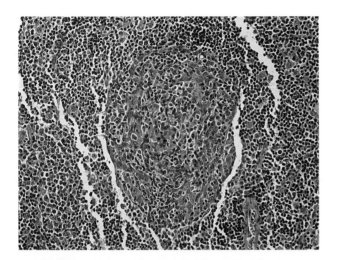

Fig. 14-2. Photomicrograph of an epimyoepithelial island resulting from squamous metaplasia of the ductal epithelium in human immunodeficiency virus–related cystic lymphoepithelial disease of the parotid gland. (×200.)

Box 14-4. Cystic lymphoepithelial disease of the parotid gland

History and physical examination

Parotid swelling: stable size, nontender
Persistent generalized lymphadenopathy
No facial nerve dysfunction

Radiology

Bilateral multicystic disease of parotid glands
Persistent generalized lymphadenopathy

Histopathology

Lymphoid hyperplasia with germinal centers
Metaplasia of ductal epithelium, epimyoepithelial islands
No atypia

---

ated mediastinal adenopathy, which may indicate lymphoma or sarcoidosis. HIV serology should be recommended as part of the workup for parotid swelling, whether or not the usual HIV risk factors exist.

The differential diagnosis of parotid enlargement is narrowed by the identification of cysts on CT, MRI, or ultrasound.[36] The differential diagnosis of cystic parotid disease includes Sjogren's syndrome, cystic Warthin's tumor, and branchial cleft cysts.[188] Bilateral cystic Warthin's tumors can be radiologically differentiated from bilateral cystic lymphoepithelial disease of HIV infection by the presence of focal nodularity in the cyst wall in the former and PGL in the latter. A unilateral mass with a significant solid component is suspicious for neoplasm and ought to be cytologically or histologically evaluated.

Box 14-5. Indications for parotidectomy in the human immunodeficiency virus–infected patient

Fine-needle aspiration cytology suggestive of neoplasm
Fine-needle aspiration cytology negative for neoplasm and any of the following:
   Enlarging mass
   Unilateral parotid mass
   Significant solid component
   Mass firm and fixed
   Facial nerve dysfunction
   Tenderness despite antibiotics
   Constitutional symptoms

FNA can be useful in the diagnosis of the parotid mass and also offers relief of pressure symptoms in patients with large cysts. Aspirates taken from the cystic and solid components should be sent for cytologic and microbiologic evaluations, including fungal and mycobacterial stains and culture.

Indications for parotidectomy include a unilateral parotid mass with a significant solid component or features that are worrisome for malignancy, such as progressive growth, pain, facial nerve dysfunction, or associated constitutional symptoms (Box 14-5).

Cystic lymphoepithelial disease of the parotid glands does not require parotidectomy in most cases. Any further growth or change in parotid swelling should be closely followed up. Parotidectomy may be necessary if the size of the mass changes, if the mass is disfiguring, or to relieve pressure symptoms.

ACQUIRED IMMUNODEFICIENCY SYNDROME–DEFINING NEOPLASMS OF THE HEAD AND NECK

Non-Hodgkin's lymphoma

The strong association between NHL and advanced immunocompromise in the HIV-infected population has led the CDC to designate NHL as an AIDS-defining illness.[31] NHL is also associated with other immunocompromising diseases, such as congenital immunodeficiencies and iatrogenic immunosuppression in organ transplant recipients.[142,188]

Between 1973 and 1987, the incidence of NHL increased tenfold among 20- to 49-year-old men in San Francisco with risk factors for HIV infection.[150] NHL occurs in 10% to 15% of HIV-infected patients.[146,156] The risk of developing NHL steadily rises as the duration of HIV infection and associated immunosuppression increase and as the CD4+ count decreases.[146,166] The incidence of NHL among homosexual men has been shown to increase from 0.8% at 3 years after seroconversion to 2.6% after 8 years of HIV infection.[152] The mean CD4+ count at the diagnosis of NHL is less than 200 cells/μl, and as many as 32% of cases have been previously diagnosed as AIDS.[87] However, NHL may also occur in the setting of relative immune competence and cannot therefore be ruled out based on the absence of either a low CD4+ count or a history of AIDS. Initially, the incidence of NHL was thought to be the same for all routes of HIV infection;[87,101,102,215] however, homosexual, bisexual, and hemophiliac patients now appear to be at greater risk than heterosexual patients and IVDUs, suggesting that an infectious agent may play a role in its pathogenesis.[14]

NHL has more malignant features in HIV-infected patients compared with the general population because of greater host susceptibility and the tendency for more aggressive tumor behavior (Box 14-6). Eighty percent to 90% of NHLs in the HIV-infected population are high-grade B-cell lymphomas compared with 10% to 15% of NHLs in the HIV-negative population.[101,150] These high-grade B-cell lymphomas are most commonly B-immunoblastic or small noncleaved types, which may be of the Burkitt's or non-Burkitt's variety.[105] Burkitt's lymphomas tend to occur earlier in the course of HIV infection when CD4+ counts are relatively high, compared with the immunoblastic and large-cell lymphomas, which in 87% of cases occur in patients already diagnosed with AIDS.[14,157]

The etiology and pathogenesis of AIDS-related NHL is thought to be multifactorial. An infectious agent is thought to have a role in the genesis of these lymphomas because the incidence is higher in some life styles than in others. EBV is considered a possible agent in the pathogenesis of NHL, especially primary central nervous system (CNS) lymphoma.[79] However, 40% to 60% of patients do not have EBV DNA sequences present in lymphoma cells.

Localized nodal disease is uncommon. The prevalence of extranodal disease is high, occuring in 68% to 84% of patients with HIV-related lymphomas compared with 40% in non–HIV-infected patients.* The most prevalent NHL sub-

---

* Refs. 27, 83, 87, 101, 102, 131, 150, 215.

> **Box 14-6.** Features of malignancy in human immunodeficiency virus–infected patients compared with the general population
>
> Younger patients
> Faster regional and systemic spread
> Chemotherapy complicated by opportunistic disease
> Radiotherapy complicated by severe mucositis, exacerbated human immunodeficiency virus–associated periodontal disease
> Higher recurrence rates
> Shorter life expectancy, higher mortality rates
> High histologic grade (non-Hodgkin's lymphoma)
> Extranodal lymphoma (non-Hodgkin's lymphoma and Hodgkin's disease)

types in extranodal sites are the diffuse large-cell and immunoblastic varieties.[156] Common extranodal sites include the CNS, gastrointestinal (GI) tract, bone marrow, and liver. The CNS may be either the site of primary lymphoma or just one of many sites in disseminated disease.

In the head and neck, both nodal and extranodal disease occur. The microscopic features of HIV-related NHL in this region are similar to those in other locations, except for a relatively higher number of CD 30-positive anaplastic large-cell lymphomas.[28] Nodal lymphoma predominates in the neck, which is the most common site of disease in the head and neck region.[83] Nodal lymphoma frequently involves the submandibular, jugulo-digastric, and supraclavicular regions.[174]

The oral cavity and sinonasal region are among the most frequently affected extranodal sites, followed by the pharynx and larynx. In a series of 58 patients with lymphoma of the head and neck, 26 occurred in the neck, 13 in the CNS, 7 in the mandible, 6 in the paranasal sinuses, 3 in the larynx, 2 in the oropharynx, and 1 in the orbit.[55]

NHL of the head and neck may present as a growing mass. Sinonasal lymphoma may present with epistaxis, nasal obstruction, and progressive proptosis and oral extension (see sinonasal lymphoma, discussed later).[55,148] NHL of the oral cavity most commonly affects the gingiva and palate, manifesting as a persistent sore, an enlarging mass, or loose teeth.[113] Hoarseness, respiratory symptoms, and dysphagia may indicate laryngeal or pharyngeal disease. Nasopharyngeal lymphoma often presents with nasal obstruction and serous otitis media (OM). Of HIV-infected patients with NHL, 82% present with fever, night sweats, and unintentional weight loss greater than 10%.[102]

Although lymphoma may be diagnosed on FNA,[174] a biopsy must be performed to determine the histologic type. The search for extranodal disease must be thorough because management and prognosis depend on it. The presence of lymphoma in the CNS and other regions of the head and neck, mediastinum, and abdomen should be investigated by CT or MRI. A bone scan and bone marrow biopsy are useful in staging the lymphoma. A lumbar puncture should be routinely performed because asymptomatic leptomeningeal lymphoma occurs in as many as 60% of cases.[171]

A diagnosis of HIV infection should not be missed in a patient with lymphoma. The increasing prevalence of NHL in the HIV-infected population, which is growing, mandates that all patients newly diagnosed with lymphoma be tested for HIV infection. The prognosis and management of lymphoma are affected by the HIV status of the patient.

The prognosis of NHL is worse in the HIV-infected patient than in the HIV-negative patient because of the relatively advanced stage of the lymphoma and its more aggressive behavior. The increased susceptibility of these patients to serious opportunistic infections, especially while being treated with chemotherapy, is also a frequent cause of morbidity and mortality.[215] Clinical factors that are associated with NHL and that are predictive of short life expectancy (in the order of months) include involvement of the bone marrow, a previous diagnosis of AIDS, a Karnofsky performance status less than 70%, and a CD4$^+$ count less than 200 cells/μl.[102] Kaplan and others[27] demonstrated similar risk factors, except extranodal disease of any location and CD4$^+$ count less than 100 cells/μl were emphasized. The histologic type does not appear to be of predictive value. NHL in cervical lymph nodes respond better to management and are associated with longer survival than extranodal disease of the paranasal sinus, mandible, or other extranodal sites.[55] However, primary lymphoma of the CNS has the worse prognosis because of its association with profound immunosuppression and its tendency to recur.[101]

Multiagent chemotherapy is the primary modality for managing HIV-related NHL. Radiotherapy is useful in the management of localized lymphoma or symptomatic lesions in the head and neck. The therapy must balance the need to eradicate the neoplasm with the risk of further immunosuppression. When used at stage-appropriate doses, chemotherapeutic agents worsen immune function in AIDS patients. Short survival is partly caused by the resulting opportunistic infections[87] (Box 14-7).

Survival is maximized when complete remission is achieved and the immune system is functional. Survival has been improved with the use of low-dose chemotherapy in combination with antiretroviral therapy, *Pneumocystis carinii* pneumonia (PCP) prophylaxis, and CNS prophylaxis.[103,171] Complete remission has been attained in 46% of patients treated with a low-dose modification of M-BACOD (methotrexate, calcium leucovorin, bleomycin doxorubicin, cyclophosphamic vincristine, and dexamethasone) and intrathecal chemotherapy for CNS prophylaxis. Levine and others[103] report that the median survival of patients in whom complete remission was achieved was 15 months compared with 5.6 months for the entire group. Hematopoietic stimulating factors, such as granulocyte-macrophage colony-stimulating factor (GM-CSF), may help prevent bone marrow suppression in these patients during chemotherapy.[88]

Kaposi's sarcoma

KS is a malignant neoplasm of mesenchymal origin, which occurs in three epidemiologic settings: (1) The classic

form occurs in the lower extremities of elderly men of Mediterranean or Ashkenazic Jewish descent. (2) The African (endemic) type is divided into the cutaneous and lymphadenopathic varieties, which occur in black men aged 25 to 40 years and in children aged 2 to 13 years, respectively.[54] Epidemic KS occurs most commonly in patients who are immunocompromised from AIDS or less commonly in organ transplant recipients given immunosuppressive drug therapy.

KS is an AIDS-defining illness that is associated with infection by a new herpes virus-like organism called *KSHV*.[84] The prevalence of KS in homosexual and bisexual HIV-infected men supports the role of a sexually transmittable agent in the pathogenesis of this tumor. The risk of developing KS increases as the CD4$^+$ count decreases to less than 100 cells/μl.[60] KS is also increasingly aggressive at lower cell counts. KS occurs in about 15% of patients with AIDS, of whom 95% are homosexual and bisexual men.[15] The incidence of KS is decreasing as sexual behavior among gay men changes and as IVDU and heterosexual transmission become increasingly common.

Compared with the classic and endemic forms of KS, the epidemic form is more aggressive and responds poorly to therapy. Most patients (90%) have multiple lesions involving the skin, oral mucosa, or lymph nodes. Visceral disease, especially pulmonary KS, is unusual in early cases and tends to be a very late manifestation with a poor prognosis. When treated, it has a high rate of recurrence in the HIV-infected patient. KS is associated with a shortened life expectancy, with a median survival of 408 days after diagnosis. Most patients die of AIDS-related opportunistic infections or lymphoma and not from KS.[33] This tumor can be associated with significant morbidity, such as painful mastication and deglutition.

KS occurs in the head and neck in as many as 63% of cases, in which the skin, mucosa, and lymph nodes may be involved.[179] Cutaneous and mucosal KS occur at about equal rates. Cutaneous KS presents as multicentric purple-red macular lesions that are nontender and nonblanching and frequently progresses to violaceous nodular lesions.[68] In the head and neck, multiple lesions of the postauricular region, scalp, and neck are common. They are usually asymptomatic but may become pruritic and aesthetically displeasing when lesions coalesce.

Mucosal KS most commonly occurs in the oral cavity, which is the initial site of presentation in as many as 20%.[54,68,179] It has a predilection for attached keratinizing mucosa, occurring most frequently on the hard palate followed by the gingiva.[54] Unlike the cutaneous form, mucosal KS is more commonly symptomatic because of pain, ulceration, and bleeding. Loose teeth may impair mastication, pharyngeal disease may cause dysphagia, and laryngeal disease may cause dyspnea and stridor.[142] Furthermore, compared with cutaneous KS, oral KS is associated with increased immunocompromise and lower CD4$^+$ counts (mean, 66.6

Box 14-7. Poor prognostic factors in human immunodeficiency virus–related lymphoma

Previous diagnosis of acquired immunodeficiency syndrome
CD4$^+$ count less than 200 cells/μl
Karnofsky score less than 70%
Extranodal disease
Pancytopenia
Incomplete response to chemotherapy

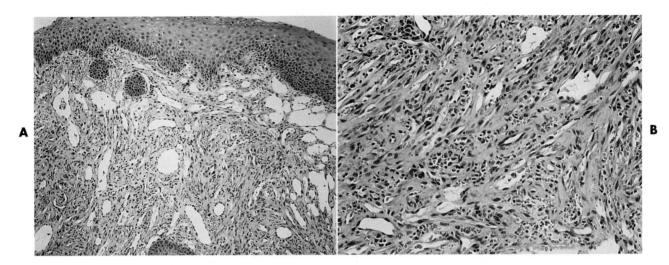

Fig. 14-3. Mucosal Kaposi's sarcoma. **A,** Photomicrograph of submucosal Kaposi's sarcoma showing slit-like vascular channels and scattered extravasation of erythrocytes. (×100.) **B,** Higher power photomicrograph of the same lesion showing characteristic spindle cell proliferation. (×200.)

cells/μl).[54,65] Pulmonary KS manifests as shortness of breath, a chronic cough, and hemoptysis.

The differential diagnosis of KS includes melanoma and bacillary angiomatosis. Bacillary angiomatosis is a capillary proliferative lesion caused by the etiologic agents of cat-scratch disease, *Rochalimaea henselae*, and *Rochalimaea quintana*.[10] Exposure to cats is a strong risk factor for the development of bacillary angiomatosis, which may present as a subcutaneous nodule or as an indurated and hyperpigmented cutaneous or mucosal lesion that is indistinguishable from KS. Bacillary angiomatosis can be locally destructive in the head and neck and may disseminate to cervical lymph nodes and the viscera, leading to significant morbidity and mortality.[66] It can be diagnosed by the presence of pleomorphic bacilli on Warthin-Starry silver stain or by the identification of *Rochalimaea sp.* DNA on biopsy using polymerase chain reaction techniques. Erythromycin, doxycycline, or rifampin is effective therapy for bacillary angiomatosis.

KS can be histologically identified by the presence of slit-like vascular channels (in contrast to the more oval-shaped vascular channels of bacillary angiomatosis), extravasated erythrocytes, and spindle-cell proliferation (Fig. 14-3). As KS progresses from the relatively early macular form to the more mature nodular form, spindle-cell proliferation and pleomorphism become more prominent.[54] More mature KS tends to ulcerate and bleed, making it particularly difficult to differentiate from other malignant tumors (Fig. 14-4). The identification of KSHV DNA is a promising new diagnostic method to distinguish KS from other vascular lesions.[85] Melanoma is not a vascular lesion but may be confused with more mature forms of KS in which spindle-cell proliferation predominates. Melanoma markers, such as HMB and S100, are helpful for diagnosis.

Although the characteristic appearance of KS often ob-

viates the need for biopsy, there should be a low threshold to biopsy especially if the color or size of the lesion changes. If biopsy is necessary, nuisance bleeding should be planned for, especially for lesions of the pharynx, airway, and tracheobronchial tree. Symptomatic KS lesions may benefit from palliative therapy, but a biopsy should be performed to confirm the diagnosis before initiating therapy.

The available therapies for KS have side effects and are of variable long-term benefit. Indications for management include disfiguring facial lesions, oral pain, impaired mastication, dysphagia, and threatened respiratory function caused by airway or pulmonary lesions.

Local therapy, including intralesional chemotherapy and cryotherapy, is effective for superficial and limited KS, whereas radiotherapy is useful for regional disease of the head and neck.[203] Intralesional injections of vinblastine have been used in cases of mucosal disease to temporize symptoms without systemic side effects. Radiotherapy is useful for the management of cutaneous and mucosal KS. Low-dose radiotherapy results in control of greater than 90% of cutaneous lesions, with a median duration of response of 21 months.[16] Single-dose therapy of 800 cGy with repetition for recurrent disease has been successfully used. Mucositis is a complication of radiotherapy of mucosal KS. This effect is diminished with good therapeutic results, by using low-dose fractions, and an accumulative dose less than 3000 cGy.[54]

Systemic chemotherapy is more appropriate for large lesions or disease of the viscera, including the lungs. However, the risk of bone marrow suppression increases the patient's vulnerability to opportunistic infections. Single-agent therapy has a role in limited disease. Etoposide may be given orally for localized KS, with as much as a 90% response rate and a median duration of response of 9 months. Single-

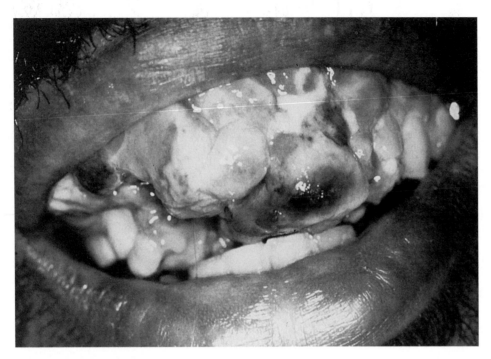

Fig. 14-4. Nodular Kaposi's sarcoma of the gingiva and palate. Given the ulcerated and fungating appearance, the differential diagnosis includes non-Hodgkin's lymphoma and squamous cell carcinoma. (Courtesy of Dr. Russel Corio.)

agent therapy with liposomal daunorubicin has limited toxicity and holds some promise, even for advanced disease.[64] Combination chemotherapy is recommended for disseminated KS. One of several proposed regimens is a combination of doxorubicin, vincristine, and bleomycin, which has a response rate of 79% but is complicated by immunosuppression and opportunistic infections.[63] Another example is doxorubicin, vinblastine, and bleomycin, which has an 84% response rate with a remission of 8 months' median duration.[98] Low-dose, long-term interferon-α-2b in combination with zidovudine has some promise as a well-tolerated effective therapy for KS, especially in patients with CD4+ counts greater than 250 cells/μl.[121]

Factors associated with decreased survival include (1) prior or present history of opportunistic infections; (2) fever greater than 100° F, greater than 10% weight loss, diarrhea, or night sweats; and (3) CD4+ count less than 300 cells/μl.[33] Tumor bulk and the number of sites involved are not risk factors. A staging system based on these risk factors is useful to determine the prognosis in patients with KS (Box 14-8).

OTHER HEAD AND NECK NEOPLASMS IN HUMAN IMMUNODEFICIENCY VIRUS–INFECTED PATIENTS

The incidence of carcinomas and other tumors is known to be higher in the organ transplant population than in the general population after several years of immunosuppression.[143] However, until recently, an increase in the incidence of malignancies other than KS, NHL, and anogenital carci-

---

Box 14-8. Staging system for patients with Kaposi's sarcoma[33]

Stage	*Characteristics*
I	No history of opportunistic infections, no constitutional symptoms, CD4+ greater than 300 cells/μl
II	No history of opportunistic infections, no constitutional symptoms, CD4+ less than 300 cells/μl
III	No history of opportunistic infections, constitutional symptoms
IV	History of prior or coexistent opportunistic infections (median survival, 7 months)

---

noma has not been shown in AIDS patients, possibly because of the short life expectancy of these patients. For example, although the incidence of NHL was markedly increased among men at risk for HIV in San Francisco between 1973 and 1987, the incidence of carcinomas of the oral cavity and pharynx and melanoma did not appreciably change in these patients (incidence rates were the same in the age-matched general population).[150,151] However, the overall incidence of non–AIDS-defining malignancies, may be increasing as improved antiretroviral therapy and prophylactic regimens progressively prolong the survival and the period of immunosuppression in AIDS patients.[115,156]

Proving an increase in the incidence of individual non–AIDS-defining tumors is difficult in HIV infection because of the small numbers. However, when malignancies occur in the HIV-infected patient, disease occurs in younger age groups and is more extensively disseminated because of poorly understood host and tumor factors (see Box 14-6). In general, these patients are younger and succumb to malignancy at an increased rate compared with non–HIV-infected counterparts. HD, cutaneous malignancies, and head and neck squamous cell carcinoma (SCC) are presenting an increasing challenge to the otolaryngologist and other clinicians who treat patients with head and neck malignancies.

Hodgkin's disease

Recent evidence shows that the incidence of HD is increasing in the HIV-positive population.[115] Whereas NHL usually occurs in patients with severely impaired immunity, HD occurs in HIV-infected patients with a wide range of immune function. Only approximately 20% of cases have AIDS, and a wide range of CD4+ counts are found.[172]

In the setting of HIV infection, HD has a more virulent course and is associated with a poorer outcome. For unclear reasons, this finding appears to be particularly true among IVDUs.[156] In the HIV-infected patient, extranodal HD is common with bone marrow involvement, seen in as many as 50% of cases compared with 10% of cases of non–HIV infection.[5,27,131,173] As a result, up to 91% of HIV-positive patients with HD present with stage III and IV disease compared with 46% of HIV-negative patients.[172] The unfavorable histologic subtypes of HD—mixed cellularity and lymphocyte depletion—predominate, partially explaining the aggressive nature of these tumors and the poor outcomes.

Poor survival is explained by a combination of increased malignant behavior of the tumor and increased host susceptibility to opportunistic infections. The survival at 1 year is 30% in HIV infected patients, whereas in the general population it is greater than 80% at 9 years.[40] In another series, the 5-year actuarial survival was 0% for HIV-infected patients with HD compared with 80% for HIV-negative patients.[173] The dismal prognosis of HD in these patients mandates that the clinician make as early a diagnosis as possible by maintaining a high level of suspicion when confronted with lesions in the head and neck.

HIV-related HD frequently presents as a mass in the head and neck region. It is more often associated with fever, night sweats, and weight loss in the HIV-infected patient than in the general population.[172] Once the histologic diagnosis has been made, the staging workup should consist of brain, thoracic, and abdominal CAT scans or MRI. Bone scanning, bone marrow biopsy, and staging laparotomy are required to plan management.

Multiagent chemotherapy is the mainstay of management. Radiotherapy is used to manage local disease or symptomatic lesions in the setting of disseminated HD. Bone marrow suppression secondary to chemotherapy leads to significant morbidity in the HIV-infected patient. Complete remission by chemotherapy results in increased disease-free survival. However, these patients often eventually die of opportunistic infections secondary to AIDS or bone marrow suppression. Poor prognostic factors include (1) a diagnosis of AIDS, (2) premanagement pancytopenia, and (3) failure of chemotherapy to result in a complete remission.[173]

Serrano and others[173] reported that HIV infection was asymptomatic in as many as 45% of patients with HIV-related HD at the time of diagnosis. Given the unfavorable prognosis and clinical behavior of HD in the HIV-infected patient and the high rate of asymptomatic HIV infection in this group, all persons diagnosed with HD should be tested for HIV.

Cutaneous neoplasms

Basal cell carcinoma (BCC) and malignant melanoma (MM) may be occurring at an increasing rate in the HIV-infected population.[201] BCC is the second most common skin neoplasm after KS, occurring in 1.8% of HIV-infected patients in a series by Smith and others.[184] MM on the other hand, is still relatively uncommon. Both tumors may occur in the setting of immunocompromise and low CD4+ counts but rarely in association with AIDS.

Of BCC lesions, 30% occur on the head and neck of HIV-positive patients compared with 85% in HIV-negative patients. The superficial subtype of BCC predominates in HIV infection, whereas the nodular type is most prevalent in the general population.[183] As in the general population, the risk factors for developing BCC include fair skin and significant sunlight exposure, but HIV-infected patients experience a more aggressive form of the disease.

The HIV-infected patient with BCC is younger than his or her counterpart in the general population. BCC is often multicentric and occasionally metastasizes.[181] Mohs' surgery is the technique of choice for resecting BCC in HIV-infected patients because of the locally aggressive behavior in this population and the proclivity for recurrence.[81]

MM also has more aggressive features in the setting of HIV infection. The thickness of the skin lesion appears to be inversely proportional to the CD4+ count,[124] and the risk of disseminated MM increases as the CD4+ count decreases.[201]

The increased incidence of BCC and MM[201] in HIV infection, and the tendency for early dissemination require that there be a low threshold to biopsy new and suspicious skin lesions. HIV-infected patients with fair skin should also be counseled to minimize sun exposure and to use sun screen when outdoors.

Carcinomas of the upper aerodigestive tract

No evidence thus far proves that the incidence of head and neck SCC is increased in HIV-infected patients. However, HIV-infected patients with these tumors experience a more virulent clinical course than HIV-negative patients, presumably because of differences in host and tumor biology. When associated with HIV infection, head and neck

SCC afflicts patients who are, on average, in their fourth decade of life.[56,158,180] These patients often present with more advanced tumors than their HIV-negative counterparts.[56,158] In a report by Singh and others,[180] HIV-infected patients presented with primary lesions of median size T3 and median stage IV, whereas non–HIV-infected patients presented with lesions of median size T2 and median stage III. In this clinical series, HIV-associated head and neck SCC had a significantly reduced tumor-related survival after adjusting for stage and site. Tumor-related survival at 1 and 2 years was 57% and 32%, respectively, whereas for HIV-negative patients it was 74% and 59%, respectively. The presentation of SCC at more advanced stages may indicate an accelerated pathogenesis of malignancy in association with HIV infection.[56] However, morbidity caused by HIV infection and chemotherapy are also likely to be important factors underlying the poor rates of survival in these patients.

The high rate of tobacco and alcohol use in HIV-infected patients with head and neck SCC suggests that the underlying oncogenesis of this tumor is similar to that in the general population.[56,150,180] However, the identification of human papillomavirus (HPV) DNA in some lesions raises the possibility that HIV-related immunocompromise increases the infection rate of oncogenic viruses, which when combined with impaired host immune surveillance results in an accelerated disease course in younger patients.[56,158] HIV-related SCC appears to have a predilection for the larynx over other sites in the head and neck.[59,158,180] As in the anogenital region, HPV has a similar predisposition to cause pathology including papillomas in the larynx, and may be a player in the oncogenesis of head and neck SCC, particularly laryngeal SCC.[139]

The diagnosis of head and neck SCC is often delayed by prolonged management of presumed benign pathology.[56] The oral cavity and pharynx are common sites of various manifestations of HIV infection. Missing the occasional malignancy that arises in the upper aerodigestive tract is easy because lesions in this region are usually benign and of infectious origin. Malignancies in this region are unlikely to be missed if a high level of suspicion is maintained, if new lesions are closely followed, and if biopsies are taken early.

A history of heavy tobacco and alcohol use by an HIV-infected patient mandates that a thorough head and neck examination be performed on a regular basis. Effective surveillance for neoplasms in this high-risk group depends on close communication with primary care providers, who should be alerted of the importance of the head and neck examination and of early referral for evaluation of suspicious lesions. All such lesions should undergo biopsy on presentation or if persistent after a short trial of therapy.

SINONASAL DISEASE

Sinonasal lymphoma

Sinonasal NHL is a disease of advanced HIV infection that is most common in patients with a CD4$^+$ count of less than 200 cells/μl and a history of AIDS-defining opportunistic disease.[148] The presence of rhinorrhea and maxillary pain may lead to a misdiagnosis of infection. However, the diagnosis of malignancy is often suggested by persistent unilateral sinonasal disease, an oral mass, tooth mobility and pain, and orbital pain or diplopia. Patients with isolated sinonasal NHL only occasionally present with constitutional symptoms.

Physical examination findings include an intranasal or paranasal mass, an intraoral mass, and subcutaneous swelling over the maxilla. Eye findings include proptosis, restricted extraocular motion, and periorbital edema. On sinus CT, a unilateral destructive sinonasal process is seen, usually involving the maxillary sinus and sometimes extending into other sinuses, the orbit, the intracranial compartment, or the soft tissues of the face. Biopsy of the nasal mass can be easily performed in the office if the lesion does not enhance with intravenous contrast on CT, indicating that the tumor is not vascular.

The prognosis of HIV-related NHL of the sinonasal region is poor. The mean life expectancy for HIV-infected patients with sinonasal NHL is 3.5 months compared with 4.2 months for patients with HIV-associated NHL of other sites and 9.3 months for non–HIV-infected patients.[148] The incidence of bony destruction and multiple sinus involvement by NHL is higher when associated with AIDS. Proptosis, ophthalmoplegia, and systemic dissemination of the lymphoma can progress very rapidly. Systemic chemotherapy is often required because of the high incidence of dissemination, but it must be individualized to the patient's medical condition. Local radiotherapy has a role in palliating orbital and oral symptoms.

Sinonasal infection

Sinonasal infections and allergies are increasingly common in HIV-infected patients.[18] Up to 95% of randomly chosen AIDS patients have MRI findings consistent with sinus disease.[39] As many as 68% of HIV-infected patients develop sinus infections.[97,162] The maxillary and ethmoid sinuses are most frequently involved;[217] however, sphenoid sinusitis is present in as many as 57% of patients, which is about twice the incidence in the general population.[6,67]

Sinusitis should be suspected in an AIDS patient with fever of unknown origin or headache. The pathogenesis of rhinosinusitis in HIV infection is influenced by a combination of local and systemic factors (Box 14-9). As a result,

---

Box 14-9. Pathogenesis of sinusitis in human immunodeficiency virus infection

Impaired systemic and local immunity
Mucociliary dysfunction
Increased atopy

the spectrum of organisms is wider and the rate of complications is increased.

The pathogenesis of sinusitis is influenced by systemic immunity and local factors, including mucociliary function, osteomeatal patency, and mucosal immunity. Mucociliary transport time is significantly prolonged in HIV-infected patients, especially when the CD4[+] count is less than 280 cells/μl.[128] A history of nasal congestion or sinusitis closely correlates with longer mucociliary transport times. The etiology of slowed mucociliary clearance in HIV infection is likely to be multifactorial and may include ciliary dysfunction and the production of more teniceous mucus as a result of chronic viral infections of the mucosa and increased regional atopy.

An increased susceptibility to sinusitis is partially explained by a higher rate of atopy in the HIV-infected population, resulting in mucociliary dysfunction and obstruction of sinus ostia. New or increased allergic symptoms (e.g., allergic rhinitis, drug allergies, and asthma) are experienced by as many as 87% of HIV-infected patients.[165] HIV-infected patients have positive skin tests at a much higher rate than HIV-negative patients, although both groups share similar patterns of allergen sensitivity.[182]

The increased atopy associated with HIV infection results from the polyclonal activation of B cells and the increased production of immunoglobulins, including immunoglobin E (IgE).[193] IgE levels increase as HIV infection progresses to AIDS,[182] and the incidence and chronicity of sinus infections increase. The management of allergic rhinitis with nasal corticosteroid sprays and antihistamines therefore plays an important role in the management and prevention of sinusitis in HIV infection.

The clinical characteristics of sinusitis closely correlate with the clinical stage of HIV infection and therefore with the status of host immunity. Acute sinusitis is more likely to completely resolve with medical management if the CD4[+] count is greater than 200 cells/μl. However, a decrease in the CD4[+] count to less than 200 cells/μl is associated with a greater number of involved sinuses and a greater likelihood that chronic sinusitis will result.[67,193,217]

A wider spectrum of organisms cause sinusitis in the HIV-infected patient. The most commonly cultured organisms in acute sinusitis are *Streptococcus pneumoniae* (19%), *Streptococcus viridans* (19%), coagulase-negative staphylococci (13%), *Staphylococcus aureus* (9%), and *Haemophilus influenzae* (13%).[67,129] However, with worsening immunocompromise, gram-negative bacteria and fungi can cause life-threatening infections.

Unusual organisms cultured from HIV-infected patients with sinusitis include *Cryptococcus neoformans*,[38] *Legionella pneumophilia*,[170] *Acanthamoeba*,[69] *Mycobacterium kansasii*, and CMV.[199] CMV may act as a primary cause of an erosive sinusitis[210] or as a cofactor in the pathogenesis of bacterial and fungal sinusitis through local effects on the mucosa and systemic effects on neutrophil function.[214] *Pseu-*

domonas aeroginosa and *Aspergillus fumigatus* are of special interest because they cause the most clinically significant cases of atypical sinusitis in the HIV-infected patient.

P. aeruginosa causes sinusitis at much higher rates in the HIV-infected population and is rarely encountered in the HIV-negative population.[67,129,193] *P. aeruginosa* has been cultured in up to 17% of HIV-positive patients with sinusitis.[129] A combination of impaired humoral immunity, neutrophil dysfunction, and abnormal complement activation is likely to be responsible for this high incidence. Risk factors for *Pseudomonas* infection include frequent and prolonged hospitalizations and the administration of corticosteroids and medications (e.g., ganciclovir, zidovudine, and antineoplastic chemotherapy) which may cause neutrophil dysfunction.[137,176]

There should be a high index of suspicion for sinus infection by *P. aeruginosa* because this infection can be life-threatening. *P. aeruginosa* can cause vasculitis leading to avascular necrosis.[37,128] Orbital and intracranial complications may occur as a result of a necrotizing sinusitis, with direct extension of infection and vasculitis to these adjacent sites. Fungal infections exhibit similar angiocentric spread and a predilection for extension beyond the boundaries of the sinonasal region.

Fungal sinusitis most commonly occurs in late-stage AIDS when the CD4[+] count is less than 150 cells/μl.[127] Fungi, including *Candida albicans*, *Cryptococcus neoformans*, *Rhizopus arrhizus*,[20] *Pseudallescheria boydii*, and *Schizophyllum commune*, reportedly cause complicated sinusitis.[127] However, *A. fumigatus* is the fungus most commonly reported to infect the paranasal sinuses.

Aspergillus has a predilection to infect the sinuses of patients with CD4[+] counts less than 50 cells/μL.[112,127] Neutrophils and macrophages form the primary defense against *Aspergillus* infection.[168] Neutropenia and neutrophil dysfunction caused by HIV infection or by the effects of medications have been identified as risk factors for invasive pulmonary and sinonasal aspergillosis.[46,112,127]

Early diagnosis of fungal disease is important to prevent life-threatening complications (Box 14-10). Fungal sinusitis should be suspected in a patient with a low CD4[+] count; unilateral symptoms, including facial paresthesias, swelling, and pain; and fever despite broad-spectrum antibiotics. Proptosis, decreased extraocular motion, and decreased vision suggest orbital extension. Meningismus and mental status changes are ominous signs of intracranial involvement.

The endoscopic appearance of nasal aspergillosis, which often accompanies and may precede sinus involvement, ranges from pale ischemic mucosa to well-circumscribed necrotic plaques with a yellow-white shaggy surface. Perforations of the nasal septum and hard palate may be present. Fungal sinusitis in the HIV-infected patient is often associated with suppuration, making its distinction from bacterial sinusitis quite difficult.[127] Fungal sinusitis, however, is more likely to be unilateral. Suspicious lesions should undergo

<table>
<tr><td>

Box 14-10. Clinical features of fungal sinonasal disease

History

Sinusitis refractory to antibiotics
Unilateral nasal congestion, facial pain
Visual changes, facial paresthesias (with intracranial extension)
Recent therapy with corticosteroids, chemotherapy
Diagnosis of acquired immunodeficiency syndrome

Physical examination

Nasal mucosa ischemic or necrotic
Septum, hard palate eroded or perforated
Cranial nerve abnormalities (with intracranial extension)

Radiology

Computed tomography: sinus wall erosion
Magnetic resonance imaging: nasal or sinus process with one of the following:
    T1-weighted isointense signal
    T2-weighted hypointense signal

Laboratory

CD4$^+$ less than 150 cells/μl
Neutropenia, positive or negative

Histopathology

Hyphae
    Aspergillus: septate, 45° branching
    Mucor: aseptate, 90° branching, bulbous endings
Angioinvasion

</td></tr>
</table>

biopsy and should be submitted for histopathology, silver staining, and culture. Middle meatal discharge should also be sampled and sent for bacterial and fungal cultures and stains. A diagnostic antrostomy and lavage should be performed early in the workup of persistent sinusitis (Fig. 14-5). However, the absence of fungal elements on antral tap does not rule out fungal sinusitis.[127] A definitive diagnosis of fungal sinusitis is best made by submitting a biopsy of sinus mucosa for histopathology, culture, and stains.

Fungal sinusitis can extend to the orbital and intracranial compartments in the absence of histologic evidence of mucosal invasion.[112,127] Therefore, when *Aspergillus* is identified by stains or culture in a sinonasal sample, amphotericin and surgical débridement should not await histologic confirmation of mucosal invasion. The occasional absence of bone erosion on CT, despite orbital and intracranial complications of invasive *Aspergillus* sinusitis, can be explained by the angiocentric extension of disease beyond the confines of the sinuses.[127]

Unilateral disease and bony erosion on radiography of the paranasal sinuses should lead to suspicion of a neoplasm or fungal sinusitis (Fig. 14-6, *A*). MRI can help differentiate

fungal from bacterial sinusitis. In fungal disease, the signal of sinus contents on T1-weighted image is isointense to hypointense, whereas on T2-weighted image, the signal intensity remains low or is further decreased.[218] In bacterial sinusitis, the signal intensity on T1-weighted image is also isointense, but on T2-weighted image the signal intensity significantly increases (Fig. 14-6, *B*). If extension of disease to the orbits and intracranial compartments is suspected, MRI or CT of the orbits and brain should be performed with intravenous contrast.

Management of sinusitis

Sinonasal disease in the HIV-infected patient should be addressed with a combination of clinical assessment and empiric therapy (see Fig. 14-5). The aim of this approach is early resolution of cases of bacterial origin and early diagnosis and management of other causes of sinonasal disease, especially neoplasms and fungal infection.

The initial evaluation of an HIV-infected patient suspected of having sinusitis should include nasal endoscopy. The primary goal of this procedure is to identify mucosal and structural abnormalities that may indicate the nature of the underlying process. Discharge from the middle meati and sphenoethmoid recesses should be collected and submitted for bacterial and fungal cultures and stains. Mucosal lesions should be sampled and sent for histopathologic and microbiologic evaluation. CT of the paranasal sinuses is useful in the workup of a fever or headache of unknown etiology. Otherwise CT should be reserved for patients who continue to have signs and symptoms of sinusitis despite antibiotic therapy and for cases in which complications are suspected.

There should be a low threshold for performing an antral tap for bacterial, fungal, and viral cultures, especially when the CD4$^+$ count is less than 200 cells/μl. This diagnostic test is required when fever or symptoms of sinusitis are refractory to antibiotic therapy. Antral lavage should also be performed because it has shown some therapeutic value.[67]

Initial medical management of sinusitis consists of broad-spectrum antibiotics, decongestants, and mucolytics. Patients with AIDS and CD4$^+$ counts less than 200 cells/μl are especially vulnerable to gram-negative sinusitis. Patients presenting with their first episode of sinusitis or an occasional recurrence should be started on an antibiotic regimen effective against *Streptococcus* and *H. influenzae*. Amoxicillin or cefuroxime axetil are examples of good first-line agents for sinusitis in the HIV-infected population. Decongestants and high-dose guaifenesin enhance sinus drainage and provide symptomatic improvement.[203] Close contact should be kept with patients, and antibiotics changed if improvement does not occur within 72 hours. If a patient presents with persistent fever after 3 days of first-line therapy or local symptoms after 10 days or if a history of frequent recurrences is present, antibiotic coverage should be ex-

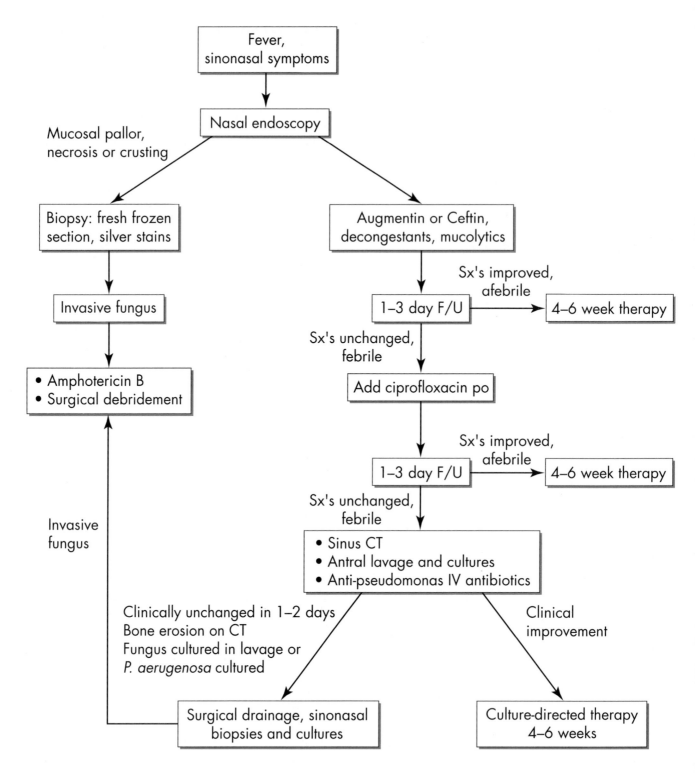

Fig. 14-5. The evaluation and management of sinusitis in human immunodeficiency virus infection.

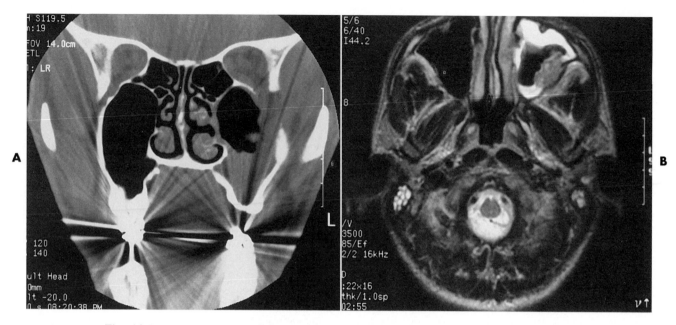

Fig. 14-6. Computed tomography and magnetic resonance imaging of *Aspergillus* sinusitis. **A,** Coronal computed tomography of the paranasal sinuses shows left maxillary sinusitis with erosion of the superior lateral bony wall. **B,** T2-weighted axial magnetic resonance imaging of the same case shows thickened left maxillary sinus mucosa with a hyperintense signal consistent with inflammation and a transmural process of the lateral wall with a hypointense signal corresponding to the region of bone destruction on computed tomography. Differential diagnosis includes invasive fungal disease, lymphoma, and squamous cell carcinoma.

panded to include *P. aeruginosa*. Oral ciprofloxacin with clindamycin is reasonable under these circumstances.

The more toxic cases should undergo early sinus imaging, early antral aspiration for culture, and broad-spectrum parenteral antibiotic therapy. As culture and biopsy results become available, antibiotic coverage can be adjusted to address the organisms of concern. At least 4 to 6 weeks of antibiotic therapy should be administered.

The patient with persistent fever after 2 to 3 days of antibiotic therapy that includes antipseudomonal drugs should undergo CT of the paranasal sinuses. An antral tap should be performed to culture sinus contents if sinus disease is seen on radiographs, followed by antral lavage to facilitate sinus drainage. Pseudomonal infection should be suspected, and broad-spectrum intravenous antibiotics with adequate coverage against *Pseudomonas* should be instituted. An antipseudomonal penicillin or third-generation cephalosporin given with an aminoglycoside is standard therapy, although combinations containing quinolones can also be used. The patient must be closely monitored for septicemia or regional complications of a pseudomonal sinusitis, including orbital cellulitis and cavernous sinus thrombophlebitis. Prompt surgical drainage should be performed if antral aspirates grow *P. aeruginosa*, if fever persists, or if there is evidence of extension of infection beyond the confines of the sinuses.[58]

Fungal sinusitis must be suspected when fever and other symptoms of sinusitis persist despite antral lavage and broad-spectrum antibiotics, including parenteral antipseudomonal agents. Sinusotomy and débridement should be pursued to establish drainage and to obtain mucosa and sinus contents for histopathologic and microbiologic evaluation, especially when risk factors of fungal disease are present, including a very low CD4$^+$ count ($<$150 cells/μl), neutropenia, or corticosteroid therapy. External and transnasal approaches to the sinuses may be used depending on the clinical scenario and the surgeon's preference.

Transnasal sinusotomies provide an opportunity to examine the sinus mucosa, assess the integrity of the bony walls, and take multiple biopsies without oral or facial incisions. Fresh frozen section should be performed on suspicious mucosa for rapid diagnosis because timely débridement of tissue infected with *Aspergillus* may be life-saving, especially in the profoundly immunocompromised host.

The goal of therapy for fungal sinusitis in the HIV-infected patient is to minimize the fungal load that the impaired immune system should clear. This goal is achieved with medical and surgical therapy. High-dose amphotericin B ($>$1 mg/kg/day) should be administered intravenously in all cases of sinusitis in which *Aspergillus* or *Rhizopus* has been cultured, whether or not there is histologic evidence of invasion because this feature does not correlate well with the risk of complications in the HIV-infected patient.[46,112,127] Itraconazole has shown some promise as an alternative to amphotericin B, especially in patients with poor renal function. Surgery is an important component of therapy because medical management is often ineffective as the sole modality for invasive fungal disease.

The severity of infection and the level of immune impairment should be considered when planning the surgical management of fungal sinusitis (see Fig. 14-5). Sinusotomy for drainage is not sufficient for fungal sinusitis. Rather, the surgical débridement of as much infected tissue as possible is necessary to minimize the fungal burden that the immune system should clear. Depending on the location and extent of disease, endoscopic or open approaches may be used. Fungal disease limited to the turbinates, septum, medial maxillary wall, and anterior ethmoids can be débrided by transnasal endoscopy. Lateral rhinotomy or other transfacial approaches may be considered in the setting of more extensive disease requiring partial or total maxillectomy, enucleation, or craniofacial resection. Intraoperative fresh frozen section is useful for defining the limits of resection where angioinvasion is absent.

Fungal sinusitis can be successfully managed without *en bloc* resection of all infected tissue in the patient whose immune system is only moderately impaired.[20] Endoscopic débridement of grossly infected tissue may be curative in combination with amphotericin B in a patient who, for example, has a CD4+ count greater than 200 cells/μl, does not have AIDS, is not neutropenic or receiving corticosteroids, and can be relied on to comply with frequent follow-up endoscopy and débridement in the office (as often as twice per week). However, the criteria for selecting these patients are not well established. It is unclear if the increase in neutrophil count experienced by AIDS patients taking recombinant human GM-CSF will translate into better outcomes for this limited surgical approach.[117] Close follow-up with frequent sinonasal endoscopy should be performed in the clinic or operating room, and biopsies of suspicious areas should be taken for frozen section, culture, and silver stains. There should be a low threshold for returning to the operating room for further débridement or *en bloc* resection if fungal disease is persistent.

OTOLOGIC AND NEUROTOLOGIC MANIFESTATIONS

The incidence of otologic symptoms in patients with HIV has been reported to be as high as 56%.[17] Hearing loss, otalgia, and otorrhea are the most common presenting symptoms,[92] whereas sensorineural hearing loss (SNHL), otitis externa (OE), acute otitis media (AOM), and serous otitis media (SOM) are the most common otologic diagnoses in the HIV-infected population.

Human immunodeficiency virus–related diseases of the outer and middle ear

The risk of OE and malignant OE is increased in patients with AIDS.[205] As in the general population, *P. aeruginosa* is the primary etiologic agent of both disease entities. The

susceptibility of the HIV-infected patient to *P. aeruginosa* is heightened by a combination of impaired humoral immunity, neutrophil function, and complement activation.[90] The pathogenesis of OE is further facilitated by the breakdown of the local cutaneous barrier in the external auditory canal (EAC) secondary to dermatologic lesions (e.g., eczema, seborrhea) and self-induced trauma caused by pruritis. OE will progress to necrotizing and malignant OE if not managed aggressively and in a timely fashion. Therapy should consist of frequent cleaning of the EAC by the clinician and topical instillation of aminoglycoside-containing drops. Oral ciprofloxacin should be considered in the severely immunocompromised patient, or when early auricular perichondritis is present. Malignant OE should be suspected when otalgia, swelling, and otorrhea persist despite therapy or when there is onset of facial nerve paralysis or other cranial nerve dysfunction (Box 14-11).

Early diagnosis and management of malignant OE is essential because osteomyelitis of the skull base is a life-threatening complication, especially in patients with low CD4+ counts and neutropenia.[205] Otoscopy reveals granulation tissue at the bony cartilagenous junction of the EAC. The diagnosis is confirmed by increased uptake of technetium-99 by the temporal bone on a bone scan. CT may show erosion of the EAC bone. EAC debris should be cultured and stained for bacteria, fungi, acid-fast bacilli (AFB), and pneumocystis. Management of malignant OE consists of 6 weeks of broad-spectrum intravenous antibiotics with adequate coverage against *P. aeruginosa*. An antipseudomonal penicillin or third-generation cephalosporin given with an aminoglycoside is standard therapy, although combinations containing quinolones can also be used. Serial gallium-67 bone scans help monitor the response to therapy.

Eustachian tube obstruction caused by adenoidal hypertrophy or sinonasal disease is prevalent in HIV-infected children and adults. It is therefore not surprising that OM commonly occurs in the HIV-infected population, particularly in children.[74,211] SOM and conductive hearing loss (CHL) are more prevalent in adults and older children, whereas AOM frequently occurs in young children.[8,47] The frequency

---

Box 14-11. Differential diagnosis of chronic otorrhea and otalgia in human immunodeficiency virus infection

Chronic bacterial otomastoiditis with or without cholesteatoma
Malignant otitis externa
Invasive *Aspergillosis:* otomastoiditis or otitis externa
Pneumocystis infection: otomastoiditis or otitis externa
Mycobacterial infection: otomastoiditis
Neoplasm: non-Hodgkin's lymphoma or Kaposi's sarcoma of the temporal bone

of recurrent AOM increases as immune function deteriorates. During the first 3 years of life, HIV-infected children with CD4$^+$ counts less than 1500 cells/μl have up to twice the incidence of AOM as children with CD4$^+$ counts greater than 1500 cells/μl in the first 3 years of life.[8] The bacteriology of acute OM parallels that in non–HIV-infected patients, with *S. pneumoniae, H. influenzae,* Group A *Streptococcus,* and *Moraxella catarrhalis* predominating.[96,118] An exception to this is the severely immunocompromised child in whom *S. aureus* causes OM at a significantly higher rate. Therefore, initial therapy for acute OM is the same as that for the non–HIV-infected patient. However, in the severely immunocompromised child who does not respond to first-line therapy within 3 days, antibiotic coverage should be expanded to include *S. aureus.* If OM persists, tympanocentesis should be performed and therapy guided by culture and sensitivity results.

The role of tympanostomy tube placement and adenoidectomy in the management of recurrent OM and persistent SOM is poorly established in HIV-infected patients. Despite the placement of tympanostomy tubes, OM with otorrhea frequently occurs in many cases.[8] Persistent tympanic membrane (TM) perforation with intermittent otorrhea has also been the experience of some clinicians on placing tubes in adults with SOM. Each case must be judged separately, but in general, the threshold for the placement of tympanostomy tubes in HIV-infected patients should be higher than in the general population. The severity of hearing loss and morbidity associated with OM should be taken into account when deciding whether to place tympanostomy tubes.

Petrous apicitis, cranial neuropathies (VII and VIII), temporal bone osteomyelitis, and intracranial sepsis are uncommon but are more likely to complicate OM in the setting of advanced immunocompromise.[109] Patients with suppurative OM refractory to antibiotics should undergo early tympanocentesis for culture and special stains, and granulation tissue, polyps, and other masses should be carefully biopsied to rule out neoplasms and atypical infections. *A. fumigatus* and *P. carinii* are examples of organisms that cause otomastoiditis refractory to standard antibiotic therapy.

Otomastoiditis and OE caused by *P. carinii* usually occur in the absence of pulmonary disease.[22,61,92,202] Like KS of the middle ear and EAC, pneumocystis infections of the temporal bone only occur in HIV infection. Patients with pneumocystis otomastoiditis commonly present with unilateral otalgia, otorrhea, and hearing loss and demonstrate a mass arising in the middle ear or EAC on otoscopy. CT of the temporal bones reveals bony sclerosis without erosions and opacification of the middle ear and mastoid air spaces.

A persistent aural polyp accompanied by signs and symptoms of OM despite otic drops and systemic antibiotics, should undergo biopsy for histopathology and special stains. Silver stains should be requested and will reveal *P. carinii* organisms surrounded by a foamy granular exudate. *P. carinii* otitis is resolved with recovery of hearing using oral tri-

methoprim-sulfamethoxazole (15 mg/kg/day trimethoprim) in three to four divided doses for 10 to 14 days.[22] Other regimens have been used successfully, including trimethoprim and dapsone[61] and pentamidine.[140] The route of transmission of *P. carinii* to the temporal bone is not clear. Retrograde spread from the nasopharynx through the Eustachian tube and hematogenous spread have been proposed.

A. fumigatus infection of the EAC may be superficial in the relatively immunocompetent HIV-infected patient, causing a chronic OE. However, in severely immunocompromised patients, invasive *Aspergillus* infection of the temporal bone can cause malignant OE and otomastoiditis with skull base and intracranial extension.[155] Risk factors for invasive aspergillosis of the temporal bone include a low CD4$^+$ count, AIDS diagnosis, neutropenia, corticosteroid therapy, antineoplastic therapy, and prolonged antibiotic therapy (Box 14-12).

Invasive OE caused by *A. fumigatus* presents with otalgia, otorrhea, and hearing loss. Otoscopy usually reveals white debris in the EAC, which may be mistaken for cholesteatoma. Facial nerve weakness indicates bone invasion, which

---

Box 14-12. *Aspergillus* of the temporal bone

History

Persistent otorrhea, otalgia despite antibiotics
Rapid and severe hearing loss
Dizziness
Facial nerve weakness

Physical examination

White fungal debris in external auditory canal
Enlarging, multiple tympanic membrane perforation
Middle ear mucosa ischemic, necrotic, or insensate

Audiology

Maximal conductive hearing loss
Mixed hearing loss

Radiology

Computed tomography
  Bony destruction
  Absent ossicles
Magnetic resonance imaging
  Intracranial extension
    Lateral sinus thrombosis
    Middle lobe, cerebellar invasion

Histopathology

Biopsy of middle ear mucosa shows septate hyphae with 45° branching and the following:
  Mucosal invasion
  Angioinvasion

can often be confirmed by the presence of bony erosion on temporal bone CT.

Otomastoiditis caused by *A. fumigatus* may start in the middle ear space or extend from the EAC.[75] Invasive disease results in destruction of ossicles, erosion of the facial canal with nerve invasion, and destruction of dural plates with possible extension to the dural sinuses and other intracranial structures.[192] Patients often have a history of worsening otalgia, otorrhea, and hearing loss despite antibiotic therapy.[114] Vertigo indicates labyrinthine invasion by *Aspergillus*, whereas meningismus and mental status changes indicate intracranial extension. Otoscopy often reveals a pale tympanic membrane with enlarging single or multiple perforations. The middle ear mucosa may be pale or necrotic, and white fungal debris resembling cholesteatoma may also be seen.

There should be a high index of suspicion for the presence of invasive *Aspergillus* of the temporal bone, particularly in the AIDS patient with persistent OE or OM and new cranial nerve findings. Otorrhea should be routinely cultured and stained for bacterial and fungal organisms and for pneumocystis. If the TM is intact, tympanocentesis should be performed when antibiotic therapy is ineffective. If *Aspergillus* is identified on stain or culture, invasive disease can be implied by the presence of bone erosion on CT. The presence of fungal invasion in a mucosal biopsy from the middle ear is diagnostic for *Aspergillus* otomastoiditis. Brain MRI should be performed if extensive mastoid disease or dural plate erosion is present on CT. Lateral sinus blood flow should be assessed and other clues of intracranial extension sought.

OE and OM caused by invasive *A. fumigatus* require prompt surgical and drug therapy.[192] High-dose amphotericin B should be started immediately. As much *Aspergillus*-infected tissue as possible should be removed to slow down extension of disease to vital structures and to facilitate the ameliorating effects of drug therapy and host immunity. In the case of OE caused by invasive *Aspergillus*, infected soft tissue and bone of the EAC should be débrided. Limited disease may be addressed by a transcanal approach, but a transmastoid approach with removal of the canal wall will provide more complete débridement and less risk to the facial nerve. Otomastoiditis should be managed with a radical mastoidectomy if middle ear contents and mastoid air cells are to be removed. The management of the facial nerve in these cases is controversial because invasion of the nerve by *Aspergillus* is not easily proven without biopsy. When the facial nerve is paralyzed and gross evidence of invasion and necrosis is present, the nerve should be resected.

The absence of tissue invasion on histopathology and the absence of bone erosion on CT do not rule out the diagnosis of invasive *Aspergillus* of the temporal bone. The clinician should maintain a high index of suspicion for invasive aspergillosis in the HIV-infected patient with severe immunocompromise, despite the absence of these findings. Therefore,

the patient with early HIV infection may first be treated with topical clotrimazole and seen up to several times per week for frequent cleaning of EAC debris. If symptoms persist or cranial nerve deficits occur, surgery and amphotericin B should be considered after biopsies are taken and CT studies repeated.

Cranial nerve and central nervous system effects

Neurologic disorders are a common manifestation of HIV infection resulting from the neurotropic and immunosuppressive properties of the virus. As many as 40% of HIV-infected adults have clinical signs of neurologic disease, and 70% to 80% show neuropathologic abnormalities at autopsy.[50,107] Peripheral neuropathy comprises 5% to 20% of all neurologic complications in HIV infection.[141] Of AIDS patients, 2% to 3% develop cranial neuropathies. The most commonly affected are the facial, trigeminal, optic, and cochleovestibular nerves.[107,196]

Neuropathy associated with early-stage HIV infection exhibits a tendency for motor nerve involvement, whereas sensory nerves are more likely to be affected in later stages.[141] Neuropathies associated with HIV seroconversion and asymptomatic HIV infection tend to result from autoimmune demyelination as demonstrated by common pathologic findings and electrophysiologic correlates.[50,62,109,141] An autoimmune etiology is supported by the presence of increased titers of circulating antibodies against peripheral nerve antigens, subperineural deposition of IgM, and improvement in nerve function with plasmapheresis. Neuropathies associated with symptomatic HIV infection and AIDS are characterized by distal symmetric polyneuropathy and axonal degeneration. A similar pattern of neuropathy selectively affects cranial nerves in the form of a mononeuritis multiplex resulting in a transient mononeuropathy or progressive sensorimotor polyneuropathy.[41] Axonal degeneration induced by necrotizing vasculitis may be the underlying pathologic process.

In later stages of HIV infection, cranial nerve dysfunction is often associated with CNS disease.[107,187] AIDS dementia (subacute encephalitis) is the most common neurologic manifestation of HIV infection and is sometimes associated with focal motor deficits. Aseptic meningitis is thought to be a less fulminant form of subacute encephalitis, occurring in the less immunocompromised patient and occasionally associated with dysfunction of cranial nerves V, VII, and VIII. Progressive multifocal leukoencephalopathy (PML) is a demyelinating disease of the CNS associated with papovavirus infection. In PML, there is progressive deterioration of mentation and other neurologic functions, including cranial nerve weakness. *Toxoplasma gondii* infection of the brain produces large areas of coagulation necrosis. The resulting mass lesion causes altered levels of consciousness and focal deficits, including cranial nerve dysfunction. Toxoplasmosis is definitively diagnosed by brain biopsy but is usually diagnosed presumptively by the presence of an enhancing lesion on MRI or CT, and a clinical and radiographic response to empiric management with pyrimethamine and either sulfadiazine or clindamycin. Cranial nerve deficits are rare complications of primary CNS lymphoma, occurring at a rate of only 8% according to Levy and others.[107] On the other hand, cranial nerve abnormalities occur in as many as 40% of patients with secondary involvement of the CNS by systemic lymphoma probably resulting from secondary involvement of the basal meninges. Other neurologic complications of HIV infection include cryptococcal meningitis, which is associated with cranial neuropathies in the presence of increased intracranial pressure, tuberculous meningitis, and toxic neuropathy caused by therapy with didanosine, zalcitabine, stavudine, and other agents.[62] Multiple pathologic processes may be present at the same time in the CNS and peripheral nervous system.

Hearing loss

Various degrees of SNHL can be found in as many as 49% of HIV-infected patients, although vestibular symptoms are relatively uncommon.[96,153] Audiometry most commonly demonstrates a high-frequency SNHL.[7,73,96,153,194]

Cochleovestibular dysfunction increases with the duration of HIV infection.[7,17,77] For example, in a group of asymptomatic HIV-infected men, the prevalence of audiometric abnormalities increased over 6 to 9 months.[93] The pure-tone average (PTA) gradually increases as the T-cell ratio falls in an AIDS patient, possibly because of an accumulation of insults to the CNS by opportunistic diseases and HIV itself.[17,93,107]

The differential diagnosis of SNHL in the HIV-infected patient is influenced by the level of immunocompromise (Box 14-13). Peripheral auditory pathology caused by drug-induced ototoxicity and otosyphilis and by idiopathic processes may produce SNHL at any stage in HIV infection, whereas central causes of hearing loss are more likely to occur in later stages of the disease.

Progressive central auditory dysfunction appears to be a common cause of SNHL associated with HIV infection and is shown by the results of auditory brainstem response testing. Auditory brainstem response testing of asymptomatic HIV-infected patients commonly shows a delayed and poorly defined wave V suggesting auditory brainstem conduction abnormalities.[7,17,160,186,206] These auditory brainstem response abnormalities occur in early HIV infection, often preceding the onset of symptoms of hearing loss or elevation of hearing thresholds.[57,78] The central auditory pathway in the upper brainstem is dysfunctional in earlier stages of HIV infection as indicated by prolonged I-V and III-V intervals, whereas the lower brainstem is affected in advanced HIV infection as indicated by a prolonged I-III interval.[137] Positive stapedial reflex decay, increased interaural time delay, and the absence of recruitment are common findings in HIV-related SNHL, supporting retrocochlear pathology.[76,152,205] Central auditory processing can

---

> **Box 14-13.** Differential diagnosis of sensory neural hearing loss in human immunodeficiency virus (HIV) infection
>
> Otosyphilis
> Cryptococcal meningitis*
> Central nervous system toxoplasmosis*
> Mycobacterial meningitis*
> Central effects of HIV infection
>   Aseptic meningitis
>   Autoimmune demyelination of the cochlear nerve
>   Subacute encephalitis*
> Progressive multifocal leukoencephalopathy*
> Hodgkin's lymphoma
> NHL of the brain and meninges*
> Mass lesions of the cerebellopontine angle/internal auditory canal and petrous apex
> Ototoxic medications
>   Cerebrovascular accident
>   Ideopathic

* Associated with late HIV infection, including acquired immunodeficiency syndrome.

---

also be impaired in the absence of auditory brainstem response abnormalities because of HIV-related cortical pathology and dementia.[7]

The causes of central auditory pathology include the direct effects of HIV and secondary effects of immunosuppression. Early demyelination of the central auditory tract is suggested by prolonged wave latencies when faster click rates are used in auditory brainstem response studies of asymptomatic HIV-infected subjects.[7,57] The progressive demyelination of the central auditory pathway may be a direct effect of HIV on neuroglia, as part of the pathogenesis of subacute encephalitis.[141] Multiple cranial nerve abnormalities, including deafness may also result from central demyelination associated with PML of the brainstem.[95] Opportunistic diseases including CNS toxoplasmosis, TB meningitis, cryptococcal meningitis, and NHL may also cause SNHL in the AIDS patient.

The labyrinth is not as common a site of HIV-related pathology as is the central auditory system. Few abnormal findings are present on temporal bone histopathology,[35] even on specimens from which viruses have been cultured.[43] Sudden deafness and vestibular hypofunction have occurred in association with acute HIV infection and aseptic meningitis possibly as a result of a viral labyrinthitis or cochleovestibular neuropathy.[73] The ototoxic effects of new antiretroviral drugs and the long-term effects of various drug combinations are not well established. Medications that have potential ototoxic effects when used for long periods of time include acyclovir, aminoglycosides, amphotericin B, azidothymidine, flucytosine, pentamidine, azithromycin, and trimethoprim-sulfamethoxazole.[3,91,200] Chemotherapy and radiotherapy for the management of malignancy can also lead to ototoxicity and hearing loss. Syphilis and cryptococcal meningitis are manageable causes of temporal bone pathology and SNHL, which can cause significant morbidity in the HIV-infected patient if they are not discovered and managed in a timely fashion.

Otosyphilis

HIV is most frequently contracted through sexual contact, accounting for a high coincidence of other sexually transmitted diseases, including syphilis.[185] Otosyphilis should be suspected in any HIV-infected patient who presents with cochleovestibular complaints (Box 14-14). In turn, HIV infection should be suspected in patients diagnosed with syphilis. Hearing loss resulting from syphilis is often bilateral, may be progressive or fluctuate, or may have a sudden onset.[42,111,209] Tinnitus, aural fullness, and dysequilibrium occasionally occur. The audiometric curve often shows a low-frequency hearing loss in association with diminished speech discrimination scores.

The fluorescent treponemal antibody absorption test (FTA-ABS) is a treponeme-specific serologic test that remains positive for life, even after eradication of the infection. The Venereal Disease Research Laboratory test (VDRL) indicates active infection when it is positive along with the FTA-ABS. However, the VDRL can be negative in primary and tertiary disease. Although a useful screening tool in low-risk populations, VDRL is not sufficiently sensitive to the study of high-risk groups. In the HIV-infected population as many as 63% of patients have a history of syphilis.[149,178] In this population, a positive FTA-ABS and cochleovestibular abnormalities are strongly predictive of otosyphilis.[84] These patients should undergo therapy for otosyphilis even if the VDRL is negative.

Progression of primary syphilis to otosyphilis and neuro-syphilis is accelerated, even after appropriate management has been given.[185] The interval between primary infection and otosyphilis appears to be shortened to 2 to 5 years in HIV infection compared to 15 to 30 years in the general population. Viable treponemes have been found in perilymph[209] and in temporal bone tissue[116] of patients clinically cured of syphilis. Smith and Canalis[185] hypothesized that residual treponemes, which remain dormant in the temporal bone, are reactivated as cell-mediated immunity deteriorates because of HIV infection. Otosyphilis should therefore be suspected in an HIV-infected patient with cochleovestibular abnormalities and a previous history of treated syphilis because labyrinthine disease may result from reactivation, reinfection, or persistent treponemal infection.

The mainstay of management of otosyphilis is penicillin and corticosteroids. Use of corticosteroids in the HIV-infected patient may be associated with a risk of further immunocompromise, leading to infectious complications. Corticosteroid therapy should be of short duration and be given in close consultation with the patient's primary care provider. Higher than usual doses of penicillin and longer management times have been suggested for otosyphilis because organisms tend to persist in the temporal bone. A more aggressive management regimen may be especially necessary in HIV-infected patients who cannot take corticosteroids. Therefore, these patients will not benefit from the proposed salutary effects of corticosteroids on endarteritis, which increase vessel patency for improved delivery of antibiotics to the temporal bone.[42,185] Smith and Canalis[185] propose a 3-week course of up to 24 million units/day of penicillin G in HIV-infected patients. Further studies are needed to determine the most effective management of otosyphilis in the HIV-infected patient.

Sensorineural hearing loss caused by cryptococcal meningitis

Cryptoccal meningitis is an opportunistic infection by the fungus *C. neoformans*, and is considered an AIDS-defining illness that rarely occurs when the CD4$^+$ count is greater than 100 cells/μl. Permanent SNHL occurs in as many as 27% of patients with non–HIV-related cryptococcal meningitis (Box 14-15).[108] Deafness may be sudden or rapidly

---

Box 14-14. Otosyphilis and human immunodeficiency virus (HIV) infection

There is an increased rate of syphilis in persons at risk for HIV infection
Syphilis in association with HIV infection:
  tends to persist or reactivate despite previous therapy
  tends to progress more rapidly to otosyphilis and neuro-syphilis
  requires a prolonged course of high-dose penicillin
Otosyphilis should be suspected if:
  Auditory and vestibular symptoms are present
  The fluorescent treponemal antibody absorption test is positive
A previous history of syphilis exists
A negative Venereal Disease Research Laboratory test does not rule out otosyphilis

---

Box 14-15. Cryptococcal meningitis and sensorineural hearing loss (SNHL)

Associated with low CD4$^+$ counts (<100 cells/μl)
Common presenting symptoms: frontal headache, cranial nerve abnormalities, disorientation
Sudden or rapidly progressive SNHL may be the only symptom
Rule out cryptococcal meningitis by lumbar puncture before treating with corticosteroids for sudden SNHL

progressive, and is often bilateral.[120] Audiometry, including discrimination scores and auditory brainstem response studies, demonstrate predominantly retrocochlear pathology.[77,120] Cryptococcal meningitis may also be associated with facial nerve weakness and dysequilibrium, which usually occurs after the onset of hearing loss.[96,120]

Temporal bone histopathology supports the retrocochlear audiometric features of cryptococcus-induced hearing loss. *C. neoformans* causes extensive invasion and destruction of the fibers and spiral ganglion of the cochlear nerve. Relative sparing of cochlear structures and vestibular nerves occurs in most cases of cryptococcal meningitis, except in fulminant infections.[77,82,95,123] Less prominent involvement of the vestibular nerve on temporal bone histopathology is consistent with less dominant vestibular signs and symptoms.[77,120]

The diagnosis of cryptococcal meningitis may be delayed because of its sometimes indolent course. The most common presenting symptoms are frontal headache (71%), cranial nerve abnormalities (66%), disorientation (52%), and nausea and vomiting (50%).[108,120] Meningeal signs and fever may be found in one half of patients. However, patients with cryptococcal meningitis may only complain of sudden hearing loss.[123] Hearing loss is the most common cranial nerve manifestation followed by abnormal pupillary reflexes, extraocular muscle paralysis, facial nerve paralysis, and blurred vision. Intracranial hypertension is thought to be the primary cause of visual and extraocular abnormalities associated with cryptococcal meningitis.[86,89]

If SNHL resulting from cryptococcal meningitis is misdiagnosed as idiopathic sudden hearing loss or autoimmune inner ear disease, management with corticosteroids places the patient at risk of developing fulminant life-threatening cryptococcal infection. Sudden and rapidly progressive hearing loss in an immunocompromised HIV-infected patient should therefore include serum cryptococcal antigen and a lumbar puncture before corticosteroid therapy is considered. The cerebrospinal fluid (CSF) abnormalities, which are most commonly associated with cryptococcal meningitis, are an elevated cell count (may be normal in severe cases), an increased protein level, and a high opening pressure.[108] The diagnosis is made by the detection of cryptococcal antigen and by the identification of *C. neoformans* on culture. Visualization of the encapsulated budding yeast using India ink is a quick and easy but less sensitive test. The current standard therapy is at least 2 weeks of amphotericin B (0.7 mg/kg/day) with or without 5-fluorocytosine, followed by high-dose fluconazole (at least 400 mg/day) for approximately 6 weeks, followed by life-long suppression therapy with fluconazole (200 mg/day).[208] Persistent intracranial hypertension may require serial lumbar punctures, acetazolamide, or ventricular-peritoneal shunt placement.[86]

Evaluation of sensorineural hearing loss

The first priority in the evaluation of SNHL in a patient with HIV infection is to rule out potentially life-threatening disease. A thorough history should include a description of

the rate of progression of hearing loss and the presence of dysequilibrium, other neurologic symptoms, headache, fever or neck stiffness. A complete list of all medications should be obtained and ototoxic drugs discontinued if medically feasible. A complete head and neck and neurologic examination should be performed. An audiometric evaluation should include a pure tone audiogram, stapedial reflex testing, and speech discrimination scores. Electronystagmography is useful in the evaluation of dysequilibrium to assess peripheral function. Laboratory studies, including VDRL, FTA-ABS, serum cryptococcus antigen, antinuclear antibodies (ANA), erythrocyte sedimentation rate (ESR), and rheumatoid factor (RF) titres should be routine in the evaluation of patients with SNHL. If SNHL is accompanied by headache, fever, meningeal signs, or other neurologic abnormalities, head CT or MRI should be followed by lumbar puncture (LP). Patients with advanced immunocompromise and progressive or sudden SNHL should also undergo brain imaging followed by CSF examination. Cryptococcal antigen and fungal, mycobacterial, and bacterial cultures should be performed. CSF should also be examined for cytology, VDRL and cell count, protein, and glucose. MRI of the cerebellopontine angle (CPA) with gadolinium should be considered in patients with asymmetric hearing loss and an otherwise negative workup to rule out acoustic neuromas or other lesions of this region. Auditory brainstem response abnormalities are common in the HIV-infected population, rendering this test insensitive for the detection of cochlear nerve pathology caused by mass lesions in the CPA and internal auditory canal.

Management of hearing loss in the HIV-infected population should focus on the underlying cause. As mentioned above, indiscriminate administration of corticosteroids in the setting of HIV infection is risky. There may be multiple causes of hearing loss during the course of HIV infection. As a result, the clinician should be prepared to repeat the evaluation in search for new causes of SNHL in cases of sudden and rapid deterioration of residual hearing. Finally, auditory rehabilitation with hearing aids has an important role in maintaining the quality of life in an otherwise disabling and isolating disease.

Facial nerve paralysis

Unilateral and bilateral idiopathic facial nerve paralyses occur with greater frequency in the HIV-infected population: 4.1%[169] versus about 0.04% in the general population.

Isolated facial nerve paralysis more commonly occurs in early-stage HIV infection,[11,13,23] whereas facial nerve paralysis in AIDS may be accompanied by other cranial neuropathies and neurologic abnormalities.[196]

Facial nerve palsy may be one of several neurologic abnormalities resulting from AIDS-related CNS disease.[12,96,106] Lalwani and Sooy[95] reported that facial nerve paralysis was present in 7.2% of AIDS patients with neurologic disease.[96] Facial nerve paralysis occurred in 30% of patients with toxoplasmosis, in 22% of patients with AIDS encephalopathy, in 13% of patients with CNS lymphoma, and in 8.7% of patients with cryptococcal meningitis.[96] Facial nerve paralysis may also be one of several neurologic deficits caused by progressive multifocal leukoencephalopathy, the progressive demyelinating disease of the CNS.[12,98,110] There is strong evidence that on crossing the blood–brain barrier, HIV incites a host-mediated autoimmune demyelination of cranial nerves similar to Guillain-Barré syndrome.[2,41] Increased immunoglobulins and lymphocyte pleocytosis in CSF often occurs in association with facial nerve and other cranial neuropathies, supporting an autoimmune etiology in some cases of cranial polyneuropathy.[11,62]

Isolated facial nerve paralysis may be the first symptom of HIV infection occurring in association with the acute infection or thereafter.[13,49,135,169,213] An exception to this is Ramsey-Hunt syndrome, which occurs more frequently in the setting of impaired cell-mediated immunity in later stages of HIV infection. When associated with acute HIV infection, transient facial nerve paralysis precedes seroconversion by 4 to 6 weeks.[207] Aseptic meningitis is commonly associated with facial nerve paralysis in this setting.[94,145] A flu-like illness marked by fever, myalgia, lymphadenopathy, diarrhea, and a rash usually precedes the onset of facial palsy by 3 weeks.[94,135,169,207]

The pathogenesis of isolated facial nerve weakness in HIV infection is similar to that in the general population but is likely to be influenced by the neurotropic effects of HIV and the increased susceptibility of the host to other infectious agents (Box 14-16). Nerve conduction measurements using magnetic stimulation reveal normal function of the intracranial portion of the nerve and its cortical and bulbar connections.[161] However, the intratemporal portion of the nerve shows abnormal conduction properties and clinical evidence of complete axonotmesis in most cases. This is supported by MRI findings of increased enhancement of the facial nerve in the labyrinthine portion of the fallopian canal, especially in the perigeniculate region.[49,166]

The underlying mechanisms of HIV-related isolated facial nerve paralysis therefore appear to be similar to those of Bell's palsy and zoster oticus. Inflammation of the nerve leads to intraneural edema and nerve compression at the meatal foramen and the narrow labyrinthine segment of the canal. A viscous cycle of nerve ischemia is followed by further swelling and compression, resulting in progression from neuropraxia to axonotmesis and degeneration. The viral agents that produce facial nerve dysfunction are ambiguous.[136] Inciting events leading to this cascade are likely to occur in the geniculate ganglion where herpes simplex[195] or herpes zoster[11,130] may be reactivated in the immunocompromised patient, or there may be primary infection by CMV, EBV, or HIV. Zoster oticus is a relatively infrequent cause of facial nerve paralysis in association with HIV infection. However, when it occurs in a patient diagnosed with

---

Box 14-16. Differential diagnosis of facial nerve paralysis in human immunodeficiency virus (HIV) infection

Isolated facial nerve paralysis

Geniculate ganglionitis
  Herpes zoster
  Herpes simplex, cytomegalovirus, Epstein-Barr virus, or HIV
Neuritis
  HIV
  Autoimmune demyelination
  Mononeuritis multiplex
Malignant otitis externa
Complicated otomastoiditis
Space-occupying lesion of cerebellopontine angle/internal auditory canal
Malignancy of parotid gland or temporal bone
Ideopathic

Facial nerve paralysis associated with other neurologic abnormalities

Effects of HIV infection
  Autoimmune demyelination
  Mononeuritis multiplex
  Subacute encephalitis
Central nervous system infections
  Toxoplasmosis
  Cryptococcal meningitis
  Progressive multifocal leukoencephalopathy
  Mycobacterial meningitis
Central nervous system neoplasms
  Non-Hodgkin's lymphoma
  Metastatic Kaposi's sarcoma
Skull base neoplasm
Cerebrovascular accident

---

or at risk for HIV infection, it is a predictor of deteriorating immune function and impending AIDS.[125] The prevalence of HIV infection among patients with idiopathic facial nerve paralysis is disproportionately high in endemic populations of Africa, accounting for 25% of cases in Kenya[4] and 69% of cases in Central Africa.[13] This variation in the prevalence of HIV-related facial nerve paralysis in different parts of the world suggests that either different endemic organisms are involved or there are several strains of the same organism with different neurotropic properties. HIV strains for instance are known to differ in their neurotropism.[106]

The often reported association among acute HIV infection, aseptic meningitis, and acute facial paralysis supports a direct role by HIV in some cases.[169,196] HIV may directly infect the geniculate ganglion or Schwann cells. Alternatively, inflammation associated with autoimmune demyelination of the nerve in response to infection of the CNS by HIV may result in facial nerve compression in the narrow segments of the fallopian canal. Etiologic agents thought to be involved in the pathogenesis of Bell's palsy in the general population (e.g., herpes simplex),[24,133] may infect the geniculate ganglion, or latent infection may be reactivated at an increased rate in the HIV-infected population.

Evaluation and management

The workup of facial nerve weakness may provide the initial diagnosis of HIV infection. Belec and others[13] reported that 15 of 16 patients with HIV-related facial palsy were diagnosed with HIV in the course of their evaluation for facial weakness. However, because HIV-related facial nerve paralysis can occur prior to HIV seroconversion and symptom onset of HIV infection, the true diagnosis can be easily missed.[94] Facial nerve paralysis has a high predictive value for HIV infection in populations with high rates of seroconversion.[4,13] HIV serology should therefore be included in the routine evaluation of facial nerve paralysis, especially in patients with high-risk behavior. The clinician's suspicion for HIV infection should be further increased by the presence of bilateral facial nerve paralysis, a recent flu-like illness, and Ramsay Hunt syndrome with disseminated herpes zoster.[129] Because the onset of facial weakness may precede HIV seroconversion, a negative HIV test should be followed by a repeat test 6 weeks later.[94]

Evaluation of facial nerve paralysis in HIV-infected patients should include a search for potentially life-threatening and treatable causes, such as malignant OE, temporal bone and parotid tumors, cryptococcal meningitis, and toxoplasmosis or NHL of the CNS. The history should include an account of other symptoms associated with facial nerve paralysis, including neurologic symptoms, headache, meningismus, and fever. A recent history of a flu-like illness may indicate acute HIV infection. The physical examination should include a complete neurologic examination. Otoscopy should be routinely performed to rule out middle ear and EAC pathology. Vesicles in the concha and EAC, especially when associated with otalgia, are diagnostic of zoster oticus. The parotid glands should be palpated for masses. Audiometry should be routinely performed as part of the cranial nerve evaluation. Blood should be tested for cryptococcal antigen, VDRL, FTA-ABS, ESR, and ANA.

Subsequent tests should be directed by the level of immunocompromise, results of the neurologic evaluation, and time course of the facial paralysis. The presence of other neurologic abnormalities along with facial nerve dysfunction, especially in the setting of AIDS, should raise the clinician's suspicion of an intracranial process. A brain MRI or CT with contrast should be performed in search for toxoplasmosis, NHL, and PML.[107,187] A LP should be performed and CSF sent for cell counts; glucose; protein; immunoglobulin panel to evaluate for demyelinating process; VDRL; fungal, viral, and bacterial cultures; cryptococcal antigen; and cytology for lymphoma. Unfortunately, lymphomatous meningitis is not always detected on brain imaging or CSF cytology.

Serial CSF cytology may have to be performed in the setting of persistent or progressive cranial polyneuropathy and other neurologic findings. A presumptive diagnosis of CNS lymphoma may be made in some patients based on a previous history of systemic NHL, and empiric management of the brain with radiotherapy considered.[187] Isolated and idiopathic facial nerve palsy in the asymptomatic and relatively immunocompetent HIV-infected patient may be followed clinically, similar to Bell's palsy in the general population. The absence of improvement in facial function by 4 to 6 weeks should lead to MRI or CT of the brain, temporal bones, and parotids to rule out pathology in these locations, followed by examination of the CSF.

HIV-infected patients with facial nerve paralysis, especially those with bilateral disease, are at increased risk for exposure keratitis because of poor eye closure. HIV-related periodontitis may also be exacerbated because of impaired oral sphincter function and oral dryness, leading to tooth and gum loss and poor nutrition.[49] When eye closure is insufficient to protect the cornea, artificial tears should be used throughout the day and a moisture chamber placed over each involved eye at bedtime. Frequent oral rinses and effective dental hygiene should be instituted. Ophthalmology and dentistry consultations should be requested early in the course of bilateral facial nerve dysfunction.

Medical therapy may be beneficial in some cases of HIV-related facial nerve paralysis, whereas other cases resolve spontaneously. Zidovudine has been proposed for early HIV-related paralysis, but there are no well-controlled studies to demonstrate efficacy. Corticosteroids, the mainstay of management of Bell's palsy in the immunocompetent patient, may increase the risks of life-threatening infection in the HIV-infected patient. However, in early HIV infection, especially in cases of bilateral facial paralysis, a short course of corticosteroids should be given because the risks of management are outweighed by the possible ophthalmologic and dental complications of the neuropathy. High-dose acyclovir may be beneficial in HIV-infected patients with an idiopathic facial palsy, although this has not been systematically studied.[95] Plasmapheresis may be considered for the patient who is significantly disabled by multiple cranial nerve deficits resulting from autoimmune demyelination similar to Guillain-Barré syndrome and in whom corticosteroid therapy is too risky.[107] The role of surgical decompression of the entrapped facial nerve in HIV infection is unknown. However, the potential benefit of improved nerve recovery should be weighed against the risks of craniotomy in the presence of immunocompromise.

The literature on the quality of facial nerve recovery in HIV infection is sparse. Complete recovery is more commonly reported than is incomplete recovery. The duration of weakness ranges from days to months and tends to be shorter and associated with a better outcome in early HIV infection.[94]

ORAL MANIFESTATIONS

Oral lesions (Boxes 14-17 and 14-18) occur in almost all patients during the course of HIV infection.[48] The most commonly encountered oral manifestations include candidiasis, oral hairy leukoplakia (OHL), KS, periodontal and gingival infections, aphthous ulcers, herpes simplex stomatitis, and xerostomia. The presence of one or more of these oral lesions in a patient who is at risk for HIV infection is highly predictive for HIV seroconversion.[126] KS and NHL are the most prevalent malignancies occurring in the oral cavity and pharynx. However, as the longevity of AIDS patients increases, so does their risk of developing other malignancies. The clinician should be prepared to handle this increasing challenge (1) by being familiar with the oral lesions that commonly occur in this patient population, (2) by performing biopsies of all lesions that are suspicious or that do not respond to a short course of empiric therapy, and (3) by not assuming that multiple concurrent lesions have the same pathogenesis.

Multiple different pathologic processes can occur at the same time, especially when the CD4[+] count falls to less than 200 cells/μl. In fact, identification of two or three different lesions has a predictive value of 75% and 100%, respectively. The CD4[+] count is less than 200 cells/μl.

Oral candidiasis

Candidal infection is the most common oral manifestation of HIV infection. The prevalence of oral candidiasis is 54.2%,[65] but it occurs in 70% to 90% of patients with symptomatic HIV infection and AIDS.[177] Oral candidiasis appears to be presenting in increasingly advanced stages of HIV infection according to a report by Glick and others,[65] who demonstrated a mean CD4[+] count of 149.5 cells/μl at diagnosis. These patients have a poorer-than-average prognosis and progress rapidly to AIDS.

Candidal infection of the oral mucosa can take four forms:[71] (1) Pseudomembranous candidiasis presents as a smooth white plaque that can occur on any mucosal surface (Fig. 14-7, *A*). When the plaque is wiped off, an erythematous and bleeding base remains. (2) Atrophic candidiasis presents as zones of hyperemia and tenderness on the dorsum of the tongue or the hard palate. (3) Hyperplastic candidiasis most commonly involves the buccal mucosa to produce raised white plaques that cannot be scraped off. The differential diagnosis of this lesion includes leukoplakia, carcinoma in situ, and oral hairy leukoplakia. Diagnosis is made by biopsy or potassium hydroxide preparation, which reveals hyphae and yeast. (4) Angular cheilitis presents as tender and erythematous fissures and ulcers at the oral commissure (Fig. 14-7, *B*).

Candidal infection can be diagnosed based on the resolution of these lesions with empiric anticandidal therapy. More definitive diagnosis can be made by a potassium hydroxide preparation or Gram's stain of a scraping or by periodic acid-schiff stain of a biopsy specimen.

Topical therapy is effective for oral candidiasis in early HIV infection. Nystatin solution 200,000 to 400,000 units five times per day or clotrimazole 10 mg five times per day are commonly used. Angular cheilitis can be managed with topical antifungal creams, such as nystatin, clotrimazole, or ketoconazole. Oral candidiasis can also be effectively managed with systemic therapy, including ketaconazole 200 mg/day or fluconazole 50 mg/day. A combination of topical and systemic therapy should be used in patients with severe immunocompromise.

Oral hairy leukoplakia

OHL is a white lesion with a corrugated and shaggy surface; it most frequently occurs on the lateral surface of the tongue. This lesion only occurs in the setting of HIV infection, affecting 17% to 25% of patients.[65,177] OHL appears to result from a local opportunistic infection by EBV.[72] Its presence in an otherwise asymptomatic patient is a strong indicator of a diagnosis of HIV infection and moderate to severe immunosuppression. In one series, the mean CD4[+] count of patients with OHL was 143 cells/μl.[65] OHL indicates a poor prognosis for progression to AIDS.[71] Within 3

Box 14-17. Differential diagnosis of oral lesions in human immunodeficiency virus infection

Oral candidiasis
Oral hairy leukoplakia
Herpes stomatitis
Gingival and periodontal disease
    Acute necrotizing ulcerative gingivitis*
    Necrotizing stomatitis
Aphthous ulcers
Bacillary angiomatosis*
Squamous cell carcinoma*
Leukoplakia
Non-Hodgkin's lymphoma*
Kaposi's sarcoma

* May be associated with bone erosion.

Box 14-18. Oral disease and human immunodeficiency virus infection

More than two different HIV-related oral lesions suggest a CD4[+] count of less than 200 cells/μl
Presence of major aphthous ulcer suggests CD4[+] count less than 200 cells/μl
Rule out malignancy with early biopsy of new lesions
Complications of gingival and periodontal disease can be prevented by early periodontal consultation

years of the appearance of OHL 86% of cases progress to AIDS.[19]

When an oral lesion persists despite a short course of anticandidal therapy, a biopsy is indicated to rule out a malignant or premalignant lesion. The differential diagnosis of OHL includes leukoplakia, carcinoma in situ, hypertrophic candidiasis, and lichen planus. OHL is diagnosed on biopsy by the presence of hyperkeratosis, acanthosis, and clear or ''balloon'' cells in the upper spinous cell layer with minimal inflammation (Fig. 14-8). Once the diagnosis is made, further management is rarely needed because OHL is asymptomatic and does not undergo malignant transformation. No single medication has been consistently successful in pro-

ducing a remission of OHL. Occasional success has been reported with the use of acyclovir, zidovudine, and sulfa drugs, but the recurrence rate is high.[19,71]

Herpes simplex stomatitis

Infections of the oral cavity by herpes simplex virus increase in all stages of HIV infection. The overall incidence is 5%, whereas in late-stage HIV infection it is 9% to 29%.[65,177] Herpetic lesions are particularly persistent when the CD4[+] count is less than 100 cells/μl.

Herpes labialis is the most common manifestation of herpes simplex infection of the oral cavity. When they occur in the HIV-infected patient, these ''fever blisters'' are gener-

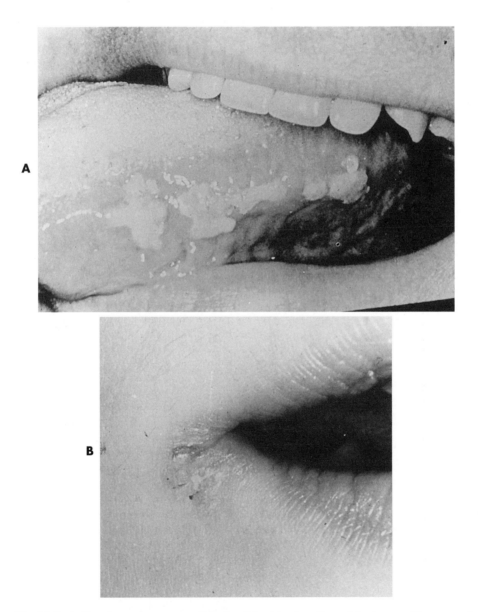

Fig. 14-7. A, Pseudomembranous candidiasis of the lateral surface of the tongue. These smooth white plaques are easily scraped from the mucosa, leaving an erythematous and bleeding base. **B,** Angular cheilitis characterized by tender ulcers and fissures of the oral commissure as a result of candidal infection. (Courtesy of Dr. Steven Ashman.)

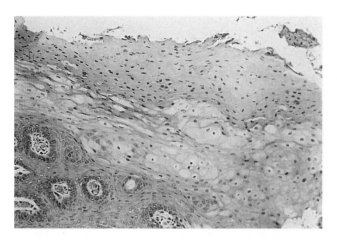

Fig. 14-8. Photomicrograph of oral hairy leukoplakia. Characteristic hyperparakeratosis is present, as is a layer of "balloon cells" in the upper spinous cell layer. (Courtesy of Dr. Russel Corio.)

ally larger, are more numerous, persist longer, and recur more frequently than in the general population.

Intraoral infection by herpes simplex usually affects the keratinized and attached mucosa of the hard palate and gingiva and the dorsum of the tongue. The characteristic appearance is that of small round ulcers without an erythematous halo. Multiple ulcers can produce significant discomfort with mastication and swallowing, threatening nutrition. Herpes simplex virus (HSV) infection in the HIV-infected patient is likely to be prolonged and less localized than in the general population.

Herpes simplex infection can be diagnosed by culturing the virus from vesicles or by showing HSV in cells scraped from the base of the lesion using monoclonal anti–HSV antibodies (Tzanck test). As soon as vesicles consistent with HSV infection appear, topical acyclovir therapy should be instituted five times per day for 5 days. In the severely immunocompromised patient or in the patient with a generalized vesicular rash, topical therapy should be combined with systemic therapy for 5 days, with acyclovir at 200 mg five times per day.[71]

Gingivitis and periodontal disease

Infection of the gingiva and periodontal structures in the HIV-infected patient can produce a spectrum of pathology ranging from gingivitis to necrotizing stomatitis. Despite good oral hygiene and timely therapy, gingivitis and periodontal disease commonly recur in the HIV-infected patient.

Gingivitis presents as a red line at the free gingival margin, and the gums bleed with minimal trauma.[71] Periodontitis results from the extension of infection to the peridontium and resorption of alveolar bone, resulting in loosening and loss of teeth and deep dental pain.

A rapidly progressive and necrotizing form of gingivitis is known as acute necrotizing ulcerative gingivitis (ANUG). Gingivitis progresses to ANUG within 4 weeks, resulting in the necrosis of gingival tissue and alveolar bone.[71] Symptoms include deep jaw pain, bleeding, halitosis, and loose teeth. The tissue above the interdental papillae is typically yellow-grey and bleeds easily. Necrotizing stomatitis is a complication of ANUG resulting from extensive soft-tissue destruction and the exposure of bone with significant bone destruction and sequestration.[71] Gram-negative anaerobes appear to play an important role in the pathogenesis of ANUG and necrotizing stomatitis.

The risk of progression from gingivitis to periodontitis and then to ANUG increases as immune function deteriorates and the CD4+ count falls. Patients with HIV-related gingivitis tend to have T4:T8 ratios greater than 1, whereas those with periodontitis have significantly reduced ratios.[212] The incidence of HIV-related ANUG increases as the CD4+ count falls to less than 200 cells/μl. The mean CD4+ count at diagnosis is approximately 50 cells/μl.[65]

The differential diagnosis of a destructive process that involves the soft tissue and bone of the alveolar crests includes lymphoma, SCC, KS, bacillary angiomatosis, fungal infection, and mycobacterial infection. The presence of bone destruction out of proportion with the soft-tissue changes is more likely to be caused by bacillary angiomatosis than ANUG.[66] Tissue should be sent for histopathology and microbiology. Periodontal consultation should be requested for appropriate and expeditious management of periodontal disease.

The mainstay of therapy for HIV-related gingivitis and periodontitis includes dental plaque removal and oral rinses with 10% povidone-iodine with 0.1% to 0.2% chlorhexidine gluconate.[71] Management of ANUG and necrotizing stomatitis includes a combination of local care and systemic antianaerobic drug therapy. The necrotic tissue should be débrided, the teeth scaled, and parenteral antibiotic therapy with clindamycin or flagyl instituted.

Aphthous ulcers

Aphthous ulcers are of three types, all of which affect unattached oral mucosa. Herpetiform ulcers are smaller than 0.2 mm in diameter and are self-limited with minimal morbidity. Minor aphthous ulcers are well-circumscribed, painful ulcers less than 6 mm in diameter with an erythematous halo. In the HIV-infected patient, ulcers frequently coalesce to form larger lesions lasting about 2 weeks.

Major aphthous ulcers (Sutton's disease) are larger than 6 mm in diameter (Fig. 14-9). They are painful, persist for weeks, and threaten nutritional intake. They are difficult to grossly differentiate from malignancy. The incidence of major aphthous ulcers is as high as 14% in association with HIV infection.[177]

Glick and others[65] have shown that major aphthous ulcers are highly predictive of a CD4+ count less than 200 cells/μl presenting in patients with a mean CD4+ count of 33.7 cells/μl.

Management should focus on ruling out malignancy, pro-

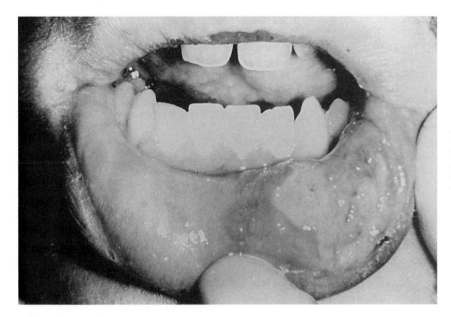

Fig. 14-9. Major aphthous ulcer (Sutton's disease) of the lower lip. This lesion is indistinguishable from lymphoma or squamous cell carcinoma and should undergo biopsy. (Courtesy of Dr. Steven Ashman.)

viding symptomatic relief, and monitoring nutritional status. The edge of the ulcer should be biopsied and submitted for histopathology to rule out lymphoma and SCC. The size, chronicity, and exquisite tenderness of major aphthous ulcers mandate close monitoring of body weight and the provision of liquid nutritional supplements. Aphthous ulcers are treated with topical corticosteroids, such as triamcinolone or fluocinomide mixed in orobase and applied up to six times per day.[71] Other topical preparations include tetracycline, 250 mg per 5 ml used as a mouth wash four times per day for 4 days, or chlorhexidine, 0.1% to 0.2% twice per day for 7 days. The prudent use of systemic corticosteroids may be necessary in major aphthous ulcers.

Xerostomia

Of HIV-infected patients, 7% to 14% complain of xerostomia.[65,177] Some cases are iatrogenically induced by the use of antidepressants and other drugs, whereas other cases are caused by chronic mouth breathing secondary to sinonasal disease or adenoidal hypertrophy. HIV-related xerostomia is associated with parotid enlargement in 33% of cases possibly because of autoimmune or infectious disease of the salivary glands.

The incidence of dental caries is increased and deglutition is often impaired. Salivary substitutes, frequent saline rinses, and sialogogues help alleviate these problems. Dental caries can be prevented with fluoride.

REFERENCES

1. Abrams DI: AIDS-related lymphadenopathy: the role of biopsy, *J Clin Oncol* 4:126, 1986.
2. Abrams DI and others: Persistent diffuse lymphadenopathy in homosexual men: endpoint or prodrome, *Ann Intern Med* 100:801, 1984.
3. AHFS, McEvoy GK, editor: Drug information, Bethesda, Md, 1996, American Society of Health-Systems Pharmacists, Inc.
4. Amayo EO, Kwasa TOO: HIV and acute peripheral facial nerve palsy, *East Afr Med J* 68:948, 1991.
5. Ames ED and others: Hodgkin's disease and AIDS, *Hematol Oncol Clin North Am* 5:343, 1991.
6. Armstrong M and others: Radiographic imaging of sinusitis in HIV infection, *Otolaryngol Head Neck Surg* 108:36, 1993.
7. Bankaitis AE, Keith RW: Audiological changes associated with HIV infection, *Ear Nose Throat J* 74:353, 1995.
8. Barnett E and others: Otitis media in children born to human immunodeficiency virus–infected mothers, *Pediatr Infect Dis J* 11:360, 1992.
9. Baroni CD, Uccini S: The lymphadenopathy of HIV infection, *Am J Clin Pathol* 99:397, 1993.
10. Batsakis J and others: Bacillary angiomatosis, *Ann Otol Rhinol Laryngol* 104:668, 1995.
11. Belec L and others: Peripheral facial nerve palsy related to HIV infection: relationship with the immunological status and the HIV staging in Central Africa, *Cent Afr J Med* 37:88, 1991.
12. Belec L and others: Peripheral facial paralysis and HIV infection: report of four African cases and review of the literature, *J Neurol* 236:411, 1989.
13. Belec L and others: Peripheral facial paralysis indicating HIV infection, *Lancet* ii:1421, 1988.
14. Beral V and others: AIDS-associated non-Hodgkin lymphoma, *Lancet* 337:805, 1991.
15. Beral V and others: Kaposi's sarcoma among persons with AIDS: a sexually transmitted infection? *Lancet* 335:123, 1990.
16. Berson A and others: Radiation therapy for AIDS-related Kaposi's sarcoma, *Int J Radiat Oncol Biol Phys* 19:569, 1990.
17. Birchall MA and others: Auditory function in patients infected with the human immunodeficiency virus, *Clin Otolaryngol* 17:117, 1992.
18. Birchall MA and others: Changing patterns of HIV infection in otolaryngology, *Clin Otolaryngol* 19:473, 1994.
19. Birchall M, Murphy S: *HIV infection and AIDS*, Edinburgh, Scotland, 1992, Churchill Livingstone.
20. Blatt SP and others: Rhinocerebral zygomycosis in a patient with AIDS, *J Infect Dis* 164:215, 1991.
21. Bottles K and others: Fine-needle aspiration biopsy of patients with the acquired immunodeficiency syndrome (AIDS): experience in an outpatient clinic, *Ann Intern Med* 108:42, 1988.
22. Breda SD and others: Pneumocystis carinii in the temporal bone as

a primary manifestation of the acquired immunodeficiency syndrome, *Ann Otol Rhinol Laryngol* 97:427, 1988.

23. Brown MM and others: Bell's palsy and HIV infection, *J Neurol Neurosurg Psychiatry* 51:425, 1988.

24. Burgess R and others: Polymerase chain reaction amplification of herpes simplex viral DNA from the geniculate ganglion of a patient with Bell's palsy, *Ann Otol Rhinol Laryngol* 103:775, 1994.

25. Burke AP and others: Systemic lymphadenopathic histology in human immunodeficiency virus-1 seropositive drug addicts without apparent acquired immunodeficiency syndrome, *Hum Pathol* 25:248, 1994.

26. Burton F and others: Open cervical node biopsy in HIV-positive patients, *Otolaryngol Head Neck Surg* 107:367, 1992.

27. Carbone A and others: A clinicopathologic study of lymphoid neoplasms associated with human immunodeficiency virus infection in Italy, *Cancer* 68:842, 1991.

28. Carbone A and others: Morphologic patterns and molecular pathways of AIDS-related head and neck and other systemic lymphomas, *Ann Otol Rhinol Laryngol* 105:495, 1996.

29. Carson PJ and others: Antibody class and subclass responses to pneumococcal polysaccharides following immunization of human immunodeficiency virus–infected patients, *J Infect Dis* 172:340, 1995.

30. Centers for Disease Control: 1993 Revised classification system for HIV infection and expanded surveillance case definition for AIDS among adolescents and adults, *MMWR Morb Mortal Wkly Rep* 41:1, 1992.

31. Centers for Disease Control: Revision classification of acquired immunodeficiency syndrome for national reporting: United States, *MMWR Morb Mortal Wkly Rep* 34:373, 1985.

32. Centers for Disease Control: US HIV and AIDS cases reported through June 1994, *HIV/AIDS Surveillance Report* 6, 1994.

33. Chachoua A and others: Prognostic factors and staging classification of patients with epidemic Kaposi's sarcoma, *J Clin Oncol* 7:774, 1989.

34. Chadburn A and others: Progressive lymph node histology and its prognostic value in patients with acquired immunodeficiency syndrome and AIDS-related complex, *Hum Pathol* 20:579, 1989.

35. Chandra Sekhar SS and others: Histopathologic and ultrastructural changes in the temporal bones of HIV-infected human adults, *Am J Otol* 13:207, 1991.

36. Chapnik JS and others: Parotid gland enlargement in HIV infection: clinical/imaging findings, *J Otolaryngol* 19:189, 1990.

37. Cheung SW and others: Orbitocerebral complications of pseudomonas sinusitis, *Laryngoscope* 102:1385, 1992.

38. Choi SS and others: Cryptococcal sinusitis: a case report and review of literature, *Otolaryngol Head Neck Surg* 99:414, 1988.

39. Chong WK and others: The prevalence of paranasal sinus disease in HIV infection and AIDS on cranial MR imaging, *Clin Radiol* 47:166, 1993.

40. Colby T and others: Hodgkin's disease: a clinicopathologic study of 659 cases, *Cancer* 49:1848, 1982.

41. Dalakas MC, Pezeshkpour GH: Neuromuscular diseases associated with human immunodeficiency virus infection, *Ann Neurol* 23(suppl): S38, 1988.

42. Darmstadt GL, Harris JP: Luetic hearing loss: clinical presentation, diagnosis and treatment, *Am J Otolaryngol* 10:410, 1989.

43. Davidson BJ and others: Lymphadenopathy in the HIV-seropositive patient, *Ear Nose Throat J* 69:478, 1990.

44. Davis JM and others: Lymph node biopsy in patients with human immunodeficiency virus infections, *Arch Surg* 123:1349, 1988.

45. Davis LE and others: Clinical viral infections and temporal bone histologic studies of patients with AIDS, *Otolaryngol Head Neck Surg* 113:695, 1995.

46. Denning DW and others: Pulmonary aspergillosis in the acquired immunodeficiency syndrome, *N Engl J Med* 324:654, 1991.

47. Desai S: Seropositivity, adenoid hypertrophy, and secretory otitis media in adults: a recognized clinical entity, *Otolaryngol Head Neck Surg* 107:755, 1992.

48. Dichtel W: *Oral manifestations of human immunodeficiency virus infection.* In Tami TA, editor: *Otolaryngologic manifestations of the acquired immunodeficiency syndrome,* Philadelphia, 1992, WB Saunders.

49. Durham TM and others: Facial nerve paralysis related to HIV disease: case report and dental considerations, *Oral Surg Oral Med Oral Pathol* 75:37, 1993.

50. Elder GA, Sever JL: AIDS and neurological disorders: an overview, *Ann Neurol* 23(suppl):S4, 1988.

51. Ellis M and others: Impaired neutrophil function in patients with AIDS or AIDS-related complex: a comprehensive evaluation, *J Infect Dis* 158:1268, 1988.

52. Fahey JL and others: The prognostic value of cellular and serologic markers in infection with human immunodeficiency virus type I, *N Engl J Med* 322:166, 1990.

53. Fauci AS: The human immunodeficiency virus: infectivity and mechanisms of pathogenesis, *Science* 239:617, 1988.

54. Ficarro G and others: Kaposi's sarcoma of the oral cavity: a study of 134 patients with a review of the pathogenesis, epidemiology, clinical aspects and treatment, *Oral Surg Oral Med Oral Pathol* 66:543, 1988.

55. Finn DG: Lymphoma of the head and neck and acquired immunodeficiency syndrome: clinical investigation and immunohistological study, *Laryngoscope* 105(suppl 68):1, 1995.

56. Flaitz CM and others: Intraoral squamous cell carcinoma in human immunodeficiency virus infection: a clinicopathologic study, *Oral Surg Oral Med Oral Pathol* 80:55, 1994.

57. Frank Y, Pahwa S: Serial brainstem auditory evoked responses in infants and children with AIDS, *Clin Electroencephalogr* 24:160, 1993.

58. Fried MP and others: Pseudomonas rhinosinusitis, *Laryngoscope* 94: 192, 1984.

59. Gachupin-Garcia A and others: Population-based study of malignancies and HIV infection among injecting drug users in a New York City methadone treatment program, 1985–1991, *AIDS* 6:843, 1992.

60. Gallant J and others: Risk factors for Kaposi's sarcoma in patients with advanced human immunodeficiency virus disease treated with zidovudine, *Arch Intern Med* 154:566, 1994.

61. Gherman CR and others: Pneumocystis carinii otitis media and mastoiditis as the initial manifestation of the acquired immunodeficiency syndrome, *Am J Med* 85:250, 1988.

62. Ghika-Schmid F and others: Diversite de l'atteinte neuromusculaire de 47 patients infectes par le virus de l'immunodeficience humaine, *Schweiz Med Wochenschr* 124:791, 1994.

63. Gill P and others: Advanced acquired immune deficiency syndrome–related Kaposi's sarcoma: results of pilot studies using combination chemotherapy, *Cancer* 65:1074, 1990.

64. Gill P and others: Phase I/II clinical and pharmacokinetic evaluation of liposomal daunorubicin, *J Clin Oncol* 13:996, 1995.

65. Glick M and others: Oral manifestations associated with HIV-related disease as markers for immune suppression and AIDS, *Oral Surg Oral Med Oral Pathol* 77:344, 1994.

66. Glick M, Cleveland D: Oral mucosal bacillary epithelioid angiomatosis in a patient with AIDS associated with rapid alveolar bone loss: case report, *J Oral Pathol Med* 22:235, 1993.

67. Godofsky EW and others: Sinusitis in HIV-infected patients: a clinical and radiographic review, *Am J Med* 93:163, 1992.

68. Goldberg AN: Kaposi's sarcoma of the head and neck in acquired immunodeficiency syndrome, *Am J Otolaryngol* 14:5, 1993.

69. Gonzalez MM and others: Acquired immunodeficiency syndrome associated with Acanthamoeba infection and other opportunistic organisms, *Arch Pathol Lab Med* 110:749, 1986.

70. Greenberg P: *Immunopathogenesis of HIV infection.* In Corey L, editor: *AIDS: problems and prospects,* New York, 1993, WW Norton & Co.

71. Greenspan D and others: *AIDS and the mouth,* Copenhagen, Denmark, 1990, Munksgaard.

72. Greenspan J and others: Replication of Epstein-Barr virus within the epithelial cells of oral hairy leukoplakia, an AIDS-associated lesion, *N Engl J Med* 313:1564, 1985.

73. Grimaldi LME and others: Bilateral eighth cranial nerve neuropathy in human immunodeficiency virus infection, *J Neurol* 240:363, 1993.

74. Hadfield P and others: The ENT manifestations of HIV infection in children, *Clin Otolaryngol* 21:30, 1996.

75. Hall P, Farrior J: Aspergillus mastoiditis, *Otolaryngol Head Neck Surg* 108:167, 1993.

76. Hamilton JC and others: Synergistic effect on mortality in mice with murine cytomegalovirus and Pseudomonas aeruginosa, Staphylococcus aureus, or Candida albicans infection, *Infect Immun* 14:982, 1976.

77. Harada T and others: Temporal bone histopathology in deafness due to cryptococcal meningitis, *Ann Otol* 88:630, 1979.

78. Hausler R and others: Neuro-otological manifestations in different stages of HIV infection, *Acta Otolaryngol (Stockh)* 481(suppl):515, 1991.

79. Herndier BG and others: Pathogenesis of AIDS lymphomas, *AIDS* 8:1025, 1994.

80. Holmes KK: *The changing epidemiology of HIV transmission.* In Corey L, editor: *AIDS: problems and prospects,* New York, 1993, WW Norton & Co.

81. Hruza GJ, Snow SN: Basal cell carcinoma in a patient with acquired immunodeficiency syndrome: treatment with Mohs micrographic surgery fixed-tissue technique, *J Dermatol Surg Oncol* 15:545, 1989.

82. Igarashi M and others: Temporal bone findings in Cryptococcal meningitis, *Arch Otolaryngol* 101:577, 1975.

83. Ioachim HL and others: Acquired immunodeficiency syndrome–associated lymphomas: clinical, pathologic, immunologic, and viral characteristics of 111 cases, *Hum Pathol* 22:659, 1991.

84. Jaffe HW: The laboratory diagnosis of syphilis, *Ann Intern Med* 83:846, 1975.

85. Jin J and others: Detection of Kaposi's sarcoma–associated herpesvirus-like DNA sequence in vascular lesions: a reliable diagnostic marker for Kaposi's sarcoma, *Am J Clin Pathol* 105:360, 1996.

86. Johnston S and others: Raised intracranial pressure and visual complications in AIDS patients with cryptococcal meningitis, *J Infect* 24:185, 1992.

87. Kaplan LD and others: AIDS-associated non-Hodgkin's lymphoma in San Francisco, *JAMA* 261:719, 1989.

88. Kaplan LD and others: Clinical and virologic effects of recombinant human granulocyte-macrophage colony-stimulating factor in patients receiving chemotherapy for human immunodeficiency virus–associated non-Hodgkin's lymphoma: results of a randomized trial, *J Clin Oncol* 9:929, 1991.

89. Keane J: Intermittent third nerve palsy with cryptococcal meningitis, *J Clin Neuroophthalmol* 13:124, 1993.

90. Kielhofner M and others: Life-threatening Pseudomonas aeruginosa infections in patients with human immunodeficiency virus infection, *Clin Infect Dis* 14:403, 1992.

91. Kohan D and others: Otologic disease in AIDS patients: CT correlation, *Laryngoscope* 100:1326, 1990.

92. Kohan D and others: Otologic disease in patients with acquired immunodeficiency syndrome, *Ann Otol Rhinol Laryngol* 97:636, 1988.

93. Koralnik IJ and others: A controlled study of early neurologic abnormalities in men with asymptomatic human immunodeficiency virus infection, *N Engl J Med* 323:864, 1990.

94. Krasner CG, Cohen SH: Bilateral Bell's palsy and aseptic meningitis in a patient with acute human immunodeficiency virus seroconversion, *West J Med* 159:604, 1993.

95. Kwartler JA and others: Sudden hearing loss due to AIDS-related cryptococcal meningitis: a temporal bone study, *Otolaryngol Head Neck Surg* 104:265, 1991.

96. Lalwani AK, Sooy CD: Otologic and neurotologic manifestations of acquired immunodeficiency syndrome, *Otolaryngol Clin North Am* 25:1183, 1992.

97. Lamprecht J, Wiedbrauck C: Sinusitis und andere typische Erkrankungen im HNO-Bereich im rahmen des erworbenen immunodefektsyndroms (AIDS), *HNO* 36:489, 1988.

98. Langford-Kuntz A and others: Impairment of cranio-facial nerves due to AIDS, *Int J Oral Maxillofac Surg* 17:227, 1988.

99. Laubenstein L and others: Treatment of epidemic Kaposi's sarcoma with etoposide or a combination of doxorubicin, bleomycin, and vinblastine, *J Clin Oncol* 2:1115, 1984.

100. Lee K, Cheung S: Evaluation of the neck mass in human immunodeficiency virus–infected patients, *Otolaryngol Clin North Am* 25:1287, 1992.

101. Levine AM: Acquired immunodeficiency syndrome–related lymphoma, *Blood* 80:8, 1992.

102. Levine AM: Epidemiology, clinical characteristics, and management of AIDS-related lymphoma, *Hematol Oncol Clin North Am* 5:331, 1991.

103. Levine AM and others: Low-dose chemotherapy with central nervous system prophylaxis and zidovudine maintenance in AIDS-related lymphoma, *JAMA* 226:84, 1991.

104. Levine AM and others: Results of initial lymph node biopsy in homosexual men with generalized lymphadenopathy, *J Clin Oncol* 4:165, 1986.

105. Levine AM and others: Retrovirus and malignant lymphoma in homosexual men, *JAMA* 254:1921, 1985.

106. Levy JA: *The retroviruses and pathogenesis of HIV infection.* In Corey L, editor: *AIDS: problems and prospects,* New York, 1993, WW Norton & Co.

107. Levy RM and others: Neurological manifestations of the acquired immunodeficiency syndrome (AIDS): experience at UCSF and review of the literature, *J Neurosurg* 62:475, 1985.

108. Lewis JL, Rabinovich S: The wide spectrum of cryptococcal infections, *Am J Med* 53:315, 1972.

109. Linstrom CJ and others: Otologic neurotologic manifestations of HIV-related disease, *Otolaryngol Head Neck Surg* 108:680, 1993.

110. Lipton RB and others: Progressive multifocal leukoencephalopathy of the posterior fossa in an AIDS patient: clinical, radiographic and evoked potential findings, *Eur Neurol* 28:285, 1988.

111. Little JP and others: Otosyphilis in a patient with human immunodeficiency virus: internal auditory canal gumma, *Otolaryngol Head Neck Surg* 112:488, 1995.

112. Lortholary O and others: Invasive aspergillosis in patients with acquired immunodeficiency syndrome: report of 33 cases, *Am J Med* 95:177, 1993.

113. Loveday C, Hill A: Prediction of progression to AIDS with serum HIV-1 RNA and CD4 count, *Lancet* 345:790, 1995.

114. Lyos A and others: Invasive Aspergillosis of the temporal bone: an unusual manifestation of acquired immunodeficiency syndrome, *Am J Otol* 14:444, 1993.

115. Lyter DW and others: Incidence of human immunodeficiency virus–related and nonrelated malignancies in a large cohort of homosexual men, *J Clin Oncol* 13:2540, 1995.

116. Mack LW and others: Temporal bone treponemes, *Arch Otolaryngol Head Neck Surg* 90:37, 1969.

117. Manfredi R and others: Recombinant human granulocyte-macrophage colony-stimulating factor (RHUGM-CSF) in leukopenic patients with advanced HIV disease, *J Chemother* 8:214, 1996.

118. Marchisio P and others: Etiology of acute otitis media in human immunodeficiency virus–infected children, *Pediatr Infect Dis J* 15:58, 1996.

119. Mascart-Lemone F and others: Differential effect of human immunodeficiency virus infection on the IgA and IgG antibody responses to pneumococcal vaccine, *J Infect Dis* 172:1253, 1995.

120. Maslan MJ and others: Cryptococcal meningitis: presentation as sudden deafness, *Am J Otol* 6:435, 1985.

121. Mauss S, Jablonowski H: Efficacy, safety, and tolerance of low-dose, long-term interferon-alpha 2b and zidovudine in early-stage AIDS-

associated Kaposi's sarcoma, *J Acquir Immune Defic Syndr Hum Retrovirol* 10:157, 1995.

122. McChesney MB, Oldstone MBA: Virus-induced immunosuppression: infections with measles virus and human immunodeficiency virus, *Adv Immunol* 45:335, 1989.

123. McGill TJI: Mycotic infection of the temporal bone, *Arch Otolaryngol Head Neck Surg* 104:140, 1978.

124. McGregor JM and others: Cutaneous malignant melanoma and human immunodeficiency virus (HIV) infection: a report of three cases, *Br J Dermatol* 126:516, 1992.

125. Melbye M and others: Risk of AIDS after herpes zoster, *Lancet* 1: 728, 1987.

126. Melnick S and others: Oral mucosal lesions: association with the presence of antibodies to the human immunodeficiency virus, *Oral Surg Oral Med Oral Pathol* 68:37, 1989.

127. Meyer RD and others: Fungal sinusitis in patients with AIDS: report of 4 cases and review of the literature, *Medicine* 73:69, 1994.

128. Milgram LM and others: Mucociliary clearance abnormalities in the HIV-infected patient: a precursor to acute sinusitis, *Laryngoscope* 105:1202, 1995.

129. Milgram LM and others: Sinusitis in human immunodeficiency virus infection: typical and atypical organisms, *J Otolaryngol* 23:450, 1994.

130. Mishell JH, Applebaum EL: Ramsey-Hunt syndrome in a patient with HIV infection, *Otolaryngol Head Neck Surg* 102:177, 1990.

131. Monfardini S and others: Characterization of AIDS-associated tumors in Italy: report of 435 cases of an IVDA-based series, *Cancer Detect Prev* 14:391, 1990.

132. Moss AR, Bacchetti P: Natural history of HIV infection, *AIDS* 3:55, 1989.

133. Mulkens P and others: Acute facial paralysis: a virological study, *Clin Otolaryngol* 5:305, 1980.

134. Murphy PM and others: Impairment of neutrophil bactericidal capacity in patients with AIDS, *J Infect Dis* 158:627, 1988.

135. Murr AH, Benecke JE: Association of facial paralysis with HIV positivity, *Am J Otol* 12:450, 1991.

136. Niparko J: *The acute facial palsies.* In Jackler RK, Brackman O, editors: *Neurotology,* St Louis, 1994, Mosby.

137. O'Donnell JG and others: Sinusitis due to Pseudomonas aeruginosa in patients with human immunodeficiency virus infection, *Clin Infect Dis* 16:404, 1993.

138. Pagano MA and others: Brain-stem auditory evoked potentials in human immunodeficiency virus–seropositive patients with and without acquired immunodeficiency syndrome, *Arch Neurol* 49:166, 1992.

139. Palefsky J: Human papillomavirus infection among HIV-infected individuals: implications for development of malignant tumors, *Hematol Oncol Clin North Am* 5:357, 1991.

140. Park S and others: Pneumocystis carinii infection in the middle ear, *Arch Otolaryngol Head Neck Surg* 118:269, 1992.

141. Parry GJ: Peripheral neuropathies associated with human immunodeficiency virus infection, *Ann Neurol* 23(suppl):S49, 1988.

142. Patow C and others: Pharyngeal obstruction by Kaposi's sarcoma in a homosexual male with acquired immune deficiency syndrome, *Otolaryngol Head Neck Surg* 92:713, 1984.

143. Penn I: Tumor incidence in human allograft recipients, *Transplant Proc* 11:1047, 1979.

144. Peterlin BM, Luciw PA: Molecular biology of HIV, *AIDS* 2(suppl 1):S29, 1988.

145. Piette AM and others: Acute neuropathy coincident with seroconversion for anti-LAV/HTLV-III, *Lancet* 1:852, 1986.

146. Pluda JM and others: Development of non-Hodgkin lymphoma in a cohort of patients with severe human immune deficiency virus (HIV) infection on long-term antiretroviral therapy, *Ann Intern Med* 113: 276, 1990.

147. Poletti A and others: Study of AIDS-related lymphadenopathy in the intraparotid and perisubmaxillary gland lymph nodes, *J Oral Pathol* 17:164, 1988.

148. Pomilla PV and others: Sinonasal non-Hodgkin's lymphoma in patients infected with human immunodeficiency virus: report of three cases and review, *Clin Infect Dis* 21:137, 1995.

149. Quinn TC and others: Serologic and immunologic studies in patients with AIDS in North America and Africa, *JAMA* 257:2617, 1987.

150. Rabkin CS and others: Increasing incidence of cancers associated with the human immunodeficiency virus epidemic, *Int J Cancer* 47:692, 1991.

151. Rabkin CS, Blattner WA: HIV infection and cancers other than non-Hodgkin lymphoma and Kaposi's sarcoma, *Cancer Surv* 10:151, 1991.

152. Rabkin CS, Goedert JJ: Risks of non-Hodgkin lymphoma and Kaposi's sarcoma in homosexual men, *Lancet* 336:248, 1990.

153. Rarey KE: Otologic pathophysiology in patients with human immunodeficiency virus, *Am J Otolaryngol* 11:366, 1990.

154. Reath DB and others: Primary Kaposi's sarcoma of an intraparotid lymph node with AIDS, *Plast Reconstr Surg* 80:615, 1987.

155. Reiss P and others: Invasive external otitis caused by Aspergillus fumigatus in two patients with AIDS, *AIDS* 5:605, 1991.

156. Remick SC: AIDS-related non-Hodgkin's lymphoma, *Cancer Control* 2:97, 1995.

157. Roithmann S and others: AIDS-associated non-Hodgkin lymphoma, *Lancet* 338:884, 1991.

158. Roland JT and others: Squamous cell carcinoma in HIV-positive patients under age 45, *Laryngoscope* 103:509, 1993.

159. Rosenberg ZF, Fauci AS: The immunopathogenesis of HIV infection, *Adv Immunol* 47:377, 1989.

160. Rosenhall U and others: Otoneurological abnormalities in asymptomatic HIV-seropositive patients, *Acta Neurol Scand* 79:140, 1989.

161. Rosler KM and others: Electrophysiological characteristics of lesions in facial palsies of different etiologies: a study using electrical and magnetic stimulation techniques, *Electroencephalogr Clin Neurophysiol* 97:355, 1995.

162. Rubin J, Honigsberg R: Sinusitis in patients with the acquired immunodeficiency syndrome, *Ear Nose Throat J* 69:460, 1990.

163. Rubinstein A: *Pediatric AIDS.* In Lockhart JD and others, editors: *Current problems in pediatrics,* Chicago, 1986, Mosby.

164. Ryan JR and others: Acquired immune deficiency syndrome–related lymphadenopathies presenting in the salivary gland lymph nodes, *Arch Otolaryngol* 111:554, 1985.

165. Sample S and others: Elevated serum concentration of IgE antibodies to environmental antigens in HIV-seropositive male homosexuals, *J Allergy Clin Immunol* 86:876, 1990.

166. Sartoretti-Schefer S and others: Idiopathic, herpetic, and HIV-associated facial nerve palsies: abnormal MR enhancement patterns, *AJNR Am J Neuroradiol* 15:479, 1994.

167. Sattentau QJ: The role of the CD4 antigen in HIV infection and immune pathogenesis, *AIDS* 2(suppl 1):S11, 1988.

168. Schaffner and others: Protection against conidia by mononuclear and against mycelia by polymorphonuclear phagocytes in resistance to aspergillus: observations on these two lines of defense in vivo and in vitro with human and mouse phagocytes, *J Clin Invest* 69:617, 1982.

169. Schielke E and others: Peripheral facial nerve palsy associated with HIV infection, *Lancet* 1:553, 1989.

170. Schlanger G and others: Sinusitis caused by Legionella pneumophilia in a patient with the acquired immune deficiency syndrome, *Am J Med* 77:957, 1984.

171. Schurmann D and others: Intensive treatment of AIDS-related non-Hodgkin's lymphomas with the MACOP-B protocol, *Eur J Haematol* 54:73, 1995.

172. Seddon BM and others: Differential diagnosis of parotid masses in HIV positive men: report of five cases and review, *Int J STD AIDS* 7:224, 1996.

173. Serrano M and others: Hodgkin's disease in patients with antibodies to human immunodeficiency virus, *Cancer* 65:2248, 1990.

174. Shapiro AL and others: Head and neck lymphoma in patients with the acquired immune deficiency syndrome, *Otolaryngol Head Neck Surg* 106:258, 1992.

175. Shapiro AL, Pincus RL: Fine-needle aspiration of diffuse cervical lymphadenopathy, *Otolaryngol Head Neck Surg* 105:419, 1991.

176. Shepp DH and others: Serious Pseudomonas aeruginosa infection in AIDS, *J Acquir Immune Defic Syndr* 7:823, 1994.

177. Silverman S and others: Oral findings in people with or at risk for AIDS: a study of 375 homosexual males, *J Am Dent Assoc* 112:187, 1986.

178. Sindrup JH and others: Syphilis in HTLV-III infected male homosexuals, *AIDS Res Hum Retroviruses* 2:285, 1986.

179. Singh B and others: Kaposi's sarcoma of the head and neck in patients with acquired immunodeficiency syndrome, *Otolaryngol Head Neck Surg* 111:618, 1994.

180. Singh B and others: Upper aerodigestive tract squamous cell carcinoma: the human immunodeficiency virus connection, *Arch Otolaryngol Head Neck Surg* 122:639, 1996.

181. Sitz KV and others: Metastatic basal cell carcinoma in acquired immunodeficiency syndrome–related complex, *JAMA* 257:340, 1987.

182. Small CB and others: Sinusitis and atopy in human immunodeficiency virus infection, *J Infect Dis* 167:283, 1993.

183. Smith FB and others: Benign lymphoepithelial lesion of the parotid gland in intravenous drug users, *Arch Pathol Lab Med* 112:742, 1988.

184. Smith KJ and others: Cutaneous neoplasms in a military population of HIV-1 positive patients, *J Am Acad Dermatol* 29:400, 1993.

185. Smith ME, Canalis RF: Otologic manifestations of AIDS: the otosyphilis connection, *Laryngoscope* 99:365, 1989.

186. Smith T and others: Clinical and electrophysiological studies of human immunodeficiency virus-seropositive men without AIDS, *Ann Neurol* 23:295, 1988.

187. Snider WD and others: Neurological complications of acquired immune deficiency syndrome: analysis of 50 patients, *Ann Neurol* 14:403, 1983.

188. Som PM and others: Nodal inclusion cysts of the parotid gland and parapharyngeal space: a discussion of lymphoepithelial, AIDS-related parotid, and branchial cysts, cystic Warthin's tumors, and cysts in Sjogren's syndrome, *Laryngoscope* 105:1122, 1995.

189. Spector BD and others: Genetically determined immunodeficiency disease (GDID) and malignancy: report from the Immunodeficiency-Cancer Registry, *Clin Immunol Immunopathol* 11:12, 1978.

190. Sperling NM and others: Cystic parotid masses in HIV infection, *Head Neck* 12:337, 1990.

191. Sperling NM, Lin P-T: Parotid disease associated with human immunodeficiency virus infection, *Ear Nose Throat J* 69:475, 1990.

192. Strauss M, Fine E: Aspergillus otomastoiditis in acquired immunodeficiency syndrome, *Am J Otol* 12:49, 1991.

193. Tami TA: The management of sinusitis in patients infected with the human immunodeficiency virus (HIV), *Ear Nose Throat J* 74:360, 1995.

194. Timon CI, Walsh MA: Sudden sensorineural hearing loss as a presentation of HIV infection, *J Laryngol Otol* 103:1071, 1989.

195. Toma E and others: Herpes simplex type 2 pericarditis and bilateral facial palsy in a petine with AIDS, *J Infect Dis* 160:553, 1989.

196. Uldry P-A, Regli F: Paralysie faciale peripherique isolee et recidivante dans l'infection a human immunodeficiency virus (HIV), *Schweiz Med Wochenschr* 118:1029, 1988.

197. Ulirsch RC, Jaffe ES: Sjogren's syndrome–like illness associated with acquired immunodeficiency syndrome–related complex, *Hum Pathol* 18:1063, 1987.

198. Unsworth DJ and others: Defective IgG2 response to Pneumovax in HIV seropositive patients, *Genitourin Med* 69:373, 1993.

199. Upadhyay S and others: Bacteriology of sinusitis in human immunodeficiency virus–positive patients: implications for management, *Laryngoscope* 105:1058, 1995.

200. Wallace M and others: Ototoxicity with azithromycin, *Lancet* 343:241, 1994.

201. Wang C-Y and others: Skin cancers associated with acquired immunodeficiency syndrome, *Mayo Clin Proc* 70:766, 1995.

202. Wasserman L, Haghighi P: Otic and ophthalmic pneumocystosis in acquired immunodeficiency syndrome, *Arch Pathol Lab Med* 116:500, 1992.

203. Wawrose SF and others: The role of guaifenesin in the treatment of sinonasal disease in patients infected with the human immunodeficiency virus (HIV), *Laryngoscope* 102:1225, 1992.

204. Webster G: Local therapy for mucocutaneous Kaposi's sarcoma in patients with acquired immunodeficiency syndrome, *Dermatol Surg* 21:205, 1995.

205. Weinroth S and others: Malignant otitis externa in AIDS patients: case report and review of the literature, *Ear Nose Throat J* 73:772, 1994.

206. Welkoborosky H-J, Lowitzsch K: Auditory brain stem responses in patients with human immunotropic virus infection of different stages, *Ear Hear* 13:55, 1992.

207. Weschler AF, Ho DD: Bilateral Bell's palsy at the time of HIV seroconversion, *Neurology* 39:747, 1989.

208. White M, Armstrong D: Cryptococcus, *Infect Dis Clin North Am* 8:383, 1994.

209. Wiet RJ, Milko DA: Isolation of the spirochetes in the perilymph despite prior antisyphilitic therapy, *Arch Otolaryngol Head Neck Surg* 101:104, 1975.

210. Williams JD and others: Cytomegalovirus sinusitis in a patient with acquired immunodeficiency syndrome, *Otolaryngol Head Neck Surg* 112:750, 1995.

211. Williams MA: Head and neck findings in pediatric acquired immune deficiency syndrome, *Laryngoscope* 97:713, 1987.

212. Winkler J and others: *Clinical description and etiology of HIV-associated periodontal diseases.* In Robertson PB, Greenspan JS, editors: *Perspectives on oral manifestations of AIDS,* Littleton, 1988, PSG Publishing Company.

213. Wiselka MJ and others: Acute infection with human immunodeficiency virus associated with facial nerve palsy and neuralgia, *J Infect* 15:189, 1987.

214. Yourtee E and others: Neutrophil response and function during acute cytomegalovirus infection in guinea pigs, *Infect Immun* 36:11, 1982.

215. Ziegler JL and others: Non-Hodgkin's lymphoma in 90 homosexual men: relation to generalized lymphadenopathy and the acquired immunodeficiency syndrome, *N Engl J Med* 311:565, 1984.

216. Zinreich SJ and others: Fungal sinusitis: diagnosis with CT and MR imaging, *Radiology* 169:439, 1988.

217. Zurlo JJ and others: Sinusitis in HIV-1 infection, *Am J Med* 93:157, 1992.

Chapter 15

Special Considerations in Managing Geriatric Patients

W. Jarrard Goodwin, Jr.
Thomas Balkany
Roy R. Casiano

The social and economic significance of the graying of America has received a great deal of attention. Specialists in geriatric medicine are defining a general system of care that can keep elderly adults more healthy, more functional, and more independent. At the same time, otolaryngologists have taken the lead in describing and treating senescent ear, nose, and throat problems, especially those causing disorders in communication. In our role as communication specialists, otolaryngologists are a key resource in helping the elderly to avoid isolation.

BASIC PRINCIPLES OF GERIATRIC MEDICINE

Irvine[28] defined six useful basic principles in the care of elderly patients. Clinical decisions in this patient group tend to be complex and these fundamentals are worthy of review and emphasis.

1. Coexistence of multiple diseases: The unitary disease hypothesis usually does not apply; signs and symptoms are more likely to be the result of several medical problems.
2. Unique spectrum of illness: In addition to many of the diseases seen in their younger counterparts, the elderly tend to suffer certain diseases that occur only in old age. This includes a wide range of degenerative disorders and certain cancers.
3. Unusual presentation of illness: Typical symptoms, such as fever and pain, are often absent, and nonspecific symptoms, such as anorexia or falling, may herald a serious underlying disorder.
4. Proper role of the aging process: Differentiating treatable disease from the natural aging process may be difficult, particularly in the area of degenerative diseases. Most geriatric specialists believe that patients and families have a tendency to overrate the role of aging. As a result, they experience unnecessary suffering and dysfunction; specific disease processes should be sought and treated whenever possible.
5. Under reporting of health problems: Patients and families often fail to report symptoms commonly relegated to old age.
6. Function-based treatment goals: At some point, adding life to years becomes more important than adding years to life. Therapeutic goals shift toward maximizing function and independence, possibly at the expense of potential for cure.

ACCESS TO MEDICAL CARE

A decreased level of strength and confidence may limit the ability of the elderly to visit a physician's office or the hospital, especially in the absence of strong family support. Social support systems often function better for acute and more serious problems, therefore, the well-known benefits of early detection and treatment may be lost. The high cost of modern health care may also create a relative barrier.

Society and physicians share a responsibility for providing care to all segments of the population, and a point can be made for making allowances for the elderly. Physicians

REFERENCES

1. Anthonisen NR and others: Airway closure as a function of age, *Respir Physiol* 8:58, 1969/1970.
2. Avon J, Gurwitz J: *Principles of pharmacology.* In Cassel CK, Riesenberg DE, Sorensen LB, editors: *Geriatric medicine,* ed 2, New York, 1990, Springer-Verlag.
3. Benjamin BJ: Frequency variability in the aged voice, *J Gerontol* 36: 722, 1981.
4. Biever DM, Bless DM: Vibratory characteristics of the vocal folds in young adult and geriatric women, *J Voice* 3:120, 1989.
5. Bosisio E and others: Mean transit time forced expiratory volume and age in healthy male smokers and non-smokers, *Respiration* 49:23, 1986.
6. Bradsetter RD, Kazemi H: Aging and the respiratory system, *Med Clin North Am* 67:419, 1983.
7. Brown WS, Morris RJ, Michel JF: Vocal jitter in young adult and aged female voices, *J Voice* 3:113, 1989.
8. Castell DO: *Eating and swallowing disorders.* In Hazzard WR and others, editors: *Principles of geriatric medicine and gerontology,* ed 2, New York, 1990, McGraw-Hill.
9. Dawson DA, Adams PF: *National center for health statistics: current estimates from the health interview survey, United States, 1986,* Vital Health Statistics Series 10, no. 164, DHHS publication number (PHS) 87, United States Department of Health and Human Services, 1987.
10. Deems DA, Doty RL: Age-related changes in the phenyl ethylalcohol odor detection threshold, *Trans Pa Acad Ophthalmol Otolaryngol* 39: 646, 1987.
11. Doty RL: *Age-related alterations in taste and smell function.* In Goldstein JC, Kashima HK, Koopman CF Jr, editors: *Geriatric otolaryngology,* Toronto; 1989, Decker.
12. Doty RL, Reyes P, Gregor T: Presence of both odor identification and detection deficits in Alzeheimer's disease, *Brain Res Bull* 18:597, 1982.
13. Doty RL and others: Smell identification ability: changes with age, *Science* 226:1441, 1984.
14. Edelstein DR: Aging of the normal nose in adults, *Laryngoscope* 106: 1, 1996.
15. Gacek RR, Schuknecht HF: Pathology of presbycusis, *Int Audiol* 8: 199, 1969.
16. Gates GA and others: Central auditory dysfunction, cognitive dysfunction, and dementia in older people, *Arch Otolaryngol Head Neck Surg* 122:161, 1996.
17. Glorig A, Davis H: Age noise and hearing loss, *Ann Otol Rhinol Laryngol* 70:556, 1961.
18. Gracco C, Kahane JC: Age-related changes in the vestibular folds of the human larynx: a histomorphometric study, *J Voice* 3:204, 1989.
19. Granieri E: Nutrition and the older adult, *Dysphagia* 4:196, 1990.
20. Gussan R: Plugging of the vascular channels in the otic capsule, *Ann Otol Rhinol Laryngol* 78:1306, 1969.
21. Havlik RJ: *National Center for Health Statistics: aging in the eighties, impaired senses for sound and light in persons aged 65 and over: preliminary data from the supplement on aging to the national health interview survey, United States, January–June 1984: advance data from vital and health statistics,* No 125, DHHS Pub No (PHS) 86-1250, Hyattsville, Md, 1986, Public Health Service.
22. Hermel J and others: Taste sensation in aging man, *J Oral Med* 25: 39, 1970.
23. Hoeffding V, Feldman ML: Changes with advanced age in the morphology of the rat auditory nerve, *Soc Neurosci Abstr* 1987:13, 1259.
24. Hollender AR: Histopathology of the nasal mucosa of older persons, *Arch Otolaryngol Head Neck Surg* 40:92, 1994.
25. Hollien H, Shipp T: Speaking fundamental frequency and chronologic age in males, *J Speech Hear Res* 15:155, 1972.
26. Honjo I, Isshiki N: Laryngoscopic and voice characteristic of aged persons, *Arch Otolaryngol* 106:149, 1980.
27. Honrubia V: Vestibular function in the elderly, *Ear Nose Throat J* 68: 904, 1989.
28. Irvine PW: *Patterns of disease: the challenge of multiple illnesses.* In Cassel CK, Riesenberg DE, Sorensen LB, editors: *Geriatric medicine,* ed 2, New York, 1990, Springer-Verlag.
29. Isshiki N and others: Thyroplasty as a new phonosurgical technique, *Acta Otolaryngol* 78:451, 1974.
30. Johnson LG, Hawkins JE: Vascular changes in the human inner ear associated with aging, *Ann Otol* 81:364, 1972.
31. Johnson JT, Rabuzzi DD, Tucker HM: Composite resection in the elderly: a well-tolerated procedure, *Laryngoscope* 87:1509, 1977.
32. Jordanoglou J and others: Effective time of the forced expiratory spirogram in health and airways obstruction, *Thorax* 34:187, 1979.
33. Kahane JC: *A survey of age related changes in the connective tissues in the human adult larynx.* In Bless DM, Abbs JH, editors: *Vocal cord physiology,* San Diego, 1983, College-Hill Press.
34. Keil CH, Smith MC: *National Center for Health Statistics: office based ambulatory care for patients 75 years and over: national ambulatory medical care survey, 1980, advanced data from vital health statistics,* No 110. DHHS Pub No (PHS) 85. Hyattsville, Md, 1985, Public Health Service.
35. Knudson RJ and others: Changes in the normal maximal expiratory flow-volume curve with growth and aging, *Am Rev Respir Dis* 127: 725, 1983.
36. Krmpotic-Nemanic J: Presbycusis presbystatis and presbyosmia as consequences of the analogous biological process, *Acta Otolaryngol (Stockh)* 67:217, 1969.
37. Kushnick SD and others: A scanning electron microscopic study of smoking and age-related changes in human nasal epithelium, *Am J Rhinol* 6:185, 1992.
38. Larson EB and others: Adverse drug reactions associated with global cognitive impairment in elderly persons, *Ann Intern Med* 107:169, 1987.
39. LeJeeune FE, Guice CE, Samuels PM: Early experiences with vocal ligament tightening, *Am Otol Rhinol Laryngol* 92:475, 1983.
40. Levine R, Robbins J, Maser A: Periventricular white changes in oropharyngeal swallowing in normal individuals, *Dysphagia* 7:142, 1992.
41. Levitzky MG: Effects of aging on the respiratory system, *Physiologist* 27:102, 1984.
42. Linvell SE, Fisher HB: Acoustic characteristics of women's voices with advanced age, *J Gerontol* 40:324, 1985.
43. Liss JM, Weisner G, Rosenbek JC: Selected acoustic characteristics of speech production in very old males, *J Gerontology* 45:35, 1990.
44. Liss L, Gomez F: The nature of senile changes of the human olfactory bulb and tract, *Arch Otolaryngol* 67:167, 1958.
45. Logemann J: *Manual for the videofluorographic study of swallowing,* ed 2, Austin, 1993, Pro-Ed.
46. Makila E: Oral health among the inmates of old people's homes: salivary secretions, *Proc Finn Dent Soc* 73:64, 1977.
47. McGuirt WF, Davis SP: Demographic portrayal and outcome analysis of head and neck cancer surgery in the elderly, *Arch Otolaryngol Head Neck Surg* 121:150, 1995.
48. Mellert TK and others: Characterization of the immune barrier in human olfactory mucosa, *Otolaryngol Head Neck Surg* 106:181, 1992.
49. Morgan RF and others: Head and neck surgery in the aged, *Am J Surg* 144:449, 1982.
50. Mueller PB, Sweeney RJ, Baribeau LJ: Acoustic and morphologic study of the senescent voice, *Ear Nose Throat J* 63:292, 1984.
51. Murty GE, Carding PN, Kelly PJ: Combined glottographic changes in the elderly, *Clin Otolaryngol* 16:532, 1991.
52. Nadol JB, Schuknecht HF: The pathology of peripheral vestibular disorders in the elderly, *Ear Nose Throat J* 68:930, 1989.
53. Naessen R: An enquiry on the morphological characteristics and possible changes with age in the olfactory region of man, *Acta Otolaryngol (Stockh)* 71:49, 1971.
54. Nakashima T, Kimmelman CP, Snow JB Jr: Immunohistopathologic

analysis of olfactory degeneration caused by ischemia, *Otolaryngol Head Neck Surg* 93:40, 1985.

55. Nedelman CI, Bernick S: The significance of age changes in human alveolar mucosa and gum, *J Prosthet Dent* 39:495, 1978.

56. Nixon JC, Glorig A: Changes in air and bone conduction thresholds, *J Laryngol* 76:288, 1962.

57. Orma EJ, Koskenoja M: Postural dizziness in the aged, *Geriatrics* 12:49, 1957.

58. Paik SI and others: Human olfactory biopsy: the influence of age and receptor distribution, *Arch Otolaryngol Head Neck Surg* 118:731, 1982.

59. Parker DR and others: The relationship of nonspecific airway responsiveness and atopy to the rate of decline in lung function, *Am Rev Respir Dis* 141:589, 1990.

60. Patterson CN: The aging nose: characteristics and correction, *Otolaryngol Clin North Am* 13:275, 1980.

61. Pressman JJ, Keleman G: Physiology of the larynx, *Physiol Rev* 35:513, 1955.

62. Ramig LA: Effects of physiologic aging on vowel spectral noise, *J Gerontology*, 38:223, 1983.

63. Ramig LA, Ringel RL: Effects of physiologic aging on selected acoustic characteristics of voice, *J Speech Hearing* 26:22, 1983.

64. Ramig LA and others: Acoustic analysis of voice in amyotrophic lateral sclerosis: a longitudinal case study, *J Speech Hear Res* 55:2, 1990.

65. Robbins J and others: Oropharyngeal swallowing in normal adults of different ages, *Gastroenterology* 103:823, 1992.

66. Rosen S, Olin K: Hearing loss in coronary heart disease, *Arch Otolaryngol* 82:836, 1965.

67. Sakakura Y and others: Nasal mucociliary clearance under various conditions, *Acta Otolaryngol (Stockh)* 96:167, 1983.

68. Santos AL, Gelperin A: Surgical mortality in the elderly, *J Am Geriatr Soc* 23:42, 1975.

69. Schiffman SS: Taste and smell in disease, *N Engl J Med* 308(2 pt 1):1275, 1983.

70. Scott J: Quantitative age changes in the histological structure of human submandibular salivary glands, *Arch Oral Biol* 22:221, 1977.

71. Settipane GA, Chafee FH: Nasal polyps in asthma and rhinitis, a review of 6,037 patients, *J Allergy Clin Immunol*, 59:17, 1997.

72. Seymour DG, Pringle R: Post-operative complications in the elderly surgical patient, *Gerontology* 29:262, 1983.

73. Shaker R, Lang I: Effects of aging on the deglutitive oral, pharyngeal, and esophageal motor function, *Dysphagia* 9:221, 1994.

74. Shipp T and others: Acoustic and temporal correlates of perceived age, *J Voice* 6:211, 1992.

75. Simpson WJ: Thyroid malignancy in the elderly, *Geriatrics* 37:119, 1982.

76. Sinha UK and others: Temporal bone findings in Alzheimer's disease, *Laryngoscope* 106:1, 1996.

77. Smith CG: Age incidence of atrophy of olfactory nerves in man, *J Comp Neurol* 77:589, 1942.

78. Snow JB Jr: *Clinical disorders of olfaction and gustation in the aged.* In Goldstein JC and others, editors: *Geriatric otolaryngology*, Toronto, 1989, Decker.

79. Sonies BC and others: Durational aspects of the oral phase of swallow in normal aging adults, *Dysphagia* 3:1, 1988.

80. Sorbinni CA and others: Arterial oxygen tension in relation to age in healthy subjects, *Respiration* 25:3, 1986.

81. Strehler BL: *Aging in cellular level.* In Rossman I, editor: *Clinical geriatrics*, Philadelphia, 1971, Lippincott.

82. Sunberg J: *The science of the singing voice*, De Kalb, Ill, 1987, Northern Illinois University Press.

83. Tanaka S, Hirano M, Chijiwa K: Some aspects of vocal fold bowing, *Ann Otolaryngol Rhinol Laryngol* 103(5 pt 1):357, 1994.

84. Tracy JF and others: Preliminary observations on the effects of age on oropharyngeal deglutition, *Dysphagia* 4:90, 1989.

85. Trupe EH, Siebens H, Siebens A: Prevalence of feeding and swallowing disorders in a nursing home, *Arch Phys Med Rehabil* 65:651, 1984.

86. Tucker HM: Laryngeal framework surgery in the management of the aged larynx, *J Otol Rhinol Laryngol* 97:534, 1988.

87. Van der Veken PJ and others: Age related CT-scan study of the incidence of sinusitis in children, *Am J Rhinol* 6:45, 1992.

88. Wolf GT: *Aging, the immune system and head and neck cancer.* In Goldstein JC, Kashima HK, Koopmann CF, editors: *Geriatric otolaryngology*, Burlington, Vt, 1989, BC Decker.

89. Woo P and others: Dysphonia in the aging: physiology versus disease, *Laryngoscope* 102:139, 1992.

Chapter 16

Fundamentals of Molecular Biology and Gene Therapy

Bert W. O'Malley, Jr.

Molecular biology is a relatively young scientific field with its major thrust arising from the discovery of methods to study and manipulate deoxyribonucleic acid (DNA) in the 1970s. Rapid advances in this arena, however, enabled clinical application by the 1980s and 1990s. No longer does molecular biology reside solely within the research laboratory. Many diagnostic laboratory tests routinely used in clinical medicine as well as the development and mass production of pharmaceuticals employ molecular biology techniques. The surge of molecular biology and the new understanding of genes and their products has allowed the emergence of a rising field called *gene therapy*. This rapidly expanding field is founded on the ability to introduce genetic material into the body in order to treat disease or alter an ongoing pathologic process.

The purpose of this chapter is not to discuss molecular biology in detail. Rather, the purpose is to review basic molecular terminology, introduce the concept of gene therapy, and focus on the rationale and methods for clinical application of this evolving molecular therapy.

MOLECULAR BIOLOGY

Fundamentals

The basic premise of molecular biology is to study cell function and regulation at the level of the genome. With this understanding comes insight into human disease, because aberrances in cell function or regulation are the basis for most diseases. The following section reviews fundamental terminology and concepts on how information travels from the genetic code to the functional protein level. Included is a brief discussion on cell cycling, which is an important concept in tumor molecular biology.

Gene expression

The information for conducting all aspects of cellular function is contained within molecules of DNA located in the nucleus. The actual length of a human DNA strand is 1.8 M, however, it is coiled around nuclear proteins called *histones* that structure the folds and loops of DNA to allow compression into the microscopic size of the cell's nucleus. Each strand of DNA contains thousands of genes that are specific subunit sequences that code for the information required to synthesize a protein. One molecule of double-stranded DNA and its genes make up each of a cell's 46 total chromosomes. Although every cell in the human body contains the same DNA, the expression of individual genes are not the same. Gene expression will vary depending on the cell's function. These differences in gene expression result in the multiple cell and tissue phenotypes that constitute the human body as a whole.

The process by which a gene codes for a specific protein begins with *transcription*, which is the formation of a single-stranded ribonucleic acid (RNA) molecule that compliments a single strand of the DNA subunit (Fig. 16-1). This RNA molecule is subsequently modified to become the messenger that brings the genetic information or directions from the nucleus to the cell's cytoplasm where the actual synthesis of the functional protein occurs. After reaching the cytoplasm, the process of *translation* begins (see Fig. 16-1). During translation, the message from the RNA molecule directs the construction of a protein from its basic subunit, the amino

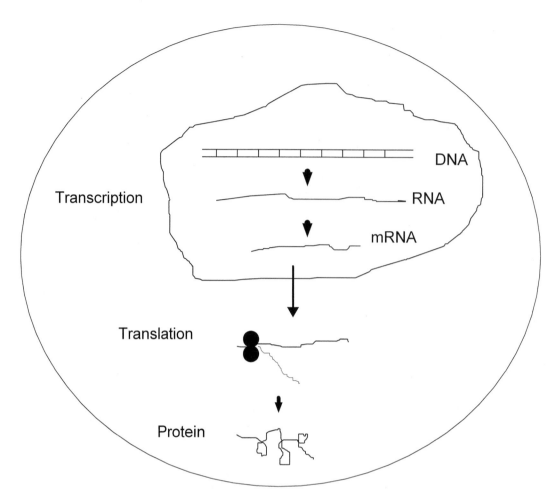

Fig. 16-1. The basic steps involved in gene expression. The *black dots* at the level of translation represent the ribosome complex that is composed of ribosomal ribonucleic acid (RNA). The ribosome orchestrates the cytoplasmic machinery required to produce the protein product. It is within this step that a transfer RNA molecule brings in a specific amino acid coded for by a three–base-pair sequence on the messenger ribosomal. The ribosomes direct the linkage of each amino acid to produce the protein molecule specific to the original deoxyribonucleic acid sequence.

acid. Once a protein is formed, it may require further modification or control steps to enable its designated function. These modifications include the addition of sugars, lipids, or phosphates to the protein backbone. These internal control steps are mediated by existing cytoplasmic enzymes, which, if defective, also may lead to defined diseases. Once a protein is formed within the cell cytoplasm, it may reside in the cell or be released to affect other tissues within the body. Depending on the original genetic program for the protein, it may serve its purpose and be rapidly degraded, it may enter the circulation, or reside in local or distant tissues for an extended period of time. Transcription and translation are complex processes that have many more modification and regulatory steps that are governed by regulatory genes and their protein products. When these delicate control mechanisms are lost, a disease state or a state of abnormal cell proliferation can ensue, as is exemplified in the development of cancer.

Cell division

Disorders in cell function may lead either to cell death or proliferation. Abnormal stimulation of cell proliferation is the basis for the development of cancer. In order for a cell to divide, it must progress through the various phases of growth and reproduction that constitute what is called the *cell cycle* (Fig. 16-2). The principal components of the cell cycle are the replication of nuclear DNA and its distribution among the progeny cells (daughter cells). The first phase of the cell cycle is called *G1*, and it is here where all the enzymes, nucleic acids, and other factors are produced that enable DNA replication or "synthesis," which occurs in the *S phase*. Once the DNA is replicated, a period of cell growth and duplication of cellular proteins and structures occurs in a period called *G2*. After this cell growth, the actual distribution of the replicated DNA and the physical division of the parent cell into two daughter cells occurs in the *M phase*, which takes approximately 1 hour. After cell division, the

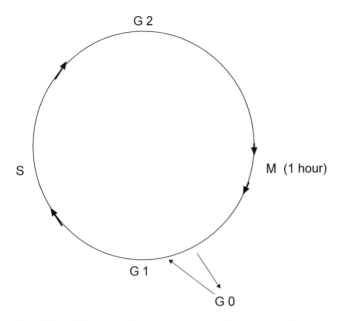

Fig. 16-2. Cell cycle. The various phases of the entire cell cycle are depicted. The cell cycle typically lasts 10 to 25 hours in animals. Only 1 hour is spent in the M phase. The longest and most variable phase is G1, which can range from 4 to 24 hours.

cell cycle process may begin again or the cell may enter a state of rest called *G0*. The signal to divide may either come from internal factors or exogenous growth factors that bind to cell-surface receptors and stimulate a cascade of events that lead to division. Important internal control mechanisms exist at the genetic level that help regulate cell cycling. The "negative regulatory" genes, which code for proteins that inhibit abnormal cell proliferation, are called *tumor suppressor genes*. A mutation or loss of a tumor suppressor gene is a basic step in the development of many human cancers. Cell cycling also can be abnormally induced by cellular *oncogenes*, which naturally exist within cells but are typically kept dormant either by tumor suppressor genes or other regulatory mechanisms. Loss of negative regulation from tumor suppressor genes or amplification or mutation of the actual oncogene also has been associated with cancer formation. Continued molecular research will provide further understanding of cell cycle regulation and may lead to novel therapies for treating human cancer.

A discussion of basic molecular biology techniques that have provided the means to understand gene expression, regulation, and cell cycling can be found in Chapter 17.

GENE THERAPY

Arising from the dramatic progress in molecular and cellular biology is an exciting new field of clinical research and human investigation. This new field of translational research, known as *gene therapy*, focuses on the transfer of therapeutic genes to normal or abnormal target cells. During the advent of gene therapy, the initial clinical targets were rare inherited diseases such as adenosine deaminase deficiency, which results in a deadly systemic immune deficiency, enzymatic deficiencies, which result in liver failure, or coagulation pathway deficiencies, which result in various types of hemophilia. In the past 5 years, however, it has become clear that gene therapy may have its most immediate and effective role in treating more common diseases such as cancer, cystic fibrosis, arthritis, and atherosclerosis.[41] As the field of gene therapy continues its rapid advancement, the techniques and therapies will not be restricted to the practice of geneticists and specialists studying rare inherited diseases. It is likely that gene therapy will be a standard regimen that may be selected by both internists and surgeons in the course of routine clinical care.

Principles and concepts

Basic principle

The basic principle of gene therapy is that normal or therapeutic genes can be introduced into body tissues to treat a disease. In many genetic diseases, this may involve introducing a normal gene into the body to carry out the function that is defective because of the inheritance of a mutant gene. Hemophilia is an example, in which individuals at the time of birth lack a normal gene for clotting factor VIII and have prolonged bleeding. The transfer of a normal factor VIII gene into the patient's endothelial cells or hepatocytes could restore the ability of these cells to secrete factor VIII and restore the bleeding time to normal. Acquired diseases such as cancer can also be treated with gene therapy. For example, one of the first clinical trials focused on the treatment of melanoma.[46] In this clinical trial, lymphocytes that had infiltrated the tumors (tumor infiltrating lymphocytes [TIL]) were purified from a tumor at the time of surgical resection. The TIL cells were grown in the laboratory, and the gene for tumor necrosis factor (TNF) was introduced into the cells. The genetically engineered cells were subsequently transfused into the patient with the expectation that they would preferentially migrate to the site of residual tumor, delivering a therapeutic dose of TNF.

The potential success of gene therapy for diseases such as hemophilia or cancer illustrates several essential points about somatic gene therapy in general as discussed below.

Somatic versus germ cell gene therapy

Gene therapy has two possible target cell types. The first and presently used target are the *somatic cells*, or those cells that constitute the organs and postnatal tissues of the body. The second potential target are the *germ cells*, or those cells that produce the sperm or ovum and are passed on to the patient's offspring. Many different organs and cell types are targets for somatic gene therapy including bone marrow, liver, tumor cells, muscle, skin, endothelium, thyroid, and others (Fig. 16-3). Genetic manipulation and therapy at these sites does not alter the inherited genetic material, and raises few novel ethical or social issues.[37] Genetic manipulation

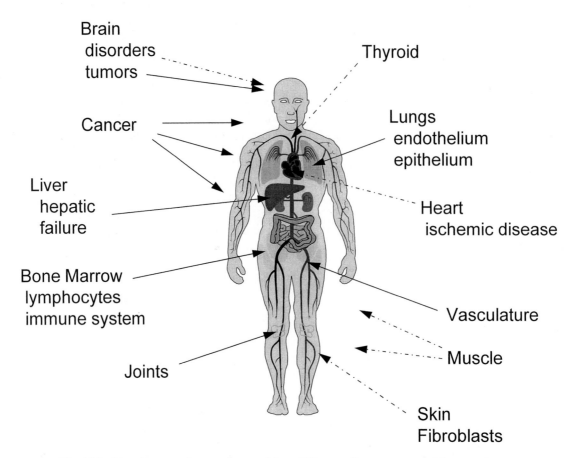

Fig. 16-3. Somatic targets for gene therapy. Many different cell types are potential targets for gene therapy. *Solid arrows* represent tissue targets presently under human clinical trial investigation and *dotted arrows* represent targets under investigation in animal models. Current gene therapy laboratory and clinical investigation explicitly excludes manipulation of germ cells (sperm and ovum) that may pass genes to future generations.

of the sperm or ovum, however, could prevent inherited diseases by altering the genetic constitution of offspring. Although an appealing idea on casual consideration, there are serious technical and safety issues, as well as profound ethical concerns. Currently, gene therapy is restricted to somatic cells, and genetic manipulation of human germ cells would be prohibited under existing recombinant DNA guidelines.[45]

Homologous recombination

It is possible to introduce a gene into a targeted cell in such a way that the defective region of the existing genetic material will be excised and replaced with a new gene sequence. This process, known as *homologous recombination*, has been used to restore mutant genes to normal in embryonic mouse cells. Homologous recombination methods, however, are presently ineffective for human gene therapy because of the low efficiency of actual gene transfer (1 of 10^5 to 10^7 targeted cells).[56] Current gene therapy strategies are much more efficient than attempts at homologous recombination and involve the introduction of new genetic material into cells to express a therapeutic gene product. Gene ther-

apy, therefore, is not only applicable for treating single gene disorders, but can be used for any disorder in which the expression of a gene product has a therapeutic effect.

Therapeutic mechanism

The gene that is delivered to a target cell is not itself therapeutic. Rather, it is the product encoded by the gene that is responsible for the resulting therapeutic effect. The gene product is typically a protein that has a specific function such as a hormone or cytokine, but could also be a bioactive RNA molecule or a regulatory molecule (RNA or protein) that alters the regulation of a pathologic process. Therefore, while gene therapy commonly focuses on methods for delivering genes to cells, it is the ability to achieve expression of the gene product at therapeutic levels that ultimately determines the effectiveness and efficacy of therapy.

Permanent versus temporary gene therapy

A common perception is that the goal of gene therapy is to ''permanently'' introduce a therapeutic gene into the patient. Permanent gene therapy, however, may not be necessary or optimal in a clinical setting. As a general principle, permanent gene therapy could prove more desirable when the methods required for introducing the gene into the patient involve significant surgical procedures or substantial risk to the patient, e.g., organ resection, cellular transplantation, or stereotactic injection under anesthesia. In order to achieve permanent gene therapy, the gene that is introduced into the patient should be expressed indefinitely. The gene also must demonstrate appropriate regulation in response to normal and pathologic situations, and there should be no detrimental consequences of this gene expression to the patient in later life. In considering diseases such as growth hormone deficiency or juvenile diabetes, correction by permanent gene transfer would require precise regulation of the gene products to ensure short-term efficacy and long-term safety. This tight control and regulation of transfered genetic material is not feasible with present techniques.

For many diseases such as cancer, cystic fibrosis, arthritis, and disorders requiring surgery, insertion of a ''temporary'' gene into a patient's tumor, residual tumor, or other target cells could produce a selected beneficial therapy over a limited period of time. For example, the treatment of a tumor or area of residual tumor after surgery only may require a one-time, limited expression of a gene that either produces a substance directly toxic to the cancer cell, or a cytokine or other factor that can initiate an antitumor immune response. Instead of permanent gene therapy, repeat gene transfer over a period of time could also prove effective, as in the case of radiotherapy or possible chemotherapy regimens. Repeat gene transfer also may play a role in the treatment of arthritis and other chronic diseases. With respect to surgical procedures, the use of gene therapy to enhance wound healing or tissue regeneration after an injury might only require gene expression for a period of days or weeks. Another new frontier on the horizon is gene therapy that can be administered repetitively by minimally or noninvasive routes such as intramuscular, intravenous, or oral routes of administration. This novel future application could allow establishment of steady state gene product levels that parallel present medical regimens and enable the physician to adjust the dose and schedule of administration to the patient's needs.

Therapeutic levels of gene expression

Effective gene therapy requires not only delivery of genes to the appropriate target cell within the body, but the expression of the therapeutic gene product at appropriate levels. It is the ability to achieve adequate gene expression that will determine the efficacy and therapeutic index of gene therapy. There are several ways to achieve appropriate expression of a therapeutic gene product.

Specific genetic elements called *promoters* and *enhancers* that normally control the rate of therapeutic product expression can be incorporated into the gene transfer vehicles. These elements also can control the level of gene expression, restrict it to specific cell types, and provide regu-

lated gene expression in response to endocrine or pharmacologic factors. For example, gene therapy for diabetes will certainly require the incorporation of genetic elements that provide normal regulation of insulin levels by glucose.

Promoter and enhancer elements derived from different genes can be combined to provide an improved effect. In this way vectors can be designed to produce gene products at high levels from a cell that normally produces only low levels, or to constitute expression of a gene product from a cell that does not normally produce that particular gene product. For example, clotting factors or peptide hormones can be expressed from muscle cells after gene transfer using vehicles that incorporate the promoter and enhancer elements from muscle-specific genes such as skeletal actin or myosin. In considering cancer gene therapy, highly efficient viral promoters can be mixed and matched with a variety of gene delivery vehicles that will result in high levels of expression of therapeutic antitumor genes directly from the targeted cancer cells.

Another important regulatory mechanism resides in the natural actions of a cell, tissue, or organ. As is the case with conventional pharmaceuticals, the basic principles of drug distribution, metabolism, and elimination within cells and tissues of the body will provide additional means for regulating the level of the gene product.

Why gene therapy?

An important universal question is what advantage does gene therapy have over presently accepted medical and surgical treatments that would warrant clinical investigation and application in routine patient care. In response to this basic question there are several reasons why gene therapy may become a first-line treatment option in clinical practice.

A new therapeutic approach

With the rapid evolution of molecular biology over the past decade, an increasing number of basic biologic phenomenon and pathologic conditions are now understood in terms of the events that take place on a molecular level between genes and their products. In experimental animal models and early human clinical trials it was possible to alter processes such as immunity, growth, development, regeneration, and malignancy on a molecular level using gene transfer. Therapeutic gene transfer provides a novel approach to diseases that are not satisfactorily managed using conventional pharmacologic or surgical intervention. As a general example, gene therapy to reconstitute deficient functions resulting from failing organs or tissues may provide an alternative to allogenic transplantation of bone marrow, solid organs, or individual cells.

Site-specific gene expression

Using the techniques and principles of gene transfer, therapeutic products can be released from specific cell types in precise locations within the body. This concept of site-specific gene expression provides a valuable advantage for gene therapy. Therapeutic proteins such as cytokines or growth factors can be expressed in precise locations, rather than administering similar products through a systemic route. The highest concentration of the therapeutic product will therefore be focused at the desired site of action. For example, gene transfer may be used to express products specifically in the epidermal or dermal layers of the skin without affecting underlying connective tissue, nerves, muscles, or vessels. Such spatial specificity will minimize untoward consequences or toxicity in organs or other vital structures outside the site being treated.

Improved efficacy and safety

Gene therapy establishes the expression of healthy, human proteins acting in a directed therapeutic fashion within the body. Based on this concept, gene therapy may prove more efficacious and safer than the application of proteins purified from microorganisms, animals, or human populations that carry the attendant risk of transmitting pathogens or inciting allergic reactions. Moreover, gene therapy can be used to achieve regulated, physiologic expression of gene products that may further improve efficacy. By altering the dose or schedule of gene administration to a patient, it is possible to optimize the level, effect, and safety of the gene product.

Improved routes of administration and compliance

The majority of standard medications have short half-lives and need to be administered by frequent oral dosing, injections, or even constant infusions to achieve an optimal therapeutic effect. Gene therapy, however, provides continuous endogenous expression of natural protein products and requires less frequent administration of the gene, ranging from one-time administration, to weekly or monthly treatments depending on the disease target and gene transfer strategy. As is known to all clinicians, decreasing the frequency of administration improves acceptance and compliance with therapeutic regimens.

Preventative medicine and a reduction in healthcare costs

As molecular and genetic research continue to identify factors that predispose individuals to diseases such as atherosclerosis, cancer, diabetes, infections, or degenerative disorders, the application of gene therapy may allow a physician to alter the expression of these factors in a preventative manner. Of particular importance is the ability to deliver therapy over a long period of time for clinically asymptomatic or minimally symptomatic patients who have inherited or acquired progressive diseases, a combination of circumstances that is traditionally associated with poor compliance. For example, treating a diabetic patient in the early stages of disease with gene therapy may prevent morbidity later in life that ensues even with conventional exogenous insulin

therapy. Also, combining the advances in molecular diagnostics of cancer may allow replacement of lost or defective critical tumor suppressor genes in normal or premalignant tissues, thereby preventing the progression of the defective tissue into cancer.

Because gene therapy can establish continuous release of a therapeutic product with one-time treatment or infrequent dosing, its use for prevention is more practical and affordable than conventional therapies. The practice of preventative gene therapy to diminish morbidity and early mortality, and the use of more affordable treatment regimens will ultimately reduce the rapidly growing cost of healthcare.

Methods for gene transfer

A major focus in the field of gene therapy is the development of vehicles for introducing genetic material into selected target cells. Two general classes of gene vehicles and transfer methods can be distinguished. *DNA-mediated gene transfer* involves the administration of DNA alone to the patient in various formulations such as in saline or lipid complex mediums. *Viral-mediated gene transfer* involves packaging a therapeutic gene into a defective virus particle and using the natural process of viral infection to introduce the gene. The purpose of viral-mediated gene transfer is to exploit the efficient and often complex mechanisms that viruses have evolved to introduce their viral genes into human cells during infections.

Deoxyribonucleic acid-mediated gene transfer

The process of DNA-mediated gene transfer is called *transfection*, and the vehicle through which a therapeutic gene is transferred into a cell is called a *vector*. Functional DNA vectors are circular molecules of DNA that contain various additional genetic elements required to achieve expression of the gene product at therapeutic levels (Fig. 16-4). Included in these are the special elements (promoter and enhancer), which direct gene expression and elements that determine the processing and persistence of genetic material within the cell.

The delivery of DNA vectors into cells is possible through a variety of techniques. One classic method is to simply microinject DNA directly into the cell nucleus.[6] This method is time consuming and inefficient for achieving large numbers of transfected cells. Although this method is common in the laboratory with *in vitro* studies, its technical limitations prohibit effective application to living animal models or human subjects. A more efficient process, which also is limited to *in vitro* application, is the process of *electroporation*, where cultured cells are exposed to DNA in the presence of a strong electrical pulse.[18] The electrical pulse creates pores in the cell membrane that allow electrophoresis of DNA into the cell.

It is possible to effectively introduce genes into muscle[59] or thyroid[52] simply by injecting DNA into these tissues *in vivo* where the process of *endocytosis* enables cellular up-

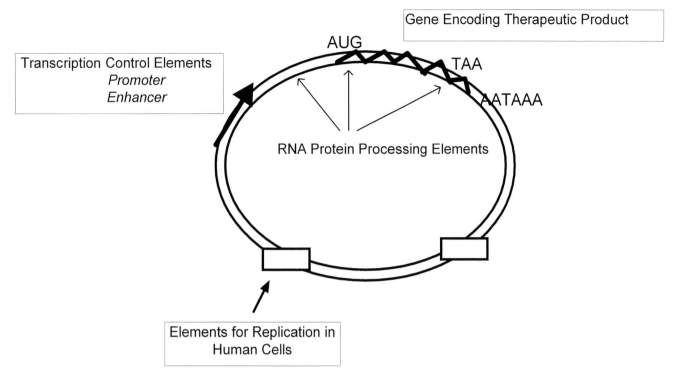

Gene Encoding Therapeutic Product

Transcription Control Elements
Promoter
Enhancer

AUG

TAA

AATAAA

RNA Protein Processing Elements

Elements for Replication in
Human Cells

Fig. 16-4. Schematic structure of a plasmid deoxyribonucleic acid (DNA) vector. Plasmid DNA vectors are circular molecules of DNA encoding a therapeutic gene product. DNA vectors contain special elements required to achieve expression of the gene product at therapeutic levels. Promoter and enhancer regions regulate the transcription of plasmid DNA into ribonucleic acid (RNA), and specific processing elements regulate the translation of RNA into protein. A DNA vector may be complexed with protein, lipids, or synthetic organic compounds that enhance vector uptake or provide cell uptake specificity.

take. This is not true of other tissues examined to date. Gene transfer into other organs requires special methods to enhance the uptake of DNA into the specific target cells. A common alternative method is the use of cationic lipids that encase DNA vectors and fuse with the target cell membrane[17] to enhance intracellular gene uptake. This process has been termed *lipofection*. Another method is to couple the DNA vector to proteins that bind to specific receptors on the target cell leading to uptake of the DNA by receptor-mediated endocytosis.[57,60] A recent technical advance is the development of the "gene gun" that uses electrical currents and magnetic properties to project DNA vectors that are coated with microscopic gold particles into the target cells.[61] Another less common technique still under early investigation involves using select viral components to enhance vector movement across the cell membrane and into the cell.[14,58]

An important point to understand is that DNA-mediated gene transfer typically results in only transient residence of the therapeutic genes in the targeted cell. DNA vectors that are introduced into cells are degraded and eliminated from the cell over time. Different cell types eliminate the introduced genetic material at different rates. In muscle, for example, DNA vectors may persist in cells for many months and continue to express gene products.[59] In contrast, DNA

vectors injected into the thyroid have a shorter half-life and the gene product is eliminated after 2 days.[52] Vectors introduced into the liver are eliminated with a half-life of approximately 1 to 2 hours and expression is significantly reduced after 6 to 24 hours.[53]

Although permanent incorporation of genes into cells occurs rarely after DNA-mediated gene transfer in cultured cells ($<1:10^5$ cells), this phenomenon has not been observed *in vivo*. DNA vectors are therefore considered "safe" because they do not incorporate into the recipient cell's chromosome *in vivo*, and therefore should not present a theoretic risk inherent to altering a cell's genome. Moreover, DNA vectors have not demonstrated significant toxicity to recipient tissues or any anti-DNA immune response. DNA vectors can, therefore, be delivered repeatedly, which overcomes the potential limitation of transient therapeutic gene expression. The transient nature of gene expression does have an advantage in certain clinical scenarios because the therapeutic gene may be administered by conventional oral, intramuscular, or intravenous routes to provide its beneficial effect over a predictable and extended period of time. In contrast to conventional medications with short half-lives, DNA-mediated gene therapy could lead to prolonged expression of a gene product at continuous levels, eliminating the need for continuous infusions, or enhancing compliance by minimizing the frequency of injections.

Viral-mediated gene transfer

The majority of research to date has focused on developing methods for using viruses as vectors. Viral-mediated gene transfer involves the construction of synthetic virus particles that lack pathogenic functions, are incapable of replication, contain a therapeutic gene within the viral genome, and can deliver this gene to cells by the process of infection. Certain viruses have the property of permanently integrating their genes into the chromosomes of the infected cell, therefore, select forms of viral-mediated gene transfer can lead to permanent gene therapy.

Retroviruses as gene transfer vehicles

The original prototypes for viral-mediated gene transfer were retroviral vectors derived from the moloney murine leukemia virus.[27,32] Retroviral vectors were chosen as vehicles because of several useful properties. First, ''defective'' virus particles can be constructed that contain therapeutic genes and are capable of infecting cells, but that contain no viral genes and express no pathogenic viral gene products. A general scheme for constructing a ''defective'' retroviral particle is illustrated in Figure 16-5. Second, retroviral vectors are capable of permanently integrating the therapeutic genes they carry into the chromosomes of the target cell.

Because of this property, retroviral vectors are well suited for treating diseases that require permanent gene expression. Third, modifications can be made in retroviral vectors and in the cell lines producing vectors that result in enhanced safety features. Previous experience in animal models[10,11] and initial experiences in clinical trials suggest that these vectors have a high margin of safety.

A major limitation of this strategy is that retroviruses only will integrate into actively dividing cells, and the efficiency of retroviral infection is relatively low. It is difficult, therefore, to generate large numbers of transduced cells that are required for effective gene expression. Perhaps the most serious problem, however, is the difficulty in achieving stable, regulated expression from retroviral vectors in cells that permanently carry these genes despite the known permanent integration. Cells are apparently able to shut off expression from retroviral vectors under certain conditions, which have not been clearly defined.

Adenoviruses as gene transfer vehicles

A recent focus of gene therapy has been the development of adenovirus vectors as powerful and effective vehicles for gene transfer.[3] An overview for the construction of a replication-defective adenoviral vector is shown in Figure 16-6. Adenoviral vectors differ from retroviral vectors in that they remain *episomal*, i.e., they do not integrate their genes into the target cell's chromosome. Compared with retroviral vec-

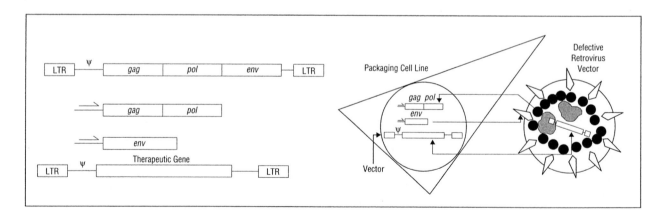

Fig. 16-5. Construction of a replication-defective retroviral vector. **Left,** The Moloney leukemia virus genome encodes three polyproteins gag, pol, and env, which together constitute a retroviral particle. The gag and pol genes encode the inner core of the retrovirus as well as enzymes required for processing the retroviral gene after infection of the target cell. The env gene forms the outer envelope of the virus and recognizes a specific receptor on target cells. Defective retroviral vectors are made using several recombinant genes: one that expresses the gag-pol polyprotein, one that encodes the env protein, and one that contains the therapeutic gene in conjunction with two long terminal repeat (promoter and enhancer) sequences and the psi (packaging) sequence. **Right,** A packaging cell line expresses gag, pol, and env from the constructs shown in the left panel. When a vector containing the therapeutic gene with the long terminal repeat and psi sequences is introduced into this cell, a nonpathogenic viral particle will be assembled from the gag, pol, and env proteins that is capable of carrying the therapeutic sequence into cells by the process of infection. (From O'Malley BW Jr, Ledley FD: Somatic gene therapy: methods for the present and future, *Arch Otolaryngol Head Neck Surg* 119:1100, 1993, Copyright 1993, American Medical Association. By permission.)

tors, adenoviral vectors demonstrate the significant advantage of infecting a wide variety of both dividing and nondividing cells *in vitro* and *in vivo* with a high level of efficiency.[4,7,38] Using adenoviral gene transfer, expression of the therapeutic gene is possible for a period of several weeks to months. Although current technologies enable the construction of adenoviral vectors that cannot proliferate, they are not completely ''defective'' and will express a series of viral gene products. Under certain conditions, adenoviral vectors remain capable of inducing an inflammatory response and subsequent cell lysis. The potential disadvantages of nonpermanent gene expression and possible limiting inflammatory responses have been addressed by further manipulation of the adenovirus genetic backbone to create new vectors that remain for months in the target cell, express less viral proteins, and have greatly reduced inflammatory responses.[16] While the safety of adenoviral vectors for gene therapy has not been studied as extensively as retroviral vectors, there is considerable experience with the use of attenuated adenovirus in animal models and in human subjects, which suggests that there is a high margin of safety.[4,7,13,38]

Other viral vectors

There exist other viruses that exhibit properties that may be useful for gene transfer, but experimentation with these vectors is still in the early stages. The herpes virus is capable of infecting cells and persisting indefinitely in a latent state. Vectors using the herpes virus have been constructed that are replication-defective and capable of expressing recombinant genes for prolonged periods of time in animal models.[21] These viruses are not completely defective, and continue to express many viral proteins that can be cytopathic, a property that severely limits the herpes virus for present gene therapy applications.

The human papillomavirus has the ability to persist indefinitely in the host cell as an independent, extrachromosomal element. This papillomavirus, however, has detrimental transforming potential that must be eliminated before it can be used as a vector for gene therapy. Another viral vector on the horizon is based on the adeno–associated virus which, like the retrovirus, can provide a completely defective vector that permanently integrates in the chromosomes of the target cell.[150] Unlike retrovirus, adeno-associated virus integrates in a predictable location within the infected cell, which could make these vectors safer than those that integrate randomly in the genome. A disadvantage of the adeno-associated virus is that a wild-type ''helper virus'' is required to help produce the therapeutic recombinant vector. The ''safe'' recombinant vector must then be purified from the potentially cytotoxic helper virus prior to amplification. Further investigation is required to define the role and safety of adeno–associated virus in clinical application. A summary of viral vector characteristics is shown in Table 16-1.

Strategies

Two general strategies exist for administering gene therapy (Fig. 16-7). The first and earliest conceived strategy is *ex vivo* gene therapy in which tissue from a patient is removed by a surgical biopsy, cells are isolated and grown in culture, genes are inserted into these cells typically using retroviral vectors, and the cells are reimplanted in the body by autologous transplantation. The second is *in vivo* gene therapy in which DNA or viral vectors (predominantly adenoviral vectors) are administered directly to patients.

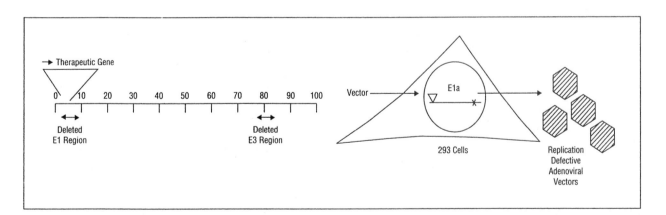

Fig. 16-6. Construction of a replication-defective adenoviral vector. **Left,** Adenoviral vectors are constructed using a deleted adenoviral genome that lacks the E3 gene as well as the E1 gene that is required for producing a proliferating adenovirus particle. Recombinant genes are inserted into the site of the E1 gene. **Right,** Adenoviral particles are produced in the 293 cell line that is able to express E1 and therefore is capable of assembling a viral particle containing only the recombinant viral genome with the therapeutic gene. (From O'Malley BW Jr, Ledley FD: Somatic gene therapy: methods for the present and future, *Arch Otolaryngol Head Neck Surg* 119:1100, 1993, Copyright 1993, American Medical Association. By permission.)

Table 16-1. Viral vectors currently used for gene therapy

	Adenovirus	Retrovirus	Adeno-associated virus	Herpes simplex virus
Infectivity	Broad	Dividing cells	Broad	Broad
Integration	Episomal	Random chromosomal integration	Specific chromosomal integration	Episomal
Viral titer	High	Low	Low	Low
Maximum insert size	Intermediate (approximately 8 kb)	Intermediate (approximately 10 kb)	Small (approximately 5 kb)	Large (approximately 36 kb)
Risks	Immune response	Mutagenesis tumorigenesis	Wild-type virus contamination	Cytopathogenicity
Viral production	Helper-free	Helper-free	Helper virus	Helper virus and helper-free vectors

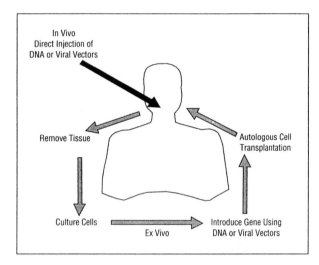

Fig. 16-7. Strategies for *ex vivo* and *in vivo* gene therapy. *In vivo* strategies for gene therapy involve the direct administration of deoxyribonucleic acid or viral vectors to patients by conventional routes of injection *(black arrows)*. *Ex vivo* strategies involve removing tissue from patients, growing cells in culture, introducing genes into these cells in the laboratory, and then returning the genetically modified cells to the patient by autologous transplantation *(shaded arrows)*. (From O'Malley BW Jr, Ledley FD: Somatic gene therapy: methods for the present and future, *Arch Otolaryngol Head Neck Surg* 119:1100, 1993, Copyright 1993, American Medical Association. By permission.)

Ex vivo *gene therapy*

Initial clinical trials of gene transfer and gene therapy employed the *ex vivo* strategy to deliver genes to lymphocytes, hepatocytes, tumor cells, fibroblasts, or bone marrow stem cells.[1,31] The intent of *ex vivo* gene therapy is to create a population of cells within the body that permanently express a therapeutic function. Therefore, *ex vivo* strategies for gene therapy commonly employ retroviral vectors because they integrate into the target cells and theoretically result in permanent therapeutic gene expression.

The initial attraction of *ex vivo* gene therapy stemmed from the concept that gene transfer could be performed in the laboratory under controlled conditions without exposing the patient directly to a viral or DNA vector. *Ex vivo* strategies, however, require methods for cellular transplantation to return the genetically manipulated cells back into the patient. Although bone marrow transplantation, lymphocyte transfusion, and skin grafting are accepted clinical procedures, there is little precedent for the transplantation of cells into solid organs. At present, this approach continues to be a difficult field of surgical research. Methods have been described for transplanting hepatocytes,[28] thyroid follicular cells,[40] myoblasts,[2] or fibroblasts,[51] although the effectiveness of these methods has not yet been established in clinical practice. In the above models, the number of cells that can be transplanted into the body may limit the amount of the therapeutic gene product that can be expressed by *ex vivo* methods.[28]

In vivo *gene therapy*

A recent major focus in gene therapy is the application of *in vivo* strategies for gene therapy in which genes are administered directly to patients using viral or DNA vectors. Investigations with retroviral vectors in animal models have demonstrated that it is possible to infect dividing cells in the liver, endothelium, lung, or tumors *in vivo*.[1,31] Studies using adenoviral vectors have demonstrated infection of both dividing and nondividing cells in the pulmonary epithelium,[30] liver,[54] muscle,[55] a variety of tumors,[7,38] and other tissues *in vivo*. Other studies have demonstrated the feasibility of delivering DNA vectors to organs including muscle,[59] thyroid,[52] liver,[60] and joints[62] *in vivo*.

Although the goal of *ex vivo* gene therapy is to permanently introduce a recombinant gene into a patient's cells, the primary goal of *in vivo* strategies may vary depending on the tissue and disease for which the treatment has been designed. *In vivo* gene therapy can be performed with single treatments for certain tumors,[7,38] be administered intermittently in response to acute disease, or be administered chronically to establish steady state levels of the therapeutic gene product. The *in vivo* strategy correlates with conventional regimens of medical therapy, however, gene therapy could provide prolonged or improved effects. Furthermore, the *in vivo* strategy facilitates the combination of conventional medical treatments or surgical procedures with gene therapy to potentially provide synergistic effects. It is the development of *in vivo* and relatively noninvasive methods for gene delivery that may allow the widespread application of gene therapy to routine problems of medicine and surgery.

Human gene therapy

Ethical and social considerations

Over the past decade there has been extensive debate over the proprietary and social implications of gene therapy.[18] It is now generally accepted that the implantation of therapeutic genes into somatic cells is conceptually similar to the implantation of cells, organs, or artificial devises for therapeutic purposes, and raises few novel ethical or social issues.[26] No governmental or religious sector in this country has raised objections to gene therapy research in somatic cells, and the public understands intent to develop novel therapies.

In designing gene therapy clinical trials, careful attention has been directed at ensuring no risk to nonsubjects, observing the conventional principles of balancing risk versus benefit, and ensuring fairness, privacy, and confidentiality. Clinical trials of gene therapy are, in fact, not significantly different than trials of nongenetic technologies.

Regulatory agencies and approval for clinical trials

Because of the unusual public and professional concern about gene therapy, a special review process has been established in which clinical trials are reviewed by both local and federal agencies. Within each medical institution or hospital, internal review boards and biosafety committees have been established to review and monitor human clinical trial proposals and progress. On a federal level, the Recombinant DNA Advisory Committee of the National Institutes of Health (NIH) and the Food and Drug Administration (FDA) also have established a strict review process as outlined in the *Points to consider in the design and submission of human somatic cell gene therapy protocols*.[45] These guidelines sanction the application of gene therapy for medical purposes only, and explicitly proscribe genetic manipulation of germ cells.

As concerns about the social implications of genetic engineering have abated, increasing attention has been focused on developing models for clinical trials and the clinical issues involved in performing such clinical trials. These issues include establishing procedures for patient selection, documents for informed consent, standards for clinical care, sources of funding, and mechanisms for long-term follow-up.[29]

The status of clinical trials

The first gene therapy clinical trials began at the NIH in 1989 and demonstrated that gene transfer could be performed safely and with public acceptance. By June, 1996 149 clinical trials had been proposed and approved by regulatory agencies.

The early gene therapy trials involved "gene marking" studies. In this type of study a gene with no therapeutic potential is introduced into various cells before they are transplanted into the body to assist in the quantitative study of these cells *in vivo*. The initial clinical trial at the NIH in 1989 used a retrovirus to introduce a "marker gene" into TIL and demonstrated that these cells would preferentially infiltrate tumors when reimplanted in the body.[47]

The first true therapeutic trial of gene therapy involved retroviral transfer of a gene for adenosine deaminase into the peripheral blood lymphocytes of patients with severe combined immunodeficiency due to mutations in this enzyme.[31] In this temporary therapy, the gene persisted for several weeks, correlating with the survival time of lymphocytes after transfusion, and resulted in significant improvement of the immune status of these patients.

The clinical targets in active gene therapy trials have broadened to include familial hypercholesterolemia, cystic fibrosis, arthritis, AIDS, Gaucher's disease, leukemia, and solid tumors.[22] The majority of clinical trials focus on novel treatments for cancer or "marking trials" of hematopoietic cells. The marking of hematopoietic cells has been applied to understanding important questions regarding the tumor selectivity of TIL and issues in bone marrow transplantation. For the direct treatment of cancer, targets include melanoma, neuroblastoma, mesothelioma, and brain, colon, breast, prostate, lung, renal, and head and neck cancer. The gene therapy strategies include gene transfer of specific cytokines, cytotoxic genes, and tumor suppressor genes into established, advanced, or recurrent tumors.

Applications of somatic gene therapy in otolaryngology

Gene therapy is relatively new to the field of otolaryngology. Its applications are broad and important, and advances in overlapping medical and surgical fields can be applied to the diseases and clinical scenarios common to the otolaryngologist. The remainder of this chapter will review the various applications arising from ongoing basic research and proposed clinical trials.

Inherited disease

A variety of inherited diseases are associated with head and neck pathology such as sinus disease in cystic fibrosis, hearing loss in Usher's, Alport's, or Pendred's syndrome, and goiter in certain forms of congenital hypothyroidism. In some of these diseases it may be possible to place a normal gene in appropriate cells to carry out the function of the inherited, mutant gene. For example, the first clinical trial of gene therapy for cystic fibrosis involved the introduction of a normal cystic fibrosis transmembrane conductance regulator (CFTR) gene into the nasal mucosa using adenoviral vectors.[63] The intention of this study was to assess expression of the CFTR gene in respiratory epithelium and determine any toxic or inflammatory side effects. This trial provided a foundation for future studies in which the CFTR gene would be replaced throughout the respiratory tract using viral or DNA vector.[12]

Head and neck oncology

Many of the initial clinical trials of somatic gene therapy are focused on the treatment of cancer. Although gene therapy specifically for the head and neck oncology patient is just emerging, the tumor targets for the original gene therapy cancer trials included melanoma, which is encountered in the head and neck cancer patient population. Various approaches for treating cancer by gene therapy have been proposed (Fig. 16-8) and are applicable to common head and neck tumors.

Genetic modification of tumor infiltrating lymphocytes

Although the first clinical trial of gene therapy involved only the introduction of marker genes into TIL cells that infiltrate solid tumors such as melanoma, this trial founded the principle, feasibility, and safety of gene transfer into human patients. The original interest in TIL cells stems from

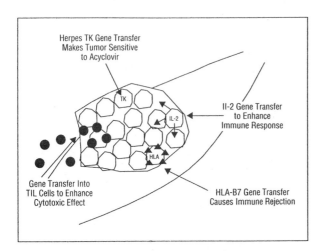

Fig. 16-8. Strategies for gene therapy of cancer. Several different strategies have been described for managing cancers with gene therapy. These strategies include: expression of cytokines such as interleukin-2 (IL-2) within tumor cells to enhance the immune response against tumor-specific antigens; introduction of a foreign transplantation antigen such as HLA-B7 to induce immune rejection; introduction of cytokines into tumor infiltrating lymphocytes (TIL cells) to enhance their cytopathic effect; and introducing genes such as herpes TK to make tumor cells sensitive to drugs such as acyclovir or ganciclovir. (From O'Malley BW Jr, Ledley FD: Somatic gene therapy: methods for the present and future, *Arch Otolaryngol Head Neck Surg* 119:1191, 1993, Copyright 1993, American Medical Association. By permission.)

prior studies demonstrating that adoptive transfer of TIL cells coupled with administration of interleukin (IL)-2 could cause significant tumor regression in some patients with malignant melanoma.[47] TIL cells, however, are relatively inefficient at destroying tumors despite their ability to selectively infiltrate tumor sites.

Gene therapy is therefore an ideal strategy to increase the antitumor potential of TIL cells by providing concurrent expression of stimulatory proteins such as cytokines. In an early melanoma trial, TIL cells were harvested from the tumors of patients, and a gene for TNF was introduced into these cells.[49] When these genetically engineered cells were transfused into the patient they were expected to target the tumor and express the antitumor TNF. The expression of high levels of TNF was expected to cause tumor cell lysis with minimal systemic exposure to this toxic protein.[15]

Another clinical trial for cancer patients uses autologous cancer cells modified with a gene that produces IL-2, a cytokine that increases the immunogenicity of cancer cells and suppresses tumor growth.[48] Using this strategy, transfer of the gene for IL-2 is performed directly into a patient's tumor that results in the local formation of tumor-specific cytolytic TIL cells. An excisional biopsy of a draining lymph node allows harvesting of sensitized TIL cells that are multiplied in culture and transfused back into the patient. The TIL cells are now sensitized to the specific tumor and when infused into the patient, will home in on any cancer tissue or cells and enact a cytolytic response. This protocol focuses on patients with primary or metastatic cancer on which standard therapy has proven ineffective.

Direct *in vivo stimulation of an antitumor immune response*

Direct *in vivo* stimulation therapy involves introducing genes for various cytokines directly into tumor cells to increase the natural immune response to tumor-specific antigens. The human body has natural cellular and humoral immune effectors that inhibit or prevent tumor cell growth. Examples of such effectors include, major histocompatibility complex (MHC)-restricted cytotoxic T cells, natural killer (NK) cells, and lymphokine-activated killer (LAK) cells. The majority of human malignancies, however, arise in immunocompetent individuals, which infers that tumor cells escape the body's natural immune defenses. Tumors are also known to lack or demonstrate deficiencies in the expression of class I MHC antigens, which prevents recognition and attack by cytotoxic T cells.[25]

In animal models, the transfer of the gene for foreign class I MHC antigen HLA-B7 into colon carcinoma, melanoma, and sarcoma cell lines has resulted in cytolytic activity from splenic lymphocytes.[36] In this immunologic gene therapy strategy, the gene for HLA-B7 expression is transferred into a cutaneous melanoma lesion of patients who have primary or recurrent tumors, or distant metastases that have not responded to conventional therapy.[36] Expression of the

HLA-B7 antigen on the melanoma cells is expected to lead to rejection of the primary tumor and metastases by the immune system. B7 gene therapy using nonviral vectors has been approved for a multitumor phase I clinical trial that includes head and neck squamous cell carcinoma.

In a head and neck cancer animal model, the use of adenoviral-mediated delivery of the cytokine IL-2 in combination with a cytotoxic gene has demonstrated synergistic effects on tumor regression.[39] The proposed mechanism is the stimulation of a cytotoxic T-cell immune response magnified by released tumor antigens and cellular debris created by the cytotoxic gene. This work will provide the foundation for future human clinical trials using combination therapy in the head and neck cancer patient.

Cytotoxic or suicide gene therapy strategies

Methods have been described for altering the response of tumor cells to chemotherapeutic agents. One experimental approach involves infecting tumor cells by direct injection with a retrovirus that encodes the thymidine kinase gene from herpesvirus.[44] Since retroviruses infect dividing cells, this virus will selectively enter growing tumor cells, causing them to express the herpes thymidine kinase gene and making them susceptible to chemotherapy with ganciclovir or acyclovir. Because these drugs are relatively nontoxic to the immune system, this treatment strategy not only eliminates the fraction of cells that are infected with the virus, but also allows for a more general immune response against tumor-specific antigens.

Based on the low efficiency of retrovirus application in animal and human model, highly efficient adenovirus vectors have been created that are capable of transferring the thymidine kinase gene directly to tumor cells.[38] This system has been effective in animal models and received FDA approval for a phase I clinical trial in 1996.

Modifying oncogenes and tumor suppressor genes

The discovery of oncogenes and tumor suppressor genes that are involved in the transformation of normal cells into tumor cells has stimulated new approaches for molecular therapy. Oncogenes are naturally present in cells and have proposed functions involving growth and differentiation until a mutation or overexpression activates them to oncogenic potential. Tumor suppressor genes also are naturally occurring, and their expression prevents unrestrained cell proliferation. A deletion or mutation that results in the loss of tumor suppressor gene function will therefore allow uncontrolled cell growth. Mutations in the tumor suppressor genes p53 and p16 have been detected in a variety of human tumors and a majority of head and neck cancers.[5] Please refer to Chapter 17 for a thorough discussion of tumor suppressor genes and their relation to head and neck cancer.

Ongoing research in these areas will provide the foundational understanding needed to develop models for screening patients for specific oncogenes and tumor suppressor genes

and allow for correction by gene transfer mechanisms. With respect to activated oncogenes, gene therapy may prove effective in blocking the production of oncogenic proteins. In lung cancer experiments, for example, cell lines containing the activated oncogene *K-ras* were transfected with a *K-ras* segment oriented in an antisense direction.[34] Transcription of the antisense DNA produced messenger RNA (mRNA) that hybridized with the activated mutant mRNA and blocked its translation into the oncogenic protein. This resulted in significant inhibition of tumor cell growth. Although encouraging, this strategy does not reverse the activated oncogene, therefore, strategies must be designed to enable permanent antisense mRNA production before any clinical benefit can be achieved.

Gene transfer of tumor suppressor genes for the treatment of head and neck cancer is another strategy currently under investigation. Using nude mouse models, adenovirus-mediated delivery of p53 has resulted in stimulation of apoptosis and subsequent squamous cell cancer regression.[9] This approach to gene therapy of cancer, however, could prove difficult because it requires the transfer of tumor suppressor genes into a majority of tumor cells. Furthermore, the expression of the suppressor gene is transient, and the tumor regression in these studies has not been permanent. Adenovirus-mediated p53 gene therapy is presently under a phase I clinical trial for squamous cell carcinoma of the head and neck.

Antiangiogenesis

An approach with future potential in cancer gene therapy involves introducing genes that inhibit angiogenesis in the vicinity of a tumor.[19] A decrease or regression of important vascular supply by the action of antiangiogenesis factors has been shown to cause significant tumor regression in mouse melanoma models. Continued development and investigation of inhibitors of growth and angiogenesis coupled with the packaging of these factors into vectors for gene transfer *in vivo* may provide alternative or adjuvant therapies for both benign vascular and malignant tumors of the head and neck.

Plastic and reconstructive surgery

Great potential for gene therapy exists in the area of plastic and reconstructive surgery. The principle concept of gene therapy as applied to this field is the expression of growth regulating factors to enhance repair or regeneration of damaged tissues, as well to induce local proliferation to fill surgical defects. By introducing genes into cells within a surgical site, local expression of growth factors can be constituted at levels that maximize the therapeutic response. The use of gene transfer to release growth factors, as opposed to simply injecting suspensions of purified factors, enables regulated expression of the product over a programmed period of time with restriction of the product to specific targeted layers of tissue. The combination of this property with the incorporation of proper regulatory elements could minimize associated toxicities or unwanted proliferation of nearby tissues.

Reconstructive tissue flaps and wound healing

A common problem encountered with the use of local or regional flaps is distal flap necrosis with atrophy or even partial loss.[35] Timely angiogenesis and neovascularization is essential for the survival of these tissues, as well as healing of the surgical wound. This process of angiogenesis is stimulated by various growth factors such as basic fibroblast growth factor (bFGF) and heparin-binding growth factor.[20] Using gene transfer techniques, a gene encoding an angiogenesis factor could be introduced into cells within a reconstructed tissue, recipient site, or primary wound defect. Subsequent to this gene therapy, an accelerated and magnified vascular response resulting from local expression of angiogenic factors could promote healing with improved tissue survival. The use of gene therapy may prove very important in free tissue flaps, where failure often occurs because of inadequate venous efflux leading to vascular engorgement and tissue destruction.

There are multiple other growth factors that influence the process of tissue repair and regeneration. Examples include transforming growth factors (TGF-α, TGF-β), insulin-like growth factors (IGF-I, IGF-II), platelet-derived growth factors (PDGF), nerve growth factors, and others. Different combinations of these factors can be used to enhance regeneration of vascular tissue, muscle, epithelium, and even nerves.[23] The factor IGF-I is especially important in maintaining muscle mass and differentiation, and may even be able to promote reinnervation of damaged muscle.

Basic FGF, epidermal growth factor (EGF), and TGF-β are potent growth stimulators in dermal layers and may prove advantageous in the management of soft tissue defects caused by trauma or resulting from surgery, a particularly difficult problem for the reconstructive surgeon. For example, the gene for a therapeutic growth factor could be transferred into the surgical defect created by a tongue-jaw-neck resection for oral squamous cell cancer. The local programmed production of healing and growth factors resulting from the direct gene therapy would then stimulate the growth of muscle, fascia, blood vessels, or dermal structures. This growth response would decrease the size of the defect and provide added strength and vascularized tissue to prevent wound dehiscence or extrusion or infection of reconstruction plates. Because of the ability to increase muscle and connective tissue mass and retard atrophy, much smaller flaps could be taken that reduce the overall morbidity and cosmetic defect at the donor site.

Skin grafting

Skin grafts are an attractive target for somatic gene therapy because of the known ability to cultivate epidermal cells *ex vivo* and subsequently engraft these cells successfully in patients. Furthermore, previous studies have established the feasibility of effective gene transfer into skin grafts in animal models.[33]

Survival of skin grafts is dependent on adequate nutrition and oxygenation of the graft, as well as removal of waste products. Until the blood supply is established, the recipient bed is responsible for the fibrous and plasma exudate through which nutrition is supplied and metabolic wastes are transferred.[42] Gene therapy to increase vascularization or provide local growth factors for the dermal or epidermal layers (depending on the thickness of the graft) could promote early graft take and overall improved strength survival. As a protective mechanism, gene transfer of various cytokines, complements, or antimicrobial factors may prove effective in preventing infection. This particular application could prove invaluable in burn patients who require extensive skin grafting, and in cases where grafting is performed over irradiated tissues, ulcers, or prostheses where survival is typically poor.

Repair and regeneration of irradiated tissue

Morbidity associated with primary or postoperative radiotherapy is common in head and neck cancer patients. Inflammation, fibrosis, pain, and even wound breakdown with infection are problems encountered in our patients receiving radiotherapy.[43] Despite efforts to narrow the x-ray field and block surrounding structures, there is still substantial damage to superficial and nearby tissues. Growth factors such as endothelial cell growth factor (ECGF)[24] have been shown to enhance viability and vascularity in irradiated soft tissue in animal models. Gene transfer of reparative factors such as ECGF may provide spatially precise and regulated expression of reparative factors within the field of radiation and result in reduced toxicity and overall morbidity.

CONCLUSION

The founding work over the past 20 years in molecular biology has enabled clinical application in the realm of gene therapy. Only 5 years have passed since the first clinical trial of gene transfer into human subjects was performed. Now there are 149 clinical trials approved by the NIH, and the pace continues rapidly. Although the majority of these early trials have not focused on efficacy, they do show that gene transfer can be performed safely and with public acceptance.

No longer is gene therapy simply a speculative approach for treating disease in the distant future. Although the methods for gene therapy are still evolving, current methods are already sufficiently advanced as to be employed in trials of gene therapy for select diseases and to be incorporated into clinically efficacious pharmaceutical products. Gene therapy has great potential not only for the treatment of inherited diseases, but also for providing new treatments for complex diseases such as cancer and for the development of novel adjuvants to standard medical or surgical interventions. Gene therapy technologies should have a significant impact on the quality of medicine and provide the additional benefit of cost reduction. As the field rapidly advances, increasing opportunities should arise for physicians to apply these technologies in clinical trials and eventually clinical practice.

REFERENCES

1. Anderson WF: Human gene therapy, *Science* 256:808, 1992.
2. Ban E, Leiden JM: Systemic delivery of recombinant proteins by genetically modified myoblasts, *Science* 254:1507, 1991.
3. Berkner KL: Development of adenovirus vectors for the expression of heterologous genes, *Biotechniques* 6:616, 1988.
4. Brody SL, Crystal RG: Adenovirus-mediated *in vivo* gene transfer, *Ann NY Acad Sci* 716:90, 1994.
5. Califano J and others: Genetic progression model for head and neck cancer: implications for field cancerization, *Cancer Res* 56:2488, 1996.
6. Capecchi MR: High efficiency transformation by direct microinjection of DNA into cultured mammalian cells, *Cell* 22:479, 1980.
7. Chen S-H and others: Gene therapy for brain tumors: regression of experimental gliomas by adenovirus-mediated gene transfer *in vitro, Proc Natl Acad Sci U S A* 91:3054, 1994.
8. Chu G and others: *Nucleic Acids Res* 15:1311, 1987.
9. Clayman GL and others: *In vivo* molecular therapy with p53 adenovirus for microscopic residual head and neck squamous carcinoma, *Cancer Res* 55:1, 1995.
10. Cornetta K and others: Amphotropic murine leukemia retrovirus is not an acute pathogen for primates, *Hum Gene Ther* 1:15, 1990.
11. Cornetta K and others: Safety issues related to retroviral mediated gene transfer in humans, *Hum Gene Ther* 2:5, 1991.
12. Crystal RG: Gene therapy strategies for pulmonary disease, *Am J Med* 92:44, 1992.
13. Crystal RG and others: Administration of an adenovirus containing the human CFTR cDNA to the respiratory tract of individuals with cystic fibrosis, *Nat Genet* 8:42, 1994.
14. Curiel DT and others: Adenovirus enhancement of transferrin-polylysine-mediated gene delivery, *Proc Natl Acad Sci U S A* 88:8850, 1991.
15. Debs RJ and others: Immunomodulatory and toxic effects of free and liposome-encapsulated tumor necrosis factor alpha in rats, *Cancer Res* 50:375, 1990.
16. Engelhardt JF and others: Ablation of E2A in recombinant adenoviruses improves transgene persistence and decreases inflammatory response in mouse liver, *Proc Natl Acad Sci U S A* 91:6196, 1994.
17. Felgner PL and others: Lipofection: a highly efficient, lipid-mediated DNA-transfection procedure, *Proc Natl Acad Sci U S A* 84:7413, 1987.
18. Fletcher JC: Evolution of ethical debate about human gene therapy, *Hum Gene Ther* 1:55, 1990.
19. Folkman J: Angiogenesis and its inhibitors. *Imp Adv Oncol* 42, 1985.
20. Folkman J, Klagsbrun M: Angiogenic factors, *Science* 235:442, 1987.
21. Geller AI and others: An efficient deletion mutant packaging system for defective herpes simplex virus vectors: potential applications to human gene therapy and neuronal physiology, *Proc Natl Acad Sci U S A* 87:8950, 1990.
22. Hanania EG and others: Recent advances in the application of gene therapy to human disease, *Am J Med* 99:537, 1995.
23. Hansson HA and others: Regenerating human nasal mucosa cells express peptide growth factors, *Arch Otolaryngol Head Neck Surg* 117:1368, 1991.
24. Hom DB, Girma A, Chang WS: Endothelial cell growth factor (ECGF) application to irradiated soft tissue, *Laryngoscope* 103:165, 1993.
25. Isakov N and others: Loss of expression of transplantation antigens encoded by H-2K locus on Lewis lung carcinoma cells and its relevance to the tumor's metastatic properties, *J Cancer Inst* 71:139, 1983.
26. Ledley FD: Clinical considerations in the design of protocols for somatic gene therapy, *Hum Gene Ther* 2:77, 1991.
27. Ledley FD: *Human gene therapy*. In Jacobson GK, Jolly SO, editors: *Biotechnology, a comprehensive treatise,* vol 7b, Weinheim, 1989, VCH Verlagsgesellschaft.
28. Ledley FD and others: Development of a clinical protocol for hepatic gene transfer: lessons learned in pre-clinical studies, *Pediatr Res* 33:313, 1993.
29. Ledley FD and others: The challenge of follow-up for clinical trials of somatic gene therapy, *Hum Gene Ther* 3:657, 1991.
30. Mastrogeli A and others: Diversity of airway epithelial cell targets for in vivo recombinant adenovirus-mediated gene therapy, *J Clin Invest* 91:225, 1993.
31. Miller AD: Human gene therapy comes of age, *Nature* 357:455, 1992.
32. Miller AD: Retrovirus packaging cells, *Hum Gene Ther* 61:5, 1990.
33. Morgan JR and others: Expression of an exogenous growth hormone gene by transplantable human epidermal cells, *Science* 237:1476, 1987.
34. Mukhopadhyay T and others: Specific inhibition of K-ras expression and tumorigenicity of lung cancer cells by antisense RNA, *Cancer Res* 51:1744, 1991.
35. Myers MB, Cherry G: Causes of necrosis in pedicle flaps, *Plast Reconstr Surg* 42:43, 1983.
36. Nabel GJ and others: Clinical protocol: immunotherapy of malignancy by *in vivo* gene transfer into tumors, *Hum Gene Ther* 3:399, 1992.
37. Office of Technology Assessment: *Human gene therapy,* background paper, Washington, DC, 1984, US Government Printing Office.
38. O'Malley BW Jr and others: Adenovirus-mediated gene therapy for head and neck cancer in a nude mouse model, *Cancer Res* 55:1080, 1995.
39. O'Malley BW Jr and others: Combination gene therapy for oral cancer in a murine model, *Cancer Res* 56:1737, 1996.
40. O'Malley BW Jr, Finegold MJ, Ledley FD: Autologous, orthotopic thyroid follicular cell transplantation: a surgical component of *ex vivo* somatic gene therapy, *Otolaryngol Head Neck Surg* 108:51, 1993.
41. O'Malley BW Jr, Ledley FD: Somatic gene therapy: methods for the present and future, *Arch Otolaryngol Head Neck Surg* 119:1100, 1993.
42. Paparella MM and others: *Otolaryngology plastic and reconstructive surgery vol IV*, Philadelphia, 1991, WB Saunders.
43. Parson JT: *The effects of radiation on normal tissues of the head and neck.* In Million RR, Cassissi NJ, editors: *Management of head and neck cancer: a multidisciplinary approach*, Philadelphia, 1984, JB Lippincott.
44. Ram Z and others: *In situ* retroviral-mediated gene transfer for the treatment of brain tumors in rats, *Cancer Res* 53:83, 1993.
45. Recombinant DNA Advisory Committee: Points to consider in the design and submission of human somatic cell gene therapy protocols, Federal register 54:no 169, 36698-36703. Reprinted in *Hum Gene Ther* 1:93, 1990.
46. Rosenberg SA: Gene therapy for cancer, *JAMA* 268:2416, 1992.
47. Rosenberg SA and others: Gene transfer into humans—immunotherapy of patients with advanced melanoma, using tumor-infiltrating lymphocytes modified by retroviral gene transduction, *N Engl J Med* 323:570, 1990.
48. Rosenberg SA and others: Clinical research project: immunization of cancer patients using autologous cancer cells modified by insertion of the gene for interleukin-2, *Hum Gene Ther* 3:75, 1992.
49. Rosenberg SA and others: Clinical research project: immunization of cancer patients using autologous cancer cells modified by insertion of the gene for tumor necrosis factor, *Hum Gene Ther* 3:57, 1992.
50. Samulski RJ and others: Helper-free stocks of recombinant adeno-associated viruses: normal integration does not require viral gene expression, *J Virol* 63:3822, 1989.
51. Scharfmann R, Axelrod JH, Verman IM: Long-term *in vivo* expression of retrovirus-mediated gene transfer in mouse fibroblast implants, *Proc Natl Acad Sci U S A* 88:4676, 1991.
52. Sikes ML and others: *In vivo* gene transfer into rabbit thyroid follicular cells by direct DNA injection, *Hum Gene Ther* 5:837, 1994.
53. Stankovics J and others: Overexpression of human methylmalonyl CoA mutase in mice after *in vivo* gene transfer with asialoglycoprotein/polylsine/DNA complexes, *Hum Gene Ther* 5:1095, 1994.
54. Stratford-Perricaudet LD and others: Evaluation of the transfer and

expression in mice of an enzyme encoding gene using a human adenovirus vector, *Hum Gene Ther* 3:241, 1990.

55. Stratford-Perricaudet LD and others: Widespread long-term gene transfer to mouse skeletal muscles and heart, *J Clin Invest* 90:626, 1992.

56. Vega MA: Prospects for ''homologous recombination'' in human gene therapy, *Hum Genet* 87:245, 1991.

57. Wagner E and others: Influenza virus hemagglutinin HA-2 N-terminal fusogenic peptides augment gene transfer by transferrin-polylysine-DNA complexes: toward a synthetic virus-like gene-transfer vehicle, *Proc Natl Acad Sci U S A* 89:7934, 1992.

58. Wagner E and others: Transferrin-polycation conjugates as carriers for DNA uptake into cells, *Proc Natl Acad Sci U S A* 87:3410, 1990.

59. Wolff JA and others: Direct gene transfer into mouse muscle *in vivo*, *Science* 247:1465, 1990.

60. Wu GY, Wu CH: Receptor-mediated *in vitro* gene transformation by a soluble DNA carrier system, *J Biol Chem* 262:4429, 1987.

61. Yang NS and others: *In vivo* and *in vitro* gene transfer to mammalian somatic cells by particle bombardment, *Proc Natl Acad Sci U S A* 87:9568, 1990.

62. Yovandich J and others: Gene transfer to synovial cells by intra-articular administration of plasmid DNA. *Hum Gene Ther* 6:603, 1995.

63. Zabner J and others: Adenovirus-mediated gene transfer transiently corrects the chloride transport defect in nasal epithelium of patients with cystic fibrosis, *Cell* 75:207, 1993.

Chapter 17

Molecular Biology of Head and Neck Tumors

Wayne Martin Koch

An explosion of information in the past decade is producing a revolution in cancer management. This revolution is made possible by technologic developments that allow for precise analysis and manipulation of genetic material in tumor cells. Physicians who care for cancer patients have long been frustrated by the failure to improve outcome despite innovations in diagnostic imaging, surgical and anesthetic techniques, radiation, chemotherapy, and immunotherapy. A better understanding of the events that take place during neoplastic transformation, invasion, and metastasis is needed to develop novel approaches to cancer diagnosis and treatment. The molecular biology revolution is providing such an understanding. But the rapidity of new developments and the complexity of molecular biologic terminology, techniques, and concepts threaten to make the fruit of the revolution inaccessible to clinical oncologists and their patients. It is imperative that we strive to stay abreast of developments in the molecular biology of cancer. We must be able to apply what is learned in the laboratory to the diagnosis and treatment of our patients.

FOUNDATIONAL CONCEPTS

What is cancer?

Cancer occurs when cells escape the controls regulating the cell cycle and are able to proliferate regardless of signals from their environment. Homeostatic mechanisms that commit one daughter cell to differentiation and senescence and the other to continued stem-cell growth are lost. Additionally, these cells develop the capability of commanding the ingrowth of new blood vessels that supply the nutritional needs of the tumor. Alterations in their interactions with the surrounding tissues permit cancer cells to invade those tissues and metastasize. Tumors vary in their ability to grow, invade, and spread, often developing greater virulence with time. Cancer cells faithfully pass on their cancer phenotype, or outward characteristics of growth, differentiation, and behavior, to their progeny.

The central dogma of molecular biology

What is the mechanism behind these fundamental, permanent, and inheritable changes in the cancer cell? Landmark discoveries during the mid-1900s form the basis of the central dogma of molecular biology—which states that the flow of information controlling cellular function is from genes (deoxyribonucleic acid [DNA]) to ribonucleic acid (RNA) to proteins.[90] A great deal of evidence exists demonstrating that cancer has a genetic basis; i.e., it is caused by alterations or mutations in DNA. For example, normal cells can adopt a cancer phenotype in the laboratory by the introduction of certain genes from cancer cells or tumorigenic viruses. On the other hand, cancer cells may revert to a normal phenotype when other genes that have lost function during malignant transformation are reintroduced. Additionally, known carcinogenic agents or their metabolites generally have been found to be mutagenic.

It is apparent from a variety of evidence that the development of cancer is a multistep process. First, experimental models of cancer produced in laboratory animals (e.g., skin cancer in mice) provided an early indication that at least two steps are necessary.[35] These studies showed that a low dose of an initiating carcinogen will not cause cancer unless it is followed by multiple treatments with a tumor-promoting

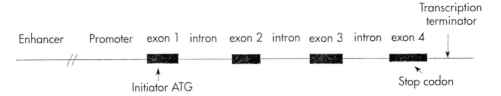

Fig. 17-1. Structural map of a typical gene. (Modified from Watson JD and others: *Recombinant DNA*, ed 2, New York, 1992, WH Freeman.)

agent. Secondly, the introduction of more than one oncogene is required for cancer transformation in *in vitro* transfection experiments.[29] Additionally, the incidence of most cancers increases with the age of the individual, suggesting the necessity of an accumulation of genetic damage over time. Most compelling of all, molecular studies of primary tumors have uncovered the presence of multiple genetic alterations in individual cancer specimens.[22]

Clonality of cancer

Clinical neoplasms are comprised of a population of identical cancer cells known as a clone derived from a common ancestor.[88] The initial genetic change in cancer transformation is thought to provide a growth advantage for the altered cell and its progeny. Although each new generation of daughter cells retains the original mutation, the opportunity exists for individual cells in the clone to sustain additional alterations that provide further growth enhancement. This results in the successive overgrowth of increasingly altered subclones that soon outnumber the less abnormal parent population, a phenomenon known as clonal expansion.

The phenomenon of field cancerization, commonly described in patients with cancer of the upper aerodigestive tract, raises interesting questions about clonality. It is possible that multiple areas of *in situ* or invasive carcinoma arise independently through unique series of mutations in separate cells after exposure to carcinogens. Alternatively, clonally related cells sharing an early mutation may migrate some distance apart before sustaining different additional alterations and developing into separate tumors. Molecular evidence discussed below may help to distinguish between these two possibilities.

Important terms that are commonly used in molecular biology are defined in Box 17-1. The structural organization of a typical gene is illustrated in Figure 17-1.

NEOPLASTIC TRANSFORMATION

Damage inflicted on DNA by a variety of mechanisms can alter the production or function of encoded proteins. Many mutations are lethal, and only occasionally will the damage result in a growth advantage for the cell. Mutations can be classified according to the type of change that occurs in the DNA molecule, the functional effect in the transformation process, or the biochemical mechanism involved.

Box 17-1. Glossary of important terms

Transcription—the production of messenger RNA (mRNA) from DNA;

Translation—the production of protein from mRNA;

Codon—group of three DNA bases encoding a single amino acid;

Exon—translated segment of a gene interrupted by intronic sequences;

Intron—untranslated DNA interspersed between exons within a gene. Introns are removed by splicing after transcription;

Promotor regions—DNA immediately upstream from a gene that includes the RNA polymerase binding site and specific transcriptional control sequences;

Enhancer regions—DNA regions further upstream from a gene that bind agents that regulate the amount of mRNA produced;

Alleles—duplicate copies of a gene (paternal and maternal) encoding the same protein;

Polymorphisms—minor variations in alleles that are inherited in a Mendelian fashion and usually do not significantly alter the function of the encoded protein;

Heterozygosity—the state in which an individual has two slightly different copies of a given allele.

Mechanisms of mutation

Exogenous mutation

Genetic damage leading to malignant transformation is thought to occur through exogenous and endogenous pathways. Many substances are known to cause mutation. Most of these have been shown to form covalent links to DNA, which result in hybrid structures called adducts. The adducts may interfere with the proper reading of the DNA sequence during replication.

Certain DNA sequences are known to be target binding sites for specific mutagens. For example, tobacco smoke contains nitropolycyclic aromatic hydrocarbons that form 7-methylguanine and 4-aminobiphenyl at guanine nucleotides. Using this type of information, analysis of the spectrum of mutations in a particular type of tumor provides evidence of a causal relationship between known carcinogens and that type of cancer.[7,34]

The susceptibility to environmental carcinogenesis varies among individuals. Patterns of susceptibility have been linked to the expression of enzymes that are involved in the biotransformation of toxic chemicals. Such variability may partially explain the prevalence of cancer in some families and the high susceptibility of some individuals to carcinogens.[36]

Deoxyribonucleic acid repair and endogenous mutations

Some endogenous mutations are attributable to the chemical instability of DNA. Depurination, the cleavage of the chemical link between a purine base and the deoxyribose backbone, produces an empty site in the DNA sequence 10,000 times each day in each cell. Deamination of cytosine to form uridine occurs somewhat less frequently. In addition, cytosine is often methylated after replication, particularly when it is located before a guanine (a CpG site).[16] Deamination of methylcytosine to thymine causes a base pair change of CmXG to AmXT. Other endogenous mutations occur because of errors made during DNA synthesis. Replication of DNA is an astoundingly accurate cellular process, with errors occurring only in 1 of 109 to 1011 bases. Exonuclease enzymes follow the polymerase in a proofreading function, replacing incorrectly matched bases before the completion of DNA synthesis. In yet another repair step, mismatch-repair enzymes can cut out incorrect bases after replication is completed.[16] Under normal circumstances, errors in replication or chemically induced alterations in the DNA sequence are repaired before cell division and growth. When errors are not corrected by repair mechanisms, the altered gene sequence is inherited by the progeny cells. DNA repair capacity may be reduced in segments of the population, as well as in certain disease states (such as xeroderma pigmentosum), and may decline with the aging process.[13,92] The susceptibility of lymphocyte DNA to breakage when exposed to bleomycin has been proposed as a measurement of individual risk for failure in DNA repair. Mutagen sensitivity in this assay was found to be associated with a 2.5-fold increased risk for head and neck squamous cell carcinoma (HNSCC)[80] and a similarly increased risk for developing a second cancer.[81]

Damaged cells may be able to repair DNA prior to replication if controls on the cell cycle are intact. A number of putative tumor suppressor genes (TSGs) are now recognized to be involved in this cell cycle control mechanism including Rb, p53, and p16. Failure to repair DNA results either in cell death or perpetuation of the mutation in progeny cells.

Types of mutations

The substitution of one nucleotide base for another may change a single amino acid in what is called a missense point mutation. Other substitutions may produce codons that do not specify any amino acid, or yield a stop signal, resulting in a truncated protein (nonsense mutation). A frameshift mutation is the deletion or insertion of one or more bases that causes a shift in the codon grouping of all the bases that follow. This results in protein truncation or the mistaken incorporation of a number of amino acids. Large deletions and insertions can also occur. Transforming mutations may occur outside the coding regions of the genes. Alterations at enhancer, promotor, and splice-site sequences can have a profound effect on the production of protein.

Oncogenes and tumor suppressor genes

Another way of classifying genetic alterations is according to the way they contribute to the cancer phenotype. The genes involved in cancer generally encode proteins involved in the key cellular pathways such as those that regulate the cell cycle, cell growth, or differentiation. Proto-oncogenes are normal cellular genes that influence cell growth in a positive way. When these genes are altered, becoming oncogenes, the corresponding protein function is increased (through a gain-of-function mutation or amplification) either through the production of a more active or more stable protein or through an increased amount of protein. TSGs, on the other hand, encode proteins that normally exert a negative regulatory control on the cell. When these genes are altered, the protein function is decreased or lost (a loss-of-function mutation or deletion), and the control on growth is lost. It now appears that loss of function of TSGs is more common than gain of oncogenic function in the development of most solid tumors.

Tumorigenic viruses provided some of the first clues to the identity of oncogenes and TSGs.[35,62] The cellular proto-oncogenes are believed to have been stably incorporated from viruses during the course of evolution. Therefore, many proto-oncogenes have been identified because they share a high percentage of their sequence (sequence homology) with retroviral genes that have transforming capability.[90] Other transforming viral proteins bind and inactivate normal cellular proteins. These cellular proteins are good TSG candidates.

For example, the large T antigen of simian virus 40 (SV40), the E1B adenoviral protein, and the E6 protein of human papillomavirus (HPV) each can form a complex with p53 protein.* T antigen, E1A adenoviral protein, and HPV E7 proteins bind to the p105 protein of the retinoblastoma (RB) gene.

Oncogenes have been identified by several other strategies besides the analysis of retroviral sequence homology. The detection of chromosomal structural changes by the evaluation of cytogenetic banding patterns has identified a variety of specific gene amplifications and rearrangements that are seen in many tumors. Growth-regulatory genes are considered to be candidate oncogenes when they are located near the breakpoint of translocations or inversions, or when they are present in increased copy number because of chromosomal amplification. The *c-myc* oncogene was first iden-

---

* Newly discovered proteins are designated by p, followed by their molecular weight in kilodaltons.

tified in this manner. It is found near a breakpoint on the long arm of chromosome 11 (11q13).* New, more sensitive measures for the detection of altered numbers of copies of chromosomal bands have recently been described. Comparative genomic hybridization and fluorescence *in situ* hybridization are useful tools to screen the genome for regions of tumor-specific amplifications or deletions.[83]

Transfection experiments have identified a number of other oncogenes. In such experiments, the genomic DNA of cancer cells is enzymatically cut, diluted, and placed into viral DNA (a transfection vector). The vector is then introduced into NIH-3T3 mouse fibroblasts, so that each cell gets one piece of DNA from a human cancer cell. Fibroblasts that develop a transformed phenotype are isolated, and the transforming human DNA is extracted and analyzed. NIH-3T3 cells are unique in their ability to be transformed by a single oncogene in this way. They probably contain some preexisting genetic alteration.

Oncogenes may be best classified according to their proteins' function and location in the cell. Those with sequence homology to known growth factors stimulate cell growth by constantly providing a growth-factor signal in an autocrine-positive feedback loop. *Int-2* is one such oncogene that is closely related to fibroblast growth factor.

Another group of oncogenes located in the cell membrane disrupts transduction of external signals involved in growth control by serving as rogue growth-factor receptors. Without requiring the actual presence of growth factors, they constantly stimulate cell growth through their intracellular tyrosine kinase activity, which mimics the normal growth-factor receptor. One example of this class is the oncogene *erbB/neu* that encodes a truncated protein resembling the epidermal growth–factor receptor (EGF-R).

A third group of oncogenes encodes protein kinases that are soluble proteins located in the cytoplasm and transported to the nucleus when activated. They transmit a growth-inducing signal from the membrane-bound receptors to the nucleus. An example of an oncogene that mimics this second-messenger function is *c-raf.*

The *ras* family is an example of the membrane-associated G-protein group of oncogenes. These proteins are constitutively active guanosine triphosphatases (GTPs) that maintain an activated GTP-bound state and serve as signal transducers for cell surface growth–factor receptors.

Within the nucleus of the cell, members of another group of oncoproteins serve as regulators of transcription. Mutations in the genes that encode these proteins allow for the unregulated transcription of other genes, causing the cell to constantly move through the cell cycle. An example of oncogenes that serve as transcription factors is the *myc* fam-

ily.[35] Oncogenes may cooperate with one another in tandem or parallel pathways to transform a cell.

Cell-fusion experiments gave early indication that the loss of a gene with cell-regulatory function might contribute to tumorigenesis. When normal cells were fused with cancer cells in these experiments, the hybrids could not cause tumors. When pieces of DNA were subsequently lost or removed from the hybrids in tissue culture, the cells regained their tumorigenic capability. Evaluation of the critical lost pieces of DNA provided some indication of the location of putative suppressor genes.[62]

Knudson's landmark analysis of familial (early-onset) cases of retinoblastoma provided an important clue leading to the discovery of the RB gene and other TSGs. He postulated that affected individuals with the familial form of RB inherit a normal allele from one parent and a mutant, nonfunctional allele from the other. When the normal allele is subsequently lost or mutated, leaving no functional gene, cancer develops. In the late-onset, spontaneous form of RB, both copies of the gene must be inactivated by mutation or deletion before the onset of disease. These multiple sequential events require more time, accounting for the later age of onset of illness in patients.[45]

An analysis of the sites of chromosomal deletions in RB patients led to the localization of the responsible gene at 13q14. A candidate gene encoding a large, 928–amino-acid nuclear phosphoprotein, p105, was identified.[62]

Knudson's idea to look for genes in areas where one copy of a DNA segment is lost in tumors has been applied as a general strategy for locating TSGs. The phenomenon of loss of a chromosomal segment in a tumor is called loss of heterozygosity (LOH). Evaluation of areas of LOH in a number of cancer types was used to identify the p53 gene on 17p. The smallest area of loss on 17p that was common to many cancers was identified. The p53 gene was known to reside within that region. The protein encoded by this gene is a 375–amino-acid phosphoprotein that resides in the nucleus. Sequence analysis of the remaining copy of p53 in human tumors that had LOH of 17p revealed single point mutations, strong evidence for the involvement of p53 in tumorigenesis.[62]

The role of p53 as a TSG was established by several observations. Some cancer cell lines and primary tumors contain deletions of both copies of p53 (homozygous deletions). This observation suggested the possibility that p53 may play a role in limiting cell growth, and that one copy of the normal gene may be sufficient p53 to exert its negative regulatory function. In this case, the loss of function of both copies would contribute to tumorigenesis. Further evidence that the contribution of p53 to cancer transformation occurs through loss-of-function comes from comparisons of oncogenic and nononcogenic HPV strains. The E6 protein of tumorigenic HPV strains (16 and 18) not only binds p53 protein but also degrades it, whereas nontumorigenic virus protein only forms stable complexes with p53.[72]

---

* The location of a genetic marker is given by the number of the chromosome, a p for the short arm or q for the long arm, and a number indicating the relative position of the corresponding cytogastric band on the arm.

More definitive evidence for the function of p53 as a tumor suppressor comes from transfection experiments in which a normal or wild type (WT) p53 gene was placed into tumor cell lines containing only a mutant gene. This approach resulted in a clear decrease in growth rate and colony-forming efficiency in a colorectal carcinoma line.[62]

Cell cycle control

In order for repair of DNA to occur before a cell divides, the cell cycle of a damaged cell must be temporarily halted. Transitions from the G1 to the S phase and from the G2 to the M phase are two critical control points in the cycle of a growing cell. At these points, DNA synthesis and mitosis begin, respectively. A group of proteins called cyclic AMP–dependent protein kinases (cdks) participates in the regulation of these transitions. These cdks form quaternary functional complexes with a cyclin protein, an inhibitory protein (p21), and the proliferating cell nuclear antigen (PCNA).[87]

The tumor suppressors p53, p16, and RB participate in the regulation of the cell cycle through interactions with the cyclin/cdk complex. Acting as a regulator of transcription, p53 protein binds to both DNA and other proteins. Among other things, it controls the expression of the cell cycle inhibitor, p21. When cells are damaged by a variety of mechanisms, normal p53 expression is increased in response to an unknown signal. Elevated p53 causes an increase in p21, which inhibits cyclin/cdk, and stops passage through the cell cycle, presumably to allow time for the cell to repair itself.[87] Similarly, p16 protein inhibits cyclin-dependent kinases 4 and 6, preventing phosphorylation of the Rb protein and causing a blockage of cell cycle progression from G1 to S phase.[54] Cells lacking functional p53 or p16 will continue to replicate DNA and divide despite damaged DNA. If the damage is not lethal but provides a growth advantage, the genetic alterations are perpetuated, and tumor progression with clonal expansion may result.

The suppressive function of RB is deactivated by phosphorylation mediated by the cdk/cyclin/PCNA/p21 complex. Active p105RB exists in a dephosphorylated form during G1 and G0. In order for a cell to enter S phase, p105RB must be phosphorylated through the action of a cdk. Phosphorylated RB participates in a further cascade of events by releasing a transcriptional factor, E2F-1, that facilitates DNA polymerase production. Mutant RB is not able to undergo phosphorylation, aborting the cyclin/cdk–induced cascade controlling the cell cycle.[51,62]

Cyclin D1 (PRAD-1) is also involved in cell cycle control. This protein binds with cdk4 and acts to phosphorylate RB. Overproduction of PRAD-1 through gene amplification may push a tumor cell through the G1 phase to the S transition, resulting in uncontrolled growth and perpetuation of other genetic alterations.

Genomic instability and the mutator phenotype

A mathematical model based on the age of onset of various types of cancer estimates that 8 to 11 mutations must accumulate for the development of HNSCC and four to seven mutations more accumulate for the induction of salivary gland neoplasms.[69] However, other mathematical estimations indicate a low probability that such an accumulation of transforming mutations will occur in a single cell. It has been suggested that the induction of a mutator phenotype, or genetic tendency for a cell to incur further DNA damage, is necessary to account for the development of cancer.[13]

Multiple genetic abnormalities have been detected in individual cancers, and the number of changes seems to increase with tumor stage. These abnormalities include cytogenetic findings such as the presence of an irregular number of chromosome copies (aneuploidy), amplifications of portions of chromosomes, chromosomal rearrangements, and chromosome loss.[13] Additionally, LOH for some chromosomal markers is seen in as many as 75% of all human cancers. For example, 17p loss often follows p53 mutation, eliminating the remaining normal allele. Errant recombination or deletion accounts for most cases of LOH after point mutation. The loss of controls on the cell cycle through the mutation of p53, RB, or other key regulatory genes may facilitate the perpetuation of many other genetic alterations.[32] Genes involved in the regulation of duplication, recombination, and distribution of chromosomes to progeny cells, as well as those involved in DNA repair, also are potential targets for mutations that lead to further genomic instability and cancer progression.

Epigenetic events

Whereas the central dogma of molecular biology states that permanent, heritable changes in cell phenotype require changes in the DNA sequence of genes, other mechanisms altering gene function may play a role. Alterations in the methylation of CpG sequences are a prime example. Such alterations have been seen at several chromosomal loci in lung and colon cancer specimens.[59] Increased methylation of CpG sites in or near a gene is a signal to normal cells to shut down transcription of the gene or chromosomal segment.[41] The normal methylation process plays a role in the inactivation of one X chromosome in every female cell, as well as in imprinting, or selecting one allele for expression during normal development. Abnormal methylation of 17p has been seen in brain, colon, and renal cancer cells, occurring either before or after p53 mutation. This increased methylation may contribute to eventual LOH of 17p.[59] In addition, methylation appears to be one mechanism in which p16 function is lost in HNSCC.[68] Some carcinogens are known to interfere with DNA methylation.[41] Since alterations in methylation can be passed on to daughter cells, these epimutational events can contribute substantially to cancer progression.[33] Another example of epigenetic control of cancer phenotype is the activity of retinoids. Retinoids are vitamin A analogues that modulate epithelial cell differentiation. They have been shown to reverse premalignant lesions, eliminate metaplasia in animal models of epithelial disease, suppress human oral premalignancy, and prevent the development of second primary cancers.[95] The mechanism of action of retinoic acid involves the regulation of expression of various genes mediated through retinoic acid receptors or RARs. A large number of genes are induced or suppressed by retinoids including collagenase, keratins, and growth factors such as transforming growth factor (TGF)-α and epithelial growth factor receptor.[28,30] The relative importance of these genes in the action of the retinoids is uncertain. Retinoic acid also has been shown to cause demethylation of DNA, accounting for altered expression of the collagen IV gene in an experimental cancer cell line.[9]

A variety of other factors may play an epigenetic role in cancer development by acting as tumor promoters. Tissues often respond to chronic irritation by hypertrophy and hyperplasia, which are mediated by underlying alterations in cell cycle control.[73] This acceleration of cell growth may result in an increased risk of mutation and thereby contribute to cancer progression. Oral hyperkeratosis in the setting of dental trauma, denture wear, lichen planus, and short-term exposure to smokeless tobacco are possible examples of this tumor-promoter phenomenon. The chronic irritations of poor dental hygiene and gastroesophageal reflux have also been implicated as contributors to cancer of the upper aerodigestive tract.

Metastatic phenotype

The ability of cancer cells to metastasize is not always proportional to the size or growth rate of the primary tumor. Invasion and metastasis must be mediated by proteins involved in tumor-cell binding and proteolysis of the extracellular matrix. Other proteins may induce extraordinary cell motility, as well as provide the ability to penetrate barriers of the target organ and establish new colonies. Only a few of the proteins that mediate the activities necessary for metastasis have been identified. For example, altered expression of the metalloproteinase collagenase IV, an enzyme that degrades a key component of basement membrane, has been shown to correlate with metastatic potential. A number of oncogenes, including *ras, c-erbB-2/neu,* and *nm 23* have been implicated in the metastatic process.[19,44,98] So far, however, the molecular mechanism of metastases and its genetic basis are poorly understood.

METHODS OF MOLECULAR BIOLOGY

The technologic revolution behind the explosion of information on the genetic basis of cancer involves a number of complex laboratory methods. Detailed information about these methods is beyond the scope of this chapter. The interested reader is encouraged to refer to several excellent texts.[16,90]

Enzymatic manipulation of DNA

The discovery of a group of proteins called restriction endonucleases has made a wide variety of molecular techniques possible. These enzymes cut DNA at specific sites comprised of four to eight bases. Enzymes that cut over 150 different target sequences are now available. Other proteins, called ligases, can rejoin cut strands of DNA. DNA polymerase produces complimentary strands by using a single-strand template in the presence of an abundance of free nucleotides and small oligonucleotide primers. These primers are manufactured chemically to match each end of the DNA segment of interest. The discovery of a heat-stable polymerase from *Thermus aquaticus* (Taq) bacteria was a key breakthrough that allowed the automation of many steps involved in the polymerase chain reaction (PCR). Reverse transcriptase is another important enzyme that makes complimentary DNA (cDNA) from a mRNA template so the active genes in a cell can be identified and studied.

Amplifying DNA

The methods of analyzing a tumor for the presence or absence of a particular gene and determining the precise mutated sequence require many identical copies of DNA. The techniques of PCR and cloning of DNA into bacteria have permitted scientists to produce the large numbers of copies needed. Fresh tumor sample and normal control tissue are the critical raw materials needed for the optimal analysis of genetic alterations in cancer. Standard histopathologic analysis is necessary to assess the purity of the tumor in the sample. Microdissection to remove necrotic tumor and surrounding normal tissue maximizes the percentage of tumors cells in the sample before DNA is extracted. This is an important step if clear, reliable data are to be generated.

The polymerase chain reaction

The PCR produces an exponentially increasing number of copies of a piece of DNA (Fig. 17-2). In PCR, a small amount of double-stranded DNA template is separated at high temperatures into single strands. Oligonucleotide primers that match sequences at either end of the DNA segment to be studied, along with Taq polymerase and an excess of free nucleotides, are added. The temperature is then lowered to allow the primers to anneal to the template. Synthesis of new strands begins at the double-stranded (primed) regions along both the sense and antisense strands of the template. After 5 minutes, the reaction mixture is heated again, the strands are separated, and synthesis is stopped. This first cycle produces new strands of DNA that also serve as templates for the next cycle. Heating and cooling steps are repeated, and each time the number of copies of DNA is doubled. The predominant DNA species in the reaction quickly becomes the specific piece of interest that is flanked by the selected primers. Thirty cycles will produce 10^9 copies of DNA. With automation, this yield can now be achieved in a few hours.

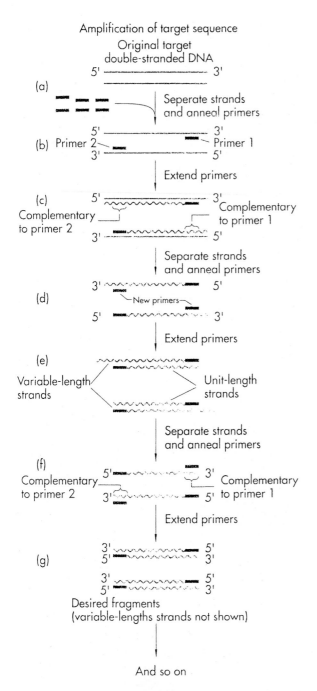

Amplification of target sequence
Original target
double-stranded DNA

(a)

Seperate strands
and anneal primers

(b) Primer 2   Primer 1

Extend primers

(c)   Complementary
Complementary   to primer 1
to primer 2

Separate strands
and anneal primers

(d)
New primers

Extend primers

(e)
Variable-length   Unit-length
strands   strands

Separate strands
and anneal primers

(f)
Complementary   Complementary
to primer 2   to primer 1

Extend primers

(g)

Desired fragments
(variable-lengths strands not shown)

And so on

Fig. 17-2. Schematic diagram of the polymerase chain reaction. *a,* Double-stranded DNA is extracted from a tumor sample and separated by heating. *b,* Primers (small, complementary DNA segments that flank the area of interest) are added as the reaction cools, allowing one primer to bind to each strand of the sample. *c,* Taq polymerase synthesizes new DNA strands complimentary to the original template. In the first cycle of the reaction, the newly synthesized fragments are variable in length. The reaction is continued long enough to overshoot the target segment of DNA. *d* through *g,* DNA produced in the second cycle is delimited by the position of the primers. This quickly becomes the predominant species, increasing in number exponentially with each cycle. (From Watson and others: *Recombinant DNA,* ed 2, New York, 1992, WH Freeman.)

The quality of the PCR product is directly dependent on the template and primers selected. It is critical to avoid contamination by outside DNA. Since the reaction has no proofreading capability, a misincorporation occurs in 1 of every 20,000 bases. Any impurity or misincorporation is perpetuated and expanded in subsequent cycles of the reaction. When the tumor sample is very small, necessitating many PCR cycles, or when it contains many contaminating cells, the PCR product may not have a single predominant DNA fragment. In this circumstance, analysis of the product will not produce clear results.

Cloning

Cloning involves the introduction of a piece of human DNA into a bacteria as a small circular piece called a plasmid. The human DNA is then replicated with the bacterial genome as the bacteria multiply in culture. This process produces many identical copies, which are then extracted and analyzed. Recent innovations in PCR technology have eliminated the need for further amplification by cloning for many applications.

Detection of genetic alterations in cancer

Southern and northern blotting

Blotting involves the detection of specific fragments of DNA or RNA that have been electrophoretically separated on an agarose gel. The separated DNA or RNA is transferred to a porous membrane. A radiolabeled probe with a sequence that is complementary to the gene of interest is added and allowed to hybridize with bands containing the target sequence. These bands are then visualized by autoradiography. Analysis of DNA in this way is called Southern blotting. Northern blotting involves detection of mRNA extracted from cells. The presence of mRNA indicates that the gene is being actively transcribed.

Blotting may be used to detect the presence or absence of a particular gene. Tumor and normal DNA must be analyzed simultaneously to demonstrate that any alteration is unique to the tumor. Blotting also can be used to detect subtle changes in a particular gene if it displays the phenomenon of restriction fragment length polymorphism (RFLP). When two copies of a gene in an individual's cells differ slightly in sequence because of an inherited polymorphism or mutation, specific restriction enzymes may cleave these alleles into fragments of slightly different sizes. Gel electrophoresis will separate these fragments and probing with an oligonucleotide that recognizes a sequence common to both alleles will label the two distinct bands. Tumors that have undergone a loss of one allele will show the complete absence of one of the bands in the tumor sample (Fig. 17-3).

Blotting can be used to detect the tumor-specific loss of pieces of DNA even when no specific target gene is available by using microsatellite alterations as chromosomal markers. Microsatellites are regions between or within genes consist-

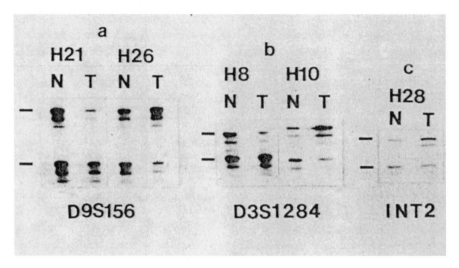

Fig. 17-3. Loss of heterozygosity displayed by autoradiography of gels containing polymerase chain reaction amplified deoxyribonucleic acid (DNA) and probed with microsatellite markers. Normal *(N)* and tumor *(T)* DNA from five representative patients are shown. The microsatellite markers D9S156, D3S1284, and INT 2 reveal loss on 9p, 3p, and either loss or amplification of 11q, respectively. (From Nawroz and others: *Cancer Res* 54:1152, 1994.)

ing of multiple repeated sequences of two or more bases. These sequences are highly polymorphic, meaning that the maternal and paternal chromosomes usually have a different number of repeated patterns. For this reason, amplified samples of DNA that include the microsatellite area will produce two bands with gel electrophoresis. Tumors may have a loss of one allele resulting in only a single band, or may have an altered number of repeats in one allele, resulting in an unique, shifted band. Both patterns are easily recognizable as different from the normal DNA sample.[60] Microsatellite analysis is commonly used to screen the genome for areas of DNA loss indicative of the location of a TSG candidate.

Gene sequencing

The most rigorous, definitive way to detect a genetic alteration is to determine the exact sequence of the gene. Several methods for DNA sequencing have been developed. Each involves reducing the gene to four collections of differently sized, radiolabeled fragments ending with each of the four nucleotide bases. The sizes of the fragments in each mixture are dictated by the relative position of one of the bases (A,C,G,T) in the gene sequence. The fragments are then separated and detected on long polyacrylamide gels, with normal and tumor DNA arranged side by side. Comparing the bands produced from normal and tumor DNA shows a different pattern if one base has been replaced by another in the mutant gene (Fig. 17-4).

Screening for mutations

Strategies to screen for base-pair substitutions in genes have been developed as an alternative to the laborious task of direct sequencing. Single-strand conformation polymor-

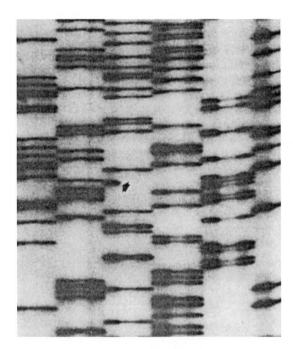

Fig. 17-4. Point mutation in p53 gene identified by direct-sequencing. A unique band in tumor deoxyribonucleic acid (DNA) *(arrow)* that is not in normal DNA is present, but a corresponding normal band is absent in the tumor sample.

phism (SSCP) analysis uses the fact that the electrophoretic mobility of a single-stranded fragment depends on its nucleotide sequence as well as it size.[16] Changes in the three-dimensional folding of the DNA that affect mobility in a gel may occur with a single base substitution. Single strands of radiolabeled DNA, including the gene or exons of interest, are produced by PCR and then run on gels. If the substitution changes the folding of the fragment sufficiently, the mutation may produce a shift in its mobility compared with control DNA.

SSCP is not as rigorous as direct sequencing in detecting mutations. Some mutations will be missed by SSCP because they fail to produce a conformational change. Furthermore, the sensitivity of the method decreases dramatically with large fragments (more than 300 nucleotides) because a single base change is less likely to alter their mobility. False-positive results occur when a fragment of DNA can exist in several stable conformational forms or when a gene is present in several normal polymorphic forms. Both of these situations may result in multiple or shifted bands without the presence of a mutation.

GENETIC ALTERATIONS IN HEAD AND NECK SQUAMOUS CELL CARCINOMA

Little is known about the identity of the multiple mutations thought to be necessary for the development of HNSCC. The available information is rapidly expanding, however, as putative oncogenes and suppressor genes are identified.

Oncogenes

Conflicting results have been reported about the importance of the *ras* family of oncogenes in this disease. Most investigators have found the mutation rate and incidence of increased expression of N-*ras*, H-*ras*, and K-*ras* in HNSCC to be quite low (|Ld10%).[15,37,74,75] However, in one report, mutations in H-*ras* codons 12 and 61 were found in 20 of 57 primary tumors in people from India with extensive smokeless tobacco exposure.[71]

Amplification of the chromosomal segment 11q13 has been reported in up to 50% of HNSCC tumors.[49,78] The PRAD-1 (cyclin D1) oncogene resides on this segment and has been shown to be amplified in 34% of primary HNSCC.[12]

Epigenetic changes in *c-myc* expression may contribute to the development of a small percentage of HNSCC.[23,26,37,79] Several small studies have reached contradictory conclusions about the clinical significance of altered *myc* expression. Amplification and increased expression of *c-erb* has also been reported in HNSCC; however, no mutations of *myc* or *erb* in HNSCC have been described.[37] Therefore, it would appear that known oncogenes other than H-*ras* and PRAD-1 play only a minor role in HNSCC.

Tumor suppressor genes

p53

By far, the most thoroughly studied genetic alteration in HNSCC is p53 mutation. Direct sequencing of primary tumor DNA is the most definitive method to assess the inci-

dence of this mutation. An overall incidence of 42% was reported in a series of 65 invasive tumors from the United States studied by direct sequencing of exons 5 through 8.[6] This incidence remained unchanged when the series was expanded to include 144 patients,[7] and it has been corroborated in independent studies using SSCP.[14,51] However, the incidence may vary in other populations. For example, only 3 of 30 oral squamous cell carcinoma (SCC) samples from betel nut chewers from Papau New Guinea had p53 mutations.[82]

Immunohistochemical staining for p53 protein overexpression is commonly employed as a means of estimating genetic alteration. WT p53 protein has a very brief half-life; therefore, normal cells generally do not stain with p53 antibody. Many, but not all, p53 alterations result in the production of protein with an unusually long half-life that can be detected by staining. However, false-positive and false-negative results are seen.[94] Tumors with deletions, splice-site mutations, or mutations that produce stop signals have absent or truncated p53 protein and do not stain. Furthermore, positive staining may not be indicative of mutation in all cases. This is apparent from the relatively high percentage of tumors that stain for p53 (> 70% in some studies), compared with the percentage of mutations seen in series that have employed PCR-based sequencing techniques. False-positive staining may be caused by the stabilization of normal p53 protein when it is bound to other cellular proteins such as heat-shock protein, HPV E6, or mdm2. In fact, a study of a large number of breast carcinoma samples analyzed by direct sequencing and immunohistochemistry demonstrated a 33% false-negative and 30% false-positive rate for immunohistochemistry detection of mutation.[77] Positive staining of cells lacking p53 mutation may still indicate an absence of p53 protein function since binding of p53 by HPV E6 may inactivate the tumor suppressor function. The presence or absence of p53 mutation in HNSCC has so far not been found to correspond to clinical parameters such as tumor site, stage, or grade. However, several investigators have found a higher incidence of p53 mutation in the tumors of smokers and drinkers than in the tumors of patients who developed HNSCC without exposure to these agents.[6,7,24] The incidence of p53 mutation also appears to be lower in patients who develop HNSCC at an older age.[48]

Direct sequencing provides a profile of specific types and locations of mutations seen in this disease. The spectrum of mutation types found in the p53 gene among smokers and drinkers is much broader that it is among nonsmokers and nondrinkers. In the latter group, most p53 mutations occur at sites typical of endogenous or spontaneous mutation. Smokers and drinkers have a spectrum of mutation that is more suggestive of exogenous mutagenesis caused by polycyclic hydrocarbons.[7] It appears that malignant transformation by an endogenous spontaneous pathway often takes longer and involves p53 less frequently than does the induction of HNSCC by known carcinogens.

Loss of heterozygosity as evidence of other putative tumor suppressor genes

According to Knudson's hypothesis, when a tumor displays LOH of a particular chromosomal segment, that segment may contain a TSG that has been inactivated in neoplastic transformation. By using markers known to be located on each chromosomal arm to screen a large number of tumors for sites of LOH, a profile of segments commonly lost in that tumor type can be derived. Such a profile, called an allelotype, has been published for HNSCC by several groups[1,65] with similar results (Fig. 17-5).

Ah-See and others[1] and Nawroz and others[65] report a high incidence of partial loss of chromosome 17p where p53 resides. However, 17p LOH does not coincide with p53 mutation in many cases, suggesting that another suppressor gene may be nearby. One candidate gene on 17p, HIC-1, has recently been identified.[89] LOH or amplification of 11q where PRAD-1 is located also was found by both groups. Chromosome 3p displays LOH in a large number of HNSCC samples, as well as in lung cancers.[1,20,50,65] Three distinct regions of LOH on 3p have been described in a population of HNSCC, suggesting the presence of three separate suppressor genes.[58,70] LOH on 6p is seen in HNSCC and in colon and ovarian carcinomas. Prostate, bladder, and hepatocellular carcinomas, along with HNSCC, have 8p LOH. LOH of chromosomes 4 and 14q are not commonly seen in other cancers. Putative TSGs on all of these chromosomal segments have yet to be identified.

The known TSG RB resides on 13q, a chromosomal arm that displays a high rate of LOH in HNSCC (56%).[65] Since the RB gene is located in the area of common loss, alterations in the RB gene were analyzed in 31 tumors showing 13q LOH.[97] When the RB gene is mutated, its protein production is completely shut off. Absence of p105RB staining was seen in only 20% of the 31 tumors. Therefore, another as yet unidentified TSG may reside near the RB locus on 13q. An excellent candidate is the BRCA2 gene that has been linked to breast carcinoma in a large number of high-risk breast cancer families.[93] This gene is located at 13q12-13. Intriguingly, families with multiple cases of breast carcinoma associated with BRCA2 mutation also have an increased rate of laryngeal cancer deaths.[67]

p16

Chromosome 9p LOH is a common genetic event in a variety of human cancers, including HNSCC.[65,86] In fact, 9p loss is the most common genetic alteration in HNSCC, occurring in nearly 80% of cases.[65] Recently, investigators have identified a putative TSG, p16, in an area of homozygous deletion found in several melanoma cell lines. The protein encoded by p16 inhibits the activity of cdk-4, a member of the cyclin complex that is involved in p53–mediated cell cycle regulation.[31,43]

It is not certain at this time whether p16 is the relevant TSG for HNSCC on 9p. Sequence analysis of the p16 gene in 75 primary tumors (including nine HNSCCs) revealed only two mutations overall, one of which was in a HNSCC sample.[10] Other researchers found homozygous deletions of p16 in 6 of 16 HNSCC cell lines, but in only 2 of 36 fresh tumors.[57] More extensive analysis of the status of p16 in

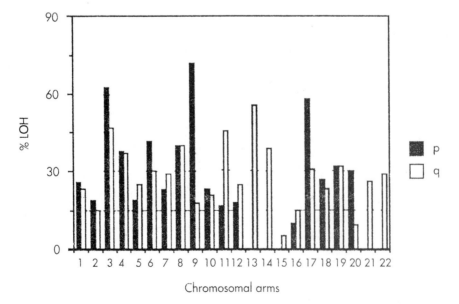

Fig. 17-5. Allelogram indicating the frequency of allelic loss for markers on each chromosomal arm in head and neck squamous cell carcinoma (HNSCC) tumors. Data shown for each chromosomal arm is for the marker with the greatest loss of heterozygosity (LOH). ''Background'' LOH of 25% to 30% is typical of HNSCC. (From Nawroz and others: *Cancer Res* 54:1152, 1994.)

HNSCC has recently been reported. Using immunohistochemistry to stain for the presence of p16 protein, 24 of 30 fresh HNSCC tumors displayed loss of function of this gene. Loss of protein was found to be due to three different mechanisms. Two thirds (16 of 24) of the samples had homozygous deletions of the p16 gene. Five others (21%) had methylated p16 genes indicating an epigenetic mechanism of inactivation. One of the other three samples that did not stain for protein was found to have a somatic mutation of the p16 gene, while the other two had 9p LOH without definitive evidence for the cause of loss of function of the second allele.[68] This study provides strong evidence that p16 is, indeed, the target gene on chromosome 9p. If confirmed in larger populations, p16 would replace p53 as the most frequently altered known specific gene in HNSCC.

As new TSGs are discovered, it will be possible to develop a more complete picture of tumor progression for HNSCC. More specific understanding about tumorigenesis in this disease will enhance the prospects for clinical applications.

Temporal order of mutations in head and neck squamous cell carcinoma: tumor progression model

It is of considerable interest to determine whether specific genetic events occur early or late in the course of HNSCC malignant transformation. This information would impact the potential usefulness of these alterations as clinical markers. For example, genetic alterations that occur early in transformation would be ideal markers for the efficacy of chemopreventive therapy, while late events would be more likely to provide prognostic information. One strategy for temporal ordering of genetic events is to compare the frequency with which they are encountered at various stages of clinical tumor progression. If a particular target is rarely altered in premalignant lesions, it would be placed later than those alterations commonly seen in early disease states. For example, in isolated premalignant lesions such as dysplasia and

carcinoma *in situ*, a significantly lower incidence of p53 mutation (19%) has been demonstrated than has been seen in invasive cancer.[6] This indicates that although p53 mutation can occur before the development of invasive capability, its incidence increases with clinical tumor progression. This suggests that p53 mutation is an intermediate event in HNSCC progression.

An equal frequency of 9p loss (71%) has been demonstrated in 29 invasive HNSCC and 17 preneoplastic lesions. This finding suggests that 9p LOH occurs very early in HNSCC tumor progression.[86] A more comprehensive analysis of allelic loss at 10 major chromosomal loci has further defined the molecular progression model for HNSCC.[11] There was a clear accumulation of allelic losses seen with histopathologic progression, with an increase in the mean number of losses from benign hyperplasia to dysplasia to carcinoma *in situ*, and finally to invasive cancer. Besides 9p21, 3p21 was found to have LOH in many early lesions. The frequency of loss of these loci plateaued in carcinoma *in situ*, and was no more common in invasive disease. Roz and others provide additional evidence for the early loss of 3p markers in oral dysplastic lesions.[70] In Califano's study,[11] losses at 8p and 4q were found only in a few *in situ* lesions and were significantly more common in invasive cancer, making them likely late events. LOH of 17p, 11q, 13q, 14q, 6p, and 8q were judged to be intermediate events. Figure 17-6 represents a model for tumor progression of HNSCC based on these studies. It is not possible to know the exact order of genetic events in any individual cancer. Indeed, the order of events probably varies from individual to individual, as has been demonstrated in colon cancer.[22]

Field cancerization: molecular clues

Slaughter proposed the concept of field cancerization to explain the observed high rate of second primary cancers seen in the upper aerodigestive tract of patients with HNSCC.[76] All mucosa exposed to carcinogens is at risk for

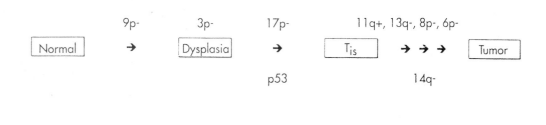

Fig. 17-6. Preliminary tumor progression model incorporating stages of clinical progression with molecular alterations. The exact sequence of events is likely to vary somewhat among tumors of similar clinical appearance. A great deal of detail remains to be discovered.

second primary cancers in this population. However, different molecular explanations can account for the phenomenon. The field cancerization concept postulates that multiple, independent transforming events take place in separate progenitor cells in the aerodigestive tract of an individual. Alternatively, a single initial event may produce a partially transformed clonal population that then separates and migrates to separate positions within the mucosa. Later, additional, unshared events may accumulate as the lesions progress toward invasive cancers.

An intriguing study focused on a group of 31 patients with multiple primary cancers of the aerodigestive tract. These patients were analyzed for p53 mutation in each of their tumors. Alterations were found in at least one tumor in 21 of these patients. In every individual, the p53 status of the tumors was discordant, with either distinctly different mutations in each tumor or the presence of mutation in only one tumor.[14] However, p53 alterations are intermediate to late events according to the tumor progression model discussed previously. To differentiate between the two explanations for multiple primary cancers, early genetic events that are more likely to be shared by both tumors must be considered.

Bedi and others have attempted to answer the field cancerization question by examining tumors from eight women with multiple HNSCC primaries.[4] They studied patterns of X chromosome inactivation, microsatellite alterations, and specific breakpoints for LOH on chromosomal arms 3p and 9p, early targets in HNSCC tumorigenesis. (X chromosome inactivation occurs randomly as a result of methylation during embryogenesis in females. The inactivation is passed on to daughter cells resulting in a mosaic pattern throughout the body. Therefore, independent tumors have a 50% chance of sharing the same X inactivation pattern.) The investigators were able to demonstrate identical alterations of early markers in both tumors in five of eight patients. This implies that, in at least some patients, multiple primaries may arise from a common progenitor clonal population. Another approach to the field cancerization problem is to look at regions of premalignant change around an invasive tumor, searching for differences and similarities in the genetic alterations of histologically distinct regions. If patterns of tumor initiation and progression are different within a tumor, this would argue for widespread independent neoplastic change rather than clonal expansion and migration. Two groups have demonstrated that peripheral preneoplastic regions share some patterns of LOH with the invasive tumor, but lack other areas of loss seen in the advanced disease. These results support the model of progressive accumulation of alterations within a clonal population and the overgrowth of the successively more altered subclones.[11,24]

Human papillomavirus in head and neck squamous cell carcinoma

The E6 protein of HPV types 16 and 18 binds and degrades the p53 protein, and the E7 protein forms a tight complex with the RB protein. HPV 16 and 18 DNA has been detected in HNSCC samples with a variable incidence (10% to 54%).[2,66,84,91] Interestingly, the highest frequency of HPV was seen in a population of betel quid chewers.[3] Another study demonstrated a higher frequency of HPV DNA in younger (<60 years of age) HNSCC patients.[17] These studies do not determine whether the viral DNA is integrated into the host genome. HPV DNA also has been found in normal mucosa from some cancer patients, raising the possibility that its presence indicates infection rather than a neoplastic transformational role.

CLINICAL APPLICATIONS

Although the molecular analysis of cancer is still in its infancy, it is compelling to begin searching for clinical applications to the diagnosis, prognosis, and treatment of disease.

Molecular screening

When a substitution mutation has been identified in a tumor sample, oligonucleotide probes can be used to detect the presence of single cells containing the mutated sequence among a background of normal cells.[8,46] To do this, an oligonucleotide (18 to 20 bases) radiolabeled fragment matching the mutated sequence is manufactured. DNA from clinical samples such as saliva, lymph nodes, and tumor-free surgical margins is extracted. The exon containing the tumor-specific mutation is amplified by PCR and placed into the DNA of a bacteriophage. Diluting the DNA ensures that each virus gets only one copy of the human exon, either mutant or normal, in proportion to the number of cells containing the mutation in the original sample. The phage are then diluted and plated onto a lawn of bacteria producing clear plaques, each caused by one original phage with one unique copy of the gene in question. The DNA is transferred from the culture plate to a nitrocellulose filter and allowed to hybridize with the labeled probe. The number of plaques containing mutant copies is detected autoradiographically (Fig. 17-7). One tumor cell amidst more than 5000 normal cells can be detected in this way.

Oligonucleotide probing has been used to screen histologically clean tumor margins and lymph nodes for cancer cells that are not visible by light microscopy. In a small pilot series, the potential clinical efficacy of this approach was clearly demonstrated. Twenty-five patients with HNSCC that contained p53 mutations, who had undergone surgical resection with clean histopathologic margins, were studied. Specific oligonucleotide probes designed for each tumor identified clonal cancer cells in margin tissue taken from 13 patients. These samples were taken from the patient beyond the final rim of resection that had been judged by frozen section to be free of disease.

In five patients the positive molecular data accurately heralded tumor recurrence, despite postoperative radiotherapy in four of the patients. The location of the molecularly positive tissue in each patient was predictive of the location of recurrence. None of the patients without molecular evi-

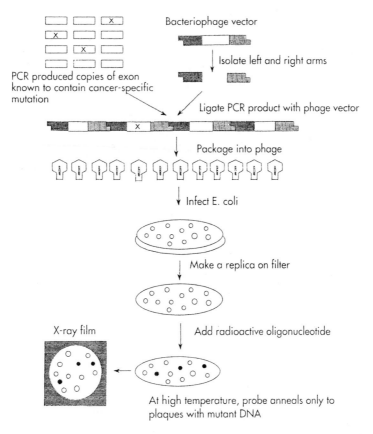

Fig. 17-7. The presence of mutated p53 deoxyribonucleic acid in rare cells from tumor-free resection margins demonstrated by oligonucleotide probing of phage plaques. (Modified from Watson JD and others: *Recombinant DNA*, ed 2, New York, 1992, WH Freeman.)

dence of cancer cells in the margins had recurrence. The clinical relevance of molecular margin analysis has yet to be confirmed in a large study.

Oligonucleotide probing has also been used to detect cancer cells that are exfoliated from mucosal surfaces and collected when the mouth is rinsed with saline or swabbed with a gloved finger or tongue blade. Cancer cells were detected by this method in 71% of saliva samples collected before treatment from cancer patients whose tumors had known p53 mutations.[5] Since the exact mutation in the p53 gene must be identified for this molecular screening method, it cannot be used to screen for occult malignancy in an at-risk population. However, the technique is immediately applicable for the surveillance of cancer recurrence after the completion of therapy. Oligonucleotide hybridization can also be used to link a metastatic or recurrent lesion with a primary tumor containing a known point mutation. Its use is limited because less than half of all HNSCCs contain p53 alterations, and some mutations are not amenable to oligonucleotide probing. Additional specific target genes must be identified so that the molecular probing methods can be extended to more patients.

Screening for cancer cells in a clinical sample may be possible even when a specific mutation in a target gene is not known by targeting tumor-specific alterations in microsatellite repeat sequences.[60] The location of a number of microsatellite markers has been described, and primers are available for their PCR amplification. If a clinical sample contains an altered number of repeats in comparison with normal tissue, a band will appear in a unique position on the gel. The presence of such a tumor-specific band in DNA isolated from a clinical sample such as saliva indicates the presence of clonal cancer cells. The intensity of this band in the test sample is proportional to the relative number of cancer cells present. As few as one tumor cell in a background of 200 normal cells can be detected using this approach.

Using a panel of nine microsatellite probes, 29% of a group of HNSCCs were detected from cells harvested by an oral rinse or swab prior to surgery. With a larger panel of probes, a larger segment of the HNSCC population could be detected using microsatellite repeat markers.[60]

Prognostication and treatment planning

Many investigators have tried to derive prognostic significance from molecular data obtained from small series of patients. HNSCC is a complex disease with a wide spectrum of clinical behavior. The molecular alterations are similarly complex. Seven or more genetic alterations are predicted to contribute to each HNSCC. Tumors can be categorized by many clinical criteria, including stage, site, metastatic activity, histologic grade, and exposure to risk factors. Therefore, the expectation that the analysis of one genetic factor in a small series of patients will produce clinically significant prognostic data seems optimistic and naive.

Many reports have been published regarding the prognostic implication of p53 gene expression with highly variable results. An analysis of 110 HNSCC patients has demonstrated an association between p53 mutation as demonstrated by gene sequencing and shortened locoregional disease-free survival. The risk of locoregional recurrence was 2.4 times greater for the p53-mutated group. This difference remained significant when controlled for site and stage in multivariant analysis. However, the presence of a p53 mutation did not correspond to a shorter overall survival.[47] This result is consistent with the role of p53 in apoptosis. All patients in the series received radiotherapy that produces tumor cell death by apoptosis. Tumors that lack functional p53 may not undergo apoptosis and therefore may survive radiation leading to tumor persistence or recurrence. Amplification of 11q13 has also been shown to be associated with an increased risk of recurrent disease and decreased survival in a group of 56 HNSCC patients.[63] Several investigators have shown that tumors with multiple areas of LOH have a poorer prognosis, an observation consistent with the tumor progression concept.[53,56] As a more complete spectrum of genetic alterations is analyzed in large, carefully constructed cohorts of HNSCC patients, more precise information predictive of treatment response and patient survival should become available.

Gene therapy

A number of interesting experimental studies have illustrated the feasibility of new strategies to treat cancer by introducing genetic material into cancer cells. This application of molecular information is considered in Chapter 16.

GENETIC ALTERATIONS IN OTHER HEAD AND NECK NEOPLASMS

Salivary gland neoplasms

Little information is available about the molecular basis of salivary gland neoplasms. Preliminary allelograms for pleomorphic adenoma, adenoid cystic carcinoma, and mucoepidermoid carcinoma have been published.[40] These allelograms are based on a small number of tumor samples. Like allelograms for HNSCC, they represent a screening of chromosomal arms for areas of LOH. As expected on the basis of its benign nature, the frequency of LOH in pleomorphic adenoma is low. 12q loss was seen in 35% of 11 cases. Cytogenetic studies have also shown 12q alterations in pleomorphic adenoma.[61] Less than a quarter of the specimens had losses at 5p, 7q, 11q, and 19q markers.[40] In a similar

study, 18 pleomorphic adenoma samples were analyzed using microsatellite markers located on chromosomes 3p, 6q, 8p, and 8q. LOH was seen most commonly on 8q (27%), with 13% and 15% LOH on 6q and 8p, respectively.[27]

Ten adenoid cystic carcinomas have also been studied for allelic loss. Again, LOH was uncommon with the highest frequency of loss seen on 19q (40%). LOH on 1p, 2p, 17p, and 20p was also seen. Only five mucoepidermoid carcinoma specimens were analyzed in Johns' study.[40] Four of these samples were high grade, and LOH was correspondingly more varied and frequent than seen in pleomorphic adenoma. Three tumors had LOH on 5p and 16q, while two tumors had losses on 2q, 5q, 11q, and 12p. This preliminary study demonstrates that LOH in salivary gland neoplasms includes some loci unique to these tumors. Furthermore, the pattern of genetic alterations mirrors the clinical virulence of disease.[40]

A few small studies have used immunohistochemical staining and blotting techniques to indicate a low percentage of *neu*, *ras*, and *myc* alterations in salivary gland neoplasms.[18,38,42] In one study, *ras*, p21, and p53 staining were found in a significantly higher number of carcinoma *ex pleomorphica* cases than in pleomorphic adenoma samples.[18]

Thyroid neoplasms

Several small series of thyroid tumors have been screened for p53 mutation using PCR-based techniques.[39,96] The incidence of p53 alterations is quite low in papillary, follicular, and medullary thyroid carcinoma, but is higher in anaplastic carcinoma. Activated *ras* mutations have been found in both benign and malignant thyroid neoplasms, with the incidence inversely related to the degree of differentiation.[52]

Studies of families with the multiple endocrine neoplasia (MEN) syndrome type IIA have revealed alterations in the proto-oncogene RET in some cases of medullary thyroid carcinoma (MTC).[64] In most instances, the mutation was also present in normal tissue of the individuals but was not found in unaffected family members. This finding suggests that it was an inherited germline mutation. Tumors from MEN type IIB families and tumors in individuals with spontaneous MTC do not often contain RET alterations, but mutations do occur in familial cases of MTC that are not associated with MEN.[64]

Nerve sheath neoplasms

Studies of individuals in families with neurofibromatosis type 2 have revealed a putative TSG called NF2 located at chromosome 22q12.[45,62] The NF2 gene encodes a protein similar to meosin that links cytoskeletal components with cell membrane proteins. Point mutations of NF2 have also been found in a minority of sporadic meningiomas and schwannomas. Linkage analysis of NF1 families has attributed this disease to alterations on chromosome 17.

Basal cell carcinoma

Individuals with Gorlin's syndrome, an autosomal dominant disorder predisposing to basal cell carcinoma (BCC), ovarian fibroma, and medulloblastoma were analyzed, and a common area of LOH was identified on 9q.[25] LOH at 9q31 was also seen in 69% of sporadic BCC tumors. The putative TSG at 9q31 has yet to be identified. A high incidence of p53 mutation (44%) was also found in BCC. In general, p53 mutation is associated with more aggressive tumor types, and the high frequency of mutation in BCC was unexpected. Interestingly, only 1 of 36 BCC samples showed LOH of 17p, and in all cases with p53 mutation, only one allele was altered.[86]

FUTURE HORIZONS

The next decade will bring a great deal of specific information about a host of new cancer-related target genes. The numerous areas of LOH seen in HNSCC allelograms may each contain one or more TSGs. Careful analysis of large groups of tumors will be necessary to establish the relative importance of each new candidate gene. It will also be necessary to compare the incidence of each genetic alteration in premalignant, early, and advanced or metastatic tumors to learn which events correspond to initiation of tumorigenesis and which are required for progression and spread.

Accurate prognostic information should become available through molecular analysis. In order to achieve this, a profile of all known genetic alterations must be compiled from a large group of patients. After adequate follow-up, careful evaluation may reveal molecular events that predict response to various therapeutic modalities and overall outcome.

Gene therapy may eventually play a significant role in the treatment of disease. Molecular screening methods should soon permit early diagnosis and enhanced evaluation of the adequacy of treatment. Although a great deal of work lies ahead, there has never been a more profound revolution in the fundamental understanding and approach to malignancy of the upper aerodigestive tract.

REFERENCES

1. Ah-See KW and others: An allelotype of squamous carcinoma of the head and neck using microsatellite markers, *Cancer Res* 54:1617, 1994.
2. Anwar K and others: ras gene mutations and HPV infection are common in human laryngeal carcinoma, *Int J Cancer* 53:22, 1993.
3. Balaram P and others: Human papillomavirus in 91 oral cancers from Indian betel quid chewers—high prevalence and multiplicity of infections, *Int J Cancer* 61:450, 1995.
4. Bedi GC and others: Multiple head and neck tumors: evidence for a common clonal origin, *Cancer Res* 56:2484, 1996.
5. Boyle JO and others: Gene mutations in saliva as molecular markers for head and neck squamous cell carcinomas, *Am J Surg* 168:429, 1994.
6. Boyle JO and others: The incidence of p53 mutations increases with progression of head and neck cancer, *Cancer Res* 53:4477, 1993.
7. Brennan JA and others: Association between cigarette smoking and mutation of the p53 gene in head and neck squamous carcinoma, *N Engl J Med* 332:712, 1995.
8. Brennan JA and others: Molecular assessment of histopathologic staging, *N Engl J Med* 332:429, 1995.
9. Burbelo PD, Horikoshi S, Yamada Y: DNA methylation and collagen IV gene expression in F9 teratocarcinoma cells, *J Biol Chem* 265:4839, 1990.
10. Cairns P and others: Rates of p16 (MTS 1) mutations in primary tumors with 9p loss, *Science* 265:415, 1994.
11. Califano J and others: A genetic progression model for head and neck cancer: implications for field cancerization, *Cancer Res* 56:2488, 1996.
12. Callender T and others: PRAD-1 (CCND1)/Cyclin D1 oncogene amplification in primary head and neck squamous cell carcinoma, *Cancer* 74:152, 1994.
13. Cheng KC, Loeb LA: Genomic instability and tumor progression: mechanistic considerations, *Adv Cancer Res* 60:121, 1993.
14. Chung KY and others: Discordant p53 gene mutations in primary head and neck cancers and corresponding second primary cancers of the upper aerodigestive tract, *Cancer Res* 53:1676, 1993.
15. Clark LJ and others: The absence of Harvey ras mutations during the development and progression of squamous cell carcinomas of the head and neck, *Br J Cancer* 68:617, 1993.
16. Cooper DN, Krawczak M: *Human gene mutation*, Oxford, Great Britain, 1993, BIOS Scientific.
17. Cruz IBF and others: Age-dependence of human papillomavirus DNA presence in oral squamous cell carcinomas, *Oral Oncol Eur J Cancer* 32B:55, 1996.
18. Deguchi H, Hamano H, Hayashi Y: c-myc, ras p21 and p53 expression in pleomorphic adenomas and its malignant form of the human salivary glands, *Acta Pathol Jpn* 43:413, 1993.
19. Egan SE and others: Transformation by oncogenes encoding protein kinases induces the metastatic phenotype, *Science* 238:202, 1987.
20. El-Nagger AK and others: Polymerase chain reaction-based restriction fragment length polymorphism analysis of the short arm of chromosome 3 in primary head and neck squamous carcinoma, *Cancer* 72:881, 1993.
21. El-Naggar AK and others: Sequential loss of heterozygosity at microsatellite motifs in preinvasive and invasive head and neck squamous carcinomas, *Cancer Res* 55:2656, 1995.
22. Fearon ER, Vogelstein B: A genetic model for colorectal tumorigenesis, *Cell* 61:759, 1990.
23. Field JK and others: Elevated expression of the c-myc oncoprotein correlates with poor prognosis in head neck squamous cell carcinoma, *Oncogene* 4:1463, 1989.
24. Field JK and others: Elevated p53 expression correlates with a history of heavy smoking in squamous cell carcinoma of the head and neck, *Br J Cancer* 64:573, 1991.
25. Gailani MR and others: Developmental defects in Gorlin Syndrome related to a putative tumor suppressor gene on chromosome 9, *Cell* 69:111, 1992.
26. Gapany M and others: Immunohistochemical detection of c-myc protein in head and neck tumors, *Arch Otolaryngol Head Neck Surg* 120:255, 1994.
27. Gillenwater AM and others: Chromosomal abnormalities in pleomorphic adenoma, *Otolaryngol Head Neck Surg* 113:83, 1995.
28. Grandis JR and others: Retinoic acid normalizes the increased transcription rate of TGF-a and EGFR in head and neck cancer cell lines, *Nature Med* 2:237, 1996.
29. Greenhalgh DA and others: Cooperation between v-fos and v-rasHA induces autonomous papillomas in transgenic epidermis but not malignant conversion, *Cancer Res* 5:5071, 1993.
30. Gudas LJ: Retinoids, retinoid-responsive genes, cell differentiation, and cancer, *Cell Growth Diff* 3:655, 1992.
31. Hannon GJ, Beach D: p15INK4B is a potential effector of TGF-b-induced cell cycle arrest, *Nature* 371:257, 1994.
32. Hartwell L: Defects in a cell cycle checkpoint may be responsible for the genomic instability of cancer cells, *Cell* 71:543, 1992.

33. Holliday R, Grigg GW: DNA methylation and mutation, *Mutat Res* 285:61, 1993.

34. Hollstein M and others: p53 mutations in human cancers, *Science* 253:49, 1991.

35. Hunter T: Cooperation between oncogenes, *Cell* 64:249, 1991.

36. Idle JR: Is environmental carcinogenesis modulated by host polymorphism? *Mutat Res* 247:259, 1991.

37. Irish JC, Bernstein A: Oncogenes in head and neck cancer, *Laryngoscope* 103:42, 1993.

38. Issing WJ and others: erbB-2/Her-2 gene amplification and over expression in parotid gland tumors, *Eur Arch Otorhinolaryngol* 250:150, 1993.

39. Ito T and others: Unique association of p53 mutations with undifferentiated but not with undifferentiated carcinomas of the thyroid gland, *Cancer Res* 52:1369, 1992.

40. Johns ME and others: Allelotype of salivary gland tumors, *Cancer Res* 56:1151, 1996.

41. Jones PA, Buckley JD: The role of DNA methylation in cancer, *Adv Cancer Res* 54:1, 1990.

42. Kahn HJ and others: Expression and amplification of neu oncogene in pleomorphic adenomas of salivary gland, *Arch Pathol Lab Med* 116:80, 1992.

43. Kamb A and others: A cell cycle regulator potentially involved in genesis of many tumor types, *Science* 264:436, 1994.

44. Kantor JD and others: Inhibition of cell motility after nm23 transfection of human and murine tumor cells, *Cancer Res* 53:1971, 1993.

45. Knudson AG: Antioncogenes and human cancer, *Proc Natl Acad Sci U S A* 90:10914, 1993.

46. Koch WM and others: p53 gene mutations as markers of tumor spread in synchronous oral cancers, *Arch Otolaryngol Head Neck Surg*, 120:943, 1994.

47. Koch WM and others: p53 mutation is associated with locoregional recurrence but not decreased survival in head and neck squamous cell carcinoma, *J Natl Cancer Inst*, 88:173, 1996.

48. Koch WM and others: Squamous cell carcinoma of the head and neck in the elderly, *Arch Otolaryngol Head Neck Surg* 121:262, 1995.

49. Lammie GA and others: D11S287, a putative oncogene on chromosome 11q13, is amplified and expressed in squamous cell and mammary carcinomas and linked to BCL-1, *Oncogene* 6:439, 1991.

50. Latif F and others: Chromosome 3p deletions in head and neck carcinomas: statistical ascertainment of allelic loss, *Cancer Res* 52:1451, 1992.

51. Lee NK: Tumor suppressor genes, *Head Neck* 14:407, 1992.

52. Lemoine NR and others: High frequency of ras oncogene activation in all stages of human thyroid tumorigenesis, *Oncogene* 4:159, 1989.

53. Li X and others: Allelic loss at chromosomes 3p, 8p, 13q, and 17p associated with poor prognosis in head and neck cancer, *J Natl Cancer Inst* 86:1524, 1994.

54. Lukas JD and others: Retinoblastoma-protein dependent cell-cycle inhibition by the tumour suppressor p16, *Nature* 375:503, 1995.

55. Reference deleted in pages.

56. Lydiatt WM and others: The relationship of loss of heterozygosity to tobacco exposure and early recurrence in head and neck squamous cell carcinoma, *Am J Surg* 168:437, 1994.

57. Lydiatt WM and others: Homozygous deletions and loss of expression of the CDKN2 gene occur frequently in head and neck squamous cell carcinoma cell lines but infrequently in primary tumors, *Genes, Chromosomes Cancer* 13:94, 1995.

58. Maestro R and others: Three discrete regions of deletion at 3p in head and neck cancers, *Cancer Res* 53:5775, 1993.

59. Makos M and others: Distinct hypermethylation patterns occur at altered chromosome loci in human lung and colon cancer, *Proc Natl Acad Sci U S A* 89:1929, 1992.

60. Mao L and others: Microsatellite alterations as clonal markers for the detection of human cancer, *Proc Natl Acad Sci U S A* 91:9871, 1994.

61. Mark J, Dahlenfors F: Cytogenetical observations in 100 human benign pleomorphic adenomas: specificity of the chromosomal aberrations and their relationship to sites of localized oncogenes, *Anticancer Res* 6:299, 1986.

62. Marshall CJ: Tumor suppressor genes, *Cell* 64:313, 1991.

63. Meredith SD and others: Chromosome 11q13 amplification in head and neck squamous cell carcinoma, *Arch Otolaryngol Head Neck Surg* 121:790, 1995.

64. Mulligan LM and others: Germ-line mutations of the RET proto-oncogene in multiple endocrine neoplasia type 2A, *Nature* 363:458, 1993.

65. Nawroz H and others: Allelotype of head and neck squamous cell carcinoma, *Cancer Res* 54:1152, 1994.

66. Perez-Ayala M and others: Presence of HPV 16 sequences in laryngeal carcinomas, *Int J Cancer* 46:8, 1990.

67. Peto J and others: Cancer mortality in relatives of women with breast cancer: the OPCS study, *Int J Cancer* 65:275, 1996.

68. Reed A and others: High frequency of p16 (CDKN2/MTS-1/INK-4A) inactivation in head and neck squamous cell carcinoma, *Cancer Res* 56:3630, 1996.

69. Renan MJ: How many mutations are required for tumorigenesis? Implications from human cancer data, *Mol Carcinog* 7:139, 1993.

70. Roz L and others: Allelic imbalance on chromosome 3p in oral dysplastic lesions: an early event in oral carcinogenesis, *Cancer Res* 56:1228, 1996.

71. Saranath D and others: High frequency mutations in codons 12 and 61 of H-ras oncogene in chewing tobacco-related human oral carcinoma in India, *Br J Cancer* 63:573, 1991.

72. Scheffner M and others: The E6 oncoprotein encoded by human papillomavirus types 16 and 18 promotes the degradation of p53, *Cell* 63:1129, 1990.

73. Schuller HM: The signal transduction model of carcinogenesis, *Biochem Pharmacol* 42:1511, 1991.

74. Sheng ZM and others: Analysis of the c-Ha-ras-1 gene for deletion, mutation, amplification and expression in lymph node metastases of human head and neck carcinomas, *Br J Cancer* 62:398, 1990.

75. Shidara K and others: Lack of synergistic association between human papillomavirus and ras gene point mutation in laryngeal carcinoma, *Laryngoscope* 104:1008, 1994.

76. Slaughter DP, Southwick HW, Smejkal W: Field cancerization in oral stratified squamous epithelium, *Cancer* 6:963, 1953.

77. Sjogren S and others: The p53 gene in breast cancer: prognostic value of complementary DNA sequencing versus immunohistochemistry, *J Natl Cancer Inst* 88:173, 1996.

78. Somers KD, Cartwright SL, Schechter GL: Amplification of the int-2 gene in human head and neck squamous cell carcinomas, *Oncogene* 5:915, 1990.

79. Spandidos DA, Lamothe A, Field JK: Multiple transcriptional activation of cellular oncogenes in human head and neck solid tumours, *Anticancer Res* 5:221, 1985.

80. Spitz MR and others: Mutagen sensitivity in upper aerodigestive tract cancer: a case-control analysis, *Cancer Epidemiol Biomarkers Prev* 2:329, 1993.

81. Spitz and others: Mutagen sensitivity as a risk factor for second malignant tumors following malignancies of the upper aerodigestive tract, *J Natl Cancer Inst* 86:1681, 1994.

82. Thomas S and others: Mutations in the conserved regions of p53 are infrequent in betel-associated oral cancers from Papau New Guinea, *Cancer Res* 54:3588, 1994.

83. Thompson CT, Gray JW: Cytogenetic profiling using fluorescence in situ hybridization (FISH) and comparative genomic hybridization (CGH), *J Cell Biochem* 17G (suppl):139, 1993.

84. Tsuchiya H and others: Detection of human papillomavirus in head and neck tumors with DNA hybridization and immunohistochemical analysis, *Oral Surg Oral Med Oral Pathol* 71:721, 1991.

85. van der Riet P and others: Frequent loss of chromosome 9p21-22 early in head and neck cancer progression, *Cancer Res* 54:1156, 1994.

86. van der Riet P and others: Progression of basal cell carcinoma through

loss of chromosome 9q and inactivation of a single p53 allele, *Cancer Res* 54:25, 1994.

87. Waga S and others: The p21 inhibitor of cyclin-dependent kinases controls DNA replication by interaction with PCNA, *Nature* 369:574, 1994.

88. Wainscoat JS, Fey MF: Assessment of clonality in human tumors, *Cancer Res* 50:1355, 1990.

89. Wales MM and others: p53 activates expression of HIC-1, a new candidate tumour suppressor gene on 17p13.3, *Nature Med* 1:570, 1995.

90. Watson JD and others: *Recombinant DNA*, ed 2, New York, 1992, WH Freeman.

91. Watts SL, Brewer EE, Fry TL: Human papillomavirus DNA types in squamous cell carcinoma of the head and neck, *Oral Surg Oral Med Oral Pathol* 71:701, 1991.

92. Wei Q and others: DNA repair and aging in basal cell carcinoma: a molecular epidemiology study, *Proc Natl Acad Sci U S A* 90:1614, 1993.

93. Wooster R and others: Localization of breast cancer susceptibility gene, BRCA2, to chromosome 13q12-13, *Science* 265:2088, 1994.

94. Wynford-Thomas D: p53 in tumor pathology: can we trust immunocytochemistry? *J Pathol* 166:329, 1992.

95. Xu XC and others: Anti-retinoic acid (RA) antibody binding to human premalignant oral lesions, which occurs less frequently than binding to normal tissue, increases after 13-cis-RA treatment in vivo and is related to RA receptor b expression, *Cancer Res* 55:5507, 1995.

96. Yana I and others: Inactivation of the p53 gene is not required for tumorigenesis of medullary thyroid carcinoma or pheochromocytoma, *Jpn J Cancer Res* 83:1113, 1992.

97. Yoo GH and others: Infrequent inactivation of the retinoblastoma gene despite frequent loss of chromosome 13q in head and neck squamous cell carcinoma, *Cancer Res* 54:4603, 1994.

98. Yu D and others: c-erb B-2/neu overexpression enhances metastatic potential of human lung cancer cells by induction of metastasis-associated properties, *Cancer Res* 54:3260, 1994.

Chapter 18

Outcomes Research

Frederic A. Pugliano
Jay F. Piccirillo

Outcomes research is the scientific study of the outcomes of diverse therapies used for a particular disease, condition, or illness.[98] The goal of outcomes research is to document treatment effectiveness.[30,37,75] Treatment effectiveness implies that therapies have a positive impact on aspects of care that are important to both clinicians and patients. Identifying the most effective treatment strategies through outcomes research has gained increasing importance due to the cost-conscious environment of health care in the United States.[125] The following are key features of outcomes research: the nonrandomized study of diverse therapies for a particular illness, the expanded definition of outcome, and the central role of the patient in treatment selection.[28,46]

This chapter examines the development of outcomes research from geographic variation studies and appropriateness research. The methodology of outcomes research and the importance of expanded definitions of outcome are then presented. Finally, the requirements for conducting sound outcomes research and its importance to clinical practice are discussed.

BACKGROUND

Geographic variation studies

Beginning in the early 1970s, Wennberg and others investigated the wide variation in the use of surgical procedures across small geographic areas.[124,126] For example, within counties of the state of Vermont, fivefold differences in tonsillectomy rates were found without clear evidence of differences in illness severity. The observed variations in the use rates for these various procedures were not explained by the differences in the prevalence or severity of the disorders, and were more likely related to the individual physician's beliefs in the efficacy of and indications for the procedure.

Appropriateness research

In an effort to explain the geographic variation in the use of medical and surgical treatment, investigators at the Rand Corporation initiated a series of Appropriateness Research studies during the 1980s.[16,17,70] Appropriateness Research is conducted by first performing a thorough literature review for a therapy of interest. A detailed set of preliminary indications for the procedure are then developed based on the literature review. An expert panel is asked to consider and modify the list of preliminary indications and rate the degree of appropriateness for a wide range of clinical scenarios. The expert panel consists of a diverse mix of practitioners from all parts of the country familiar with the condition under study. Finally, a structured medical record review is performed to determine the proportion of patients whose procedures were judged to be appropriate, equivocal, or inappropriate.[10] Although the original goal of appropriateness research was to explain geographic variation, the same methodology is now used by a variety of organizations to create guidelines for use review by insurance companies and other third-party payers.

Initial studies examined appropriateness of coronary angiography and carotid endarterectomy.[17,78] The results of these studies indicated that a surprisingly high number of procedures were performed for inappropriate indications, i.e., 17% of coronary angiographies[17] and 32% of carotid endarterectomies.[78] Interestingly, the amount of inappropriate use was approximately the same across different geographic areas regardless of use rates. Within otolaryngology, Kleinman and others studied the appropriateness of tympanostomy tube placement and found a 27% rate of inappropriate tube insertions.[65] Work by Piccirillo and others demonstrated 16% of endoscopic sinus surgeries were performed for inappropriate indications.[93]

When interpreting the conclusions of appropriateness research, it must be remembered that the determination of appropriateness was made by a select panel of experts after a review of the published literature. This research is complicated by the lack of controlled studies on treatment effectiveness. The consensus of experts, based on clinical experience, may only serve to reinforce mistaken beliefs about the efficacy of a treatment.[88,90] For instance, a review of the published literature on the efficacy of surgical treatments for obstructive sleep apnea revealed poor quality of the available information.[105,106]

OUTCOMES RESEARCH METHODOLOGIES

Outcomes research differs from traditional clinical research by addressing a wide variety of issues pertaining to healthcare delivery, strategy, and policy. The goal of a randomized clinical trial is to study treatment *efficacy* while the goal of outcomes research is to study treatment *effectiveness*. Treatment effectiveness implies the value or strength of a treatment as used in daily practice by the community. To achieve these goals, outcomes research uses two principal methodologic strategies: (1) nonrandomized research methodologies, and (2) expanded descriptions of patient outcomes. There are three separate nonrandomized research methodologies within outcomes research: (1) prospective, observational studies of multiple therapies for a specific disease; (2) secondary data analysis of results of therapy from large computerized, administrative, and financial data bases; and (3) meta-analysis, literature review, and consensus technique for establishment of optimal treatment guidelines.

Prospective observational studies

The term *prospective* means relating to the future, and *observational* means that participants in the study are observed with no treatment intervention prescribed by the study protocol. New patients presenting for care can be studied as a part of routine clinical practice. Subject accrual is typically high, because the inclusion criteria are kept simple and no randomization is required. Excluding randomization, the observational method uses many of the scientific techniques developed for randomized clinical trials to reduce bias and ensure validity, e.g., identification of inception cohort, explicit definition of outcome measure, and identification and control of confounding factors. Through the use of precise research methods, scientific accuracy and avoidance of bias can be achieved in observational research.[36,59] For these reasons, the prospective observational trial has proved to be a scientifically sound and efficient form of clinical research.

Several prospective observational studies have been published in various areas of otolaryngology in recent years including otitis media,[76] hearing disorders,[86,133] cochlear implants,[51,127] balance,[68,132] sinusitis,[58] and head and neck cancer.[13,49,52] A multiinstitutional, prospective observational study of obstructive sleep apnea has been conducted under the sponsorship of the American Academy of Otolaryngology-Head and Neck Surgery (AAO-HNS) Foundation.[95] Recently, two studies have used the Surveillance, Epidemiology and End Results (SEER) program of the National Cancer Institute to supplement institutional databases in the study of head and neck cancer. One study examined the association of head and neck cancer and cervical cancer,[109] and a second study examined the survival rate of patients with head and neck cancer as a function of alcohol consumption.[23]

Secondary data analysis

The secondary data contained within the administrative and financial databases maintained by third-party payers, particularly Medicare, describe the results of treatments of a large number of patients over wide geographic areas.[79,123] Sophisticated techniques have been developed to control disease severity and comorbidities, and to select appropriate endpoints to study from these databases. The fundamental problem with analyzing secondary data is that the data are used for purposes for which they were not originally intended. Although useful medical and research data are contained in these databases, the statistical reprocessing required for such analyses can create many problems.[33]

Secondary data analysis is particularly useful when evaluating the cost of care across different geographic regions, and examining the financial impact of an illness on a particular population. A recent study of treatment costs for colon, breast, and prostate cancers in patients enrolled in a Health Maintenance Organization (HMO) was performed using administrative data.[113] Data from a national use review firm were also used to assess the appropriateness of tympanostomy tubes in children.[65] These databases provide a resource for future studies in many areas of otolaryngology.

Meta-analysis, literature review, and consensus conferences

The third type of methodology actually involves three separate processes: meta-analysis,[69,116] literature review,[41,83] and consensus conferences.[80,89] Meta-analysis is the process of combining study results to draw conclusions about treatment effectiveness or to plan new studies. Meta-analysis is particularly helpful in the following situations: when several studies disagree with regard to the magnitude or direction of an effect; when sample sizes are individually too small to detect an effect; or when a large trial is too costly and time consuming to perform. Meta-analysis applies a more structured quantitative approach to the review than the qualitative literature review. The final product of a meta-analysis has both quantitative and qualitative elements.[199]

Several studies have used meta-analysis to investigate treatment effectiveness of children with otitis media.[9,100,101,128] These studies have examined the use of oral steroids, antibiotics, and tympanostomy tubes in the treatment of middle ear effusions. A large meta-analysis of

7443 head and neck cancer patients showed a survival advantage when single-agent chemotherapy was given simultaneously with radiotherapy.[81] Synderman and D'Amico examined the neurologic morbidity and oncologic effectiveness of carotid artery resection.[107] In patients with head and neck cancer, meta-analysis was used to determine the incidence of second malignant tumors[54] and also to study the effect of blood transfusion on the development of locoregional recurrence.[129]

Literature review is the process of reviewing a collection of published articles on a particular topic with the intent of drawing some general qualitative conclusions about the topic. The preparation of literature reviews has experienced a transformation in recent years with the use of new techniques that make these reviews more objective, scientific, and efficient at extracting useful information.[71] Sher and others performed an extensive review of the published literature on the efficacy of surgical treatment of obstructive sleep apnea.[106] Among the more than 100 articles reviewed, not one used a randomized design. A literature review of surgical treatment of squamous cell carcinoma of the temporal bone identified 96 studies, all employing a case-control design.[99] The authors concluded that the addition of radiotherapy to the surgical resection of dura mater did not improve survival, but stated that randomized, controlled studies were required to answer specific questions.

The use of consensus techniques has become more common since the creation of the National Institutes of Health (NIH) Consensus Development Program.[89] This program brings together scientists, medical practitioners, and informed citizens to conduct public evaluation of scientific information about biomedical technologies. The findings are presented in the form of a consensus statement that contains recommendations for medical practice. At present, over 60 consensus development conferences have been held covering a wide range of topics. One recent conference examined the diagnostic workup of patients with suspected acoustic neuroma, and the care of patients with documented acoustic neuroma.[1] Another conference studied screening for hearing loss in newborns.[25] Despite wide acclaim for the concept of the NIH Consensus Development Program, empiric evidence suggests that the care provided by practitioners may not substantially change as a result of the recommendations of these programs.[67]

In addition to the consensus statement, clinical practice guidelines have been created according to the methods outlined by the Agency for Health Care Policy and Research (AHCPR). The AHCPR developed the *Clinical practice guidelines on the management of otitis media with effusion in children* in conjunction with a multidisciplinary panel of physicians, nurses, audiologists, and speech pathologists.[74] Despite the influence of the membership of the expert panel on the acceptance of the guidelines,[57] the publication of the practice guidelines still produced varied responses from practitioners.[8,85]

EXPANDED DESCRIPTIONS OF PATIENT OUTCOMES

Expanded patient outcomes have been described in a hierarchical fashion by Fries and Spitz.[38] In this arrangement, mortality and morbidity form the first two levels of description of patient outcome. The next level of patient outcome is described by the health status of the patient. Health status can be described by the physical, functional, and emotional limitations experienced by an individual.[56,61] Health-related quality-of-life (HRQOL) represents the fourth level of patient outcome. Patient satisfaction with medical care is viewed as the final level of patient outcome.

Outcome measures used in traditional clinical research include mortality, morbidity, and changes in objective laboratory measures. However, these measures do not capture the essence of clinical practice and human illness. In fact, they may obscure the true clinical experience. Nevertheless, these "hard" biologic variables continue to form the basis of clinical research, instead of information collected routinely in the practice of medicine (i.e., patient-based measures of symptoms, functional capacity, social and emotional consequences of disease and its treatment, and satisfaction with care). Traditionally, these "hard" variables were felt to be more objective, scientific, and easier to collect.[34] Unfortunately, the scientific, objective, and "hard" data often can be quite unreliable due to measurement error and observer variability.[29] More importantly, the information is often extraneous to the actual practice of medicine and patient care.

Outcomes research introduces patient-based measures of outcome such as relief of symptoms, health status, health-related quality-of-life, and satisfaction with care.[84] Patients and physicians recognize these additional outcome measures as critically important to the evaluation of treatment. With the increased pressure from managed care companies to control cost, cost effectiveness has become increasingly important in the evaluation of treatment effectiveness.[26]

Functional status and health-related quality-of-life

Health status is a description of the physical, functional, and emotional impairments experienced by the patient. A definition of HRQOL which all patients, physicians, and researchers can agree on, may be impossible to obtain. However, during the past decade, a sufficient amount of research has been conducted by a large number of investigators over a wide range of conditions, therefore, a common core description of health-related quality-of-life may now be possible.[48,64] Health-related quality-of-life includes a suitable description of the health status of the patient and the value placed on that condition by the patient.[21,40] Functional status and health-related quality-of-life instruments have been developed and validated for several otolaryngologic illnesses, including dizziness,[62] sinusitis,[44,96] and hearing impairment.[118]

Development of health-related quality-of-life instruments has been a active area of research in head and neck cancer.[7,11,14,20,53] These instruments provide reliable measures of treatment outcome. A recent review provides an excellent overview of Health-related quality-of-life in head and neck cancer.[22] Health-related quality-of-life studies have also been conducted in obstructive sleep apnea,[18,39] cochlear implant surgery,[73,110] hearing aids,[4] middle ear surgery,[12] and sinusitis.[43,72]

Patient satisfaction

Although laboratory tests and patient-based functional status and health-related quality-of-life measures after treatment can provide important outcome information, many authors argue that the degree of satisfaction a patient gains from their medical care should serve as the essential measure of treatment effectiveness.[5,94,102,103,119] The collection of patient satisfaction scores on a routine basis is now a fundamental aspect of certification programs for hospitals and outpatient facilities. Rubin and others presented results on the measurement of patient satisfaction with outpatient medical care using a nine-item questionnaire used in the Medical Outcomes Study.[104,114] The questionnaire measures overall satisfaction with visits; technical skills, manner, and explanations given by the healthcare providers convenience; time wait for an appointment; and time wait in the office. Piccirillo published results showing improvement in patient satisfaction scores after an academic otolaryngology department instituted a quality improvement program.[92]

Cost-effectiveness

The monetary cost of care for a particular illness and the associated indirect costs, such as number of lost work days, can also be used as an outcome measure. The actual cost of care is usually not studied but rather the cost effectiveness or cost benefit of the intervention is analyzed.[26,117] There are three different dimensions in which to consider the economic analysis of medical care: (1) type of analysis, (2) point of view, and (3) types of costs and benefits. The three types of analyses are cost identification, cost effectiveness, and cost benefit.[102] There are four points of view associated with economic analysis: provider, payer, patient, and society. The four types of costs and benefits are direct medical, direct nonmedical, indirect morbidity and mortality, and intangible.[26]

Recent studies in the treatment of T1 carcinoma have demonstrated a cost benefit of surgical treatment over radiotherapy.[19,82] The cost benefit for treatment options in retromolar trigone carcinoma has also been examined.[42] Wyatt and others examined the cost-effectiveness of cochlear implantation using cost utility analysis and determined that the cost-effectiveness of cochlear implantation was comparable with other medical interventions.[130,131]

RELATED AREAS OF HEALTH SERVICES RESEARCH

Decision analysis

Decision analysis is a methodology that provides a quantitative framework for describing the options, potential consequences, and tradeoffs inherent in making decisions when information is imperfect.[77,87] In decision analysis, "trees" are created that correspond to treatment options for the clinical problem under study. Probabilities are assigned at each "branch" point and the relative value of the outcome at the end of each "branch" is obtained from the literature or from discussions with experts or patients. The stability of the analysis is determined by performing a sensitivity analysis, which alters the probabilities and the utilities of the outcome. Decision analysis can provide an organized approach to complex clinical problems.

Decision analysis has been used to examine treatment options for both pyriform sinus carcinoma[97] and the clinically negative (N0) neck.[122] In pyriform sinus carcinoma, quality-of-life issues were shown to have an important role in treatment planning as determined by sensitivity analysis.[97] Management of the N0 neck is a complex clinical problem. By employing decision analysis, watchful waiting was found to be indicated when the risk of occult metastasis was less than 20%. When the risk was greater than 20%, a single-modality treatment provided the optimal outcome.[122]

Health utility assessment

Health utility assessment is a method for determining the utility or importance the patient places on their health status. A utility is a quantified measure of a person's preference for a specific health state.[108,121] Several metrics have been developed to quantify a person's preference. The "Time Trade-Off" determines the number of years a patient is willing to trade in exchange for perfect health. The "Standard Gamble" technique determines the amount of risk the patient is willing to assume in order to obtain perfect health. The third technique, known as "Willingness To Pay," correlates desired health states with relative monetary amounts. The amount a patient is willing to pay, in relative terms, reflects the strength of their desire for the health state. At Washington University, a computerized utility assessment program called *U-titer*[111,112] is being used to measure hearing-aid benefit. In the utility assessment, patients are asked how many years of life they would trade for perfect hearing before and after hearing-aid use. Trading less time of life for perfect hearing after hearing-aid fitting demonstrates benefit from the hearing aid over unaided hearing.

METHODOLOGIC REQUIREMENTS

There are four methodologic requirements for the conduct of scientifically sound outcomes research:

1. Establish diagnostic criteria for the disease under study.

2. Create a clinical-severity index for prognostic stratification.
3. Identify and measure comorbidities.
4. Establish outcome measures that incorporate:
    a) standard outcome measures (e.g., survival rates);
    b) patient's subjective assessments (e.g., quality-of-life, satisfaction with medical care);
    c) monetary costs of care.

The first three requirements form the scientific standards for the description of the baseline, or pretreatment, condition of the patient. The fourth requirement is necessary for the accurate and complete description of a patient's health status following therapy.[6] Each requirement is discussed separately in the following sections.

Establishing diagnostic criteria for disease

The first step in outcomes research is the establishment of the necessary diagnostic criteria for the proper identification of eligible patients. Diagnostic criteria for many diseases within otolaryngology are well established. These criteria are generally based on the combination of clinical presentation and findings on laboratory and radiographic testing. Where diagnostic criteria do not exist, or there is disagreement, consensus conferences, literature reviews, and clinical research may be used to establish the needed criteria.

After a disease is selected for study, appropriate methods are employed to identify all patients who have the disease and present for care. Inclusion of all eligible patients at the beginning of the study is necessary to eliminate bias in the inception cohort. When evaluating treatment effectiveness, patients should be studied at an early phase of their disease to observe the clinical manifestations of the disease and the impact of treatment.

Creating a clinical-severity index for prognostic stratification

Clinical severity defines the seriousness of a disease and is an important measurement in both clinical practice and research.[32,35,45,60] Correction for differences in the pretreatment severity of a disease must be made before evaluating the effect of treatment on outcome. Thus, clinical-severity indices are a convenient method for controlling for severity of illness when studying treatment effectiveness. Examples of commonly used clinical-severity indices for describing illness are the Apgar Index,[3] Glasgow Coma Scale,[115] the Acute Physiology and Chronic Health Evaluation (APACHE),[66] and the American Joint Committee TNM Staging System for cancer.[2] The use of a staging system that divides patients into stages based on the severity of their illness is necessary for the evaluation of therapy and the estimation of prognosis. Unfortunately, for many diseases in otolaryngology, no such indices exist. Fundamental clinical research is required for the creation of clinical staging systems to stratify patients based on the severity of their otolaryngologic illness.

Identifying and measuring comorbidity

Comorbidity refers to the presence of concomitant disease, not related to the index disease, which may affect the diagnosis, treatment, and prognosis of the patient.[15,32,63] Although patients with more than one diagnosed disease are frequently encountered in modern practice, the interrelationships and effects of multiple diseases have not been adequately studied in clinical medicine. The neglect of comorbidity has many detrimental effects on statistics of disease and the evaluation of treatment.[47]

Comorbidity can affect the time of detection, prognostic anticipation, therapeutic plans, and posttherapeutic outcome of the index disease. Severe comorbidity predisposes the patient to the development of adverse outcomes either by itself or in combination with the index disease. In clinical trials and daily medical practice, these adverse outcomes are often the outcome of interest and form the basis of statistical analyses. Examples of severe comorbidity include malignant hypertension, congestive heart failure, recent myocardial infarction, stroke with residua, hepatic failure, uncontrolled malignancy, and severely decompensated alcoholism. The identification of prognostic comorbidity is important in estimating outcome, because death or decline in functional status may be due to the comorbidity rather than the index disease.[91]

Establishing appropriate definitions of outcome

The fourth requirement for prospective outcomes research is the establishment of appropriate outcome measures. As discussed earlier, the measures used in outcomes research are multidimensional and include patient-based descriptions of illness. The classic list of outcome measures include "the five Ds": death, disease, disability, discomfort, and dissatisfaction.[27] These five conditions can be stated in the positive using more current terminology: mortality, morbidity, health status, quality of life, and satisfaction with medical care. Outcomes research uses all five descriptions of outcomes, as well as economic costs of care.[34]

OUTCOMES RESEARCH IN ROUTINE CLINICAL PRACTICE

Incorporating outcomes research into routine clinical practice provides an excellent means for evaluating medical practice, as well as enhancing efforts to improve quality of care with outcomes research information. Additionally, outcomes research helps fulfill the demands of third-party payers to provide evidence of treatment effectiveness. Outcomes research information can build a stronger and more successful practice by identifying more effective treatment strategies that are likely to increase patient satisfaction.

The first requirement for the successful integration of outcomes research within a practice is the presence of a motivated medical staff. The medical and administrative support staff should be willing to collect the additional data. Secondly, the method of data collection must be brief and transparent to the physician. The third requirement is to create data collection forms that are simple and self-explanatory, because the majority of data for outcomes research is obtained directly from the patient. Well-designed forms, clear instructions, and physicians and office staff who display interest in the patient's responses will increase patient participation.

The choice of which disease, condition, or illness to study should be based on the particular disease mix of the medical practice. For instance, a practice that has a large pediatric population may wish to focus research efforts on treatment outcomes for otitis media and tonsillitis. A practice with a large volume of otology work might wish to focus on outcomes of treatment for hearing loss. Conditions that have several different treatment modalities without a clearly superior option are amenable to study.

The data collected should include the following information: (1) demographics, (2) general health status, (3) disease-specific health status or staging information, (4) comorbidity, (5) directed physical examination findings, (6) results of diagnostic laboratory tests, (7) treatment results, (8) follow-up, and (9) outcome condition. Demographic information should include age, sex, and race. Many validated instruments for measuring general health status are available.[5,120] Few validated disease-specific health status measures or staging systems exist in otolaryngology. Correct staging information is included when a staging system is available for a particular disease. Otherwise, the baseline information needed for creating a novel classification index is collected. When the baseline information is collected, an experimental staging system can be created.[31,50] Several comorbidity instruments have been validated for use in general medical practice.[15,63] The physician should record pertinent physical examination abnormalities and results of important diagnostic tests. Information should be collected on the type of initial treatment used, complications, and subsequent treatments. Outcome information collected should address the five levels of patient outcomes described earlier (mortality, morbidity, health status, quality of life, and satisfaction with care). Data analysis determines the effect of different treatments on the outcome of interest, and controls for severity of illness. The goal is to describe the best treatment within each category of illness severity.

SUMMARY

Outcomes research is an innovative clinical methodology designed to identify the most effective treatment for a particular disease, condition, or illness among the potential treatment options currently available. As technology advances, treatment options increase and the cost of treatment rises. As a result, the need to identify the most effective treatment becomes increasingly important. The methodology of outcomes research is derived from more traditional clinical research methods and uses an expanded description of patient outcome.

Outcomes research uses new methods for the evaluation of the effects of diverse therapies presently in use in the community and introduces new areas of research not traditionally included in evaluation of medical care. Outcomes research focuses more on the outcomes of healthcare services and less on the process.

Many areas within otolaryngology are appropriate for outcomes research, including obstructive sleep apnea, sinusitis, chronic tonsillitis, otitis media, head and neck cancer, and vestibular and auditory disorders in the elderly. Because the prospective, observational trial uses patients in their "natural" clinical setting, it is ideal, and in fact necessary, to involve community-based physicians. The AAO-HNS can continue to lead in this effort by playing a fundamental role in the development, coordination, analysis, and dissemination of findings from outcomes research.

REFERENCES

1. *Acoustic neuroma consensus statement*, Bethesda, Md, 1991, National Institute of Health.
2. American Joint Committee on Cancer: *Manual for staging of cancer*, Philadelphia, 1992, JB Lippincott.
3. Apgar V: A proposal for a new method of evaluation of the newborn infant, *Anesth Analg* 32:260, 1953.
4. Appollonio I and others: Effects of sensory aids on the quality of life and mortality of elderly people: a multivariate analysis, *Age Ageing* 25:89, 1996.
5. Bergner M and others: The sickness impact profile: development and final revision of a health status measure, *Med Care* 19:787, 1981.
6. Bergner M: Measurement of health status, *Med Care* 23:696, 1985.
7. Bjordal K, Kassa S: Psychometric validation of the EORTC Core Quality of Life questionnaire, 30-item version and a diagnosis-specific module for head and neck cancer patients, *Acta Oncol* 31:311, 1992.
8. Bluestone CD, Klein JO: Clinical practice guideline on otitis media with effusion in young children: strengths and weaknesses, *Otolaryngol Head Neck Surg* 112:507, 1995 (editorial).
9. Bodner EE and others: Can meta-analysis help uncertainty in surgery for otitis media in children, *J Laryngol Otol* 105:812, 1991.
10. Brook RH, McGlynn EA: *Maintaining quality of care.* In Ginzberg E, editor: *Health services research. Key to health policy*, Cambridge, Mass, 1991, Harvard University Press.
11. Browman GP and others: The Head and Neck Radiotherapy Questionnaire: a morbidity/quality-of-life instrument for clinical trials of radiation therapy in locally advanced head and neck cancer, *J Clin Oncol* 11:863, 1993.
12. Browning GG: Reporting the benefits from middle ear surgery using the Glasgow Benefit Plot, *Am J Otol* 14:135, 1993.
13. Cano E, Flickinger J, Johnson J: Multivariate analysis results of radiotherapy for laryngeal cancer, *Head Neck* 15:382, 1993.
14. Cella DF and others: The Functional Assessment of Cancer Therapy Scale development and validation of the general measure, *J Clin Oncol* 11:570, 1993.
15. Charlson ME and others: A new method of classifying prognostic comorbidity in longitudinal studies: development and validation, *J Chron Dis* 40:373, 1987.
16. Chassin MR and others: Does inappropriate use explain geographic variations in the use of health care services? *JAMA* 258:2533, 1987.
17. Chassin MR and others: How coronary angiography is used. Clinical determinants of appropriateness, *JAMA* 258:2543, 1987.

18. Chua W, Chediak AD: Obstructive sleep apnea. Treatment improves quality of life—and may prevent death, *Postgrad Med* 95:123, 131, 135, 1994 (review).

19. Cragle SP, Brandenburg JH: Laser cordectomy or radiotherapy: cure rates, communication, and cost, *Otolaryngol Head Neck Surg* 108: 648, 1993.

20. D'Antonio LL and others: Quality of life and functional status measures in patients with head and neck cancer, *Arch Otolaryngol Head Neck Surg* 122:482, 1996.

21. de Haes JCJM, van Knippenberg FCE: *Quality of life of cancer patients: review of the literature.* In Aaronson NK, Beckmann J, editors: *The quality of life of cancer patients,* New York, 1987, Raven Press.

22. Deleyiannis FW-B, Weymuller EA: *Quality of life in patients with head and neck cancer.* In Myers EN, Suen JY, editors: *Cancer of the head and neck,* ed 3, Philadelphia, 1996, WB Saunders.

23. Deleyiannis FW and others: Alcoholism: independent predictor of survival in patients with head and neck cancer, *J Nat Cancer Inst* 88: 542, 1996.

24. Detsky AS, Naglie IG: A clinician's guide to cost-effectiveness analysis, *Ann Intern Med* 113:147, 1996.

25. NIH Consensus: Early identification of hearing impairment in infants and young children, *NIH Consensus Statement* 11:1, 1993.

26. Eisenberg JM: Clinical economics. A guide to the economic analysis of clinical practice. *JAMA* 262:2879, 1989.

27. Elinson J and others: Advances in health assessment conference discussion panel, *J Chron Dis* 40(suppl 1):183S, 1987.

28. Ellwood PM: Shattuck lecture—outcomes management. A technology of patient experience, *N Engl J Med* 318:1549, 1988.

29. Elmore JG, Feinstein AR: A bibliography of publications on observer variability (final installment), *J Clin Epidemiol* 45:567, 1992.

30. Epstein AM: The outcomes movement—will it get us where we want to go? *N Engl J Med* 323:266, 1990.

31. Feinstein AR: Clinical biostatistics. XLI. Hard science, soft data, and the challenges of choosing clinical variables in research, *Clin Pharmacol Ther* 22:485, 1977.

32. Feinstein AR: Clinical biostatistics. XV. The process of prognostic stratification. I. *Clin Pharmacol Ther* 13:442, 1972.

33. Feinstein AR: Clinical biostatistics. XVI. The process of prognostic stratification, part 2, *Clin Pharmacol Ther* 13:609, 1972.

34. Feinstein AR: Para-analysis, faute de mieux, and the perils of riding on a data barge, *J Clin Epidemiol* 42:929, 1989.

35. Feinstein AR: The pre-therapeutic classification of co-morbidity in chronic disease, *J Chron Dis* 23:455, 1970.

36. Feinstein AR, Wells CK: Randomized trials vs. historical controls: the scientific plagues of both houses, *Trans Assoc Am Physicians* 90: 239, 1977.

37. Foundation for Health Services Research: *Health outcomes research: a primer,* Washington, DC, 1993.

38. Fries JF, Spitz PW: *The hierarchy of patient outcome.* In Spilker B, editor: *Quality of life assessments in clinical trials,* New York, 1990, Raven Press.

39. Gall R, Isaac L, Kryger M: Quality of life in mild obstructive sleep apnea, *Sleep* 16:S59, 1993.

40. Gill TM, Feinstein AR: A critical appraisal of the quality of quality-of-life measurements, *JAMA* 272:619, 1994.

41. Glaser EM: Using behavioral science strategies for defining the state-of-the-art, *J Applied Behav Sci* 16:79, 1980.

42. Glenn MG, Komisar A, Laramore GE: Cost-benefit management decisions for carcinoma of the retromolar trigone, *Head Neck* 17:419, 1995.

43. Gliklich RE, Hilinski JM: Longitudinal sensitivity of generic and specific health measures in chronic sinusitis, *Quality of Life Research* 4: 27, 1995.

44. Gliklich RE, Metson R: Techniques for outcomes research in chronic sinusitis, *Laryngoscope* 105:387, 1995.

45. Gonella JS, Hornbrook MC, Louis DZ: Staging of disease. A case-mix measurement, *JAMA* 251:637, 1984.

46. Greenfield S and others: Flaws in mortality data. The hazards of ignoring comorbid disease, *JAMA* 260:2253, 1988.

47. Greenfield S: The state of outcomes research: are we on target? *N Engl J Med* 320:1142, 1989 (editorial).

48. Guyatt G, Feeny D, Patrick D: Issues in quality of life measurement in clinical trials, *Controlled Clin Trials* 12:81S, 1991.

49. Hall SF, Dixon PF: What we learn from a clinical database, *J Otolaryngol* 23:184, 1994.

50. Harrell FE and others: Regression modelling strategies for improved prognostic prediction, *Stat Med* 3:143, 1984.

51. Harris JP, Anderson JP, Novak R: An outcomes study of cochlear implants in deaf patients: audiologic, economic, and quality-of-life changes, *Arch Otolaryngol Head Neck Surg* 121:398, 1995.

52. Harrison LB and others: Performance status after treatment for squamous cell cancer of the base of tongue—a comparison of primary radiation therapy versus primary surgery, *Int J Radiat Oncol Biol Physics* 30:953, 1994.

53. Hassan SJ, Weymuller EA Jr: Assessment of quality of life in head and neck cancer patients, *Head Neck* 15:485, 1993.

54. Haughey BH and others: Meta-analysis of second malignant tumors in head and neck cancer: the case for an endoscopic screening protocol, *Ann Otol Rhinol Laryngol* 101:105, 1992.

55. Health Services Research Group: A guide to direct measures of patient satisfaction in clinical practice, *Can Med Assoc J* 146:1727, 1992.

56. *Healthy People 2000,* Washington, DC, 1991, Public Health Service, US Department of Health and Human Services Publication DHHS 91-50212.

57. Healy GB: Quick reference guide for clinicians. Managing otitis media with effusion in young children: a commentary (see comments), *Arch Otolaryngol Head Neck Surg* 120:1049, 1994.

58. Hoffman SR and others: Symptom relief after endoscopic sinus surgery: an outcomes-based study, *Ear Nose Throat J* 72:413, 1993.

59. Horwitz RI, Feinstein AR: Improved observational method for studying therapeutic efficacy. Suggestive evidence that lidocaine prophylaxis prevents death in acute myocardial infarction, *JAMA* 246:2455, 1981.

60. Iezzoni LI: Severity of illness measures. Comments and caveats, *Med Care* 28:757, 1990.

61. Institute of Medicine: *Disability in America. Toward a national agenda for prevention,* Washington, DC, 1991, National Academy Press.

62. Jacobson GP, Newman CW: The development of the dizziness handicap inventory, *Arch Otolaryngol Head Neck Surg* 116:424, 1990.

63. Kaplan MH, Feinstein AR: The importance of classifying initial co-morbidity in evaluating the outcome of diabetes mellitus, *J Chronic Dis* 27:387, 1974.

64. Katz S: The Portugal Conference: measuring quality of life and functional status in clinical and epidemiological research, *J Chron Dis* 40: 459, 1987.

65. Kleinman LC and others: The medical appropriateness of tympanostomy tubes proposed for children younger than 16 years in the United States, *JAMA* 271:1250, 1994.

66. Knaus WA and others: APACHE II: a severity of disease classification system, *Crit Care Med* 13:818, 1985.

67. Kosecoff J and others: Effects of the National Institutes of Health Consensus Development Program on physician practice, *JAMA* 258: 2708, 1987.

68. Kroenke K and others: One-year outcome for patients with a chief complaint of dizziness, *J Gen Intern Med* 9:684, 1994.

69. L'Abbe KA, Detsky AS, O'Rourke K: Meta-analysis in clinical research, *Ann Intern Med* 107:224, 1987.

70. Leape LL and others: Does inappropriate use explain small-area variations in the use of health care services? *JAMA* 263:669, 1990.

71. Light RJ, Pillemer DB: *Summing up. The science of reviewing research*, Cambridge, Mass, 1984, Harvard University Press.

72. Lund VJ, Mackay IS: Outcome assessment of endoscopic sinus surgery, *J Roy Soc Med* 87:70, 1994.

73. Maillet CJ, Tyler RS, Jordan HN: Change in the quality of life of adult cochlear implant patients, *Ann Otol Rhinol Laryngol* 165(suppl): 31, 1995.

74. Agency for Health Care Policy and Research: *Clinical practice guideline - quick reference guide for clinicians, Managing otitis media with effusion in young children*, Bethesda, Md, 1994.

75. Marwick C: Federal agency focuses on outcomes research: medical news and perspectives, *JAMA* 270:164, 1993.

76. Maw AR, Bawden R: The long term outcome of secretory otitis media in children and the effects of surgical treatment: a ten year study, *Acta Oto Rhino Laryngologica Belgica* 48:317, 1994.

77. McNeil BJ, Pauker SG: Decision analysis for public health: principles and illustrations, *Ann Rev Public Health* 5:135, 1984.

78. Merrick NJ and others: *Indications for selected medical and surgical procedures: a literature review and ratings of appropriateness: carotid endarterectomy*, Publication R-3204/6-CWJ-HF-HCFA-PMT-RWJ, Santa Monica, Calif, 1986, The Rand Corp.

79. Mitchell JB and others: Using medicare claims for outcomes research, *Med Care* 32(suppl):JS38, 1994.

80. Mullan F, Jacoby I: The town meeting for technology: the maturation of Consensus Conferences, *JAMA* 254:1068, 1985.

81. Munro AJ: An overview of randomized controlled trials of adjuvant chemotherapy in head and neck cancer, *Br J Cancer* 71:83, 1995.

82. Myers EN, Wagner RL, Johnson JT: Microlaryngoscopic surgery for T1 glottic lesions: a cost-effective option, *Ann Otol Rhinol Larynol* 103:28, 1994.

83. Neely JG: Literature review articles as a research form, *Otolaryngol Head Neck Surg* 108:743, 1993.

84. O'Young J, McPeek B: Quality of life variables in surgical trials, *J Chron Dis* 40:513, 1987.

85. Paradise JL: Treatment guidelines for otitis media: the need for breadth and flexibility *Pediatr Infect Dis J* 14:429, 1995 (review).

86. Parving A: Intervention and the hearing-impaired child—an evaluation of outcome, *Int J Pediatr Otorhinolaryngol* 23:151, 1992.

87. Pauker SG, Kassirer JP: Decision analysis, *N Engl J Med* 316:250, 1996.

88. Payer L: *Medicine and culture*, New York, 1988, Penguin Books.

89. Perry S: The NIH consensus development program: a decade later, *N Engl J Med* 317:485, 1987.

90. Phelps CE: The methodologic foundations of studies of the appropriateness of medical care, *N Engl J Med* 329:1241, 1993.

91. Piccirillo JF and others: Psychometric and clinimetric validity of the 31 item rhinosinusitis outcome measure (RSOM-31), *Am J Rhinol* 9: 297, 1996.

92. Piccirillo JF and others: Obstructive sleep apnea treatment outcomes pilot study, *Otolaryngol Head Neck Surg* 1997, (in press).

93. Piccirillo JF: Patients' ratings of visits to an academic otolaryngology department, *Otolaryngol Head Neck Surg* 122:1405, 1996.

94. Piccirillo JF and others: Indications for sinus surgery: how appropriate are the guidelines? *Laryngoscope* 1997 (in press).

95. Piccirillo JF: The use of patient satisfaction data to assess the impact of continuous quality improvement efforts, *Arch Otolaryngol Head Neck Surg* 122:1045, 1996.

96. Piccirillo JF and others: New clinical severity staging system for cancer of the larynx: five-year survival rates, *Ann Otol Rhinol Larynol* 103:83, 1994.

97. Plante DA, Piccirillo JF, Sofferman RA: Decision analysis of treatment options in pyriform sinus carcinoma, *Med Decis Making* 7:74, 1987.

98. Roper WL and others: Effectiveness in health care: an initiative to evaluate and improve medical practice, *N Engl J Med* 319:1197, 1988.

99. Rosenfeld RM: How to systematically review the medical literature, *Otolaryngol Head Neck Surg* 115:53, 1996.

100. Rosenfeld RM, Mandel EM, Bluestone CD: Systemic steroids for otitis media with effusion in children, *Arch Otolaryngol Head Neck Surg* 117:984, 1991.

101. Rosenfeld RM, Post JC: Meta-analysis of antibiotics for the treatment of otitis media with effusion, *Otolaryngol Head Neck Surg* 106:378, 1992.

102. Ross CK, Steward CA, Sinacore JM: A comparative study of seven measures of patient satisfaction, *Med Care* 33:392, 1995.

103. Rubin HR and others: Patients' ratings of outpatient visits in different practice settings: results from the medical outcomes study, *JAMA* 270: 835, 1993.

104. Rubin HR, Wu AW: *Patient satisfaction: its importance and how to measure it*. In Gitnick G, editor: *The business of medicine: a physician's guide*, New York, 1991, Elsevier Science Publishing.

105. Schechtman KB, Sher AE, Piccirillo JF: Methodological and statistical problems in sleep apnea research: the literature on uvulopalatopharyngoplasty, *Sleep* 18:659, 1995 (review).

106. Sher AE, Schechtman KB, Piccirillo JF: The efficacy of surgical treatments for obstructive sleep apnea, *Sleep* 19:156, 1996.

107. Snyderman CH, D'Amico F: Outcome of carotid artery resection for neoplastic disease: a meta-analysis, *Am J Otolaryngol* 13:373, 1992.

108. Sox H and others: *Medical decision making*, Boston, 1988, Butterworths.

109. Spitz MR and others: Association between malignancies of the upper aerodigestive tract and uterine cervix, *Head Neck* 14:347, 1992.

110. Summerfield AQ, Marshall DH: Preoperative predictors of outcomes from cochlear implantation in adults: performance and quality of life, *Ann Otol Rhinol Laryngol* 166(suppl):105, 1995.

111. Sumner W and others: Status report on automated utility assessment with U-Titer, *Med Decis Making* 13:399, 1993.

112. Sumner W, Nease R, Littenberg B: *U-Titer: a utility assessment tool*, Proceedings of the Fifteenth Annual Symposium on Computer Applications in Medical Care 701, Washington, DC 1991.

113. Taplin SH and others: Stage, age, comorbidity, and direct costs of colon, prostate, and breast cancer care, *J Natl Cancer Inst* 87:417, 1995.

114. Tarlov AR and others: The Medical Outcomes Study: an application of methods for monitoring the results of medical care, *JAMA* 262: 925, 1989.

115. Teasdale G, Jennett B: Assessment of coma and impaired consciousness: a practical scale, *Lancet* 2:81, 1974.

116. Thacker SB: Meta-analysis. a quantitative approach to research integration *JAMA* 259:1685, 1988 (review).

117. Torrance GW: Measurement of health state utilities for economic appraisal: a review, *J Health Econ* 5:1, 1986.

118. Ventry IM, Weinstein B: The Hearing Handicap Inventory for the elderly: a new tool, *Ear Hear* 3:128, 1982.

119. Ware JE, Hays RD: Methods for measuring patient satisfaction with specific medical encounters, *Med Care* 26:393, 1988.

120. Ware JE, Sherbourne CD: The MOS 36 Item Short-Form Health Survey (SF-36):I. conceptual framework and item selection, *Med Care* 30:473, 1992.

121. Weinstein M, Fineberg H: *Clinical decision analysis*, Philadelphia, 1980, WB Saunders.

122. Weiss MH, Harrison LB, Isaacs RS: Use of decision analysis in planning a management strategy for the stage N0 neck, *Arch Otolaryngol Head Neck Surg* 120:699, 1994 (review).

123. Wennberg JE: Outcomes research, cost containment, and the fear of health care rationing, *N Engl J Med* 323:1202, 1990.

124. Wennberg JE and others: Use of claims data systems to evaluate health care outcomes: mortality and reoperation following prostatectomy, *JAMA* 257:933, 1987.

125. Wennberg J, Gittelsohn A: Variations in medical care among small areas, *Sci Am* 246:120, 1982.

126. Wennberg J, Gittelsohn A: Small area variations in health care delivery, *Science* 182:1102, 1973.

127. Weston SC, Waltzman SB: Performance as a function of time: a study of three cochlear implant devices, *Ann Otol Rhinol Laryngol* 165(suppl):19, 1995.

128. Williams RL and others: Use of antibiotics in preventing recurrent acute otitis media and in treating otitis media with effusion, A meta-analytic attempt to resolve the brouhaha (published erratum), *JAMA* 271:430, 1994.

129. Woolley AL and others: Effect of blood transfusion on recurrence of head and neck carcinoma: retrospective review and meta-analysis, *Ann Otol Rhinol Laryngol* 101:724, 1992.

130. Wyatt JR and others: Cost effectiveness of the multichannel cochlear implant, *Am J Otol* 16:52, 1995 (review).

131. Wyatt JR and others: Cost utility of the multichannel cochlear implants in 258 profoundly deaf individuals, *Laryngoscope* 106:816, 1996.

132. Yardley L, Luxon LM, Haacke NP: A longitudinal study of symptoms, anxiety and subjective well-being in patients with vertigo, *Clin Otolaryngol* 19:109, 1994.

133. Zazove P and others: The health status and health care utilization of deaf and hard-of-hearing persons, *Arch Fam Med* 2:745, 1993.

Chapter 19

Ethics and the Otolaryngologist

Carl Patow
Ruth Gaare

" 'Would you tell me please which way I ought to go from here?' asked Alice. 'That depends a good deal on where you want to go,' said the Cat."[10]

FROM *ALICE IN WONDERLAND* BY LEWIS CARROLL

Ethical issues are everywhere in medicine, and a professional ethic built on trust has always been the very cornerstone of the doctor-patient relationship. Yet in the course of everyday medical practice, ethics often have not been consciously considered. Because the field of ethics has been perceived as "academic" and remote from general clinical practice, its interest for many physicians has been limited. However, the unrelenting pace and magnitude of contemporary technologic development, along with the dramatic changes in healthcare management and financing, are changing these attitudes. Physicians at the bedside are beginning to encounter ethical dilemmas which until recently, were "hypothetical" situations posed only for philosophic discussion. Increasingly complex ethical concerns are emerging about access to healthcare services, the limits of physician responsibility and advocacy, genetic testing and counseling, and so on.

In otolaryngology, issues of increasing concern include head and neck cancer staging,[32] experimental procedures such as laryngeal transplantation,[36] sleep apnea therapy,[38] cost effectiveness of laryngeal cancer treatment,[28] practice guidelines for otitis media,[7,35] the efficacy of adenoid surgery,[16] and cochlear implantation safety[9,41] and outcomes.[19] Underlying these issues are ethical concerns that include patient preferences, physician autonomy, resource allocation, and informed consent.[12]

These concerns lead us to ask, like Alice, "Would you tell us please which way we ought to go from here?" A growing awareness that the answer to this question requires moral sensitivity and analysis has led to a growing interest in medical ethics over the past 25 years and to the emergence of a new discipline called "bioethics." Scholars with backgrounds in medicine, philosophy, law, social sciences, and the humanities all contribute to the field of bioethics, which has its own faculty, academic scholarship, journals, and research centers. This new discipline has become a vehicle for clinicians and society to gain an understanding of the rapid advancements in medicine and of how they stretch the traditional understandings of life and death.

CLINICAL ETHICS

One particular focus of bioethics is clinical ethics, which examines professional behavior and ethical dilemmas that arise in patient care. Its roots can be traced to the 2500-year-old Hippocratic tradition. Although clinical ethics does consider professional codes of conduct and ethical statements from professional societies, the discipline also has produced various methods and case studies that serve as practical models for examining and resolving ethical issues at the bedside. These models are proving useful to physicians who reason through problems on their own, and to ethics committees and consultants, by providing a framework for analysis and discussion.

In this chapter a number of ethical frameworks are introduced that facilitate ethical analysis in clinical cases. No matter what ethics model or framework is used, however, four major themes are addressed in every real-world ethics case and form the basis of moral inquiry in clinical ethics:

1. The appropriateness of the medical intervention (balancing benefits and harms, and considerations of quality of life).
2. The quality of the informed consent and shared decision making process (respect for patient autonomy and patient preferences).
3. The professional obligations (including considerations

about the goals of medicine, the goals of treatment for any individual patient, and professional responsibilities to others beside the patient).

4. The extrinsic considerations, such as the cultural context, family norms, religious values, economic factors, and allocation of scarce resources.

These themes will be illustrated by a series of cases relevant to the field of otolaryngology after a brief introduction to moral reasoning.

MORAL REASONING

Each scholarly discipline, whether engineering, mathematics, or literary criticism, has its own language and methods to analyze and resolve questions in that particular field of study. Recent literature suggests that the process of medical diagnosis requires not only an underlying knowledge of the medical sciences and diseases, but also a combination of analytic logical reasoning with an intuitive, nonlinear mental process that includes assessing nonverbal patient cues. Both abilities assist the physician in: ''(1) assessing the severity of illness; (2) forming an impression about the credibility of data; (3) generating hypotheses about the causes and complications of diseases; and (4) providing confirmatory data for diagnostic hypothesis.''[31]

Similarly, an ethical ''diagnosis'' or analysis in clinical medicine is informed by a knowledge of philosophic theories and historic cases, and has a method for moral deliberation that combines analytic logical reasoning and an assessment of our intuitions about right and wrong that come from our history and culture. Especially relevant to medical ethics is the medical tradition and culture, which provides the background not only for our understanding of the body, illness, and death, but also for our beliefs about the roles of medicine and the healthcare professional in society.

The process of moral deliberation, like medical diagnosis, is one of careful examination, interpretation, analysis, and justification.

Moral deliberation involves:

- *examining* the facts and contextual features of the case
- *interpreting* and understanding the relevant features
- *assessing* alternative solutions to the dispute
- *justifying* the preferred resolution by, for example, using analogous cases, formulating arguments based on ethical theories and principles, analyzing arguments, and appealing to professional codes.

As with medical diagnosis, the goals of moral deliberation are to increase our understanding of a particular patient's situation, and to help us articulate reasons (justification) for what seems to be the best resolution.

ETHICAL THEORY

Although clinical ethics focus on practical deliberations about specific situations and particular cases, the more abstract ethical theories and traditions play an important role in moral deliberation. They are part of the cultural background or environment and provide the foundation for how many individuals and groups approach ethical dilemmas.

Innumerable, diverse ethical theories and visions of the ''good'' are alive and well in our contemporary, pluralistic society. These ethical traditions include:

- *Character or virtue-based ethics*, which follow the traditions of Plato and Aristotle and focus on the motivation and character of the agent who performs the act.[14]
- *Utilitarianism*, which judges rightness and wrongness of an action by its consequences.[34]
- *Kantian ethics*, which maintain that intrinsic features of an act, not consequences, carry moral weight and that the rightness of an action can be understood by whether it conforms with the categorical imperative, i.e., ''I ought never to act except in such a way that I can also will that my maxim become a universal law.''[16]
- *Rights-based analysis*, which emphasizes the justified claims that individuals or groups can make on others or on society.[4]
- *Communitarian approaches*, which emphasize the common good and traditional social values.[33]
- *Ethics of care*, which evolve from a feminist orientation, and hold that morality is contextual and grows out of our relationships and connections with others, and therefore, our responsibility to nurture and care for each other.[17]
- *Casuistry or a ''case-based'' approach*, which focuses on the particulars of individual cases and looks for guidance to the social consensus found in similar precedent cases.[23]
- *Principle-based ethics*, which identifies one or several principles that are then used to analyze and discuss the moral dimensions of cases, or policies.[4]

Whether one is a utilitarian, a communitarian, or influenced by another ethical tradition, deep disagreements about these traditions often do not interfere with agreement and resolution in specific cases. Instead, different ethical traditions can provide unique and complementary ''lenses'' or frameworks through which to view a real-world case, with each illuminating different features of the case.

As Beauchamp and Childress point out, in moral deliberation about real world cases ''we often blend appeals to principles, rules, rights, virtues, passions, analogies, paradigms, parables, and interpretations. To assign priority to one of these factors as the key ingredient is a dubious project, as is the attempt to dispense with ethical theory altogether. The more general (principles, rules, theories, etc.) and the more particular (feelings, perceptions, case judgments, practices, parables, etc.) should be linked together in our moral thinking.''[4]

Moral problems and moral deliberation involve considerable complexity. There are no easy cookbook recipes to make the right decision, nor are there simple, ready-made answers. Decision making requires clinical judgement, practical wisdom, and moral argument. Ethical theories and traditions provide a rich resource for this process and serve as a source for moral justification.

We turn now to a discussion of ethical issues and cases on four topics of interest to otolaryngologists: the human immunodeficiency virus (HIV) epidemic, confidentiality, managed care, and genetics. A number of different ethical approaches will be introduced.

CARE OF THE HUMAN IMMUNODEFICIENCY VIRUS-POSITIVE PATIENT

An ethical analysis of physician responsibility to treat HIV-positive patients by Dr. Edmund Pellegrino illustrates an ethical analysis that appeals to various ethical traditions, although it particularly focuses on character ethics and the role of the healthcare professional.[30]

Issue

During the 1980s, the HIV epidemic became a focus for intense ethical debate.[25] The uniformly fatal nature of the infection and the fear of inadvertent inoculation during invasive procedures fostered a re-examination of the role of health care providers and patients. In his classic article, Pellegrino raises three questions regarding treatment of HIV-positive patients: (1) Is there a moral obligation that compels physicians to treat patients with HIV infections, even at risk to themselves? (2) If there is such a duty, in what ways, if any, is it modified by the universally fatal outcome of the disease? (3) How does a diagnosis of HIV infection affect treatment decisions and the vigor with which they are pursued?

Discussion

Pellegrino argues that physicians have an obligation to treat HIV-infected patients, based on the moral identity of physicians found in six sources: professional ethics, the traditions of the profession, the character of the physician, general ethical principles, socially-defined roles, and the internal morality of medicine.

In addition, Pellegrino cites the Kantian categorical imperative, which states that one should follow only those individual guidelines in individual instances that one would make into a universal law. Refusal to treat HIV-infected patients, using this viewpoint, is unacceptable; universal refusal to treat HIV-infected patients would leave patients without access to necessary treatment.

Pellegrino addresses the question of the fatal risk of the disease by examining the likelihood of healthcare providers becoming infected. Because the risk of transmission is small, he argues that physicians do have an obligation to treat. Surgeons are at special risk for transmission,[40] but also have a special covenant with society in the training and perfection of necessary skills. The surgeon, therefore, may reasonably be expected to assume more risks. Pellegrino suggests that surgeons who are unwilling to accept these special risks may wish to change professions or may need temporary relief from high-risk procedures to recover from emotional strain.[24]

The question of the extent of treatment of HIV-infected patients is addressed by Pellegrino with the recommendation that treatment be delivered, withheld, or withdrawn on the basis of prognosis, effectiveness, benefit of treatment, and the patient's consent, rather than on the ultimate outcome of the disease. He states that there is no justification to treat HIV-infected patients differently than patients with other fatal diseases.

Pellegrino also refers to policy statements from professional organizations and legal factors. The refusal to treat a patient based solely on HIV infection has been condemned by most major medical societies and associations.[27] The Council on Ethical and Judicial Affairs of the American Medical Association has written, ''A physician may not ethically refuse to treat a patient whose condition is within the physician's realm of competence solely because the patient is seropositive.''[3]

Pellegrino cites a legal standard set by the 1990 passage of the Americans with Disabilities Act (ADA), which provides a minimum federal standard of antidiscrimination. The ADA does not list the specific disabilities included under its coverage, but instead provides protection for people with ''handicaps,'' which are broadly defined as a ''physical or mental impairment'' that ''substantially limits one or more . . . major life activities.'' Subsequent court rulings suggest that the ADA protects not only those who are seropositive, but also those who are presumed to be seropositive (e.g., people participating in high-risk behavior).[13]

This analysis addresses one of the four major themes in clinical ethics—professional obligation. It justifies its position on the care of HIV patients by drawing on ethical traditions, such as character or virtue ethics, and on statements by professional organizations like the Council on Ethical and Judicial Affairs of the American Medical Association.

CONFIDENTIALITY AND A PATIENT WITH VERTIGO

The following analysis about confidentiality illustrates a ''principles'' approach to clinical analysis. Developed originally by Beauchamp and Childress in their seminal book, *Principles of Biomedical Ethics*,[4] the principles approach has been a dominant way of ''doing bioethics'' since the late 1970s and has been used by a number of influential government commissions.

The method of principlism begins with the identification of the central norms or principles of obligation that permeate our common moral experience and that are embedded in the institutions of this culture. While there are several varieties of principlism, the Beauchamp and Childress approach identifies four principles for biomedical ethics. Those principles are autonomy (respecting an individual's choices, preferences, and goals), beneficence (fostering the interests of others), nonmaleficence (preventing or avoiding harm to others), and justice (acting fairly, giving persons what they are "due"). A fifth principle of proportionality (i.e., balancing benefits and burdens) is also identified.

These principles do not constitute an overarching ethical system or theory. Instead, they provide a starting point and a framework within which to identify, discuss, and analyze the moral features in specific cases. The principles help us organize our thinking and discussion, yet they are broad enough to allow the details and contexts of each case to shape the meaning of the principles appropriately.

In the Beauchamp and Childress approach, none of the principles are absolute and there is no hierarchical ordering of the principles. Each of the four principles are *prima facie* or presumptively binding, which means that principles must not be violated unless there are compelling reasons for doing so. In real-world cases, when two principles collide and pull us in different directions, the claims of competing principles must be weighed and balanced to determine which exerts a stronger pull and which must yield.

Case

"G.J." is a 48-year-old man and a heavy crane operator who is referred to you by his primary care physician for evaluation of vertigo. Over the past 6 months, the patient has noted multiple episodes of imbalance that at first were barely noticeable, but are increasing in frequency and severity. His supervisor at the construction site noticed that the patient was unsteady while walking, and jokingly remarked that "he should see a doctor or stop drinking." The patient has recently noticed the onset of a pulsatile noise in his left ear. It is barely audible, except at night. He has had no loss of hearing of which he is aware, although on questioning he notes that when he places his right ear on the pillow he cannot hear his wife snore.

The patient is otherwise in good health and takes no medications. He has worked around heavy equipment and noisy generators for 20 years. He is a skilled crane operator, and one of the few in the area who is competent to use a new advanced crane with bimanual controls. His primary responsibility is lifting steel girders and concrete to upper stories of buildings under construction. He has good union benefits and has plans to retire in 2 years. He is at the top of his pay scale. He has never had an on-the-job reportable safety incident.

The patient has been married for nearly 25 years. His wife accompanied him to your office today, and is in the waiting room. She is also a patient of yours, and you have a close, friendly, professional relationship with her. The patient has three sons, all of whom have graduated from college and live in the area. He and his wife recently purchased a lakefront retirement cottage. The patient is heavy-set, with a close-cropped beard, denim overalls, and a red kerchief in his pocket. He describes himself as "the man-of-the-house."

The physical examination is remarkable for a slight left facial paresis, present in all branches of the facial nerve. The remainder of the cranial nerve examination is unremarkable. Tissue deep in the left external auditory canal completely obscures the tympanic membrane. The right tympanic membrane is normal in appearance. The audiogram is remarkable for a severe left mixed hearing loss, and a right moderate high-frequency sensorineural hearing loss.

The primary care physician ordered a computed tomography (CT) scan of the head as part of his workup. The patient had the scan performed just prior to his visit to you. On reviewing the films you discover a mass extending from the middle ear space to the skull base. There is an extensive mass effect in the external auditory canal and mesotympanum. The medial extent of the mass pushes against but does not seem to extend beyond the dura. The tumor involves the hypotympanum and jugular bulb. The bony features of the carotid canal at the genu of the carotid and perilabyrinthine bone appear eroded.

You explain to the patient that based on your examination and the results of the CT, he has a moderately large glomus jugulare tumor that has become symptomatic. You explain that the mass will slowly become larger with time and that additional symptoms will arise. Given enough time the mass may be fatal. He asks whether it is a cancer, and you reassure him that, as far as you can tell, it is not. In your opinion the mass is probably resectable, however, you would like some additional tests prior to surgery. He asks what surgery would be involved, and you describe an infratemporal fossa dissection. As you describe the risks of the surgery, including bleeding, cranial nerve deficits, and possible cerebrospinal fluid leakage, you notice that the patient becomes quite uneasy. He asks when he would be able to return to work. When you respond that he may never be able to safely operate a crane again, he quietly responds that he is capable of dealing with this condition now, that he is not going to have any treatment at this point, and that he does not want you to discuss his condition with his wife or employer. On follow-up calls to his home and work, he has the same response.

Ethical issues

Should the physician agree not to tell the wife about his findings and the potentially important medical treatment the patient is refusing?

Does the physician have ethical obligations to the patient's employer or to those who work with the patient to warn them that the patient's medical condition puts other employees at risk?

Discussion

The moral tension in this case can be characterized as a pull between two principles of medical ethics. On one side is the time-honored obligation of medical confidentiality, which is grounded in both the principle of autonomy (respecting patients' rights to control information about themselves), and the principle of beneficence (fostering the interests of patients who will seek more medical attention if they trust physicians not to reveal private information). On the other side is the physician's duty to prevent and protect others from harm, which is grounded in the principle of beneficence.

A strong case for respecting patient confidentiality can be made in this case. The concept of medical confidentiality and the clinician's duty to protect the privacy of patients was addressed as long ago as the fourth century BC in the *Hippocratic Corpus*, which states in part, "Whatsoever things I shall see or hear concerning the life of men, in my attendance on the sick or even apart therefrom, which ought not to be noised abroad, I will keep silence thereon, counting such things to be as holy secrets."[21]

Contemporary restatements of the obligation to protect patient confidentiality are often cast in terms of patient autonomy and rights and can be found in numerous professional codes and statements, including the American Medical Association's (AMA) Principles of Ethics, the American Nurses' Association's Code for Nurses, and the American Hospital Association's Patients' Bill of Rights.[18] Beauchamp and Childress point out that our contemporary interpretations of respect for autonomy can be traced back to Immanuel Kant, who argued that it "flows from the recognition that all persons have unconditional worth, each having the capacity to determine his or her own destiny," and to John Stuart Mill, a utilitarian, who believed that individuals should be allowed to shape their own lives.[4]

These notions offer strong support for allowing G.J. the opportunity to assume his own risks for refusing medical treatment in this case and determine his own destiny without having his medical information revealed to others, even his wife.

As strong as it is, however, the principle of autonomy is not absolute, and legitimate breaches are recognized. As understood by Beauchamp and Childress, respect for the principle of autonomy "has only *prima facie* standing and can be overridden by competing moral considerations. Typical examples are the following: If our choices endanger the public health, potentially harm innocent others, or require a scarce resource for which no funds are available, others can justifiably restrict our exercises of autonomy."[4] Justification to override the principle of autonomy and the claims of confidentiality must be based on competing and overriding moral principles, in this case the prevention of harm to innocent identifiable others. Such decisions to override confidentiality are subject to intense ethical scrutiny.

In this case, G.J.'s right to refuse medical treatment is not in question, because capable patients have a right to refuse any treatment when the elements of informed consent have been met. The ethical issue is whether his demands for confidentiality also must be respected. A decision to override confidentiality and tell G.J.'s wife or employer about his medical condition depends on the physician's assessment of the following factors: (1) the likelihood that G.J.'s physical symptoms could lead to the harm of his wife or coworkers (e.g., the likelihood that he might suffer physical impairment to such a degree that he might not be capable of operating a crane or an automobile safely); (2) the magnitude of the potential harm to others; and (3) alternative ways to protect against the possible harm short of breaching confidentiality (e.g., convincing G.J. to explain his situation to others himself or to take steps to protect others). Alternate steps G.J. could take to protect others from harm might include deciding not to drive an automobile or confiding in a coworker who could help him when his symptoms became severe.

If the likelihood of harm to G.J.'s wife or coworkers is low, then the physician does not have a strong case for breaching confidentiality. Although G.J.'s wife arguably does have a right to know of her husband's condition, it is G.J.'s duty to inform her, not the physician's duty. The physician should encourage G.J. to tell his wife, since his condition does and will continue to have a great effect on her life and on their marriage.

However, as the severity of G.J.'s symptoms increase, and with it the likelihood of proximate harm to his wife, his coworkers, and himself, there is a stronger obligation for the physician to try to convince G.J. to inform his wife and employer and to request a different job that does not pose a risk to others. The physician should explain to G.J. that his condition and actions impose grave risks of harm on others. The physician also should point out the potential harm to G.J. if his condition results in an occupational accident. G.J. might be putting himself at legal and financial risk. If the physician still can not convince G.J., the physician might suggest a second medical opinion and counseling to help the patient understand and accept the severity of his condition and its consequences for others. Counseling sessions would be an appropriate place to explore issues such as G.J.'s perception of risk and why he is willing to subject himself and others to harm. Other issues to explore include the dissonance between his appraisal of his abilities and the medical determination of disability in this case. Even with a "principles" approach to clinical cases, enhancing the communication between healthcare providers and the patient is an important part of the process of moral deliberation to ensure shared decision making, and to understand how the current situation fits in with the patient's life history.

When the risk to others becomes great, G.J.'s decision not to reveal his condition and seek different employment becomes morally deficient. This does not justify the physician's breach of confidentiality, however. The burden would be on the clinician to overcome the strong presumption for respecting autonomy and confidentiality with even stronger claims and justification. Although a much-cited case, Tarasoff versus Regents,[37] has suggested that there may be a duty to warn or to take steps to protect identifiable third parties from great harm in some situations, it is unclear how this case law would apply in the case of G.J. On the issue of HIV-notification, a number of professional organizations have advised physicians to inform identifiable parties who are at risk for HIV infection when their partners will not reveal their condition.[26] However, the harm of HIV infection is known to be fatal and the risk of transmission is great. The closer G.J.'s situation comes to the HIV case in terms of risk and gravity of harm, the stronger the justification for breaching confidentiality in some way. The physician would need a clear understanding of the details of G.J.'s job and of the effects and severity of G.J.'s physical symptoms. The physician might also consider whether the employer already was put "on notice" of G.J.'s condition when his supervisor noticed and commented on his staggering. This might place the burden of responsibility on the employer to seek further information about G.J.'s condition and arguably lessen the physician's duty to protect the other employees by breaching confidentiality.

If the physician believes the risk and gravity of harm to others is great enough to justify some type of active intervention, a "principles" approach requires that the infringement of autonomy and confidentiality be the least possible in the circumstance, and that the physician should minimize the effects of the infringement. Therefore, after persuasion and counseling fail to convince the patient, the physician might offer to include the patient in the discussion and meet privately with G.J. and his employer and together help determine another appropriate job, rather than revealing the information to the employer without warning the patient. The physician also should take steps to ensure that only those persons necessary to prevent the risk of harm to others are told, and these persons should understand that the information being imparted is confidential medical information. Physicians who consider breaching confidentiality also should seek legal advice to ascertain if there are reporting requirements under public health law or, in this case, if there are occupational safety regulations or protocols from federal or state offices that establish procedures or mechanisms for warning of occupational risks.

To summarize, a "principles" approach to case analysis structures the ethical discussion around four widely accepted norms or principles of obligation in health care: autonomy, beneficence, nonmaleficence, and justice. The complexities and details of each case are explored and the ethical tensions and pulls of the different obligations are identified. Analysis then seeks to understand what, for example, respecting the principle of autonomy or the principle of beneficence requires in each particular case.

MANAGED CARE CHALLENGES

Before examining a managed care case and introducing another framework for ethical analysis, a brief introduction to some of the ethical issues in managed care and some policy statements by professional organizations are presented to provide a context for the discussion.

Managed care was designed to promote cost-efficient, quality medical care for a defined population of enrollees. Managed care raises a host of complicated ethical issues, not the least of which involves potential conflicts of interest between physicians and their patients that strike at the very heart of this traditionally sacred relationship.

Many of the ethical issues arise because healthcare delivery in the era of managed care is often challenged by containment and limits, a sharp contrast and perhaps reaction to the healthcare system of the previous 30 years, which was characterized by unparalleled growth in technology, therapeutic management, patient choices, patient rights, and physician reimbursement and power. Current statements from professional societies and other analysts focus on two areas of concern: (1) the changing role and responsibilities of the physician, and (2) financial conflicts of interest, particularly between physicians and patients.

The physician in the era of managed care

In the not-so-distant past the physician and patient were an isolated twosome outside of any organizational context, whereas physicians in the era of managed care are challenged to redefine their role as they struggle to negotiate and understand contracts that make their medical practice essentially a threesome: physician, patient, and the corporate entity.

Many of the ethical dilemmas at issue in managed care are due to inherent conflicts between the managed care plan's responsibility to provide cost-effective medical care for a group and the traditional physician role to advocate for each patient. The Woodstock Theological Center's report, *Ethical Considerations in the Business Aspects of Health Care*,[39] describes this conflict: "Physicians and other practitioners in the group are under pressures to control costs, and often are required to abide by practice guidelines and standards of treatment designed to limit the use of resources in cases where the benefits are expected to be marginal relative to costs. These rules and standards may at times be at odds with what the patient wants, and even with what the practitioner judges to be in the patient's best interest."[39] Other similar constraints, (e.g., limitations on the specialists or laboratories to whom physicians can refer) can cause ethical conflicts, such as when primary care physicians have concerns about the quality of services offered by those on the managed care plan's approved referral list.

Professional reports and guidelines have begun to address these issues and generally argue strongly for continuing the primacy of the physician-patient relationship. Physicians also are urged to be strong advocates for individual patients in the corporate structure when necessary, as well as to be actively involved in corporate policy making. The AMA's Council on Ethical and Judicial Affairs published guidelines for *Ethical Issues in Managed Care*,[11] which include the following edited statements.

- Physicians should be given an active role in contributing their expertise to any allocation process and should advocate for guidelines that are sensitive to differences among patients.

- In cases in which the physician thinks care has been denied that would ''materially benefit the patient,'' the physician's duty as patient advocate requires not only a challenge to any denials of management from the guideline, but also advocacy at the health plan's policy making level to seek an elimination or modification of the guideline.
- Physicians should assist patients who wish to seek additional appropriate care outside the plan when the physician believes the care is in the patient's best interests.
- Physicians should promote full disclosure to patients enrolled in managed care organizations. Physicians must tell patients of all their management options, regardless of the cost and regardless of whether they are covered by the insurance plan.

The Woodstock Report also issued guidelines that propose an aggressive role for physicians and healthcare professionals when rules and regulations conflict with their professional judgement.

- If a third party refuses funding for a course of treatment deemed by the provider to be indispensable for the health or survival of a patient, it is ethically proper for the healthcare provider to express strong disagreement, carry out the treatment, and strive to justify this decision after the event in order to secure funding. Failing successful resolution, the healthcare provider or the healthcare institution may have to absorb the cost, if it is entirely beyond the means of the patient.[39]

Compensation packages and conflicts of interest

Another major source of ethical concern is the reimbursement arrangements offered by managed care groups to physicians, who often are compensated by a fixed-fee salary, by a share in the profits of the plan, or by bonuses. This can create financial incentives for physicians to undertreat, cut corners, or reduce the services they provide. Such incentives to withhold care are generally believed to pose more of a threat to the patient than the traditional fee-for-service incentives to overtreat because a patient has no way of knowing when a management option has been withheld, and therefore, would not realize the need for a second opinion.

The AMA guidelines also address financial incentives:[11]

- Financial incentives are permissible only if they promote the cost-effective delivery of healthcare and not the withholding of medically necessary care.
- Any incentive to limit care must be disclosed fully to patients by the managed care plan on enrollment and at least annually thereafter.
- The amount of fee withholds, bonuses, and other financial incentives should be limited.
- Payments should be calculated according to the perfor-

mance of a sizable group of physicians, rather than on an individual basis.

- Health plans should develop financial incentives based on quality of care to complement financial incentives based on the quantity of services used.

Case introduction

An example of a ''case-based'' approach to clinical ethics is illustrated in the following case discussion about a managed care issue. The framework is outlined in Box 19-1.[15] The method is built on the premise that ethical considerations are deeply embedded in the details of each patient's case and therefore best addressed by developing an overall plan of care with the patient. This approach helps to anticipate and prevent ethical problems and promotes good clinical practice by integrating ethics with a practical model for care planning and management.

Case

''P.B.'' is a 34-year-old secretary for a fashion design studio who makes an appointment for an evaluation of her nose. She was referred by one of the operating room nurses in your hospital who raved about your operative technique and bedside manner. The patient's chief complaint is that her nose seems crooked to her, and that the tip is uneven. She also repeats frequently during the evaluation that her nose seems constantly blocked and that she must breathe through her mouth to get enough air. Her nocturnal nasal airway obstruction seems to change from side to side. She thinks she might have broken her nose as a child when she fell from a bicycle. She has no allergies and no history of sinusitis. She has no other significant health conditions.

When asked what she would like to have changed about her nose she states that she would like to have the top of her nose straight and less prominent and the tip refined. She also wonders if the nasal breathing could be improved.

She has plans to marry in 6 months and says her boyfriend often teases her about her nose, which really upsets her. She believes that her employment opportunities in the fashion world are limited until she has a rhinoplasty. She describes bouts of depression due, she says, to her appearance. She understands from her friend, the operating room nurse, that you might be able to help her get the nasal breathing and the external deformity improved in one operation, and that the procedure might be covered under her health plan. Her friend has also given her the name of a plastic surgeon at another hospital. She states that she will only consider having surgery if both the external and internal problems can be addressed during the same operative procedure.

Through her employer she is a member of managed care organization with whom you have a relationship. Your arrangement is that you are paid a negotiated reduced fee, from a usual and customary fee schedule determined by the managed care organization. You opened your practice 3

Box 19-1. A case method in planning for care of patients

Short outline

I. Assessment
   A. What are the relevant contextual factors?
   B. What is the patient's medical condition? Indications for treatment?
   C. Is the patient capable of decision making?
   D. What are the patient's preferences?
   E. What are the preferences of family/surrogate decision makers?
   F. What are the needs of the patient as a person?
   G. Are there interests other than, and potentially competing with, those of the patient which need to be considered?
   H. Are there institutional or legal factors contributing to the ethical problem in the case?
   I. Are there issues of power in the interactions of the key actors in the case that need to be addressed?
   J. Are there issues associated with the goals or processes of a healthcare "system" or managed care organization that need to be addressed?

II. Identification of ethical problems and considerations
   A. What are the ethical problems (and their ranking) in the case?
   B. What are the ethically relevant considerations in the case?
   C. Are there similar cases in the literature?
   D. Are there institutional policies relevant to the case?
   E. Are there ethically relevant guidelines or recommendations for clinicians from commissions, specialty groups, interdisciplinary groups?

III. Decision making and implementation
   A. What are the ethically acceptable options?
   B. What justification can be given for the preferred resolution of the case?
   C. How is a satisfactory resolution of the case to be accomplished?
   D. Is ethics consultation necessary or desirable?
   E. Is legal consultation necessary or desirable? Judicial review?

IV. Evaluation
   A. Current: is the plan working? If not, why not?
   B. Retrospective: How might the problem have been prevented or managed better?

From Fletcher J and others: *Introduction to clinical ethics*, Frederick, Md, 1996, University Publishing Group. Reprinted with permission.

months ago and are interested in eventually building a predominantly facial plastics practice.

On physical examination the nose is found to be relatively narrow considering the patient's other facial features. The nasal dorsum is asymmetric, with a prominent hump. The tip also is asymmetric, with slight prominence of the left inferior lateral cartilage. The septum is slightly curved to the left anteriorly and is somewhat wide in its superior portion. At the junction of the perpendicular plate of the ethmoid and the cartilaginous portion of the septum there is a small septal spur that continues posteriorly. The turbinates are slightly enlarged. The nasal airway, in general, appears adequate but slightly narrow. When the patient is asked to sniff, there is no collapse of the lateral nasal tissues and the nasal airflow seems unimpeded.

As you discuss the possible procedures with her, rhinoplasty and septoplasty, you become concerned that the symptoms of nasal airway obstruction seem out of proportion with the physical findings. You suspect that she may have discussed her condition with the operating room nurse, and that her complaints may in part be the result of some coaching by her friend. You are aware that the managed care organization will not consider the rhinoplasty portion of the procedure as a covered benefit of the member's policy. She does, however, have physical findings of septal deformity. She has requested that, if at all possible, you repair the septum and that the entire procedure be billed to the managed care organization.

Case discussion

The case method in Box 19-1 is used for the following case analysis (Box 19-2), with only those sections of the box relevant for a surgical consultation included.

GENETICS: A DEAF COUPLE WANTS A CHILD

The ability to discern genetic variation in individual patients is readily available for a growing number of disorders. It is estimated that the Human Genome Project and rapid private sector advances in mapping and sequencing the human genome will result in "a plethora of population screens, diagnostic tests, and therapies (that) will be available—perhaps commonplace—in the next decade. Conservative estimates are that some 50,000 gene markers will be developed as a result of molecular biology and translated into easy-to-employ biochemical assays, genetic tests, new drugs, and genetic therapies."[8] Knowledge of genetic composition and its potential for causing disease places the physician, the patient, and the patient's family into social, legal, ethical, and medical situations that can be unanticipated and threatening.

The National Center for Human Genome Research[22] has recognized four areas of high priority raised by the most immediate potential applications or consequences of genome research: ethical issues surrounding the conduct of genetics research, responsible clinical integration of new genetic technologies, privacy and fair use of genetic information, and professional and public education about these issues. For most clinical otolaryngologists, the issues of clinical integration and privacy will be most commonly encountered.

The following case developed by Dr. Walter Nance, Chairman of the Department of Genetics at the Medical College of Virginia, is hypothetical, although it is based on his

Box 19-2. Case Method

I. Assessment
  A. Contextual factors
    1. Patient's impending marriage.
    2. Patient's desire for improved appearance.
    3. Patient's employment in the fashion industry is dependent on an attractive appearance.
    4. Patient's complaints of psychologic stress and depression may be due to the appearance of her nose.
    5. Patient has a knowledgeable friend, with whom the physician will have a continuing professional relationship. The preference of the patient's friend, the operating room nurse, is that the procedure be performed at her institution.
    6. Patient is not willing or able to pay for the rhinoplasty.
    7. The physician has a contract with the managed care organization and as part of the contract has agreed to follow accepted standards of medical practice.
    9. The physician's residency training included a special year of training in facial plastic surgery and he has an interest in becoming known within the medical community as an expert in this field.
  B. Patient's medical condition
    1. Good general medical health. No medical contraindications for the procedure.
    2. Although the patient has physical findings of nasal septal deviation, the nasal airway appears patent.
    3. There is deformity on examination of the external nose.
    4. The patient has severe complaints of nasal obstruction.
    5. The procedures proposed are not without risk, including surgical and anesthetic complications and the patient's possible dissatisfaction with the final appearance and function of her nose.
    6. Patient complains of psychologic stress and depression due to appearance of nose.
  C. Capacity of patient
    1. Patient is competent.
  D. Patient preferences and quality of life
    1. Strong preference for having a procedure that will improve the appearance of her nose.
    2. Strong preference for having the managed care organization take responsibility for the entire cost of the operation.
  E. Preferences of family
    1. The patient's boyfriend has remarked about the appearance of her nose, although the boyfriend's opinion about any surgery is unknown.
  F. Needs of the patient as a person
    1. Her sense of attractiveness is important to her personal and professional life.
    2. Her emotional responses to her boyfriend's comments and her poor self-image have an effect on her psychologic well-being.
    3. Limited financial resources.
    4. Specific time frame, with an approaching wedding.

  G. Competing interests
    1. Interest of the managed care organization to limit liability for procedures that are not medically indicated.
    2. The rights and expectations of the other plan members that healthcare costs be contained so that premiums are kept low. The expectation of members that medical resources will be allocated fairly and equitably.
  H. Institutional or legal factors
    1. The contractual agreement that the physician has with the managed care organization.
    2. The institutional expectation that the physician's documentation accurately represents the procedures that he or she is performing.
  I. Issues of power
    1. Because of the physician's continuing professional relationship with the operating room nurse, he might have concerns about what she might relate to other colleagues. She may be a source for further referrals.
    2. The patient is a potential source for other facial plastic surgery referrals because of her employment in the fashion industry, or alternately, for negative comments to possible referrals.
II. Identification of ethical problems
  A. What are the ethical problems
    1. The patient desires to have a procedure performed to improve her appearance that is not covered by her medical plan. Should the physician perform a procedure (septoplasty) that is probably not medically indicated?
    2. To what extent should consideration for building the physician's practice through future potential referrals from the patient and her friend be considered in the decision to operate?
    3. The physician believes that other physicians bend the rules and might be persuaded to perform the septoplasty and rhinoplasty because there are some physical findings of septal abnormality, despite the fact that they are not severe enough to technically qualify as "medically necessary" in his opinion. Is it unfair to this patient that the physician does not bend the rules, given some medical evidence? (The physician is convinced that she will probably find anther physician for the surgery if he declines.)
    4. Should the physician advocate, on the patient's behalf, to the managed care organization that the rhinoplasty should be considered in her case "medically necessary" on the basis of the complaints of depression and psychologic stress?
  B. Ethically relevant considerations
    1. Medical benefit to the patient is marginal
    2. Professional integrity
    3. Justice for other enrollees
    4. Complicity with patient's attempt to circumvent the contractual agreement with her managed care plan

Continued

Box 19-2. Case Method—cont'd

C. Similar cases in the literature
  1. Unknown
D. Institutional policies
  1. Only general policies to follow standard medical practices
E. Guidelines or recommendations from commissions or groups
  1. A number of guidelines, such as those issued by the AMA and the Woodstock Theological Center contain strong recommendations to avoid conflicts of interest and to diligently uphold standards of professional integrity. The Woodstock Theological Center report speaks explicitly to the issue of deceitful reporting and states, ''Health care professionals have an ethical obligation to report truthfully all relevant information about a patient's condition, appropriate treatments, and their associated costs. . . . They also have a professional obligation to keep accurate and truthful medical records, and to provide truthful and accurate information on official forms and documents required by third-party payers.''[39]
III. Decision making
A. Options
  1. Because the physical findings do not meet the indications for septoplasty, the physician could refuse to do the septoplasty. The physician might offer to perform the rhinoplasty and explain that the patient would be responsible for all charges, since her insurance plan provides no coverage for cosmetic procedures.
  2. The physician could refuse to do the septoplasty, but offer to perform the rhinoplasty and waive the professional fee, with the understanding that the patient would bear personal responsibility for hospital and anesthesia charges.
  3. The physician could offer to advocate, on the patient's behalf, to the managed care organization that the rhinoplasty should be covered due to psychologic symptoms.
B. Justification for the preferred solution
  1. To justify the preferred solution, Fletcher and others[15] suggest looking to ethical principles and other resources from ethical theory for support. In this case, strong reasons can be given to support option 1 above the other options based on the principles of promise keeping and truth telling (professional integrity) and justice. The patient and physician have entered into contractual agreements with the managed care organization that define the type of medical care that will be reimbursed. Providers have a legal and ethical duty to present information honestly and are obligated to honor commitments. The physician in this case is required to follow the accepted standards of medical practice and not allow his medical judgement to be influenced by how others may bend the rules in similar circumstances. He must particularly guard against this influence when he serves to gain financially, as he does in this case because of the fee-for-service payment to him and potential referrals that may flow from this case. The principle of justice also supports option 1. Managed care organizations allocate resources among their members in part on the basis of standard medical practice, and they depend on physician integrity for determinations of medical necessity. Bending the rules or ''gaming the system'' for one patient is unfair to other enrollees in the managed care organization.
C. How and by whom is a satisfactory resolution of the case to be done?
  1. Fletcher and others[15] ask us to consider what dialogue or interactions between clinicians and the patient or family are needed to develop and implement a satisfactory plan for the care of the patient. In this case, when the physician tells the patient that he will not perform the septoplasty at this time (and only the rhinoplasty if the patient assumes personal financial responsibility), this conversation would take place within a larger discussion of the plan of care for the patient. Physician and patient might discuss and agree that she should be followed for a period of time to see if her breathing difficulties could be managed in other ways, or to see if continuing or worsening symptoms justify a septoplasty in the future. Given that the patient's personal finances precluded paying for a rhinoplasty now, the physician might also address the issue of her psychological symptoms and depression, and how she might seek help for these, if necessary.

''real-world'' counseling experience with many deaf couples. The case raises some of the complex questions with respect to genetic testing, and shows the importance of understanding the cultural context of ethical dilemmas.

Case

A deaf couple, here referred to as Cindy and Ray, have been married for 4 years. Cindy, a teacher in a school for the deaf, has inherited two copies of a recessive gene that is the cause of her deafness. Her one brother and one sister are also deaf. Her parents were first cousins, and consanguinity increases the risk of genetic disease, including genes that cause deafness.

Ray is a computer programmer, whose social life is centered around the deaf students and teachers at the school where his wife teaches. Ray has a dominantly inherited form of deafness, which was transmitted from his grandfather to Ray's mother to Ray. His mother, one of his brothers, and one of his sisters are deaf. Ray has one sister who can hear. The dominant gene for Ray's deafness has been mapped to chromosome 2.

Cindy and Ray consider themselves members of the deaf culture; they use American Sign Language in preference to English and do not consider their lack of hearing a disability. Both feel strongly enough about their connection with the deaf community to want any children they have to be deaf. They believe that they can raise a deaf child more successfully than a hearing child. Cindy and Ray have no children, but as part of their planning for a child they have consulted a pediatric otolaryngologist and a geneticist about genetic testing. They understand that if they have a child there will be a 50% chance that the child will be deaf. Specifically they are interested in *in utero* testing of the fetus early in development to assure that the fetus has the genetic characteristics that result in deafness. They are willing to use selective abortion after prenatal diagnosis to achieve their goal.

Discussion: genetic testing

Dr. Walter Nance, in *Prescribing Our Future*,[29] describes the challenges inherent in integrating the latest genetic technology into clinical practice and genetic counseling. Before the advent of gene identification in individual patients, much counseling was based on family history and educated guesses about the behavior of the inherited genes. With genetic testing of individuals there is improved specificity in diagnosing genetic disorders, but there is also a reduction in a sense of chance, and perhaps of hope, in affected families. At the same time society is changing rapidly; diversity is often tolerated or even embraced where once it was anathema. Assessing the power of the testing methodology, the needs and capabilities of the individual, and the cultural milieu in which the information is used is a new challenging role for the clinician.[5]

The case study of Cindy and Ray clearly shows how important it is that clinicians be sensitive to the cultural context in which ethical dilemmas are raised. Respecting the unique preferences of individuals, grounded in the principle of autonomy, must be informed by an understanding and appreciation of different world views. When belief systems of various cultures are not familiar or easily understood, the requests or actions of believers may seem inappropriate when taken out of context. In this case, understanding the unique culture of the deaf frames the ethical discussion. The deaf culture has changed dramatically over the past few decades, and to Cindy and Ray and many other deaf persons, their request for genetic testing for the purpose of having a deaf child is appropriate. For society at large, however, their request may raise serious ethical issues. Understanding the life experience and values of the deaf becomes paramount in weighing the strength and validity of their arguments for preferring a deaf child. Ethical discussions about cases such as Cindy and Ray's, which focus on increasing our understanding of the experience of others rather than on moral

argument, may contribute to important shifts in cultural awareness and respect.

Another issue complicating genetic testing is that not all patients may benefit from the additional information provided, despite their desire to have the testing performed. Because of issues of stigmatization, ostracism, and labeling of tested persons, the psychologic response to such testing can be unanticipated. Some patients, on learning they have a significant risk of acquiring a disease, may stop preventive measures and necessary clinical examinations for fear of finally having a dreaded illness diagnosed. Genetic diagnosis of heritable conditions may create great tension within families, because certain members prefer full disclosure to all possibly affected members, while others demand complete privacy. Ownership of genetic information and the consent for disclosure of genetic information are extremely sensitive issues, especially with respect to the current system of medical insurance.

Use of genetic information as a discriminating factor in insurance underwriting has occurred, although examples are relatively rare considering the number of policies generated.[6] A particularly serious question arises when insurers deny coverage for medical expenses incurred by a genetic disorder on the grounds that it represents a preexisting condition.[1] For example, an individual who is genetically determined to develop a degenerative disease late in life might be characterized as having a condition that is present, albeit in latent form, as soon as the individual acquired, or knew that he or she acquired, the abnormal gene. Alternatively, it could be argued that the person only has the predisposition to develop the condition, and not the condition itself. The legal issues regarding the use of genetic information by competitive insurance companies to deny coverage are complex.[2] Interpretations of the law are particularly uncertain regarding genetic discrimination by insurers and employers under the Americans with Disabilities Act and under the regulations of the Equal Employment Opportunities Commission. Despite the lack of clarity in the legal statutes, Dr. Bernadine Healy, as director of the National Institutes of Health in 1992, made it clear that "in order to allow those who choose to do so to benefit from our new genetic tools, discrimination based on genotype must be prohibited as a matter of basic human rights."[20] The ethical and legal challenge for the future is to ensure that this vision prevails.

CONCLUSION

Clinical ethics, which focus on "real-world" dilemmas, look to many sources for guidance, including our philosophic traditions. One of its goals is to facilitate and encourage conversations between providers and patients, between different professionals, between providers at the bedside and policy makers, and between different ethical traditions. A number of different ethical approaches that can provide a framework for these conversations are introduced in this chapter. But, as Dr. Edward Spencer writes, "There are no magic lists of 'virtues' or 'principles' or 'case studies' which will guarantee success. The search for the ethics of clinical care is a continuing process which can never be totally completed, so looking for an 'answer' should be discouraged."[53]

The process of ethical inquiry, however, does offer clinicians a unique perspective on the four major themes in clinical ethics presented in this chapter: (1) the appropriateness of the medical intervention (see Managed care challenges); (2) the quality of the shared decision-making process (see Confidentiality and a patient with vertigo); (3) professional obligations (see Care of the human immunodeficiency virus-positive patient); and (4) extrinsic considerations and cultural issues (see Genetics: a deaf couple wants a child). Ethical reflection may not always yield a simple answer to Alice's question, "Would you tell me please which way I ought to go from here?," but it ensures we take the thoughtful path.

REFERENCES

1. The Ad Hoc Committee on Genetic Testing/Insurance Issues: Background statement: genetic testing and insurance, *Am J Hum Genet* 56: 327, 1995.
2. Allen W, Ostrer H: Anticipating unfair uses of genetic information, *Am J Hum Gen* 53:16, 1993.
3. American Medical Association, Report of the Council on Ethical and Judicial Affairs: *Ethical issues involved in the growing AIDS crisis*, Chicago, 1987, American Medical Association.
4. Beauchamp T, Childress J: *Principles of biomedical ethics,* ed 4, New York, 1994, Oxford University Press.
5. Bedway B: Are you prepared for these new ethical dilemmas? *Med Econ* 72:81, 1996.
6. Billings PR and others: Discrimination as a consequence of genetic screening, *Am J Hum Gen* 50:476, 1992.
7. Bluestone CD, Klein JO: Clinical practice guideline on otitis media with effusion in young children: strengths and weaknesses, *Otolaryngol Head Neck Surg* 112:507, 1995.
8. Boyle PJ: Shaping priorities in genetic medicine. *Hastings Cent Rep* 25(3):52, 1995.
9. Burgio P: Safety considerations of cochlear implantation, *Otolaryngol Clin North Am* 19:237, 1986.
10. Carroll L: *Alice in wonderland.* In *The best of Lewis Carroll*, New York, 1865, Castle Publishing.
11. Council on Ethical and Judicial Affairs, American Medical Association: *Ethical issues in managed care, JAMA* 273(4):330, 1995.
12. Dupuis HM and others: Moral dilemmas in pediatric otorhinolaryngology, *Int J Ped Otolaryngol* 32(suppl):S209, 1995.
13. Feldblum C: *Workplace issues: HIV and discrimination.* In Hunter N, Rubinstein W, editors: *AIDS agenda: emerging issues in civil rights,* New York, 1992, The New York Press.
14. Flanagan O, Rorty AO, editors: *Identity, character, and morality,* 1990, Cambridge, Mass, MIT Press Bradford Books. A MacIntyre, editor: *After virtue,* 1981, Notre Dame, University of Notre Dame Press. E Pellegrino, D Thomasma, editors: *For the patient's good,* New York, 1988, Oxford University Press.
15. Fletcher J and others: *Introduction to clinical ethics,* Frederick, Md, 1995, University Publishing Group.
16. Gates GA: Sizing up the adenoid, *Arch Otolaryngol Head Neck Surg* 122:239, 1996.
17. Gilligan C: *In a different voice,* Cambridge, Mass, 1982, Harvard University Press. *Mapping the moral domain,* Cambridge, Mass, 1988, Harvard University Press. Baier A, editor: *Postures of the mind,* Minneapolis, 1985, University of Minnesota Press. Sherman N, editor: *The fabric of character,* Oxford, 1989, Oxford University Press.
18. Gorlin R: *Codes of professional responsibility,* ed 2, Washington, DC, 1990, The Bureau of National Affairs.
19. Harris JP, Anderson JP, Novak R: An outcomes study of cochlear implants in deaf patients, *Arch Otolaryngol Head Neck Surg* 121:398, 1995.
20. Healy B: Hearing on the possible uses and misuses of genetic information, *Hum Genome Ther* 3:51, 1992.
21. *Hippocratic Corpus,* 4th century BC.
22. *The human genome project, progress report, fiscal years 1993-1994,* National Center for Human Genome Research, Division of Extramural Research, Bethesda, National Institutes of Health.
23. Jonsen A, Toulmin S: *The abuse of casuistry: a history of moral reasoning,* Berkeley, Calif, 1988, University of California Press.
24. Lucente F: The HIV-positive physician—1992, *Laryngoscope* 103: 333, 1993.
25. Lucente F: Impact of the acquired immunodeficiency syndrome epidemic on the practice of laryngology, *Ann Otol Rhinol Laryngol* 102(8 pt2):1, 1993.
26. Marshall MF: *Respecting privacy and confidentiality.* In Fletcher J and others, editors: *Introduction to clinical ethics,* Frederick, Md, 1995, University Publishing Group.
27. Mass C, Sussman S, Hewett J: The human immunodeficiency virus and facial plastic surgery, *ENT J* 75(5):364, 1995.
28. Myers EN, Wagner RL, Johnson JT: Microlaryngoscopic surgery for TI glottic lesions: a cost-effective option, *Ann Otol Rhinol Laryngol* 103:28, 1994.
29. Nance W: *Parables.* In Bartels D, Le Roy B, Caplan A, editors, *Prescribing our future: ethical challenges in genetic counseling,* New York, 1993, Aldine De Gruyter Press.
30. Pellegrino E: HIV infection and the ethics of clinical care, *J Leg Med* 10:29, 1989.
31. Peters M: The role of intuitive thinking in the diagnostic process, *Arch Fam Med* 4:939, 1995.
32. Picarillo JF: Purposes, problems, and proposals for progress in cancer staging, *Arch Otolaryngol Head Neck Surg* 121:143, 1995.
33. Sandel M: *Liberalism and its critics,* New York, 1984, University Press. Walzer M: *The Communitarian Critique of Liberalism, Political Theory* 18, 1990.
34. Singer P, editor: *Practical ethics,* ed 2, Cambridge, England, 1993, Cambridge University Press. Brandt R, editor: *Morality, utilitarianism and rights,* Cambridge, England, 1992, 1994, Cambridge University Press.
35. Stool SE and others: *Otitis media with effusion in young children,* Clinical practice guideline no. 12 AHCPR Pub No. 94-0622. Rockville, Md, Agency for Health Care Policy and Research, Public Health Service, U.S. Department of Health and Human Services.
36. Strome S, Strome M: Laryngeal transplantation: ethical considerations, *Am J Otolaryngol* 13:75, 1992.
37. Tarasoff V: *Regents of the University of California,* 529 P2d 118 (Cal. 1974); 551 P2d 334 (Cal. 1976).
38. Weymuller EA: *Ethical issues in clinical research.* In *Outcomes research in otolaryngology head and neck surgery,* American Academy of Otolaryngology Head and Neck Surgery, Washington, DC, 1995.
39. Woodstock Theological Center: *Ethical considerations in the business aspects of health care,* Washington, DC, 1995, Georgetown University Press.
40. Wright J and others: Mechanisms of glove tears and sharp injuries among surgical personnel, *JAMA* 266:1668, 1991.
41. Yin LY, Segerson DA: Cochlear implants: overview of safety and effectiveness, *Otolaryngol Clin North Am* 19:423, 1986.

Chapter 20

Interpreting Medical Data

Richard M. Rosenfeld

Congratulations! By turning to this chapter you have taken the first step in acknowledging the fundamental importance of properly interpreting medical data. In every chapter of this text, whether it relates to clinical medicine or basic science, the authors draw on their own experience and the experience of others to form systematic conclusions. Experience yields data, and interpreting data is the heart and soul of the cumulative process called science. Learning how to interpret medical data will make you a better clinician, researcher, and teacher.

Effective data interpretation is a habit: a combination of knowledge, skill, and desire.[9] My goal is primarily to light the fires of desire, because I cannot possibly convey all the knowledge and skill in the space of a book chapter. Instead, I will focus on the fundamental principles that underlie *all* data interpretation, regardless of the specific situation or statistical test to which they are applied. If you understand and apply these principles, you will be able to tackle the most complex data set or analytic problem.

By applying the seven habits (Table 20-1) outlined in this chapter, any otolaryngologist—regardless of their level of statistical knowledge or lack thereof—can interpret data. The numerous tables that accompany the text are designed as stand-alone reminders, and often contain keywords with definitions endorsed by the International Epidemiological Association.[24] I will also discuss the practice of data interpretation, including specific hypothesis tests, sample size determination, and common statistical deceptions encountered in the otolaryngology literature. You do not have to be a numerical wizard to understand data; all you need are patience, persistence, and a few good habits that will help settle the dust following the clash of statistics with the human mind.

THE SEVEN HABITS OF HIGHLY EFFECTIVE DATA USERS

The seven habits that follow are the keys to understanding data. They embody fundamental principles of epidemiology and biostatistics that are developed in a logical and sequential fashion. Table 20-1 gives an overview of the seven habits, and the corresponding principles and keywords that comprise them.

Habit one: check quality before quantity

Bias is a four-letter word that is easy to ignore, but difficult to avoid.[37] A clinician who ignores bias when interpreting data is like a prospective employer who takes an applicant's resume at face value. Similarly, being the world's fastest ladder climber matters little if you get to the top only to find the ladder resting against the wrong wall. Checking quality before quantity means checking the data for *bias*—systematic error—before plunging ahead with statistical analysis. It also means checking references before believing a resume and checking the wall before climbing the ladder.

Data collected specifically for research (Table 20-2) are likely to be accurate and unbiased—they reflect the true value of the attribute being measured. In contrast, data collected during routine clinical care will vary in quality depending on the specific methodology applied. For example, data in a medical record review are often tainted by unintentional systematic errors from the reviewer abstracting the data. Errors, however, can be reduced by attention to detail; a protocol with unambiguous data extraction forms, a data dictionary for precise definitions, and attention to inter-rater reliability will maximize accuracy. Consequently, the method of data collection must always be scrutinized.

Table 20-1. The seven habits of highly effective data users

Habit	Underlying principles	Keywords
1. Check quality before quantity	All data are not created equal; fancy statistics cannot salvage biased data from a poorly designed and executed study	Bias, accuracy, research design, confounding, causality
2. Describe before you analyze	Special data require special tests; improper analysis of small samples or data with an asymmetric distribution gives deceptive results	Measurement scale, frequency distribution, descriptive statistics
3. Accept the uncertainty of all data	All observations have some degree of random error; interpretation requires estimating the associated level of precision or confidence	Precision, random error, confidence intervals
4. Measure error with the right statistical test	Uncertainty in observation implies certainty of error; positive results must be qualified by the chance of being wrong; negative results by the chance of having missed a true difference	Statistical test, type I error, P value, type II error, power
5. Put clinical importance before statistical significance	Statistical tests measure error, not importance; an appropriate measure of clinical importance must be checked	Effect size, statistical significance, clinical importance
6. Seek the sample source	Results from one data set do not necessarily apply to another; findings can be generalized only for a random and representative sample	Population, sample, selection criteria, external validity
7. View science as a cumulative process	A single study is rarely definitive; data must be interpreted relative to past efforts, and by their implications for future efforts	Research integration, level of evidence, meta-analysis

Table 20-2. Effect of data quality on data interpretation

Aspect of data quality	Effect on data interpretation
How were the data originally collected?	
Specifically for research	Interpretation is facilitated by quality data collected according to an *a priori* protocol
During routine clinical care	Interpretation is limited by the consistency, accuracy, availability, and completeness of the source records
Is the study experimental or observational?	
Experimental study with conditions under direct control of the investigator	Low potential for bias; randomization reduces allocation bias and blinding reduces ascertainment bias
Observational study without intervention other than to record, classify, and analyze	High potential for bias; systematic errors may occur during sample selection, treatment assignment, and measurement of exposures and outcomes
Is there a comparison or control group?	
Comparative or controlled study with two or more groups	Permits analytic statements concerning efficacy, effectiveness, and association
No comparison group present	Permits descriptive statements only, because of natural history, placebo effect, and regression to the mean
What is the direction of study inquiry?	
Prospective study in which subjects are identified and followed prior to developing an outcome or disease	Measures incidence; time-span component permits assessment of causality when a comparison group is included; must check adequacy of follow-up
Retrospective study in which subjects are identified after developing an outcome or disease and their past histories are then examined	Measures prevalence; time-span component permits assessment of causality when a comparison group is included
Cross-sectional study of a defined population at a single point in time	Measures associations; cannot assess causality because there is no time-span component

Data from experimental studies are generally of higher quality than data from observational investigations.[19] *Experiments* are performed under carefully controlled conditions for the sole purpose of increasing knowledge. Common examples include animal research, basic science studies, and randomized controlled trials. In an *observational study*, however, the compared treatment options or exposures are not under the control of the investigator. This introduces numerous hidden biases, many of which cannot be estimated. Observational studies may be improved through well-defined inclusion and exclusion criteria, data collection by impartial observers, and adequate measurement of important baseline variables relevant to the effect under study (confounders).[10]

The presence or absence of a *control group* has a profound influence on data interpretation (see Table 20-2). An uncontrolled study—no matter how elegant—is purely descriptive. Nonetheless, authors of case series often find delight in unjustified musings on efficacy, effectiveness, association, and causality. As shown in Table 20-4, potential explanations for favorable treatment outcomes in a case series include chance, natural history, placebo effect, and the halo effect. The placebo and halo effects alone may account for on average 70% of good to excellent outcomes seen in medical and surgical case series.[42] Furthermore, patients with chronic disease typically have fluctuating symptoms and seek medical care (and enroll in research studies) when symptoms are at their worst. Therefore, the next change is likely to be an improvement (independent of therapy), a phenomenon called regression to the mean. Therefore, do not waste any time interpreting data from a case series that purports to assess efficacy.[29]

When data from a comparison or control group are available, inferential statistics may be used to test hypotheses and measure associations. Causality also may be assessed when the study has a time-span component, either retrospective or prospective (see Table 20-2). Prospective studies measure *incidence* (new events), whereas retrospective studies measure *prevalence* (existing events). Unlike time-span studies, cross-sectional inquiries measure association not causality. Examples include surveys, screening programs, and evaluation of diagnostic tests. Experimentally planned interventions are ideal for assessing cause-effect relationships, because observational studies are prone to innate distortions or biases caused by individual judgments and other selective decisions.[13]

Another clue to data quality is study type,[30] but this cannot replace the four questions in Table 20-2. Note the variability in data quality for the study types listed in Table 20-3, particularly the observational designs. Randomization balances baseline prognostic factors (known and unknown) among groups, including severity of illness and the presence of comorbid conditions. Because these factors also influence a clinician's decision to offer treatment, nonrandomized studies are prone to allocation (susceptibility) bias (Table 20-4) and false-positive results.[12] A typical example occurs when the survival of surgically treated cancer patients is compared with nonsurgical controls (e.g., radiation or chemotherapy). Without randomization, the surgical group will generally have a more favorable prognosis—independent of therapy—because the customary criteria for operability (special anatomic conditions and no major comorbidity) also predispose to favorable results.

The relationship between data quality and interpretation is illustrated in Table 20-5 using hypothetical studies to determine if tonsillectomy causes baldness. Note how a case series (study designs 1 and 2) can have either a prospective or retrospective direction of inquiry depending on how subjects are identified; contrary to common usage, all cases series are not "retrospective reviews." Only the controlled studies (study designs 3 through 7) can measure associations, and only the controlled studies with a time-span component (study designs 4 through 7) can assess causality. The nonrandomized studies (study designs 3 through 6), however, require adjustment for potential confounding variables: base-

Table 20-3. Relationship of data quality to study design

Study type	How were the data originally collected?	Is there a control or comparison group?	What is the direction of study inquiry?
Experimental studies			
Basic science study	Research	No or yes	Prospective or cross-sectional
Clinical trial	Research	No or yes	Prospective or cross-sectional
Randomized trial	Research	Yes	Prospective
Observational studies			
Cohort study	Research or clinical care	No or yes	Prospective
Historic cohort study	Clinical care	Yes	Prospective
Outcomes research	Research or clinical care	No or yes	Prospective
Case-control study	Clinical care	Yes	Retrospective
Case series	Clinical care	No or yes	Retrospective or prospective
Survey study	Research or clinical care	No or yes	Cross-sectional
Diagnostic test study	Research or clinical care	No or yes	Cross-sectional

Table 20-4. Explanations for favorable outcomes in treatment studies

Explanation	Definition	Solution
Bias	Systematic variation of measurements from their true values; may be intentional or unintentional	Accurate, protocol-driven data collection
Chance	Random variation without apparent relation to other measurements or variables; e.g., getting lucky	Control or comparison group
Natural history	Course of a disease from onset to resolution; may include relapse, remission, and spontaneous recovery	Control or comparison group
Placebo effect	Beneficial effect caused by the expectation that the regimen will have an effect; e.g., power of suggestion	Control or comparison group with placebo
Halo effect	Beneficial effect caused by the manner, attention, and caring of a provider during a medical encounter	Control or comparison group treated similarly
Confounding	Distortion of an effect by other prognostic factors or variables for which adjustments have not been made	Randomization or multivariate analysis
Allocation (susceptibility) bias	Beneficial effect caused by allocating subjects with less severe disease or better prognosis to treatment group	Randomization or comorbidity analysis
Ascertainment (detection) bias	Favoring the treatment group during outcome analysis; e.g., rounding up for treated subjects, down for controls	Blinded outcome assessment

Table 20-5. Determining if tonsillectomy causes baldness: study design versus interpretation*

Study design	Study execution	Interpretation
1. Case series, retrospective	A group of bald subjects are questioned as to whether or not they ever had tonsillectomy	Measures prevalence of tonsillectomy in bald subjects; cannot assess association or causality
2. Case series, prospective	A group of subjects who had, or who are about to have, tonsillectomy are examined later for baldness	Measures incidence of baldness after tonsillectomy; cannot assess association or causality
3. Cross-sectional study	A group of subjects are examined for baldness and for presence or absence of tonsils at the same time	Measures prevalence of baldness and tonsillectomy and their association; cannot assess causality
4. Case-control study	A group of bald subjects and a group of nonbald subjects are questioned about prior tonsillectomy	Measures prevalence of baldness and association with tonsillectomy; limited ability to assess causality
5. Historic cohort study	A group of subjects who had prior tonsillectomy and a comparison group with intact tonsils are examined later for baldness	Measures incidence of baldness and association with tonsillectomy; can assess causality when adjusted for confounding variables
6. Cohort study (longitudinal)	A group of nonbald subjects about to have tonsillectomy and a nonbald comparison group with intact tonsils are examined later for baldness	Measures incidence of baldness and association with tonsillectomy; can assess causality when adjusted for confounding variables
7. Randomized controlled trial	A group of nonbald subjects with intact tonsils are randomly assigned to tonsillectomy or observation and examined later for baldness	Measures incidence of baldness and association with tonsillectomy; can assess causality despite baseline confounding variables

* Studies are listed in order of increasing ability to establish a causal relationship.

line prognostic factors that may be associated with both tonsillectomy and baldness and, therefore, influence results. As noted previously, adequate randomization ensures balanced allocation of prognostic factors among groups, thereby avoiding the issue of confounding.

By checking quality before quantity, you will not waste any time interpreting uninterpretable data. I urge you to review Tables 20-2 through 20-5 before proceeding, with particular attention to the study designs in Table 20-5. Understanding the profound influence of data quality on data interpretation must precede any attempt to describe or analyze the data set.

Habit two: describe before you analyze

Statistical tests often make assumptions about the underlying data. Unless these assumptions are met, the test will be invalid. Describing before you analyze avoids trying to unlock the mysteries of square data with a round key.

Describing data begins by defining the *measurement scale* that best suits the observations. Categorical (qualitative) observations fall into one or more categories and include dichotomous, nominal, and ordinal scales (Table 20-6). Numerical (quantitative) observations are measured on a continuous scale, and are further classified by the underlying *frequency distribution* (plot of observed values versus the frequency of each value). Numerical data with a symmetric (normal) distribution are symmetrically placed around a central crest or trough (bell-shaped curve). Numerical data with an asymmetric distribution are skewed (shifted) to one side of the center, have a sloping "exponential" shape that resembles a forward or backward J, or contain some unusually high or low outlier values.

Depending on the measurement scale, data may be summarized using one or more of the descriptive statistics in Table 20-7. Note that when summarizing numerical data, the descriptive method varies according to the underlying distribution. Numerical data with a symmetric distribution are best summarized with the mean and standard deviation (SD), because 68% of the observations fall within the mean $\pm$ 1 SD and 95% fall within the mean $\pm$ 2 SD. By contrast, asymmetric numerical data are best summarized with the median, because even a single outlier can strongly influence the mean. If a series of five patients are followed after sinus surgery for 10, 12, 15, 16, and 48 months, the mean duration of follow-up is 20 months, but the median is only 15 months. In this case a single outlier, 48 months, distorts the mean.

Although the mean is appropriate only for numerical data with a symmetric distribution, it is often applied regardless of the underlying symmetry. An easy way to determine whether the mean or median is appropriate for numerical data is to calculate both; if they differ significantly, the median should be used. Another way is to examine the SD; when it is very large (e.g., larger than the mean value with which it is associated), the data often have an asymmetric distribution and should be described by the median and interquartile range. When in doubt, the median should always be used over the mean.[14]

A special form of numerical data is called *censored* (see Table 20-6). Data are censored when three conditions apply: (1) the direction of study inquiry is prospective, (2) the outcome of interest is time-related, and (3) some subjects die, are lost, or have not yet had the outcome of interest when the study ends. Interpreting censored data is called *survival analysis*, because of its use in cancer studies where survival is the outcome of interest. Survival analysis permits full use of censored observations by including them in the analysis up to the time the censoring occurred. If censored observations are instead excluded from analysis (e.g., exclude all patients with less than 3 years follow-up in a cancer study), the resulting survival rates will be biased and sample size will be unnecessarily reduced.

Although censored observations are common in biomedical studies, survival analysis is underused by otolaryngologists.[36] Censored data occur in most studies where time to event is the outcome of interest, unless 100% follow-up occurs over a prolonged period. Effective use of survival analy-

Table 20-6. Measurement scales for describing and analyzing data

Scale	Definition	Examples
Dichotomous	Classification into either of two mutually exclusive categories	Obese (yes/no), sex (male/female)
Nominal	Classification into unordered qualitative categories	Race, religion, country of origin
Ordinal	Classification into ordered qualitative categories, but with no natural (numerical) distance between their possible values	TNM* stage (I, II, III, IV), patient satisfaction (low, medium, high), age group (1-5, 6-10, and so on)
Numerical	Measurements with a continuous scale, or a large number of discrete ordered values	Temperature, age in years, hearing level in decibels
Numerical (censored)	Measurements on subjects lost to follow-up, or in whom a specified event has not yet occurred by the end of a study	Survival rate, recurrence rate, or any time-to-event outcome in a prospective study

* *TNM*—Primary tumor, regional nodes, metastasis.

Table 20-7. Describing data

Descriptive measure	Definition	When to use it
Central tendency		
Mean	Arithmetic average	Numerical data that are symmetric
Median	Middle observation; one half the values are smaller and half are larger	Ordinal data; numerical data with an asymmetric distribution
Mode	Most frequent value	Nominal data; bimodal distribution
Dispersion		
Range	Largest value minus smallest value	Emphasizes extreme values
Standard deviation	Spread of data about their mean	Numerical data that are symmetric
Percentile	Percentage of values that are equal to or below that number	Ordinal data; numerical data with an asymmetric distribution
Interquartile range	Difference between the 25th percentile and 75th percentile	Ordinal data; numerical data with an asymmetric distribution
Outcome		
Survival rate	Proportion of subjects surviving, or with some other outcome, after a time interval (1-year, 5-year, and so on)	Numerical (censored) data in a prospective study
Odds ratio	Prevalence of a risk factor in subjects with a disease or outcome divided by prevalence in controls	Dichotomous data in a retrospective, controlled study
Relative risk	Incidence of a disease or outcome in subjects with a risk factor divided by incidence in controls	Dichotomous data in a prospective, controlled study
Rate difference	Event rate in management group minus event rate in control group	Compares success or failure rates in clinical trial groups
Correlation coefficient	Degree to which two variables have a linear relationship; ranges -1 to $+1$ with zero indicating no relationship	Numerical data (Pearson correlation); ordinal data (Spearman rank correlation)

sis in noncancer studies includes estimating the recurrence rate for surgically treated cholesteatoma (censored patients are lost to follow-up or disease-free when the study ends),[35] estimating the time to natural resolution of congenital subglottic stenosis (censored patients are lost, have surgical correction, or have not yet resolved when the study ends),[33] or comparing the bacteriologic efficacy of antibiotics for pneumococcal otitis media in chinchillas (censored animals die or remain culture-positive when the study ends).[34] In each of these examples, survival analysis could estimate the median time to event, as well as time-related event rates for any desired interval (e.g., 7-day, 1-year, 10-year, and so on). Censored data should never be described using the mean, because they tend to have a strongly asymmetric distribution.

The odds ratio, relative risk, and rate difference (see Table 20-7) are useful ways of comparing two groups of dichotomous data.[5] A retrospective (case-control) study of tonsillectomy and baldness might report an *odds ratio* of 1.6, indicating that bald subjects were 1.6 times more likely to have had tonsillectomy than were nonbald controls. In contrast, a prospective study would report results using *relative risk*. A relative risk of 1.6 means that baldness was 1.6 times more likely to develop in tonsillectomy subjects than in nonsurgical controls. Finally, a *rate difference* of 30% in a prospective trial or experiment reflects the increase in baldness caused by tonsillectomy, above and beyond what occurred in controls. No association exists between groups when the rate difference equals zero, or the odds ratio or relative risk equals one (unity).

Two groups of ordinal or numerical data are compared with a *correlation coefficient* (see Table 20-7). A coefficient (R) from 0 to .25 indicates minimal or no relationship, from .25 to .50 a fair relationship, from .50 to .75 a moderate to good relationship, and greater than .75 a good to excellent relationship. A perfect linear relationship would yield a coefficient of 1.00. When one variable differs from the other, the coefficient is positive; a negative coefficient implies an inverse association. Sometimes the correlation coefficient is squared (R^2) to form the *coefficient of determination*, which estimates the percentage of variability in one measure that is predicted by the other.

When interpreting a large number of observations, the easiest way to describe the data is by using a statistical computer program. Any statistical package can describe data graphically or numerically, making it easy to assess the underlying distribution and choose appropriate descriptive measures (see Table 20-7). For interpreting biomedical data, I highly recommend TRUE EPISTAT (Epistat Services, Richardson, TX), a personal computer program written by a physician for other physicians. The package includes many functions that are difficult (or impossible) to perform in general statistical programs, such as survival analysis, epidemiologic outcome measures (e.g., relative risk, odds ratio, rate difference), confidence intervals, power curves, sample size estimation, logistic regression, meta-analysis, and decision-analysis.

Habit three: accept the uncertainty of all data

Uncertainty is present in all data, because of the inherent variability in biologic systems and in our ability to assess them in a reproducible fashion. If you measure hearing in 20 healthy volunteers on five different days, how likely would it be to get the same mean result each time? Very unlikely, because audiometry has a variable behavioral component that depends on the subject's response to a stimulus and the examiner's perception of that response. Similarly, if you measured hearing in five groups of 20 healthy volunteers each, how likely would it be to get the same mean hearing level in each group? Again, unlikely, because of variations between individuals. We would get a range of similar results, but rarely the exact same result on repetitive trials.

Uncertainty must be dealt with when interpreting data, unless the results are meant to apply only to the particular group of patients, animals, cell cultures, deoxyribonucleic acid (DNA) strands, and so on, in which the observations were initially made. Recognizing this uncertainty, we call each of the descriptive measures in Table 20-7 a *point estimate*, specific to the data that generated it. In medicine, however, we seek to pass from observations to generalizations, from point estimates to estimates about other populations. When this process occurs with calculated degrees of uncertainty, we call it *inference*.

Here is a brief example of clinical inference. After treating five vertiginous patients with vitamin C, you remark to a colleague that four patients had excellent relief of their vertigo. She asks, "how confident are you of your results?" "Quite confident," you reply, "there were five patients, four got better, and that's 80%." "Maybe I wasn't clear," she interjects, "how confident are you that 80% of vertiginous patients you see in the next few weeks will respond favorably, or that 80% of similar patients in my practice will do well with vitamin C?" "In other words," she continues, "can you *infer* anything about the real effect of vitamin C on vertigo from only five patients?" Hesitatingly you retort "I'm pretty confident about that number 80%, but maybe I'll have to see a few more patients to be sure."

The real issue, of course, is that a sample of only five patients offers low *precision* (repeatability). How likely is it that the same results would be found if five new patients were studied? Actually, we can state with 95% confidence that 4 of 5 successes in a single trial is consistent with a range of results from 28% to 99% in future trials. This *95% confidence interval* may be calculated manually or with a statistical program,[17,20,28] and tells us the range of results consistent with the observed data. Therefore, if this trial were repeated we could obtain a success rate as low as 28%, not very encouraging compared with the original point estimate of 80%. To make an analogy to a mutual fund prospectus, past performance is no guarantee of future results. Statistics,

however, allow us to estimate future performance with a calculated degree of uncertainty.

Precision may be increased (uncertainty may be decreased) by using a more reproducible measure, by increasing the number of observations (sample size), or by decreasing the variability among the observations. The most common method is to increase the sample size, because we can rarely reduce the variability inherent in the subjects we study. Even a huge sample of perhaps 50,000 subjects still has some degree of uncertainty, but the 95% confidence interval will be quite small. Realizing that uncertainty can never completely be avoided, we use statistics to estimate precision. Therefore, when data are described using the summary measures listed in Table 20-7, a corresponding 95% confidence interval should accompany each point estimate.

Precision differs from accuracy. Precision relates to random error and measures repeatability, accuracy relates to systematic error (bias), and measures nearness to the truth. A precise otologist may always perform a superb mastoidectomy, but an accurate otologist performs it on the right patient. A precise surgeon cuts on the exact center of the line, but an accurate surgeon first checks the line to be sure it is in the right place. Succinctly put, precision is doing things right and accuracy is doing the right thing. Precise data include a large enough sample of carefully measured observations to yield repeatable estimates; accurate data are measured in an unbiased manner so that they reflect what is truly purported to be measured. When we interpret data, we must estimate both precision and accuracy.

Before moving on to habit four, let me briefly summarize habits one, two, and three. Habit one, "check quality before quantity," determines whether or not the data are worth interpreting. Assuming they are, we move to habit two, "describe before you analyze," and summarize the data using appropriate measures of central tendency, dispersion, and outcome for the particular measurement scales involved. Next, we "accept the uncertainty of all data" as noted in habit three, and qualify the point estimates in habit two with 95% confidence intervals to measure precision. When precision is low (e.g., the confidence interval is wide) we proceed with caution. Otherwise, we proceed with habits four, five, and six, which deal with errors and inference.

Habit four: measure error with the right statistical test

To err is human—and statistical. When comparing two or more groups of uncertain data, errors in inference are inevitable. If we conclude the groups are different, they may actually be equivalent. If we conclude they are the same, we may have missed a true difference. Data interpretation is an exercise in modesty, not pretense—any conclusion we reach may be wrong. The ignorant data analyst ignores the possibility of error; the savvy analyst estimates this possibility by using the right statistical test.[6]

Now that we've stated the problem in English, let's restate it in thoroughly confusing statistical jargon (Table

Table 20-8. Glossary of statistical terms encountered when testing hypotheses

Term	Definition
Hypothesis	A supposition, arrived at from observation or reflection, that leads to predictions that can be tested and refuted
Null hypothesis	Results observed in a study, experiment, or test are no different from what might have occurred due to chance alone
Statistical test	Procedure used to reject or accept a null hypothesis; statistical tests may be parametric or nonparametric (distribution-free)
Parametric test	Requires either normally distributed data or a sample size of about 30 or more, e.g., t-test and analysis of variance (ANOVA)
Nonparametric test	Makes no assumptions regarding data distribution, e.g., Mann-Whitney U test and Kruskal-Wallis ANOVA
Type I (α) error	Rejecting a true null hypothesis; declaring that a difference exists when in fact it does not
P value	Probability of making a type I error; $P < .05$ indicates a statistically significant result that is unlikely to be caused by chance
Type II (β) error	Accepting a false null hypothesis; declaring that a difference does not exist when in fact it does
Power	Probability that the null hypothesis will be rejected if it is indeed false; mathematically, power is 1.00 minus type II error

20-8). We begin with some testable *hypothesis* about the groups we are studying, such as "gibberish levels in group A differ from those in group B." Rather than keep it simple, we now invert this to form a *null hypothesis*: "gibberish levels in group A are equal to those in group B." Next we fire up our personal computer, enter the gibberish levels for the subjects in both groups, choose an appropriate statistical test, and wait for the omnipotent P value to emerge.

The *P value* tells us the probability of making a type I error: rejecting a true null hypothesis. In other words, if $P = .10$ we have a 10% chance of being wrong when we declare group A differs from group B. Alternatively, there is a 10% probability that the difference in gibberish levels is explainable by random error: we can't be certain that uncertainty isn't the cause. In medicine, $P < .05$ is generally considered low enough to safely reject the null hypothesis. Conversely, when $P > .05$ we accept the null hypothesis of equivalent gibberish levels. Nonetheless, we may be making a type II error by accepting a false null hypothesis. Rather than state the probability of a type II error directly (which would make too much sense), we state it indirectly by specifying *power* (see Table 20-8). Clear as mud, right?

Now let's digress from principles to practice. We'll use two hypothetical studies for this purpose. The first is an observational, prospective study to determine if tonsillectomy causes baldness: 20 patients undergoing tonsillectomy and 20 controls are examined 40 years later and the incidence of baldness is compared. The second study will use the same groups, but will determine if tonsillectomy causes hearing loss. This will allow us to explore statistical error from the perspective of a dichotomous outcome (bald versus nonbald) and a numerical outcome (hearing level in decibels [dB]).

Suppose that baldness develops in 80% of tonsillectomy patients (16 of 20) but in only 50% of controls (10 of 20). If we infer that, based on these results in 40 specific patients, tonsillectomy predisposes to baldness *in general*, what is

our probability of being wrong (type I error)? Because $P = 10$ (Fisher's exact test) there is a 10% chance of a type I error, so we are reluctant to associate tonsillectomy with baldness based on this single study. Intuitively, however, a rate difference of 30% seems like a big difference, so what is our chance of being wrong when we conclude it is not significant (type II error)? The probability of a type II error (false-negative result) is actually 48% (same as saying 52% power), which means we may indeed be wrong in accepting the null hypothesis. Therefore, we need a larger study before any definitive conclusions can be drawn.

Intrigued by our initial findings, we repeat the tonsillectomy study with twice as many patients in each group. Suppose that baldness again develops in 80% of tonsillectomy patients (32 of 40), but only 50% of controls (20 of 40). The rate difference is still 30%, but now $P = .01$ (Fisher's exact test). We therefore conclude that tonsillectomy is associated with baldness, with only a 1% chance of making a type I error (false-positive result). By increasing the number of subjects studied, we increased precision to a level where we could move from observation to generalization with a tolerable level of uncertainty.

Returning to our earlier study of 20 tonsillectomy patients and 20 controls, we find that the hearing levels for the groups are 25 ± 9 dB and 20 ± 9 dB, respectively (mean value $\pm$ standard deviation [SD]). What is our chance of being wrong if we infer that posttonsillectomy patients have hearing levels 5 dB lower than controls? Because $P = .09$ (t-test), there is a 9% probability of a type I error. If, however, we conclude there is no true difference between the groups, we have a 58% chance of making a type II error. Therefore, we can say little about the impact of tonsillectomy on hearing based on this study, because power is only 42%. In general, studies with "negative" findings should be interpreted by power not P values.

When making inferences about numerical data, precision

Table 20-9. Statistical tests for independent samples

Situation	Parametric test	Nonparametric test
Comparing two groups of data		
Numerical scale	t-test	Mann Whitney U,* median test
Numerical (censored) scale	Mantel-Haenszel life table	Wilcoxon, Logrank, Mantel-Cox
Ordinal scale	—	Mann Whitney U,* median test, chi-squared test for trend
Nominal scale	—	chi-squared, log-likelihood ratio
Dichotomous scale	—	chi-squared, Fisher's exact test, odds ratio, relative risk
Comparing three or more groups of data		
Numerical scale	One-way ANOVA	Kruskal-Wallis ANOVA
Ordinal scale	—	Kruskal-Wallis ANOVA, chi-squared test for trend
Dichotomous or nominal scale	—	chi-squared, log-likelihood ratio
Associating an outcome with predictor variables		
Numerical outcome, one predictor	Pearson correlation	Spearman rank correlation
Numerical outcome, two or more predictor variables	Multiple linear regression, two-way ANOVA	—
Numerical (censored) outcome	Proportional hazards (Cox) regression	—
Nominal outcome	—	Log-linear
Dichotomous outcome	Discriminant analysis	Multiple logistic regression

* The Mann Whitney U test is equivalent to the Wilcoxon rank-sum test.
ANOVA—Analysis of variance.

Table 20-10. Statistical tests for related (matched, paired, or repeated) samples

Situation	Parametric test	Nonparametric test
Comparing two groups of data		
Dichotomous scale	—	McNemar's test
Ordinal scale	—	Sign test, Wilcoxon signed rank test
Numerical scale	Paired t-test	Sign test, Wilcoxon signed rank test
Comparing three or more groups of data		
Dichotomous scale	—	Cochran Q test, Mantel-Haenszel chi-squared
Ordinal scale	—	Friedman ANOVA
Numerical scale	Repeated measures ANOVA	Friedman ANOVA

ANOVA—Analysis of variance.

may be increased by studying more subjects or subjects with less variability in their responses. For example, suppose that we again study 20 tonsillectomy patients and 20 controls, but this time the hearing levels are 25 ± 3 dB and 20 ± 3 dB. Although the difference remains 5 dB, the SD is only 3 for this study compared with 9 for the study in the preceding paragraph. The second subjects had more consistent (less variable) responses. What effect does this reduced variability have on our ability to make inferences? We now obtain $P < .001$ (t-test), indicating less than a 1 : 1000 probability of a type I error if we conclude that the hearing levels truly differ.

All statistical tests measure error. Choosing the right test for a particular situation (Tables 20-9 and 20-10) is determined by (1) whether the observations come from independent or related samples, (2) whether the purpose is to compare groups or to associate an outcome with one or more predictor variables, and (3) the measurement scale of the variables. Despite the myriad of tests available, the principles underlying each remain constant.

Two events are independent if the occurrence of one is in no way predictable from the occurrence of the other. A common example of *independent samples* is two or more parallel (concurrent) groups in a clinical trial or observational study. Conversely, *related samples* include paired organ studies, subjects matched by age and sex, and repeated measures on the same subjects (e.g., before and after treatment). Measurement scales have been previously discussed, but the issue of frequency distribution deserves reemphasis. The tests in Tables 20-9 and 20-10 labeled as ''parametric'' assume an underlying symmetric distribution for data. If the data are sparse, asymmetric, or plagued with outliers, then a ''nonparametric'' test must be used.

Using the wrong statistical test to estimate error invalidates results. For example, suppose we measure intelligence quotient (IQ) in 20 subjects before and after tonsillectomy, and find that the mean IQ increases from 125 to 128. For this three-point increase $P = .29$ (t-test, independent samples), suggesting a high probability (29%) of reaching a false-positive conclusion. However, the observations in this example are related, before and after IQ tests in the same subjects. What is really of interest is the mean *change* in IQ for each subject (related samples), not how the mean IQ of all subjects before surgery compares with the mean IQ of all subjects postoperatively (independent samples). When the proper statistical test is used (t-test, paired samples), $P = .05$ suggests a true association. Related (matched) samples are common in biomedical studies, and should never be analyzed as though they were independent.

Habit five: put clinical importance before statistical significance

Results are *statistically significant* when the probability of a type I error is low enough ($P < .05$) to safely reject the null hypothesis. If the statistical test compared two groups, we conclude that the groups differ. If the statistical test compared three or more groups, we conclude that there are global differences among them. If the statistical test related predictor and outcome variables (regression analysis), we conclude that the predictor variables explain more variation in the outcome than would be expected by chance alone. These generalizations apply to all the statistical tests in Tables 20-9 and 20-10.

The next logical question after ''is there a difference?'' (statistical significance) is ''how big a difference is there?'' (*clinical importance*). Unfortunately, most data interpretation stops with the P value, and the second question is never asked. For example, a recent clinical trial of nonsevere acute otitis media found amoxicillin superior to placebo as initial treatment ($P = .009$).[23] Before we agree with the author's recommendation for routine amoxicillin therapy, let's look more closely at the magnitude of clinical effect. Initial treatment success occurred in 96% of amoxicillin-treated children versus 92% of controls, yielding a 4% rate difference favoring drug therapy. Alternatively, we must treat 25 subjects (100/4) with amoxicillin to increase the success rate by one subject over what would occur from placebo alone. Is this clinically important? Maybe, or maybe not.

Statistically significant results must be accompanied by a measure of *effect size,* which reflects the magnitude of difference between groups.[25] Otherwise, findings with minimal clinical importance may become statistically significant when a large number of subjects are studied. In the above example, the 4% difference in success rates was highly statistically significant because over 1000 episodes of otitis media contributed to this finding. Large numbers provide high precision (repeatability), which in turn reduces the likelihood of error. The final result is a hypnotically small P value, which may reflect a clinical difference of trivial importance.

Common measures of effect size when comparing groups include the odds ratio, relative risk, and rate difference (see Table 20-7). For example, in the hypothetical study of tonsillectomy and baldness noted above, the rate difference was 30% ($P = .01$), with a 95% confidence interval of 10% to 50%. Therefore, we are 95% confident that tonsillectomy increases the rate of baldness between 10% and 50%, with only 1% chance of a type I error (false-positive). Alternatively, results could be expressed in terms of relative risk. For the tonsillectomy study, relative risk is 1.6 (the incidence of baldness was 1.6 times higher after surgery), with a 95% confidence interval of 1.1 to 2.3. Effect size and 95% confidence limits may be calculated manually[11,41] or with a computer program.[20]

Effect size is measured by the correlation coefficient (R) when an outcome variable is associated with one or more predictor variables in a regression analysis (see Table 20-9). Suppose that a study of thyroid surgery reports that shoe size had a statistically significant association with intraoperative blood loss (multiple linear regression, $P = .04$, R $= .10$). A correlation of only .10 implies little or no relationship (see ''describe before you analyze''), and an R^2 of .01 means that only 1% of the variance in survival is explainable by shoe size. Who cares if the results are ''significant'' when the effect size is clinically irrelevant, not to mention nonsensical. Besides, when $P = .04$ we have a 4% chance of being wrong when we reject the null hypothesis, which may in fact be the case here. A nonsensical result should prompt a search for confounding factors that may not have been included in the regression, such as TNM (primary tumor, regional nodes, metastasis) stage, comorbid conditions, duration of surgery, and so on.

Confidence intervals are more appropriate measures of clinical importance than P values, because they reflect *both* magnitude and precision.[4,17] For example, a recent clinical practice guideline on otitis media with effusion discouraged steroid-antibiotic therapy because the combined results from three randomized trials were not statistically significant.[32] Nonetheless, therapy boosted cure rates by 25% (rate difference) with a 95% confidence interval of -1% to 50%. Although not statistically significant (the confidence interval contains zero), the data are consistent with a rate difference up to 50%, a potentially important result. The broad confidence interval suggests low precision and a high probability of a type II error (low power). Therefore, rather than discard steroid-antibiotic therapy as useless because $P > .05$, we conclude that more studies are needed to determine if an important clinical benefit may have been missed.

Habit six: seek the sample source

When we interpret medical data, we ultimately seek to make inferences about some target population based on results in a smaller sample (Table 20-11). Rarely is it possible to study every patient, medical record, DNA strand, or fruit fly with the condition of interest. Nor is it necessary, inferential statistics allow us to generalize from the few to the many, provided that the few we study are a *random and representative* sample of the many. However, random and representative samples rarely arise from divine providence. Therefore, you must always seek the sample source before generalizing your interpretation of the data beyond the confines of the study that produced it.

As an example of sampling, consider a new antibiotic that is touted as superior to an established standard for treating acute otitis media. When you review that data on which this statement is based, you learn that the study endpoint was bacteriologic efficacy: the ability to sterilize the middle ear after treatment. Furthermore, the only patients included in the study were those whose initial tympanocentesis revealed an organism with *in vitro* sensitivity to the new antibiotic; patients with no growth or resistant bacteria were excluded. Can you apply these results to your clinical practice? Most likely not, because you probably don't limit your practice to patients with sensitive bacteria. In other words, the sample of patients included in the study is not representative of the target population in your practice.

A statistical test is valid only when the study sample is *random* and *representative*. Unfortunately, these assumptions are frequently violated or overlooked. A random sample is necessary because most statistical tests are based on probability theory or playing the odds. The odds apply only if the deck is not stacked and the dice are not rigged; i.e., all members of the target population have an equal chance of being sampled for study. Investigators, however, typically have access to only a small subset of the target population because of geographic or temporal constraints. When they choose an even smaller subset of this *accessible population* to study, the method of choosing (sampling method) affects our ability to make inferences about the original target population.

Of the sampling methods listed in Table 20-12, only a random sample is theoretically suitable for statistical analysis. Nonetheless, a consecutive or systematic sample offers a relatively good approximation, and provides data of sufficient quality for most statistical tests. The worst sampling method occurs when subjects are chosen based on convenience or subjective judgments about eligibility. Applying statistical tests to the resulting convenience (grab) sample is the equivalent of asking a professional card counter to help you win a blackjack game when the deck is stacked and cards are missing: all bets are off because probability theory will not apply. A brute force sample of the entire population is also unsatisfactory because lost, missing, or incomplete units tend to differ systematically from those that are readily accessible.

''Seek the sample source'' means identifying the sampling method and selection criteria (inclusion and exclusion

Table 20-11. Glossary of statistical terms related to sampling and validity

Term	Definition
Target population	Entire collection of items, subjects, patients, observations, and so on, about which we want to make inferences; defined by the selection criteria (inclusion and exclusion criteria) for the study
Accessible population	Subset of the target population that is accessible for study, generally because of geographic or temporal considerations
Study sample	Subset of the accessible population that is chosen for study
Sampling method	Process of choosing a sample from a larger population; the method may be random or nonrandom, representative or nonrepresentative
Selection bias	Error caused by systematic differences between a study sample and target population; examples include studies on volunteers and those conducted in clinics or tertiary care settings
Sample size determination	Process of deciding, before a study begins, how many subjects should be studied; based on the incidence or prevalence of the condition under study, anticipated differences between groups, the power that is desired, and the allowable level of type I error
Internal study validity	Degree to which conclusions drawn from a study are valid for the study sample; results from proper study design, unbiased measurements, and sound statistical analysis
External study validity (generalizability)	Degree to which conclusions drawn from a study are valid for a target population (beyond the subjects in the study); results from representative sampling and appropriate selection criteria

criteria) that were applied to the target population to obtain the study sample. When the process appears sound, we conclude that the results are generalizable and *externally valid* (see Table 20-11). If the process appears flawed, we cannot interpret or extrapolate the results beyond the confines of the study sample. For example, a nasal spray that is effective for tree pollen allergy in patients referred to a tertiary rhinology center would offer uncertain benefit for patients with dust mite allergy treated by a family practitioner. Similarly, patients studied by otolaryngologists generally have more severe and chronic disease than the population at large, or the population seen by primary care physicians. Volunteers and hospital-based patients are further examples of biased samples with potentially low generalizability.

The impact of sampling on generalizability is particularly important when interpreting a diagnostic test.[38] For instance, suppose an audiologist develops a new test for diagnosing middle ear effusion (MEE). After testing 1000 children, she reports that 90% of children with a positive result did in fact have MEE (positive predictive value of 90%). Yet when you screen unselected kindergarten children for MEE, the positive predictive value of the test is only 50%. Why does this occur? Because the baseline prevalence of MEE is lower in the kindergarten class (10% have MEE) than in the referral-based audiology population in which the test was developed (50% have MEE). Whereas the sensitivity and specificity of the test are unchanged in both situations, the predictive value is related to baseline prevalence (Bayes' theorem). Therefore, the ultimate use of the test depends on the sample to which it will be applied.

Habit seven: view science as a cumulative process

A single study—no matter how elegant or seductive—is rarely definitive. Science is a cumulative process that requires a large body of consistent and reproducible evidence before conclusions can be formed.[26] When interpreting an exciting set of data, the cumulative basis of science is often overshadowed by the seemingly irrefutable evidence at hand at least until a new study, by different investigators in a different environment, adds a new twist.

Habit seven is the process of *integration*: reconciling our findings with the existing corpus of known similar research. It is the natural consequence of habits one through three that deal with *description*, and habits four through six that deal with *analysis*. Thus, we can summarize data interpretation with three words: describe, analyze, and integrate. This is a sequential process in which each step lays the foundation for subsequent ones, just as occurs for the six habits that underlie them.

Research integration begins by asking ''do the results make sense?'' Statistically significant findings that are biologically implausible, or that are inconsistent with other known studies, can often be explained by hidden biases or design flaws that were initially unsuspected (habit one). Improbable results can become statistically significant through biased data collection, natural history, placebo effects, unidentified confounding variables, or improper statistical analysis. A study with design flaws or improper statistical analysis is said to have low *internal validity* (see Table 20-11) and should be reanalyzed or discarded.

At the next level of integration we compare the study design that produced the current data with the design of other published studies. The *level of evidence* generally increases as we progress from uncontrolled observational studies (case reports, case series), to controlled observational studies (cross-sectional, retrospective, prospective), to controlled experiments (randomized trials). For example, if several randomized efficacy trials have already been published about the topic of interest, an uncontrolled study is unlikely to provide any new insights. When a certain level of evidence has been accumulated, causation may be inferred. *Causation* is an epidemiologic concept based on the consistency, strength, specificity, temporal relationship, and dose-re-

Table 20-12. Methods for sampling a population

Method	How it is performed	Comments
Brute force sample	Includes all units of study (charts, patients, laboratory animals, or journal articles) accessible to the researchers	Time-consuming and unsophisticated; bias-prone because missing units are seldom randomly distributed
Convenience (grab) sample	Units are selected on the basis of accessibility, convenience, or subjective judgments about eligibility	Assume this method when none is specified; study results cannot be generalized because of selection bias
Consecutive sample	Every unit is included over a specified time interval, or until a specified number is reached	Excellent method when intake period is long enough to adequately represent seasonal and other temporal factors
Systematic sample	Units are selected using some simple, systematic rule, such as first letter of last name, date of birth, or day of week	Less biased than a grab sample, but problems may still occur because of unequal selection probabilities
Random sample	Units are assigned numbers then selected at random until a desired sample size is attained	Best method; bias is minimized because all units have a known (and equal) probability of selection

sponse relationship of the association between a factor and a particular disease or outcome.[21]

Quantitative data integration ranges from simple tabular listings to sophisticated health services studies suitable for publication as original research. A simple table summarizing results of the current study and related studies is a good starting point. Unfortunately, authors of a new and exciting randomized trial often view their results as the "bottom line," and spend little time reconciling it with other prior studies. Systematic reviews or *meta-analyses* are an ideal way to synthesize results from a group of logically related randomized trials or, less commonly, observational studies.[31] The "bottom line" in a systematic review typically includes a summary measure of effect size (e.g., rate difference), a 95% confidence interval, and a statistical test for heterogeneity among source articles. Other types of integrative studies include practice guidelines, decision analysis, and economic analysis.

At this point I urge you to review the seven habits outlined in Table 20-1. The same fundamental principles apply when interpreting your own data, interpreting someone else's data (e.g., a journal article), reviewing an unpublished manuscript for a journal, and reviewing a grant application for a funding agency. I have purposely avoided listing specific formulae and calculations throughout this presentation to keep you focused on the forest, not the trees. For the tree lovers among you, I recommend the basic book by Dawson-Saunders and Trapp.[11]

POPULAR STATISTICAL TESTS USED BY OTOLARYNGOLOGISTS

Over the past 20 years, the prevalence of inferential statistics in otolaryngology journals has quadrupled, with one or more *P* values present in about approximately 30% of clinical studies.[36] Familiarity with only six statistical techniques, however, will provide access to over 90% of published articles. Salient features of the most popular tests in otolaryngology journals are listed below and summarized in Table 20-13. Note that each test is simply an alternative way to mea-

sure error (habit four), not a self-contained method of data interpretation.

t-test

Description

The t-test is a classic parametric test for comparing the means of two independent or matched (related) samples of numerical data. t-Tests are found in nearly 30% of analytic clinical research articles in otolaryngology journals.

Interpretation

A significant *P* value for independent samples implies a low probability that the mean values for the two groups are equal. When the samples are matched, a significant *P* value implies that the mean differences of the paired values are unlikely to be zero. Because valid results depend on relatively equal variances (SD) within each group, a statistical test is required to verify this assumption (F-test).

Precautions

T-tests will produce an artificially low *P* value if the groups are small (less than 10 observations) or have an asymmetric distribution; instead, a nonparametric test (Mann-Whitney U or Wilcoxon rank sum test) should be used. If, however, each group contains over 30 observations, the underlying distribution can deviate substantially from normality without invalidating results. t-Tests should *never* be used to compare more than two groups; ANOVA is required.[18] When the outcome of interest is time related (e.g., cancer survival, duration of hospital stay, disease recurrence), survival analysis (see below) is more appropriate than a t-test.

Analysis of variance

Description

ANOVA tests if the means of *three or more* independent groups of continuous data differ significantly with regard to a single factor (one-way ANOVA) or two factors (two-way ANOVA). ANOVA is found in only 9% of analytic clinical

Table 20-13. Popular statistical tests in otolaryngology journals

Statistical test	What it can do	What it cannot do
t-test	Compare the means of two groups of numerical data	Compare three or more groups; analyze sparse or asymmetric data
Analysis of variance	Compare the means of three or more groups of numerical data	Compare subgroups when there are no significant overall differences
Contingency table (chi-square)	Test for an association among two groups of categorical data	Compare subgroups when there are no significant overall differences
Survival analysis	Estimate the time-related probability of an event adjusted for censored data	Compensate for inadequate periods of follow-up
Multivariate analysis	Examine the simultaneous effect of multiple variables on an outcome	Adjust for biased data; make valid predictions unless model fit is assessed
Nonparametric analysis	Analyze small data sets with an underlying asymmetric distribution	Analyze very sparse data

research articles in otolaryngology journals, but is more common in basic research.

Interpretation

A significant P value implies a low probability that the mean values for all groups are equal. From a statistical standpoint, we say that the variance between groups is larger than the variance within each group. Note that ANOVA provides no information on whether *individual* pairs of groups differ significantly; it only tests for an overall global difference. For example, when comparing four groups of data (A, B, C, and D), the finding $P < .05$, ANOVA means there is less than a 5% chance that the statement "A = B = C = D" is true; however, it says nothing about whether A ≠ B or C ≠ D or D ≠ A, and so on. Once the investigators demonstrate a significant global difference ($P < .05$) using ANOVA, they can then use *multiple comparison* procedures (Bonferroni, Tukey, Newman-Keuls, Scheffe, Dunnett) for individual group comparisons.

Precautions

ANOVA will produce an artificially low P value if the groups contain small samples (less than five observations per group, or 20 in all groups combined) with asymmetric distributions; instead, a nonparametric test (Kruskal-Wallis ANOVA) should be used. A nonparametric test is also preferred if the groups have unequal variance as determined by an F-test. Multiple pairwise t-tests cannot substitute for ANOVA; the effect is to greatly increase the odds of a false-positive result (type I statistical error).

Contingency tables

Description

Contingency tables test for an association between two categorical variables by using the chi-square statistic. A modification, called the McNemar test, can be used for two groups of paired data. Contingency tables are found in 20% of analytic clinical research articles in otolaryngology journals.

Interpretation

A significant P value implies a significant association between the two variables whose categorical values form the rows and columns of the contingency table. However, even a very small P value provides no information about the strength of the association (effect size). Therefore, effect size can be measured with the odds ratio (two-by-two table) or by Pearson's contingency coefficient (tables with more than two rows or columns). The chi-square statistic compares the observed values for each cell (row-column intersection) with the expected values that would occur if chance alone were operating.

Precautions

As with t-tests and ANOVA, small samples can produce an artificially small P value. If the *expected* frequency for any cell is less than 5, an alternate test must be used (e.g.,

Fisher's exact test or the log-likelihood ratio). Beware of authors who overinterpret a "significant" chi-square result. As with ANOVA, when $P < .05$ we claim a *global* association between variables; we cannot specify which particular subgroups of rows and columns are or are not associated.

Survival analysis

Description

Survival analysis estimates the probability of an event (typically, but not necessarily, survival) based on the total period of observation, and tests for associations with other variables of interest. Survival analysis permits maximum use of data from *censored* observations, which occur when a subject is lost to follow-up, or if the study ends before the outcome of interest has occurred.

Interpretation

There are two main ways of analyzing survival data: the life table method divides the time into intervals and calculates survival at each interval; the Kaplan-Meier method calculates survival each time an event occurs. Both methods produce a graph (survival curve) showing the cumulative probability of the event versus total period of observation. Authors sometimes eliminate the curve, and instead give the event rates only for specific time periods (e.g., 1-year, 3-year, 10-year, and so on). When two or more survival curves are compared, and the P value is low, a probable association exists between time to event and the factor used to stratify the curves.

Precautions

When you see a "survival curve," be sure that it has been calculated using survival analysis (life table or Kaplan-Meier), not by simply dividing cumulative events at a given time by the total subjects still around at that time. The latter method mistreats censored observations, yielding artificially low estimates. Nor is it desirable to simply exclude from analysis all subjects not meeting some arbitrary cut-off for observation time; resulting rates may be artificially high. Whereas the life table method requires a minimum sample size of 20 uncensored observations, Kaplan-Meier analysis requires only five uncensored observations for valid results.

Multivariate (regression) procedures

Description

Multivariate (regression) procedures examine the *simultaneous* effect of multiple predictor variables (generally three or more) on an outcome of interest. In contrast, t-tests, one-way ANOVA, chi-square, and survival analysis examine the *univariate* effect of variables on an outcome one at a time. Different multivariate procedures are used depending on the measurement scale of the outcome variable (see Table 20-9).

Interpretation

Multivariate analysis produces a statistical model that predicts outcomes based on combinations of individual variables. The adequacy of the model as a whole is determined by the coefficient of determination (R^2) and its associated *P* value. Each predictor variable also has an associated coefficient, whose magnitude represents the relative effect of the variable on outcome when adjusted for all the other variables in the model. A positive coefficient implies a positive association; a negative coefficient implies a negative association. When the coefficient's *P* value is small, the association is significant.

Precautions

Biased results may occur if the data set has outliers, or if variables in the model are highly correlated with each other (R > .90). Although a model may precisely fit the investigator's data, there is no guarantee that it will predict outcomes for subjects outside the study with equal precision. As with any statistical test, garbage in, garbage out. No degree of multivariate analysis can adjust for confounding variables that were not recorded at the start of the study.

Nonparametric tests

Description

Nonparametric tests check hypotheses without requiring that the data have a normal distribution. The nonparametric equivalents of the t-test, paired t-test, and one-way ANOVA are the Mann-Whitney U, Wilcoxon signed rank, and Kruskal-Wallis tests, respectively (see Tables 20-9 and 20-10).

Interpretation

When an author uses a parametric test (e.g., t-test or ANOVA), the data must be either normally distributed or come from a large enough sample (about 30 or more subjects) such that this assumption may be relaxed. Nonparametric tests avoid this requirement by ranking the data in each group, and then comparing rank sums instead of the actual values of individual observations. Whereas the parametric tests discussed above make inferences about *means*, nonparametric tests make inferences about *medians*. When there is doubt as to whether a nonparametric test is necessary, the *P* value should be calculated both ways; parametric and nonparametric. If the results differ significantly, the nonparametric test is preferred.

Precautions

Sparse data sets are suitable for neither parametric nor nonparametric analysis; more sophisticated exact significance tests must be used. Fisher's exact test is a well-known exact procedure for two by two contingency tables. Exact tests for other situations require special computer software.[28]

COMMON STATISTICAL DECEPTIONS

Over a century ago, Benjamin Disraeli noted: ''There are three kinds of lies: lies, damn lies and statistics.'' Although such consummate skepticism is rarely justified, statistics can undoubtedly be misused—either by intent, or through ignorance or carelessness—to produce incorrect conclusions.[2] Because most physicians are either amateur statisticians, or have no recollection of statistics beyond bad memories in medical school, misuse is common. Reviews of clinical research indicate that about 50% of published articles contain statistical flaws serious enough to question the validity of the conclusions.

How does statistical misuse slip by editors, peer reviewers, and journal readers? Because of the ''dazzle'' phenomenon observed by Darrell Huff, author of *How to Lie with Statistics*: ''If you can't prove what you want to prove, demonstrate something else and pretend that they are the same thing. In the daze that follows the collision of statistics with the human mind, hardly anybody will notice the difference.''[22] Be particularly wary of the following dazzling phenomena (Table 20-14).

Standard error switcheroo

When you see results reported as ''mean value ± X'' don't assume that X is the SD unless specifically stated. Sometimes X is actually the standard error (SE), a number that is always smaller than SD. Actually, SD and SE are very different, so understanding why many authors report the latter is difficult, unless they are enamored by the smaller value. When describing a set of data, SD is always preferred, because it measures how variable individual observations are within a sample.[8] If the data have a symmetric distribution, the mean ± 2 SD describes about 95% of observations. In contrast, the SE is an inferential, not a descriptive, statistic; it measures how variable the mean is from one sample to another.

Consider a study of 25 patients undergoing rhinoplasty that reports a mean blood loss of 150 ± 30 ml where 30 is the SD. We now know that 95% of subjects had a blood loss of 150 ± 60 ml (assuming the data are normally distributed). To obtain the SE, we divide the SD by the square root of the sample size. In this example the square root is 5, giving the SE five times smaller than the SD: 6 versus 30. The mean blood loss now is written as 150 ± 6 ml, where 6 is the SE. Obviously this ''looks'' better than the SD, but what exactly does it mean? It means ''based on our results, if we extrapolate to the general population of rhinoplasty patients, we estimate with 95% confidence that the mean blood loss will be 150 ± 12 ml.'' This statement no longer describes the study data, but makes an inference about some hypothetical population. Unless the authors clearly state that this is their intent, the SD should have been used.

Small sample whitewash

Because medical research is costly and time consuming, we rarely have the luxury of studying large samples. Fortu-

Table 20-14. Statistical deceptions used in journal articles

Deception	Problem	Solution
Standard error is used instead of standard deviation	Range is artificially low, making data look better than they are	Always use standard deviation when summarizing data
Small sample study results are taken at face value	Results are imprecise and would likely vary if study were repeated; uncertainty is ignored	Determine the range of results consistent with data by using a 95% confidence interval
Post hoc P values are used for statistical inference	Statistical tests are valid only when hypotheses are formulated prior to examining the data	*Post hoc P* values must be viewed as hypothesis-generating, not hypothesis-testing
Some results are "significant" but there are too many *P* values to count in a lifetime	"Significant" results may be false-positives because each *P* value has a 5% error rate*	Reduce the number of *P* values through multivariate analysis or analysis of variance
Subgroups are compared until statistically significant results are found	If you torture the data sufficiently, they will eventually confess to something	Subgroup comparisons are valid only when all groups as a whole are significantly different
No significant difference is found between groups in a small sample study	A significant difference may have been missed because of inadequate sample size	Be sure the authors discuss power and sample size before believing study results
Significant *P* values are crafted through improper use of hypothesis tests	Small studies with asymmetrically distributed data require special methods of analysis	Don't believe results unless a nonparametric or exact statistical test was used

* Assuming that .05 is selected as the level of statistical significance.

nately, we can derive meaningful conclusions from small samples by estimating uncertainty (precision) with a 95% confidence interval. Remember, statistics is the art and science of dealing with uncertain data; the smaller the sample, the greater the uncertainty. Beware when authors claim their sample is "too small for statistical analysis;" that is when they need it most.

For example, while perusing the *Journal of Low Budget Research* an article on an innovative new surgical procedure captures your attention. The authors operate successfully on four of four elephants (100% success rate) and conclude that "testing in humans is indicated based on these superb results." Do you agree? Actually, the range of results (95% confidence interval) consistent with this single experiment on four elephants is 47% to 100%![28] Knowing that the "true" success rate may be as low as 47% you may now disagree with the need for human testing. Conversely, if the investigators succeeded in 40 of 40 elephants, the 95% confidence interval would be 93% to 100%, a much greater level of confidence, secondary to the tenfold increase in sample size.

Post hoc *P* values

A fundamental assumption underlying all statistical tests is that the hypothesis under study was fully developed before the data were examined in any way. When hypotheses are formulated *post hoc*—after even the briefest glance at the data—the basis for probability statements is invalidated. Unfortunately, we have no way of knowing at which stage of the research process a hypothesis was developed. Therefore,

unless the investigators state specifically that the test was planned *a priori*, you should infer with caution.

As physician-friendly computer programs for statistical analysis continue to proliferate, more physicians are likely to analyze their own data. Unless the probability framework underlying hypothesis tests is understood and appreciated (habits three and four), the risk of *post hoc P* values will increase dramatically as they become easier to produce. When the primary research purpose is to test an *a priori* hypothesis, the *P* value will aid in statistical inference. When hypotheses are generated after the study, however, *P* values cannot be used to make inferences. Instead, they become a means of identifying promising associations that might form the new *a priori* hypotheses in a follow-up investigation.

Multiple *P* value phenomenon

P values have a momentum of their own; once you start churning them out, it's hard to stop (especially if you have a nifty computer program that chums them out for you). When you see a journal article or data table that is chock full of *P* values, realize that some "significant" *P* values ($P < .05$) are likely to occur by chance alone.[6] Consider, for example, a researcher who performs 20 individual hypothesis tests on a group of observations (e.g., calculates 20 *P* values). If we assume that the subjects studied do not differ beyond random variation, there is only a 36% chance that none of the *P* values will be significant! Furthermore, the chance of getting one, two, or three, significant *P* values is 38%, 19%, and 6%, respectively.

What accounts for the multiple *P* value phenomenon?

The problem arises because each test is based on a cut-off of $P < .05$ as a measure of significance; the effect of performing multiple tests is to inflate this 5% error level for the study as a whole. The probability of getting at least one spurious result is: $1-(1-\alpha)^n$ where α is the level of significance for each individual test (generally .05) and n is number of tests performed.

Multiple P values can arise when pairwise comparisons are made between several groups of data, or when numerous hypothesis tests are applied to a single data set. When several groups are compared, ANOVA overcomes the multiple P value problem created by repeated t-tests. Furthermore, special multiple comparison tests are available with ANOVA that can search for subgroup differences provided a global difference exists between groups. When a single data set is being studied, multivariate analysis will eliminate the multiple P value problem induced by repeated univariate tests (e.g., t-test, chi-square).

Selective analysis of results

Check for selective analysis of results in every study that compares three or more groups of subjects, including animal research. Authors may pluck out a few groups for pairwise comparisons and then pontificate on the "statistically significant" findings they discover. Unfortunately, this violates a basic tenet of statistics: you cannot compare subgroups of your data unless you first check for statistically significant differences between all groups considered simultaneously. For categorical data, a chi-square is first calculated for the entire contingency table; if $P < .05$, the authors can then extract subsets of the table for selective analysis provided they adjust for multiple comparisons. For continuous data, ANOVA should be used (not multiple pairwise t-tests) as described previously.

Powerless equalities

Some authors would like to convince you that a new treatment or diagnostic test is equivalent to an established standard. In particular, support for the use of a new antibiotic or antihistamine often arises from a randomized trial claiming "no significant difference $(P > .05)$" from another drug. When interpreting these results, look not at the P value but at the statistical power; the size of the P value is pertinent only when a statistically significant result is given. Power tells you the probability that the investigators would have detected a true difference, given that one really existed. With small samples, power is usually inadequate $(< 80\%)$ to state confidently that the investigators didn't miss a real difference. Because very few articles calculate power you may need to calculate it yourself (habit four).

Nonparametric nihilism

When sample sizes are modest—less than 10 to 15 observations per group—a nonparametric hypothesis test should generally be used unless the authors specifically examine the data and determine that they have symmetric distribution. However, despite the small and asymmetrically distributed samples common in clinical research, only 7% of articles from 1989 in otolaryngology journals contained nonparametric methods.[36]

Using a garden variety t-test for small samples with an asymmetric distribution can produce deceptive results through artificially low P values. Even a single outlier (data that differs markedly from the rest of the values) can invalidate a parametric test result. In general, beware of conclusions drawn from small data sets analyzed with conventional parametric tests. Although nonparametric tests provide more meaningful results under these circumstances, very sparse data (less than five observations per group) require more complicated exact techniques for analysis.[28]

UNDERSTANDING SAMPLE SIZE

As noted throughout this chapter, the number of observations in a data set (sample size) must be taken into account when interpreting results. Small samples may produce low precision, inadequate statistical power, and asymmetric distributions requiring nonparametric or exact techniques for proper analysis. Large samples offer high precision, but can waste resources and make results of trivial clinical importance appear statistically significant. Recognizing these problems, the American Academy of Otolaryngology—Head & Neck Surgery Foundation has made a sample size calculation a mandatory component of all grant applications for research funding. This section will summarize the essential concepts of sample size calculations in a nontechnical format.

A sample size calculation before beginning a study ensures that the planned number of observations will offer a reasonable chance of obtaining a clear answer at the end.[16] This is of paramount importance in animal studies, where sample size is limited by financial constraints, concerns over animal welfare, and limited laboratory space.[27] For example, a ground-breaking experiment in 10 giraffes is of little value when a sample size of 20 is needed for adequate power or precision. Similarly, why experiment on 200 chinchillas when only 100 are adequate to test an hypothesis? Such considerations are by no means limited to basic science studies. Why devote endless hours to abstracting data from 500 patient charts when only 150 observations may be needed?

The basic ingredients needed in a statistical recipe of sample size vary slightly according to the measurement scale (see Table 20-6). Ingredients common to all scales include estimates of (1) the smallest difference you want to be able to detect between the groups, (2) how confident you must be that any difference you detect is not simply due to chance (typically 95% or 99%), and (3) how confident you must be that you can detect a difference as small as what was specified earlier (typically 80% or 90%), assuming that such a difference truly exists. In addition, sample size calculations for numerical data require some estimate of the variability (variance) among observations.

Determining the minimally important difference you wish to detect is based solely on clinical judgment. When comparing categorical data, the difference of interest is between proportions (rate difference, see Table 20-7). For example, you may wish to know if success rates for two drugs differ by at least 20% for otitis media, but a difference of perhaps 5% may be important when treating cancer. In contrast, differences in numerical data are expressed as a difference in means. For example, you may wish to know if a potentially ototoxic drug decreases mean hearing by at least 5 dB, or if a new surgical technique decreases blood loss by at least 200 ml.

Outcomes measured on a numerical scale require an estimate of variance to calculate sample size. Because variance is defined as the square of the SD, we need a method to estimate SD to derive variance. If pilot data are available, some estimate of SD may already exist. Alternatively, you can "guess" the SD by realizing that the mean value ± 2 SD typically encompasses 95% of the observations. In other words, the SD of a set of measurements can be approximated as one fourth of the range of that set of measurements. Suppose you are interested in detecting a 200 ml difference in blood loss between two procedures, and based on your clinical experience expect that about 95% of the time you will see a difference ranging from 100 ml and 500 ml. Subtracting 100 from 500 and dividing by 4 gives 100 as an estimate of SD. Squaring the SD yields 10,000, which estimates variance.

The remaining elements of a sample size calculation reflect basic principles of statistical error (habit four). Recognizing that errors are unavoidable (see Table 20-8), we specify in advance our levels of tolerance and then calculate a sample size that will accomplish this goal. Tolerating a 5% probability of type I error (false-positive) is the same as being 95% certain that any difference you detect is not simply due to chance. Tolerating a 20% probability of a type II error (false-negative) is the same as being 80% certain that you do not miss a true difference of the magnitude already specified (80% statistical power).

The size of the sample needed in a given study will increase when the difference of interest is small, the variance of the observations is high (applies to numerical data only, not proportions), and the tolerance for error is low. More subjects are also required to determine if any difference at all exists between groups (two-tailed statistical test) than if one group fares either better or worse than another (one-tailed statistical test). A two-tailed test is considered more conservative, and should always be used unless it was determined *a priori*—before examining the data—that a one-tailed test was appropriate. A one-tailed test requires about half the sample size as a two-tailed test to show significance, and produces P values about half as small when applied to the data.

Sample size calculations may be performed manually,[7,11,16] with nomograms,[27,40] or with a computer program.[20] A computer program is optimal because of the flexibility in seeing how different assumptions alter results. Specific formulae are required based on whether the samples are independent or related, the number of groups involved, and the measurement scale of the data (note the similarity to selecting a statistical test, Tables 20-9 and 20-10). When the research purpose is to demonstrate that groups are equivalent (e.g., to prove the null hypothesis), sample size requirements increase and special formulae apply.[3] Special formulae also apply to regression analysis, although a rough guide is that 10 subjects with the outcome of interest are required for each predictor variable included in the model.

PUTTING PRINCIPLES INTO PRACTICE

My goal throughout this chapter has been to convince you that effective interpretation of medical data involves much more than statistics or numerical formulae. Rather, it is a systematic process of moving from observations to generalizations with predictable degrees of certainty (and uncertainty). Every physician is involved in this process to some extent, whether a solo practitioner in a rural community, or a full-time academician in a large university. Moving from observations to generalizations is the foundation for all scientific progress, a foundation that could not exist without a systematic process for interpreting data.

The seven habits listed in Table 20-1 provide a systematic framework for interpreting data, of which statistical tests are only a small part. Although habit four—measure error with the right statistical test—generates P values, it is sandwiched between habits one through three and habits five through seven. P values are part of the process, but represent neither the beginning nor the end. We begin by verifying that the data are of sufficient quality and precision to merit statistical analysis (habits one through three). We end by seeking clinically significant findings that can be generalized beyond the study, and are consistent with prior knowledge and experience (habits five through seven). Obsession with P values, which has been called the "religion of statistics," may produce medical publications, but rarely achieves effective data interpretation.[39]

Every clinician need not be a statistician, but all should understand the fundamental principles of data analysis and interpretation. When understood and applied, the habits in Table 20-1 will permit intelligent, synergistic dialogue between clinicians and statisticians. Such dialogue ideally precedes any serious research endeavor, because even the most elegant statistics cannot adjust for biased data or confounders that were never measured.[15] The statistician excels at analyzing data the right way, but the clinician's leadership ensures that the right data are analyzed. Furthermore, clinical importance (habit five) is best determined by clinicians, not statisticians.

Having hopefully lit the fires of inferential desire, I will end by summarizing some good sources of firewood. *A Dictionary of Epidemiology* by Last[24] is an indispensable companion to reading the medical literature and understanding statistical terms. Dawson-Saunders and Trapp[11] provide a delightfully palatable overview of research methodology and biostatistics in *Basic & Clinical Biostatistics. Making Sense of Data* by Abramson[1] is a useful self-instruction manual on association, causation, odds ratios, and other rates and measures. Light and Pillemer[26] offer an engaging and lucid overview of research review in their classic book, *Summing Up*. Finally, a clinically oriented statistical program such as TRUE EPISTAT (Epistat Services, Richardson, Tx) will give you hands-on experience through its superb tutorial and physician-friendly approach to data interpretation.

REFERENCES

1. Abramson JH: *Making sense of data: a self-instructional manual on the interpretation of epidemiological data,* New York, 1988, Oxford University Press.
2. Bailar JC III: Science, statistics, and deception, *Ann Intern Med* 104:259, 1986.
3. Blackwelder WC, Chang MA: Sample size graphs for "proving the null hypothesis," *Control Clin Trials* 5:97, 1984.
4. Borenstein M: The case for confidence intervals in controlled clinical trials, *Control Clin Trials* 15:411, 1994.
5. Brown GW: 2 × 2 tables, *Am J Dis Child* 139:410, 1985.
6. Brown GW: Errors, types I and II, *Am J Dis Child* 137:58, 1983.
7. Brown GW: Sample size, *Am J Dis Child* 142:1213, 1988.
8. Brown GW: Standard deviation, standard error: which 'standard' should we use? *Am J Dis Child* 136:937, 1982.
9. Covey RC: *The seven habits of highly effective people,* New York, 1989, Fireside.
10. Datta M: You cannot exclude the explanation you have not considered, *Lancet* 342:345, 1993.
11. Dawson-Sanders B, Trapp RG: *Basic & clinical biostatistics,* ed 2, Norwalk, Conn, 1994, Appleton & Lange.
12. Feinstein AR: Epidemiologic analyses of causation: the unlearned scientific lessons of randomized trials, *J Clin Epidemiol* 42:481, 1989.
13. Feinstein AR: Fraud, distortion, delusion, and consensus: the problems of human and natural deception in epidemiologic science, *Am J Med* 84:475, 1988.
14. Feinstein AR: Median and inner-percentile range: an improved summary for scientific communication, *J Chron Dis* 40:283, 1987.
15. Finney DJ: The questioning statistician, *Stat Med* 1:5, 1982.
16. Florey C: Sample size for beginners, *BMJ* 306:1181, 1993.
17. Gardner MJ, Altman DG: Confidence intervals rather than p values: estimation rather than hypothesis testing, *BMJ* 292:746, 1980.
18. Godfrey KAM: Comparing the means of several groups, *N Engl J Med* 313:1450, 1985.
19. Gray-Donald K, Kramer MS: Causality inference in observational vs.
experimental studies: an empirical comparison, *Am J Epidemiol* 127:885, 1988.
20. Gustafson TL: *TRUE EPISTAT reference manual,* Richardson, Tex, 1994, Epistat Services.
21. Hill AB: The environment and disease: association or causation, *Proc R Soc Med* 58:295, 1965.
22. Huff D: *How to lie with statistics,* New York, 1954, WW Norton.
23. Kaleida PH and others: Amoxicillin or myringotomy or both for acute otitis media: results of a randomized clinical trial, *Pediatrics* 87:466, 1991.
24. Last JM: *A Dictionary of epidemiology,* ed 3, New York, 1995, Oxford University Press.
25. Laupacis A, Sackett DL, Roberts RS: An assessment of clinically useful measures of the consequences of treatment, *N Engl J Med* 318:1728, 1988.
26. Light RJ, Pillemer DB: *Summing up: the science of reviewing research,* Cambridge, Mass, 1984, Harvard University Press.
27. Mann MD, Crouse DA, Prentice ED: Appropriate animal numbers in biomedical research in light of animal welfare considerations, *Lab Animal Sci* 41:6, 1991.
28. Mehta C, Patel N: *StatXact: statistical software for exact nonparametric inference,* Cambridge, Mass, 1991, Cytel Software Corporation.
29. Moses LE: The series of consecutive cases as a device for assessing outcome of intervention, *N Engl J Med* 311:705, 1984.
30. Rosenfeld RM: Clinical research in otolaryngology journals, *Arch Otolaryngol Head Neck Surg* 117:164, 1991.
31. Rosenfeld RM: How to systematically review the medical literature, *Otolaryngol Head Neck Surg* 115:53, 1996.
32. Rosenfeld RM: What to expect from medical treatment of otitis media, *Pediatr Infect Dis J* 14:731, 1995.
33. Rosenfeld RM, Bluestone CD: Does early expansion surgery have a role in the management of congenital subglottic stenosis?, *Laryngoscope* 103:286, 1993.
34. Rosenfeld RM and others: Third generation cephalosporins in the treatment of acute pneumococcal otitis media: an animal study, *Arch Otolaryngol Head Neck Surg* 118:49, 1992.
35. Rosenfeld RM, Moura RL, Bluestone CD: Predictors of residual-recurrent cholesteatoma in children, *Arch Otolaryngol Head Neck Surg* 106:378, 1992.
36. Rosenfeld RM, Rockette HE: Biostatistics in otolaryngology journals, *Arch Otolaryngol Head Neck Surg* 117:1172, 1991.
37. Sackett DL: Bias in analytic research, *J Chron Dis* 32:51, 1979.
38. Sackett DL: A primer on the precision and accuracy of the clinical examination, *JAMA* 267:2638, 1992.
39. Salsburg DS: The religion of statistics as practiced in medical journals, *Am Stat* 39:220, 1985.
40. Young NJ, Bresnitz EA, Strom BL. Sample size nomograms for interpreting negative clinical studies, *Ann Intern Med* 99:248, 1983.
41. Thomas DG, Gart JJ: A table of exact confidence limits for differences and ratios of two proportions and their odds ratios, *J Am Stat Assoc* 72:73, 1977.
42. Turner JA and others: The importance of placebo effects in pain treatment and research, *JAMA* 271:1609, 1994.

PART TWO

FACE

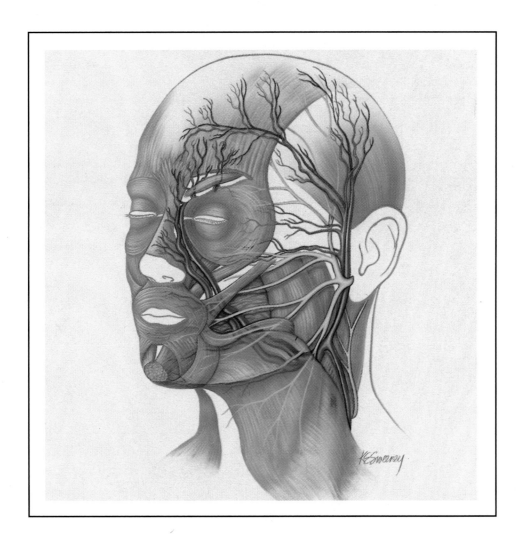

Chapter 21

Anatomy

Daniel O. Graney
Shan R. Baker

In this first chapter on anatomy a few remarks are appropriate regarding the general approach to the anatomy of the head and neck that is used in this and subsequent chapters. In each chapter the essential anatomic terms, relations, and concepts of the particular topographic region are reviewed. The goal of these chapters is to provide a reasonable review of the pertinent anatomy rather than duplicate existing encyclopedic texts of anatomy. It follows, therefore, that the definition of ''essential'' is the individual author's, and that the reader may find certain subjects fragmentary or omitted.

FACIAL MUSCLES

The muscles of the face differ from the usual concept of muscles as joint movers. The role of the facial muscles is to move the skin and in effect regulate the apertures of the orbit, nasal cavity, and oral cavity. A simplified view is that one end of the muscle is attached to bone and the other is attached to skin. This arrangement produces tension lines on the skin that are directed at right angles to the plane of the muscle fiber. These tension lines (Langer's cleavage lines) deepen with the aging process as the skin loses its elasticity. Obvious examples are the ''frown lines'' of the forehead, the nasolabial fold, and the ''crow's feet'' of the orbital region. These cleavage lines can provide camouflage for surgical incisions or in fact may be the reason for the surgery.

Scalp and forehead

The scalp contains a series of muscles that allow it to be moved in an upward or downward direction. Movement of the skin of the forehead in this manner functions to serve as shading for the eyes, such as in squinting or in elevating the skin during upward gaze. For these purposes the following muscles are located within the scalp: the frontal and occipital bellies of the occipitofrontal muscle and the corrugator supercilii (Fig. 21-1). The frontal belly fibers of the occipitofrontal muscle have no bony attachment. They are continuous with the procerus, corrugator, and orbicularis oculi. The fibers are directed vertically, thinning before inserting into an aponeurosis termed the *galea aponeurotica*, which they share with the occipital belly fibers. The occipital belly arises from bone and periosteum along the superior nuchal line before its fibers join into the aponeurosis.

The occipital frontal muscles acting together draw the scalp backward, raising the eyebrows and wrinkling the forehead. The frontal bellies, acting alone, raise the eyebrows.

The other muscle of this region, the corrugator supercilii, arises from the orbital rim near the medial canthus and then directs its fibers superiorly and laterally to insert into the deep surface of the frontal belly of the occipitofrontal muscle (Fig. 21-2). Contraction of the corrugator supercilii draws the brow medially, producing the oblique frown lines over the glabellar region. During forehead lifts, a section of this muscle is resected in an attempt to reduce or eliminate the glabellar frown lines. Likewise, the central portion of the frontal belly fibers of the occipital frontal muscle, located between the two supraorbital nerves, is frequently sectioned in a grid-like pattern to weaken this portion of the muscle for the purpose of reducing the horizontal creases of the forehead.

The other small muscles in the scalp relate to the ear, and because they are not important, they are not considered in this chapter. Another aspect of the scalp, however, that is germane to the otolaryngologist is the layering of the scalp tissues. The letters of the word *scalp* are a familiar acronym to medical students for remembering the five individual layers of the scalp structure: skin, connective tissue, aponeuro-

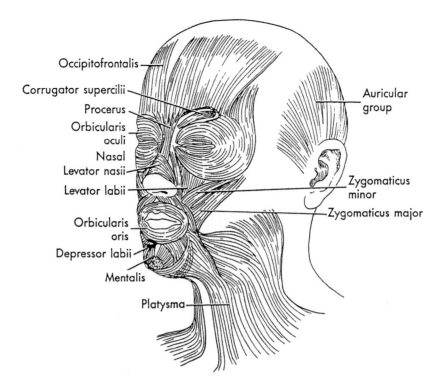

Fig. 21-1. Scalp and facial mimetic muscles.

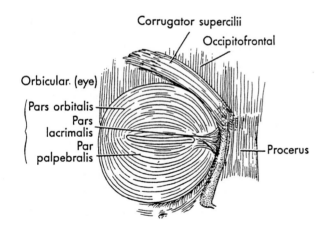

Fig. 21-2. Corrugator supercilii arises from orbital rim and inserts superiorly and laterally into the frontal belly of occipitofrontal muscle.

sis, loose connective tissue, and periosteum. The first three layers of the scalp—the skin, dense connective tissue, and aponeurosis—do not readily separate. The majority of blood vessels and cutaneous nerves are located in the dense connective tissue space superficial to the galea aponeurotica. An important exception to this rule is the origin of the supraorbital and supratrochlear neurovascular bundle at the rim of the orbit. As these vessels emerge from the orbit, they must traverse the loose connective space and galea aponeurotica before penetrating into the dense connective tissue

plane. At this point they are vulnerable during brow- or forehead-lifting procedures. Similarly, lacerations of the brow at the supraorbital rim may result in anesthetized areas of the scalp when the supraorbital or supratrochlear nerves are severed. These nerves are cutaneous and have no role in the innervation of the scalp muscles, which are supplied by branches of the seventh cranial nerve (CN VII). These are discussed in the following section after the description of the facial muscles.

Separation of the scalp from the skull in avulsion injuries usually occurs at the plane of the loose connective tissue layer. The term *danger space* as applied to the loose connective tissue layer refers not to this particular traumatic event but to the fact that infection may spread readily in this space and be subsequently transmitted intracranially by emissary veins.

Orbital region and eyelid

The orbicular eye muscle, a series of concentric rings, originates either from the medial palpebral ligament or from bone on the medial orbital wall. Three parts of the muscle are usually described: the large orbital region, which covers the superior and inferior limits of the orbit; the palpebral part, which is adjacent to the upper or lower eyelids, and the lacrimal portion attached to the posterior lacrimal crest. Closure of the entire orbital region and lid is accomplished by coordinated contraction of the entire muscle group, whereas blinking is limited to the palpebral region of the muscle covering the lid. The palpebral portion of the muscle passes posterior to the medial palpebral ligament adjacent to the lacrimal sac (see Fig. 21-2). When the eye is closed, these fibers can exert traction on the lacrimal sac, serving as a pump to aid in the drainage of the tears.[2,3] The orbital portion is attached to the skin where it broadens over the anterior temporal and malar region. These skin attachments give rise in the aging face to the radially oriented skin creases known as *crow's feet*. The palpebral portion does not attach to the overlying skin or underlying orbital septum, but rather is separated from these structures by a layer of areolar connective tissue. This relationship accounts for the ease in developing a cutaneous or musculocutaneous flap during blepharoplasty.

The eyelid is best viewed structurally from a sagittal section, which illustrates the central tarsal region versus the peripheral septal region (Fig. 21-3). In the central part of the upper lid just above the margin of the eyelash, the layers of the eyelid are skin, orbicular eye muscle, tarsal plate, and conjunctival sac. More peripherally the layers are skin, orbicular eye muscle, orbital septum, preaponeurotic space, levator aponeurosis, postaponeurotic space, superior tarsal muscle, and conjunctival layer. Three muscles, therefore, are represented in the upper lid. The orbicular eye muscle is a striated muscle supplied by CN VII, which is responsible for lid closure. The levator palpebrae superioris muscle, also striated, functions to elevate the upper lid and is supplied by CN III. In contrast, the superior tarsal muscle is smooth muscle supplied by the sympathetic nervous system and has only a minor role in supporting the lid. Nevertheless, loss of function in either CN III or the sympathetic nervous system can result in ptosis of the upper lid.

The pathway of sympathetic fibers to the superior tarsal muscle begins in the lateral gray matter of the spinal cord at the level of T1. These preganglionic fibers pass through the first thoracic spinal nerve and its white ramus communicantes. After entering the sympathetic trunk, the preganglionic fibers ascend in the cervical chain, where they synapse in the superior cervical sympathetic ganglion. Postganglionic fibers form a plexus on the surface of the internal carotid artery and in this way are distributed via branches of the internal carotid system (ophthalmic artery) ultimately to the superior tarsal muscle in the upper eyelid.

Interruption of these fibers along any point from the spinal cord to the point of innervation of the muscle will result in ptosis and myosis, which are part of Horner's syndrome. The additional clinical findings of Horner's syndrome, anhidrosis and vasodilatation of the ipsilateral face, occur only if the fibers are disrupted in the neck at the level of the superior cervical sympathetic ganglion. Metastatic masses, whether derived from primary tumors in the head and neck or thorax (e.g., Pancoast's tumor of the lung), can erode the sympathetic trunk and cause Horner's syndrome. Likewise, trauma or surgery performed in the vicinity of the sympathetic cervical ganglion can produce a similar finding.

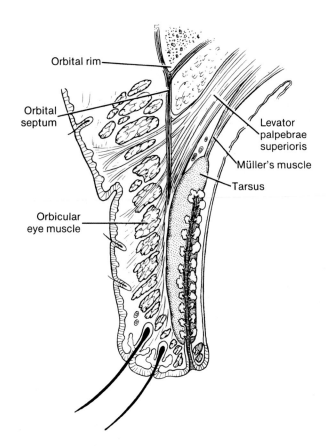

Fig. 21-3. The sagittal section of an eyelid illustrating central tarsal region.

In contrast, CN III palsy, while also producing ptosis, results in mydriasis because of the loss of the constrictor pupili muscle. The severity of ptosis is usually gravest with CN III palsy, whereas in Horner's syndrome it is more moderate. In fact, in some cases it is almost imperceptible.

The levator palpebrae superioris extends foward from the lesser wing of the sphenoid to form a broad aponeurosis that attaches to the entire anterior surface of the tarsal plate of the upper eyelid. At the junction of the levator's muscle belly with its aponeurosis, two "check ligaments" are formed by thickenings of the connective tissue sheath of the muscle. These ligaments assist in tensing the levator at the level of the supratarsal fold, thus creating the fold.

Clinically, the septum orbitale is a particularly important structure in that it represents a line of continuity between periosteum and periorbita, and technically separates the intraorbital contents from the extraorbital structures. Preseptal infections of the eyelid are known as *periorbital cellulitis*, and are more common and less serious than postseptal orbital cellulitis. However, preseptal infections may expand posteriorly through the septum to produce orbital cellulitis and abscess formation, resulting in rapid deterioration of vision and even complete, permanent blindness. The orbital septum also represents an important landmark for the cosmetic surgeon performing blepharoplasties in that the septum must be penetrated to remove orbital fat where required as part of the surgical procedure. In the case of upper lid blepharoplasty, the surgeon must take care in removing the fat located between the orbital septum and the levator aponeurosis so as not to injure the latter structure, causing iatrogenic ptosis.

Nose

The muscles of the nose include the procerus muscle and the nasal muscle. The procerus muscle is a small muscle overlying the bridge of the nose and in part continuous with the frontal belly fibers of the occipitofrontal muscle. This muscle actually works with the frontal belly fibers in drawing the skin of the forehead downward during the act of squinting. Because of its vertically arranged muscle fibers, it forms transverse frown lines in the skin between the eyes. During rhinoplasty, avulsion of the procerus muscle is sometimes performed in attempts to deepen the nasofrontal angle.

The nasal muscle is frequently described as having two portions: a transverse portion and an alar portion. The transverse fibers, also termed the *compressor naris*, form an inverted U over the bridge of the nose. As the name implies, these fibers compress the naris by compressing or flexing the upper lateral nasal cartilage at its joint with the alar or lower lateral nasal cartilage. Dilatation of the naris is accomplished by the alar portion, which elevates the lower lateral or alar cartilage.

Mouth region (cheek and lips)

The buccinator muscle arises from the pterygomandibular raphe and the tuberosity of the maxilla. The fibers of the muscle cross anteriorly in the substance of the cheek and then blend at the corner of the mouth with the fibers of the orbicular mouth muscle. The essential function of the bucinator muscle is to maintain food between the teeth during the masticatory process. In this regard, it is more a muscle of mastication than a muscle of facial expression. Tension in this muscle also maintains the cheek against the teeth when one forcibly blows into a wind instrument, such as a trumpet, and thus prevents the cheeks from "ballooning out."

The buccal space is located immediately lateral to the buccal muscle, and includes the buccal fat pad and the parotid duct. The space is limited above by the attachment of the buccal muscle to the alveolar process of the maxilla, and below by the attachment to the mandible. In most adults, the molar apices are not beyond the muscle attachments, so that an apical abscess presents in the oral vestibule medial to the muscle. In contrast, younger individuals frequently have tooth roots that extend beyond the muscle attachment. Apical abscess formation in these individuals, as well as in adults with exceptionally long roots, often will result in extension of the infective process to the buccal space. Infections ascending along the parotid duct toward the gland from the mouth can also involve the buccal space. Patients with an abscess of the buccal space may present with marked swelling of the cheek without abnormalities visible intraorally.

The muscles of the lips include the orbicular mouth muscle, which is primarily a contractor or constrictor of the mouth region, and several muscles that open the mouth by elevating or depressing the lip. The orbicular mouth muscle is a series of concentric rings surrounding the mouth, which, when contracted, purse the lips. Many of the fibers interlace with the buccinator muscle, as well as with muscles that elevate or depress the lip. Elevation of the upper lip is accomplished by either the levator labii or the levator anguli oris muscle. The levator labii muscle elevates the lip itself, whereas the levator anguli oris muscle moves the angle of the lip. A complementary pair of muscles is found in the lower lip: the depressor labii and depressor anguli oris muscles.

The elevators of the lip arise from the infraorbital portion of the maxilla, whereas the depressors arise from the anterior aspect of the body of the mandible. The muscle fibers of the buccinator muscle, orbicular mouth muscle, and the elevators and depressors of the lip are substantially interlaced. The greater and lesser zygomatic muscles are located more superficially than the levators of the lip. Both the greater and lesser zygomatic muscles arise from the zygomatic bone lateral to the infraorbital foramen. The lesser zygomatic attaches into the orbicular mouth muscle near the ala of the nose, whereas the greater zygomatic attaches at the corner of the mouth. Both are elevators of the lip, although the lesser zygomatic muscle is important in producing the melolabial fold.

Chin and neck

The mentalis (levator labii inferioris) is a flat band of fibers arising from the mandible near the roots of the incisors and inserting into the skin near the midline. The action of these fibers is to tense the skin of the chin as well as aid in protruding the lower lip.

Although the platysma may be thought of as a muscle of the neck region, it is in fact part of the facial musculature. The muscle arises from the inferior margin of the body of the mandible as a broad sheet from the mental symphysis anteriorly, to the area of the parotid gland at the angle of the mandible. The fibers descend over the neck, crossing the clavicle superficially and inserting into the skin over the upper portion of the breast area. The platysma is an important landmark for many surgical procedures performed in the region of the upper neck, such as facelift surgery and excision of the submandibular gland. In this region the mandibular branch of the facial nerve is located immediately deep to the muscle.

FACIAL NERVE AND INNERVATION OF THE FACIAL MUSCLES

The muscles discussed previously, from the occipitofrontal to the platysma, are supplied by CN VII, the facial nerve. The embryologic origin of these muscles is from mesodermal components in the second branchial arch. The position of this arch in the embryo is adjacent to the developing brainstem and the emerging nerve fibers, which will become CN VII. Axons growing from cell bodies in the motor nucleus of CN VII innervate the primitive muscle cells in the second branchial arch. Regardless of the migration of these future muscle cells, whether cranial or caudal to their original position in the branchial arch, the basic pattern of innervation by CN VII is thus established.

Because a sensory element accompanies CN VII, mostly taste fibers that are distributed to the tongue, neural crest cells become associated with the developing CN VII. These cells send central processes into the brainstem to synapse with neurons in the nucleus solitarius. Peripheral processes growing from these same neural crest cells join with the motor fibers to be distributed to taste buds in the oral cavity. In this manner, the neural crest cells form the geniculate ganglion of CN II, a homologue of the sensory dorsal root ganglion of the spinal nerves.

The intracranial course of the facial nerve within the temporal bone is discussed in Chapter 132, and a discussion of the nervus intermedius appears in Chapter 63. Innervation of the lacrimal gland by the great petrosal branch of the geniculate ganglion is discussed in Chapter 40.

CN VII exits the skull via the stylomastoid foramen. The first branch to arise from CN VII after it emerges from the stylomastoid foramen is the posterior auricular nerve. This nerve courses inferior to the auricle, ascending superficially on the mastoid process to supply eventually the occipital belly of the occipitofrontal muscle. In relation to the auricle, some sensory fibers may supply the skin of the external auditory meatus. The evidence for this is the clinical presentation of vesicles in herpes zoster oticus (Ramsay-Hunt syndrome). Also arising from the major trunk of CN VII in this region are direct motor branches to the posterior belly of the diagastric muscle and to the stylohyoid muscle. The remaining trunk of CN VII forms two or three divisions with five major branches: temporal, zygomatic, buccal, mandibular, and cervical (Fig. 21-4).

The temporal branch of CN VII arises from the anterior aspect of the parotid gland and courses superficial to the zygomatic arch. It provides motor innervation to the frontal belly of the occipitofrontal muscle, as well as to the orbicular eye muscle and the corrugator supercilii muscle. The zygomatic branch ascends to the lateral canthus, where it also supplies the orbicular eye muscle and forms an anastomotic network with the temporal branch. The buccal branch crosses transversely on the face to supply the central muscles of the face, including the greater and lesser zygomatic muscles, the levator anguli oris and levator labii superioris muscles, and all the small muscles associated with the surface of the nose. The buccal branch overlaps with the zygomatic branch in its supply of muscles in the central part of the face. Principally, it supplies the buccinator muscle and the orbicular eye muscle. The mandibular branch (marginal

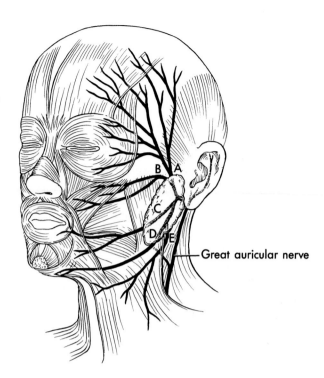

Fig. 21-4. The branches of a facial nerve: *A,* temporal; *B,* zygomatic; *C,* buccal; *D,* mandibular; *E,* cervical.

mandibular) crosses inferior to the angle of the mandible into the submandibular triangle and then ascends, crossing the mandible a second time to supply the muscles over the surface of the chin. The cervical branch of CN VII emerges from the inferior tip of the the parotid gland, following the deep surface of the platysma muscle, which it innervates.

In review, three areas of CN VII may be delineated on a general topographic basis: an intraparotid portion, an exposed area, and a submuscular portion. Clearly, the most vulnerable part of CN VII is the part between the parotid gland and the muscles it innervates. Dissection superficial to either the parotid fascia or superficial to any of the facial muscles is a safe plane with respect to the branches of CN VII.

As the individual branches leave the substance of the parotid gland and course distal to the muscles, they gain an increasingly superficial plane in relation to the skin. For instance, the area where the temporal branch crosses the zygomatic arch represents the most superficial location of any of the major divisions of the facial nerve, and is considered a ''danger zone'' for facelift surgery. Terminals of the zygomatic branch at the point where they innervate the orbicular eye muscle are essentially at the level of the dermis. Even shallow incisions (for removal of moles, for example) may divide these nerves, producing paralysis of the orbicular eye muscle and an inability to close the eye. Another particularly vulnerable site is the region of the submandibular triangle. Although the mandibular branch of CN VII is under the cover of the platysma, the site is a common surgical approach to the submandibular gland. Interruption of the mandibular branch of CN VII results in an inability to depress the lower lip. In these patients the angle of the lip on the affected side is slightly elevated, whereas the lower portion of the lip on the affected side is pulled to the opposite side by tonic activity of the nonparalyzed muscles.

There are certain anatomic relationships between branches of CN VII and adjacent structures that are important to the surgeon performing parotidectomy, repairing cheek lacerations that have injured branches of the nerve, or performing other types of facial surgery. The zygomatic branch lies approximately 1 cm below the zygomatic arch in the region of the parotid gland, a fact that can be used as a guide in identifying this branch. The buccal branch crosses the parotid duct on its superficial surface, running from superior to inferior before turning anteriorly to be distributed to the facial musculature. By virtue of this relationship, injuries usually involve both structures concomitantly. The mandibular branch usually lies below the point at which the facial artery and vein emerge from the submandibular gland. In such instances, the commonly used maneuver in which the vascular structures are identified, divided, and elevated along with the overlying platysma and skin, does not represent a safe method of protecting the mandibular nerve. The nerve does, however, lie external to the fascial capsule of the submandibular gland and rarely extends below its inferior margin. Incising the capsular fascia at the inferior margin of the gland and elevating it along with the overlying tissues will provide protection for the nerve. The cervical branch of CN VII has an important relationship to the posterior division of the retromandibular vein, which, together with the posterior auricular vein, forms the external jugular vein. The nerve lies immediately on the lateral aspect of the posterior division of the retromandibular vein. Knowledge of this relationship can be used in performing retrograde dissection to the main trunk of CN VII. This is accomplished by identifying the external jugular vein, which is an easily located surgical landmark in the neck, and dissecting the vein upward to the posterior division of the retromandibular vein, at which point the cervical branch is encountered. The branch can be dissected retrograde to the inferior division of CN VII.

Lesions of the seventh cranial nerve

It is important to realize the differences between CN VII lesions that affect the upper motor neurons and those that involve the lower motor neurons. A lower motor neuron lesion is a deficit of the motor neuron in the CN VII nucleus or at any point distal to the nucleus. Thus, all motor branches, whether from the intracranial or facial parts of CN VII, would be affected. If the lesion is complete, a total hemiparesis of the face will result. Bell's palsy is an example of such a lesion, although in this case the site of injury is the bony facial canal in the temporal bone. In contrast, should a lesion affect the upper motor neuron at any point from the motor cortex or along the length of the axon before it synapses with the facial nucleus, a different set of physical findings will result. Paralysis as a result of this type of lesion spares the muscles of the upper portion of the face (that is, the orbicular eye and occipitofrontal muscles). However, the muscles of the central and lower portions of the face are paralyzed. This sparing occurs because the muscles of the upper part of the face receive motor supply from both cerebral cortices. Thus in a patient with a stroke lesion in the cerebral cortex or internal capsule, the orbicular eye and occipitofrontal muscles will be spared on the contralateral side because they receive secondary innervation from the ipsilateral cerebral cortex. Thus, the usual finding in stroke patients is paralysis of the muscles of the nose and mouth on the contralateral side of the cortical lesion.

CUTANEOUS FACIAL INNERVATION

A line projected from the tip of the chin to the vertex of the skull will define a plane in which the trigeminal nerve supplies all skin lying anterior to this plane. In contrast, the cervical plexus innervates all skin lying posterior to this plane (Fig. 21-5). The distribution of cervical fibers to the skin of the posterior aspect of the face and neck is discussed in Chapter 86. Distribution of trigeminal nerve fibers is topographically arranged according to the three divisions of the trigeminal. The ophthalmic division of the trigeminal supplies the forehead and bridge of the nose, the maxillary division supplies the area of the cheek, and the mandibular division supplies the area of skin overlying the mandible and the temporal region.

The ophthalmic division of the trigeminal begins at the semilunar ganglion of CN V in the middle cranial fossa. After traversing the cavernous sinus, it enters the orbital cavity through the supraorbital fissure. At this point it divides into several branches, some of which eventually reach the skin of the nose and periorbital region. The three subdivisions of the ophthalmic branch within the orbit are the lacrimal, the nasociliary, and the frontal. The lacrimal nerve follows along the lateral and superior wall of the orbit and supplies a small area of skin near the upper lateral portion of the eyelid. The nasociliary nerve supplies two areas of skin: one via the infratrochlear nerve to the skin near the medial canthus of the upper lid and the other via the external nasal branch to the skin over the bridge of the nose. The external nasal nerve is not a direct branch of the nasociliary nerve; rather, it is the terminal branch of the anterior ethmoidal nerve after it supplies the ethmoid sinuses. The lacrimal, infratrochlear, and external nasal nerves supply only small areas of skin on the face. The major area of skin in the periorbital and frontal regions is supplied via branches of the frontal nerve from the ophthalmic division. The frontal nerve is given off soon after the ophthalmic division enters the orbit. Traversing the superior part of the orbital wall, the frontal division divides into the supraorbital and supratrochlear nerves, which emerge from the orbit through the supra-

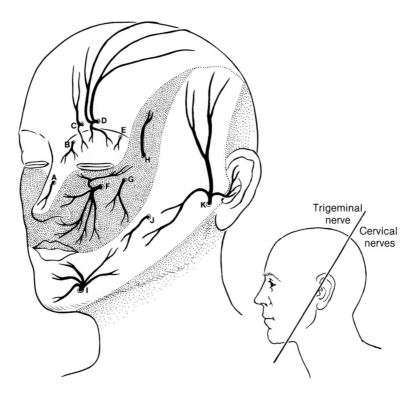

Fig. 21-5. The cutaneous branches of a trigeminal nerve: *A,* external nasal; *B,* infratrochlear; *C,* supratrochlear; *D,* supraorbital; *E,* lacrimal; *F,* infraorbital; *G,* zygomaticofacial; *H,* zygomaticotemporal; *I,* mental; *J,* buccal; *K,* auriculotemporal.

orbital notch. In some individuals the notch is closed to form a bony foramen. From this point the nerve pierces the loose connective tissue and aponeurotic layers of the scalp to travel upward in the dense connective tissue layer of the scalp.

The maxillary division of the trigeminal nerve begins at the semilunar ganglion and enters the orbital region via the round foramen. As it enters the floor of the orbit, a zygomatic branch is given off that abruptly subdivides into two branches: the zygomaticotemporal and the zygomaticofacial. These nerves supply skin over the temporal and malar regions, respectively. After the zygomatic branch is given off, the maxillary nerve enters the infraorbital groove and traverses the infraorbital canal, emerging on the face via the infraorbital foramen. At this point three named branches of the infraorbital nerve appear (see Fig. 21-5): the palpebral branch, which supplies the lower lid; the external nasal branch, which supplies the lateral and alar portions of the nasal skin; and the labial branch, which supplies the upper lid and cheek skin. In orbital blow-out fractures that disrupt the orbital floor, the zygomatic branch of the maxillary nerve is usually spared, because the injury is distal to its origin. However, the infraorbital branch of the maxillary nerve can be completely involved, leaving the patient with an anesthetized area over the lower lid, side of the nose, and upper lip and cheek. Furthermore, because the anterosuperior alveolar nerves arise from the infraorbital nerve, the anterior teeth (incisors and canines) are also numb. These nerves descend

from the infraorbital nerve through small bony canals located in the anterior wall of the maxillary sinus. Caldwell-Luc and other surgical procedures that remove part or all of the anterior wall of the maxillary sinus will result in some numbness of these teeth as well.

After leaving the semilunar ganglion, the mandibular nerve exits the middle cranial fossa via the oval foramen. Here the nerve enters the infratemporal fossa and divides into several named branches, three of which are important to the innervation of the face. One is the auriculotemporal nerve, which courses laterally around the neck of the mandible and ascends the side of the skull in the skin of the scalp anterior to the ear. In addition to being a sensory nerve, the auriculotemporal nerve carries both parasympathetic postganglionic fibers from the otic ganglion to the parotid gland, and sympathetic fibers distributed via the carotid artery to innervate sweat glands of the skin in the area of the nerve distribution. Parotidectomy results in division of some of the branches of the auriculotemporal nerve, and may give rise to faulty reinnervation of sweat gland secretomotor receptors by parotid gland secretomotor fibers, resulting in the auriculotemporal (Frey) syndrome of gustatory sweating.

The second important sensory branch of the mandibular nerve is the buccal branch, which traverses the infratemporal fossa and supplies part of the buccal mucosa, as well as the skin over the cheek region. The third branch is the inferior alveolar nerve, which, after entering the mandibular canal and supplying all of the mandibular teeth, emerges as the mental nerve, supplying skin over the point of the chin. While all of these nerves may be affected by lesions involving the proximal trunk of the mandibular division, each of these nerves individually may be injured by operative procedures or trauma. In the case of the auriculotemporal nerve, it may be injured by fractures of the neck of the mandible or during face-lifting procedures when the skin anterior to the ear is being elevated over the path of the nerve. Mandibular fractures through the mandibular canal almost always produce impairment of the mental nerve, as well as numbness of the teeth. Injury to the mental nerve can also occur during the elevation of skin or mucosal flaps in the region of the mental foramen. Another consideration with respect to the anatomy of the trigeminal nerve is in regard to herpes zoster. The distribution of vesicles on the skin usually follows the pattern of one of the trigeminal divisions. Herpetic involvement of the ophthalmic division often causes more discomfort to patients because of the distribution of the nasociliary branch to the cornea and conjunctiva, resulting in excessive tearing, burning sensations, and shooting pains over the eye.

FACIAL BLOOD SUPPLY

Both the internal and external carotid branches supply the face. The internal carotid gives off an ophthalmic branch at the level of the circle of Willis. This vessel traverses the optic canal, where it enters the orbit and is concerned principally with supplying the eye and intraorbital tissues. From this plexus of intraorbital arteries, two branches emerge; the supraorbital and the supratrochlear emerge at the orbital rim to parallel the course of the supraorbital and supratrochlear nerves (Fig. 21-6). These form a neurovascular bundle in the dense connective layer of the scalp. In summary, the internal carotid supplies the periorbital and scalp tissues of the forehead.

Two branches of the external carotid contribute to the blood supply of the face along with the internal carotid. These are the superficial temporal artery and the facial artery itself (see Fig. 21-6). The superficial temporal artery is the terminal branch of the external carotid. It begins in the substance of the parotid, exiting at the superior pole of the gland, where it joins the auriculotemporal nerve to lie just under the skin anterior to the tragus of the ear. It is also vulnerable during the elevation of skin flaps for face-lifting procedures. After entering the upper portion of the scalp, the superficial temporal artery anastomoses in the region of the forehead with the supraorbital and supratrochlear branches of the ophthalmic artery. There is also an anastomotic pattern over the occipital area with posterior auricular branches of the external carotid.

The facial artery, a branch of the external carotid artery, supplies the major portion of the face. After its origin from the external carotid, the facial artery ascends deep to the posterior belly of the digastric muscle and crosses the mandi-

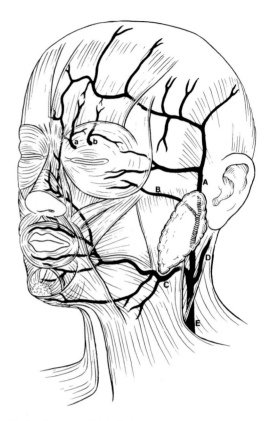

Fig. 21-6. The superficial facial arteries: *a,* supratrochlear; *b,* supraorbital. External carotid system: *A,* superficial temporal; *B,* transverse facial; *C,* facial; *D,* posterior auricular; *E,* external carotid.

ble at the anterior margin of the masseter muscle. Here, the artery lies deep to the plane of the facial muscles and is protected by them until it reaches the angle of the mouth, where the artery divides into inferior and superior labial arteries. The main trunk continues into the nasolabial angle and, after coursing deep to the lesser zygomatic muscle, is no longer covered by a muscle sheath. The artery terminates by sending small branches to the lateral aspect of the nose and finally anastomosing in small networks with the plexus of vessels about the orbital region. This effectively provides an anastomotic link between the facial and ophthalmic arteries (external and internal carotid systems, respectively). In some individuals the facial artery may end effectively at the angle of the mouth. In this case the transverse facial artery originates from the superficial temporal artery within the parotid gland. This vessel exits the parotid, following a course similar to the zygomatic branch of the facial nerve. When this vessel is large, it replaces the angular portion of the facial artery.

In summary, three major trunks supply blood to the face. The first is the ophthalmic artery through its orbital branches. The second is the superficial temporal artery, which supplies most of the forehead and lateral scalp tissues. The third is the facial artery, which supplies the central and lower portions of the face. All these vessels have anastomotic connections, not only on the side of their origins, but also across the midline with their corresponding vessel. Furthermore, superficial vessels anastomose with vessels in the deep portion of the face, such as the intraorbital artery. The infraorbital artery, the terminal branch of the maxillary, is another example of an anastomosis between the internal carotid branches about the orbit with the external carotid system.

In the region of the orbit, the normal flow of blood is from ophthalmic arterial branches into the periorbital arterial plexus. In patients with occlusive disease of the internal carotid, the direction of this flow may be reversed because of the pressure differential between the internal carotid system (low) and the external carotid system (high). Anatomic and Doppler flow studies by Berthelot and Hureau[1] have shown that, depending on the dominant pattern of anastomosis, blood can enter the ophthalmic vessels via either the superficial temporal, the infraorbital, or the angular branch of the facial artery in patients in whom the internal carotid is occluded.

FACIAL VENOUS DRAINAGE

The principal venous drainage of the face occurs via the facial and retromandibular veins. The facial vein begins as the angular vein near the medial canthus of the eye, coursing inferiorly in the nasolabial angle (Fig. 21-7). The vessel receives branches from the nose and region of the lip. Paralleling the course of the facial artery, it descends on the face, crossing the angle of the mandible, where it joins the common facial vein, which empties into the internal jugular vein. The common facial vein also receives the retromandibular vein, which begins in the scalp as the superficial temporal vein. When the superficial temporal vein enters the superior portion of the parotid gland, it is joined by the maxillary vein from the infratemporal fossa. The union of these two vessels forms the retromandibular vein before it exits the parotid at its inferior pole to join the common facial vein at the angle of the mandible. In addition to joining the common facial vein, the retromandibular vein also anastomoses with the external jugular vein. In this manner the anterior and more lateral aspects of the face drain to both the internal and external jugular veins. The veins of the orbital region and lower portion of the forehead-scalp are tributaries of the ophthalmic veins within the orbital cavity. Usually there are superior and inferior branches of the orbital vein, which collect blood from the orbital region. These veins usually drain posteriorly through the apex of the orbit, becoming tributaries of the cavernous sinus.

The clinical significance of the venous drainage of the face is primarily the anastomosis of the superficial veins with vessels in the deep parts of the face and skull. Clearly, the anastomosis of vessels about the orbit with the cavernous sinus poses the potential for bacterial infection of the cavernous sinus and its disastrous sequela: cavernous sinus thrombosis. Scalp vessels may also anastomose via emissary veins with other veins within the diploic space or with meningeal

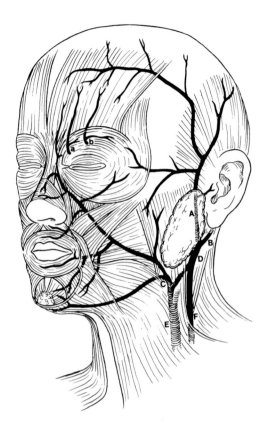

Fig. 21-7. The superficial facial veins. Ophthalmic vein tributaries: *a,* supratrochlear; *b,* supraorbital. Jugular system: *A,* superficial temporal; *B,* posterior auricular; *C,* anterior facial; *D,* posterior facial; *E,* internal jugular; *F,* external jugular.

veins. Hence the possibility of osteomyelitis or meningitis exists from infections tracking along these particular vessels. In the central region of the face, the superficial veins also anastomose with vessels that are tributaries of the pterygoid venous plexus. While much of the blood flow in this plexus ultimately reaches the internal jugular veins, some of it may enter the base of the skull via emissary veins and, when bacteria are present, produce encephalitis or meningitis. While surface infections of the skin of the face or scalp may be the focus of such events, another common mechanism is sinusitis. The complications of meningitis following frontal sinusitis, or of orbital cellulitis following ethmoid sinusitis, are all well documented in the clinical literature.

FACIAL LYMPHATICS

The lymphatic drainage of the face occurs via several routes. The lower lip and skin of the chin drain inferiorly to submental and submandibular nodes that drain to second eschalon nodes located in the superior aspect of the internal jugular chain. Lymphatic channels from the medial central face, such as the upper lip, nasal vestibule, external nose, medial cheek, canthus, and the skin of the glabellar, drain to submandibular lymph nodes and then to second eschalon nodes in the internal jugular chain. The most prominent lymphatic channel draining the medial central face is the facial chain, which parallels the facial artery. This chain contains the perifacial lymph nodes located on either side of the facial artery located along the inner aspect of the body of the mandible. These nodes may become involved with metastases from midfacial skin cancer, and their enlargement may be missed on clinical examination if bimanual palpation of the floor of the mouth is not done. The forehead, the frontal and temporal scalp, the skin of the temple, the eyelids, and the lateral cheek drain into periparotid lymph nodes and then to second eschalon nodes in the internal jugular vein. The parotid nodes are located both superficial and deep to the parotid fascia, and a few are in intraglandular locations. Reactive and neoplastic enlargement of the parotid nodes may occur and thus must be considered in the differential diagnosis of a parotid mass.

The lymphatics of the parietal and occipital scalp and postauricular skin drain to postauricular and suboccipital lymph nodes with secondary drainage to the upper spinal accessory chain. The auricle represents a ''watershed'' area, draining anteriorly to the parotid nodes and posteriorly to the postauricular nodes. Thus, melanomas or other cutaneous malignancies of the external ear may drain to either or both of the nodal groups.

REFERENCES

1. Berthelot JL, Hureau J: Clinical anatomical study of the macroscopic anastomoses of the ophthalmic artery in the periorbital region, *Anat Clin* 3:271, 1982.
2. Jones LT: Epiphora. II. Its relation to the anatomic structures and surgery of medical canthal region, *Am J Ophthalmol* 49:29, 1957.
3. Reeh MJ, Wobig JL, Wirtschafter JD: *Ophthalmic anatomy*, San Francisco, 1982, American Academy of Ophthalmology.

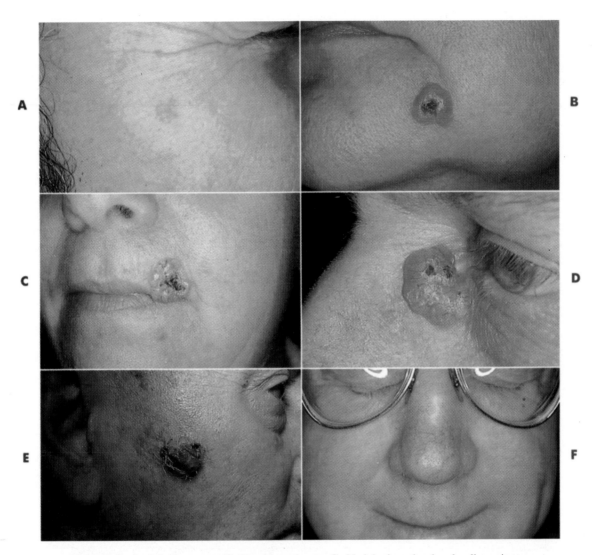

Plate 1. A, Actinic keratoses. **B,** Keratoacanthoma. **C,** Noduloulcerative basal cell carcinoma. **D,** Nodular basal cell carcinoma. **E,** Pigmented basal cell carcinoma. **F,** Morpheaform basal cell carcinoma.

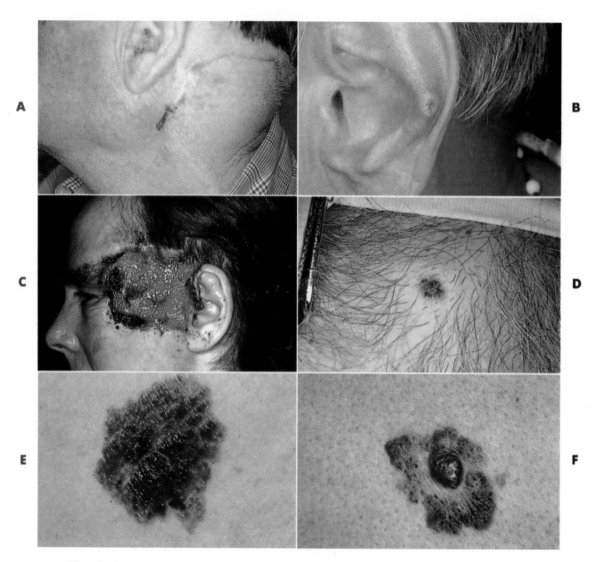

Plate 2. A, Recurrent basal cell carcinoma. **B,** Chondrodermatitis nodularis helicis. **C,** Squamous cell carcinoma. **D,** Pigmented squamous cell carcinoma. **E,** Superficial spreading melanoma. **F,** Irregular border of superficial spreading melanoma.

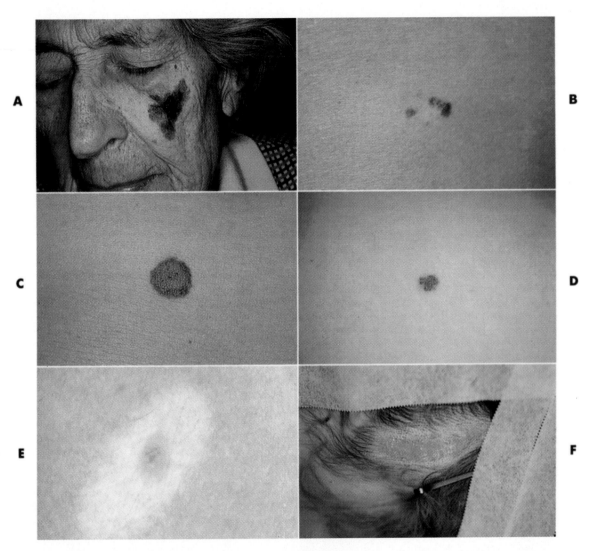

Plate 3. A, Lentigo maligna melanoma. **B,** Junctional nevus. **C,** Intradermal nevus. **D,** Blue nevus. **E,** Halo nevus. **F,** Nevus sebaceus.

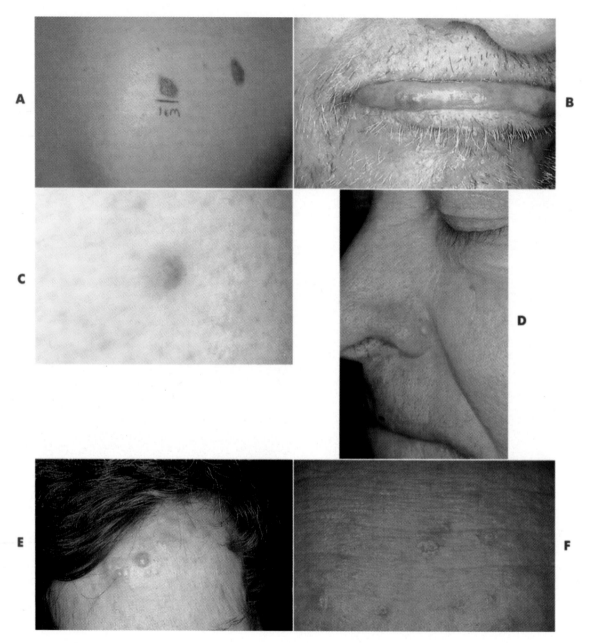

Plate 4. A, Dysplastic nevus. **B,** Venous lakes. **C,** Dermatofibroma. **D,** Fibrous papule. **E,** Cylindroma. **F,** Sebaceous hyperplasia.

Chapter 22

Recognition and Treatment of Skin Lesions

Neil A. Swanson
Roy C. Grekin

Cutaneous lesions are often the first entity the otolaryngologist encounters. They may be visible in even the most cursory examination, or the patient may bring them to the attention of the physician. To the untrained eye, they can often provide a challenging diagnosis. Even to the experienced eye, the diagnosis must often be confirmed histologically. Treatment of cutaneous lesions can be performed with confidence, skill, and success. Several "tricks" to the treatment of these lesions can help ensure a satisfactory outcome.

This chapter is structured to provide the otolaryngologist with practical knowledge concerning the differential diagnosis of cutaneous tumors by the physician, including epidermal tumors, melanocytic tumors, cystic lesions, vascular tumors, and fibroadnexal tumors. Within the discussions of the various tumor categories are reviews of the preferred therapeutic options for each specific tumor. At the end of the chapter is a discussion of treatment methods and biopsy techniques commonly used by the dermatologist and cutaneous surgeon that can easily be applied by the otolaryngologist. The details of various biopsy techniques used to establish a histologic diagnosis are stressed, as the pathologist's ability to establish a definitive diagnosis depends directly on the clinical specimen obtained for histopathologic review.

An in-depth discussion of all cutaneous tumors (benign and malignant) is beyond the scope of this chapter. The recognition of the three most common cutaneous malignancies will be discussed, with detailed chapters concerning these tumors to follow. The treatment of basal cell carcinoma and squamous cell carcinoma is discussed in Chapter 25. Chapter 26 details the current status of the treatment of malignant melanoma. This chapter will serve only to introduce these three tumors.

EPIDERMAL NEOPLASMS

The epidermis is a highly differentiated tissue, which is limited in its possible response to stimuli. Epithelial neoplasms of the skin can range from entirely benign to highly malignant tumors. Epidermal tumors are so common that few people go through life without acquiring at least one. A great assortment of epidermal tumors have been described, under a wide variety of names. The more common and important ones will be discussed in this chapter.

Three important factors relevant to epidermal tumors should be noted. First, the epidermis in the healthy person is a relatively thin structure and is the outermost layer of the skin. Hyperproliferation of the epidermis or its layers results in tumors that usually are superficial appearing and often are associated with scale. Dermal tumors and tumors of the cutaneous appendages (adnexal tumors) are usually deeper and, therefore, more nodular in appearance. Recognizing these differences is one general way of differentiating between the two tumor groups. Second, three types of lesions occur within epidermal tumors: benign, cancerous, and precancerous. The precise nature of precancerous lesions has been debated widely, but the term persists in the literature; it refers to a group of epidermal lesions of which a small percentage can go on to become malignant neoplasms. Finally, because the epidermis is limited in the number of ways it can respond to stimuli, the clinical presentations of many tumors will be similar. Even the most experienced dermatologist often has to resort to a biopsy for the definitive diagnosis of an epidermal tumor.

Seborrheic keratoses

Seborrheic keratoses, which are very common lesions, usually begin around the fourth decade of life. They can be single or multiple and can occur anywhere on the body with the exception of palms and soles. Clinically they are sharply demarcated and slightly raised, appearing as if they were stuck on the skin surface (Fig. 22-1). Many have a verrucous surface with a soft, friable consistency. However, others may have a smooth surface. Characteristically, all seborrheic keratoses show keratotic plugs on careful surface inspection. Their color is usually brownish to brown-black, although it can vary from flesh color to deep black. The color within an individual lesion is usually uniform. Lesions can measure from a few millimeters to several centimeters. When subjected to trauma they can become irritated, causing an inflammatory base and occasional bleeding. Occasionally, seborrheic keratoses are pedunculate, especially on the neck.

The etiology of seborrheic keratoses is unknown, although they may be dominantly inherited. They are benign with no malignant potential, although the appearance of hundreds in rapid "showers" may be a sign of internal malignancy. This is the much-debated Leser-Trélat sign. The most common tumor seen in this association is colonic adenocarcinoma.

All seborrheic keratoses share histologic evidence of hyperkeratosis, acanthosis, and papillomatosis. The acanthosis in most instances is due entirely to upward extension of the tumor. Therefore, the lower border of the tumor often lies at the same level as the normal, well-demarcated epithelium on either side of the tumor.

In the head and neck, the most common mistaken diagnosis is melanoma; therefore, the pathologist frequently receives a widely excised seborrheic keratosis that had been mistaken for melanoma. If the diagnosis is in doubt, a biopsy before definitive treatment should be performed.

Treatment of these lesions varies. Because these lesions are so superficial, they often can be excised flush with the skin, using any of the shaving techniques described at the end of this chapter. These lesions also are amenable to a light liquid nitrogen freezing, creating an intraepidermal blister and allowing removal of the keratosis with the blister. A nice trick with these tumors is to freeze them with one of the prepared refrigerants commonly used for dermabrasion (Frigiderm, Floro Ethyl, Cryosthesia). The lesion can then be literally "flicked" off with a curette in a cosmetically elegant manner. Because these are truly benign lesions, the best treatment is often no treatment, unless they are cosmetically disfiguring.

Dermatosis papulosa nigra (DPN) is a condition found in approximately 35% of black adults often with its onset during adolescence. The lesions are located predominantly on the face, especially in the malar region. They may also infrequently occur on the neck and upper trunk. They consist of small (1- to 3-mm), smooth, pigmented, stuck-on hyperkeratotic papules. They have the histologic appearance of seborrheic keratoses but are smaller. Most clinicians consider them a true variant of seborrheic keratoses.

The treatment of DPN is difficult because of pigmentary problems in treating black skin. Options that have been tried include fine-needle electrosurgery followed by use of a small curette, light freezing with liquid nitrogen, and dermabrasion. If the lesions are few, the authors prefer the first method. Cryosurgery can produce spotted hypopigmentation in blacks and should be avoided unless other treatment modalities are not available. Dermabrasion can be of two types. By means of either a 2-mm wheel or a small cone or pear diamond fraise, the lesions can be removed singly, very quickly and easily. Dermabrasion also can result in mottled pigmentation on healing, which usually will fade with time. If the lesions are multiple and confluent, total regional dermabrasion may be the treatment of choice to offer the best cosmetic blend.

Warts

Warts, very common lesions, are the only tumors definitively known to be caused by a virus—the human papillomavirus (HPV), which is a deoxyribonucleic acid (DNA) virus. Warts can be classified in three ways. The traditional classification, based on the clinical appearance and location, is as follows: (1) verruca vulgaris, or common wart, including the filiform wart; (2) deep hyperkeratotic palmar-plantar wart; (3) superficial mosaic-type palmar-plantar wart; (4) verruca plana; (5) epidermodysplasia verruciform; and (6) condyloma acuminatum. The second classification is based on histology. The third, and most recent classification, is based on the presence of several antigenic types of papilloma viruses, each with a distinct DNA genome and type-specific antigen. Serotypes have been added.

The most definitively characterized types include the following. Papillomavirus type 1, or HPV-1, is specifically associated with deep, hyperkeratotic palmar-plantar warts.

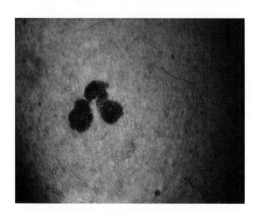

Fig. 22-1. Seborrheic keratoses.

HPV-2 is associated with superficial mosaic palmar-plantar warts as well as with common and filiform warts. HPV-3 is associated with verruca plana and the benign variant of epidermodysplasia verruciformis. HPV-5, initially called HPV-4, is associated with the dysplastic type of epidermodysplasia verruciformis. These four are the most highly specific serotypes. Less specific serotypes include HPV-4, largely associated with superficial mosaic palmar-plantar warts and some common warts; HPV-6, largely associated with condyloma acuminatum; and HPV-7, warts detected on the hands of nine butchers.

The most common facial warts include common warts, flat warts (verruca plana), and filiform warts. These warts would be most commonly associated with the antigenic serotypes HPV-2 and HPV-3. Clinically these lesions are hyperkeratotic. The filiform wart is often a pedunculate lesion occurring in isolation on the cheek, nasal tip or columella, or eyelid (Fig. 22-2). Common warts can occur anywhere on the face. Flat warts usually occur in younger patients; they are small (1- to 2-mm), flat-topped, hyperkeratotic lesions, which can coalesce (Fig. 22-3).

Treatment of these warts is at times difficult. The filiform wart can be anesthetized at its base and with scissors excised, with the base being lightly curetted and fulgurated under low current. This approach affords the best chance for cure. Filiform warts often are too verrucous and hyperkeratotic to be effectively treated with cryosurgery. Common warts, when not too verrucous, can be treated effectively with liquid nitrogen cryotherapy. Flat warts present a difficult problem. At times, they can be effectively treated with liquid nitrogen. Perhaps the best method is to individually scrape each small wart off the skin with a small curette, treating, when possible, all the flat warts in an area at one time. In young children who do not tolerate surgical therapy well, one may use topical retinoic acid (Retin-A) at a concentration sufficient to produce erythema and irritation in an attempt to stimulate the body's own immunity against the wart virus. At times, avoiding treatment is best, as the vast majority of warts will spontaneously involute once the patient's immune system recognizes the virus.

Related to the poxvirus family is a group of viruses known as the molluscum contagiosum virus family (EM-2). An infection with one of these viruses appears clinically as a variable number of small, discrete, waxy, skin-colored, dome-shaped papillomas, 2 to 4 mm in diameter, with umbilicated centers (Fig. 22-4). Like all viral lesions, they ultimately will involute spontaneously. Histologically, they have a classic appearance of cytoplasmic inclusion bodies, the so-called molluscum bodies. The best treatment is usually superficial cryotherapy or curettage, as with common warts.

Actinic keratoses

Actinic keratoses, sometimes called solar keratoses, are precancerous lesions. Studies indicate that from 5% to 20% of persons with solar keratoses will develop squamous cell carcinoma or basal cell carcinoma in one or more of the

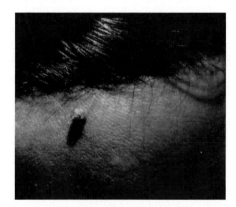

Fig. 22-2. Filiform warts.

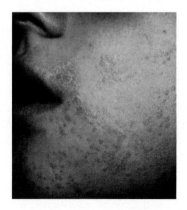

Fig. 22-3. Flat warts.

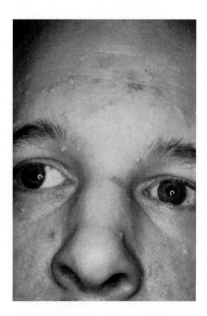

Fig. 22-4. Molluscum contagiosum.

lesions. As the name implies, actinic keratoses result solely from solar damage. They are seen on sun-exposed areas of the skin, usually in persons after the fourth decade of life. They are seen most commonly in fair individuals who frequently burn (Celts with type I skin). Clinically, these lesions are usually erythematous with covering adherent scale and show little or no infiltration (being very superficial) (Plate 1, *A*). A patient often can feel the rough, adherent scale before the lesion is clinically visible. Solar keratoses can be flesh colored or pigmented. They often do not have a sharp demarcation from surrounding skin and can spread peripherally. Occasionally these lesions develop marked hyperkeratosis, giving a clinical appearance of a cutaneous horn. On the vermilion border of the lip, actinic keratosis is known as solar or actinic cheilitis.

Actinic keratoses lesions are best removed and not watched. The most commonly used method for removing discrete lesions is cryosurgery. Shave excision can also be performed. However, in the milieu of sun-damaged skin, new lesions may frequently appear. In persons with severe sun damage to the face or with diffuse actinic keratoses, topical 5-fluorouracil (Efudex) is effective for treatment of a region, or the entire face. Because proper use results in severe irritation, sound patient understanding and education and physician reassurance are necessary to ensure adequate compliance. A full-face dermabrasion is also a good method of treatment for severe, diffuse cases.

Keratoacanthoma

A keratoacanthoma is a rapidly growing tumor usually seen on sun-damaged skin (Plate 1, *B*). Two types of keratoacanthomas exist—solitary and multiple. The solitary keratoacanthoma was first recognized as a distinct entity in 1950. Before then, this lesion was thought to be a form of squamous cell carcinoma. This common lesion is now recognized as an entity that is clinically and histologically different from squamous cell carcinoma. The solitary keratoacanthoma occurs in elderly persons, usually as a single rapidly growing tumor with three classic phases: growth, plateau, and involution. During the growth phase, the tumor begins as a firm, dome-shaped papule, which grows to become a nodule, usually peaking at 1 to 2.5 cm in diameter, with a central horn-filled crater (Plate 1, *C*). Sites of predilection are the sun-exposed areas, where up to 95% of solitary keratoacanthomas have been reported. They have not been reported on palms, soles, or mucosal surfaces. A keratoacanthoma will classically reach full size within 6 to 8 weeks and then enter the plateau stage. It then will generally involute spontaneously within 6 months, often healing with a slightly depressed scar. However, keratoacanthomas may grow for more than 2 months and take up to 1 year to involute.

Of the three rare clinical forms of solitary keratoacanthoma, two are pertinent to the physician: the giant keratoacanthoma presents with a rapid growth, reaching a size of 5 cm or more, and may cause destruction of underlying tissues.

Nevertheless, spontaneous involution will usually occur. The most common site for this lesion is the nose. The keratoacanthoma centrificum marginata, may reach 20 cm in diameter, with little tendency toward spontaneous involution and with peripheral extension. This lesion is most commonly located over the dorsum of the hand.

Claims have been made that keratoacanthomas may undergo transformation to squamous cell carcinoma in the setting of immunosuppression. Debate continues as to whether this transformation actually occurs or whether a ''transformed'' lesion has been a squamous cell carcinoma from the beginning. The most common site, in the authors' experience, for this malignant transformation to occur is the nose. The authors have seen three lesions with the histologic diagnosis of keratoacanthoma destroy the entire nose as well as upper palate. The authors have also seen two ''keratoacanthomas'' metastasize. Therefore, especially in dealing with central facial keratoacanthomas, care must be taken in interpreting the histologic report and correlating it with the clinical behavior of the tumor.

The second type of keratoacanthoma is the multiple variety, of which there are two forms. The first is the multiple, self-healing epithelioma of the skin. Such lesions usually begin to occur in childhood or adolescence and can be located anywhere, including palms, soles, and head and neck. Generally, no more than a dozen lesions exist at any one time, and they behave clinically the same as solitary keratoacanthomas, regressing after a few months with a depressed scar. The second form of multiple keratoacanthoma is the eruptive keratoacanthoma. Eruptive keratoacanthomas do not usually appear until adult life, often presenting as many hundreds of characteristic papules measuring 2 to 3 mm in diameter. The oral mucosa and larynx may be involved.

Treatment of keratoacanthomas can be difficult. Surgical excision is probably the treatment of choice for most lesions when they cannot be left to spontaneously involute. Intralesional injection of cytotoxic agents, the most common being 5-fluorouracil and methotrexate, has induced involution, after which healing occurs similarly to spontaneous involution. We favor methotrexate, at a dose of 12.5 to 25 mg/ml, with approximately 1 ml being injected into the lesion at 3- to 4-week intervals. Large keratoacanthomas—those in which the distinction from squamous cell carcinoma is difficult clinically and histologically—especially when they occur in the central facial area, are best treated using Mohs' surgery. This technique is detailed in Chapter 25.

Basal cell carcinoma

Basal cell carcinoma is the most common malignancy in humans. It comprises approximately 65% of all epithelioid tumors, and accounts for 20% of all cancers in men and 10% to 15% of all cancers in women. Depending on the study cited, approximately 86% of lesions occur initially in the head and neck, with 25% of all primary lesions occurring on the nose. Approximately 96% of recurrences are in the head and neck, with 38% being on the nose.[2] Emmet[3] reported that 75.5% of previously untreated basal cell carcinomas found in Australia occurred in the head and neck, 8.4% on the chest and back, and 16% on the arms and legs. When looking at recurrent tumors, Emmet found that 91% occurred on the head and neck, 7.5% on the chest and back, and 1.5% on the arms and legs. In this discussion, we will outline the epidemiology and clinical and histologic variations of basal cell carcinoma. Treatment of basal cell carcinoma and squamous cell carcinoma is dealt with in detail in Chapter 25.

Basal cell carcinoma, more common in men than in women, is seen most frequently between the ages of 40 and 60 years. With the aging of the sunbathing generation, however, basal cell carcinomas are occurring with increasing frequency in younger people. Scandinavians and people of Celtic extraction (in particular, Irish), who frequently have type I or type II skin, appear to be more prone to basal cell carcinoma than persons with more darkly pigmented skin. Exposure to sunlight, primarily in the ultraviolet B (UVB) spectrum, is the primary factor causing basal cell carcinoma. This has been shown experimentally and reproduced clinically. The tumor is more common as one proceeds toward the equator and is also more common at high altitudes. The head and neck area is the most common site for basal cell carcinoma. On the head and neck, the nose is the most common site, with the nasal tip and the nasal ala being the most common locations on the nose itself. The cheeks and the forehead are the next most common sites. Basal cell carcinoma is more common on the left side of the body than on the right, perhaps because of selective sun exposure in individuals whose occupation preferentially exposes the left side.

Although sun exposure is the primary etiologic agent in producing basal cell carcinoma, other risk factors include occupation, genetic conditions, immunosuppression, and former injury. Farmers, sailors, and fishermen, because of their heavy occupational actinic exposure, have a higher than average incidence of skin cancer. Genetic syndromes include the autosomal-dominant nevoid basal cell carcinoma syndrome and xeroderma pigmentosum. In the former, basal cell carcinomas can arise on any area of the body, with the predilection being toward sun-exposed sites, beginning at an early age and continuing throughout life. These patients also have skeletal abnormalities, including bifid ribs, jaw cysts, and frontal bossing, as well as calcified cerebra as shown on skull radiograph. Xeroderma pigmentosum, autosomal recessive in inheritance, is a defect in DNA repair, which can result in the formation of basal cell carcinoma and other cutaneous neoplasms at a very early age, usually in response to sun exposure. Immunosuppression, either iatrogenic or in patients with leukemias or lymphomas, has been shown to increase the incidence and aggressiveness of basal cell carcinomas. Chemical carcinogens, notably arsenic, play a tumorigenic role. The arsenic usually comes from well water contaminated with arsenic; or patients with

asthma, hay fever, or psoriasis may have taken arsenic as Fowler's solution. Arsenic-induced basal cell carcinomas tend to be primarily on the trunk and are accompanied by keratoses of the palms and soles, pigmentary changes, and nail changes (Mees' lines) associated with arsenic ingestion. Exposure to ionizing radiation is also an important etiologic factor; tumors can arise in areas of radiation damage, often many years after superficial radiotherapy for acne or tinea, or as a depilatory, at an early age. Basal cell carcinoma can arise at the edge of a scar or area of trauma. The injury may possibly have acted as a cofactor, adding to the effect of already existing factors such as sunlight and racial susceptibility. Smallpox vaccinations and burn scars have been associated with basal cell carcinoma.

To the trained and curious eye, the clinical recognition of basal cell carcinoma is not difficult. Typically, there is a raised, nodular lesion with a smooth, clear (pearly) border, and telangiectasia (Plate 1, *D*). The lesion can ulcerate and form a crust (see Plate 1, *C*). A typical history involves a pimplelike lesion that bleeds and does not heal. Pruritus is a common early symptom.

There are, however, several different clinical presentations and distinctive histologic pictures. The nodular or noduloulcerative basal cell carcinoma is the most common of clinical presentations (see Plate 1, *C* and *D*). This lesion has a well-formed clinical border, with the histologic features of basal cell carcinoma usually being confined within the clinical border. It is, therefore, one of the easiest variants of basal cell carcinoma to treat. Basal cell carcinoma can be pigmented (Plate 1, *E*). Even when it is pigmented, the lesion maintains the clinical features of a pearly, translucent border and telangiectasia. The superficial multicentric basal cell carcinoma is often present in the setting of actinic damage, with differing, intercommunicating extensions of tumor in a superficial histologic field. The lesion may contain cystic spaces appearing as very ill-defined clinical margins, which make treatment difficult. Some sources separate a cystic basal cell carcinoma from the nodular and multicentric types. This is mostly a histologic separation.

Three forms of basal cell carcinoma are often more subtle clinically, more aggressive histologically, and more difficult to treat. Clinically, the morpheaform basal cell carcinoma (Plate 1, *F*) presents as a yellowish plaque, which develops telangiectasia, may ulcerate, and may form a sclerotic or scarlike appearance. The margins are often indistinct; histologically, this tumor extends subclinical, fingerlike projections intradermally, making complete excision difficult. This tumor has a scarlike, stromal matrix, which gives it a very fibrous, sclerotic appearance and nature. Another aggressive tumor is the *keratotic* basal cell carcinoma (*basosquamous carcinoma* or *metatypical carcinoma*). The term "keratotic" is gaining rapid acceptance, replacing the terms in parenthesis. With the advent of monoclonal antibody staining, it has become evident that basal cell carcinoma and squamous cell carcinoma are individual neoplasms; a true intermediate tumor probably does not exist. Therefore, the keratotic tumor represents a basal cell carcinoma that keratinizes and is aggressive clinically. Histologically, within the same field typical basal cell carcinoma exists in association with cells that appear squamous and keratinize. *Recurrent* basal cell carcinoma (Plate 2, *A*) presents a varying clinical appearance, depending on the type of initial treatment. It may appear at the edge of a skin graft, within a scar created by electrosurgery, under a scar created by cryosurgery, or as a nodule developing within a suture line. Recurrent basal cell carcinoma is often nodular and accompanied by a morpheaform or sclerotic histologic picture in the deeper portions of the tumor. This picture may represent an aggressive histologic dedifferentiation of the tumor, a factor that may partially account for its clinically aggressive behavior and resistance to treatment.

The typical basal cell carcinoma occurring in the middle-aged or elderly, fair-skinned person in the head and neck is not difficult to diagnose. One must be aware, however, that this tumor has a variety of clinical appearances, can appear in young people, and can occur in areas other than the head and neck. Any suspicious, nonhealing, pruritic, scaly lesion, especially one occurring in a sun-exposed area on a fair-skinned individual, should be investigated by biopsy.

Biopsy techniques for basal cell carcinoma are simple. It has been well documented that implantation metastases from basal cell carcinoma do not occur, as the tumor needs a stroma to provide an environment in which to grow. The most appropriate technique is a medium-depth shave biopsy. The depth of the biopsy ideally should be mid-dermis. This depth gives a dermal collagen network that is amenable to any form of therapy. If a morpheaform basal cell carcinoma is suspected, the biopsy specimen often must extend deeper, perhaps through a punch or incisional biopsy. In cases of recurrent or superficial multicentric lesions or large clinical lesions, biopsy specimens should be obtained in multiple sites to assess the true clinical nature and size of the tumor. Biopsies of recurrent deep nodular lesions should be performed in an appropriate fashion to ensure an adequately deep specimen from the dermal nodule. This maneuver can be accomplished by means of an incisional biopsy or a deep-punch biopsy. As a rule of thumb, if the biopsy does not confirm the clinical opinion of basal cell carcinoma and the lesion remains suspicious, an additional biopsy of the lesion is indicated.

Chondrodermatitis nodularis helicis (Plate 2, *B*) is an inflammatory disease of underlying helical cartilage that can mimic and be mistaken for basal cell carcinoma. The condition usually results from chronic trauma. The entire diseased cartilage (which will appear yellow) must be excised for a surgical cure.

Squamous cell carcinoma

Squamous cell carcinoma, though less common than basal cell carcinoma, is still a common neoplasm. Many of the etiologic factors are the same as for basal cell carcinoma, the most important of which is long-standing, chronic sun exposure—especially if a person has lived close to the equator or at high altitudes. For example, in Michigan the ratio of basal cell carcinoma to squamous cell carcinoma is approximately 8:1, whereas in Texas the ratio approaches 2:1. Squamous cell carcinoma is more common in men than women and is more likely to present with multiple cutaneous carcinomas. It often is found in skin adjacent to basal cell carcinomas, a fact that is indicative of similar etiologic factors for both tumors. These include actinic (solar) damage, irradiation, trauma (scars), genetic susceptibility (nevoid basal cell carcinoma syndrome and xeroderma pigmentosum), occupation, and exposure to chemicals (especially arsenic).

Clinically, squamous cell carcinomas can often be separated into actinically induced squamous cell carcinomas and *de novo* squamous cell carcinomas. The former are the more common, arise on sunexposed areas, and are associated with a low incidence of metastasis (less than 1% in most series). The *de novo* lesions can be associated with some of the nonsolar etiologies for squamous cell carcinomas. Some studies suggest that *de novo* lesions have a higher metastatic potential (approximately 2% to 3%) than the actinically induced squamous cell carcinomas. The mucosal variant of squamous cell carcinoma, seen clinically as carcinoma of the lip, has the highest metastatic potential, approaching 11% to 12% in some series. Therefore, these distinctions are important in prognosis. Carcinoma of the lip is discussed in detail in Chapter 25.

Squamous cell carcinoma may present clinically in any of several ways. It can present as a thick and scaly hyperkeratonic patch on the exposed surface of the body, in particular the ear, lip, or nose (Plate 2, *C*). The lesion may change slowly over a period of time. If the crust is removed, the base is often ulcerated and has a rolled margin. The lesion may also present as a persistent ulcer, particularly in an old scar, or as a superficial multifocal change in generally sun-damaged skin. The latter is often the most difficult lesion to diagnose, requiring several biopsies at different points. Occasionally, a squamous cell carcinoma will become a vegetative nodular lesion. This lesion often has a cystic feel and can ulcerate and progressively enlarge. Often these exophytic lesions have not invaded deeply. They all have a tendency to ulcerate and become more erosive in appearance than a basal cell carcinoma. As with basal cell carcinoma, they can become pigmented (Plate 2, *D*) and often appear very similar clinically to keratoacanthomas, especially when the latter are in the growth phase. However, these lesions usually grow more slowly than keratoacanthomas, thus allowing distinction on clinical as well as histologic grounds. When this occurs, biopsy is always indicated.

Squamous cell carcinoma of the skin can be divided histologically into five groups. *Adenoid* squamous cell carcinoma is the most common. It is the classic nodular, ulcerative lesion, often appearing periauricularly. A second group is the *bowenoid* squamous cell carcinoma. This variant has the histologic appearance of Bowen's disease but can invade through the basement membrane and can become invasive carcinoma. A third group, *generic* squamous cell carcinoma, is the most common histologic group and carries the highest (still less than 1%) risk of metastasis. As the name implies, *verrucous* squamous cell carcinoma is a verruciform lesion that invades by blunt, pseudopod-type growth. The last group, *spindle* squamous cell carcinoma, is the least common and most indistinct clinically. The treatment of cutaneous squamous cell carcinoma, very similar to that of basal cell carcinoma, is discussed in depth in Chapter 25.

Bowen's disease is a variant of a squamous cell carcinoma. By definition it is a full-thickness dysplasia of the epidermis, thereby being noninvasive; however invasion can occur. Clinically Bowen's disease presents as a well-demarcated, erythematous, scaly patch or plaque in sun-exposed areas. It may be very psoriasiform in nature, psoriasis being one of the most common mistaken diagnoses. Bowen's disease carries the same etiologic implications as basal cell carcinoma and squamous cell carcinoma; it is probably the most common tumor found in patients with histories of long-term arsenic ingestion. Some studies have suggested an increased incidence of internal malignancy when Bowen's disease occurs in non-sun exposed areas. However, reports are conflicting, and the definitive word is not in at this time.

MELANOCYTIC NEOPLASMS

The melanocyte is the pigment-producing cell of the epidermis. However, many tumors of this cell line, the neural crest cells embryologically, occur in the dermis either by migration or because crest cells fail to reach the epidermis during embryogenesis. The most common of these tumors are nevocellular nevi and melanoma. This section discusses the clinical manifestations of melanoma and nevocellular nevi and other tumors of melanocytes included in the differential diagnosis of melanoma. Chapter 26 discusses in detail the behavior and treatment of melanoma.

Malignant melanoma

Malignant melanoma, the third most common skin cancer, is increasing in incidence throughout the world. This disease is important because it is a lethal cutaneous neoplasm. With sophistication of the physician and patient, however, this disease can be recognized early and cured. Every effort, therefore, should be made to diagnose melanoma at its earliest stage (stage I—less than 0.85 mm thick or level I or II of Clark). The clinical recognition of melanoma depends on four major criteria: color, border, topography, and surrounding tissue. To a lesser degree, symptoms including pruritus, tingling, and bleeding are important. Changes in any of the four major criteria in connection with a preexisting mole or the continued growth of a new lesion should signal the clinician to suspect melanoma. The most significant change is one that occurs over time (weeks or months) rather than over a few days. A fairly rapid change is rarely due to malignancy but more commonly to infection or trauma.

1. *Color.* Melanoma is said to be a patriotic tumor, exhibiting shades and hues of red, white, and blue. Melanoma is rarely uniform in color but often has differing hues within the same lesion (Plate 2, *E*). Blue in a lesion signifies dermal melanin. The more blue the lesion, the deeper the dermal melanin because of the refractile properties of the skin. One can often see shades of blue, blue-black, or blue-green within a melanoma. Red in a melanoma often indicates inflammation. White areas indicate sites of regression within a melanoma.

2. *Border.* The border of a melanoma is classically irregular and scalloped, often bending diffusely into the normal skin (Plate 2, *F*). Changes in the border of a preexisting mole are sometimes the earliest signs of transformation to melanoma, reflecting an early radial growth phase of the melanoma.

3. *Topography.* Topography is critical to the diagnosis of melanoma (see Plate 2, *F*). Rarely are melanomas macular (flat) lesions. Surface characteristics include nodularity, ulceration, verrucousness, and irregular undulations. Development of nodularity within a melanoma usually suggests invasion and vertical growth. Ulceration within a melanoma is one of the clinically poor prognostic signs.

4. *Surrounding tissue.* Changes in surrounding tissue suggest development of satellite pigmented lesions, which are often melanoma or at least atypical melanocytic hyperplasia.

Changes in one or more of these important clinical criteria, as well as the other symptoms and signs, should alert one to suspect melanoma and to perform a biopsy for diagnosis.

The biopsy of a melanoma is important. As will be suggested in Chapter 26, the most critical determination in judging the treatment and prognosis of stage I melanoma is the depth of invasion as defined in millimeters by Breslow or in levels by Clark. The most elevated portion of a melanoma clinically is not always the deepest portion of the melanoma histologically. To give the pathologist (and therefore the patient) the best chance for an accurate diagnosis and treatment recommendation, an excisional biopsy of the entire suspicious lesion should, therefore, be performed. This approach allows the pathologist to step or serial section the entire specimen to determine the maximum vertical depth of the lesion. When excisional biopsy is impossible, multiple biopsies, including the most nodular area of the melanoma, are the next best choice.

There are two phases of growth noted in a melanoma: a radial growth phase (centripetal growth) and a vertical growth phase. The radial growth phase involves the circumferential growth of the tumor; this type of growth is confined to the dermoepidermal junction before actual invasion. The vertical growth phase involves the invasive growth of the tumor.

The four common types of melanoma fall within a spectrum. *Lentigo maligna melanoma* occurs in the head and neck (sun-exposed areas) of elderly patients and exhibits the longest radial growth phase. It makes up approximately 7% of the melanomas and often carries the best prognosis. It classically begins as an irregularly pigmented, flat macule, which grows very slowly over a period of several years (often a decade or more) (Plate 3, *A*). Malignant changes are evidenced by thickening and the development of discrete tumor nodules. The lesion may ultimately grow to a diameter of several centimeters because of its extensive radial growth. The precursor lesion is called lentigo maligna or (in older terminology) Hutchinson's freckle. It becomes melanoma once invasion or a vertical growth phase has developed.

The second type in the continuum is *superficial spreading melanoma*, the most common form of melanoma, representing approximately 65% of cases. This tumor has variable radial and vertical growth phases, with the radial phase often existing for a period of time before nodularity and vertical growth develop. This type of melanoma occurs most commonly in the fourth and fifth decades of life, although the age is declining as with other cutaneous neoplasms, possibly because of increased sun exposure. This is the classic melanoma of multiple colors, irregular border, and nodularity (see Plate 2, *E* and *F*).

Next along the continuum of growth is the *acfral lentiginous melanoma*. This most recently described melanoma also has variable radial and vertical growth phases. It is the most common type of melanoma seen in blacks. As implied by the name, these tumors are seen in acral areas, including hands, feet, and oral and anogenital mucosa. They carry a poorer prognosis than other forms of melanoma, perhaps because of the rich vascular supply and early angiolymphatic spread or because they are not easily or often seen early in their development. These lesions make up approximately 5% to 7% of melanomas.

The last form of melanoma is the *nodular melanoma*, which develops a very early vertical growth phase. It constitutes approximately 7% to 8% of melanomas and is the most invasive form. It often presents as a blue-black, polypoid, smooth surface nodule that may bleed and has a tendency toward early ulceration. By definition, it is deeply invasive and has a vertical growth phase from its inception, leading to a poor prognosis.

Other melanocytic tumors fall into the differential diagnosis of melanoma and will be discussed in that light. They are for the most part nevocellular nevi, very common tumors that can appear shortly after birth to late in life.

Junctional nevus

Junctional nevi are tan to brownish macules (flat lesions) of uniform color and smooth border (Plate 3, *B*). Dots of black pigment may be present, but unlike melanoma, the normal skin markings are preserved. The lesion varies from a few millimeters to a centimeter or more in diameter. The melanocytes or nevus cells are located at the junction of the epidermis and the dermis (dermoepidermal junction). The lesion can occur anywhere on the body and is the nevus most commonly mistaken for melanoma. When in doubt, one should perform a biopsy of the lesion. Junctional nevi occur anytime after birth and are the common moles in children before puberty. Their importance lies in their ability to develop into malignant melanoma, although this rarely occurs before puberty. The vast majority of junctional nevi remain benign throughout life and can evolve over time into either compound or intradermal nevi. Their treatment is often dictated by suspicion of melanoma or cosmetic reasons and usually includes a roll shave in noncosmetic areas or a fusiform excision with closure in cosmetically important areas. Melanocytes are very cold sensitive, and a strictly junctional nevus can be removed with deep cryotherapy.

Intradermal nevus

The intradermal nevus is the common mature mole of adults, occurring anywhere on the body but rarely on the palms and soles. It is most common on the scalp or face in adults, varying in size from a few millimeters to several centimeters. It may be flat and smooth or raised and warty, pigmented or nonpigmented, sessile or pedunculate (Plate 3, *C*). It often contains coarse hairs, reflecting the depth within the dermis of the nevus cells. It is quite benign and rarely becomes malignant. By definition, all of the nevus cells occur within the dermis. This mole is best treated by shave excision when it is pedunculate and hairless. When it is on the head or neck and contains hair, it is necessary to excise this mole using either the punch excision technique (described later) or routine excision to remove the complete depth of the hair follicles within the nevus.

Compound nevus

The compound nevus, a combination of junctional and intradermal elements is found most commonly in adults. It is a brown to black mole, usually less than 1 cm in diameter. A brown, macular ring is frequently around the periphery of the lesion. It can contain hair and is often clinically indistinguishable from an intradermal nevus. Although the compound nevus, like any mole, can develop into a malignant melanoma, it usually remains benign and matures into an intradermal nevus. Treatment usually consists of shave or excision and closure. As with intradermal nevi, the choice of treatment depends on location and on the presence or absence of hair.

Blue nevus

Blue nevi may be flat or raised. These uncommon nevi present as dark blue or black hairless lesions that are less than 0.5 cm in diameter. They are usually indurated and palpable. The overlying epidermis is remarkably smooth and the outline regular (Plate 3, *D*). Blue nevi most commonly occur on the head and neck, the dorsa of the hands and feet, and the buttocks. They are more common in women than men and usually undergo very little change after their initial presentation. The treatment of these lesions is excision or observation. The excision must be deep because the pigment often extends deep into the subcutaneous fat, resulting in the deep blue color of the lesion.

Halo nevus

The halo nevus is a phenomenon usually associated with a junctional nevus in children or adolescents. Most commonly found on the back, it is often a benign-looking, brown papular lesion in the center of a well-circumscribed, pale white circle of depigmented skin (Plate 3, *E*). This appearance reflects the body's rejection of the nevus cells, as an inflammatory response ensues in which the melanocytes of the nevus and those of the immediately surrounding epidermis are destroyed. If left alone, these nevi will often disappear, which is rarely a sign of malignant change.

Spitz nevus

The spitz nevus is also known as a juvenile melanoma or a compound melanocytoma. This rapidly growing pigmented lesion occurs principally in children, although it can occur in adults. It is usually less than 1 cm in size and is pink or red; occasionally it can be brown or black. A Spitz nevus may be soft or hard but is usually dome-shaped and can be either sessile or pedunculated. It can occur anywhere on the body and is often difficult to diagnose clinically. Its main importance is its histologic resemblance to melanoma, with even experienced pathologists having difficulty distinguishing between the two. Very few, however, progress to malignancy. Treatment of a Spitz nevus is the same as that for an intradermal or compound nevus.

Congenital nevus

Congenital nevi are present at birth. They are not easily distinguished histologically from compound or intradermal nevi, although an expert can diagnose them. They often are dark brown to black and contain hair. They appear to be associated with an increased risk of developing a malignant melanoma, especially when they are large. Most studies define ''large'' as lesions greater than 1.5 cm, in which case the risk of melanoma ranges from 8% to 20%. The most quoted figure is about 10%, and the highest chance of melanoma developing exists in the first two decades of life. Whether this malignant potential is due to the increased number of melanocytes or to some inherited premalignant tendency in the cells themselves is not clear. Most clinicians recommend removal during early childhood, often a difficult task when a lesion is very large. The treatment of choice is surgical excision, which often must be performed in stages to remove a large lesion. Dermabrasion of the lesion within the first 6 weeks of life has been proposed by some, but recent evidence suggests that such early removal is of cosmetic importance only, as a repeat biopsy of the area will show residual neural crest nevus cells.

Nevus sebaceus

Not a true nevocellular nevus, the nevus sebaceus presents clinically as a warty, pebbly, flesh-colored, hairless, well-demarcated lesion in the scalp (Plate 3, *F*). It can also present in other areas of the head and neck. Off the scalp, the lesion can be linear, closely resembling a linear epidermal nevus. The full name is nevus sebaceus of Jodassohn. Its size varies from 0.5 cm to several centimeters. Histologically these tumors appear in three stages. In the first few months of life, the sebaceous glands in the lesion are well developed. Thereafter, through childhood, the sebaceous glands in a nevus sebaceus are underdeveloped and, therefore, greatly reduced in size and number. In this phase, the diagnosis may be missed. At puberty the lesions assume a diagnostic appearance, histologically characterized by the presence of large numbers of mature or nearly mature sebaceous glands and by papillomatous hyperplasia of the epidermis. During this stage various types of appendical tumors develop secondarily within the lesion. A syringocystadenoma papilliferum has been found in 8% to 19% of lesions. Less commonly found tumors include nodular hidradenoma, syringoma, and sebaceous epithelioma. Of primary importance is the occurrence of basal cell carcinoma in 5% to 7% of cases of nevus sebaceus. A nevus sebaceus is often small and clinically not apparent, showing no aggressive growth pattern. Therefore, full-thickness excision of a nevus sebaceus is warranted before puberty as a preventive measure.

Nevoid pseudomelanoma

Pseudomelanomatotic changes in melanocytic nevi occur after trauma and in nevi recurring after incomplete removal. The resulting lesions can look clinically and histologically like melanomas. Such a lesion often must be diagnosed histologically and on the basis of the clinical history of a previously removed nevus. Usually these lesions are reexcised full thickness for the purpose of diagnosis and treatment.

Lentigo senilis

Lentigo senilis is not a nevocellular lesion but is an important entity in the diagnosis of pigmented lesions of the head and neck. Lentigo senilis commonly occurs as multiple lesions in areas exposed to sun, often being referred to as a solar or actinic lentigo. The lesions rarely occur before the fifth decade of life, slowly increase in size and number, and form in more than 90% of whites over 70 years old, most commonly on the dorsa of the hands and on the face. They are not infiltrative, and they possess a uniform dark brown color and an irregular outline. Varying in size from minute to greater than 2 cm, they may coalesce to form larger lesions. Malignant degeneration does not occur. These lesions may resemble seborrheic keratoses in clinical appearance, and both conditions are referred to in lay terms as ''liver spots.'' Lentigo senilis lesions, however, are much less hyperkeratotic than seborrheic keratoses and have no areas of follicular prominence. They are best treated using a chemical peelant such as trichloroacetic acid or phenol or by cryosurgery using liquid nitrogen.

Dysplastic nevus syndrome

Dysplastic nevus syndrome, recently described by Clark, is also known as the B-K mole syndrome. It consists of the association of familial malignant melanoma, often occurring in multiple lesions, with ''dysplastic nevi'' in both the melanoma patients and many of their relatives. Dysplastic nevi are usually larger than ordinary melanocytic nevi, measuring from 5 to 15 mm; they present with an irregular border and a haphazard mixture of tan, brown, black, and pink. Centrally there is often a small, palpable component (Plate 4, *A*). Dysplastic nevi are located on either exposed or nonexposed skin and form throughout adult life.

Because a dysplastic nevus may transform itself into a malignant melanoma, its recognition is critical. Dysplastic nevi occur in two forms—familial and sporadic. It is important to note that melanomas arising in patients with dysplastic nevi have more of a tendency to arise *de novo* than within a preexisting dysplastic nevus, although the latter can occur. The treatment consists of careful observation after histologic confirmation of the diagnosis in the most suspicious lesions. Patients are then followed with careful photography at 4- to 6-month intervals, with biopsy and removal of any nevi that undergo change or any new, clinically bothersome nevi. Patients with the dysplastic nevus syndrome, especially those with familial variant, have a significantly higher chance than the general population of developing malignant melanoma.

CYSTS

Cutaneous cysts may be located either intradermally or within subcutaneous tissue. These generally spherical growths contain a cavity that may be fluid filled or contain cellular products or debris. A true cyst has an epithelial lining, whereas a pseudocyst lacks such an organized epithelium. Cysts are generally classified according to the pattern of differentiation they exhibit on histologic examination. Many are difficult to differentiate clinically. As a rule, malignant degeneration is rare for all of the cysts described here.

Epidermoid cysts

Epidermoid cysts are true cysts. The lining of these common tumors consists of a stratified squamous epithelium that resembles that of normal epidermis. This lining produces fully matured, keratinized cellular debris, which fills the cavity of the cyst. In a series of 125 consecutively excised epidermoid cysts at the University of Michigan, 60% occurred in the head and neck, and men were affected twice as often as women. Epidermoid cysts are thought to originate from the follicular infundibulum of hair shafts and may arise either spontaneously or as a result of inflammation or trauma to the area. Injection of surface epidermal material to deeper dermal or subcutaneous layers as a result of penetrating trauma or the use of needles has also been postulated. These cysts are rarely found before puberty, but have been found in all age groups after this period. Should these cysts appear before puberty or in large numbers, they may be an indication of Gardner's syndrome, an autosomal dominant condition that predisposes the patient to intestinal cancer.

Although malignant degeneration is uncommon, epidermoid cysts can present a cosmetic problem, and should they rupture or become infected, they may cause severe pain and scarring. Whereas some of these lesions will occasionally respond to intracystic injections of triamcinolone, surgical excision is the most effective treatment. It is necessary to carefully dissect and remove the entire cyst wall, as retained segments may lead to recurrent growth of the cyst.

Pilar cysts

Pilar cysts, also known as trichilemmal cysts or wens, are also true cysts. They are clinically indistinguishable from epidermal cysts. The tendency to form such cysts appears to be inherited as an autosomal dominant trait. The lining of the cyst differentiates in a manner analogous to that of the outer root sheath of the hair follicle. This fact allows for its differentiation from epidermal cysts. In a series of 100 consecutive cases of pilar cysts studied at the University of Michigan, 80% were on the scalp. They are uncommon before puberty. Multiple cysts are often present. If a pilar cyst ruptures or becomes infected, considerable pain and scarring may result. On the scalp, rupture may lead to areas of alopecia. As with epidermal cysts, the best treatment is complete surgical excision.

Dermoid cysts

Dermoid cysts are rare tumors that are frequently present at birth. They may measure up to 4 cm in diameter, although they are generally less than 2 cm. They may occur anywhere but are most common on the face, particularly in the area of the lateral eyebrow, the orbit, and the nose. Dermoid cysts appear to result from the inclusion of embryonic epidermis within embryonal fusion planes. Histologically these cysts are lined by an epithelium that resembles normal epidermis. They can be differentiated from epidermal cysts by their attachment to adnexal structures, which include hair, sebaceous glands, eccrine glands, and apocrine glands. Treatment is by surgical excision. If a dermoid cyst is located over the nasal root, however, care must be taken because this tumor may be confused with a nasal glioma.

Steatocystoma multiplex

Steatocystoma multiplex, an uncommon condition, is often familial, representing an autosomal dominant mode of inheritance. Although lesions can be discovered at any age, they most commonly occur shortly after puberty. The condition represents as multiple 1- to 2-cm cysts, generally located intradermally. They are most commonly found on the anterior chest but are also found on the face, forehead, ears, eyelids, and scalp. When punctured, these lesions exude a yellowish, oily fluid and occasionally hairs. On histologic examination these cysts contain a highly corrugated wall of epithelial cells. Embedded within the wall are multiple sebaceous gland lobules, which may be partially responsible for the contents of the cyst. The mode of keratinization of the epithelial lining appears to resemble that of the outer root sheath, and indeed invaginations are often present within the cyst wall that appear similar to hair follicles. Infection with pain and subsequent scarring is a major problem associated with this condition. Treatment is disappointing because of the large number of lesions present, although individual lesions can easily be excised. On the face, cosmetically acceptable improvement has been reported with dermabrasion.

Milia

Milia are small, usually 1- to 2-mm, cysts that differ histologically from epidermal cysts only in their small size. Clinically they are whitish, smooth globules, most commonly seen on the face. They may arise spontaneously, but are also frequently present as a result of trauma such as dermabrasion or burns or as a result of bullous diseases. When they arise after trauma or disease as a result of the occlusion of the pilosebaceous unit, they represent a retention cyst. Treatment is the same, whether milia arise spontaneously or secondarily, and is necessary only for cosmetic reasons. The lesion can easily be shelled out with a hypodermic needle or a comedo extractor. Because they may occasionally number in the hundreds, this treatment can be a considerably tedious chore.

Mucous cysts

Mucous cysts are pseudocysts, as no true lining is present. They are also called mucous retention cysts or mucoceles. These lesions are usually located on the mucous surface of the lower lip and are asymptomatic. They are generally less than 1 cm in diameter and, if superficial, may appear slightly bluish and translucent. They appear to be the result of traumatic rupture of the ducts of minor salivary glands. With leakage of the contents into the tissue, an inflammatory process ensues, with the resultant formation of granulation tissue surrounding the cystic space. Mucous cysts may resolve spontaneously or can otherwise be treated by intralesional injection of low-dose triamcinolone (2.5 mg/ml), excision, or marsupialization.

VASCULAR TUMORS

Cutaneous tumors of vascular origin may be true neoplasms or may be ectatic vascular systems present in either the dermis or the subcutaneous tissue. Differentiation may be toward blood vessels, lymph vessels, or both. They may be congenital or arise later in life. Most are benign. They may cause serious psychologic or physical problems (because of impingement on important anatomic structures), or they may be markers for more serious underlying diseases or syndromes. In general these can be classified histologically according to the size and nature of the vessels present. This discussion classifies the lesion as capillary angiomas, cavernous angiomas, or lesions of vascular dilation.

Capillary angiomas

Capillary hemangioma

The capillary hemangioma, commonly known as a strawberry hemangioma, is present in as many as 2.6% of all newborns. Histologically such lesions represent capillary hamartomas, although occasionally they may have cavernous spaces. Capillary hemangiomas most often occur on the head and neck, although any portion of the skin may be affected. When first noted at or shortly after birth, they are generally macular, pink to red lesions. During the first year of life, they exhibit a rapid growth phase, and the lesions become raised, dome-shaped to polypoid, and bright red to deep purple. After the first year of life, they enter a quiescent phase, followed by a period of spontaneous involution. By the age of 5, about 50% of these lesions have spontaneously resolved; 70% resolve by the age of 7 years. If they have not involuted by 7 years of age, they are unlikely to do so. Lesions located on the mucous membranes of the lip appear to exhibit the poorest chance of spontaneous resolution.

Although these tumors are benign, they may present significant problems to the patient if they impinge upon important anatomic structures, especially the eye or the respiratory tract. Other complications include ulceration and infection, which occur most commonly during the rapid growth phase. An uncommon complication, occurring in particularly large capillary hemangiomas with cavernous components, is called the Kasabach-Merritt syndrome. This syndrome involves entrapment of platelets with partial thrombosis of the capillaries, leading to rapid consumption of the body's clotting factors. With very large lesions, this development may actually lead to production of disseminated intravascular coagulation.

Because approximately 70% of capillary hemangiomas involute spontaneously, treatment is often not necessary. Unless the lesion is growing extremely rapidly and threatens an important anatomic structure or is ulcerating, treatment is not indicated until at least the age of 7 years. Rapidly growing lesions can be treated with systemic steroids. A dose of 0.5 to 1 mg/kg of prednisone daily often results in marked regression. Treatment of the Kasabach-Merritt syndrome includes heparin, blood products, and systemic steroids. If a lesion fails to involute spontaneously, surgery is indicated. Cryotherapy and sclerosing agents are generally not successful, and radiotherapy is contraindicated because of long-term sequelae related to the radiation. Laser therapy, although helpful in port-wine stains, is generally not beneficial because of the depth of these lesions.

Cherry hemangioma

Cherry hemangiomas are also called senile hemangiomas or De Morgan's spots. They may occur anywhere on the body but most are commonly on the trunk. They usually appear during young adulthood. They are generally 1- to 3-mm, bright red, slightly raised, dome-shaped lesions. The lesions consist of multiple dilated capillaries found in the upper dermis. Cherry hemangiomas are benign and unrelated to systemic or congenital disease. Treatment is not necessary but may be desired for cosmetic reasons. They respond to both superficial electrodesiccation and laser surgery.

Pyogenic granuloma

Pyogenic granuloma, a common tumor, has several synonyms, including granuloma pyogenicum, bloody wart, and pregnancy tumor. It can occur at all ages, but is most common in young children and young adults and also in pregnant women. The etiology of pyogenic granuloma is unclear, although it tends to occur at sites of trauma or infection. There may also be a hormonal factor involved, which would explain the increased incidence during pregnancy. Histologically, the lesion presents as a polypoid, lobulated mass of newly formed capillary blood vessels surrounded by an edematous stroma. An inflammatory infiltrate is generally present. Clinically, pyogenic granuloma appears as a dark red, pedunculated or dome-shaped lesion that ranges from several millimeters to centimeters in diameter. It commonly ulcerates and becomes crusted. It most commonly occurs on the distal extremities and the face but can present on any part of the body. Oral cavity lesions are common; the gingiva is the site most often involved. There is frequently a collarette of epidermis around the base of the lesion. Because of their rapid and exuberant growth, they are sometimes thought to be malignant lesions. The differential diagnosis often includes malignant melanoma, Kaposi's sarcoma, metastatic carcinoma, and angiolymphoid hyperplasia with eosinophilia.

Occasionally the lesion spontaneously resolves. Lesions associated with pregnancy frequently involute after delivery. Most often, however, the lesion must be treated surgically. This treatment is easily accomplished by surgical excision or curettage with electrodesiccation.

Angiolymphoid hyperplasia with eosinophilia

Angiolymphoid hyperplasia with eosinophilia presents in adults as single or multiple nodules commonly on the face, ears, or scalp. Intradermal lesions are generally 0.5 to 1 cm in diameter, although subcutaneous lesions may measure several centimeters. This condition appears to represent a reactive vascular hyperproliferative response, although the exact etiology and pathogenesis are unclear. Histologically the lesions consist of two components. The first is vascular: thick-walled, well-differentiated capillaries lined by very plump and prominent endothelial cells. The second component is a cellular infiltrate, which includes lymphocytes, histiocytes, and many eosinophils. The lesions appear as erythematous to purple nodules, which may ulcerate and become crusted. The condition is frequently called pseudopyogenic granuloma. Despite the fact that the lesions histologically may resemble Kaposi's sarcoma or malignant angiosarcoma, they are benign lesions. Surgical excision may be performed, but if multiple tumors are present, no therapy is warranted.

Cavernous hemangiomas

Cavernous hemangiomas consist of large venous channels or sinusoidal blood spaces situated in the deep dermis or underlying subcutaneous tissues. They are about one-tenth as common as capillary hemangiomas but may often occur in conjunction with them. Although congenital, cavernous hemangiomas are often not apparent at birth. Like capillary hemangiomas, they may undergo a rapid growth phase during the first 6 months of life; but unlike capillary hemangiomas, they are much less likely to undergo spontaneous involution and rarely completely resolve. Because of the depth of these lesions, they are poorly defined and often present with a bluish to reddish-blue color. Although they are generally smooth, more superficial lesions may be nodular and occasionally exhibit a hyperkeratotic epidermis. The lesions may feel cystic and are quite easily compressed. They are most commonly seen on extremities, where they may involve underlying muscle. Histologically, these lesions are composed of dilated, thin-walled vascular spaces lined by a flattened endothelium. Multiple thrombi may be present, with some being calcified. There is a fine, loose-surrounding stroma.

Cavernous hemangiomas may be associated with several congenital conditions. The Klippel-Trenaunay-Weber syndrome is characterized by large vascular malformations of the extremities, which may result in massive hypertrophy of an affected limb. Maffucci's syndrome is characterized by the combination of dyschondroplasia and cavernous hemangiomas, also usually appearing on the extremities. The patient may have marked bony deformities as well as pathologic fractures. In the blue rubber bleb nevus syndrome, multiple, soft, compressible cavernous hemangiomas are present, not only on the skin but also within the gastrointestinal tract, which may result in severe gastrointestinal bleeding.

Cavernous hemangiomas may result in complications related to their location. Involvement of articular spaces, oral and respiratory structures, or periocular tissues may result in impairment of function of these important systems. As with capillary hemangiomas, the Kasabach-Merritt syndrome may complicate these tumors.

Treatment of cavernous hemangiomas is very disappointing. Because of their size, depth, and the size of the individual vessels, surgery is often difficult and may result in severe hemorrhage. Treatment with radiotherapy or cryotherapy is usually not successful. In cases of Kasabach-Merritt syndrome, anticoagulation therapy with heparin is the treatment of choice. During periods of rapid enlargement, particularly when vital structures of the head and neck are in danger of being compromised, systemic steroids may be of some value in slowing the growth or shrinking the lesions. Pressure and surgery can be used where indicated.

Vascular ectasias

Vascular ectasias are actually telangiectasias or areas of vascular dilatation rather than true tumors. They may involve a significant portion of the skin and swell with time to become quite nodular. They may also cause significant problems for the patient because of secondary bleeding. Finally, these lesions may be an indication of serious underlying disease.

Nevus flammeus

A nevus flammeus is generally present at birth. The lesion presents in two general forms. The first is extremely common and may be present in up to one third of newborn babies. Located on the nape of the neck, it is referred to as a salmon patch or stork bite. It may also be present on the eyelid or glabella. Eyelid lesions generally resolve within the first year of life, and the glabellar lesions also spontaneously involute but take somewhat longer. The nuchal lesions may persist into adult life, although most will spontaneously fade.

The second, less common presentation of nevus flammeus occurs on the face and is called the port-wine stain. This lesion is present in approximately 0.3% of newborns. Port-wine stains show no tendency to fade, and in fact will generally darken and enlarge with age, becoming deeply violaceous and nodular in adult life. These lesions are generally unilateral and may follow a trigeminal distribution on the face. They may involve extensive areas of the skin of the face as well as oral mucous membranes and conjunctival membranes. Less commonly, they may involve other parts of the body.

Although most of these lesions represent only cosmetic problems to the patient, a small percentage may be indicators of serious underlying disease. One such disease is the Sturge-Weber syndrome (leptomeningeal nevus flammeus), in which a port-wine stain is located along the distribution of the trigeminal nerve. Patients with this syndrome may have angiomas within the meninges, with progressive calcification in these areas. Abnormalities associated with this condition include seizures (reported as early as 3 weeks of age but generally occurring later in infancy), mental retardation, hemiplegia, and ocular abnormalities such as glaucoma (in up to 40% of patients). Another syndrome associated with port-wine stain is the Klippel-Trenaunay-Weber syndrome (osteohypertrophic nevus flammeus), in which hypertropy of the soft tissues and bones of extremities is accompanied by an overlying nevus flammeus.

Histologic examination of these lesions may reveal no changes early in life. With time, however, the ectatic or dilated vessels become more prominent. They will vary in degree of dilatation and in depth among patients. The capillaries are otherwise normal. There may be overlying acanthosis.

Although nevus flammeus is usually an isolated cosmetic defect, its significance to the patient may be great. The natural history of these lesions is to present initially as pink or pale red patches, which, with time, progress through deepening shades of red to take on a deeply violaceous hue. Also with increasing age, the ectatic vessels become progressively more dilated and may become nodular and protuberant. Their prominent location on the face may cause significant psychologic trauma for the patient. These large nodular lesions may also tend to bleed and become crusted.

Treatment has always been difficult. Surgery, radiotherapy, and cryosurgery are not successful and may result in serious complications. Tattooing, while without significant risk to the patient, gives unsatisfactory results because of difficulty in matching skin color. The recent use of laser therapy, especially the argon laser, has provided the best results to date. It has emission bands that are close to the absorption spectra of hemoglobin. It was initially believed that selective absorption by the hemoglobin of the argon laser beam led to selective destruction of the ectatic vessels. This selectivity has not actually been borne out.

Hereditary hemorrhagic telangiectasia (Rendu-Osler-Weber syndrome)

Hereditary hemorrhagic telangiectasia is a dominantly inherited condition that affects blood vessels throughout the body. It is characterized by ectatic vessels of the skin, mucous membranes, and viscera. Often the presenting symptom is spontaneous epistaxis, which may begin in early childhood but more likely appears at puberty or in adult life. Telangiectasia begins generally around and after puberty. The superficial telangiectasia assumes three morphologic forms; the most common lesions are punctate, but they may also be linear or spiderlike. The mucous membranes are almost always involved, with lesions occurring on the nasal septum, mouth, nasopharynx, and also throughout the gastrointestinal tract. The lesions may ulcerate and frequently bleed. The condition is associated with pulmonary arteriovenous fistulas. Other viscera may also be affected, as well as the retina. Bleeding may occur from any of the vascular lesions throughout the body and may be fatal. The diagnosis is generally made when the combination of frequent hemorrhagic episodes, vascular ectasias, and a family history is recognized. Treatment is aimed at control of specific hemorrhages and of anemia if it arises. Individual lesions may be treated by electrocauterization and photocoagulation. Complete replacement of the nasal mucous membrane with a split-thickness skin graft has also been reported, but this operation may be somewhat hazardous.

Generalized essential telangiectasia (benign familial telangiectasia)

Generalized essential telangiectasia may be misdiagnosed as hereditary hemorrhagic telangiectasia. However, the lesions are somewhat different from those seen in the latter condition in that they present as extensive sheets of telangiectasias and in particular are not associated with internal hemorrhage. There may be recurrent mucosal or skin hemorrhages, but these rarely produce clinical problems, and the condition is essentially only a cosmetic nuisance.

Ataxia-telangiectasia (Louis-Bar syndrome)

Ataxia-telangiectasia is an autosomal recessive disease that includes telangiectasia, cerebellar ataxia, and recurrent respiratory infections. Telangiectasias involve the eyeball, conjunctiva, ear, face, and neck, as well as flexural areas of the limbs. Ataxia is often the initial symptom, occurring during early childhood and progressing to involve deficits in speech, ocular motility, and control of large muscle groups. There is an associated hypogammaglobulinemia, particularly of IgA, and more than one half of patients die of recurrent pulmonary infection.

Spider telangiectasia

Spider telangiectasia may be present in up to 15% of healthy people. The lesions are more frequent during pregnancy, during which they occur early and increase until delivery. They generally resolve spontaneously during the postpartum period. They may also be associated with liver disease or estrogen therapy. They tend to persist when seen in nonpregnant healthy persons. Clinically the condition presents as a central, raised, small body that may be pulsatile. Fanning out from this central area are multiple fine telangiectases. In otherwise healthy people the lesions are only a cosmetic problem. They may occur on mucous membranes, in which case the differentiation from hereditary hemorrhagic telangiectasia must be made. Treatment is by obliteration of the central feeding arterial, which can be accomplished with electrocautery or photocoagulation.

Venous lakes (venous varices)

Venous lakes present as deep blue, cutaneous nodules, occurring most frequently on the face, lips, and ears of elderly patients (see Plate 4, B). Sometimes called senile angiomas, they are composed of dilated thick- and thin-walled, otherwise normal-appearing vessels. The lesions may thrombose and involute but frequently persist. They are of no significance other than as a cosmetic nuisance.

Fibroadnexal tumors

Fibroadnexal tumors are derived from components of the deeper layers of the skin. They generally show differentiation toward the specific cell or tissue of origination and may be derived from any of the neurogenous, fibrillar, glandular, or pilar components of the dermis as well as the subcutaneous tissue.

Acrochordon (skin tag, fibroepithelial papilloma)

Acrochordons are extremely common lesions, occurring most often in middle to late life. They are flesh colored, pedunculate tumors, generally up to about 2 mm in diameter. They are soft and most commonly occur in flexural regions such as the axillae, sides of the neck, inframammary areas, and upper eyelids. The lesions are composed of mostly loose fibrous tissue, similar to that of the superficial dermis, and are covered by a thin epidermis. No adnexal structures are present. The lesions are easily removed by simple sharpscissors excision or light electrodesiccation.

Keloids and hypertrophic scars

Keloids and hypertrophic scars are generally considered to be located at different points along the same spectrum and represent uncontrolled proliferative responses to trauma by the fibrous tissue of the dermis. The difference between the two is one of degree. One definition currently in use is that a hypertrophic scar is a thickened scar that does not extend beyond the margins of the original injury, whereas a keloid is an exuberant growth extending beyond the borders of the initial scar. Keloids are most commonly seen in blacks. In certain African cultures, they are artistically induced and used as cutaneous decoration and status symbols. The epithelium overlying the tumor is frequently thinned and shiny, and the tumor may be tender and pruritic. The areas of predilection for keloids include the sternal area, the shoulders, and the upper back. They are also frequently seen on the earlobes after ear piercing and on the face. These tumors may be flat or extremely protuberant, dome shaped, or bosselated. They are most common in the second and third decades of life, becoming less common with age.

Hypertrophic scars and keloids are difficult to differentiate histologically, as both show a proliferation of fibroblasts in a whirling and nodular pattern. In hypertrophic scars, the pattern of fibroblast proliferation eventually flattens out and becomes more parallel to the epidermal surface, whereas the whirling nodular pattern tends to persist in keloids.

Until recently, treatment has been very unsatisfactory. Excision of these tumors generally has resulted in regrowth. Some success has resulted from the injection of very potent corticosteroids (triamcinolone, 40 mg/ml). Pressure also seems to stimulate involution, although the pressure must be maintained daily for up to 1 year. Special pressure earrings can be applied to the lobes, and Jobst body suits can be constructed. Preliminary experience with the use of the carbon dioxide laser to excise keloids, followed by highdose intralesional steroid injections, has been promising.

Dermatofibroma

The common tumors known as dermatofibromas fall into the class of fibrous histiocytomas and can occur anywhere on the body (Plate 4, *C*). They range in size up to 1 cm, and frequently are slightly hyperpigmented and hyperkeratotic. Dermatofibromas are benign and may persist for many years, although regression is not uncommon. On microscopic examination, these tumors are composed of spindle-shaped cells arranged in a whorled fashion with very ill-defined margins. No treatment is necessary, but if it is desired, excision is the best approach. Some dermatofibromas may respond to cryosurgery, which may at least flatten the lesion.

Dermatofibrosarcoma protuberans

Dermatofibrosarcoma protuberans is probably derived from fibroblasts. It is a rare, locally invasive, "malignant" tumor that most commonly occurs on the trunk but may occur on the scalp, face, or neck; it seldom metastasizes. It presents as a recurrent or persistently enlarging and protuberant mass, which may vary in color from flesh toned to bluish or reddish. Treatment is excision. Because incomplete removal invariably results in regrowth, microscopically controlled excision using the Mohs' technique may offer a distinct advantage in the treatment of this tumor.

Atypical fibroxanthoma

Atypical fibroxanthoma most commonly occurs in sun-exposed areas of elderly people, where it presents as a rapidly growing nodule. A less common presentation is in persons in the third or fourth decade of life, in which case growth is less rapid. The lesion is a pink to translucent asymptomatic nodule, generally 1 to 2 cm in diameter. Ulceration is not uncommon. The nodules may be mistaken for basal cell carcinomas because of their translucent appearance, the ulceration, and their location in sun-exposed areas of elderly people.

Histologically, these lesions have a very bizarre appearance, with large and atypical epithelioid and spindle cells. Multinucleate giant cells are also present. These tumors have been misdiagnosed as several different types of malignancies, including sarcomas, squamous cell carcinomas, and melanomas. Paradoxically, their course is quite benign and local excision is curative.

Neurofibroma

Neurofibromas are soft, dome-shaped, flesh-colored lesions that may be located anywhere on the body; they may vary greatly in size, from quite small to large pedunculate lesions. Neurofibromas are derived from the Schwann cells of cutaneous nerves. On histologic examination they present as nonencapsulated, loose, spindeloid tumors. Solitary lesions may be easily excised.

These tumors may be indicative of the genetic neurofibromatosis syndrome, which may be associated with severe neurologic problems as well as a risk of malignant degeneration of the tumor. When a neurofibroma is found, a careful search for other manifestations, which include cafe-au-lait spots and axillary freckling, as well as a family history, should be carried out to rule out the syndrome.

Angiofibroma (adenoma sebaceum)

Angiofibroma, formerly called adenoma sebaceum, is present as part of the genetic syndrome tuberous sclerosis. This autosomal dominant syndrome has variable expressivity; the finding of even one angiofibroma requires genetic counseling because the patient may pass on a much more severe form of the disease to offspring. Angiofibromas present as small dome-shaped papules, 2 to 3 mm in diameter, that are flesh colored or reddish brown. They are most commonly present on the sides of the nose and the medial cheeks. The original name is a misnomer, because on histologic examination no sebaceous components are noted. The tumors are composed mostly of fibrous tissue, with an angioid component. When the lesions are solitary or few in number, simple excision is curative.

Fibrous papule

The fibrous papule is a common lesion, generally occurring on the nose, especially the alae, in older persons (Plate 4, *D*). However, it can also be seen on the medial cheeks. These lesions present as small, 0.5-cm, dome-shaped, flesh-colored papules. Although they are rather common, some confusion persists as to their origin and histologic nature. Indeed, Lever questions whether these are an entity at all. They have been regarded as perifollicular fibromas, involuting melanocytic nevi, angiofibromas, or as simply the result of trauma, such as folliculitis or excoriating pimples. Histologically, the lesion presents as a papule composed of numerous spindle-shaped and stellate cells, with occasional multinucleate cells present. Once the lesions have grown, they are generally quite stable and may be present for years. They may be treated by excision or curettage and electrodesiccation. They are of no significance unless related to tuberous sclerosis.

Trichoepithelioma

A trichoepithelioma is an uncommon entity, most often presenting as small rounded nodules on the cheeks, eyelids, and nose. It appears to be dominantly inherited; however, pedigrees indicate a greater preponderance of affected females. The lesions are skin colored to slightly pink and gradually increase in both number and size with time. A few telangiectatic vessels may be present, and there may be a slightly translucent quality to the lesions, which may lead to confusion with basal cell carcinoma; however, the lesions rarely ulcerate. If ulceration does occur, basal cell carcinoma should be considered. The histologic appearance of these lesions also closely resembles basal cell carcinoma. Distinguishing between the two is often difficult. There are basophilic cells similar to those seen in basal cell carcinoma. The cells are arranged in masses, which may have fully keratinized centers. Abortive attempts at hair growth may also be noted, in which case differentiation from basal cell carcinoma is easy.

Occasionally, the presence of a solitary lesion makes differentiation from basal cell carcinoma somewhat more difficult, and unless definite differentiation toward hairlike structures is present, the tumor should be treated as a carcinoma. In the cases in which multiple lesions are present, treatment is difficult because of the large number of tumors. Some success has been obtained with dermabrasion of the entire affected area.

Cylindroma

Cylindromas may be single or multiple. When multiple, they appear to be dominantly inherited and may literally cover the scalp, a syndrome termed ''turban tumors'' (Plate 4, *E*). The condition affects females twice as often as males. It appears to originate from apocrine glands, and the tumors may be associated with trichoepitheliomas. The tumors generally appear in adult life and are most common on the face or scalp. They present as smooth, dome-shaped, or pedunculate lesions, which may be pink to red and are firm. They grow slowly and can reach 2 to 3 cm in diameter. Histologically, these tumors are composed of nests of darkly staining epithelial cells surrounded by a narrow band of hyaline material. The solitary lesion must be differentiated from basal cell carcinoma. Surgical excision is the only treatment. When large areas of the scalp are involved, this may be quite difficult and may require grafting.

Hidrocystoma

A hidrocystoma may be either eccrine or apocrine in origin. In either case, the tumor usually presents as a solitary lesion and is most frequently seen on the face. The lesion consists of translucent nodules with a firm, cystic consistency. The eccrine hidrocystoma is generally from 1 to 3 mm in diameter, whereas the apocrine may attain a diameter of 1 cm. Both may have a bluish hue. The two types are distinguishable by histologic criteria. Microscopic examination reveals differing cellular detail and secretion patterns for the two types. Treatment is excisional in either case.

Syringoma

Syringomas are benign tumors originating from the eccrine sweat gland duct. They appear more often in women than in men. Syringomas are most commonly located on the face, with the lower eyelids being the most common site. They generally occur in adolescence or early adulthood and may be eruptive or occur in crops. They present as small, 1- to 5-mm papules that are usually flesh colored but may be slightly translucent or yellowish. They may resemble trichoepitheliomas, but their location and histology help to differentiate them. Histologically, these tumors appear as small nests of cystic ductal structures as well as solid epithelial strands, many of which have a characteristic tail-like projection. They are not associated with underlying abnormality.

They do not tend to involute, however, and may present a cosmetic problem when located on the face. Treatment is difficult, but light electrocoagulation with a fine epilating needle appears to be the most successful modality at this time.

Sebaceous hyperplasia

Sebaceous hyperplasia occurs mainly on the face, particularly the forehead, and represents benign enlargement of the normal sebaceous gland (Plate 4, *F*). It is frequently called senile sebaceous hyperplasia because it is usually seen in older persons. One or hundreds of lesions may be present. They may be from 2 to 5 mm in diameter, and there is usually a central umbilication. These lesions are soft and yellowish and must be differentiated from basal cell carcinoma. Histologically they present as hyperplastic sebaceous lobules that are otherwise normal in appearance. They are only a cosmetic problem; and solitary lesions can easily be treated by shave excision, electrodesiccation and curettage, or cryosurgery. When the lesions are quite numerous, surgical excision is unwarranted. Therapy with systemic 13-cis retinoic acid has also been described.

Xanthelasma

Xanthelasmas present on the eyelids, or close by, as soft yellowish irregular plaques. They usually appear in middle age and affect either sex. They are not often associated with xanthomas elsewhere on the body. Frequently they are an isolated finding and do not always signify elevated serum triglyceride levels, although each patient should be examined for the existence of such a systemic problem. Histologically these lesions present as an accumulation of xanthoma cells, although giant cells and fibrosis are uncommon. Treatment is application of 20% to 35% trichloroacetic acid, light cautery, or excision.

Lipoma

Lipomas are benign tumors composed of adipose tissue and may be single or multiple. They are soft and may be lobulated or rounded and cystic in nature. They are generally freely movable. Except in rare syndromes, lipomas are nontender. They generally occur on the trunk but may also occur on the neck or any other part of the body. Histologically they present as proliferations of normal-appearing fat cells that may be surrounded by a thin connective-tissue capsule. Single lesions present only cosmetic problems, and they are generally easily excised. Despite attaining sizes of more than 1 inch in diameter, they may often be expressed through a small, 4-mm punch hole.

TREATMENT METHODS AND BIOPSY TECHNIQUES

Scalpel surgery

The *shave* excision or biopsy is one of the most common performed on cutaneous lesions. It is a rapid means of removing tissue either as part of therapy or to establish a diagnosis. A shave can be performed using various techniques, with the depth of the shave dependent on the angle of the blade as it enters the skin. Usually either a No. 15 or No. 10 Bard-Parker blade is used. One should remember that the sharpest point of the No. 15 blade is the rounded tip, whereas the No. 10 has its sharpest edge along the belly of the blade. The shave should be performed using the sharpest portion of the blade. The sharpest blade is a Gillette Blue Blade; it is excellent for shaving lesions. A blade breaker or hemostat can break the Blue Blade into any size or shape desired. The blade can then be held between thumb and forefinger and flexed, allowing the performance of a superficial shave in which the blade sculpts along the contour of the surface being excised (such as the ala of the nose or the helix of the ear). Hemostasis can then be obtained with aluminum chloride. Monsel's solution (ferric subsulfate) should be avoided on the face or cosmetic areas because of the ability of macrophages to phagocytose the iron, causing a tattoo.

The *punch*, a fixed-diameter surgical knife, is an extremely valuable tool to a dermatologist for excision or biopsy. It comes in various sizes, from 2 mm to 1 cm, with 0.5-mm increments. Punches can be purchased as disposable instruments (Baker) or as permanent, sterilizable instruments. The commonest sizes used for biopsy are 3 mm and 4 mm. However, a 2-mm punch can provide a cosmetically elegant biopsy of sufficient size for the pathologist. Whenever possible, the 4-mm punch should be used. All punch-biopsy incisions should be closed.

Some tricks help in the use of a punch. By putting tension on the skin perpendicular to the anticipated line of closure (skin tension lines), one can cause the circular punch to leave an oval or ellipse for easier closure. The incision is usually closed with sutures or the recently introduced single-shot staple. A valuable trick is to use a punch to excise intradermal nevi. By selecting a punch that just fits around the nevus, one can easily excise it to the depth necessary to remove the entire lesion. Another trick, which can be used when nevi occur in areas of neutral skin tension or where skin tension lines are not obvious (e.g., the chin), is to use the punch to help determine the best lines of closure. If the surgeon uses a punch excision with no tension placed on the skin, the resulting circle will usually form itself into an oval along lines of facial expression and help determine skin closure lines. Often the skin closure lines can occur at an angle perpendicular to what one might expect.

The *wedge* excision or biopsy, a variation of the fusiform excision (ellipse), can be used to remove lesions cosmetically or to perform biopsies. As a biopsy technique, it is either incisional or excisional. Whenever possible, especially in dealing with pigmented lesions, the excisional biopsy is preferred to give the pathologist the best chance for an accurate diagnosis. When the wedge procedure is performed as an incisional biopsy of a large, nodular lesion, the narrowest possible wedge (greater than the classic 3:1 length-width ratio) is made at the edge of the lesion so that one end of the wedge is through normal skin. Then, one side of normal skin is available through which to pass suture. This is an especially important advantage if the other side of the wedge is within friable tissue.

Scissors excision is a valuable method of cosmetically removing benign skin tumors. In experienced hands, scissors can be used to produce an often elegant cosmetic result very quickly. They are best used on raised, pedunculate skin lesions in which the pedicle can be easily and rapidly cut with scissors. Our preference is to use fine-tipped, curved Iris or Gradle scissors. Tricks similar to those for the shave apply to scissors excisions. Raising a bleb of anesthesia under a pedunculate lesion will allow for better scissors access to the base. Scissors are an excellent tool around eyelids. Often a small chalazion clamp can be placed around a lesion, permitting easy excision with fine scissors. Filiform or pedunculate lesions on eyelids can be lifted with fine forceps and then cut with curved scissors held with the tips up. This procedure will produce a small ellipse upon release of the eyelid skin, which will either heal by itself or by the placement of one small stitch. Scissors can also be used for biopsies of the oral mucosa. Again, a chalazion clamp can be placed on the lip, or a stitch can be placed around the area of the biopsy. One can then pull up on the stitch, creating a tent of tissue that can be scissors excised at the base to obtain a biopsy specimen.

A curette is a valuable tool to the skin surgeon. One should have a variety of sizes of curettes available; larger curettes are used to debulk or remove larger tumors, and smaller curettes are used to do the same for small tumors or to help track small extensions of cutaneous tumors such as basal cell carcinoma. A curette is held like a pencil, with the ring finger or small finger placed on the skin to anchor and stabilize the hand. Normal skin has a "gritty" feel with the curette, whereas abnormal skin or tumor often feels mushy or soft. One way to remove multiple molluscum contagiosum lesions on the face, for example, is to individually curette each small lesion (a small curette is used). If anesthesia is required, one can use either the usual local anesthetic or one of the refrigerant anesthetics, which will induce some anesthesia in the skin as well as harden the lesion. Hardening allows the lesion to be easily flicked off with a curette. A curette is often used in conjunction with electrosurgery.

Electrosurgery

Electrosurgery is a useful way to remove small benign lesions, to assist the curette in removing malignant lesions, and to assist the surgeon in obtaining hemostasis. Most electrosurgery performed in the office requires nothing more than a Hyfrecator-like unit. This versatile instrument is easy to use because the patient does not need to be grounded, and the electrodesiccation or fulguration is at a more superficial depth than the electrocoagulation or cutting seen when a patient is grounded. Most of these electrosurgical units have two current settings. The low current is best for light electrodesiccation of benign lesions. One also can purchase a fine steel tip or place a 30-gauge needle on the standard tip. This tip can then be threaded down adnexal structures to treat benign adnexal tumors or to coagulate arterial vessels feeding vascular lesions. The high setting, a destructive mode, is used to burn tumor and surrounding tissue, as in electro-desiccation or fulguration of basal cell carcinomas. Bipolar units, with the patient grounded, can be used in the cutting mode with a loop to remove benign lesions and to help sculpt lesions, such as in the case of a rhinophymatous nose.

Cryosurgery

Cryosurgical removal is the treatment of choice for many lesions. Systems vary from elaborate cryospray and cryoprobe units to something as simple as a Styrofoam cup containing liquid nitrogen to be applied with a cotton-tipped applicator. Most physicians prefer the latter method because of its simplicity. Use of the cryospray and cryoprobe machines is often reserved for treatment of malignant lesions. The superficial use of cryosurgery destroys tumor tissue, often with excellent cosmetic results. Hypopigmentation and other sequelae can develop, however, which make the use of cryosurgery in darker skin more difficult.

Chemical or abrasive surgery

Many superficial cutaneous lesions of the head and neck can be removed by application of a chemical or by abrasion. The chemicals most commonly used as peeling agents are trichloroacetic acid and phenol. The concentration of trichloroacetic acid used varies from 35% to 70%. Phenol is usually used as a concentrated solution (88%) or mixed as Baker's solution. These chemicals can be used to peel benign pigmented or melanotic lesions with good success.

The most common form of abrasion is spot dermabrasion. Our favorite tool is the Bell hand engine with the diamond fraise or wire brush. The fraise can be purchased in varying sizes and shapes; small, 2-mm wheel, cone, or cylindrical fraises are excellent tools for removing multiple small epithelial tumors.

Laser surgery

The use of lasers has gained increasing popularity in the treatment of many lesions of the head and neck. Laser surgery was first used in the treatment of vascular tumors—in particular, port-wine stains and hemangiomas. The argon laser was the first type used on such lesions, and its current use meets with a good degree of success. Because it seals lymphatics and vessels as well as nerve endings, the argon laser can be used in highly vascular areas or for the excision of lesions such as keloids, in cases of which minimal surgical trauma seems to play a role in preventing re-formation. The carbon dioxide laser followed and has been used in the treatment of vascular lesions as well as other cutaneous lesions. Its value is that it can be defocused and used as a destructive instrument or focused and used as a cutting unit.

Other lasers, including the tunable dye unit and the Nd: YAG unit, await further refinements for cutaneous applications. One interesting use of the tunable laser set at the correct focal length (630 nm) is to photoactivate a hematoporphyrin derivative that becomes attached to neoplastic tissue, thus causing the destruction of the cutaneous neoplasm.

Chapter 23

Lacerations and Scar Revision

Terence M. Davidson

LACERATIONS

Wound classifications

The standard first aid text of the American Red Cross classifies wounds as open or closed and defines an open wound as any wound involving a break in the skin or the mucous membrane.

The Red Cross further classifies open wounds into five types: abrasions, incisions, lacerations, punctures, and avulsions. An incision is a clean wound such as a knife makes, whereas a laceration has a jagged edge such as a traumatic shearing injury would cause.

First aid

First aid for open wounds requires stopping the bleeding, protecting the wound from contamination and infection, providing care for shock, and obtaining medical attention. Bleeding is best controlled by direct pressure and can be lessened by elevating the injured tissue. Applying pressure to the supplying artery is useful in some cases; only rarely should a constricting tourniquet be necessary. The wound is kept clean with a dressing, and the patient is treated for shock and transported to an emergency room. At this point a physician begins the medical evaluation and institutes proper medical treatment.

Diagnostic assessment

The medical evaluation always begins with an overall patient assessment to ensure that the patient is breathing, has a beating heart, and is not severely bleeding. The physician looks for other major, more important injuries such as head trauma or a fractured cervical spine. Convinced that no other matter is more pressing, the physician can investigate the wound. No matter how slight the wound, it should be evaluated for injury to bones, nerves, ducts, vessels, muscles, mucosa, and skin. Bony injury is detected by (1) observing hypesthesia, asymmetry or deformity or change in function (e.g., diplopia or trismus), (2) by palpation, and (3) by radiographic evaluation. The primary nervous functions of the face are sensation by cranial nerve (CN) V and facial movement under the control of CN VII. To some degree the astute physician suspects nerve injury. For example, if an infraorbital rim fracture exists, the experienced physician knows that these fractures invariably course through the infraorbital nerve canal, resulting in decreased sensation over that cheek. The facial nerve is at particular risk with penetrating injuries and lacerations in the region of the parotid gland. With injuries of this area, the physician must carefully assess and document the level of function of all branches of the facial nerve.

The two ducts in the head and neck which, if injured, cause dysfunction are the lacrimal duct and the parotid duct. Injury to the submandibular ducts is usually intraoral and rarely causes dysfunction. Such an injury must be suspected whenever trauma occurs in the vicinity of these ducts, and proper evaluation requires cannulating the respective ducts and determining that they are intact and functioning.

Although a myriad of small vessels in the head and neck bleed profusely when cut, only injury to the internal carotid arteries, the vertebral arteries, and the intracranial vessels causes dysfunction. Therefore, if the external carotid artery, the facial artery, or the angular artery has been lacerated, it can simply be ligated. In general, if a vessel is large enough to be specifically named, ligating it with a suture is probably best. Smaller vessels can be controlled by cautery. Detecting muscle injury at the time of wound examination is important. Mucosal and skin injuries are detected simply by examination and palpation.

432   FACE

Management

Figure 23-1 is an overview of wound repair and scar revision. Management of lacerations begins with wound cleaning. If the wound is a clean laceration such as one made by a knife or broken glass, the wound and surrounding tissues are adequately cleaned with a 2- to 5-minute gentle povidone-iodine (Betadine) scrub. A potentially contaminated wound, such as an older wound or one made by a dirty object, should be scrubbed vigorously and irrigated with povidone-iodine and may on occasion need débridement. Any foreign material in the wound, such as dirt and road particles, must

be thoroughly removed. Removal may require scrubbing the skin vigorously with a brush, dermabrading it, or even cutting out bits of dirt and other foreign material with a No. 11 scalpel blade. Removal of all foreign material at the time of the initial repair is imperative, because if left it may cause a tattoo that will be very difficult to remove later.

Guidelines and rules exist as to which wounds can be closed and what the timing of such closure should be. Most of these rules are for wounds involving the trunk and extremities and do not apply to the head and neck. The blood supply to the face and neck is so rich that the risk of infection in

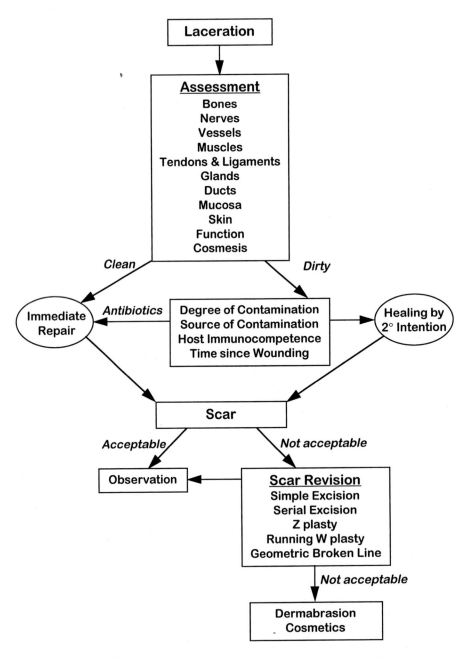

Fig. 23-1. Summary of evaluation and treatment for lacerations and scars.

almost any wound is small. Therefore any wound in the head and neck can be closed primarily unless gross contamination is obvious. Dog bites, human bites, and wounds as old as 24 hours can all be closed, and while increased risk of infection exists, that risk is small. If infection does occur, it can usually be recognized and effectively treated before any serious sequelae occur. Wounds closed by secondary or tertiary intention leave unsightly scars that are unacceptable on the face.

The indications for the use of antibiotics are rapidly changing. The majority of clean facial wounds do not require antibiotics. If the wound is a dog bite or a human bite or involves the oral or nasal mucosa, it is best to give the patient antibiotics for 5 to 10 days. Amoxicillin or amoxicillin with clavulonic acid are the drugs of choice for wounds with oral anaerobes. Cutaneous wounds without anaerobic contamination are treated with staphylococcus-active cephalosporins, pending culture and sensitivity results. There is nothing wrong with beginning with cephalexin and adjusting as needed. While the temptation to treat patients with antibiotics always exists, this temptation must be resisted unless there are bona fide indications. The consequences of injudicious use of antibiotics affect us all and include increases in the cost of medicine, increase of antibiotic-resistant bacteria, and increase of patients with allergy to antibiotics.

Anesthesia

Most facial wounds can be closed while the patient is under local anesthesia. Lidocaine is a safe and effective anesthetic agent. Doses up to 300 mg are usually safe for the average adult. Concentrations of 0.5% to 1% are effective. Unfortunately, lidocaine is a vasodilator in the head and neck, which causes substantial wound edge bleeding because of the rich vasculature. Therefore epinephrine is normally added to lidocaine solutions. The most commonly used preparation is 1% lidocaine with 1:100,000 epinephrine. For patients with large wounds or with a sensitivity to epinephrine, 0.5% lidocaine with 1:200,000 epinephrine is equally effective. Using a sharp, small-bore needle to inject the anesthetic reduces the volume of anesthetic injected and causes the patient less discomfort. Most physicians inject more anesthetic than is necessary. It is best to use a 1-inch 30-gauge siliconized needle in most situations. The pain associated with an injection comes from (1) the insertion of the needle through the skin, (2) the tissue distortion caused by the volume of anesthetic agent used, and (3) a burning sensation caused by the epinephrine. Injecting 0.5% lidocaine with 1:200,000 epinephrine slowly through a 30-gauge needle causes minimal discomfort.

Nerve blocks can be used where possible, but local infiltration is employed for most wounds to provide both anesthesia and hemostasis. Lidocaine is effective for only 30 to 60 minutes. If a longer period of time is required, supplemental anesthetic can be given with bupivacaine (Marcaine). Bupivacaine is not ideal as a single agent because its onset is much slower than lidocaine and the completeness of the an-

esthesia it provides is sometimes inadequate. The total dose of bupivacaine permissible for an average adult is around 120 mg. A 0.5% concentration should be used, since the 0.25% concentration does not seem to give effective anesthesia. The 0.75% solution is more than is needed and increases the risk of toxicity.

Bupivacaine can be injected separately after anesthesia with lidocaine. Alternatively the bupivacaine can be mixed with the lidocaine by mixing equal volumes of 2% lidocaine with 1:50,000 epinephrine and 0.75% bupivacaine. This solution containing 1% lidocaine, 0.375% bupivacaine, and 1:100,000 epinephrine provides excellent, rapid onset anesthesia with all the long-acting benefits of the bupivacaine.

There is a certain art to obtaining anesthesia for a laceration or scar with minimum patient discomfort. Some of this involves comforting and reassurance and some involves using small needles, small volumes, and the least irritating solutions. There is a format for injecting an area and typically this begins with a nerve block, followed by a field block, followed by local infiltration. Figure 23-2 depicts the sequence of injections. Nerve blocks are not always possible and field blocks are not always optimal, but local blocks are virtually always required. Nonetheless, when possible the sequence makes it a smoother process.

Internal repairs

In most instances hemostasis is readily achieved by direct pressure. Large named vessels such as the facial artery or angular vessels should be ligated with 4-0 chromic, 4-0 Vi-

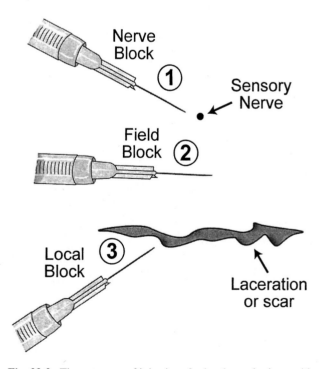

Fig. 23-2. The sequence of injections for local anesthesia providing optimal anesthesia with the least patient discomfort.

cryl, or 4-0 silk suture. All other bleeding points are easily controlled with cautery.

Skeletal injuries should be repaired before the soft tissues are repaired. The principles of skeletal repair are discussed in Chapter 24.

Injuries to large motor nerves such as the trunk or major branches of the facial nerve must be repaired. Fortunately, the facial nerve carries only motor fibers, and fascicular repair is unnecessary. Equally good results should be obtained with most gentle nerve suture techniques. Concern exists about the optimal timing of this repair. Although some studies have suggested that waiting 3 weeks may be preferable in cats, this benefit has not been substantiated in humans, nor is the delay practical. The common practice is to repair nerves at the time of initial treatment. The surgeon should repair motor nerves under a microscope, using several epineural stitches (Fig. 23-3). If the surgeon is skilled in microscopic anastomosis, 10-0 monofilament nylon is recommended. However, if the proper instruments are not available or the surgeon is not practiced in microanastomotic surgery, using 8-0 monofilament nylon is best. For large nerves such as the trunk of the facial nerve, four or five individual epineural sutures are required; for smaller nerve branches, two stitches may be sufficient. Silastic sleeving has no proven benefit, although it makes it easier to return later to find the neurorrhaphy. Therefore placing a small thin, preferably blue, piece of silastic around the neurorrhaphy may be helpful.

Wounds of the lacrimal system, the parotid and the submandibular duct should be repaired. The repair is made by cannulating the duct with an appropriate-sized silicone cannula and then repairing the injured duct over the cannula. If a portion of the duct is missing, the cannula should be left in place for 6 weeks and often the endothelium will bridge the gap. If the lacrimal system is totally avulsed and destroyed, performing a dacryocystorhinostomy will be necessary. This is best done 3 to 6 weeks after the initial injury. If the parotid or submandibular duct is not easily repaired and can be easily marsupialized into the oral cavity, this functions as well as a primary repair.

Repair of lost or damaged tissue. If extensive tissue damage or tissue loss occurs, several important factors must be considered. Skin that has been abraded will heal with an abnormal texture and color. The degree of deformity is proportional to the depth of abrasion. If this represents a small amount of tissue that can easily be excised, doing so is best. If it represents a substantial area of skin, letting this heal and then performing a scar revision at a later date is preferred. Jagged wound edges should not be trimmed, and the surgeon should do the best possible job of reapproximating the respective jagged edges. This often gives a superior result as will be evidenced in later sections dealing with running W-plasties and geometric broken-line closures. However, if some of the irregular edges contain devitalized tissue, they should be trimmed at the time of the primary repair. A defect resulting from tissue loss, as is seen in an avulsion wound, must be closed. If the loss is small, the wound can be closed by undermining and advancing local tissue. If the defect is larger, using a local skin flap may be necessary. In even larger wounds, more involved techniques such as skin grafts or regional flaps may be necessary. If in doubt, the surgeon should cover the wound with a skin graft and perform a revision later when all the different reconstructive methods can be considered.

If supporting tissue such as cartilage from the nose or ear has been lost, autogenous or homologous cartilage may be used for the reconstruction. For very small cartilaginous defects, cartilage can be taken from the patient's nasal septum or ear, or on rare occasions, costal cartilage can be used. If the avulsed tissue is brought to the emergency room with the patient and can be cleaned, it can be put back in place in an effort to have it accepted as a free graft. Small segments of skin heal easily, but larger tissue grafts heal with difficulty. If vessels are available for microvascular anastomosis, the chance of survival will certainly improve.

Three theories of repairing an avulsed ear exist. The first is simply to sew the ear back in place in the hope that it will take. When this is done, multiple cutaneous incisions should be made on both surfaces of the ear to allow drainage of serous exudate. In addition, if a hyperbaric oxygen chamber is available, hyperbaric oxygen treatments for a week or two will improve the chance of survival. Without hyperbaric oxygenation the success rate for this method is poor, and many surgeons prefer taking the skin off the cartilage and banking the cartilage underneath the skin of the abdomen until reconstruction can be performed. The author has had success and failure with both of these techniques. Recently,

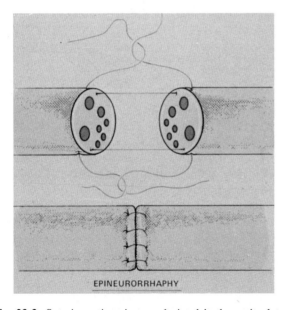

EPINEURORRHAPHY

Fig. 23-3. Suturing epineurium as depicted is the optimal technique for repairing facial nerve.

sporadic success has been reported with microvascular anastomosis. If microvascular expertise is available, the avulsed tissue is maintained in iced saline and the microvascular team performs the repair in the operating room. Microvascular repair probably has the highest success rate and should be considered whenever available.

If a portion of the nose or ear is avulsed, the segment should be sutured in place and treated as a composite graft. If a piece of soft tissue has been avulsed from the cheek or lip as in a bite injury, that tissue should not be replaced because it will have neither sensory nor motor innervation, and most such defects can be closed by rearranging local tissues.

Occasionally the physician sees an injury in which the entire scalp is avulsed. This occurs most commonly in a person whose long hair is caught in a rapidly revolving wheel and whose scalp is literally jerked from the head. Simply suturing the scalp back in place is doomed to failure. Fortunately, the scalp is supplied by four major vessels, and if any of these can be reanastomosed by microvascular surgical technique, the scalp has a good chance of surviving. Therefore, if a patient has a scalping injury the best treatment is to ask a surgeon who performs microvascular anastomoses to repair the scalp.

The vessels of the head and neck, other than the common and internal carotid arteries, do not need to be repaired.

Muscle and tendon repair

If the patient is to regain normal facial function, all muscles should be reunited. In areas such as the corner of the mouth where numerous small muscles pull in different directions, realigning them precisely is particularly important. However, in the neck and most areas of the face such as the forehead and cheek, general realignment is adequate. When muscle bundles are being repaired, 4-0 Vicryl or Dexon is effective. However, if a fascial system exists with the muscle, a permanent suture such as 4-0 nylon to approximate the fascia is preferred. Because how muscles are sutured does not seem to matter, at least on the face, a single stitch is employed, passing the needle through the fascia on one side, through the muscle, and out the fascia on the other side. The suture must be placed identically through muscle and fascia on both sides. Several sutures should be used for each muscle in case a suture pulls loose. In complex areas such as the corner of the mouth, the lips, and about the eyes, failure to reapproximate the muscles will cause a significant deformity.

The most important tendons in the face are those of the medial and lateral canthi. These must be repaired with a permanent suture such as 4-0 nylon.

Mucosal lacerations are closed with absorbable sutures. Chromic catgut or polyglycolic acid sutures seem to be equally effective. For large lacerations, interrupted vertical mattress sutures give the safest closure. For small lacerations and when a watertight closure is needed, a simple running or running locking stitch does well. If a large potential dead space exists, it should be obliterated with interrupted absorbable suture.

Skin closure

The principles of skin closure are simple, although the practice is never perfected. Deep stitches approximate the dermis. The purpose of these stitches is to take the tension off the wound edge and to align the skin for the surface closure. This step is followed by any of several techniques for closing the skin. The goal is to align the epidermis carefully to provide the best opportunity for an aesthetically acceptable scar. The standard training today for the deep sutures is to use a 4-0 Vicryl or Dexon suture that is passed through dermis and subcutaneous tissue as in Figure 23-4. A number of these are placed along the wound edge; some surgeons believe that the more stitches placed, the better the result. The author believes that each one of these strangulates the local blood flow and adversely affects wound healing when pulled tight. Therefore the fewer sutures used to achieve approximation, the better. In addition, if these sutures are placed too near the surface, they may not provide the best opportunity to create an everted wound. For these reasons, whenever possible the subcutaneous dermal stitches should be placed approximately 1 cm from the wound edge

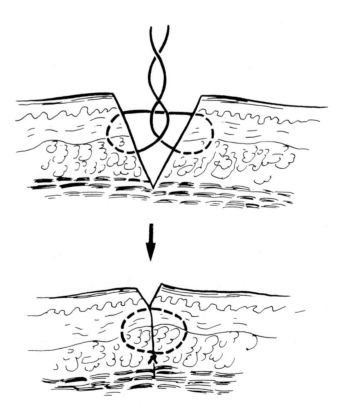

Fig. 23-4. The traditional technique for subcutaneous dermal stitches.

(Fig. 23-5). By so doing, fewer stitches are needed, the blood supply to the wound edge is less compromised, and the wound edges are easily everted with the superficial stitches.

Using an absorbable suture is important because a permanent material such as nylon, silk, or teflon can be extruded from the skin as a foreign body. Surgeons who place 20 to 50 of these in a patient may be required to see the patient 20 to 50 times postoperatively to remove each extruding stitch. Plain and chromic catgut are not ideal in the face because they may be absorbed too quickly. Polyglycolic acid sutures maintain good strength for 3 months and cause minimal inflammation. They are eventually absorbed completely and are now preferred by otolaryngologists.

Skin closure techniques. Many different techniques may be used for the superficial cutaneous closure, and it is doubtful that a single best technique for all physicians will ever exist.

Figure 23-6 illustrates the five most frequently-used stitches. A certain amount of eversion is desirable, and for this purpose interrupted *vertical mattress sutures* are optimal. Unfortunately, placing a vertical mattress suture takes twice as long as most other methods, so these sutures are not always practical. Tissue trauma is an important factor in the ultimate result. Whether the surgeon uses skin hooks or fine forceps is irrelevant, but how these instruments are used is relevant. The tissue must be handled as gently and infrequently as possible. When the sutures are removed, the

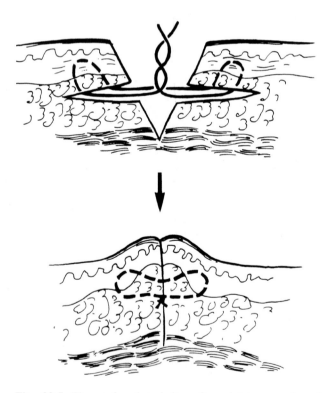

Fig. 23-5. The preferred technique for subcutaneous dermal stitches.

tissue suffers additional trauma, and the patient may experience some additional discomfort.

Another excellent stitch (but certainly a more difficult one to place) is the *running subcuticular suture*. For surgeons who frequently perform meticulous wound repairs, this technique gives excellent results, once it is perfected.

Because interrupted sutures take longer to place and may cause unneeded tissue trauma and suture marks, many surgeons prefer to use *running stitches*. The *simple running stitch* is the most commonly used, with the *running locking stitch* also frequently used. The latter usually allows a more precise alignment of skin, but can jeopardize blood supply to the wound edge if pulled too tight. A technique the author uses for most wounds, particularly those in children, in whom suture removal is difficult, is a running locking stitch of 5-0 or 6-0 fast-acting gut. This suture material is rapidly absorbed and is gone in 3 to 5 days. The added inflammation caused by the catgut does not seem to adversely affect wound healing. The author has never seen suture marks left by this material, even if strands of suture persist for 1 or 2 weeks. Because the suture may dissolve in some areas in as little as 2 to 3 days, the running locking suture is preferred so the entire stitch does not come loose.

Whatever technique is chosen, it should be performed with small superficial bites that approximate the wound margins without tension. The stitch should include only 25% to 50% of the thickness of the skin except where the skin is very thin. In these locations the suture should include the full skin thickness. Sutures should not be pulled too tight because they could strangulate tissue and cause suture marks.

Drains and dressings. If the wound is large with much oozing or if the potential for infection is high, a small drain can be left in the wound. Generally a small Penrose or even a rubberband drain will suffice.

All wounds should be dressed. Normally an occlusive dressing is applied, since this improves epidermal healing and therefore the final appearance. The wound can be covered with a nonadherent dressing such as a Telfa pad or with Steri-Strips. The second layer of the dressing should contain absorbent material such as gauze. The third layer should place gentle pressure on the wound and may be applied in such a way that it decreases tension across the wound. Properly applied Steri-Strips do this on the first dressing layer, but if a Telfa-paper tape dressing is used, the antitension effect is achieved with the paper tape layer. The second and third layers of the dressing are changed after 24 hours, and all three layers are removed after 3 or 4 days. The sutures are removed on the third or the fourth postoperative day. If they are not removed until the fifth postoperative day or later, the risk of epithelial growth down the suture increases, resulting in a permanent suture mark. If fast acting gut sutures are used, Steri-Strips are imperative because they enhance the suture breakdown. The Steri-Strips are removed after 3 or 4 days and then are reapplied for an additional 3 to 5 days. If some suture material persists after 6 or 7 days, it can be gently cut and pulled free.

All wounds should be observed by a physician, initially to be sure they do not become infected and then to be sure they do not form hypertrophic scar. If hypertrophic scar or keloid is formed, the earlier it is recognized and treated, the better the outcome.

Problems. Four potential problems are associated with traumatic wounds: (1) wound infection, (2) hypertrophic scar and keloid formation, (3) aesthetically unacceptable scar, and (4) psychologic nonacceptance. Wound infection is more common with dirty wounds, particularly in animal or human bites, and infection becomes more likely the greater the time between wounding and wound closure. In addition, infection is more likely in a patient with impaired resistance or poor blood supply to the tissues (e.g., a diabetic patient or a patient with multiple injuries who is hypertensive and hypoxic). Generally a wound infection becomes apparent 24 to 72 hours after wound closure and appears as a reddened, painful swelling. Cellulitis, a superficial spreading infection most commonly caused by *Streptococcus*, is treated with penicillin. An abscess is most commonly caused by *Staphylococcus*. If the wound has been exposed to oral cavity anaerobes, a mixed anaerobic abscess may form. When an abscess

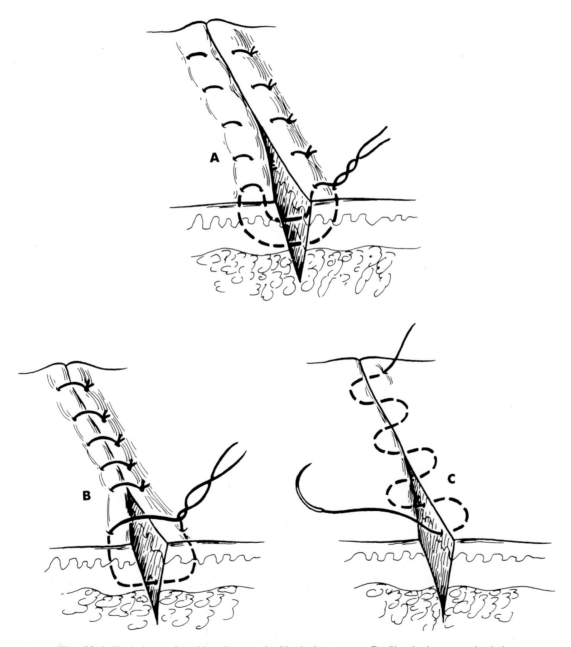

Fig. 23-6. Techniques for skin closure. **A,** Vertical mattress. **B,** Simple interrupted stitches. **C,** Running subcuticular stitches.

Continued

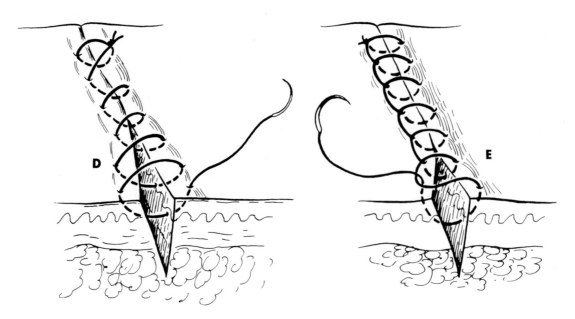

Fig. 23-6, cont'd. D, Simple running stitches. **E,** Running locking stitches.

occurs, the wound must be opened sufficiently to drain all of the exudate. A sample should be sent for culture and sensitivity testing. The wound should be irrigated with povidone-iodine solution and drained. If the bacterial agent is most likely staphylococcal, dicloxacillin should be administered. If it is uncertain which bacterium is causing the infection, a Gram stain should be taken. If gram-positive cocci are present in clumps, the patient can be given dicloxacillin; if other bacteria, particularly those associated with anaerobic infections, are present, the patient should be given amoxicillin. The antibiotic regimen is then adjusted when the culture and sensitivity results are available. The wound should be examined and irrigated daily, and the drain changed or examined for patency. When the wound is clearly healing and the drainage has subsided (normally within 3 days after incision and drainage), the drain can be removed. However, the antibiotics should be continued for at least 10 days.

Hypertrophic scar and keloid formation is the result of overzealous wound healing. Some physicians believe that hypertrophic scar and keloid are different entities, whereas others view them as points on a continuum. Both hypertrophic scar and keloid appear initially as red, inflamed excessive scar tissue commonly associated with itching. As soon as this begins (as early as 4 weeks after the wound repair or as late as a year or two after repair), the abnormal scar should be injected with a long-acting steroid preparation. Triamcinolone (Kenalog-40) is the most commonly used steroid. It can be injected into the wound with a Dermajet or with a needle and syringe. If a needle and syringe are used, a 25- or 27-gauge needle is necessary. The triamcinolone should be injected into the scar and not the normal tissue surrounding the scar. The preferred concentration is 40

mg/ml, and if delivered through a Dermajet, 0.1 ml can be deposited every 5 to 10 mm along the wound. This is repeated at 2- to 3-week intervals until the hypertrophic scar or keloid disappears.

Hypertrophic scar usually disappears after one or at the most three applications of steroids. Keloids can be more resistant and may require multiple applications. For difficult keloids, the Dermajet does not deliver sufficient volumes of triamcinolone. After the wound has been softened with two or three doses of triamcinolone delivered through the Dermajet, subsequent injections should be given into the keloid with a 27-gauge needle. Only very large keloids require excision or irradiation. Most keloids can be treated successfully with multiple injections of triamcinolone. If the keloid is large and mature, as many as 20 or 30 injections may be necessary. A keloid detected and treated early would be unlikely to require more than 10 injections. The maximum acceptable dosage of triamcinolone per month is 120 mg for adults, 80 mg for children 6 to 10 years of age, and 40 mg for children 1 to 5 years.

The third problem sometimes associated with a facial wound is an aesthetically unacceptable scar. All wounds leave some scar tissue, and every patient must recognize that even with revision a scar will remain. All scars fade with time and with scar maturation. Coaching the patient to wait and see how the scar develops is important. The scar that may look unacceptable at 6 weeks or even 6 months may mature and be perfectly acceptable after 1 or 2 years. This is dealt with further in the section on scar revision. A recent clinical review on keloids by Berman and Bieby in the *Journal of the American Academy of Dermatology* is highly recommended. They discuss numerous treatment options. Intralesional corticosteroids are the first treatment option with reported successes of 50% to 100%. Radiotherapy is used for larger and/or refractory lesions and has a variable success rate of 16% to 94%. Other reported treatment methods include pressure, excision with or without radiotherapy, topically applied silicone gel sheeting, laser vaporization, cryotherapy, and interferon therapy.

The fourth problem is the psychologic damage that can occur from a traumatic wound of the face. Since no one wants to be injured or deformed, some psychologic trauma is related to every wound. Wounds resulting from one's own follies seem to be less stressful than those inflicted by someone else. For example, an inebriated person who falls and cuts himself on the kitchen table has no one to blame but himself and tends to be psychologically more accepting of the wound. In contrast, a person who suffers a facial laceration while sitting in a parked car that is hit by another car, whose driver is inebriated and has a history of multiple arrests for drunk driving, will be angry and difficult to deal with psychologically. Similarities exist between the psychologic response to death and dying and the response to traumatic wounding. The elements of grief, anger, denial, bargaining, and ultimate acceptance are common to both. The surgeon should never perform a scar revision on a patient who is still angry and refuses to accept the fact that he has a deforming scar. The angry patient will never be pleased unless the blemish is entirely removed from his face, an impossible goal to achieve. No matter how skilled the scar revision, the patient will be unhappy and will turn his anger toward his physician. Once a patient accepts the scar, he will be grateful for any improvement and is a good candidate psychologically for scar revision. Sometimes getting a psychiatric evaluation is necessary before doing a scar revision. Finally, as a general rule, a patient involved in litigation relating to his scar will not be a good candidate until the litigation is resolved. It is amazing how many patients who show great anger over a scar completely forget about the scar and its deformity when the lawsuit is settled.

SCAR REVISION

Any scar that is longer than 2 cm, is wider than 2 mm, distorts normal anatomy, or does not lie in a favorable skin tension line may be improved by scar revision.

Scar revision carries four requirements: (1) that the patient desires having the scar revised, (2) that the patient is in a state of mind allowing him to benefit from scar revision, (3) that the scar is mature, and (4) that revision can reasonably be expected to improve the appearance of the scar.

Timing is important. First, the patient must be psychologically prepared. That is, he is no longer angry about having a scar and will be satisfied with a degree of improvement. The patient cannot expect the ultimate result to be perfect. Second, the scar should be mature, since whether or not a scar needs revision may not be known until it has had the opportunity to mature. The healing of the initial wound gives

the surgeon valuable information as to what to expect with the healing of the scar revision. Waiting for scar maturation forces the patient to become comfortable with the scar and psychologically prepared to benefit from scar revision. Generally the waiting period is 1 year. It should rarely be less than 6 months, even if the tissues are physiologically ready, since the patient will probably not be psychologically prepared.

Correcting underlying deformities

Before beginning scar revision, the surgeon must correct all underlying deformities. For example, reconstruction of the lacrimal system or of the medial canthal tendon or correction of a skeletal deformity may be necessary before the scar revision.

Sites for incision

Before beginning scar revision, the surgeon must understand the most favorable sites for incision. These are (1) inside an orifice such as the nose, mouth, or ear, (2) in a place that may be covered by hair, (3) at the junction of two aesthetic areas, and (4) in or paralleling favorable skin tension lines. While the first two may be useful in designing elective surgery, they are rarely useful in scar revision unless the surgeon can move a scar from an unfavorable site into an orifice or the hairline. Sometimes a scar can be moved into the junction of two aesthetic areas. These include the junction of the forehead with the nose, the forehead with the temple, the temple with the cheek, the temple and the cheek with the eyelid, the cheek with the nose, the cheek with the lip, the cheek with the chin, and the chin with the lip. An incision placed exactly in the boundary or junction of two areas generally forms a less obvious scar than one placed even a millimeter or two away from that boundary.

The lines that naturally occur on a person's face as a result of gravity, aging, and facial expression have been given a number of names, and to date no name is universally accepted. As early as the 1800s, these lines were of interest to surgeons, and Langer described a series of them. Other surgeons have described similarly oriented lines in relation to underlying musculature and have suggested a variety of names such as ''relaxed skin tension lines.'' In an older patient on whom these lines have already formed as wrinkles, crow's feet, and smile lines, identifying the favorable skin tension lines is easy. However, in a young patient guessing where the favorable skin tension lines lie and where wrinkles will lie later in life may be difficult. The easiest way to do this is to ask the patient to go through a number of facial movements such as smiling, frowning, and wrinkling the nose. The skin creases that form indicate the favorable skin tension lines. Even a young child when asked to squinch his nose will wrinkle the skin along the favorable tension lines. The orientation of these lines is similar from one patient to another but is also unique in each patient. The precise positions of the lines are extremely important because they dictate the preferred geometry for each scar revision.

Techniques

Simple excision

Simple excision is the least complicated scar revision technique but is rarely the technique of choice. If the scar parallels a favorable skin tension line, lies within a wrinkle or at the junction of two aesthetic areas and for some reason did not heal well initially, it is reasonable to expect that simple excision and approximation will result in a better scar. Often incisions have been closed primarily in an emergency room. The surgeon performing the scar revision may think that with excision and closure, under more favorable conditions, with more meticulous suture technique, a better result will be obtained. All too often this plan fails. Thus, simple excision should be reserved for scars that have initially healed with a complication that has caused a less favorable appearance. In addition, it may be an adequate technique for some scars that parallel favorable skin tension lines and are shorter than 2 cm.

Simple excision is easy to perform. The surgeon merely excises the scar, undermines the wound edges for about 1 cm, and closes the wound as described earlier in the section dealing with wound repair. It is important to take all tension off the wound closure, to avoid tissue injury and to evert the wound edges. If the initial scar was depressed, the surgeon may remove the epithelium from the scar, leaving the dermal scar tissue in place. The edges of the wound are then advanced over this dermal scar, which acts as a filler.

Serial excision

Removal of a large scar resulting from the excision of a large hairy nevus, an area of tissue loss that has been closed with a skin graft, or a burn injury can be accomplished by serially excising it in several operations. The technique of serial excision involves making an incision at one side of the scar, undermining the wound edges, excising the scarred area or a portion of it, and closing the wound edges under moderate tension. Over the next 6 to 12 weeks the skin stretches. The surgeon can then repeat the procedure. Skin has a tremendous potential to stretch as long as it is pulled slowly in this fashion, and even large defects such as covering 30% to 40% of the forehead can be closed by serial excision. All initial incisions and closures must be made within the scar tissue to avoid sacrificing nonscarred, healthy tissue. In the last operation the remaining bit of scar tissue is excised and normal, healthy tissue is approximated to normal, healthy tissue on the opposing side. This last procedure is sometimes done in a straight line but more often is done as a brokenline closure as discussed later in this chapter. In addition to excising large scarred areas, serial excision is used to move a scar into a hairline, into the junction of two aesthetic areas, or to a less visible site.

New methods for stretching the skin include techniques for tissue expansion. The daily growth of a fetus does a wonderful job of expanding anterior abdominal skin, and the slow acquisition of fat can stretch almost any skin. Tissue expanders have been less than desired for facial skin. Tissue expansion is expensive and time consuming. For most facial defects, serial excision remains the preferred method.

Z-plasty

Z-plasty is another important and useful technique in scar revision. A Z-plasty accomplishes two things: lengthening the scar and changing its direction. It does so, however, at a significant price. To whatever degree it lengthens in one direction, it shortens or tightens the tissue in the perpendicular direction, and if this tissue is already tight or is vascularly compromised, additional stretching can be dangerous. Furthermore, a Z-plasty requires two extra incisions, so rather than one scar, albeit less than perfect, three scars will now exist.

The most useful application for a Z-plasty is to correct a linear incision that crosses the junction of two aesthetic areas where the natural tissues are concave and therefore the contracted scar is causing a web that crosses the junction or an important favorable skin tension line.

Designing and transposing the triangular flaps of a Z-plasty can be difficult. A Z-plasty is simply two flaps that are transposed one over the other in such a way that tissue is borrowed from areas of excess and transposed into areas of deficiency. At the same time, the orientation of the revised scar is changed about 90° (Fig. 23-7). Assuming that a scar exists (indicated by the line 1-2 in Fig. 23-7), has contracted, and lies in an unfavorable direction, the goal would be to lengthen the scar and change its orientation to a more favorable one. This is begun by excising the scar (1-2) to form the central limb. Two triangular flaps are now created by making

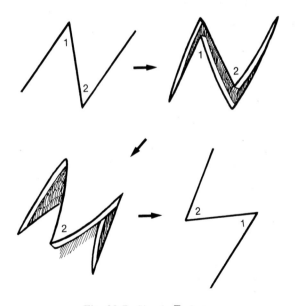

Fig. 23-7. Simple Z-plasty.

two parallel incisions, one beginning at 1 and the other beginning at 2. These incisions are called the lateral limbs. The angles between the central limb and the lateral limbs should be equal at 1 and 2. This angle is used to define the Z-plasty: that is, if the angle is 60°, the Z-plasty is called a 60-degree Z-plasty. The triangular flaps and the surrounding tissues are undermined and the flaps are transposed, one over

and one under. In so doing, the distance 1-2 is lengthened and the orientation of the central limb is changed. The amount of lengthening achieved is a function of the length of the central and lateral limbs and of the angle of the Z-plasty. The greater the angle, the greater the lengthening. Figure 23-8 indicates the theoretic degree of lengthening achieved with classic 30°, 45°, and 60° Z-plasties.

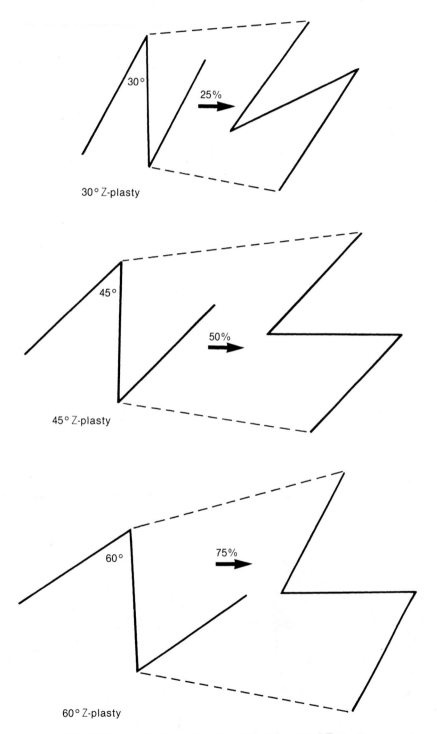

Fig. 23-8. Lengthening achieved by 30°, 45°, and 60° Z-plasties.

Surgeons most commonly employ 60° angles because they provide a reasonable balance between lengthening and local tissue distortion. Theoretically the surgeon could use 120° or 150° Z-plasties and achieve a high degree of lengthening, but the cost would be a tremendous local tissue distortion and protrusion.

In designing a Z-plasty as shown in Figure 23-9, the surgeon must pay attention to the orientation of the lateral limbs. Every Z-plasty has four different possible designs for the lateral limbs. Only one design is optimal. In most Z-plasties the central limb lies perpendicular to the favorable skin tension lines. In one orientation the lateral limbs parallel the favorable skin tension lines, and in other orientations the lateral limbs cross favorable skin tension lines. The correctly designed Z-plasty employs lateral limbs that parallel the favorable skin tension lines. This is so important that, if the favorable skin tension lines in a given area are not parallel, the surgeon would even use different angles for the two transposing flaps to keep the lateral limbs in and parallel to favorable skin tension lines. It is also important that the ends of the lateral limbs lie precisely in the line where the new central limb will be placed. Figure 23-10 shows two Z-plasties. The dotted lines joining the ends of the lateral limb lie where the new central limb will lie. The second Z-plasty

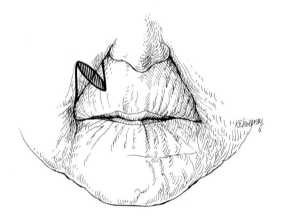

Fig. 23-9. The proper orientation of lateral limbs for Z-plasty.

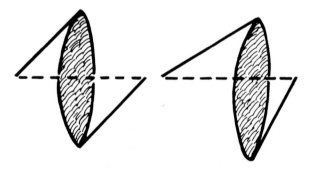

Fig. 23-10. The correct orientation and design of lateral limbs to control the ultimate position of the new central limb.

employs different angle transposition flaps. This trick is often used to ensure that the lateral limbs parallel favorable skin tension lines and that the new central limb lies precisely where it is desired.

Compound Z-plasty

Compound Z-plasty (Fig. 23-11, *A*) may be necessary to lengthen a long linear scar in situations where doing this as a single Z-plasty is disadvantageous. A large single Z-plasty is undesirable if it would necessitate incising and transposing very large flaps. The wide angles used cause undesirable tissue protrusions. One alternative is to incise and transpose a series of smaller flaps. This procedure, called serial Z-plasty, is diagrammed in Figure 23-11, *B*. An alternative to serial Z-plasty is multiple Z-plasty as depicted in Figure 23-11, *C*. Multiple Z-plasty may cause unnecessary tissue protrusions if not done properly. Therefore, before performing these techniques on a patient, the surgeon is strongly encouraged to draw the designs and closures of many different types of Z-plasty on a piece of pliant rubber. Alternatively, the surgeon can take squares of elastoplast and stick them back to back in such a way that they are rotated 90° before pasting them back to back. This creates a field that is uniformly elastic in most directions, making an excellent model for practicing Z-plasty and local skin flaps.

Broken-line closure

The techniques discussed so far provide the surgeon with a limited ability to improve the majority of facial scars. Not until the concepts of running W-plasty and geometric broken-line closure were developed could the surgeon make real improvements in most facial scars.

The concept of a broken line is simple. The eye easily perceives a straight line. Once the eye sees any portion of a straight line, it easily follows that line. For this reason a linear scar, no matter how carefully created, is never truly inconspicuous. The broken-line techniques of scar revision address this problem. By creating a scar that is a series of short, broken lines, the surgeon can fool the eye. The first attempts at broken-line closures used serial Z-plasties, but these sometimes were disadvantageous because of the lengthening created by the Z-plasties. The next pattern used was the running W-plasty, and the last pattern developed is called a geometric broken line. Figure 23-12 compares simple excision, Z-plasty, running W-plasty, and a geometric broken line.

The running W-plasty is a useful and simple scar revision technique. The scar is excised with a minimal amount of normal tissue, using the design shown in Figure 23-13. The scar is then excised. The two wound edges are undermined and advanced together, and the small triangular flaps and defects are interdigitated as shown. When properly done, this technique creates a less conspicuous scar. To be effective, each straight line must be no longer than 5 mm and

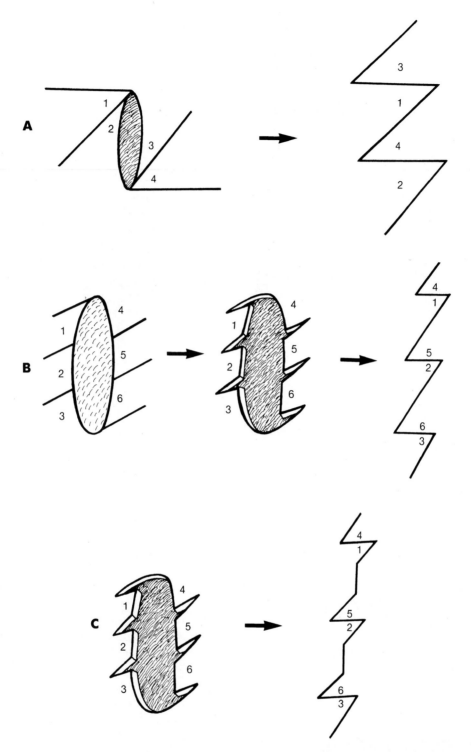

Fig. 23-11. Techniques of compound Z-plasty. **A,** Basic compound Z-plasty. **B,** Serial Z-plasty. **C,** Multiple Z-plasty.

each of the angles connecting the straight-line segments must be 90° or less. The human eye perceives one of the short segments and follows it. When it comes to the end of the segment, the eye sees normal tissue. The eye returns, picks up the next segment, and follows it. Because the angles are acute, the eye does not readily follow from one broken seg-

ment to the next. Thus a broken-line scar is less noticeable than is a straight or curvilinear scar.

Figure 23-14 shows how a running W-plasty can be adapted to a curvilinear scar, and Figure 23-15 shows how the orientation of the triangular flaps is tailored to the orientation of surrounding favorable skin tension lines.

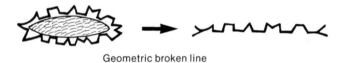

Simple excision

Serial Z-plasty

Running W-plasty

Geometric broken line

Fig. 23-12. Comparison of four techniques of scar revision.

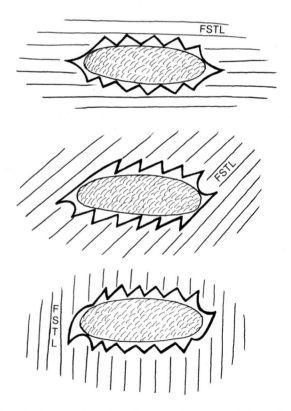

Fig. 23-14. Use of a running W-plasty on a curvilinear scar.

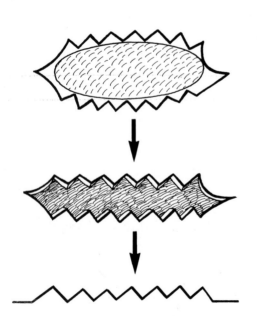

Fig. 23-13. The design for a standard running W-plasty.

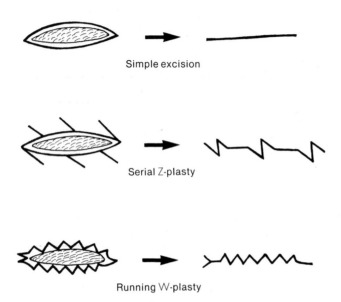

FSTL

FSTL

FSTL

Fig. 23-15. The orientation of running W-plasty relative to local favorable skin tension lines.

Often the end of a scar is wide so that bringing the end to a 30° angle to prevent tissue protrusion may create a longer linear scar and may necessitate excising excessive normal tissue. Using an M-plasty (Fig. 23-16) saves tissue, decreases the length of linear scar, and prevents tissue protrusion as effectively as a single 30° angle. Advancing or retarding the tip of the M-plasty during wound closure further controls the orientation and length of the final scar (Fig. 23-17).

Figure 23-18 shows a typical scar revision problem. An M-plasty is used at the left end of the scar. A running W-plasty adapts well to the curved portion of the scar, and a 60° transposition flap is used at the wide end of the scar. This fits nicely into the pattern of the running W-plasty.

Unfortunately, with longer scar revision a running W-plasty develops a pattern that can be recognized, and for this reason the geometric broken line was developed as an improvement. Figure 23-19 depicts a geometric broken-line design excision and closure. The only difference is that each flap is of a slightly different size and shape than those around it so the ultimate pattern is completely unpredictable. When properly done the geometric broken line is a superior technique for scar revision.

Refining technique

Several tricks will improve the surgeon's ability to use scar revision techniques. A running W-plasty and a geometric broken line must be properly designed. As many of the

short segments as possible should lie parallel to favorable skin tension lines, and as few as possible should lie perpendicular to favorable skin tension lines. As with the running W-plasty (see Fig. 23-15), the design of a geometric broken line is tailored to fit the favorable skin tension lines. Because the flaps on either side of the wound must be interdigitated,

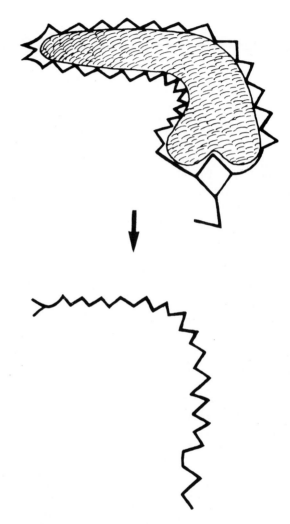

Fig. 23-18. Scar revision using running W-plasty and transposition flap.

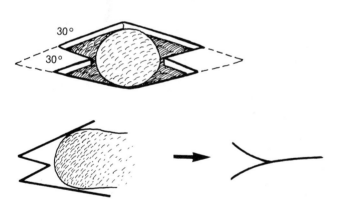

Fig. 23-16. M-plasty.

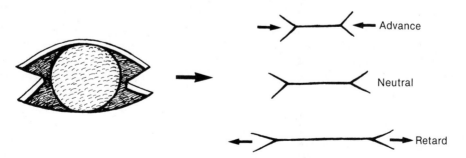

Fig. 23-17. Possible closures for M-plasty.

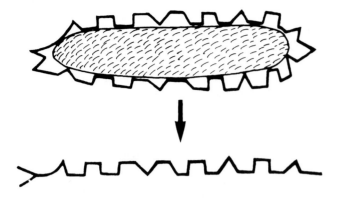

Fig. 23-19. Geometric broken line closure.

the height of the flaps and respective defects must be the same. Beginning at either end of the scar, the surgeon creates very short flaps, with the first flap 2 mm, the next flap 3 mm, the next 4 mm, and the rest between 4 and 5 mm (Fig. 23-20). The width of the flaps should vary between 3 and 5 mm. The difficulty, of course, is to make each flap and its recipient site similar in all aspects. By drawing a series of lines perpendicular to the scar, the surgeon defines the limits for each flap and recipient site. Then respective flaps and recipient sites for each box are simply filled in. This is particularly useful when the scar courses around a curve, since the design on the concave side is significantly smaller than the design on the convex side. Although designing square, trapezoid, and rectangular flaps and defects around a curve is possible, using triangular flaps for these areas is easiest. Whenever a scar goes around a curve, across a concavity, or over a convexity, triangular flaps are best.

If lengthening is required in the scar revision, interrupting the geometric broken line or the running W-plasty and putting in one or several Z-plasties is easy. Creating length with a running W-plasty by designing a series of Y to V maneuvers is also easy (Fig. 23-21). This design is particularly useful for tracheal scar revision. The disadvantage of using the Y to V maneuvers is that the flaps ultimately become 7 to 10 mm in length and are therefore more conspicuous than shorter flaps.

Closing a broken-line excision should be simple. The wound edges on either side are undermined for a distance of 1 to 2 cm, and the wound edges are brought together with interrupted absorbable sutures placed at least 5 mm back from each wound edge. This preserves blood supply to the flaps, relieves the tension from the wound edges, and allows the wound edges to be closed with eversion. To close a geometric broken line or even a running W-plasty with interrupted, monofilament permanent suture would be time consuming. A preferred and much quicker technique is to use a fast acting gut stitch sutured in a running, locking technique, catching all of the flap corners on one side of a wound, crossing over to the other side of the wound, catching all of

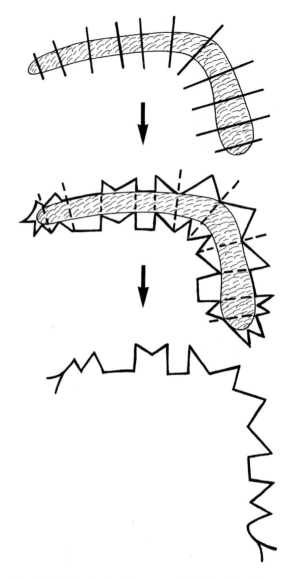

Fig. 23-20. The design for geometric broken-line closure.

the flap corners on the second side of the wound, and ultimately tying the suture to itself (Fig. 23-22).

The inexperienced surgeon may have difficulty cutting small angulated flaps. They are most easily incised with a No. 11 blade held vertically (Fig. 23-23). On delicate skin such as the upper lip or the eyelid, using flaps that are only 2 to 3 mm in length will be necessary, whereas in larger, less delicate surfaces such as the cheek and the forehead, larger flaps (5 to 6 mm) are permissible. After the wound is sutured, it is immobilized by criss-crossing it with Steri-Strips to prevent tension on the closure for at least 3 months. If the subcutaneous intradermal sutures are properly placed, they will carry most of the tension. The scar is then allowed to heal and mature. Six to twelve months later, when the scar is fully mature, it can often be further improved with dermabrasion.

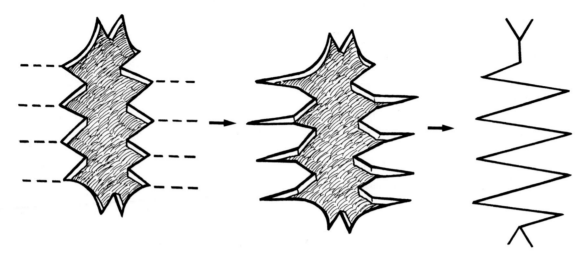

Fig. 23-21. Modified running W-plasty to achieve lengthening.

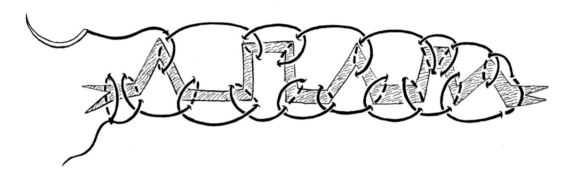

Fig. 23-22. Running locking closure for geometric broken-line design.

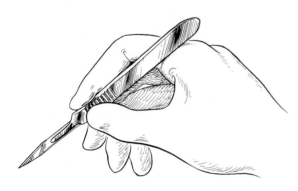

Fig. 23-23. Technique for using No. 11 scalpel to cut running W-plasty or geometric broken-line pattern.

The scar is visible because, when the scar edge is sharply vertical, it creates a shadow. In poorly or brightly lit environments, scars are generally less visible. By saucerizing the scar with dermabrasion, the edges are smoothed and no shadow is created. In addition, most scar tissue has a slightly glassy appearance. The dermabrasion removes the epidermis of the scar and the adjacent skin as well. When the epidermis regrows, it blends into that of the surrounding normal tissue.

Case Studies

The patient is a 26-year-old woman who was involved in an automobile accident and when first evaluated had the appearance shown in Figure 23-24, A. The injuries included bony fractures of the right malar bone and orbital floor. The eye was enophthalmic and was inferiorly displaced into the maxillary sinus. The cheek bone was depressed. All of the soft tissues of the right medial canthus had been avulsed, and the medial canthal ligament and lacrimal system were disrupted. The laceration at the corner of the mouth involved skin, muscle, and some mucous membrane. The laceration beneath the lower lip extended through the mucosa into the mouth. The skin was abraded and contained a moderate amount of road dirt.

After the patient was stabilized and other, more serious injuries were excluded, she was brought to the operating room. Under general endotracheal anesthesia the wounds were cleaned and all the dirt was meticulously scrubbed from her face. The medial canthal ligament was identified and sutured to the periosteum of the nasal bone with a 4-0 nylon suture. The malar and orbital floor fractures were explored, reduced, and wired in position. The orbital floor was reconstructed with a piece of Silastic sheeting. All the mucosal wounds were closed with 4-0 Vicryl, and all the muscles were reapproximated with 4-0 Vicryl. The skin was closed with 4-

0 Vicryl placed in the subcutaneous tissue and with 6-0 Davis and Geck mild chromic for the superficial sutures.

The patient healed well but had a persistent epiphora. A dacryocystorhinostomy using a Lester Jones glass tube was performed. Figure 23-24, B, shows the patient approximately 3 months after the initial repair, and Figure 23-24, C, shows the patient the same day after professional cosmetic consultation. Further scar revisions are planned but will not be performed until all the scar tissue has had an opportunity to mature.

The patient shown in Figure 23-25 is a 19-year-old girl who was involved in an automobile accident in Mexico. She did not receive medical care until approximately 10 days after the injury. Figure 23-25, A, shows the patient at the time of initial examination. She was given a general anesthetic, and the wounds were meticulously scrubbed. Unfortunately, removing all of the road dirt from her face was impossible. In addition, there was substantial tissue loss, most evident around the right lateral canthus. The wounds were closed as well as possible, and the patient is shown in Figure 23-25, B, shortly after this surgery. Figure 23-25, C, shows her approximately 3 months after the accident. Some hypertrophic scar, some obvious pigmentation, and some obvious scar and deformity were present. While she waited for the scar tissue to mature, a professional cosmetic consultation was obtained. Figure 23-25, D, shows the improvement resulting from this consultation.

Several scar revisions were carried out; Figure 23-25, E to H, shows some of these. Her appearance several years later, a year after the last of multiple surgical procedures, is shown in Figure 23-25, I to K. She was at this time a college student and refused to wear makeup but fortunately had undergone scar revision and had a very acceptable appearance.

The young man shown in Figure 23-26 was involved in a motorcycle accident in which his nose was essentially avulsed from his

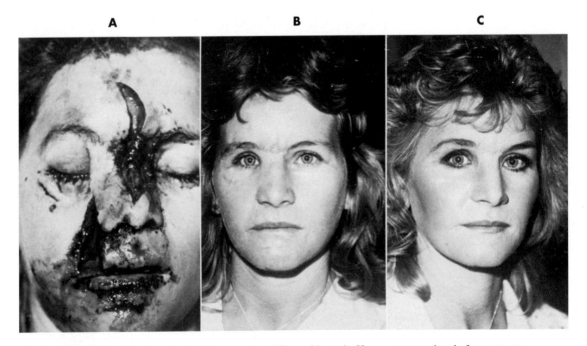

Fig. 23-24. A patient involved in an automobile accident. **A,** Her appearance just before surgery. **B,** Her appearance without makeup 3 months later. **C,** Her appearance after professional cosmetic consultation.

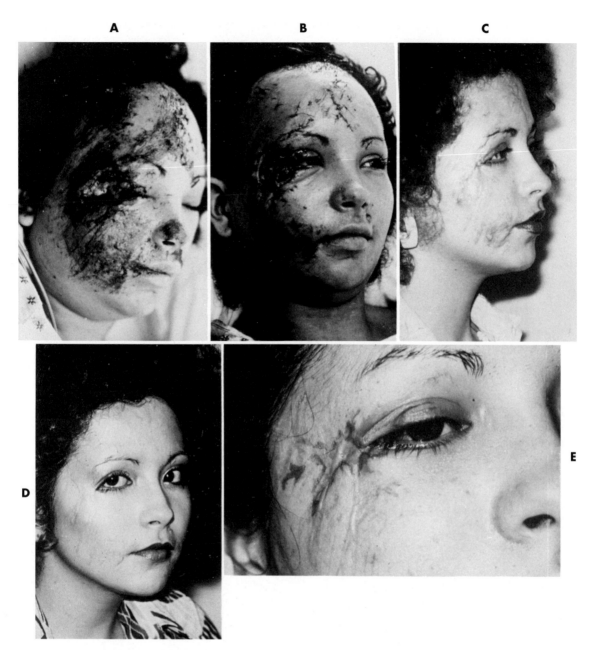

Fig. 23-25. A patient involved in an automobile accident initially seen 10 days after the injury. **A,** Her appearance at presentation. **B,** Her appearance several days later, after wounds had been closed and débrided as well as possible. **C,** Her appearance 3 months later. **D,** Her appearance the same day as in **C** but after professional cosmetic consultation. **E,** Scar revision planned around lateral canthus to excise and repair hypertrophic scar tissue in the area of previous tissue loss.

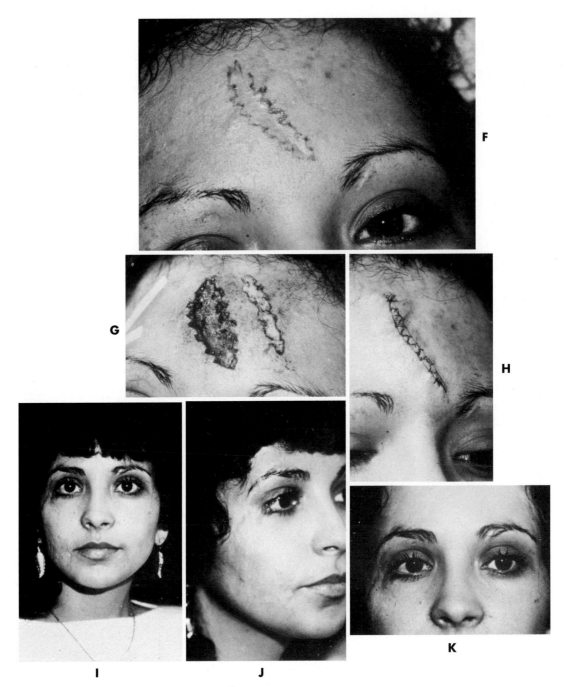

Fig. 23-25, cont'd. F, Geometric broken-line design for forehead. **G,** Geometric broken line excised. **H,** Geometric broken line closed. **I, J,** and **K,** Appearance 1 year after the final scar revision and approximately 3 years after the initial surgery.

face. The bones and cartilages of the nose were severely traumatized. All this material was packed into some sort of anatomic realignment, and all the incisions inside and outside the nose were closed. Figure 23-26 B and C, shows the result of this injury and repair 1 year later. The major deformity was the loss of support for the nose. This was repaired with a rhinoplasty (Fig. 23-26, D and E). Tip projection was augmented and reinforced with a septal cartilage strut placed in the columella. The dorsum of the nose

was augmented with Supramid mesh graft, and the tip of the nose was better defined with a cartilage graft as described by Sheen (1978). Figure 23-26, F and G, shows the patient's appearance 1 year after the rhinoplasty.

The principles of wound repair and scar revision are simple. The practice requires a full knowledge of the basic principles, a creative surgeon, a psychologically receptive patient, patience, and a little bit of luck.

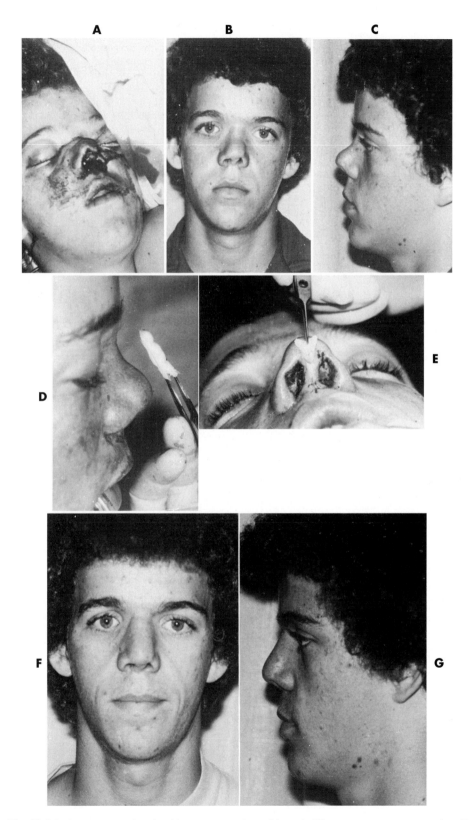

Fig. 23-26. A young man involved in a motorcycle accident. **A,** His appearance at presentation. **B** and **C,** His appearance 1 year later. **D** and **E,** Intraoperative photographs during rhinoplasty. **F** and **G,** Appearance 1 year after nasal surgery.

SUGGESTED READINGS

Berman B, Bieby HC: Keloids, *J Am Acad Dermatol* 33:117, 1995.

Bernstein L: Z-plasty in head and neck surgery, *Arch Otolaryngol* 89:574, 1969.

Borgus FA: *Elective incisions in scar revision*, Boston, 1973, Little, Brown.

Davidson TM, Sevel D: Management of facial trauma, Washington DC, 1986 (available from the American Academy of Otolaryngology—Head and Neck Surgery) (videotape).

Davidson TM, Webster RC: *Scar revision: self instructional package*, ed 2, Washington, DC, 1983, American Academy of Otolaryngology.

Ketchum LD and others: Treatment of hypertrophic scar, keloid and scar contracture by triamcinolone acetonide, *Plast Reconstr Surg* 38:209, 1966.

Peacock EE Jr, Van Winkle W: *Wound repair*, ed 3, Philadelphia, 1984, WB Saunders.

Sheen JH: *Aesthetic rhinoplasty*, ed 2, St Louis, 1987, Mosby.

Vallis CP: Intralesional injection of keloids and hypertrophic scars with the Dermo-Jet, *Plast Reconstr Surg* 40:255, 1967.

Webster RC, Davidson TM, Nahum AM, producers: Scar revision, parts I to III. San Diego, 1976, San Diego Classics in Soft Tissue and cosmetic surgery (available from the American Academy of Facial Plastic and Reconstructive Surgery) (videotape).

Wolfe D, Davidson TM: Scar revision, *Arch Otolaryngol Head Neck Surg* 117:200, 1991.

Chapter 24

Maxillofacial Trauma

Robert B. Stanley, Jr.

Traditionally, fractures of the facial skeleton have been evaluated and treated in a segmentalized fashion, even if complex injuries were obvious on the initial evaluation. It has become increasingly evident that discussion of facial injuries in terms of fractures of the upper, middle, and lower thirds of the facial skeleton is illogical and most likely is based on an arbitrary division of responsibilities among various surgical specialties that might consider treating such injuries. Although the segmentalized approach produced acceptable results in many injuries that were caused by low-velocity impact forces, such as those which might occur in sporting events or fist fights, similar success often was not achieved in victims of high-velocity impact injuries, such as those seen with high-speed motor vehicle deceleration crashes or interpersonal violence involving blunt instruments and gunshot wounds. Experienced maxillofacial trauma surgeons have recognized that suboptimal results cannot always be attributed to the severity of the injury itself, but rather in some instances they are a result of a segmentalized approach to treatment.

Advances in diagnostic imaging, surgical instrumentation, and surgical techniques have confirmed that no facial fracture should be evaluated as an "isolated" bony injury and should not be approached without regard to all surrounding structures. Not only do all bones of the face have numerous superficial articulations, but also, all relate in some fashion directly with the skull base. Therefore, the maxillofacial trauma surgeon should be familiar with the anatomy of the entire skull and be skilled in surgical procedures that involve bone immediately adjacent to the brain, eyes, cranial nerves, salivary glands, major vessels, oropharyngeal soft tissues, and teeth. In some patient, a team approach may be required for management of injuries to these associated structures. Treatment of the fractures should be coordinated by the sur-

geon who can best conceptualize the injuries to the parts and to the whole of the facial skeleton.

ANATOMY

Frontal bone

Superiorly, the frontal bone provides the gentle convex contours of the forehead, the frontal bar, and the orbital roofs (Fig. 24-1). The frontal bar is the thickened bone that bridges between the zygomaticofrontal (ZF) sutures to give structure and strength to the superciliary and glabellar areas. The frontal sinus orifices lie protected behind the glabellar bone and the stout maxillary processes of the frontal bar. The frontal bar forms the superior-most horizontal buttress of the intricate lattice-like structure that maintains dimensions of the face and surrounds and protects the orbits, nasal cavity, paranasal sinuses, and oral cavity. The orbital roofs project superiorly and posteriorly from the frontal bar to separate the anterior cranial fossa from the orbits. Structural integrity of the frontal bar is essential for reconstruction of fractures that involve the frontal bone, zygomata, orbits, nasoorbitoethmoidal (NOE) complex, and maxilla.

Maxilla

The maxilla is related superiorly to the frontal, ethmoid, and zygomatic bones and posteriorly to the pterygoid plates of the sphenoid bone within a system of relatively strong, vertically oriented struts or buttresses. These include the well-defined, paired nasomaxillary (NM), zygomaticomaxillary (ZM), and pterygomaxillary buttresses, which originate in the maxillary alveolar process and project superiorly to the skull base (see Fig. 24-1).[48] All of these buttresses have developed as a mechanical adaptation of the skull to masticatory forces. The greatest occlusal load appears to be borne by the ZM buttress, which originates in the lateral antral wall immediately above the first molar and continues superiorly through the zygoma to the ZF suture. Although the bone of the maxilla is thin overall, its lateral wall is formed by a V-shaped thickened area of compact bone that provides strength for the lower end of this strut.

The vertical buttresses are, for the most part, curved structures and should be reinforced by horizontal struts. These reinforcing connections include the frontal bar, inferior orbital rims, the maxillary alveolus and palate, the zygomatic process of the temporal bone, and the serrated edge of the greater wing of the sphenoid bone. Posteriorly, the medial and lateral pterygoid plates are suspended from the body of the sphenoid at a 45° angle to each other, creating a reinforced "angle iron" configuration that resists horizontal movement at the level of the maxillary tuberosity.[60] Additionally, the cranial base, which is almost at a 45° angle to the occlusal plane of the maxilla, is resistant to horizontal compressive forces and thus acts as a horizontal buttress itself.[48]

Zygoma

The zygoma, which forms the cornerstone of the buttress system and provides the aesthetically important malar prominence, is related to the surrounding craniofacial skeleton through four superficial and two deep projections. The superficial projections contribute to two critical external arcs of contour (Fig. 24-2). The vertical arc defines the course of the ZM buttress, running from the zygomatic process of the frontal bone over the zygoma to the lateral antral wall. The longer horizontal arc runs from the maxilla in the area of the lacrimal fossa around the zygoma to the zygomatic process of the temporal bone. It is parallel to, but slightly below, the Frankfort horizontal plane.[55] Because the height of contour of the malar prominence also is just at or slightly inferior to the Frankfort plane,[36] the point of intersection of these arcs of contour defines the position of the malar prominence (see Fig. 24-2). The two deep projections are the sphenoid projection, which articulates along the lateral orbital wall with the orbital plate of the sphenoid bone, and the orbital projection, which articulates with the orbital surface of the maxilla in the extreme lateral aspect of the orbital floor. The sphenoid and orbital projections lie beneath and

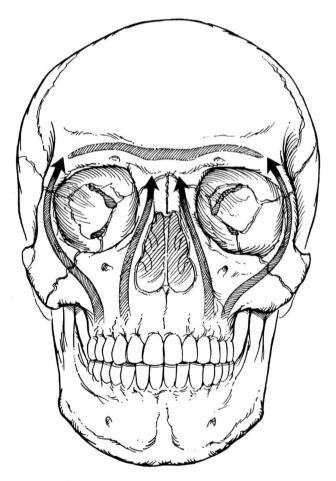

Fig. 24-1. The lattice-like structure of the middle third of the face is suspended from the frontal bar. The paired nasomaxillary and zygomaticomaxillary buttresses are the major vertical buttresses within the lattice.

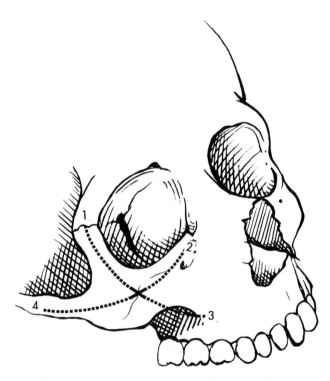

Fig. 24-2. External arcs of contour of the zygomatic complex. Intersection of vertical (*1* to *3*) and horizontal (*2* to *4*) arcs at "X" marks the position of the malar prominence. (With permission from Stanley RB: The zygomatic arch as a guide to reconstruction of comminuted malar fractures, *Arch Otolaryngol Head Neck Surg* 115:1459, 1989.)

perpendicular to the external arcs of contour in the area of the inferolateral orbital rim, thus strengthening this portion of the rim.

Medial canthal complex

The bony prominences forming the superior, lateral, and inferior portions of the orbital rim usually are palpable and often visible through their soft-tissue covering. No true medial rim exists in the area of confluence of the orbit, frontal process of the maxilla, and nasal dorsum, although this critical area serves as the attachment point for the medial canthal ligament (MCL) and as the receptacle for the lacrimal collecting system. The ligament attaches in a tripartite configuration with horizontal and vertical components anteriorly and a deeper horizontal element posteriorly (Fig. 24-3).[40] The anterior horizontal component is the strongest and is firmly attached to the anterior lacrimal crest, i.e., the frontal process of the maxilla. The anterior vertical component is less firmly attached along a line several millimeters above the insertion of the horizontal ligament. The posterior component has the weakest attachment to the posterior lacrimal crest. Although these three components surround the lacrimal sac within the lacrimal fossa, the palpable border of the ligament actually is over the bone of the anterior lacrimal crest, not the lacrimal sac. In the undisturbed state, the MCL anchors the eyelid structures to the medial orbital wall, thus maintaining the configuration of the palpebral opening, maintaining contact of the lids to the globe, and facilitating the lacrimal pump that ensures flow of tears from the lid puncta through the lacrimal system.[30]

Orbit

Within the orbit, the greatest diameter is found approximately 1.5 cm posterior to the inferior orbital rim. The orbital roof has an upward convexity that places it approximately 5 to 7 mm above the superior orbital rim, and the orbital floor is concave, with a depth of approximately 3 mm in relation to the inferior orbital rim. The globe itself rests within this concavity. Posteriorly the floor is convex, and posteromedially it slopes upward into the medial orbital wall without a sharp demarcation (Fig. 24-4). Laterally and posteriorly the floor is separated from the greater sphenoid wing by the inferior orbital fissure. The optic foramen actually lies posteriorly in the plane of the medial orbital wall, thus placing it medial and superior to the true orbital apex.

Mandible

The mandible is a rigid bone that has a U-shaped body that is extended at each end by vertically directed rami. Because the body is cantilevered off the ramus, masticatory forces can create considerable structural demands on all parts of the mandible. Tension and compression loads occur in a complex pattern throughout the body.[43] The lower border of the body is smooth, round, and thickened by dense bone to help the outer and inner cortical plates resist these forces, but the lower border in the angle region becomes thinner and more irregular. Overall, the height of the mandible is the primary determinant of strength of the horizontal portion, particularly at the critical angle. After extraction of the mandibular teeth, vertical height is lost as the alveolar process atrophies. Partially and fully edentulous mandibles therefore lose strength proportionate to this loss of bone.

The vertical rami, although relatively thin, are totally embedded in a muscle sling formed by the masseter and internal pterygoid muscles and are perfectly aligned with the compressive forces created by these muscles. The condylar neck also is a thin area and, like the angle, is not entirely protected by this muscle sling. It is fortunate that the trajectories of the masticatory and muscular stresses on the bony

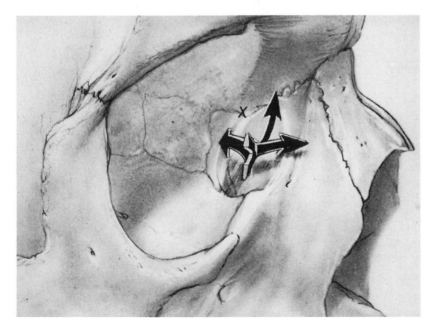

Fig. 24-3. The three components (*arrows*) of the medial canthal ligament. Total avulsion requires replacement of the tendon at the location marked X. (With permission from Rodriguez RL, Zide BM: Reconstruction of the medial canthus, *Clin Plast Surg* 15:255, 1988.)

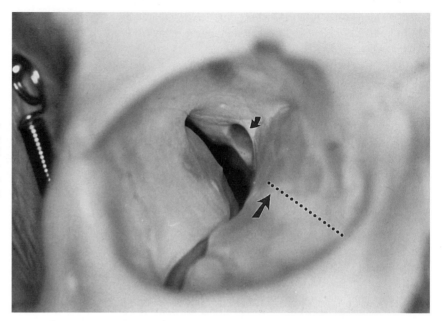

Fig. 24-4. Posterior-medial orbital floor (*large arrow*). Although the globe rests anterior to this convexity, reconstruction of this area and adjacent medial wall is critical. The optic foramen (*small arrow*) is medial and superior to the posterior limit of the required 35 to 40 mm dissection (*dotted line*) from the orbital rim.

trabeculae of the mandible have molded the orientation of the trabeculae into crests, ridges, and lines of strength that provide additional reinforcement to the thin, unprotected angle and condylar neck regions (Fig. 24-5).[48] It is unfortunate that although these reinforcements resist the normal tension, compression, and rotational forces of mastication, they do not offer serious resistance to the lateral stress forces created by external blunt trauma.

Temporomandibular joint

The mandible articulates with the skull base through the ginglymoarthroidal (hinge and sliding) temporomandibular joints. The joint is formed by the condyle of the mandible, the glendoid fossa of the temporal bone, and an interposed fibrocartilaginous disk known as the *meniscus*. The meniscus divides the joint into two compartments, with the gliding motion occurring in the upper compartment and the hinge-like action occurring in the lower compartment. A ligamentous capsule surrounds the joint space and attaches around the condylar neck just below the head. When each condylar head is maximally seated against the joint meniscus in the bottom of the glenoid fossae, the mandible is in the centric relation position, which is a retruded position, and the teeth should not be in maximal interdigitation. When the cusps of the maxillary and mandibular teeth are maximally interdigitated, the mandible is in the centric occlusion position, a position usually more than 1 mm anterior to centric relation.[38] Therefore, the relationship of the condylar head to the glenoid fossa, and thus the relationship of the mandible to the skull base, has normal range of variability. It is obvious that any form of jaw-to-jaw fracture fixation should be designed to place the jaws into the centric occlusion position.

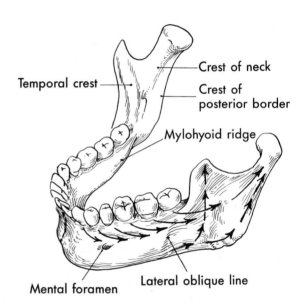

Fig. 24-5. The mandible with trajectories of stress that cause orientation of bony trabeculae into lines, crests, and ridges of strength in the body and vertical rami to resist normal occlusal forces. (With permission from Stanley RB: *Pathogenesis and evaluation of mandibular fractures.* In Mathog RH, editor: *Maxillofacial trauma,* Baltimore, 1984, Williams & Wilkins.)

PATHOPHYSIOLOGY

Orbitozygomaticomaxillary (Le Fort's) fractures

The honeycomb construction of the middle third of the facial skeleton provides excellent stability as long as it is loaded in the application for which it was intended—to resist predominantly vertical masticatory forces—and as long as the lattice remains intact.[37] Although the relatively strong vertical buttresses bear the load of mastication, the "weaker" horizontal reinforcing buttresses should absorb external impact force centered over the lower forehead, orbits, zygomata, or maxilla. The initial disruption of a buttress may weaken the entire lattice and may lead to its collapse, but a random collapse under anterior or lateral impact forces usually is prevented by the strength of the horizontal buttresses combined with the relationship to the skull base.[58] Instead, reoccurring fracture patterns are seen, and these tend to follow the three great weak lines of the midfacial skeleton, as described by Le Fort in 1901 (Fig. 24-6).

Anterior impact forces angled obliquely to the horizontal buttresses from above the Frankfort plane usually produce a separation of the vertical buttresses from the skull base, with inferior and posterior displacement of the maxilla. The maxilla may be separated from the zygomatic bodies. Impacts directed at the same level, but head-on to the horizontal buttresses, not only may separate the buttresses from the skull base, but also nearly always produce fractures that cross the lower aspects of the buttresses at near right angles through the anterior lateral walls of the maxillary antrum. This allows for a downward rotation of the anterior end of the maxilla around an axis approximating the lower end of the pterygoid plates. This organized collapse prevents total destruction of the orbits, nose, tooth-bearing segments of the maxilla, and skull base by high-velocity external impact forces.[58]

Impact forces delivered to the face in motor vehicle accidents or interpersonal confrontations usually are not perfectly centered over the face, and Le Fort's fractures usually occur in unpredictable combinations. Most often, the patterns are asymmetric, with the level of injury being higher on one side than on the other.[24] The spectrum ranges from isolated, minimally displaced Le Fort's I, II, or III fractures to multiple, widely displaced fracture–dislocations that cause gross malalignment of the buttresses. This malalignment will be evident clinically as a variable combination of maxillary retrusion or rotation, midfacial elongation, and malocclusion. An actual reduction in midfacial height is a rare occurrence caused by a severe impact force that drives the mandible superiorly into the maxilla to shatter the vertical struts and shorten midfacial vertical dimension.

Orbitozygomatic fractures

Unlike anterior impact forces, lateral forces tend to be centered over a convenient target—the prominent convex outer surface of the zygoma. The sturdy zygoma is the main buttress between the maxilla and the cranium, and strong impact forces directed to the zygoma usually are absorbed by the fragmentation of the weaker bones with which the zygoma articulates at the inferior orbital rim, orbital floor, and lateral antral wall. The exceptions to this are the stout zygomatic process of the frontal bone, which almost always is spared by the typical clean separation of the ZF suture, and the zygomatic arch, which usually suffers a single frac-

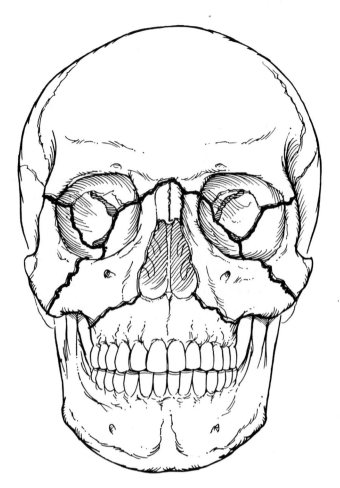

Fig. 24-6. Le Fort's fracture levels. These may be used for a general description of midfacial fractures, although they most likely will not describe the full length or exact nature of the injuries.

ture near its midpoint or a double fracture that produces a displaced, large central fragment. Therefore, fracture–dislocations of the zygoma may fragment both ends of the horizontal arc of contour and the lower end of the vertical arc. Restoration of the anterior and lateral projection of the cheek will require reconstruction of the horizontal arc, and restoration of the height of the malar prominence in relation to the Frankfort plane will require reconstruction of the vertical arc.[55] The degree of disruption and the amount of displacement of the zygoma (and thus the complexity of the needed repair) depend on the velocity of the impact force. Even comminuted Le Fort's fractures can occur from the crossfacial transmission of high-velocity lateral impact forces.

Deep orbital fractures

Within the orbit, impact forces are transmitted through the zygoma by the sphenoidal and orbital processes to the deeper structures. Any impact centered over the lateral orbital rim should be absorbed by the relatively weak sphenotemporal buttress that is formed by the zygoma, orbital plate of the greater wing of the sphenoid, and squamous portion of the temporal bone. If the ability of this buttress to absorb an impact force is exceeded, fracture–dislocations of the lateral orbital wall will result with impaction of the orbital plate of the sphenoid bone into the orbital apex or even into the middle cranial fossa. This impaction may cause injuries to the structures within the orbit, superior orbital fissure, and optic canal. Reduction of the bony injuries may be necessitated not only by the need to restore the volume of the orbit and the contour of the orbital rim, but also by the need to remove bony impingement on vital neurologic structures.[13]

Impact forces centered over the body of the zygoma are transmitted medially through the orbital process to the inferior rim and the floor of the orbit. Both structures often will suffer a comminuted fracture, the severity of which varies with the strength of the impact force. The floor fracture usually involves the concave central portion of the floor, starting at and extending medially from the groove and canal of the infraorbital nerve. High-velocity periorbital impact forces may be transmitted to the convex posterior floor and even to the medial wall, causing serious displacement of the bone in these areas. Although the globe itself rests anterior to the convexity, evaluation and reconstruction of this area and the adjacent medial wall are of equal importance to repair of the more accessible concave anterior portion of the floor.[27]

The classic blow-out fracture of the orbital floor and the less common medial wall blow-out fracture have been the subject of numerous discussions in the maxillofacial trauma literature.[31] Both are thought to result from impact forces that are centered over the globe, producing a rapid increase in the intraorbital pressure that "blows out" the thin bone of the concave portion of the orbital floor or the lamina papyracea. These isolated injuries may be occurring less frequently relative to other periorbital fractures in this time of high-velocity impact injuries. Orbital roof fractures are being seen more often and usually occur as part of a severe frontobasilar fracture caused by impact forces centered immediately above the orbit. These patients may have associated panfacial fractures, including unilateral or bilateral orbitozygomatic fractures.

The position of the globe is determined by the integrity of the orbital walls and by the extensive network of ligaments that suspends it.[22] Recession or depression of the globe within the orbit may result from an injury that pushes one or more orbital walls outward or that damages the network of suspensory ligaments. The orbital soft tissues then are displaced by gravitational forces and the remodeling forces of fibrous scar contracture, which usually changes the shape of the orbital soft tissues from a modified cone to a sphere, and the globe sinks backward and downward.[28] Probably the most common causes of posttraumatic enophthalmos are the incomplete repair of a defect in the normally convex posterior aspect of the floor or failure to recognize and correct a medial wall component of the injury.

Nasoorbitoethmoidal fractures

NOE fractures are true orbital wall injuries that result from the unilateral or bilateral impaction of the frontal processes of the maxilla and the nasal bones into the orbital space, with secondary comminution of the ethmoid air cells and out-fracturing of the medial wall of the orbit.[45] The fractures may be associated with panfacial injuries caused by broad-surface impact forces that separate the middle third of the face from the skull base or less commonly with a narrow-impact force centered in the nasal or frontonasal area. The nasal dorsum will be flattened, but more importantly, the attachments of the three components of the MCL may be partially or totally disrupted. The resultant deformity of the inner canthus becomes progressively more obvious as the number of disrupted components increases. Loss of attachment of the posterior component allows interior movement of the medial canthus; loss of attachment of the anterior horizontal component allows lateral movement; and disruption of the anterior vertical component allows inferior displacement. Symptoms and findings resulting from MCL injury may range from epiphora with minimal deformity to noticeable telecanthus and gross dystopia of the medial canthus with narrowing of the palpebral fissure.[40]

Mandibular fractures

The area of the mandible that fractures is determined by the interaction of the nature of the external force and the anatomic predisposition of the mandible to fracture at specific locations. A fracture may occur directly under the point of impact, or the force may be transmitted indirectly across the mandible to create a contralateral fracture. A blow to the body usually will cause an ipsilateral body fracture through the mental foramen (a naturally weak area) and either a contralateral angle fracture or a subcondylar fracture. The presence of a tooth at the angle seems to favor a fracture of the angle, and an unerupted third molar creates an even more favorable condition for fracture to occur.[61] Ramus fractures occur much less frequently than condylar, angle, and body fractures, most likely because of the reinforcing ridges that naturally transmit forces through the ramus to the condylar neck and also because of the muscle sling that envelopes the ramus and cushions direct blows. Impacts centered over the lower anterior alveolar ridge may cause alveolar fractures, leaving the lower incisors floating in the fragment of bone. Posterior alveolar fractures are less common because of the longer, more stable posterior tooth roots and because of the increased amount of spongy bone in the posterior alveolus to absorb fracture forces.

The velocity of the impact force also is a factor. A low-velocity blow to the mandibular body usually causes a body fracture with little or no displacement at the point of contact and a contralateral subcondylar fracture. A high-velocity blow may cause a displaced, comminuted fracture at the point of impact but not a contralateral fracture. A moderate

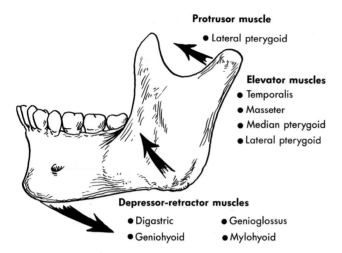

Fig. 24-7. Muscle groups that exert forces on the mandible to potentially distract fractures. (With permission from Stanley RB: *Pathogenesis and evaluation of mandibular fractures.* In Mathog RH, editor: *Maxillofacial trauma,* Baltimore, 1984, Williams & Wilkins.)

blow to the symphysis may cause a parasymphaseal fracture or bilateral condylar fractures. A violent blow to the chin may create a flail mandible with a fracture of the symphaseal or paraysmphaseal area combined with either bilateral angle or subcondylar fractures. This type of condylar fracture actually is a safety mechanism that prevents the condylar head from being driven into the middle cranial fossa or through the tympanic plate into the external auditory canal.

Displacement of the mandibular fragments also is influenced greatly by two closely related factors: muscle pull and direction of angulation of the fracture line. Muscle pull includes the relatively weak anterior depressor group and the stronger posterior elevator group (Fig. 24-7). Direction and angulation of body and angle fractures have been used to classify these fractures as either favorable or unfavorable in relation to the muscle forces in the angle and body areas (Fig. 24-8). Displacement of fractures through the condyle or condylar neck is determined by the relationship of the fracture to the insertion of the lateral pterygoid muscle. This muscle inserts into the neck of the condyle and into the articular disk of the joint through the anterior wall of the joint capsule. A fracture above the insertion into the neck

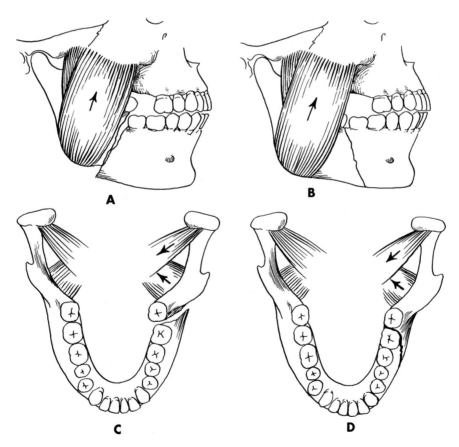

Fig. 24-8. Mandibular fracture angulations and their relationship to muscle pulls. **A,** Horizontally unfavorable; **B,** horizontally favorable; **C,** vertically unfavorable; **D,** vertically favorable. (With permission from Stanley RB: *Pathogenesis and evaluation of mandibular fractures.* In Mathog RH, editor: *Maxillofacial trauma,* Baltimore, 1984, Williams & Wilkins.)

will cause little displacement of the condylar head because of the lack of muscle pull. A fracture below the muscle insertion, i.e., a subcondylar fracture, will lead to displacement of the condylar head medially and forward because of the force of the lateral pterygoid muscle. If the segment is displaced entirely out of the joint capsule, it is called a *dislocated fracture*. Forces generated by muscle pull are thought to be more important in creating displacement of mandibular fractures than the direction and amount of the force that caused the fractures.[3]

PATIENT EVALUATION

General considerations

Examination of the patient with facial trauma has been enhanced with the use of computed tomography (CT). Axial and coronal scans can be used to show in detail fracture lines through all aspects of the facial skeleton. It now is recognized that information gained from CT scans is of greater value than that gained from a combination of clinical examination and routine radiography for all facial fractures, with the exception of mandibular fractures in patients with no clinical evidence of other injuries.[25] In these patients, a panoramic radiograph (Panorex), a form of tomogram of the mandible, adequately shows the entire lower jaw from condyle to condyle. It accurately displays fractures of the condylar area and is particularly suited to show most fractures of the ramus, angle, and body. In some instances, symphaseal and parasymphaseal fractures may be difficult to evaluate because of the poor imaging in midline as a result of the mechanics of panoramic machines. However, these fractures of this area usually are evident, clinically and detailed radiographic analysis is not necessary.

Specific areas that should be thoroughly inspected with the high-resolution scan include the frontal bone, NOE complex, orbits, and the entire craniofacial horizontal and vertical buttress systems. Although all information necessary for evaluating most facial fractures can be seen on standard axial and coronal CT views, three-dimensional reconstructions may help less-experienced surgeons conceptualize the overall injury. In addition, such reconstructions may prove valuable in patients who cannot be positioned for a coronal CT scan. In this time of cost-conscious medicine, the expense of CT examination of patients suffering facial fractures other than simple nasal fractures and mandibular fractures appears justified. It is no longer acceptable to adopt a wait-and-see attitude regarding possible delayed trauma sequelae such as enophthalmos, just as it is no longer acceptable to perform procedures such as orbital exploration simply to evaluate the status of the orbital floor and in doing so place the patient at risk for complications.

Frontal bone

External appearance and routine radiographic examination may be inconsistent with the actual severity of fractures of the frontal bone and supraorbital ridges. Because edema of the skin, subcutaneous tissue, and muscle overlying depressed fractures of the glabella and supraorbital areas may persist for several months, the surgeon should be able to relate the amount of bony displacement shown by CT scan to the flattening that subsequently will become obvious if the fracture fragments are not properly realigned.[56] Although some of the depression may be camouflaged by variations in facial features (such as the position and density of the eyebrows; the skin thickness, texture, and color; and the size and overall bony configuration of the face), the forehead asymmetry may be distressing to the patient. Early open reduction and internal fixation of the fractures are preferable to more complex delayed reconstructive techniques,[46] even if the decision to proceed with early surgery must by necessity be based on a subjective CT prediction of a future deformity.

Any fracture of the frontal bone carries the risk of an associated injury of the frontal sinus. CT scanning is critical for the direct evaluation of the walls of the sinus. The scans also will provide indirect evidence of damage to frontonasal orifices that might lead to chronic obstruction of sinus drainage.[56]

Orbit

A detailed picture of the location of orbital fracture lines can be obtained with CT scans. Of greater importance, the scans also show the amount of displacement of the malar eminence and of the four walls, which result in volume changes of the orbit. The choice of the most appropriate surgical approach for treatment of all but the most minimally displaced orbital or orbitozygomatic fractures can be made only if the integrity of the zygoma and the orbital walls is thoroughly evaluated. In particular, CT demonstration of a comminution or dislocation of both ends of the horizontal arc of contour indicates an exact reconstruction of the orbitozygomatic complex can be achieved only if the zygomatic arch is exposed and repaired (Fig. 24-9). Within the orbit itself, evaluation of the floor and medial wall is critical, especially in the areas of the convex posterior floor and the gentle slope of the floor into the medial wall. This evaluation requires either a true coronal CT scan or a three-dimensional reconstruction from an axial scan.

High-resolution studies have allowed relatively accurate calculation of orbital volume changes related to specific defects of the orbital walls. Orbital injuries that involve greater than 50% of the surface area of the floor are likely to produce enophthalmos.[42] More specifically, enophthalmos occurs when orbital floor disruption exceeds a total area of 2 cm^2, the bone volume changes exceed 1.5 ml (5% of orbital volume), or major fat and soft-tissue displacement occurs.[29] Additionally, 3 mm of displacement of either the inferior or medial wall causes an orbital volume change of 7% to 12%. These changes can produce from 2.5 to 4.0 mm of globe displacement if no change in orbital content occurs.[33]

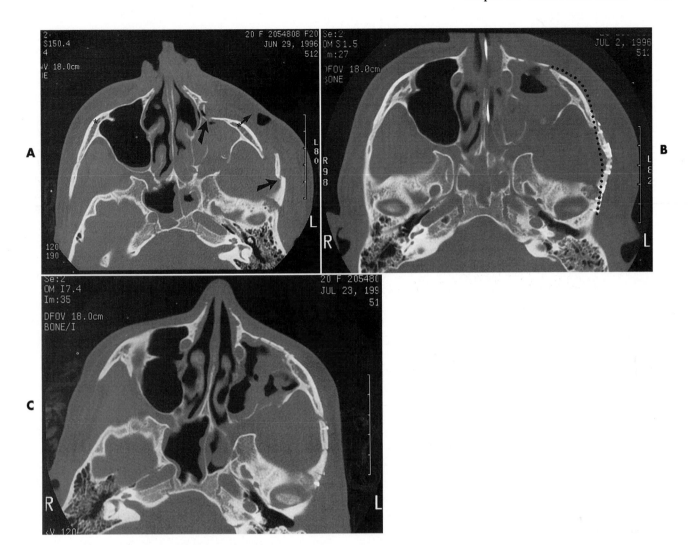

Fig. 24-9. A, Axial computed tomography (CT) scan showing fracture–dislocation of the left zygoma with comminution of the medial aspect of the inferior orbital rim and zygomatic arch (*large arrows*). Complex movement (*small arrow*) of the zygoma required to move the malar prominence (*asterisk*) back to its normal position. **B,** Postoperative CT scan of same patient showing failure to realign arch even with open reduction. *Dotted line* represents correct configuration of zygoma and the arch with its relatively straight central segment. With resolution of edema, the cheek would have appeared to be flat and the face too wide. **C,** Postoperative CT scan showing revised reconstruction that moved the malar prominence to its normal position.

The surgeon always should consider that enophthalmos may not be seen acutely with even severe orbitozygomatic fractures because of the orbital soft-tissue swelling. In addition, if the body of the zygoma has remained intact, it may be impacted medially to compensate for the increased orbital volume caused by blow-out fractures of other walls, and the globe may appear to have normal anterior projection and vertical position. Reduction of the zygomatic component of the injury to restore the malar prominence unmasks the traumatic increase in orbital volume and leads to "delayed-onset" enophthalmos if the other fractures are not treated. Careful review of the axial and coronal CT scans prevents this error.

Nasoorbitoethmoidal complex

The diagnosis of NOE fracture may be made on physical examination alone if gross posterior telescoping of the nasal bones has occurred and if the intercanthal distance has become greater than one half of the interpupillary distance.[40] In addition, a bimanual examination can be performed by placing a Kelly clamp intranasally beneath the frontal process of the maxilla and a finger directly over the MCL insertion. Any movement of the frontal process differentiates this severe injury from a simple comminuted nasal fracture.[34] However, edema may obscure posterior nasal telescoping and intercanthal widening, and bimanual palpation may not reveal the degree of fragmentation of the bones onto which the three components of the MCL attach, specifically the posterior lacrimal crest attachment of the posterior horizontal component. Diagnosis and accurate portrayal of the extent of bone fragmentation are readily available with the CT scan. Although MCL disruption cannot be seen on CT, indirect evidence exists if the bone in the area of the attachment is found to be fragmented rather than a single displaced segment.[25]

Craniofacial buttress system

This buttress system, particularly the vertical struts, should be systematically inspected preoperatively to document the degree of malalignment that has resulted from fracture displacement. Fracture lines themselves through the buttresses do not mandate open reduction, but comminution and gross malalignment strongly suggest the need for reduction of the fractures under direct visualization so that facial length and projection are accurately restored (Fig. 24-10). The hard palate also should be evaluated for fractures (usually parasagittal) that might cause widening of the maxilla and prevent accurate interdigitation of the maxillary and mandibular teeth when the jaws are placed into maxillomandibular fixation (MMF). In addition, the CT scans display fractures of the condylar head, condylar neck, and vertical ramus of the mandible (see Fig. 24-10). The status of these structures should be known before a patient with fracture–dislocations of the maxilla is placed into MMF. Although displaced fractures of the mandibular symphysis, body, or angle usually are readily apparent on clinical examination, displaced fractures closer to the temporomandibular joint may be overlooked in panfacial injuries because they are in areas not readily accessible for direct inspection and palpation. The status of these structures should be known before a patient with fracture–dislocations of the maxilla is placed into occlusion with MMF. A meticulous and time-consuming reconstruction of fractures extending from the frontal bar to the maxillary palatoalveolar complex may be totally inaccurate if condylar, condylar neck, or high ramus mandibular fractures are not recognized and appropriately addressed.

OPHTHALMOLOGIC CONSIDERATIONS

General evaluation

A complete preoperative ophthalmologic evaluation of every victim of maxillofacial trauma who suffers a fracture in the orbitozygomatic area is an unrealistic expectation and by no means mandatory. The surgeon always should be sensitive to the possibility of direct ocular trauma and should obtain proper consultation when indicated. A minimum preoperative examination should include testing of visual acuity (subjective and objective in both eyes), pupillary function, ocular motility, inspection of the anterior chamber for hyphema, and visualization of the fundus for gross disruptions. A decrease in visual acuity or any abnormality noted on the other phases of this screening examination warrants a more detailed examination by an ophthalmologist before reconstruction of the bony injuries is undertaken. The need for forced-deduction testing for muscle entrapment has decreased with use of improved CT scans to document the status of the orbital walls.

Orbital apex injuries

Located in the orbital apex are the optic canal and superior orbital fissure (SOF), both of which have a fairly protected position within the thick bone of the lesser sphenoid wing and sphenoid body.[35] Typically, impact forces centered over the orbital rims or globe are absorbed by fractures of the thin walls of the orbit itself before they can be transmitted to the posterior orbit. However, orbital trauma that does involve the optic canal usually causes an injury to the intracanalicular portion of the optic nerve and at least a partial loss of vision. Damage to the SOF and its contents is known to cause a syndrome consisting of ophthalmoplegia, ptosis, pupillary dilation, and anesthesia of the upper eyelid and forehead.[14] A combined injury to the optic nerve and SOF contents is known as the *orbital apex syndrome*.

Treatment of intracanalicular optic nerve injuries remains controversial. Traditional teaching emphasizes that immediate loss of vision associated with an injury to the intracanalicular portion of the nerve is an irreversible injury, and thus surgical intervention to decompress the nerve in the optic canal is not warranted. Delayed or progressive loss of vision implies that the nerve has remained viable after the initial insult and that decompression may prevent total necrosis of the nerve. Additionally, the response of the visual loss to massive doses of steroids has been proposed as a possible indicator for selective nerve decompression.[5] The steroids are given for a 12- to 24-hour period, and if no response is seen or if an initial response begins to deteriorate, decompression is considered. The morbidity associated with decompression of the intracanalicular portion of the nerve has been greatly reduced with the development of anterior surgical approaches through the paranasal sinuses,[39,49] and restoration of vision has been described after decompression in a patient who suffered immediate total visual loss not responsive to 5 days of megadose steroid therapy.[52]

Treatment of the injuries to the intraorbital portion of the optic nerve caused by impaction of orbital wall bone fragments into the orbital apex has been less controversial. If high-resolution CT documents the presence of an offending fragment in the orbital apex of a patient with decreased vision, early surgical reduction should be considered.[13] Although the exact injury to the nerve caused by the impaction of such fragments is unknown, it is possible that a reversible decompressive phenomenon (either incomplete ischemia or blocked axonal transport) is involved, and a certain time interval may exist before the transition to irreversible damage occurs. The role of steroid therapy in treatment of this type of optic nerve injury is undefined.

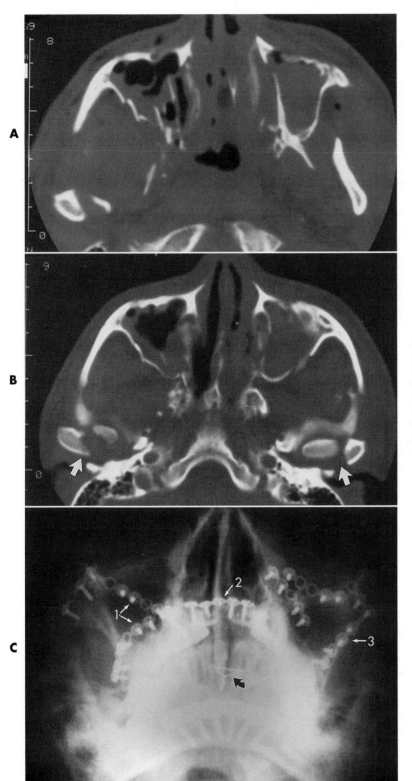

Fig. 24-10. A, Axial computed tomography scan at the level of the lower maxilla in a patient with bilateral LeFort fractures and a parasagittal fracture of the palate. **B,** Bilateral condylar head fractures (*arrows*) in same patient prevent accurate restoration of position of maxilla with MMF alone. **C,** Postoperative radiograph showing palatal reduction wire (*arrow*) and triangular pattern of plates over ZM buttresses (*1* and *3*) and anterior pyriform aperature (*2*).

Continued

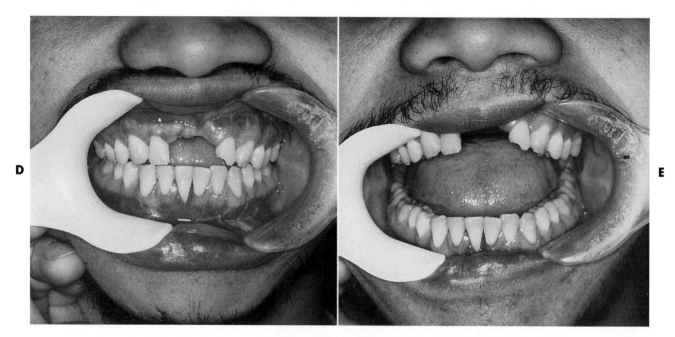

Fig. 24-10, cont'd. D, Occlusion with no lingual tipping of teeth at 3 months follow-up evaluation.
E, Very mild trismus related to condylar injuries has remained stable. The patient had been allowed
to mobilize the mandible immediately after fracture fixation.

Typically patients with bone fragments impacted into the orbital apex also will have an SOF syndrome, and removal of the offending bone fragments may speed the resolution of the problem. It has been recognized that the chance for partial, if not complete, recovery of the motor and sensory components of any SOF syndrome is good with or without surgical intervention.[62] If surgery is undertaken, the lateral or temporal approach to the orbital apex offers a safe route that minimizes the chances of further damage to the optic nerve.[54] Although this procedure technically requires a mini-craniotomy, it is an extension of the approach to severe orbitozygomatic fractures that will be described in the upcoming section on surgical techniques.

MANAGEMENT PHILOSOPHY FOR IMMEDIATE RECONSTRUCTION

The goal of modern fracture management is total reconstruction of the bony architecture of the injured facial skeleton. Immediate reconstructions generally are less difficult and more successful than are delayed reconstructions. This is mainly because of cicatricial contraction of the facial soft-tissue envelope if the underlying skeletal support collapses or is lost.[19] During the acute phase of the injury, the soft tissues (although possibly injured themselves) are pliable enough to allow restoration of the underlying bony configurations with local bone fragments or autogenous bone grafts. If the soft tissues are allowed to contract into a bone defect, restoration of the supporting bone invariably produces a less desirable result. If revision surgery for minor residual bone defects or lacerations is required, this surgery is greatly facil-

itated if the overall soft-tissue envelope has been maintained in a normal position. These principles apply to most frontal, orbitozygomatic, NOE, and maxillary injuries. Efforts also should be made to reconstruct mandibular injuries primarily (short of bone grafting) so that skin, lower lip, and tongue positions are maintained.

SURGICAL TECHNIQUES

Frontal bone

Poor aesthetic results can be the result of a failure to recognize a fracture–dislocation within the frontal and supraorbital regions and a failure to achieve proper reduction and stable fixation of fracture fragments. Problems with reduction and fixation have been lessened with the use of the coronal incision for access, rigid fixation devices (microplates and screws), and autogenous bone grafts. Visualization of the entire frontal injury and of surrounding intact structures through the coronal approach enables the surgeon to perform a more accurate reconstruction of the frontal contours than can be accomplished through smaller and less cosmetically acceptable facial incisions. The use of incisions placed above or below the brows should be restricted to men with unstable hairlines.

Once the fracture fragments have been realigned, maintenance of edge-to-edge contact and, to a certain extent, of the convex contours of the forehead and supraorbital ridges can be achieved with interosseous wires. Flattening caused by collapse of fragments across the forehead span (particularly across the span of the thin anterior wall of the frontal sinus) may occur when wire fixation alone is used. More stable fixation can be obtained with low-profile plates and screws. Even if the frontal bone reconstruction is part of the overall repair of a panfacial injury, the frontal bar usually can be stabilized adequately with microplates and 1.0- or 1.3-mm screws before the reconstructed buttress system of the middle third of the face is suspended from it. The outline of thicker plates may become visible through the skin, necessitating a second procedure for hardware removal. Small frontal bone fragments are more difficult to stabilize, even with microplate fixation, and may be lost quickly to resorption processes. Larger, split-thickness cranial bone grafts can be used to replace numerous smaller fracture fragments, greatly facilitating fixation device application and providing a thicker scaffolding that will better maintain soft-tissue contour during remodeling and new bone formation.

Although a consensus on optimal management of frontal sinus fractures does not exist, the treatment scheme shown in Figure 24-11 offers a step-wise approach to this difficult problem.[41] Obliteration of a sinus requires removal of all vestiges of the sinus mucosa and a complete occlusion of the frontonasal orifices with fascia, muscle, or bone. The sinus then is allowed to obliterate itself through neoosteogenesis, or the sinus is filled with fat or cancellous bone.[47] Removal of the posterior table to cranialize the sinus[10] usually is reserved for severe frontobasilar skull fractures.

Zygoma

The precise relocation of the displaced zygoma can be greatly simplified if the surgeon concentrates on reconstruction of the two main external arcs of contour. Restoration of the horizontal arc reestablishes anterior and lateral projection of the cheek, and restoration of the vertical arc reestablishes height of the malar prominence in relation to the middle third of the face. The repositioned zygoma then can be used as a framework for repair of any associated orbital wall fractures. Treatment required to attain multidimensional restoration of the position of the zygoma becomes increasingly complex as the injury to each arc of contour worsens (Fig. 24-12). Exposure of the inferior orbital rim through the lower eyelid invariably will be needed in these patients. The traditional approach through a subciliary incision often produces increased scleral show, if not gross lid eversion and retraction, even when done by an experienced surgeon. The risk of this iatrogenic complication can be decreased with the use of a transconjunctival incision.[2] The addition of a lysis of the inferior limb of the lateral canthal ligament allows for exposure of the medial-most aspect of the rim fracture and of the floor and medial wall of the orbit for repair of fractures in these areas. The globe, in particular the cornea, can be adequately protected during placement of rim fixation devices or large orbital implants by retracting the conjunctiva superiorly over the cornea (Fig. 24-13).

The progression to more complex fractures usually involves comminution of the lateral antral wall and the medial aspect of the inferior orbital rim, thus making traditional three-point reduction inadequate for accurate restoration of the position of the malar prominence. Typically, the prominence is displaced posterior and lateral to its normal location, and failure to recognize the amount and direction of the displacement at the time of reduction leaves a flattened cheek and widened face. In these patients, the fourth point of alignment—the zygomatic arch—should be used to accurately reposition the point of intersection of the arcs of contour.[55]

If the arch has been noted on CT scan to have a single minimally displaced or angulated fracture or two greenstick fractures with bending of the arch, dissection may be carried out over the malar eminence through the sublabial or transconjunctival incision to expose the arch fractures. Although internal fixation cannot be applied through this approach, alignment of the arch can be evaluated. If the arch has been noted to have a displaced central segment, access to the full length of the horizontal arc is required, and a coronal, hemicoronal, or extended pretragal incision is necessary for evaluation of alignment and application of internal fixation. Dissection toward the lateral orbital rim and the zygomatic arch should be in a plane deep to the superficial layer of the deep temporal fascia so that the frontal and orbital branches of the facial nerve are elevated with the flap. The periosteum then is incised along the orbital rim and along the arch fragments deep to the attachment of the superficial layer of the fascia. A subperiostial dissection is carried over the body of the zygoma to connect with the anterior dissection, and all of the components of the zygomatic arch are exposed. The arch fragments are elevated and realigned; it is important to remember that the bone of the middle portion of the arch actually is straight and should be reconstructed as such to properly reestablish anterior projection of the malar prominence (see Fig. 24-9). Stable internal fixation that will resist the downward pull of the masseter muscle after the zygoma is repositioned usually can be obtained with 1.0- or 1.3-mm plates and screws. This is true even in cases of single point fixation at the lateral antral wall. Although a 1.5- or even 2.0-mm plate can be used at this one particular site for added strength, the profile of these larger plates may become visible through the skin if they are used at the ZF suture, inferior orbital rim, or zygomatic arch.

Repair of fractures of the zygoma may be delayed for 5 to 7 days to allow for resolution of edema, which facilitates the necessary exposures of fracture lines, as will the use of preoperative steroids to reduce intraoperative edema. The repair should not be delayed more than 10 days because the masseter muscle begins to shorten after this time, making elevation of the zygoma more difficult. If extreme difficulty is encountered in mobilizing the zygoma to its correct position even with the extended access approaches, the masseter muscle can be detached from the zygoma and the arch. This often is necessary in those patients not treated within the recommended 5 to 7 days. This maneuver should not have long-term effects on jaw mobility or masticatory function,

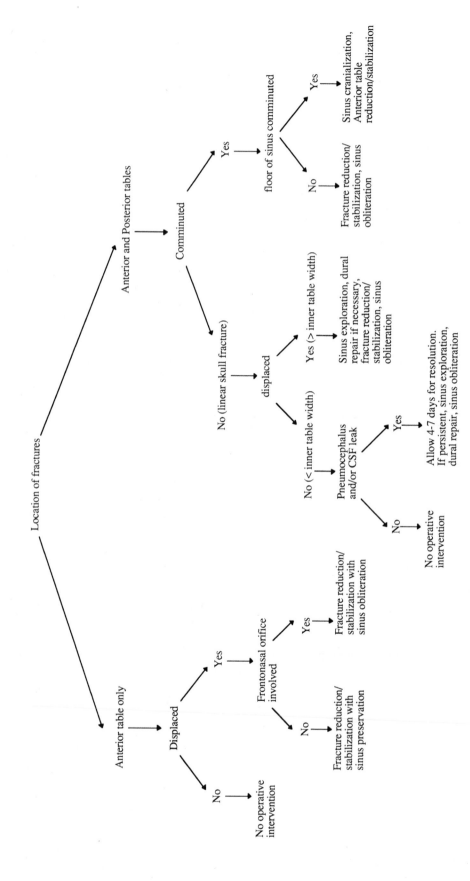

Fig. 24-11. Treatment algorithm for frontal sinus fractures.

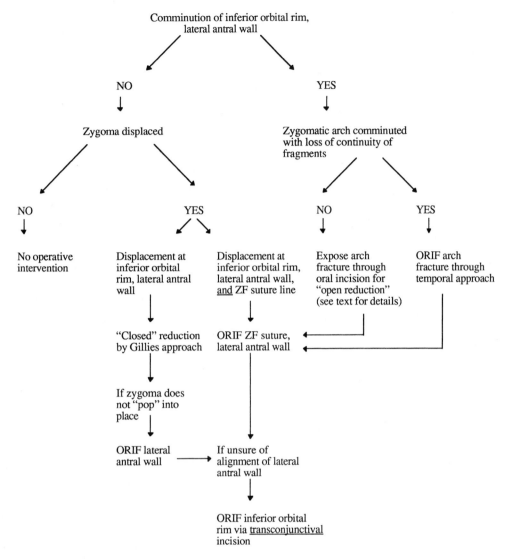

Fig. 24-12. Treatment algorithm for zygoma fractures. ORIF—Open reduction with internal fixation.

but the additional soft-tissue trauma and subsequent scarring may cause accentuation of the prominence of the reconstructed arch. Accurate draping of the soft tissues over the reconstructed arch helps to lessen this. Simultaneous upward traction on the skin flap and incised temporal fascia allows for a tight closure that holds the periosteum in correct position over the arch and zygoma.

Maxilla

Traditional treatment of most fractures involving tooth-bearing segments of the maxilla included the triad of closed reduction, MMF, and craniofacial or circumzygomatic suspension. Closed manipulation of the maxilla so that maximum interdigitation of the teeth was obtained before application of MMF would restore the position of the maxilla in the horizontal plane, if the mandible was correctly related to the skull. It would not automatically reestablish midfacial

height if the vertical buttresses were disrupted by fracture–dislocations. Closed reduction and MMF are adequate treatment for only less complex, minimally displaced maxillary fractures. MMF simply puts the jaw at rest for the 4 to 6 weeks required for fracture healing. Internal suspension wires play no useful role in the treatment of maxillary fractures and may introduce iatrogenic shortening of the midfacial vertical dimension. Internal suspension, which exerts a posteriorly and superiorly directed force, was designed to prevent elongation of the face after closed reduction of the maxillary fragments. Clinical and experimental evidence has documented that elongation caused by muscle pull does not occur after fracture reduction. Instead, internal suspension actually may telescope unstable maxillary segments on each other to shorten the vertical dimension of the middle third of the face.[20,50] Maxillary fractures that are shown on CT scans to be displaced are best treated by extended-access

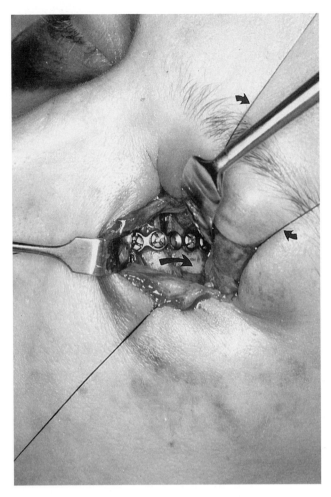

Fig. 24-13. Transconjunctival incision with cantholysis of lower tarsal plate attachment to lateral canthal ligament. Traction sutures (*small arrows*) are used to pull conjunctival superiorly to protect the cornea. A split cranial bone graft (*large arrow*) has been cantilevered from the inferior orbital rim to repair a large blow-out fracture of the floor.

approaches that allow for direct visualization and an anatomic reconstruction of the buttress system.[16,26] The buttresses should be totally exposed through extended sublabial incisions that essentially deglove the maxilla. Although this frequently removes all residual external periosteal attachments to displaced maxillary fracture fragments, bony union should proceed in a timely fashion if the fragments are stabilized adequately and if the periosteum is redraped over them. This is important because clinical evidence now indicates that maxillary fractures heal by osseous rather than fibrous reunion (as once thought).[59] Adequate stabilization can be obtained with the use of multiple interosseous wires if the patient also is maintained in MMF for 4 to 6 weeks. This prolonged period of jaw immobilization can be eliminated if plates and screws are used to stabilize the maxillary fracture fragments. Although the term *rigid* is used to describe the fixation achieved with these implants, it is somewhat inaccu-

rate when applied to maxillary fractures. Rigidity sufficient to allow for removal of the MMF can be obtained but not sufficient to allow the patient to return immediately to a normal diet. Rather, the fixation devices will maintain the position of the maxillary dentalveolar complex under the stresses of forces generated by mastication of soft foods and deglutition.

Restoration of the pretrauma relationships of the tooth-bearing segments of the maxilla to the mandible and skull base requires reestablishment of the occlusal relationship that existed in the patient before the injury (Fig. 24-14). Few people have perfect occlusion. The patient should be asked about preexisting occlusal abnormalities such as a premature occlusal contact that caused the teeth to slide into maximum interdigitation or an anterior open bite or posterior crossbite. Matching the corresponding wear facets of the maxillary with the mandibular teeth shows the preexisting occlusion of that patient. If the mandible also is fractured, i.e., a panfacial injury, the lower dental arch should first be accurately reduced and stabilized in proper relationship to the skull base, and proper alignment of the mandibular condyles in the glenoid fossae is an absolute requirement. The anteroposterior position of the maxilla then can be set by occluding the teeth in stable MMF. The midfacial vertical dimension is stabilized by reduction and fixation of any fracture line between the palatoalveolar complex and the frontal bone. In those patients with subcondylar or condylar head fractures that cannot or should not be treated with open reduction, the midfacial buttress system can be reconstructed first, using the maxilla to establish the proper vertical and horizontal position of the occlusal plane. Although this sequence may not restore the relationship of the occlusal plane to the skull base with the same accuracy as that achieved if it is related to an intact or totally reconstructed mandibular arch, it is the preferred sequence if mandibular vertical ramus height cannot be accurately restored because of the condylar head injury.

The stepwise repair of the buttress system begins with an accurate anatomic reconstruction of the frontal bar, if necessary, including the zygomatic processes of the frontal bone, the supraorbital rims, and the glabellar region.[17] Once this has been accomplished, the orbitozygomatic complexes can be reattached to the lateral ends of the bar, and reconstruction is continued inferiorly to the palatoalveolar complex, deep into the orbit, and medially to the nose and NOE complex. Although not a part of the maxilla, each zygoma should be accurately repositioned and stabilized before reattachment of the maxilla to the upper ends of the vertical buttresses. Often, zygomatic fractures associated with Le Fort's fractures of the middle third of the facial skeleton require open reduction and internal fixation of the zygomatic arch to position the zygoma correctly before reattachment of the maxilla. This is particularly critical in those patients in whom mandibular condyle fractures necessitate reconstruction of the upper jaw first. Failure to recognize and

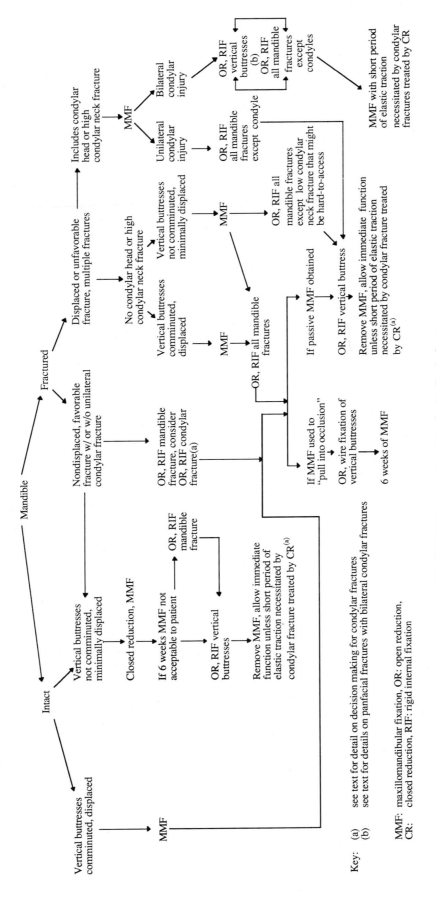

Fig 24-14. Treatment algorithm for Le Fort's fractures.

correct the amount and direction of the displacement of the zygoma at the time of reduction in these patients not only will leave a flattened cheek and widened face, but also may produce a rotated and possibly tilted maxilla when it is reattached to a malpositioned zygoma. The bone of the middle portion of the zygomatic arch actually is straight and should be reconstructed as such to properly reestablish anterior projection of the maxilla when it is reattached to the zygomata.

In addition to the accurate repositioning of both zygomata before final positioning and fixation of the maxillary segments, the integrity of the palate should be reestablished if necessary. Palatal fractures, most commonly parasagittal splits, should be reduced anteriorly at the inferior rim of the piriform aperture and posteriorly so that a solid, structurally accurate dentoalveolar complex can be related to the mandibular teeth. Open reduction and internal fixation of the anterior extent of a palatal fracture can be accomplished through the same extended gingivobuccal incision that is used to expose and repair the vertical buttresses. The bone above the anterior teeth is thick enough to place a miniadaptation plate with multiple screws. Occasionally, a small amount of bone needs to be removed immediately below the anterior nasal spine to facilitate placement of the plate on a flat contour.

The posterior extent of a palatal fracture usually can be reduced in a closed fashion if the overlying palatal mucoperiosteum is intact, although difficulty may be encountered if it is necessary to overtighten the MMF wires to pull the lingual cusp tips of the maxillary molars and premolars into the central fossae of the mandibular teeth. In such patients, an incision can be made over the posterior end of the palatal fracture to place a transosseous wire across the fracture. This wire will not serve as a point of rigid fixation of the palatal fracture, but rather it will serve to reduce the fracture gap posteriorly when it is tightened. Stable fixation is obtained from plates and screws placed across the anterior extent of the palatal fracture and across both ZM buttress areas (see Fig. 24-10).

Palatal fractures that are exposed in a laceration of the mucoperiosteum almost always are widely separated and impossible to reduce without using a transosseous wire to pull the palatal shelves together posteriorly. If this method of reduction is not used, when the MMF wire is tightened to pull the teeth into occlusion, the maxillary teeth most likely will be lingually tipped or will remain in a posterior crossbite deformity. The exposure through the laceration may be adequate to allow for placement of a plate across the split palate, although this may be technically difficult, and the plates frequently become exposed in the mouth later and have to be removed.

Acrylic palatal splints are an adjunct for stabilization of teeth in a segment of fractured alveolar bone. Even if a rigid fixation device cannot be used to attach the isolated alveolar segment to the surrounding maxillary bone, the combination of a sturdy buccal arch bar, a palatal splint, and circumdental wires to cinch the involved teeth between the bar and the splint usually provide stability sufficient to allow for removal of MMF and a soft diet.

Only when the zygomatic and palatal fractures have been repaired can the maxillary complex be reattached superiorly. The reattachment should begin with the side on which the injury is less severe. Unlike the anterior wall of the maxilla, which often is severely comminuted, the ZM buttress often is transversed by a single fracture line that can be easily reduced, or there may be a single free-floating fragment that can be accurately related to the zygoma above and the lower maxilla below. At least one ZM buttress usually can be reduced in this fashion to set the correct vertical dimension of the middle third of the face. After stabilization of this buttress, reduction and fixation of the other ZM buttress and the NM buttresses can proceed.

Comminution of the lower ends of the vertical buttresses severe enough to require bone grafting for stabilization is fortunately uncommon, although occasionally patients will be seen in whom 1- to 2-cm gaps of missing bone occur. Onlay split cranial bone grafts can be attached across these gaps with lag screws to serve the same function as a plate across reduced fracture lines. Reconstruction of vertical dimension cannot be done with the same precision in these patients as when there is edge-to-edge approximation of fracture fragments. Reconstruction of the NM buttresses may facilitate reestablishment of the vertical dimension is some patients. If the ZM buttresses are comminuted, the NM buttresses invariably are even more fragmented and difficult to realign.

Stability of the maxillary complex is established mainly through the reconstruction of the ZM buttresses. Reconstruction of the NM buttresses may provide some supplementary vertical stability to the overall reconstruction but only if the upper confluence of these struts, (the NOE complex) is relatively intact. If plates and screws are used for fixation and if the patient is allowed to function early, a delicate NOE repair should not be depended on to tolerate occlusal forces. Instead, the ZM buttress reconstructions should be relied on to hold the repositioned maxilla in place during healing. Plates should be positioned to overlie the ZM buttresses as closely as possible, and preferably three screws should be used to anchor the plate to the zygoma above and the maxilla below. Placement of screws into the lower end of a plate or a bone graft may be difficult if the fracture line is close to the apices of the molar and premolar teeth. This problem can be overcome easily by using L-shaped plates that allow for placement of more screws close to, but not through, the root tips. Bone grafts can be contoured and positioned to allow for similar placement of lag screws.

Rigid fixation is a nonforgiving technique that will not allow for an adjustment of the position of the maxilla postoperatively by the patient's own muscle pulls or with orthodontic traction on archbars. Therefore, any error in adaptation or application of the plates and screws to the bone will permanently fix the maxilla in an undesirable relationship to the skull base superiorly and the mandible inferiorly.[57] This may lead to occlusal and cosmetic disturbances unless recognized and revised immediately. Assuming that the correct interdigitation of the teeth is established by the temporary MMF, malunion of maxillary fractures treated with rigid fixation devices may result from either inaccurate adaptation of the plates to the midfacial bony contours or failure to have one or both mandibular condyles seated in the glenoid fossa in the correct centric occlusion position when the plates were applied. If the plates are not perfectly adapted to the bone, tightening of the screws may produce torque in the system, and the fragments may move to produce a malocclusion when the MMF is removed. This potential problem has been all but eliminated with the replacement of the stiff, hard-to-bend stainless steel plates with more malleable, easier to adapt plates such as the 1.3-, 1.5-, and 2.0-mm AO/ASIF titanium craniofacial plates.

The potential problem of inaccurate condylar seating in the glenoid fossa should be considered by the surgeon in all cases. Patients with complex maxillary injuries may suffer a deranged occlusal relationship that is difficult to correct. Invariably, one or both mandibular condylar heads will be displaced from their normal centric occlusion position in the glenoid fossa if the MMF is used to "pull the patient into occlusion." In such a patient, even though the plates are accurately adapted to the malpositioned maxillary fragments, a malocclusion develops when the MMF is removed and when the patient's normal muscle balances return the mandible to its correct position (Fig. 24-15). Even if a gross malocclusion does not result and if the patient learns to function in this altered position, chronic joint discomfort is likely to develop.

An altered relationship within the temporomandibular joint also may be a problem in patients who have associated mandibular injuries. Edema, effusion, or hematoma may be present within the joint structures, displacing the condylar head to an abnormal position. This produces a risky situation in the use of rigid fixation on the maxillary fractures. In patients in whom doubt exists regarding the position of the condylar heads within the glenoid fossa, plates and screws should be used to rigidly fix any Le Fort III's or zygomatic fractures, and wire osteosynthesis should be used for the Le Fort's I and II components. Although the patient must endure MMF for 4 to 6 weeks, the semirigid fixation of the buttresses at the maxillary level allows a shift of the occlusal plane into a proper relationship with the skull base during the early postsurgical period.

Orbital walls

Reconstruction of the orbital walls can begin only after total reconstruction of the zygoma and any other injuries of the horizontal and vertical buttress system, including an accurate anatomic reconstruction of the frontal bar. Orbital roof fractures are repaired with the surgeon considering that

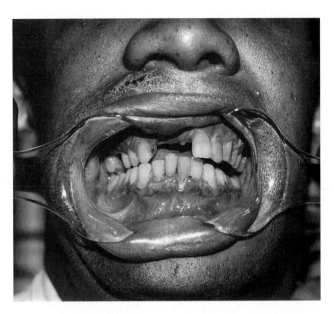

Fig. 24-15. Crossbite deformity resulting from use of maxillomandibular fixation (MMF) wires to pull patient into occlusion before application of maxillary plates. Evidence of this problem usually can be seen 7 to 10 days after surgery, and correction requires removal of the lower maxillary plates, mobilization of the palaoalveolar complex, and application of arch bars and MMF (for 4 to 6 weeks).

the normal upward convexity of the roof is difficult to duplicate, and a reconstructed roof that appears to be at the correct level often will be too flat later, thus pushing the globe inferiorly. This problem is avoided if the rebuilt roof is attached to the frontal bar at a level approximating the maximum height of the convexity of the roof rather than at the lower edge of the superior orbital rim itself.

The zygomatic contribution to the lateral orbital wall most often remains attached to the body of the zygoma and is correctly rearticulated to the greater sphenoid wing with proper reduction to the zygoma. In the unlikely event of a displaced sphenoid wing fracture, the intact lateral wall component of the zygoma can be used as a landmark for repositioning the orbital plate of the sphenoid bone. Only rarely will an alloplastic or autogenous graft be needed to reconstruct a lateral wall defect to correct herniation of orbital soft tissues into the temporal and infratemporal fossae. If a high-impact injury produces comminution and displacement of the lateral orbital wall, a split calvarial graft is the ideal choice for graft material. Because a lateral approach should be used to safely expose these retrobulbar bone injuries, the calvarial donor sight already is in the surgical field. Additionally, a relatively flat area of the skull usually can be found to produce a graft that closely matches the contour of the lateral orbital wall. Once inserted, the graft can be stabilized to the frontal bone or the zygoma with 1.0-mm plates and screws.

The orbital floor projection of the zygoma usually remains intact and is restored to a normal position when the zygoma itself is repositioned. The medial floor (orbital plate of the maxilla) then can be reconstructed using the intact lateral floor as a stable landmark. Reconstruction of a defect involving only the concave anterior aspect of the floor usually can be adequately accomplished with an alloplastic implant. Dissection of the floor should expose the entire circumference of the defect so that a 360° ledge is present to support the implant. Of the various alloplasts available, Marlex mesh has many properties that make it an ideal choice. It is readily available, is easily trimmable, and may be inserted in a layered fashion to create additional strength without inadvertently elevating the globe. Most importantly, clotted blood and eventually fibrous tissue fill the mesh to prevent implant migration, without the need for fixation of the implant to the orbital rim or residual floor.

Reconstruction of defects that involve the concave anterior and convex posterior floor requires an implant with rigidity greater than that offered by Marlex. This is because of a frequent lack of a ledge of residual floor to stabilize the implant posteriorly or medially, even when the orbital floor dissection is carried well into the posterior third of the orbit. A split calvarial graft is ideally suited for reconstruction of these larger defects. This bone is easily contoured to match most large floor defects, and its rigidity eliminates the need for medial and posterior support. The graft may be stabilized by attaching it to the reconstructed orbital rim in a cantilevered fashion with 1.3-mm plates and screws (see Fig. 24-13). It should be emphasized that not even a calvarial bone graft restores accurate position of the globe if the surgeon is hesitant in floor dissection and does not venture the sometimes necessary 35 to 40 mm into the posterior third of the orbit to allow for maximal reconstruction of the convex posterior floor (Fig. 24-16).

Reconstruction of defects that involve the concave anterior floor, convex posterior floor, and medial orbital wall (lamina papyracea) offer the greatest challenge. Although the severe orbital injuries usually are seen as part of a panfacial fracture, they may occur with isolated orbitozygomatic injuries. Complete exposure of the medial wall of the orbit is mandatory and is best accomplished through a coronal incision. Reconstruction is made difficult by the need to restore not only the integrity of walls themselves but also the exact relationship of the medial wall to the floor. Cranial bone grafts are joined together by microplates to recreate a relatively correct medial wall-to-floor relationship (Fig. 24-17). Prefabricated titanium orbital floor plates also may be used to reconstruct large defects either alone or as a cradle to facilitate placement and stabilization of bone implants.[15,44]

An ocular injury occasionally may prevent repair of orbital wall fractures if manipulation of the globe may worsen the injury. If the involved orbit houses the patient's only seeing eye, reconstruction probably is best restricted to returning the globe to a functional position if the orbital injury is severe and if the globe has sunk into the maxillary sinus.

Bone grafting should be directed toward providing basic support for the globe. Intraoperative tonometry may be helpful in these and all other patients in whom large implants are placed into the posterior orbit. Forward positioning of the globe by an oversized implant occasionally causes an acute increase in intraocular pressure. Should this occur, the implant should be removed and reduced in size.

Nasoorbitoethmoidal complex

Repair of NOE fractures requires reconstruction of the medial orbital area and nasal dorsum in preparation for redraping the overlying soft tissues and reattachment of the MCL. The reattachment of this complex ligament with its delicate functional and aesthetic roles is not a simple matter of realigning bony fragments and grossly reattaching the end of the ligament to its approximate site of insertion. It should be remembered that in the undisturbed state, the MCL has three components that surround the lacrimal sac in the lacrimal fossa and that each component has a different vector of attachment. Disruption of each vector adds a different feature to the resultant dysfunction of the MCL, particularly in its aesthetic role. Although it is impossible to reattach each component individually, understanding the vector analysis of the MCL allows the surgeon to design compensatory maneuvers to more precisely restore the appearance of the medial canthal area.[40]

Impact velocity appears to be a major determinant of the severity of the NOE injury and the needed repair.[25] Low-velocity injuries often will be unilateral and create a minimally-to-moderately displaced large fragment composed of the frontal process of the maxilla, lacrimal bone, and interiormost portion of the lamina papyracea (Fig. 24-18). The attachment of all three components of the MCL should remain intact, and repair consists of realignment and fixation of the bone fragment. The approach to the injury usually requires only a transconjunctival incision, but a sublabial incision may be necessary to allow for application of instrumentation needed to completely rotate the fragment into position. Occasionally, transnasal wiring will be necessary to pull the posterior edge of the fragment into exact alignment. Fixation can be accomplished with microplates and screws. Closed reduction and external splint stabilization often are all that are needed for the nasal bone aspect of the NOE fracture.

Medium-velocity injuries may be unilateral but more often are bilateral and similarly create a moderately displaced large fragment in the area of the MCL attachment. This fragment usually will be composed of only the frontal process of the maxilla and a portion of the lacrimal fossa, with the site of attachment of the posterior horizontal component MCL destroyed (see Fig. 24-18). The anterior horizontal and vertical components usually will remain attached to the frontal process of the maxilla, but a partial avulsion is common. Realignment and fixation of the bony fragments require a combination of transconjunctival, sublabial, and coronal incisions. Local incisions are used only when lacera-

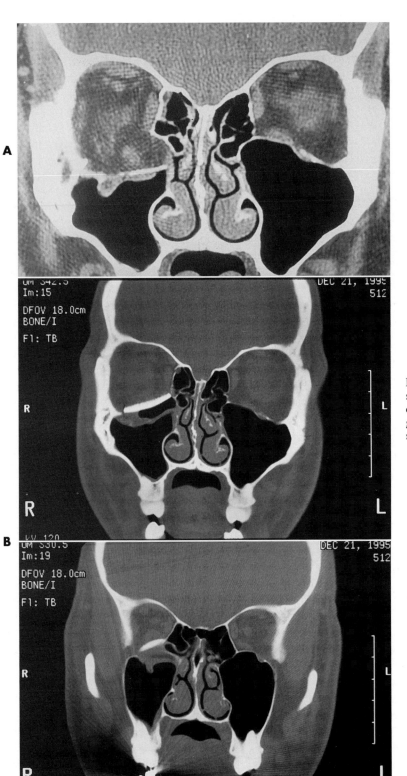

Fig. 24-16. A, Coronal computed tomography (CT) scan showing large blow-out type fracture of the right orbital floor. **B,** *Top* CT scan shows split cranial bone graft bridging defect at mid-orbital level. *Bottom* scan shows extension of bone graft into posterior orbit.

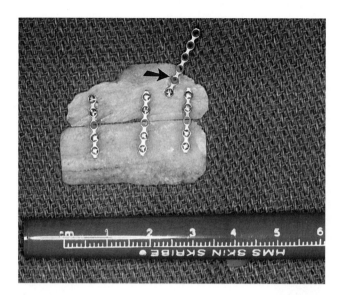

Fig. 24-17. Split cranial bone grafts that have been joined by 1.0-mm microplates. Angle of bend of plates at the joint can be adjusted to recreate the transition from orbital floor to medial wall. The graft would be inserted through the transconjunctival incision and its position adjusted through a coronal or medial orbital incision. Peripheral plate (*arrow*) is for fixation to orbital rim.

tions have occurred in the area or in men with an unstable hairline. Fixation again is accomplished with microplates and screws.

Although reduction and fixation at this point should have returned two of the three components of the MCL to their correct positions, the posterior horizontal component detachment has not been addressed. If no further MCL repair is performed, the inner canthus is left slightly forward of its normal position, and it may have a noticeably blunted appearance. Also, the medial-most aspect of the lower eyelid may stand away from the lacrimal lake. The vector of pull of the posterior horizontal component is recreated with a transnasal 28-gauge wire that is initially passed around the anterior horizontal component of the tendon (see Fig. 24-18). Access to the tendon is obtained through a small skin incision made 2 mm medial to the inner canthus.[40] A small curved needle then is used to carefully pass the wire above and below the tendon to loop the tendon just medial to the lacrimal sac. Both ends of the wire then are passed transnasally through a spinal needle that has been pushed through a hole drilled with a long 2.0-mm drill bit. The drill is aimed from the superomedial aspect of the contralateral orbit across to the presumed pretrauma location of the ipsilateral posterior lacrimal crest. The spinal needle is removed, and both ends of the wire are pulled equally taut. While the position of the medial canthus is being directly visualized, the ends of the wires are tied around a 1.3-mm screw placed into the thick cortex of the nasal process of the frontal bone, just above the passage hole of the transnasal wires (Fig. 24-19).

Bilateral injuries are treated in the same fashion, with the transnasal wire from each side being anchored independently in the contralateral orbit. This greatly facilitates tightening of the wires and eliminates the possible need to redo both repairs if one transnasal wire is broken during the tightening process. The tightening of these wires is not done until reconstruction of the deeper aspect of the medial orbital wall is completed. Closed reduction and external splint stabilization usually are sufficient for the nasal bone injuries in these patients, although severe comminution of these bones combined with posterior telescoping of the nasal septum can be present, necessitating placement of a dorsal nasal bone graft that can be cantilevered from the frontal bone with lag screws or a microplate and screws.

High-velocity force produces severe comminution of the entire NOE complex with unilateral if not bilateral detachment of all three components of each MCL (see Fig. 24-18). Repair is started with reconstruction of the frontal processes of the maxilla and medial orbital walls with available bone fragments or bone grafts if necessary. In these patients, microplates and screws facilitate the repair and provide greater stability for the subsequent MCL repair than do multiple interosseous wires. A hole is left in both medial walls immediately above and behind the normal location of the posterior lacrimal crest. The location of these holes is determined by the vector analysis of a completely detached MCL complex, which shows that the tendon should be repositioned posterior and superior to its location in the undisturbed state to stimulate the combined pull of the three components (see Fig. 24-3).[40] Transnasal wires are used to pull the tendons into the holes (see Fig. 24-19). Each wire should be anchored in the contralateral orbit while the medial canthal areas are being observed for symmetry. It is virtually impossible to overcorrect a totally detached MCL complex.[45] A patient who appears to be properly positioned in the operating room frequently appears undercorrected when the edema resolves. Bone grafts cantilevered from the frontal bone may be used in these patients to reconstruct the frontonasal angle and nasal dorsum.

A lacrimal collection system injury with subsequent dysfunction is a surprisingly uncommon sequela of all but the most severe NOE fractures. If such an injury is suspected or recognized at the time of the initial fracture reduction and fixation, insertion of silastic tubing (crawford tube) through the injured canaliculi or sac into the nose may be performed, but a complex repair probably is best delayed in favor of the optimum MCL repair that can be achieved.[18] An attempt at simultaneous lacrimal system repair invariably leads to a compromised MCL repair. A secondary reconstruction of the MCL complex usually is more difficult and less successful than a primary repair, whereas secondary lacrimal repairs have proven to be efficacious. Iatrogenic injury to the lacrimal sac is a possibility, but a thorough understanding of the tripartite structure of the MCL and its relationship to the medial orbital wall should prevent this.

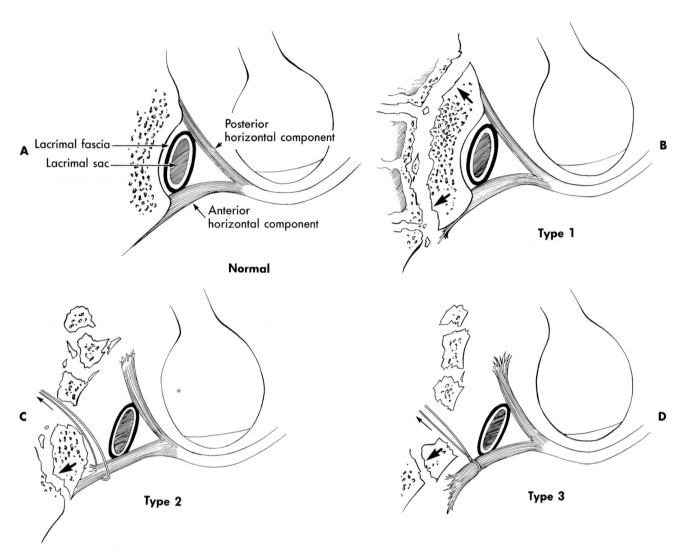

Fig. 24-18. Types of medial canthal tendon (MCT) injuries. **A,** Simplified schematic showing the relationship of anterior and posterior horizontal components of MCT to the lacrimal fossa and lacrimal sac. **B,** Type 1: *arrows* indicate the required movement of the large bone fragments to reestablish vectors of the MCT components. A transnasal wire through the bone in the area of the posterior component may be necessary to reestablish this vector. **C,** Type II: the transnasal wire looped around the anterior horizontal component simulates the vector of the posterior component. Direct wiring of the posterior component is difficult and endangers the lacrimal sac. Partial avulsion of the anterior component may require treatment as if total avulsion has occurred. **D,** Type III: the transnasal wire should be tied securely around the anterior horizontal component of the MCT.

Continued

Mandible

Traditional treatment of most mandibular fractures included a 6-week period of total jaw immobilization with MMF. This was true whether the fracture was considered to be favorable and nondisplaced (not requiring open reduction) or unfavorable and displaced (requiring open reduction and probably fixation with a transosseous wire).[7] Because the mandible resembles the long bones of the extremities in that it is a sturdy, bicortical structure, it only was natural that rigid fixation techniques used for long bone fractures eventually would be adapted for mandibular fractures.[51] Initially, relatively thick plates and large (2.7 mm) bicortical screws (with a minimum of two screws on both sides of the fracture) were used to provide a stable and rigid form of fixation for the mandible. In addition, the fixation devices most often were designed so that compression forces between the bone ends would be generated through a specifically engineered interaction of the screws with the plates. This compression allowed the bone to share the functional forces with the metallic devices and thus reduced the chances of implant failure. Because these compression plates by anatomic necessity had to be placed on the lower border of the

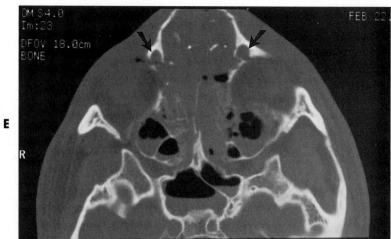

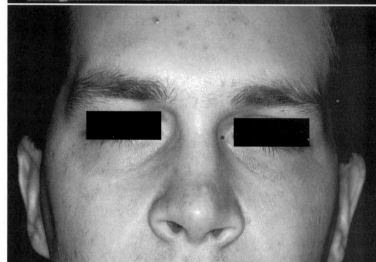

Fig. 24-18, cont'd. E, Axial computed tomography showing displaced lacrimal fossae (*arrows*) in a patient who suffered a gunshot wound to the face. Intercanthal distance measured 49 mm. **F,** Postoperative result in the same patient after repair of bilateral type II injuries with transnasal wires.

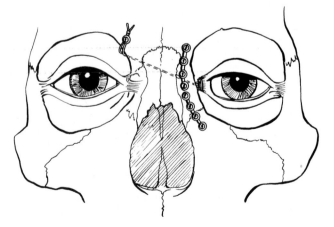

Fig. 24-19. Schematic of transnasal wire tied around left medial canthal ligament (MCL) before final tightening around screw placed above right orbit. This tightening will pull MCL posteriorly and superiorly to correct blunting of inner canthus. Bony repair is with microplates.

mandible, it was necessary to maintain additional fixation along the upper border to prevent separation of the fracture. This additional fixation was either an archbar (tension band splint) attached to the teeth across the fracture line if the fracture occurred between the teeth or a smaller plate (tension band plate) if it occurred posterior to the teeth. This form of fixation facilitated primary bone healing and allowed for immediate removal of MMF, thus allowing the patient to function with the stabilized mandible in the early postoperative period.

Subsequent modification of the rigid fixation techniques features the use of smaller, more easily bendable plates and smaller (2.0-mm) screws, sometimes placed in a monocortical fashion. This less rigid form of fixation often is used with a 2- to 4-week period of MMF. Also, lag screws across the fracture line have been used for certain strategically located fractures, providing adequate stability to allow for immediate mobilization of the mandible (Fig. 24-20).[11,32] It is well recognized that no matter which rigid fixation technique

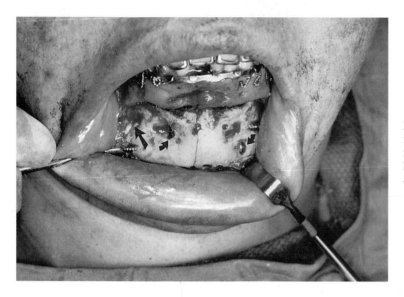

Fig. 24-20. Transoral rigid fixation of parasymphyseal fracture of mandible with two lag screws placed across fracture line in opposite directions. *Small arrows* indicate heads of screws. Mental nerve (*large arrow*) is identified and protected during the procedure.

is used, the incidence of complications, including infection, nonunion, malunion, and malocclusion, will increase disastrously if the surgeon is not thoroughly trained in the indications and instrumentation for the technique.

Treatment of isolated mandibular fractures (Fig. 24-21), whether with closed reduction or open reduction and internal fixation, is greatly facilitated by an intact maxilla. As previously mentioned, in patients with two-jaw injuries, the variable position of the condylar heads in the glenoid fossae comes into play, and MMF does not guarantee that maximal intercuspation of the teeth will restore the occlusal plane to its correct relationship to the skull base. This is particularly problematic when the mandibular injuries include fractures of the head or neck of one or both condyles. In patients with an intact maxilla, the relationship of the occlusal plane to the skull base remains undisturbed, and MMF wires can be used to "pull the patient into occlusion." Again, a knowledge of the pretrauma occlusion is helpful so that inadvertent and time-consuming attempts to correct preexisting malocclusions will not occur.

Because of the importance of MMF in setting and maintaining occlusion, application of a secure set of arch bars is critical. A malleable bar should be firmly attached to both dental arches using prestretched 25-gauge circumdental wires. If possible, a ligature should be placed around each first molar, premolar, and canine. If teeth are missing, the bars can be expanded posteriorly so that second molars can be ligated or the incisors can be used. Use of the incisors to resist MMF pulls on a long-term basis is not advisable because the slender, conical, uniroot incisor structure predisposes the maxillary and mandibular incisors to loosening in their sockets. Circumdental attachment of the arch bars can be greatly reinforced with circummandibular wires and piriform aperture suspension wires (Fig. 24-22) if rigid fixation is not being used, and the patient remains in MMF for 6 weeks. The MMF, whether wire itself or orthodontic elastics,

can be applied around the curved hooks of the arch bars, but the actual resistance to the MMF forces is carried out by the circummandibular and piriform wires. This maintains a solid jaw-to-jaw fixation even in a partially edentulous situation.

If rigid fixation is to be used and if MMF is only a temporary intraoperative condition, application of a stable set of arch bars is essential. During fixation of the fractures with plates and screws, the interocclusal relationship set by the temporary MMF should remain undisturbed if iatrogenic occlusal discrepancies are to be avoided. Ivy loops and Essig wires may be an excellent means for temporary stabilization of the jaws before surgery, but they do not offer adequate stability during surgery.

In most patients, the arch bars can be applied, and all circumdental wires can be tightened before exploration of the fracture site, although occasionally the fracture fragments will be locked in a displaced position by overlapping bone edges or interposed soft tissue, and closed reduction to allow for alignment of the occlusal plane is not possible. Exposure of the fractures to allow for direct manipulation of the fragments before final application of the archbars and MMF is necessary in these patients. Such simultaneous intraoral and external open manipulation of a mandibular fracture has been thought to increase the risk of wound infection and nonunion of the fracture. All mandibular fractures involving the tooth-bearing body already are contaminated through lacerations in the gingiva and periodontal ligaments of involved teeth. Also, fractures can be widely exposed and repaired through transoral approaches without an increased risk of infectious complications. Although infectious complications usually involve oral organisms, contamination of the wound at the time of surgery usually is not the principal cause, but rather a delay in treatment (antibiotic and surgical) or failure to adequately stabilize the fracture fragments is primarily responsible for infections.

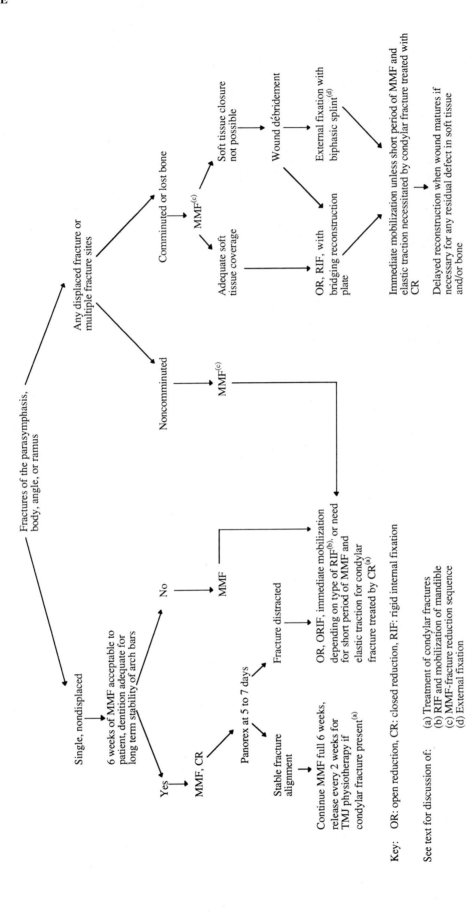

Fig. 24-21. Treatment algorithm for mandible fractures.

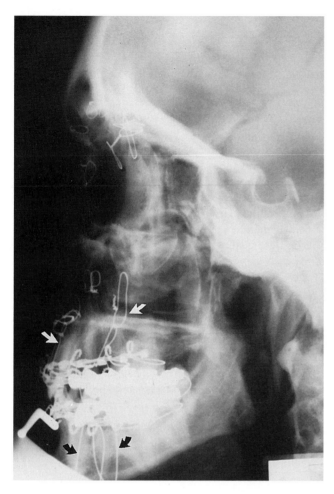

Fig. 24-22. Circummandibular wires (*black arrows*) and short maxillary suspension wires (*white arrows*). These wires serve only to stabilize arch bars under the pull of maxillomandibular fixation wires or elastics and do not stabilize fracture reductions directly.

Broad-spectrum antibiotic therapy (penicillin or cephalosporin) should be started, and a form of jaw immobilization (preferably arch bars and MMF) should be applied as soon after the injury as possible. Nondisplaced, favorable fractures treated with closed reduction then can be managed on an outpatient basis, with a follow-up panoramic tomograph to be obtained 1 week later to confirm that fracture alignment has been maintained. Patients with displaced fractures are best treated as inpatients with intravenous antibiotics begun immediately and definitive open reduction with a form of internal fixation accomplished within 3 to 5 days. Longer delays, especially in patients with severely comminuted fractures and large oral lacerations, increase the chances that the fracture site will become infected, with a resultant increase in the difficulty of the surgery and a higher complication rate.

A tooth in a fracture line and teeth immediately adjacent to the fracture should be evaluated and treated individually. It should be determined whether the root of the tooth is fractured, whether it is firmly attached to one of the bone fragments by residual periodontal ligament, and whether the tooth will aid in reduction and immobilization of the fracture. A single molar tooth in a posterior fragment may be essential to prevent superior displacement by the elevator muscle group. The canine tooth positioned at the corner of the dental arch may be essential in stabilizing parasymphaseal and anterior body fractures. A tooth that is salvageable, possibly with endodontic therapy, and that will be an important factor in stabilizing the fracture reduction should be retained. A tooth that has questionable prognosis, even with immediate or delayed endodontic therapy and with minimal contribution to stabilization, should be considered nonessential. Such teeth probably should be removed if the extraction can be performed without seriously distracting the fracture.[53] The need for extraction should be assessed for each patient and placed in the context of the likelihood that the patient actually will seek out and receive the dental care necessary for the long-term preservation of the tooth.[9]

Once unsalvageable teeth have been extracted and stable MMF established, a decision should be made regarding the use of intraoral or extraoral approach to the fracture. Fractures that occur in the anterior mandible between the mental foramina are ideal for reduction and fixation through a transoral approach. Although fractures in this area do not fit into the favorable–unfavorable classification system for lateral fractures, most should be considered unstable because of the bilateral muscle pulls to which they are subjected. Internal fixation therefore usually is indicated. An incision is made several millimeters below the junction of the attached and free gingiva, low enough to leave sufficient tissue attachment to bone to accommodate sutures when the mucoperiosteal flap is repositioned, but high enough to prevent damage to the buccal sulcus. The entire anterior surface of the mandible can be exposed, with direct visualization of both mental nerves possible (see Fig. 24-20).

Fixation can be obtained with an interosseous wire (and 6 weeks of MMF) or with a compression plate placed along the lower border using bicortical 2.4-mm screws. Successful fixation allowing for immediate jaw mobilization also has been reported with long lag screws[11] and smaller plates attached with monocortical 2.0-mm screws.[6] These latter two techniques are made possible because the fixation devices are being attached to the mandible anterior to the mental foramina, and the inferior alveolar neurovascular bundles are not at risk for damage. The level of attachment can be moved superiorly on the mandible to lie within the tension zone of fracture distraction, and therefore less sturdy devices can be used. A knowledge of the average length of each anterior mandibular tooth (available in all dental anatomy texts) is required to safely perform these techniques.

The transoral approach to anterior fractures eliminates the need for a submental incision, and also the risk of damage to one or both marginal nerves if the incision must be extended into the submandibular triangle area for adequate exposure. Treatment of fractures near or through the mental foramen by way of the intraoral approach presents the increased risk of damage to this sensory nerve from excessive traction or direct trauma during drilling, tapping, and screw insertion. The status of this nerve should be documented before surgery, and the patient should be warned to expect a transient decrease in function postoperatively if sensation has remained intact after the fracture.

The transoral approach also prevents direct inspection of the lingual surface of the mandible to ensure the accuracy of reduction. If the patient is only partially dentulous and if the number of stable occlusal contacts is limited or if there are associated maxillary and palatal fractures, failure to close the lingual cortical displacement may produce widening of the face at the level of the mandibular angles. Also, a butterfly-type fracture with a single linear defect in the buccal cortical plate and a large free-floating fragment in the lingual cortical plate may be overlooked, and attempts to insert bicortical screws for attachment of a compression plate actually may produce fracture line displacement or inadequate fixation stability. If a comminuted fracture is recognized, a compression plate cannot be used, but a more rigid reconstruction type of plate should be applied if immediate mobilization is desired. With these possible problems in mind, the surgeon may find with experience that the transoral approach to anterior fractures is preferable to an external approach in most patients. The application of plates across fracture lines actually is easier than complex figure-of-eight wiring because a lingual dissection and retrograde passing of the wire are avoided.

A second type of fracture that should be considered for a transoral approach is the minimally-to-moderately displaced noncomminuted angle fracture. This fracture usually can be adequately exposed, reduced, and stabilized through a vertical incision along the anterior border of the ascending ramus of the mandible extending for a short distance down the lateral oblique line of the buccal surface of the mandibular body. Subperiosteal dissection is carried over the buccal surface of the proximal and distal fracture edges, and soft tissue is freed from the fracture line. A bone-holding forcep can be applied to the ramus, and the fracture is pulled into reduction. Third molars in the line of fracture are evaluated and managed by the previously described criteria. Fixation can be obtained with an upper border buccal wire through the third molar socket if the tooth is extracted (along with 6 weeks of MMF), a long lag screw,[12,32] or small plates attached along the ascending ramus and oblique line with 2.0-mm monocortical screws.[6] Controversy exists whether patients treated with the smaller plates should be allowed to function immediately or whether a shortened period (2 to 4 weeks) of MMF is needed. Larger compression plates also can be placed transorally along the lower border of the mandible with 2.4-mm screws in conjunction with a smaller upper border tension-hard plate to allow for immediate mobilization. This technique should not be attempted by inexperi-

enced surgeons because the screws must be placed transbuccally and because the lower border plate may be difficult to position properly, which increases the risk of placing a screw through the inferior alveolar neurovascular bundle.

Reduction of moderately-to-severely displaced angle fractures also can be problematic through the transoral approach. An external approach offers greater access to the fragments in these patients and greatly facilitates correct application of large compression plates. Access to the angle can be achieved through a standard Risdon approach or through a modified Risdon approach (Fig. 24-23).[4] The combination of the two approaches creates a gently curving incision that follows natural skin lines to produce wide exposure of the ascending ramus, angle, and posterior body of the mandible. During deep dissection, the anterior border of the sternocleidomastoid muscle is identified, and the tail of the parotid gland is retracted forward. The lateral aspect of the platysma is incised well away from the lower border of the mandible, and the marginal branch of the facial nerve is retracted upward with the gland and upper cervical flap.

Elevation of the masseter muscle is necessary for drilling the holes and placement of a transosseous wire or a compression plate. Dissection on the lingual surface of the mandible is unnecessary if plates and screws are to be used other than

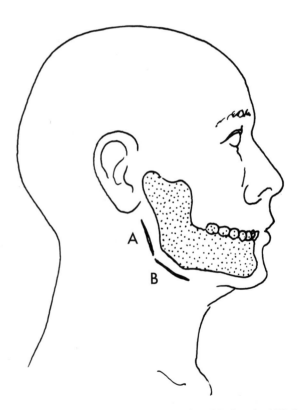

Fig. 24-23. *A,* Modified Risdon approach and *B,* Standard Risdon approach can be joined to give excellent exposure to the ramus, angle, and posterior body of the mandible. (With permission from Ardray WC: Plate and screw fixation in the management of mandible fractures, *Clin Plast Surg* 16:61, 1989.)

a blunt dissection over the major vessels to allow for placement of a protective malleable retractor. After fixation is completed, the masseter muscle is reattached with slowly absorbing sutures placed through its lower border and carried around the mandible to the fascia of the lateral pterygoid muscle. A small drain that can be attached to bulb suction is positioned in the depths of the wound in each patient and brought out through a small separate stab incision. A meticulous layered closure of the wound then is carried out.

Displaced, unfavorable fractures of the body of the mandible posterior to the mental foramen usually require an external approach. Although it is possible to apply even large compression plates to fractures in this area by way of a transoral approach combined with the transbuccal insertion of screws, the location of the mental nerve places it exactly in the way of visualization, manipulation, and stabilization of the fragments. An external approach greatly facilitates repair of body fractures, and it typically is done through a transverse upper neck incision placed approximately 2.5 cm below the lower border of the mandible, centered below the fracture line. The marginal mandibular nerve is protected during elevation of the upper skin flap by either using the facial nerve stimulator during the subplatysmal dissection or by maintaining the level of the dissection on the lateral surface of the submandibular gland up to the lower border of the mandible. A longer incision is required for application of a compression plate than for insertion of a figure-of-eight wire across the fracture site. Closure and drainage are accomplished in the same fashion that was described for angle fractures.

Treatment of condylar fractures has remained one of the most complex and controversial issues in mandibular fracture management. Although there is general agreement about conservative, closed management with early mobilization for intracapsular (condylar head) fractures, numerous series now argue against the across-the-board use of this management for all extracapsular (condylar neck) fractures.[21] The standard treatment for most unilateral condylar neck fractures is a short period of MMF (10 to 14 days) followed by progressive mobilization and placement of elastics at night for an additional 2 weeks. Rigid fixation techniques should be applied to any accompanying body or angle fractures to ensure that early mobilization is possible. If rigid fixation is not used on these fractures, thus necessitating a 6-week period of MMF, the MMF should be briefly released every 2 weeks to allow for jaw-opening exercises. This helps to reduce intra- and pericapsular fibrosis that accompanies any condylar fracture, particularly those with an intracapsular component.

Indications for consideration of open reduction and internal fixation of condylar neck fractures might include (1) displacement of the condylar head from the glenoid fossa, (2) mechanical obstruction of jaw opening caused by a displaced condylar head, (3) telescoping of the proximal and distal fragments with the loss of vertical ramus height resulting in

malocclusion, (4) displaced bilateral subcondylar fractures with malocclusion, (5) a unilateral or bilateral condylar fracture with severely comminuted midfacial fractures (see the discussion on maxillary fractures), (6) a comminuted symphysis fracture and condyle fracture with associated tooth loss, (7) a displaced condyle fracture in mentally retarded or medically compromised adults (i.e., those for whom MMF would not be desirable) with evidence of open bite or retrusion, and (8) an edentulous or partially edentulous mandible with posterior bite collapse and a displaced condyle.[4,63] Of note, these indications make no mention of attempting to prevent future dysfunction within the temporomandibular joint itself, with the possible exception of the condylar head completely displaced from the fossa. To date, there is no proof that any form of surgical therapy to realign a fractured condylar neck decreases the incidence of future degenerative problems within the joint, and surgical exploration of the joint may worsen the damage if done injudiciously.

The approach to the condylar neck, when indicated, is through the incision used for an angle fracture, although it does not have to be carried as far inferiorly. The submasseteric dissection should be carried higher on the ramus to allow adequate exposure of the proximal fragment, but specific identification of the main truck of the facial nerve[21] usually is not necessary. The mandible may be grasped at the angle and pulled away from the condyle with a bone-holding forcep or with a transosseous wire to facilitate identification and mobilization of the condylar neck segment. Plate and screw (2.0-mm) fixation offers the most effective method of holding an anatomic reduction, and the patient should be able to mobilize the mandible immediately. As with all rigid fixation implants, a minimum of two screws should be placed above and below the fracture line. Preoperative evaluation should establish that the fracture is not as high as the level of attachment of the joint capsule to the condyle neck. Occasionally, a percutaneous transparotid approach may be required for placement of the screws into the proximal fragment. If plate and screw fixation is done with careful, blunt dissection, and appropriate transbuccal instrumentation, there should be little risk of injury to the branches of the facial nerve.

Comminuted fractures of the mandible, whether the result of blunt trauma or gunshot wounds, usually are associated with serious intraoral soft-tissue injuries. These fractures are at great risk for infection, sequestration, and nonunion. This particularly is true for body fractures, whereas angle or ramus and parasymphaseal comminuted fractures tend to do well. Comminution is an absolute contraindication to the use of plates and screws to apply compression across the fracture lines. If rigid internal fixation is to be used to allow for early function, thicker and stronger reconstruction plates that are capable of bearing all of the functional forces should be applied to bridge the area of comminution or actual bone loss.

Angle or ramus comminuted injuries are particularly well

suited for open reduction and internal fixation with a sturdy reconstruction plate if the proximal condylar segment is large enough to accommodate a minimum of two 2.4-mm screws. This is an ideal treatment for gunshot wounds with associated injury to the muscles of mastication, since early mobilization usually will avoid trismus later (Fig. 24-24). Facial nerve injuries can be repaired concurrently. Sequestration of devascularized fragments of the ascending ramus usually does not occur because they are covered by the masticatory muscle sling and are not in a dependent area that will be bathed by saliva if the oral wound closure dehisces. Comminuted parasymphaseal fractures also tend to do well, although they are in a dependent area. There are numerous muscle attachments in the area that usually remain closely

adherent to the bone fragments to maintain some vascularity. Also, the most severe comminution generally involves the alveolus, which usually is vigorously débrided to reduce the chances of sequestration and infection.

Comminuted body fractures usually contain large devascularized fragments with vital molar or premolar teeth. An attempt should be made to salvage all fragments if possible, knowing that some may later sequester and require débridement. Reduction of these fragments requires an open approach, and fixation with plates and screws actually may carry less risk of further devascularization than does the placement of transosseous wires. Less additional devascularization occurs because the lingual periosteum does not have to be elevated for insertion of screws. A sturdy reconstruc-

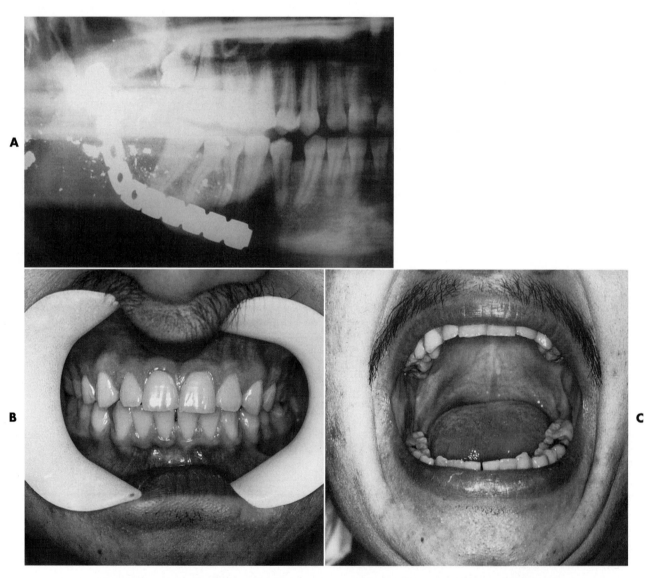

Fig. 24-24. A, The postoperative view of a severely comminuted gunshot injury of the mandibular angle and ascending ramus, treated with a reconstruction plate attached to the condylar stump above and body below. **B,** Follow-up at 6 months with normal occlusion. **C,** No trismus has resulted despite severe injury to muscles of mastication.

tion plate that bridges across the comminuted area from stable proximal segment to stable distal segment is the preferred way to manage these injuries. The plate maintains the dimensions of the mandible even if some bone is eventually lost and if a secondary reconstruction is required.

A proven alternative to internal fixation in the management of comminuted fractures and fractures with loss of bone is the Joe Hall Morris biphase system (Fig. 24-25). This form of external fixation can be cumbersome and unpleasant for the patient. Its use now generally is restricted to those with gunshot wounds that cause loss of not only bone but also of overlying soft tissue.

Edentulous mandible

Fractures of the edentulous mandible often are treated with closed reduction and immobilization using the patient's dentures or a preformed Gunning splint. The dentures or splints are attached to the mandible with circummandibular wires and to the maxilla with piriform or circumzygomatic wires. MMF then is established between the dentures or splints. Although this form of treatment leads to successful healing in most patients, it may be uncomfortable and severely restricts oral intake in patients who already may be nutritionally compromised. Open reduction and internal fixation using compression plates has been shown to be successful in jaws with a vertical height of at least 2 cm.[23] Atrophic mandibles less than 2 cm in height also can be treated with rigid fixation, but longer reconstruction plates with more screws to resist distractive forces should be used. Also, simultaneous bone grafting to augment the atrophic mandible should be considered if no violations of the oral mucosa have occurred.

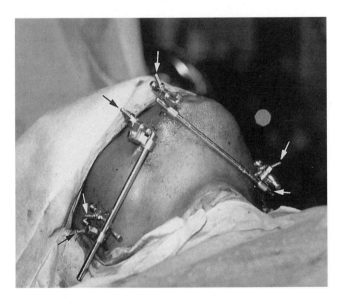

Fig. 24-25. The first phase of biphasic external fixation of bilateral comminuted mandibular body fractures. Second phase is molding of stabilizing bar of self-curing acrylic between pins (*arrows*), followed by removal of metal rods and clips.

LATE MANIFESTATIONS

Posttreatment facial asymmetry and malocclusion have been previously discussed in terms of lack of recognition or inadequate treatment of the full extent of the facial skeletal injuries. Imperfect results also may be seen in appropriately managed patients, and all patients should be informed that revision surgery may be necessary before the final result is obtained. This is particularly true for patients who suffer panfacial injuries with bilateral fractures that eliminate stable landmarks that can be used as a starting point for the reconstruction. Such revisions hopefully will be relatively minor if the goal of the original surgery was the total anatomic reconstruction of the facial skeletal unit.

Posttreatment asymmetry usually involves the orbital and periorbital structures, in particular the globes, malar prominences, and medial canthal ligaments. Subtle differences in position typically become recognizable within the first week after surgery as postsurgical edema resolves. Follow-up axial and coronal CT scans should be obtained at this time to allow for comparison of orbital wall configuration, orbital volumes, and zygomatic arch alignment (see Fig. 24-9). Assuming that gross asymmetries are not seen on the CT scans, revision surgery can be delayed if the problem involves globe or malar prominence position. A delay of more than 6 weeks may necessitate osteotomies, new bone grafts or alloplastic implants, or selective burring of overly prominent surfaces rather than simple repositioning of bony segments and readaptation of fixation hardware.

Revision surgery for asymmetry of MCL position should not be delayed. Patients with adequate corrections should look "overcorrected" for the first 2 or 3 postsurgical weeks, and if not, further relaxation of the pull of the transnasal wire that always occurs will lead to a more obvious discrepancy. Revision surgery should be performed before any cicatricial shortening of the soft tissues has occurred. If soft-tissue contracture occurs, delayed repair of MCL position may necessitate total mobilization of the lower eyelid and detachment of the lateral canthal ligament to allow for any movement of the inner canthal angle. Movement may be further restricted by scarring around a functional lacrimal system. Early revision may be as simple as retightening of a transnasal wire that was not pulled as taut as originally thought or as difficult as replacement of a wire that has cut through a MCL that was partially transected by the original injury. If the second situation is encountered, repair requires passing a wire through the residual lateral stump of the ligament as close to the inner canthal angle as possible, rather than around the ligament. This allows for a more forceful pull with the transnasal wire, but it unfortunately places the lacrimal system at higher risk for iatrogenic injury when the needle is passed through the ligament.

Malocclusion may occur in appropriately treated patients who have suffered unilateral or more often bilateral intracapsular condylar fractures of the mandible. When the MMF is removed in these patients, the mandible may drift to the side of a unilateral injury or it may assume a retruded position, creating an anterior open bite deformity in patients with bilateral injuries. Corrections usually is not a simple matter of replacing the MMF or performing an osteotomy through the condylar neck. Instead, a vertical ramus osteotomy or even bilateral sagittal split osteotomies are required to allow for correction of the malocclusion. True posttraumatic temporomandibular joint ankylosis is unusual even in patients with the more severe condylar head injuries. The actual incidence of joint dysfunction is unknown because symptoms can be somewhat subjective and because there often is a delay between injury and onset of symptomatic joint degeneration.

SUMMARY

The intent of treating fractures of the facial skeleton is to restore appearance and function. The use of newly developed diagnostic and surgical methods does not automatically ensure improved results and may increase the risk of iatrogenic injuries if they are incorrectly applied. The surgeon should be skilled in the selection and use of traditional techniques and the newer rigid fixation methods for all types of fractures. A surgeon may be hesitant to perform the extended access approaches in hopes that any facial asymmetry resulting from incomplete fracture reduction will be imperceptible. The range of imperceptible asymmetry is small, and the surgeon should not accept suboptimal results that may have been improved with a more aggressive reconstruction.

Reduction and fixation of each individual fracture line or fracture–dislocation should not be viewed in a segmentalized fashion but rather as a step in the progressive reconstruction of the entire facial skeletal complex. It is important that the trauma surgeon possess an ability to conceptualize the reconstruction three dimensionally as it is proceeding and to work safely around all of the vital soft-tissue structures contained within this complex skeletal unit.

REFERENCES

1. Anderson RL, Pange WR, Gross CE: Optic nerve blindness following blunt forehead trauma, *Ophthalmology* 89:445, 1982.
2. Appling WD, Patrinely JR, Salzer TA: Transconjunctival approach vs subcilliary skin-muscle flap approach for orbital fracture repair, *Arch Otolaryngol Head Neck Surg* 119:1000, 1993.
3. Archer WH: *Fractures of the facial bones and their treatment.* In Archer WH, editor: *Oral and maxillofacial surgery*, ed 5, vol 2, Philadelphia, 1975, WB Saunders.
4. Ardrary WC: Plate and screw fixation in the management of mandible fractures, *Clin Plast Surg* 16:61, 1989.
5. Bilyk JR, Joseph MP: Traumatic optic neuropathy, *Semin Ophthalmol* 9:200, 1994.
6. Champy M and others: Mandibular osteosynthesis by miniature screwed plates via a buccal approach, *J Maxillofac Surg* 6:14, 1978.
7. Clark WD, Bailey B: *Management of fractures of the mandible.* In Mathog RH, editor: *Maxillofacial trauma*, Baltimore, 1984, Williams & Wilkins.
8. Reference deleted in pages.
9. Dierks EJ: Management of associated dental injuries in maxillofacial trauma, *Otolaryngol Clin North Am* 24:165, 1991.
10. Donald PJ: Frontal sinus ablation by cranialization: a report of 21 cases, *Arch Otolaryngol* 108:142, 1982.
11. Ellis E, Ghali GE: Lag screw fixation of anterior mandibular fractures, *J Oral Maxillofac Surg* 49:13, 1991.
12. Ellis E, Ghali GE: Lag screw fixation of mandibular angle fractures, *J Oral Maxillofac Surg* 49:234, 1991.
13. Funk GF, Stanley RB, Becker TS: Reversible visual loss due to impacted lateral orbital wall fractures, *Head Neck Surg* 11:295, 1989.
14. Ghobrial W, Amstutz S, Mathog RH: Fractures of the sphenoid bone, *Head Neck Surg* 8:447, 1986.
15. Glassman RD and others: Rigid fixation of internal orbital fractures, *Plast Reconstr Surg* 86:1103, 1990.
16. Gruss JS, MacKinnon SE: Complex maxillary fractures: the role of buttress reconstruction and immediate bone grafting, *Plast Reconstr Surg* 78:9, 1986.
17. Gruss JS, Phillips JH: Complex facial trauma: the evolving role of rigid fixation and immediate bone grafting reconstruction, *Clin Plast Surg* 16:93, 1989.
18. Gruss JS and others: The pattern and incidence of nasolacrimal injury in naso-orbito-ethmoid fractures: the role of delayed assessment and dacrocystorhinostomy, *Br J Plast Surg* 38:116, 1985.
19. Gruss JS and others: The role of primary bone grafting in complex craniomaxillofacial trauma, *Plast Reconstr Surg* 75:17, 1985.
20. Joy ED, McGaha LE, Bear SE: Facial elongation after treatment of horizontal fracture of the maxilla without vertical stabilization, *J Oral Surg* 27:560, 1969.
21. Klotch OW, Lundy LB: Condylar neck fractures of the mandible, *Otolaryngol Clin North Am* 24:181, 1991.
22. Koorneef L: Current concepts on the management of orbital blow-out fractures, *Ann Plast Surg* 9:185, 1982.
23. Levine PA: AD compression plating technique for treating fractures of the adentulous mandible, *Otolaryngol Clin North Am* 20:457, 1987.
24. Manson PN: Some thoughts on the classification and treatment of Le Fort fractures, *Ann Plast Surg* 17:356, 1986.
25. Manson PN: *Dimensional analysis of the facial skeleton.* In Manson PH, editor: *Cranio-maxillofacial trauma: problems in plastic and reconstructive surgery*, Philadelphia, 1991, JB Lippincott.
26. Manson PN, Hoopes JE, Su CT: Structural pillars of the facial skeleton: an approach to the management of Le Fort fractures, *Plast Reconstr Surg* 66:54, 1980.
27. Manson PN, Ruas EJ, Iliff NT: Deep orbital reconstruction for correction of posttraumatic enophthalmos, *Clin Plast Surg* 14:113, 1987.
28. Manson PN and others: Mechanisms of global support and post-traumatic enophthalmos. I. The anatomy of the ligament sling and its relationship to intramuscular cone orbital fat, *Plast Reconstr Surg* 77:193, 1986.
29. Manson PN and others: Studies on enophthalmos. II. The measurement of orbital injuries and their treatment by quantitative computed tomography, *Plast Reconstr Surg* 77:203, 1986.
30. Mathog RH: *Posttraumatic telecanthus.* In Mathog RH, editor: *Maxillofacial trauma*, Baltimore, 1984, William & Wilkins.
31. Mathog RH: Management of orbital blow-out fractures. *Otolaryngol Clin North Am* 24:79, 1991.
32. Niederdellmann H, Shetty V: Solitary lag screw osteosynthesis in treatment of fractures of the angle of the mandible: a retrospective study, *Plast Reconstr Surg* 80:68, 1987.
33. Parsons GS, Mathog RH: Orbital wall and volume relationships, *Arch Otolaryngol Head Neck Surg* 114:743, 1988.
34. Paskert JP, Manson PN: The bimanual examination for assessing instability in naso-orbitoethmoid injuries, *Plast Reconstr Surg* 83:165, 1989.
35. Paskert JP, Manson, PN, Iliff NT: Nasoethmoidal and orbital fractures, *Clin Plast Surg* 15:209, 1988.
36. Powell NB, Riley RW, Lamb DR: A new approach to evaluation and surgery of the malar complex, *Ann Plast Surg* 20:206, 1988.
37. Rahn BA: Theoretical considerations in rigid fixation of facial bones, *Clin Plast Surg* 16:21, 1989.

38. Ramfjord SP, Ash MM: *Occlusion,* Philadelphia, 1969, WB Saunders.

39. Ramsey JM: Optic nerve injury in fracture of the canal, *Br J Ophthalmol* 63:607, 1979.

40. Rodriguez RL, Zide BM: Reconstruction of the medial canthus, *Clin Plast Surg* 15:255, 1988.

41. Rohrich RJ, Hollier LH: Management of frontal sinus fractures, *Clin Plast Surg* 19:219, 1992.

42. Rubin PAD, Bilyk JR, Shore JW: Management of orbital trauma: fractures, hemorrhage, and traumatic optic neuropathy. Focal points, *American Academy of Ophthalmology,* 12:1, 1994.

43. Rudderman RH, Mullen RL: Biomechanics of the facial skeleton, *Clin Plast Surg* 19:11, 1992.

44. Sargent LA, Fulks KD: Reconstruction of internal orbital fractures with vitallium mesh, *Plast Reconstr Surg* 88:31, 1991.

45. Sargent LA: *Nasoethmoid orbital fractures.* In Manson PH, editor: *Craniomaxillofacial trauma: problems in plastic and reconstructive surgery,* Philadelphia, 1991, JB Lippincott.

46. Schultz RC: Frontal sinus and supraorbital fractures from vehicle accidents, *Clin Plast Surg* 2:93, 1975.

47. Shumrick KE, Smith CP: The use of cancellous bone for frontal sinus obliteration and reconstruction of frontal bone defects, *Arch Otolaryngol Head Neck Surg* 120:1003, 1994.

48. Sicher H, Dubrul EL: *Oral anatomy,* St Louis, 1970, Mosby.

49. Sofferman RA: Sphenoethmoid approach to the optic nerve, *Laryngoscope* 91:184, 1981.

50. Sofferman RA and others: Retrospective analysis of surgically treated Le Fort fractures, *Arch Otolaryngol* 109:446, 1983.

51. Spiessl B, editor: *New concepts in maxillofacial bone surgery,* New York, 1976, Springer-Verlag.

52. Spoor TC, Mathog RH: Restoration of vision after optic canal decompression, *Arch Ophthalmol* 104:804, 1986.

53. Stanley RB: *Pathogenesis and evaluation of mandibular fractures.* In Mathog RH, editor: *Maxillofacial trauma,* Baltimore, 1984, Williams & Wilkins.

54. Stanley RB: The temporal approach to impacted lateral orbital wall fractures, *Arch Otolaryngol Head Neck Surg* 114:550, 1988.

55. Stanley RB: The zygomatic arch as a guide to reconstruction of comminuted malar fractures, *Arch Otolaryngol Head Neck Surg* 115:1459, 1989.

56. Stanley RB: *Complications and problems in the management of injuries of the frontal bone and frontal sinus.* In Manson PH, editor: *Craniomaxillofacial trauma: problems in plastic and reconstructive surgery,* Philadelphia, 1991, JB Lippincott.

57. Stanley RB, Funk GF: Rigid internal fixation for fractures involving tooth-bearing maxillary segments, *Arch Otolaryngol Head Neck Surg* 114:1295, 1988.

58. Stanley RB, Nowak GM: Midfacial fractures: importance of angle of impact to horizontal craniofacial buttresses, *Otolaryngol Head Neck Surg* 93:186, 1985.

59. Thaller SR, Kawamoto HK: A histologic evaluation of fracture repair in the midface, *Plast Reconstr Surg* 85:196, 1990.

60. Toomey JM: *Le Fort fractures.* In English GM, editor: *Otolaryngology,* Philadelphia, 1981, Harper and Row.

61. Wolujewicz MA: Fractures of the mandible involving the impacted third molar tooth: an analysis of 47 cases, *Br J Oral Surg* 18:125, 1980.

62. Zachariades N and others: The superior orbital fissure syndrome, *J Maxillofac Surg* 13:125, 1985.

63. Zide MF: Open reduction of mandibular condyle fractures, *Clin Plast Surg* 16:69, 1989.

Chapter 25

Management of Basal and Squamous Cell Carcinoma

Neil A. Swanson
Timothy M. Johnson

The clinical presentations, differential diagnosis, and etiologic factors for basal cell carcinoma (BCC) and squamous cell carcinoma (SCC) are detailed elsewhere in this text. This chapter defines the treatment modalities that are effective in extirpating cutaneous BCC and SCC, including electrodesiccation and curettage (ED&C), excisional surgery, cryosurgery, irradiation, and Mohs' surgery. Mohs' surgery, also known as microscopically controlled excision, will be discussed, including its historic evolution, the technique itself, indications for use, and a brief discussion of options for reconstruction of defects. Once the modalities have been discussed, a section dealing with the choice of the appropriate modality will follow. For the most part, BCC and SCC will be dealt with in the same fashion, since the treatment modalities are similar.

TREATMENT MODALITIES

Electrodesiccation and Curettage

ED&C is an invaluable treatment modality used primarily by the dermatologist.[1,88] It can yield 92% to 98% success rates for small, primary, properly selected tumors in skilled hands.* In a review of 2314 primary BCCs treated with ED&C, Silverman[81] showed that lesion size and tumor location were independent risk factors for recurrence following ED&C. For low-risk sites (trunk, neck, extremities) lesions of all sizes were associated with an overall 3.3% 5-year recurrence rate. For lesions located on middle-risk sites (scalp, forehead, malar region) less than 1 cm in diameter, ED&C

* Refs. 18, 21, 24, 40, 41, 81.

yielded a 5.3% 5-year recurrence rate. For lesions greater than 1 cm in diameter, the 5-year recurrence rate was 22.7%. For BCCs located in high-risk sites (central face, ears, chin, mandible), the 5-year recurrence rate for lesions less than 6 mm in diameter was 4.5%; for lesions greater than 6 mm in diameter it was 17.6%. The keys to success with this technique include (1) the skill and experience of the operator, (2) appropriate use of sharp large and small curettes, (3) appropriate selection of tumor, and (4) detailed instructions to the patient for wound healing.

Technique

The curette comes in varying sizes, from 1 to 8 mm. BCC and SCC have a soft feel that can be differentiated from uninvolved normal surrounding tissue that feels smooth and firm.[88] By first using a large curette to debulk the majority of the soft tumor–containing tissue followed by a small curette to remove any small nests and projections of tumor, the surgeon can selectively remove the cancerous tissue and spare the normal surrounding skin.

A recommended technique for ED&C follows.[88] (1) The skin is cleansed with alcohol or other antibacterial scrub and rinse, the clinical margins of the tumor are outlined, and local anesthesia is obtained. (2) With a large curette, the surgeon removes the bulk of tumor until normal-feeling surrounding tissue is reached. (3) Electrodesiccation of the periphery and base of the wound with 1- to 2-mm margins is performed to destroy residual tumor cells. (4) The surgeon again performs curettage of the base and periphery of the wound with a large curette and then a small curette. This is

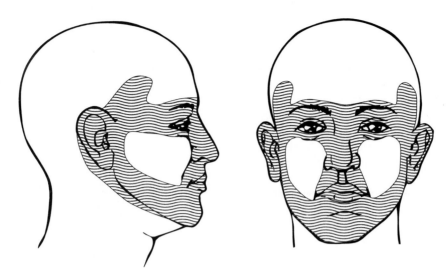

Fig. 25-1. The high risk zone of the face; problem areas in treatment of basal cell carcinoma.

again followed by electrodesiccation of the wound with 1-to 2-mm deep and peripheral margins. (5) This sequence is repeated until normal tissue is felt with both sizes of curettes. Once this occurs, electrodesiccation follows once more. Therefore, this sequence may occur twice or as many as five or six times depending on the size and feel of the lesion. (6) After final electrodesiccation, a light curetting is performed to remove excessive tissue char, and a dressing is placed.

Wound care consists of hydrogen peroxide two to three times daily, soap and water rinsing, and the application of antibacterial ointment and a Telfa bandage. Once tissue char is removed and a healthy granulating wound base is achieved, this regimen should be repeated daily. The patient is carefully instructed not to let an eschar form, since a wound granulating from the base will fill in its depth under moist occlusion and leave a more cosmetically acceptable scar.

With this technique, a high cure rate for properly selected tumors can be achieved ranging from 92% to 98%.* The treatment is appropriate for uncomplicated, small, previously untreated, nonaggressive growth histologic pattern tumors with clearly defined borders, especially in low-risk sites (trunk, neck, extremities). ED&C also yields good cure rates (95%) for lesions less than 1 cm in diameter on middle-risk sites (scalp, forehead, cheeks), and lesions less than 6 mm in diameter for high-risk sites (central face, ears, chin, mandible).

Advantages and disadvantages

The major advantage of ED&C is that in an outpatient office setting, rapid treatment of a cutaneous neoplasm can be achieved with high cure rates. Disadvantages include scarring, a delay in wound healing, and occasional bleeding.

The scar can be minimized by proper wound care. ED&C may be avoided in many patients with lesions in cosmetically important areas because a better cosmetic result can usually be obtained in these patients with excisional surgery. ED&C offers a good cosmetic result when used to treat superficial lesions on the bridge of the nose or nasal tip, small lesions on the temple, and lesions on the ear and postauricular area that have well-defined clinical borders and are smaller than 2 to 5 mm in diameter. The wound often takes 3 to 6 weeks to heal completely.

Contraindications

Relative contraindications to ED&C include large tumors (greater than 0.5 cm in diameter in high-risk areas, 1 cm in diameter in middle-risk areas, and 2 cm in diameter in low-risk areas) and those extending deeply into the dermis or fat. If the curette reaches fat, the surgeon should stop and consider a different treatment modality. Anatomic locations of high risk are shown in Figure 25-1. Other anatomic areas may yield a poorer scar compared with excisional surgery. Aggressive growth histologic patterns (morpheaform or sclerotic BCCs) have a scarlike stroma that removes the "feel" of the curette from the surgeon and should not be treated with this modality. Lastly, except for unusual circumstances, recurrent tumors are best treated by Mohs' surgery or other excisional modalities. Patients with modern pacemakers can be treated with current, short, interrupted 3- to 5-second bursts. Pulse should be monitored before and after ED&C in patients with pacemakers.

Excisional surgery

Excisional surgery also offers a high success rate for the treatment of small, low-risk primary BCC and SCC in experienced hands.* Excisional surgery can be performed with

---

* Refs. 18, 21, 24, 40, 41, 75, 81.

* Refs. 4, 17, 18, 21, 24, 25, 41, 75, 82.

a simple side-to-side closure, or the defect may be closed with a local flap or skin graft. Careful marginal control is necessary regardless of which closure modality is used. Several methods are available to check histologic margins, and the surgeon should become familiar with the method that the person processing the tissue specimens uses. Both lateral and deep margins should be checked. Proper specimen orientation for presentation to the pathologist is critical and may be accomplished by marking one end of the incision with suture, an M-plasty, dyes, or other methods worked out between the pathologist and surgeon.

Surgical margins are a debated topic. For the small, primary, well-demarcated nodular BCC, a 3- to 5-mm margin is usually sufficient. For multicentric, large, or recurrent tumors, aggressive growth pattern BCCs, and SCC, the excisional margins should be greater.[8,25,78] In a review of 588 primary BCCs treated with surgical excision, Silverman and others[82] showed that the 5-year recurrence rate for low-risk primary lesions on the neck, trunk, and extremities was 1% compared with 3.2% for BCCs less than 6 mm in diameter on the head, and 9% for lesions greater than 1 cm in diameter on the head. Unfortunately, margins of excision in this series were not reported. Rowe, Carroll, and Day,[75] reported a 5- to 10-year recurrence rate of 10% for primary BCC following excision based on all studies reported in the literature.

Technique

Excisional surgery may be performed on primary BCCs usually on an outpatient basis with the use of local anesthesia. First, the clinically apparent tumor may be curetted. Often this step will yield a clinical tumor margin outside that visible with the naked eye. The excision is then outlined and the lesion is excised with 3- to 4-mm margins for small, low-risk BCC.[33] The surgical specimen is carefully oriented and sent to the pathologist for careful examination. Margins for larger tumors (1 cm on the face, 2 cm on the trunk and extremities), aggressive growth histologic pattern BCCs, and recurrent lesions usually vary from 1 to 2 cm in diameter. Regardless of the margin size chosen, careful histopathologic interpretation is required to obtain a tumor-free defect.

When appropriate and available, random vertical frozen sections can help with the rapid assurance of obtaining tumor-free margins. However, as will be discussed under the section on Mohs' surgery, random vertical sections are not as complete as the total horizontal sections used by the Mohs' surgeon.[17,25,87] Of importance, SCC may be implanted by improper local anesthesia techniques. Care should be taken not to pass the needle through the tumor during local anesthesia. Most SCCs should be excised with excision margins of 5 to 10 mm around the erythematous component.[8,34]

Advantages and disadvantages

A major advantage of excisional surgery is the availability of tissue for histologic sectioning and confirmation of diagnosis and completeness of excision. Another advantage is cosmesis. A better scar usually forms in a shorter time than with other nonexcisional treatment modalities. The disadvantages of excisional surgery are few. It is more time consuming and expensive than ED&C or cryosurgery and entails more skill and understanding of basic surgical techniques by the surgeon.

Indications

Excisional surgery is recommended for tumors in anatomic locations where the tissue is mobile and elastic and where cosmesis is important. Excisional surgery also is indicated when rapid healing and minimal postoperative morbidity are desired and histologic confirmation of surgical margins is critical.

Contraindications

Relative contraindications, compared with Mohs' surgery, for standard excisional surgery include large and recurrent tumors and most aggressive growth pattern (morpheaform, sclerosing, fibrosing) BCCs. If excisional surgery is used for these lesions, wider margins and careful margin control are required. Lesions that are multicentric and do not have well-demarcated clinical margins are often difficult to excise completely. This is less of a problem with excision than with some other treatment modalities since tissue is available for marginal confirmation. In anatomic sites where tissue is poorly mobile, such as the central face, ears, hands, and fingers, surgeons tend to minimize surgical margins to ensure closure. Mohs' surgery is a better management alternative in these sites. In elderly patients and those with fragile general health, the length of time needed to perform adequate excisional surgery compared with ED&C or cryosurgery may be a relative contraindication.

Cryosurgery

Cryosurgery is a treatment option with cure rates that are comparable to ED&C and excision for properly selected tumors: principally small, low-risk primary BCC. Its use is less common in the treatment of SCC. As with any procedure, the skill and experience of the surgeon are critical. A detailed discussion of cryosurgery is beyond the limits of this chapter. Several good review articles exist.[48,98,99]

The cryogen of choice and the one most commonly applied for skin cancer surgery is liquid nitrogen. It is administered by either a spray apparatus or the use of cryoprobes in a ''closed system'' with the use of temperature probes. Cryogens such as carbon dioxide, Freon, and liquid nitrous oxide do not have the ability to freeze tissue to adequate depths and temperatures and should not be used.

The temperature range between $-25°$ and $-30°$ C is lethal to cutaneous malignant tissue. Modern cryosurgeons believe that for proper cryonecrosis, a minimum temperature of $-30°$ C must be obtained throughout all cancer-containing tissue. Several cryosurgeons recommend a temperature of $-50°$ C. Tumor cryonecrosis is obtained through multiple freeze-thaw cycles with temperatures monitored by thermocouple needles or a cryometer. The experienced cryosurgeon can often monitor this visually. Cryosurgery has three critical parameters: the depth of the freeze, the width of the freeze beyond the critical margin of the tumor, and the thaw time. The thaw time is differentiated into marginal thaw time and total thaw time. The marginal thaw time is more important and should be at least 120 seconds in treating BCC. Double and triple freeze thaw cycles are strongly recommended since they have been shown experimentally to increase the thoroughness of cryonecrosis.

Technique

Cryosurgery is performed by first clinically outlining the tumor with a 2- to 5-mm border of normal-appearing tissue. The area is then anesthetized with local anesthesia. Cryoprobes or thermal couples are placed to the appropriate depth at the margin of tumor (not within the tumor) by either a spray technique or a closed system. The tumor and surrounding tissue are frozen. The tissue is then allowed to thaw, noting the marginal thaw time. The procedure is then repeated a minimum of one time. The wound is handled in the usual way, with the expectation of a good amount of tissue inflammation, necrosis, and blistering. Prefreezing curettage also can be of benefit.

Advantages

The indications and advantages of cryosurgery are similar to those of electrosurgery (ED&C). This technique is excellent on or around tissue with a fixed undersurface. Cartilage can be frozen without undergoing necrosis, and therefore cryosurgery is particularly useful for a tumor overlying cartilage. Cryosurgery is a valuable addition to the overall therapeutic plan in a patient with multiple BCCs.[48]

Disadvantages

Disadvantages of cryosurgery include a prolonged healing time of 3 to 10 weeks. During the initial 2 weeks, the wound and surrounding soft tissue exhibit marked edema and often have a considerable amount of wound necrosis and serous drainage. Although the resultant scar becomes soft and pliable with time, hypopigmentation is a common occurrence. Anatomic control is limited since cryonecrosis affects anything in its path including blood vessels and nerves. Lastly, as with electrosurgery, precise anatomic control of tumor margins is lacking.

Contraindications

Relative contraindications to cryosurgery include larger skin cancers with poorly defined borders, aggressive growth pattern BCCs, tumors in cosmetically important or high-risk areas, tumors in hair-bearing skin (since the hair follicles can be permanently destroyed), and most recurrent skin cancers.

Radiotherapy

Radiotherapy was once a popular modality primarily used by dermatologists and radiation oncologists to successfully treat skin cancers.[18,21,24,62] Today, radiation oncologists are the most skilled in radiotherapy. Several relative disadvantages and contraindications of radiotherapy have made its use less common than the three modalities previously described. Radiation chondritis and osteoradionecrosis can occur. These complications can be prevented by proper dose fractionation. Radiotherapy may be a useful modality in elderly patients who are medically debilitated and who are poor operative risks. It also is a useful form of palliative therapy for large skin cancers in elderly patients and as an adjuvant for high-risk tumors.

Radiotherapy has several disadvantages. One is the length of time required, since properly fractionated therapy usually extends over 2 to 6 weeks. Therefore, the patient must be mobile enough and have sufficient time to complete therapy. Second, the development of radiodermatitis and further aging of the skin can occur. There is also potential for secondary carcinogenesis due to radiation within the treated area. Therefore, its use in relatively young patients should be limited. Third, similar to ED&C and cryosurgery, tissue for margin control is lacking. Finally, tumors that recur after radiotherapy tend to be highly aggressive, more invasive, and destructive than recurrence not associated with irradiation.[86]

In a review of 862 primary BCCs treated with radiotherapy, Silverman and others[83] reported a 5-year recurrence rate of 4.4% for lesions less than 1 cm in diameter, and 9.5% for lesions greater than 1 cm in diameter. Additionally, the proportion of recurrence-free treatment sites with good to excellent long-term cosmetic results after irradiation was 63%, significantly less than ED&C and surgical excision from the same authors.[83] Still, radiotherapy may be the treatment option of choice for a small subset of BCC and SCC.

Mohs' surgery

While a medical student in the mid-1930s, Frederic Mohs developed a technique for extirpation of cutaneous tumors using microscopic control after chemical fixation of the tumor. After clinical trials, he published the results of his "chemosurgery technique" in 1941.[53,57] The chemical fixative, zinc chloride paste, fixed the cancer *in vivo* permitting careful serial removal with histologic examination of the entire specimen to identify pockets of residual carcinoma. The cure rates were exceptionally high, even for advanced, high-risk tumors. Despite minor modifications,* the basic technique of fixed-tissue chemosurgery has remained the same. Today, however, no chemicals are applied to the skin. Fresh tissue frozen sections are obtained in a precise horizontal fashion and the term "chemosurgery" is outdated.

---

* Refs. 54, 55, 66, 69, 72, 92-94.

Table 25-1. Comparison of fixed- and fresh-tissue Mohs' surgery

Factor	Fixed	Fresh
Success (no recurrence)	96% to 99%	96% to 99%
Pain	Often intense	Little
Efficiency	One stage achievable per operation	Multiple stages achievable per operation
Hospitalization for surgery	Frequent	Infrequent
Precise anatomic control	Difficult	Easy
Bleeding during surgery	Rare	Easy
"Mapping" of tumor	Easy	Easy
Slide interpretation	Can be difficult	Easier
Conservation of normal tissue	Good	Excellent
Repair	Must be delayed	Immediately possible

In Dr. Mohs' original technique, the fixative was made by combining zinc chloride with granulated stibmite and an extract of *Sanguinaria canadensis* (blood root), resulting in a black paste. The essential principles of the fixed-tissue technique included first debulking the tumor mass and applying a thin layer of zinc chloride paste under a moist occlusive dressing. This was left in place for 12 to 24 hours, resulting in an *in vivo* fixation of tissue. A thin layer of fixed tissue was then excised, carefully mapped, marked, and color coded with colored dyes. The entire deep margin as well as the peripheral margin epidermal edge was manipulated into one horizontal plane and was prepared by the use of horizontal sectioning. Microscopic examination of these sections pinpointed the exact location of residual tumor, which was located on the map for precise anatomic control. This process was then repeated with serial sections as necessary, one stage per day due to the chemical fixation, until total tumor extirpation was achieved. The wound was then allowed to heal by second intention due to a slough of fixed tissue that occurred 3 to 4 days after completion of surgery. This meticulous serial excision of skin cancer by the fixed technique resulted in cure rates approaching 99% for primary BCCs.*

Encouraged and intrigued by the success of this meticulous technique, those making adaptations began omitting the zinc chloride paste. Mohs himself was the first to do so in 1953 in the treatment of eyelid lesions.[67] In 1970, Tromovitch presented the first series of patients on whom the fresh-tissue technique was successfully used. He found several advantages in the omission of zinc chloride paste. These included the relief of perioperative pain from tissue fixation *in vivo*, the ability to do multiple procedures (stages) in 1 day, and the ability to have a fresh wound that could be reconstructed immediately. In 1974, Tromovitch and Stegman published the technique along with the results of long-term follow-up outcomes for patients managed with the fresh-tissue technique. For the treatment of high-risk BCCs, the success rate was similar to that reported by Mohs and others with the fixed-tissue technique. After this work, the technique of fresh-tissue Mohs' surgery developed and gradually replaced that of fixed-tissue Mohs' chemosurgery. Several authors have now proved the advantages and high success of the fresh-tissue Mohs' technique.* Table 25-1 compares the fixed- and fresh-tissue techniques.

During fellowship training, the Mohs' surgeon gains experience in the Mohs' technique, learns histologic interpretation of horizontal frozen sections for numerous skin cancers, and local flap and graft soft-tissue–reconstruction techniques. Today, Mohs' surgery is usually performed under local anesthesia in an outpatient Mohs' surgical unit.[44,52,89,100]

Technique

The surgeon begins by making a clinical outline of the tumor (a hypothetic medial canthal tumor as in Fig. 25-2). The tumor is then debulked of obvious cancer cells with a scalpel or curette. With the scalpel angled 45° to the skin to bevel the excision edge, a layer of tissue is removed in the shape of a saucer with 1- to 3-mm peripheral and deep margins. Careful anatomic orientation is maintained. The remaining skin edge and the surface of the tissue removed are scored (hatched) to preserve precise mapping and orientation. Hemostasis is obtained.

A careful map is drawn corresponding to the patient's "defect." The tissue is divided along the scored lines and inverted (turned over with the dermis side up), and the edges are color coded with stains corresponding to the carefully drawn map. By inverting and flattening a saucer of tissue, the Mohs' histotechnician can perform horizontal frozen sections of 5- to 7-μm thickness, thus including the entire deep undersurface and peripheral epidermal margin in one horizontal plane for histologic evaluation. The histologic preparation and examination is performed in an area immediately adjacent to or within the outpatient Mohs' surgical suite.

The slides are stained, usually with hematoxylin and eosin, and interpreted by the Mohs' surgeon serving as his

---

* Refs. 17, 53, 54, 66, 67, 70, 89, 92.

* Refs. 14, 17, 53, 54, 57, 66, 67, 69, 70, 72, 87, 92, 94, 95.

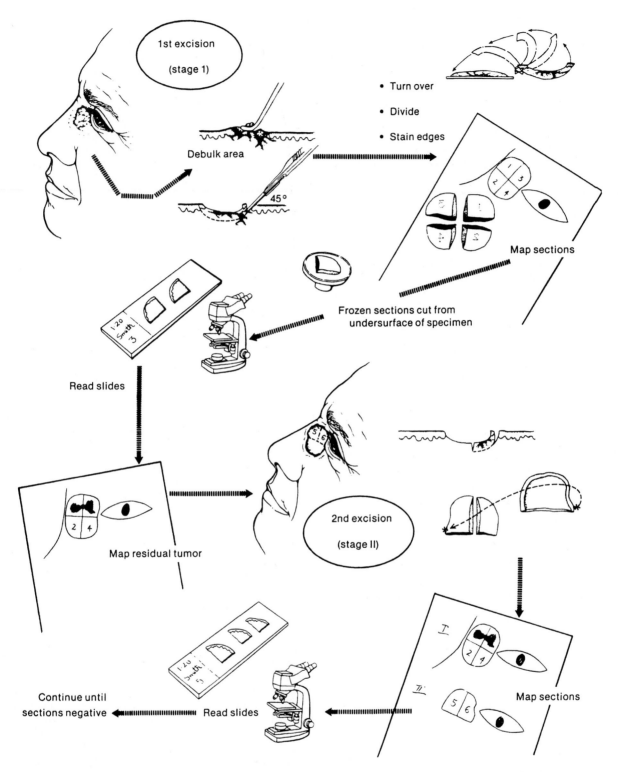

Fig. 25-2. The schematic representation of technique of Mohs' surgery. (From Swanson NA and others: *Head Neck Surg* 6:683, 1983.)

or her own on-site pathologist. Residual neoplasm can be carefully marked on the map so that the Mohs' surgeon can return to the patient and remove precisely only the tissue in which the tumor is microscopically persistent. Schematically, the superior margin of Figure 25-2 contains residual tumor, and the inferior margin of this medial canthal lesion is free of tumor. Therefore, only the superior one half must be removed in a second stage of the procedure.

The second Mohs' stage excision is performed as before with the tissue carefully handled, mapped, color coded, and processed. In our hypothetic case, this resulted in total extirpation of the tumor (see Fig. 25-2). However, the process can be repeated as often as necessary until all margins are free of tumor.

Mohs' surgery offers several obvious advantages. This precise method of removing only tissue with residual neoplasms results in high cure rates with maximal preservation of normal surrounding tissue. The defect remaining can be reconstructed immediately. In addition to precise handling of the tissue, horizontal sectioning of tissue is critical to the technique. Horizontal sectioning has been shown to be superior to vertical sectioning for the demonstration of all contiguous strands of tumor. Because surgery and handling of tissue occur within one outpatient site by one physician, the technique is both time and cost effective.

By definition, the Mohs' surgeon functions as both surgeon and pathologist, and separation of these duties is not Mohs' surgery. With proper fellowship training, the Mohs' surgeon becomes adept at microscopic interpretation of horizontally cut frozen sections of several skin cancers.[29] Separation of duties of surgeon and pathologist may result in a loss of precision and anatomic orientation, often with corresponding lower cure rates and greater amounts of normal tissue loss. Several modifications of standard surgical excision have been described that closely resemble Mohs' surgery with respect to total margin control and cure rate. These are pseudo-Mohs', slow Mohs', and peripheral section in-continuity tissue examination.[28] With these techniques, the surgeon and pathologist must work together closely as a team for optimal success with cure rates equal to Mohs' surgery. While these techniques represent improvements over excisional surgery with standard margin control, they differ from Mohs' surgery in another way.

One potential pitfall of Mohs' surgery is the quality of the frozen section slides. Good quality Mohs' frozen sections can consistently be achieved only with training and experience. Three to 6 months of training on a daily basis is necessary to develop the skill to produce high quality horizontal frozen section slides. The high cure rates associated with Mohs' surgery can only be achieved with high quality frozen section techniques.

The Mohs' surgical technique is labor intensive and requires a well-trained team. Typically, five to 10 cases are completed in 1 day. Between stages, the patient wears a temporary dressing, remains unsedated and ambulatory, and awaits the results of the frozen sections in a comfortable waiting area separate from the operative suites. Reconstruction is usually completed after each patient is tumor-free.[36]

Mohs' surgery involves the spheres of many disciplines, and close interspecialty cooperation is essential. The multi-disciplinary team approach, usually consisting of Mohs' surgeons, plastic, oculoplastic, and head and neck surgeons, is employed for extremely complex tumors and reconstructions. For deep tumors, the Mohs' surgeon removes the tumor in soft tissues and pinpoints deeper tumor to be excised by other members of the team. The other members of the surgical team then clear the remaining tumor, which may involve the facial nerve, bony ear canal, sinus, bone, brain, or orbit. The same approach is used for extensive reconstructions. The Mohs' surgeon first clears the tumor. The reconstruction is subsequently performed by other members of the team on the following day(s). At their institutions, the authors have found the multidisciplinary approach optimal and beneficial to both patients and members of the surgical team.

Indications

Mohs' surgery may be used for the measurement of many types of skin cancer* (Box 25-1). In general, Mohs' surgery should be considered for: (1) tumors associated with a higher recurrence rate following standard measurement, and (2) tumors for which conservation of adjacent normal tissue is important (Box 25-2). Tumors associated with a higher recurrence rate following traditional treatment include recurrent tumors, tumors of size greater than 0.6 to 1 cm in diameter on the face and 2 cm in diameter on the trunk and extremities, tumors located in the high-risk areas of the face (see Fig. 25-1), and those with clinically ill-defined borders.[7,8,75-77,89] Aggressive growth histologic pattern (morpheaform, sclerotic, fibrotic, keratotic, desmoplastic) BCCs have higher recurrence rates. Additionally, poorly differentiated SCC, microcystic adnexal carcinoma, dermatofibrosarcoma protuberans, and neurotropic tumors† have higher recurrence rates. SCC occurring secondary to scarring processes, chronic ulcers, osteomyelitis, and radiotherapy, or SCCs arising in immunosuppressed patients, are also more aggressive and have higher recurrence rates.[36,77] Mohs' surgery should also be considered for tumors excised with positive margins. Incompletely excised tumors result in a recurrence rate of approximately 43%.[20] Mohs' surgery in this instance allows excision around the original wound with 1- to 2-mm margins and precise location and tracking of any remaining tumor. In general, any cutaneous neoplasm that grows by contiguous spread and has a histology amenable to frozen section interpretation can be treated with high local cure rates by the Mohs' technique.

Tumors for which maximal conservation of adjacent normal tissue may be important include tumors on the eyelid,

* Refs. 9, 10, 15, 30, 43, 45, 52, 56, 61, 63, 68, 71, 74, 79, 84, 89, 95.
† Refs. 10, 30, 36, 74, 77, 79, 89.

Box 25-1. Tumors treatable with Mohs' surgery

Basal cell carcinoma
Squamous cell carcinoma
Bowen's disease
Erythroplasia of Queyrat
Keratoacanthoma
Verrucous carcinoma
Microcystic adnexal carcinoma
Other adnexal neoplasms
Dermatofibrosarcoma protuberans
Malignant fibrous histiocytoma
Atypical fibroxanthoma
Extramammary Paget's disease
Merkel cell carcinoma
Cutaneous rabdomyosarcoma

Box 25-2. Main indications for Mohs' surgery

Tumors with high recurrence rates following standard skin cancer treatment

Recurrent tumors
Size greater than 0.6 to 2 cm in diameter (depending on location)
Tumors in high-risk locations (central face, ear, chin, mandible)
Histology (aggressive growth pattern BCC)
Poorly differentiated SCC, dermatofibrosarcoma protuberans, microcystic adnexal carcinoma
Tumors with poorly-defined clinical margins
Tumors with neurotropism
Immunosuppressed patients with SCC
Incompletely excised tumors

Tumors for which maximal conservation of normal tissue may be important:

Tumors on the eyelid, nose, ear, lip, digit, genitalia
Tumors in young patients
Tumors that potentially involve vital structures (extraocular muscles, nerves, cartilage, bone, tendon)

BCC—Basal cell carcinoma; SCC—Squamous cell carcinoma.

ear, nose, lip, digits, and genitalia. Tumors in young patients, patients with public occupations, or patients concerned about scarring have important cosmetic implications.[46] In this situation, there is a tendency to reduce surgical margins with standard excisional surgery in an attempt to minimize wound size and scar.

It should be emphasized that knowledge of risk factors for skin cancer recurrence serve only as a general guideline for physicians treating skin cancer. Each and every patient and tumor should be approached individually; the physician should assess advantages and disadvantages of all available treatment options. Mohs' surgery is one option that should be considered for all tumors with high-risk factors as previously described (Fig. 25-3). If Mohs' surgery is not available or applicable for high-risk skin cancers, local excision with careful histologic margin control or a more aggressive approach with alternative treatment modalities previously described should be performed.

Verrucous carcinoma is a locally invasive, rarely metastatic tumor believed by some to be a variant of SCC, while others believe that it is a distinct entity. It can be present in one of three forms: oral or mucosal, genital, or plantar. Genital and plantar verrucous carcinomas are most amenable to Mohs' surgery, with success in preserving structure and function of the penis and foot, respectively. The same principles have been successfully applied to verrucous carcinoma of the nasal vestibule.

Dr. Mohs was the first to treat noncutaneous neoplasms of the head and neck when he used the fixed-tissue technique on parotid tumors.[56] He also used the fixed-tissue technique on some oral neoplasms and central facial paranasal sinus neoplasms. The multidisciplinary approach to large cutaneous tumors has been successful in several centers. This can be taken one step further by combining the approach of the surgeon who uses the Mohs' technique with that of the head and neck surgeon in the treatment of intraoral, paranasal sinus, and other head and neck neoplasms. In conjunction with a head and neck surgeon, the authors have used this approach in the treatment of SCC on the floor of the mouth, tongue, palate, tonsillar pillar, and paranasal sinuses. Biologically, these tumors usually present a problem of extension and recurrence locally, with metastases occurring first to the regional lymph nodes. Conventional surgery is often debilitating, resulting in the loss of mandible, tongue, or orbital structures. The interdisciplinary approach, with techniques performed simultaneously in the operating room, combines the conventional surgical management of regional metastases with total microscopically controlled excision of the primary tumor. The Mohs' technique adds more precise control than the randomly selected margins supplied by conventional frozen sections. The tissue conservation capability of Mohs' surgery has permitted the preservation of the mandible in some paranasal sinus cancer patients with tumors of the oral cavity, tongue, and orbits in whom conventional surgical methods would have sacrificed these important structures.[2,19]

Mucosal SCC of the lip warrants special discussion. These tumors are often extensive and require complex lip reconstruction after surgical ablation. These patients are often good candidates for microscopically controlled excision of the tumor. These carcinomas often have a greater metastatic potential than SCC of the skin and can be histologically more undifferentiated, particularly when they occur on the upper lip. The use of Mohs' surgery for these lesions ensures a high rate of total extirpation of the tumor with

BCC

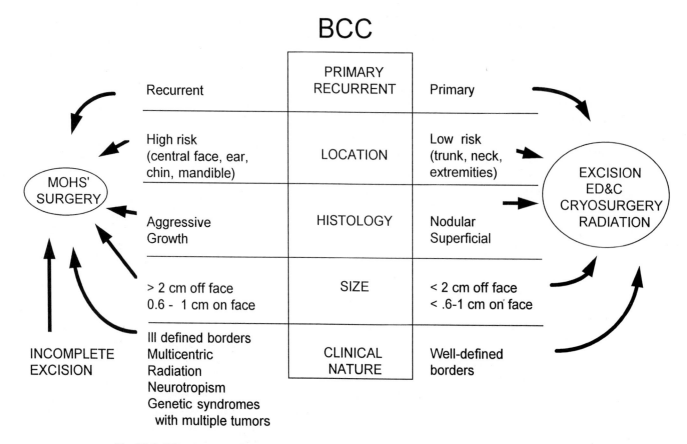

Fig. 25-3. The parameters for consideration for Mohs' surgery. Most primary basal cell carcinomas will be typed with characteristics toward the *right* side of the figure and can be effectively treated with standard treatment modalities including excision, electrosurgery, cryosurgery, or radiation. However, basal cell carcinomas with clinical characteristics toward the *left* side of figure should be approached more aggressively, with consideration of Mohs' surgery as the treatment choice. Indications for consideration of Mohs' surgery include recurrent tumors, high-risk anatomic sites, aggressive growth histologic patterns, larger tumors, multicentric tumors, neurotropic tumors, and tumors with clinically ill-defined borders. Tumors occurring in previous high-risk sites of radiation or in patients with genetic syndromes with multiple tumors in high-risk sites should be treated more aggressively. Incompletely excised tumors are also best treated by Mohs' surgery.

maximal preservation of normal surrounding skin and mucosa.

Keratoacanthoma is often aggressive and locally invasive, especially when giant or when it occurs in the central region of the face. In addition, it can often be difficult to differentiate histologically from SCC. When these tumors are larger than 1 cm in diameter, or occur in the central region of the face, are growing aggressively, or present a growth phase that seems relentless and unresponsive to routine therapy, they are amenable to and should be considered for treatment with Mohs' surgery. Large central facial keratoacanthomas may destroy an entire nose, invade the bone of the upper palate and ethmoid sinus, and metastasize to regional lymph nodes. Therefore, this subset of the keratoacanthoma needs to be differentiated and treated more aggressively than smaller lesions, and Mohs' surgery may be the treatment option of choice.

Melanoma is absent from the list of Mohs' indications in this chapter. Dr. Mohs has advocated for several years the treatment of melanoma by fixed-tissue Mohs' surgery. Many Mohs' surgeons do not agree that Mohs' surgery offers any benefit in the treatment of melanoma. The authors recommend excisional surgical management for melanoma based on contemporary knowledge.[38]

Reconstruction of defects

The Mohs' surgeon can provide the highest chance of a tumor-free defect for higher risk tumors. These surgical defects can be repaired immediately. Options for repair and criteria used in tailoring wound management to the individual patient will be discussed, but details concerning reconstruction of these defects are beyond the scope of this chapter.[3,35,36] The surgeon should always operate on the fundamental principle of tumor cure first, reconstruction second. Placing a skin flap on top of residual tumor allows tumor growth through altered deep tissue planes. Often many years elapse before tumor recurrence is noted on the skin surface that results in a deep and difficult recurrence. When soft-tissue flap reconstruction is planned, Mohs' surgery or a peripheral and deep sectioning variation of excisional surgery offers the highest chance of cure. Still, delayed definitive reconstruction should be considered for tumors that are high risk, even following Mohs' excision or surgical excision with deep and peripheral sectioning. In such a case, a split-thickness skin graft provides a "window" to monitor for recurrence.

Several factors are important for the management of Mohs' surgical defects. These include timing of the repair, the location of the defect, and the patient's occupation, age, general health, and expectations. Mohs' surgery is often used to extirpate tumors that have occurred several times, are quite large, or have occurred in areas severely damaged by prior radiotherapy. When this occurs, the chance of recurrence, even after the use of the Mohs' technique, is higher than usual. In this case, delayed reconstruction should be considered, either allowing the wound to granulate or placing a split-thickness skin graft for wound observation. Most Mohs' surgical wounds can be repaired immediately. The location of the defect is often important for both functional and cosmetic reasons.

The patient's occupation and age play a critical role in the choice of treatment. Younger patients often request and require immediate repair of their wounds so that they can return to the job market. This situation is in contrast to elderly patients who are often happy with the "acceptable" cosmetic result of granulation.

The general health of the patient is important. Patients in poor health may have difficulty tolerating either local or general anesthesia for the time necessary to perform a complex surgical repair of the defect and may do better with healing by secondary intention or repair with a split-thickness skin graft. The patient receiving chemotherapy should undergo surgery and repair at a time in the drug cycle when the leukocyte and platelet counts are not depressed so that wound healing is maximized.

Patient expectations also are of importance. Explaining the difference between total tumor ablation and reconstruction is necessary. The surgeon should emphasize and the patient must understand that these are two separate events, with the primary concern of the skin cancer surgeon being tumor extirpation. The patient can then place the cosmetic result of the repair in proper perspective, often being much happier with whatever closure option is electively performed.

Available options. There are several options for immediate repair such as granulation (secondary intention), primary or partial closure, and repair with a flap or skin graft. The list below illustrates the methods of repair used in the last 1512 Mohs' cases at the University of Michigan.

1. Granulate, 200 (13%)
2. Primary, 334 (22%)
3. Flap, 578 (38%)
4. Full-thickness skin graft, 98 (7%)
5. Split-thickness skin graft, 37 (2%)
6. Referral, 265 (18%)

Healing by granulation is still a preferred option for certain wounds and tumors. Tumors that are large, have recurred several times, or are removed from radiation-damaged skin often heal well by granulation, permitting close observation for possible recurrence and offering the option of delayed reconstruction. Some areas, particularly those over bony prominences or in concave areas, will heal as well by secondary intention as by primary closure, especially when the defect is not full thickness. Examples of this are the tip of a sebaceous nose (partial thickness wound) and the medial canthus of the eye. Often healing by secondary intention can be aided by the use of partial closure. Key sutures are used to align the wound with tension vectors that minimize distortion of free margins.

Many surgical defects can be closed by side-to-side primary closure. Often, the simplest method of closure results in the best functional and cosmetic outcome. Local flaps are the most common form of closure with the advantage of replacing lost tissue with adjacent "like" tissue. The trained Mohs' surgeon can perform local advancement, rotation, transposition, and interpolation flaps.[36,37,39] Distant flaps, large myocutaneous flaps, and other advanced techniques are closure options that the head and neck surgeon can best perform.

Finally, skin grafts are of two varieties. Split-thickness skin grafts are often used to cover wounds in which the chance of tumor recurrence is greater than usual.[35] This graft can act as a "window" through which deep tumor recurrence can be detected early. After 12 to 24 months for SCC and 5 to 10 years for BCC, during which time most tumor recurrence will occur, a definitive reconstructive procedure can be performed if the patient desires.[34,35] This type of graft can also result in good functional and cosmetic results, most often on the ears. Full-thickness skin grafts usually provide a more acceptable cosmetic result.[35] The nose, eyelid, and ear are the most common sites for the use of full-thickness skin grafts. At times, because of a patient's general health, the size of the defect, and patient expectations, a prosthesis may be the best choice for rehabilitation by camouflaging the defect. The prosthetic device can be either temporary or permanent. The nose and the ear are the most common sites for the use of prostheses. Detailed discussions of each of these types of closures are presented elsewhere in the text.

Other modalities

Interferons, a group of proteins originally identified for their antiviral properties, have been shown to demonstrate anticancer activity. Intralesional injection of recombinant interferon α-2 produces complete resolution with minimal scarring in 80% to 90% of primary, low-risk BCCs having a nonaggressive histology (superficial, nodular, well circumscribed). Injections are given three times per week for 3 weeks (nine injections), usually at a dose of 1.5 million units per injection.[27] Injections must be given superficially into the dermis and epidermis, preferably with a 30-gauge needle. Tumors that respond to intralesional interferon α-2 usually develop marked inflammation between the sixth and ninth injection. This inflammatory reaction appears to play a role in the response of BCC to intralesional interferon α-2. Long-term cure rates with this technique are presently unknown. Studies are underway to examine the effects of intralesional interferon α-2 on Bowen's disease and invasive SCC.

Topical 5-fluorouracil and other topical agents have been reported to be useful in the treatment of superficial BCC. However, a body of literature is available outlining problems with these agents and recommending discontinuing their use in the treatment of BCC and SCC.[87,88] The major problem, deep foci of tumor, can be concealed until dermal spread occurs, and then the lesion is found to be much larger than previously recognized. Topical 5-fluorouracil therapy is effective for treatment of actinically damaged skin and actinic keratoses, but should not be used for the treatment of BCC or SCC.

Lastly, another investigational treatment option is that of laser photoactivation of a porphyrin derivative that localizes in neoplastic tissue of the skin. Early reports exist of success rates of 85% to 90%. Further refinements in the porphyrin derivative (tagging the derivative to monoclonal antibody carriers), and laser physics may make this a treatment option of choice in the future. Photodynamic therapy (PDT) may be particularly useful for treatment of many low-risk lesions in one session for patients with basal cell nevus syndrome. However, PDT should not be used for high-risk lesions pending long-term outcomes results.

SELECTION OF TREATMENT

An understanding of the advantages and disadvantages of, and indications for each of the available treatment modalities discussed allows one to adopt a fairly uniform approach to the treatment of BCC and SCC. The treatment principles used for these two tumors are similar. Five major factors are related to the choice of treatment for BCC: location, histology, size, clinical nature, and recurrence (see Fig. 25-3). Factors related to the choice of treatment for high-risk cutaneous SCC are discussed at the end of this chapter.

Basal cell carcinoma

Fortunately, the majority of BCCs are small, low-risk lesions (see Fig. 25-3) that can be treated with high cure rates using standard methods such as excision, ED&C, cryosurgery, or irradiation. Combinations of these methods of therapy have been proposed, such as curettage and excision or curettage and cryotherapy. Most BCCs occur in low-risk

areas and are of a nodular or superficial histologic pattern. They are frequently small and present as slow-growing tumors with well-defined clinical margins. With radiotherapy reserved for the indications that were discussed previously, excisional surgery, electrosurgery, and cryosurgery are good treatment alternatives. Subclinical extension of small, primary, low-risk tumors is relatively predictable, and 2- to 6-mm margins result in 90% to 99% cure rates.[33,78] Unfortunately, standard treatment techniques do not result in high cure rates for higher risk skin cancers.[75-77] Skin cancers with higher risk factors represent the group of tumors that should be managed by excision with wider margins, excision with deep and peripheral sectioning, or Mohs' surgery.

Location

Local recurrence usually occurs due to an incorrect estimate of the subclinical tumor invasion. Tumors located in the central face, ear, or mandible (see Fig. 25-1) have a higher than normal recurrence rate with standard treatment.[75,80,81,89] The concept of shelving and skating, and the importance of embryonic fusion planes with respect to tumor location will be discussed later in this chapter.

Areas of cosmetic importance include nose, lip, eyelid, and helix of the ear. The nasal tip and ala are areas in which maximal preservation of normal tissue is critical because of difficulties in reconstruction. Preservation of the cartilage, alar rim, and nasal mucosa can simplify reconstructive procedures. Tissue conservation on the tip can often result in closure by simple techniques, sparing the surgeon and patient advanced and difficult reconstructive techniques. The same is true for eyelids, and preservation of normal tissue in the helical rim can often permit simple methods of repair, preserving normal auricular contour.

Figure 25-1 schematically illustrates some of the locations best suited to Mohs' surgery. These anatomic sites are important for two reasons. First, they comprise areas showing a higher recurrence rate for BCC. Second, they are important functional and cosmetic sites. Mohs' surgery, which offers maximum preservation of normal tissue and a high-cure rate, is often the preferred treatment modality in these locations.

A special area of subtle tumor spread is the nasal septum. After lateral rhinotomy for maximal surgical exposure to the septum, complete tumor ablation can be achieved while septal support structures may be preserved and the tumor observed as it tracks deeply along the septal mucosa. Excisional surgery is probably the best alternative to Mohs' surgery in these areas, with a good tissue specimen presented to the pathologist for histologic examination.

Histopathology

Aggressive growth (morpheaform, sclerotic, fibrosing, desmoplastic, keratotic) histologic pattern BCCs clinically resemble scar tissue, with ill-defined borders. Single strands of tumor islands and cells often invade lateral and deep without any evidence of clinical tumor.[33,78,80] Histopathologic characteristics of the tumor should play an important role in the management of BCC. As mentioned previously, nodular (well-circumscribed) and superficial histopathologic patterns usually present little problem in diagnosis and treatment. Numerous reports demonstrate that the aggressive growth histologic pattern BCC is a high-risk lesion for recurrence with standard non-Mohs' therapies.* Salasche and Amonette[78] found that subclinical extensions in 51 small aggressive growth pattern BCCs averaged 7.2-mm away from the clinical margin. This histologic pattern is associated with asymmetric, often extensive and destructive local subclinical invasion with a propensity for recurrence when treated with standard therapeutic modalities. Therefore, Mohs' surgery should be considered in the initial treatment of any BCC with aggressive growth pattern histologic characteristics. BCC may exhibit multiple histologic patterns within the same lesion. In this setting, the most aggressive histologic pattern determines the biologic behavior of the lesion.

Size

Tumor size is also an important consideration in the treatment of primary BCC. The success rate in treating BCC decreases with increasing tumor size, no matter what method of treatment is used.[81-83] Mohs[56] reported a cure rate of 99.8% for primary tumors smaller than 2 cm in diameter, compared with a cure rate of 98% for tumors between 2 and 3 cm in diameter and 90.5% for tumors greater than 3 cm in diameter. Robins had similar data.[71] Burg and others[11] found a greater subclinical extension of BCC with lesions larger than 2 cm in diameter. BCCs larger than 0.6 to 1 cm on the face and 2 cm on the trunk should be treated with Mohs' surgery or more aggressively with standard therapy to achieve high cure rates.

Clinical nature

The clinical nature of the tumor and the age and general health of the patient are important considerations. Because long-standing tumors tend to be more invasive, they are often best handled by Mohs' surgery. The majority of BCCs are well-circumscribed with distinct clinical borders. However, tumors may present with ill-defined, indistinct clinical borders. Also, tumors with perineural invasion may "silently" extend in a conduit fashion several centimeters from the clinical margins.[6,34,50] Mohs' surgery is usually the best treatment option for tumors with ill-defined borders or neurotropism.

Patients with multiple tumors present an unusual problem. A combination of techniques is often warranted in these patients. Multiple, small, well-defined nodular lesions can be handled appropriately by any combination of surgical

modalities. Care must be taken to maximally preserve normal surrounding skin. In patients with syndromes, such as the nevoid BCC syndrome, this concept is critical. Central facial lesions in patients with this syndrome are best approached with Mohs' surgery because of tumor aggressiveness and the need to conserve tissue. It is important to realize that skin grafts and flaps used in these patients probably will develop new tumors in the flap or graft. Side-to-side closures and granulation are often used in these patients for this reason. Often, multiple treatment modalities can be used effectively in the same treatment session.

In order to further understand which tumors are best treated by Mohs' surgery, one must understand the biology and growth characteristics of BCC and SCC.[58] These tumors locally invade via contiguous, silent extensions through the path of least resistance through the dermis, with a particular affinity for fascial planes, periosteum, perichondrium, embryonic fusion planes, nerve sheaths, and hair follicles. Affinity for the dermis is best illustrated by the stromal dependency of BCC. SCC may also invade and metastasize through lymphatic channels and blood vessels.

BCC often invades to "hard" structures such as bone, cartilage, and muscle and then spreads in shelving and skating fashion along the periosteum, perichondrium, and fascia before invading more deeply. Specific examples include spread along the muscle and fascia in the temple, medial canthus and lip region, the periosteum in the nose, forehead, and skull regions, and the perichondrium in the nose and ear regions. The temple, especially in older patients with temporal wasting, may result in more subclinical invasion because of tumor spread along facial planes. Tumors located on the scalp can readily invade in a conduit fashion down the hair follicle. Gormley and Hirsch,[26] Binstock, Stegman, and Tromovitch,[5] and Mohs and Zitelli[59] have described the aggressive nature of BCC involving the scalp. This often occurs with deep invasion and tumor extension along the periosteum. Once the bone is penetrated, tumor can extend to and invade the dura mater. BCC of the eyelid will often shelve and skate along the tarsal plate and into the conjunctival mucosa before penetrating the tarsal plate itself.

Invasion into supporting structures by BCC will occur if the tumor is neglected long enough. Robinson, Pollack, and Robins[73] demonstrated that, although rare, cartilaginous invasion does occur. Nerve sheaths, lymphatic vessels, hair follicles, and blood vessels also provide a mechanism of conduit spread for BCC.[16,49,97] Lymphatic spread from BCC is rare but has been reported. Blood vessel affinity is seen by invasion along adventitia of arteries and by permeation through the vessel wall itself. The deepest penetration of tumor often follows the most highly vascular area supplying the tumor. Perineural expansion has been widely described in both BCC and SCC.[16,49,97] This occurs by invasion of either the nerve sheath or the nerve itself. This may provide an entrance route for tumors into the maxillary sinus through the infraorbital foramen by following the infraorbital nerve.

---

* Refs. 12, 13, 22, 23, 31, 41, 47, 85, 91.

Neurotropic tumors are particularly at higher risk for local recurrence due to "silent" subclinical invasion.

Lastly, deep invasion of BCC can occur in perpendicular embryonic fusion planes.[60,64] Three important sites in which this occurs are the junction of the nasal ala with the nasolabial fold, the junction of the columella with the upper lip and floor of the nose, and the junction of the auricle with the pre- and postauricular skin. Ceilley, Bumsted, and Smith[13] have reported a higher than usual recurrence rate in the management auricular BCC. Robins[71] described the periauricular areas as having the highest recurrence rates for BCC after Mohs' surgery.

Recurrent basal cell carcinoma

Recurrent tumors have a relatively high recurrence rate when retreated with previously mentioned standard treatment techniques.[76] In an extensive review, Rowe, Carroll, and Day[76] reported a long-term recurrence rate of 5% for Mohs' surgery for recurrent BCC, and a 20% recurrence rate for all other modalities irrespective of management modality used for recurrent BCC. These tumors have already demonstrated significant subclinical extension beyond initial estimates.

Others report a success rate of greater than 96% for the retreatment of recurrent BCCs with Mohs' surgery.* This is in contrast to the success rates (approximately 50% to 80%) achieved in the management of recurrent BCCs by other methods. Menn and others[51] retrospectively studied 100 BCCs that had recurred after treatment at the New York University Skin and Cancer Hospital. These were initially treated by excision, electrosurgery, or radiation. Ninety-five recurrent BCCs were treated again by the same modality with Mohs' surgery used for five patients. Of 56 lesions treated by electrosurgery, 59% (33) recurred. Of 28 lesions treated by excision, 40% (11) recurred. Of 11 lesions treated by radiation, 27% (three) recurred. Of five lesions treated with Mohs' surgery, none recurred. Many studies support these data. Tumors that recur following radiotherapy represent a select subgroup, with a high recurrence rate following retreatment with previously mentioned standard methods.[86]

Incompletely excised basal cell carcinoma

Incompletely excised BCC is optimally treated with the Mohs' surgery technique. When tumors that have been excised (with a histopathologic report of tumor to the margins) are monitored clinically (with no reexcision), high recurrence rates result. Pascal and others[65] found that when a tumor was present within one high-power field ($\times 400$) of a surgical margin, 12% of lesions recurred. Once the tumor involved the margins itself, a 33% recurrence rate was noted. Dellon and others[20] reported a recurrence rate of 43% for incompletely excised BCCs. The mean interval between excision and recurrence in the study by Pascal and others[65]

*Refs. 17, 53-57, 66, 67, 70-72, 87, 92, 94.

was 2 years, with no difference in recurrence rate between deep and lateral margin involvement. Gooding, White, and Yatsuhashi[25] reported a recurrence rate of 35% in patients in whom the tumor involved surgical margins and who were observed for less than 2 years without reexcision. Thomas[91] reported an 82% recurrence of incompletely excised tumors around the eyes, nose, and ear. He found a 25% recurrence rate on the remainder of the head and neck. Jackson[32] reported similar findings. Retreatment of these tumors before clinical recurrence is indicated to reduce these treatment failures. Mohs' surgery represents an excellent treatment modality for inadequately excised tumors with maximal preservation of normal skin.

A modification of the Mohs' technique, the "chemocheck," is often used to treat incompletely excised skin lesions. Tromovitch, Beirne, and Beirne[93] and Swanson and others[90] have detailed this elsewhere. Briefly, the original excision scar is reexcised with 2- to 3-mm margins with the Mohs' technique. By angling the scalpel blade 45° to the skin, a triangle or wedge of tissue is removed around the entire scar, with the apex of the triangle being the deep margin. The tissue is then cut and divided along the original excisional scar so that the two noncutaneous limbs lie flat and can be horizontally sectioned to examine their entire peripheral and deep margins. When present, residual tumor can then be precisely located and ablated.

Squamous cell carcinoma

The proper selection of treatment for cutaneous SCC, like BCC, depends on an understanding of the various risk factors that identify the high-risk lesion. Based on a review of all literature since 1950, Rowe, Carroll, and Clay[77] identified nine prognostic factors that indicate a higher risk of local recurrence, metastases, and lower survival rates: (1) invasion to the reticular dermis or adipose tissue (Clark level IV or V), (2) poorly differentiated histology, (3) immunosuppressed host, (4) tumor size greater than 2 cm, (5) location on the lip or ear, (6) a lesion arising in scar tissue, irradiated skin, a chronic ulcer, or a sinus tract, (7) recurrence following treatment, (8) lesions with perineural invasion, and (9) rapid growth (Box 25-3).[18]

Box 25-3. Characteristics of high-risk squamous cell carcinoma

Invasion to reticular dermis or adipose
Poorly differentiated histology
Immunosuppressed host
Tumor size 2 cm in diameter or greater
Location on the lip or ear
Tumor arising in scar, radiated skin, or chronic ulcer/sinus tract
Recurrent tumor
Perineural invasion
Rapid growth

Fortunately, like BCC, the majority of cutaneous SCCs are small, low-risk lesions. These can be managed by excision, ED&C, cryosurgery, or radiation, with 90% to 95% cure rates. The 5-year cure rate for higher risk primary cutaneous SCC approaches 95% to 97% with Mohs' surgery compared with 85% to 87% with standard surgical excision.[77] The 5-year survival rate for higher risk recurrent cutaneous SCC is approximately 90% with Mohs' surgery compared with 50% to 75% with other methods, including standard surgical excision.[77] When available, Mohs' surgery is the management of choice for the majority of high-risk cutaneous SCCs. However, like BCC, some tumors are simply too large for Mohs' excision, mostly depending on the experience and skill of the Mohs' surgeon, general health of the patient, and location of the tumor. If Mohs' surgery is not available or applicable, local excision with careful histologic margin control should be performed.

Regional control of high-risk lesions is strongly influenced by the presence or absence of metastatic nodes. Eighty percent to ninety percent of metastases from cutaneous SCCs occur first to the regional nodes. If palpable nodes are absent, options usually include monitoring for clinical nodal disease, with prophylactic radiation to the primary site and the primary draining lymph nodes reserved for very high-risk lesions or those with neurotropism. If the primary tumor is located in a location that drains through the parotid nodes to the neck, any management of regional nodes should include the parotid bed. When adjuvant radiation is used for high-risk lesions, it is usually initiated 3 to 5 weeks after surgery. Prophylactic node dissection is usually not recommended for those patients with no clinical evidence of regional metastases. The exception to this approach is extension to the parotid capsule. Elective superficial parotidectomy should be considered in this situation.

If palpable nodes are present, therapeutic options include radiotherapy, surgical lymphadenectomy, or a combination of lymph node dissection and radiotherapy. The diagnosis of SCC should be confirmed by surgical biopsy or fine needle aspirate before definitive therapy. The survival rate may be greater using the combination of these methods. Trials using induction chemotherapy before surgical or radiation treatment may lead to higher survival rates for these patients. The outlook for distant metastatic disease is poor.

It is important to note that 70% to 85% of all local recurrences and metastases occur within the first 2 years after treatment of cutaneous SCC.[34,77] Therefore, patients with high-risk lesions should be observed every 3 to 4 months during this period. They should also be educated about clinical signs of local recurrence and about self-palpation for nodal enlargement.

SUMMARY

In summary, Figure 25-3 presents an overall approach to the current therapy for BCC of the skin. The vast majority of primary BCCs will present on the *right* side of Figure 25-3. These occur in low-risk locations, are nonaggressive histologic and clinical nature, and are small. These are fully amenable to treatment by excision, electrosurgery, cryosurgery, or radiation. The choice of technique will vary depending on the experience of the physician and the cosmetic concerns, age, and general health of the patient. BCC from the *left* side of Figure 25-3 should be treated with Mohs' surgery or more aggressive standard therapies.

Low-risk cutaneous SCC is amenable to treatment methods used for low-risk BCC. Those tumors with high-risk factors previously discussed are best treated locally with Mohs' surgery when available and applicable. Alternatively, surgical excision with good histologic margin control also may be used.

A thorough knowledge and understanding of prognostic risk factors for cutaneous BCC and SCC will enable the clinician to determine the most appropriate therapy for each individual patient and tumor. The approaches to management of skin cancers are diverse and include ED&C, cryosurgery, cold steel excisional surgery, radiation, and Mohs' surgery. The success of any of these treatment modalities depends on the proficiency of the physician performing the particular technique.

REFERENCES

1. Albright SD: Treatment of skin cancer using multiple modalities, *J Am Acad Dermatol* 7:143, 1982.
2. Baker SR, Swanson NA: Complete microscopic controlled surgery for head and neck cancer, *Head Neck Surg* 6:914, 1984.
3. Baker SR, Johnson TM, Nelson BR: The importance of maintaining the alar-facial sulcus in nasal reconstruction, *Arch Otolaryngol Head Neck Surg* 121:617, 1995.
4. Bart RS and others. Scalpel excision of basal cell carcinomas, *Arch Dermatol* 114:739, 1978.
5. Binstock JH, Stegman SJ, Tromovitch TA: Large, aggressive basal cell carcinomas of the scalp, *J Dermatol Surg Oncol* 7:565, 1981.
6. Birkby CS, Whitaker: Management considerations for cutaneous neurophilic tumors, *J Dermatol Surg Oncol* 14:731, 1988.
7. Breuninger H, Dietz K: Prediction of subclinical tumor infiltration in basal cell carcinoma, *J Dermatol Surg Oncol* 17:574, 1991.
8. Brodland DG, Zitelli JA: Surgical margins for excision of primary cutaneous squamous cell carcinoma, *J Dermatol Surg Oncol* 27:241, 1992.
9. Brown MD and others: Penile tumors: their management by Mohs micrographic surgery, *J Dermatol Surg Oncol* 13:1163, 1987.
10. Brown MD, Swanson NA: Treatment of malignant fibrous histiocytoma and atypical fibrous xanthomas with micrographic surgery, *J Dermatol Surg Oncol* 15:1287, 1989.
11. Burg and others: Histographic surgery: accuracy of visual assessment of the margins of basal-cell epithelioma, *J Dermatol Surg Oncol* 1:21, 1975.
12. Caro MR, Howell JB: Morphea-like epithelioma, *Arch Dermatol* 61:53, 1950.
13. Ceilley RI, Bumsted RM, Smith WH: Malignancies on the external ear: methods of ablation and reconstruction of defects, *J Dermatol Surg Oncol* 5:762, 1979.
14. Cobbett JR: Recurrence of rodent ulcers after radiotherapy, *Br J Surg* 52:347, 1965.
15. Coldiron BM, Goldsmith BA, Robinson JK: Surgical treatment of extramammary Paget's disease. A report of six cases and a reexamina-

tion of Mohs micrographic surgery compared with conventional surgical excision, *Cancer* 67:933, 1991.

16. Cottell WI: Perineural invasion by squamous-cell carcinoma, *J Dermatol Surg Oncol* 8:589, 1982.

17. Cottell WI, Proper S: Mohs surgery, fresh-tissue technique: our technique with a review, *J Dermatol Surg Oncol* 8:576, 1982.

18. Crissey JT: Curettage and electrodesiccation as a method of treatment for epitheliomas of the skin, *J Surg Oncol* 3:287, 1971.

19. Davidson TM, Nahum AM, Astarita RW: Microscopically controlled excision for epidermoid carcinoma of the head and neck, *Otolaryngol Head Neck Surg* 89:244, 1981.

20. Dellon AL and others: Prediction of recurrence in incompletely excised basal cell carcinoma, *Plast Reconstr Surg* 75:860, 1985.

21. Ferrar RJ: The private dermatologist and skin cancer, *Arch Dermatol* 81:225, 1960.

22. Freeman RG: Histopathologic considerations in the management of skin cancer, *J Dermatol Surg Oncol* 2:215, 1976.

23. Freeman RG, Duncan WC: Recurrent skin cancer, *Arch Dermatol* 107:395, 1973.

24. Freeman RG, Knox JM, Heaton CL: The treatment of skin cancer: a statistical study of 1341 skin tumors comparing results obtained with irradiation, surgery, and curettage following by electrodesiccation, *Cancer* 17:535, 1964.

25. Gooding C, White TG, Yatsuhashi M: Significance of marginal extension in excised basal cell carcinoma, *N Engl J Med* 273:923, 1965.

26. Gormley DE, Hirsch P: Aggressive basal cell carcinoma of the scalp, *Arch Dermatol* 114:782, 1978.

27. Greenway HT and others: Treatment of basal cell carcinoma with intralesional interferon, *J Am Acad Dermatol* 15:437, 1986.

28. Hagerty RC and others: Peripheral incontinuity tissue examination, *Plast Reconstr Surg* 83:539, 1989.

29. Headington JT: A dermatopathologist looks at Mohs micrographic surgery, *Arch Dermatol* 126:950, 1990.

30. Hobbs ER and others: Treatment of dermatofibrosarcoma protuberans with Mohs micrographic surgery, *Ann Surg* 207:102, 1988.

31. Howell JB, Caro MR: Morphea-like epithelioma, *Arch Dermatol* 76:517, 1957.

32. Jackson R: Why do basal cell carcinomas recur (or not recur) following treatment? *J Surg Oncol* 6:245, 1974.

33. Johnson TM, Tromovich TA, Swanson NA: Combined curettage and excision: a treatment method for primary basal cell carcinoma, *J Am Acad Dermatol* 24:613, 1991.

34. Johnson TM and others: Squamous cell carcinoma of the skin (excluding lip and oral mucosa), *J Am Acad Dermatol*, 1992.

35. Johnson TM, Ratner D, Nelson BR: Soft tissue reconstruction with skin grafting, *J Am Acad Dermatol* 27:151, 1992.

36. Johnson TM, Nelson BR: Aesthetic reconstruction of skin cancer defects using flaps and grafts, *Am J Cos Surg* 9:253, 1992.

37. Johnson TM, Baker S, Brown MD, and others: Utility of the subcutaneous hinge flap in nasal reconstruction, *J Am Acad Dermatol* 30:459, 1994.

38. Johnson TM and others: The Rieger flap for nasal reconstruction, *Arch Otolaryngol Head Neck Surg* 121:634, 1995.

39. Johnson TM and others: Current therapy of cutaneous melanoma, *J Am Acad Dermatol* 32:689, 1995.

40. Knox JM and others: Curettage and electrodesiccation in the treatment of skin cancer, *Arch Dermatol* 82:197, 1960.

41. Kopf AW, Bart RS: Recurring basal-cell carcinoma following Mohs' surgery, *J Dermatol Surg Oncol* 1:13, 1975.

42. Kopf AW and others: Curettage-electrodesiccation treatment of basal cell carcinomas, *Arch Dermatol* 113:439, 1977.

43. Lang PG, Metcalf JS, Maize JC: Recurrent adenoid cystic carcinoma of the skin managed by microscopically controlled surgery (Mohs surgery), *J Dermatol Surg Oncol* 12:395, 1986.

44. Lang PG: Mohs micrographic surgery: fresh-tissue technique, *Dermatol Clin* 7:613, 1989.

45. Larson PO: Keratoacanthomas treated with Mohs micrographic surgery (chemosurgery): a review of forty-three cases, *J Am Acad Dermatol* 16:1040, 1987.

46. Leffell DJ and others: Aggressive-growth basal cell carcinoma in young adults, *Arch Dermatol* 127:1663, 1991.

47. Levine JL, Bailin PL: Basal-cell carcinoma of the head and neck: identification of the high risk patient, *Laryngoscope* 90:955, 1980.

48. Lubritz RR: Cryosurgical management of multiple skin carcinomas, *J Dermatol Surg Oncol* 3:414, 1977.

49. Mark GJ: Basal cell carcinoma with intraneural invasion, *Cancer* 40:2181, 1977.

50. Matorin PA, Wagner RF: Mohs micrographic surgery: technical difficulties posed by perineural invasion, *Int J Dermatol* 31:83, 1992.

51. Menn H and others: The recurrent basal cell epithelioma, *Arch Dermatol* 103:628, 1971.

52. Mikhail GR: *Mohs micrographic surgery* ed 1, Philadelphia, 1991, WB Saunders.

53. Mohs FE: Chemosurgery: a microscopically controlled method of cancer excision, *Arch Surg* 42:279, 1941.

54. Mohs FE: Chemosurgery: a method for microscopically controlled excision of cancer of the skin and lips, *Geriatrics* 14:78, 1959.

55. Mohs FE: Chemosurgery for skin cancer: fixed-tissue and fresh-tissue technique, *Arch Dermatol* 112:211, 1976.

56. Mohs FE: *Chemosurgery: microscopically controlled surgery for skin cancer*, Springfield, Ill, 1978, Charles C Thomas.

57. Mohs FE, Guyer MF: Pre-excisional fixation of tissue in the treatment of cancer in rats, *Cancer Res* 1:49, 1941.

58. Mohs FE, Lathrop TG: Modes of spread of cancer of skin, *Arch Dermatol* 66:427, 1952.

59. Mohs FE, Zitelli JA: Microscopically controlled surgery in the treatment of carcinoma of the scalp, *Arch Dermatol* 117:764, 1982.

60. Mora CG, Robins P: Basal-cell carcinomas in the center of the face: special diagnostic, prognostic and therapeutic considerations, *J Dermatol Surg Oncol* 4:315, 1978.

61. Mora RG: Microscopically controlled surgery (Mohs chemosurgery) for treatment of verrucous squamous cell carcinoma of the foot (Epithelioma cuniculatum), *J Am Acad Dermatol* 8:354, 1983.

62. Pack G, Davis J: Radiation cancer of the skin, *Radiology* 84:436, 1965.

63. Padilla RS and others: Verrucous carcinoma of the skin and its management by Mohs surgery, *Plast Reconstr Surg* 73:442, 1984.

64. Panje WR, Ceilley RI: The influence of embryology of the mid-face on the spread of epithelial malignancies, *Laryngoscope* 89:1914, 1979.

65. Pascal RR and others: Prognosis of 'incompletely excised' versus 'completely excised' basal cell carcinoma, *Plast Reconstr Surg* 41:328, 1968.

66. Phelan JT, Milgrom H: The use of the Mohs' chemosurgery technique of the treatment of skin cancers, *Surg Gynecol Obstet* 125:549, 1967.

67. Pollack SV: Mohs' chemosurgery for skin cancer, *Prog Dermatol* 14:1, 1980.

68. Ratner D and others: Merkel cell carcinoma, *J Am Acad Dermatol* 29:143, 1993.

69. Robins P: Chemosurgery a surer method to treat basal cell epithelioma, *Consultant* 14:137, 1974.

70. Robins P: *Mohs' surgery in the treatment of basal cell and squamous cell carcinomas of the skin*. In Andrade R and others, editors: *Cancer of the skin*, Philadelphia, 1976, WB Saunders.

71. Robins P: Chemosurgery: my 15 years of experience, *J Dermatol Surg Oncol* 7:779, 1981.

72. Robins P, Menn H: Chemosurgery in the treatment of skin cancer, *Hosp Pract* 5:40, 1970.

73. Robinson JK, Pollack SV, Robins P: Invasion of cartilage by basal cell carcinoma, *J Am Acad Dermatol* 2:499, 1980.

74. Robinson JK: Dermatofibrosarcoma protuberans resected by Mohs surgery (chemosurgery): a 5-year prospective study, *J Am Acad Dermatol* 12:1093, 1985.

75. Rowe DE, Carroll RJ, Day CL: Long-term recurrence rates in previously untreated (primary) basal cell carcinoma: implications for patient follow-up, *J Dermatol Surg Oncol* 15:315, 1989.

76. Rowe DE, Carroll RJ, Day CL: Mohs surgery is the treatment of choice for recurrent (previously treated) basal cell carcinoma, *J Dermatol Surg Oncol* 15:424, 1989.

77. Rowe DE, Carroll RJ, Day CL: Prognostic factors for local recurrence, metastasis, and survival rates in squamous cell carcinoma of the skin, ear, and lip: implications for treatment modality selection, *J Am Acad Dermatol* 26:976, 1992.

78. Salasche SJ, Amonette R: Morpheaform basal-cell epitheliomas: a study of subclinical extensions in a series of 51 cases, *J Dermatol Surg Oncol* 7:387, 1981.

79. Sebastien TS and others: Microcystic adrenal carcinoma, *J Am Acad Dermatol* 29:840, 1993.

80. Siegle RJ, Schuller DE: Multidisciplinary surgical approach to the treatment of perinasal nonmelanoma skin cancer, *Dermatol Clin* 7: 711, 1989.

81. Silverman MK and others: Recurrence rates of treated basal cell carcinomas. Part 2: curettage-electrodesiccation, *J Dermatol Surg Oncol* 17:720, 1991.

82. Silverman MK and others: Recurrence rates of treated basal cell carcinomas. Part 3: surgical excision, *J Dermatol Surg Oncol* 18:471, 1992.

83. Silverman MK and others: Recurrence rates of treated basal cell carcinoma. Part 4: x-ray therapy, *J Dermatol Surg Oncol* 18:549, 1992.

84. Silvis NG and others: Spindle-cell and pleomorphic neoplasms of the skin: a clinicopathologic and immunohistochemical study of 30 cases with emphasis on "atypical fibroxanthomas," *Am J Dermatopathol* 10:9, 1988.

85. Sloane JP: The value of typing basal cell carcinomas and predicting recurrence after surgical excision, *Br J Dermatol* 96:127, 1977.

86. Smith SP, Foley EH, Grande DJ: Use of Mohs micrographic surgery to establish quantitative proof of heightened tumor spread in basal cell carcinoma recurrent following radiotherapy, *J Dermatol Surg Oncol* 16:1012, 1990.

87. Swanson NA: Mohs surgery: technique, indications, applications, and the future, *Arch Dermatol* 119:761, 1983.

88. Swanson NA: Basal cell carcinoma: treatment modalities and recommendations, *Primary Care* 10:443, 1983.

89. Swanson NA, Grekin RC, Baker SR: Mohs surgery: techniques, indications, and applications in head and neck surgery, *Head Neck Surg* 6:683, 1983.

90. Swanson NA and others: A novel method of re-excising incompletely excised basal-cell carcinomas, *J Dermatol Surg Oncol* 6:438, 1980.

91. Thomas P: Treatment of basal cell carcinomas of the head and neck, *Rev Surg* 27:293, 1970.

92. Tromovitch TA, Beirne GA, Beirne CG: Cancer chemosurgery, *Cutis* 1:523, 1965.

93. Tromovitch TA, Beirne G, Beirne C: Cancer chemosurgery (Mohs' technique): the "chemocheck," *Arch Dermatol* 92:291, 1965.

94. Tromovitch TA, Beirne G, Beirne C: Mohs' technique (cancer chemosurgery): treatment of recurrent cutaneous carcinomas, *Cancer* 19: 867, 1966.

95. Tromovitch TA, Stegman SJ: Microscopically controlled excision of skin tumors: chemosurgery (Mohs): fresh tissue technique, *Arch Dermatol* 110:231, 1974.

96. Tromovitch TA, Stegman SJ: Microscopically controlled excision of cutaneous tumors: chemosurgery, fresh tissue technique, *Cancer* 41: 653, 1978.

97. Weimar VM, Ceilley RI, Babin RW: Squamous-cell carcinoma with invasion of the facial nerve and underlying bone and muscle: report of a case, *J Dermatol Surg Oncol* 5:526, 1979.

98. Zacarian SA: Cryosurgery of skin cancer: fundamentals of technique and applications, *Cutis* 16:449, 1975.

99. Zacarian SA: *Cryosurgery of malignant tumors of the skin.* In Epstein E, editor: *Surgery,* ed 5, Springfield, Ill, 1982, Charles C Thomas.

100. Zitelli JA: Mohs micrographic surgery for skin cancer, *Principles Pract Oncol* 6:1, 1992.

Chapter 26

Management of Head and Neck Melanoma

Ross A. Clevens
Timothy M. Johnson
Gregory T. Wolf

Several important developments over the past 20 years have provided new insight into the biology of melanoma, leading to a reassessment of its clinical management. This has been particularly true in the management of melanomas arising in the head and neck. The first development was the initiation of large, cooperative, multidisciplinary efforts to study the epidemiologic, histopathologic, and clinical characteristics of melanomas arising from different sites in the body. Much of the current data reviewed in this chapter are derived from such retrospective and prospective studies. A second major development was the recognition by pathologists, most notably Clark, McGovern, and Breslow, of an association between certain histologic patterns of melanoma and the clinical behavior of the neoplasm. Regardless of histologic pattern, Breslow depth is the single most important factor in predicting outcome. Finally, it was recognized that melanoma, when diagnosed at its earliest stage of development, is as readily curable as many of its less aggressive cutaneous counterparts, such as basal cell and superficial squamous cell carcinomas. Because the incidence of melanoma is rising faster than any other human malignancy,[85] and the detection of melanoma relies primarily on visual recognition, it is important that educational efforts be directed toward primary care physicians and their patients.

Early detection and diagnosis is the single most important factor in survival. The most common early signs of melanoma are an increase in size or change in color of a pigmented lesion. The most common early symptom is persistent pruritus. Later signs and symptoms include tenderness, bleeding, and ulceration. Any lesion suspicious for melanoma should be examined and its exact location, color, configuration, border, symmetry, size, and topography recorded. The so-called *ABCDs* of melanoma are useful: A—*Asymmetry* (upon bisection, one portion of the lesion appears unlike the remaining portion); B—*border* (the border is irregular, scalloped, or poorly circumscribed); C—*color* (the color is varied from one area to another, jet black, or shades of white, red, or blue); D—*diameter* (as a rule, larger than 6 mm is suspicious. By comparison, the diameter of a pencil eraser is 6 mm). This is a valuable and convenient rule of thumb by which patients may self-assess pigmented lesions. Early melanoma, however, may lack those signs. Vigilance and self examination in the setting of appropriate patient education are important factors in early detection.[106] Wood's lamp examination may help define subclinical pigmentary changes.

Because the skin of the head and neck is one of the major exposed areas of the body, visual identification and early diagnosis of lesions suspected of being melanomas should lead to high cure rates. One half of melanomas arise from preexisting benign nevi—congenital, junctional, and especially dysplastic nevi—and malignant transformation is believed to be characterized by a change in the lesion, most commonly a change in size, color, and shape.[199] It is impossible to biopsy all pigmented cutaneous lesions, because all humans (except albinos) have a variable number of benign nevi. However, clinical signs such as characteristic coloration (shades of jet black, red, white, or blue), irregular borders, or changes in either growth, color, or morphology and the development of friability mandate the biopsy of such lesions. The cosmetic sequelae associated with major surgical resection of primary melanomas in the head and neck add importance to the early diagnosis of these lesions.

This chapter reviews the natural history of primary cutaneous melanoma of the head and neck with a major emphasis on current management principles and changing trends in management. Mucosal melanoma is also addressed, but in an abbreviated fashion. Current concepts regarding microstaging and clinical decision making based on tumor site, histology, and depth of penetration are discussed as they specifically relate to the head and neck. Excluded from in-depth review are ocular melanomas, which differ significantly from cutaneous melanomas in clinical and epidemiologic characteristics. Also excluded are acral lentiginous melanomas, because they do not occur as primary lesions in the head and neck.

EPIDEMIOLOGY

Melanomas arise from cells termed *melanocytes*, which have the ability to synthesize the pigment melanin. Melanocytes are found in the basal layer of the epidermis near the dermal-epidermal junction. Typically, melanomas occur in individuals of fair complexion, particularly those with red or blonde hair, blue eyes, and a tendency to sunburn or freckle easily after sun exposure.[23] The relationship between the development of melanoma and sun exposure is based primarily on epidemiologic studies that demonstrate higher incidence rates of melanoma in regions (such as Australia and Israel) where light-skinned individuals are exposed to intense and prolonged sunlight. These observations are further supported by geographic variations of rates (within regions) of melanoma, which increase directly with a population's proximity to the equator.[57] Queensland, Australia, with a reported rate of 40 cases per 100,000 has the highest incidence of cutaneous melanoma in the world. The Australian figures represent over seven times the incidence observed in the United States and 20 times of those reported in the United Kingdom.[91] Furthermore, lower rates of melanoma are typically reported in races having more natural skin pigmentation, such as people of African or Asian descent.[56] Sun exposure is also implicated in the development of melanoma in patients with xeroderma pigmentosum because the predilection for melanoma in these patients is limited to their sun-exposed skin.

The incidence of cutaneous melanoma is increasing worldwide at a rate faster than any other human cancer. In the United States, the age-adjusted incidence rates have more than doubled in the past 30 years.[64] Presently, 38,000 new cases develop annually in the United States resulting in 7300 deaths (one death every 1 hour and 12 minutes). Recent data from the National Cancer Institute's Surveillance Epidemiology and End Results[164] system show an 80% increase in the incidence of melanoma between 1973 and 1980.[85]

Melanoma is the most common cancer in women between the ages of 25 and 29 years. Lifetime analysis demonstrates that one in 1500 people born in 1935, one in 600 born in 1960, one in 105 born in 1990, and one in 87 born in 2000 will develop melanoma during their lifetime.[106] Overall 5-year survival rates for patients with melanoma have improved from 60% in 1963 to a current rate of 81%.[140]

The incidence rates for head and neck melanoma are changing more slowly than those for cutaneous melanoma of other anatomic sites,[75,115] whereas rates for melanoma of sun-protected areas, such as the eye and deeply pigmented skin, are not increasing.[96] Sunlight exposure is the most important predisposing factor, with ultraviolet B (280 to 320 nm) radiation being the most critical component.[109,173] Some investigators have suggested that excessive sun exposure in childhood or adolescence is a significant risk factor for later development of melanoma.[71,100,116] Others have speculated that early intermittent sun exposure and episodes of blistering sunburn may be more important than cumulative exposure. Increased recreational exposure to the sun and depletion of the earth's ozone layer with a subsequent increase in the amount of ultraviolet light reaching the earth may lead to an increase in incidence of melanoma in coming years. Despite the increasing incidence, overall mortality for head and neck melanoma has declined somewhat because of a higher percentage of patients seeking management for localized disease, and higher proportions of melanomas that are thinner. As discussed later in this chapter, these features have prognostic significance.

Primary melanoma of the head and neck accounts for 25% to 30% of all melanomas, even though the skin of the head and neck constitutes only 9% of the total body surface area.[83] The skin of the head, face, and neck is second only to the skin of the trunk in men and the trunk and the extremities in women in the prevalence of melanoma. This predilection for the head and neck has been attributed to several factors, including actinic exposure and regional variations in the distribution of melanocytes in the skin. Of note, the density of melanocytes within the epidermis of the cheek and forehead is two to three times as great as other skin regions.[19]

Natural history

The majority of patients with head and neck melanoma have a history of either recent change in a preexisting pigmented lesion or development of a new pigmented lesion. Generally 50% to 66% of melanomas arise from preexisting nevi.[19,83] McNeer and Das Gupta[128] reported that of 557 patients with melanoma, 27% of those melanomas arose in a nevus considered to have existed since birth, and 39% arose in a nevus that existed for more than 5 years. The remaining 34% of patients thought that their melanoma developed within a nevus that had appeared within the previous 5 years.

There is no strong evidence to suggest that melanoma

arising from preexisting nevi is clinically different than melanomas arising *de novo*. However, clinical and epidemiologic studies of a familial form of dysplastic nevus (B-K) mole syndrome have led to wider recognition of nonfamilial, or acquired dysplastic nevi, as potentially premalignant lesions. Familiarity with the natural history of common acquired nevi and the clinical characteristics of dysplastic nevi should enable one to diagnose and manage melanoma arising in an acquired dysplastic nevus much earlier in its natural history. The otolaryngologist should be able to differentiate among intradermal, compound, junctional, and dysplastic nevi based on clinical and pathologic examination.

Typically, common acquired nevi (i.e., junctional, compound, or intradermal) found in the skin of most white adults develop during the early years of childhood and may number from 10 to 40 lesions per person.[85] They are generally round or oval, with smooth borders sharply demarcating them from the surrounding skin. Pigmentation may vary from uniform tan or brown to less common mottled variations of these colors. They are small, generally measuring less than 6 mm. Junctional nevi tend to be light brown or tan, non-hair-bearing, and macular. Compound nevi are darkly pigmented, but not black. They are papular and typically bear hairs. Dermal nevi tend to be pink or flesh colored and may be hair-bearing. Over a period of years, nevi may undergo a characteristic and predictable series of changes. A macular junctional nevus may become elevated (compound) corresponding to the descent of the nevus into the dermis. With further descent, the lesion becomes pink or flesh-colored (dermal) and may then involute or slough. The phases of this natural evolution may be arrested at any point for a given nevus. The clinical appearance of any nevus that cannot be clinically attributed to a phase of the normal evolutionary sequence of a common acquired nevus should raise concern for an atypical nevus.[85]

Atypical (dysplastic) nevi are typically larger (6 to 15 mm in diameter) than common moles and have irregular borders and irregular tan, brown, or pink coloration. Margins tend to be indistinct and fade into the surrounding skin, virtually always maintaining some flat or macular component. The surface is usually varied, often with a central or eccentric papule surrounded by macular or nearly macular pigmentation. The development of black areas within such a lesion, as well as the onset of friability, bleeding, or ulceration should prompt an excision for pathologic examination to rule out melanoma. Acquired dysplastic nevi must be carefully followed, frequently with photographic documentation. Nevi that are changing or otherwise suspicious, or that are located in places where monitoring is difficult (e.g., the scalp) should be excised. Although the magnitude of the risk for melanoma in nonfamilial dysplastic nevi is unknown, it has been estimated that as many as 4 million people in the United States have one or more of these acquired preneoplastic nevi.[112]

The presence of a large number of benign melanocytic nevi is also a risk factor for the development of melanoma.

Case-control studies demonstrate that high total body nevus counts are closely related to the development of melanoma. In particular, high counts of common (typical) nevi on the trunk and legs in men and the legs in women were associated with the highest overall risk of melanoma. In both sexes, the presence of 20 or more common nevi on the legs increased the relative risk of melanoma twelve-fold.[155]

Giant congenital nevi (greater than 20 cm in diameter) may be considered precursors to melanoma. The lifetime risk of developing melanoma within large congenital nevi is 5% to 20%. The risk of melanoma is related to increasing size, so many doctors advocate elective resection of giant congenital nevi in childhood prior to transformation into malignancy.[107]

RISK FACTORS

The peak incidence of head and neck melanoma occurs in people 40 to 60 years of age.[48,89,91] In a review of 399 cases of melanoma of the head and neck, Gussack and others[89] found the average age at the time of diagnosis was 52 years, with a range of 16 to 93 years. Melanomas are quite uncommon in childhood or in the immediate postpubertal period. In the past, melanomas in children were thought to be associated with a favorable prognosis, however, this concept was the result of including in survival data children with certain benign nevi (Spitz nevus) that histologically simulated malignancy.[19] It is currently believed that childhood and adult melanomas share similar survival rates, though modestly improved survival in younger patients has been suggested.

Men tend to have a slightly higher incidence of head and neck melanoma than do women. Most studies report male to female ratios of 1.5:1.0,[89,180] which may be related to occupational exposure in men, particularly outdoor occupations. In a retrospective review of 660 cases, Conley and Hamaker[48] confirmed this male predominance but also noted that cheek melanomas tended to occur more frequently in women. The relative risk for developing melanoma is 4:1 for an individual with an affected first-degree relative.[99,129] Transplant recipients, as well as those patients receiving immunosuppressive therapy, do not exhibit an increased risk of developing melanoma.[106]

Anatomic location

The anatomic location of a primary melanoma affects the prognosis. Within the head and neck region, patients with scalp melanoma have a worse prognosis than those with lesions on the face or neck (Fig. 26-1).[15] These differences persist even after accounting for differences in sex or tumor thickness. In the past, the upper back, upper outer arm, and neck (the BANS region) were sites believed to carry a poor prognosis.[62] Balch and others[15] demonstrated that involvement of these sites was not associated with a worse outcome.

The cheeks, scalp, and skin of the neck, in proportion to the distribution of melanocytes, are the cutaneous sites in the head and neck most often involved by primary melanoma. Of

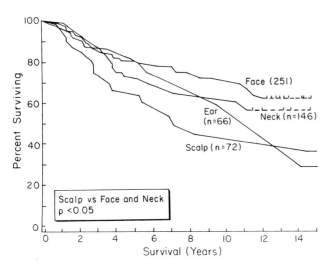

Fig. 26-1. Survival rates for patients with localized melanoma according to anatomic subsite in the head and neck. (From Balch CM and others, editors: *Cutaneous melanoma*, Philadelphia, 1985, JB Lippincott.)

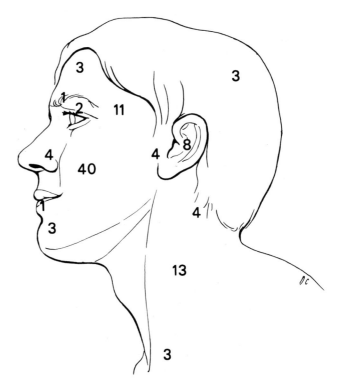

Fig. 26-2. Percentage distribution of primary head and neck melanomas according to site in 159 patients. (Modified from Harris TJ, Hinckley DM: Melanoma of the head and neck in Queensland, *Head Neck Surg* 5:197, 1983.)

399 cases reported by Gussack and others,[89] 46% had primary melanoma of the scalp and neck and 43% had primary lesions located on the face and nose. Only 11% had ear involvement. However, in the Queensland study, scalp and lip lesions were relatively uncommon, and most melanomas occurred in the skin of the cheek, temple, or neck (Fig. 26-2).[91] In 857 patients with melanoma, Fisher[77] reported that the face and neck accounted for 62% of the sites, the scalp for 26%, ear for 9%, and nose for 4%. In a study of 998 patients, O'Brien[142] found that the most common primary site was the face (47%), followed by the neck (29%), scalp (14%), and ear (10%).

Melanoma arising on the mucosal surface of the upper aerodigestive tract is uncommon. Mucosal melanoma represents 2% to 3% of all melanomas.[167,172] The majority arise in the nasal cavity or paranasal sinuses.[127,177] In the oral cavity, the areas most often involved, in descending order of frequency, are palate, upper alveolar ridge, buccal mucosa, lower alveolar ridge, lip, tongue, and floor of the mouth.[19] The age, sex, and racial distribution of patients with mucosal melanoma is similar to those for patients with melanoma elsewhere in the head and neck.

Mucosal melanoma tends to be more aggressive and to have a poorer prognosis than its cutaneous counterparts. It develops from melanocytes residing in mucous membranes and most commonly has an adjacent lentiginous component. It is unclear whether the poor prognosis associated with mucosal melanoma results from different biologic behavior or from their location in areas where blood vessels and lymphatics are much closer to the site of origin. The poor prognosis for patients with mucosal melanoma may also be explained by other factors. The relatively occult location of most mucosal melanomas of the head and neck contributes

to delay in patient presentation and diagnosis. Histologic staging based on the depth of invasion of primary mucosal melanoma has little prognostic use. Histologic factors such as blood vessel and lymphatic invasion, as well as inaccuracy in determining the level of invasion, have been reported as indicators for the poor prognosis of mucosal melanoma.[172]

Primary melanoma arising in a neck node, or metastatic from an unknown primary site is rare. Chang and Knapper[40] reported a 4.4% incidence of malignant melanoma appearing in lymph nodes in the absence of an apparent cutaneous or mucosal primary lesion. One fourth of these cases occurred in neck lymph nodes. Spontaneous regression of the primary melanoma or *de novo* development in the parenchyma of a lymph node have been offered as explanations for this rare clinical event. However, the true cause remains obscure. The peak incidence in the fifth decade is consistent with that reported for primary cutaneous or mucosal melanoma.[19,40] Management consists of radical neck dissection and radiotherapy. Survival rates of 14% to 43% are dependent on the extent of nodal disease.

DIAGNOSIS AND CLASSIFICATION

The clinical characteristics of melanoma are varied but consistent enough to make the diagnosis of a suspicious lesion fairly straightforward. The cardinal feature is change in a preexisting skin lesion or appearance of a new lesion that generally takes place over a period of months. Rapidly appearing lesions that have a duration of only days to weeks usually represent an inflammatory condition, such as a pyogenic granuloma. Lesions that have not changed over several years are unlikely to be melanomas. The differential diagnosis includes a variety of pigmented skin lesions (Table 26-1) and is discussed in more detail in Chapter 25. A variety of vascular lesions, including pyogenic granuloma, Kaposi's sarcoma, and hemangioma, look like melanoma.

Changes in growth or color are the most commonly recognized symptoms of melanoma. A melanoma's growth characteristically takes two forms, most commonly an initial horizontal or radial direction of growth as the lesion spreads superficially, followed by an invasive nodular or vertical growth phase. Infrequently, vertical growth begins *de novo*.

Hutchinson's melanotic freckle (HMF) is a premalignant, spreading, macular pigmentation that occurs most commonly in the skin of the head and neck, especially the temple and malar regions in elderly patients. It may also occur on other exposed areas of the body that characteristically show chronic solar degeneration. An HMF is a pigmented lesion with grossly irregular borders indicating regression or migration of the pigment cells. It characteristically has a smooth surface. However, malignant degeneration into lentigo maligna melanoma (LMM) is usually associated with the devel-

Table 26-1. Differential diagnosis of cutaneous melanomas

Lesion	Clinical characteristics
Seborrheic keratosis	Multiple, waxy; has long history
Nevi	
Junctional	Macular, nonpalpable, usually <1 cm, pale to dark brown, orderly color, skin markings preserved; has very slow history of change in growth
Compound	Palpable, dark brown; may occur with junctional type, may have depigmented halo
Dermal	Dome shaped, lacks pigment; has distorted skin markings
Hemangioma	Blue-black to red, slow growing; blanches with pressure unless thrombosed
Blue nevus	Usually <0.5 cm, blue-black, palpable, slow growing, rarely undergoes malignant degeneration
Pyogenic granuloma	Form of rapidly developing hemangioma, surrounded inflammation
Spitz nevus	Small, <2 cm, flat, reddish, rarely ulcerated
Pigmented basal cell carcinoma	Common, slow growing; rarely bleeds, has mottled appearance, needs biopsy to differentiate from melanoma
Squamous cell carcinoma	Rarely confused with melanoma, nonpigmented, has prominent keratin formation or ulceration

opment of a noticeable thickened or elevated nodule within the freckle. The risk of LMM grows with increasing diameter, but presence of a nodule carries a likelihood of invasion of 100%. The probability that an HMF may develop into melanoma is probably less than 5%.[45]

Lentigo maligna melanoma

LMM is the least common of the three major forms of cutaneous melanoma. It accounts for about 6% to 10% of all cases.[199] It is characterized by a slow radial growth phase that may progress for years. McGovern reported 33 cases of LMM that took from 15 months to 40 years to develop, with an average developmental period of 9 years.[83] They are very slow to invade deeply and consequently have a much better prognosis than do other forms of melanoma. Survival statistics approaching 100% have been reported for *in situ* disease.[126] LMM best exemplifies the concept of the two growth phases for melanoma popularized by Clark and others,[41] which consists of a radial phase of proliferation of melanocytes in the epidermis followed by development of a dermal invasion or a vertical growth phase. Nodular melanomas do not display these distinct growth phases.

Superficial spreading melanoma

Melanoma with an adjacent component of the superficial spreading type is most common, comprising approximately 75% of all cases. They are usually more circumscribed than LMM and start as a superficial spreading pigmentation (radial growth phase), which is seldom larger than 2 cm in diameter before ulceration and bleeding develop. Ulceration and bleeding herald dermal invasion (vertical growth phase) and are associated with a much worse prognosis. The characteristic clinical feature of a superficial spreading melanoma is a kaleidoscopic variety of colors, ranging from tan-black, brown, and blue-gray, to violaceous pink (see Plate 3, *E*). In a study of 786 cases of superficial spreading melanoma, Wick and others[199] reported that an increase in size and the presence of color changes are the most useful early clinical signs noted by patients and are present in 71% of superficial and more easily curable lesions.

The radial growth portion of a superficial spreading melanoma may consist of melanoma *in situ* or nonmalignant melanocytic dysplasia. Focal areas of spontaneous regression are also common. Lesions tend to demonstrate radial growth for 1 to 7 years before becoming deeply invasive. However, invasive radial growth pegs may coexist with the horizontal growth phase in some thin lesions. The vertical growth phase may be missed with standard histopathologic sectioning techniques. During this critical period of radial growth, superficial spreading melanomas are highly curable. As closer attention is paid to the significant features of early superficial spreading melanomas, the diagnosis will be substantiated earlier and result in improved survival rates.

Nodular melanoma

Nodular melanomas comprise only 10% to 15% of all melanomas. They tend to be much more aggressive than either the superficial spreading or the LMM types because of early vertical invasion. Both exposed and unexposed skin surfaces are affected. The color of a nodular melanoma is characteristically a shade of blue: blue-black, blue-gray, or reddish blue. The majority of mucosal melanomas tend to be of the nodular type, which is consistent with their poor prognosis. Nodular melanomas are invasive early in their development. Unlike LMM and superficial spreading melanomas, they are characterized by an early vertical growth phase, which may progress so rapidly that early surface ulceration occurs. Regardless of whether nodular melanomas arise *de novo* or from a preexisting nevus, there is little preliminary radial growth stage or peripheral spreading pigmentation. Because of its early invasive characteristics, nodular melanoma has a worse prognosis because survival rates tend to correlate inversely with the depth of invasion.

CLINICAL AND HISTOLOGIC STAGING

A variety of clinical staging systems for melanoma have been devised by both single institutions and groups of investigators. However, the resulting variation in clinical staging has significantly impaired data interpretation and standardization by which survival results or management methods can be compared among different institutions. The American Joint Committee on Cancer (AJCC) staging system is presented in Tables 26-2 and 26-3. The AJCC stage group reflects the differing prognosis for patients with localized disease according to histologic microstaging. Microsatellitoses are considered in transit metastases.

Clark's introduction of histologic microstaging with five levels of tumor involvement and the demonstration of the prognostic importance of invasion depth has allowed for the separation of patients with localized disease into groups having different prognoses and risks of metastasis.

Clark demonstrated that depth of invasion is clearly the most important characteristic in the histologic staging of melanoma.[42] Clark's microstaging classification has become widely accepted as a useful method for classifying melanomas (Fig. 26-3). However, Breslow further refined Clark's classification, relating the prognosis of a melanoma to its actual measured depth (thickness) of invasion.[31] According to this schema, lesions are divided into thin (≤1 mm), intermediate (1 to 4 mm), and thick (>4 mm) lesions (Fig. 26-4).[106] In fact, Breslow's thickness of cutaneous melanoma is the most powerful independent prognostic variable for survival. Clark's depth of invasion may be of prognostic value in lesions involving the eyelid and auricle, but generally not of other sites.

Although there are weaknesses associated with each form of histologic microstaging, the Breslow classification is a useful means of relating patient prognosis with a primary

Table 26-2. American Joint Committee on Cancer staging for melanoma

Classification	Criteria
Primary tumor (pT)	
pT0	No evidence of primary tumor
pTis	Melanoma *in situ* (atypical melanocytic hyperplasia [Clark's level I] not an invasive lesion)
pT1	Invades papillary dermis (level II) or 0.75 mm or less thick*
pT2	Invades papillary-reticular dermis interface (level III) or 0.76 mm to 1.5 mm thick*
pT3	Invades reticular dermis (level IV) or 1.51 mm to 4.0 mm thick*
pT3$_a$	Tumor 1.51 to 3.0 mm thick
pT3$_b$	Tumor 3.01 to 4.0 mm thick
pT4	Invades subcutaneous tissue (level V) or more than 4.0 mm thick or satellite within 2 cm of the primary*
pT4$_a$	Tumor >4.0 mm and/or invades subcutaneous tissue
pT4$_b$	Satellites within 2 cm of primary tumor
Nodal involvement (N)	
N0	No regional lymph node involvement
N1	Metastasis 3 cm or less in greatest dimension
N2	Metastasis greater than 3 cm in any regional node and/or in-transit metastasis
N2$_a$	Metastasis greater than 3 cm
N2$_b$	In-transit metastasis†
N2$_c$	Both N2$_a$ and N2$_b$
Distant metastasis (M)	
M0	No distant metastasis
M1	Distant metastasis
M1$_a$	In skin or subcutaneous tissue or lymph nodes beyond the regional nodes
M1$_b$	Visceral metastasis

* When thickness and level of invasion criteria do not coincide, the lesion is assigned to the higher pT classification (i.e., least favorable finding).
† In-transit metastasis involves skin or subcutaneous tissue more than 2 cm from the primary tumor but not beyond the regional lymph nodes.

Table 26-3. American Joint Committee on Cancer stage groupings for melanoma

Stage	Criteria
I	pT1, N0, M0
	pT2, N0, M0
II	pT3, N0, M0
	pT4, N0, M0
III	Any pT, N1 or N2, M0
IV	Any pT, any N, M1

pT—Primary tumor; N—Nodal involvement; M—Distant metastasis.

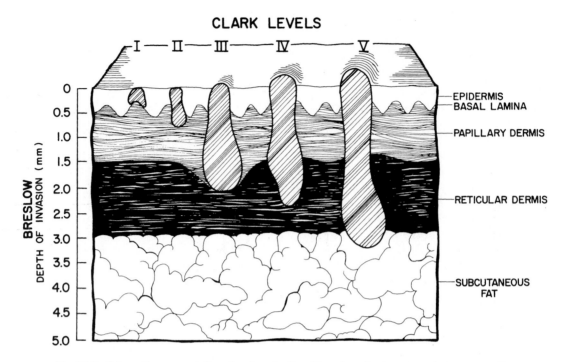

Fig. 26-3. Schematic representation of various depths of invasion of cutaneous melanoma according to Clark's and Breslow's methods of histologic microstaging.

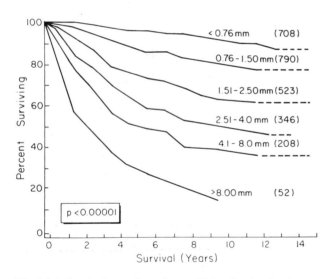

Fig. 26-4. Survival rates for patients with localized melanoma according to tumor thickness. (From Balch CM and others, editors: *Cutaneous melanoma*, Philadelphia, 1985, JB Lippincott.)

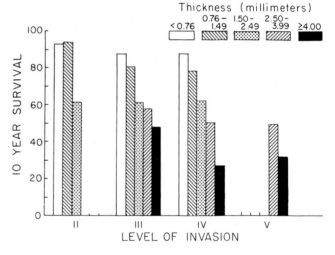

Fig. 26-5. Survival rates for patients with localized melanoma comparing tumor thickness with level of invasion (Clark's levels). Levels of invasion are subgrouped by tumor thickness. Within levels III and IV there are significant differences in survival rates according to tumor thickness. (From Balch CM and others, editors: *Cutaneous melanoma*, Philadelphia, 1985, JB Lippincott.)

melanoma's depth of invasion. Thin lesions (≤1 mm) are associated with a very low metastatic risk. Intermediate levels (1 mm to 4 mm) have a 20% to 30% risk of regional metastases and a 10% to 20% risk of distant metastases, whereas thick lesions (>4 mm) are associated with a distant metastatic rate of 60% (Fig. 26-5).[106]

Neurotropism represents a variable with unknown prognostic significance. Melanoma with neurotropism may cor-

relate with a higher risk of local recurrence thereby requiring wider margins for local control or perhaps postoperative indication.

Other factors that influence the results of melanoma management have been identified. These factors include age, sex, presence of ulceration, and various histologic parameters, such as vascular invasion, mitotic activity, and differentiation. Several other factors pertinent to head and neck melanomas also correlate with prognosis, such as the site of the melanoma and the lymph node status. These are discussed later in this chapter. The complete prognostic index must include all of the factors noted above as well as general patient factors. Given this multivariate index, the outcome of most cutaneous melanomas can be predicted.

SURGICAL MANAGEMENT

General principles

Successful management of a melanoma depends on the early recognition and accurate surgical excision of the lesion. As with most solid malignancies, the best chance to cure a melanoma is at its initial presentation, and that occasion should be used to remove all malignant cells. Traditionally this has meant wide excisions with margins of 3 to 5 cm. These excisions are cosmetically and functionally unacceptable in the head and neck. Accumulated experience with less radical excisions of primary head and neck melanoma together with the increasing percentage of patients diagnosed with earlier lesions[6,91] and the low recurrence and metastasis rates associated with thin lesions have resulted in an appreciation that wide resections are not necessary in most instances.[52,63,166,189] These observations have now been confirmed in a prospective randomized trial by Veronesi and others.[95] Only four recurrences were reported in 305 patients with trunk extremity melanomas who underwent narrow (1 cm) excision margins. No recurrences were reported in 185 of these patients who had lesions less than 1.0 mm in thickness.[192,195]

It is axiomatic that accurate surgical planning depends on adequate staging, and that for localized melanomas this requires optimal biopsy and skilled histologic interpretation. Other factors that influence planning include the size and location of the lesion, patterns of regional lymphatic drainage, type of melanoma, and the general health of the patient. Because of these factors, the biopsy of suspicious lesions is best managed by the surgeon who will be responsible for the patient's definitive care. This allows not only adequate planning for the resections of large lesions but also shorter time intervals between biopsy and resection and often more complete histologic microstaging.

For the surgeon, key considerations in decision making for a localized melanoma include (1) the type and timing of the biopsy, (2) the extent of local excision, (3) the type of closure, (4) the need for lymph node dissection, and (5) the potential that further management with adjuvant therapy may be warranted. For patients with clinically positive regional nodes, therapeutic node dissection is indicated, since significant benefit is frequently derived from local and regional tumor control, even if regional node metastases portend distant dissemination in the vast majority of such patients.[163] Locally recurrent lesions are generally managed with surgical resection and adjuvant radiotherapy.

Biopsy

Any lesion suspected of harboring a melanoma should be entirely excised. Shave excision and curettage biopsy of suspicious pigmented lesions are contraindicated.[67] The entire depth of the lesion must be excised to provide accurate microstaging. No evidence shows that incisional biopsy of melanoma is associated with an increased risk of local recurrence, nodal metastases, or death from disease.[6,150]

Regardless of technique, biopsies must be full thickness into the subcutaneous tissue to permit microstaging. Smaller lesions (<1.5 cm), especially those located on the face, can be completely excised with only a small margin (2 mm) of normal skin, so that the resulting deformity is minimal if the lesion is benign.[83,87] Associated satellite lesions should be removed at the time of definitive surgical procedure. The underlying fascia should be left intact unless it is grossly involved.

Maximal depth of invasion is generally found to be greater when techniques of serial sectioning are used.[174] The tumor biopsy specimen must be bisected through the point of maximal elevation or through the area of the most intense pigmentation to measure the thickness and level of invasion accurately. The total vertical height of the lesion must be measured at the point of minimal thickness. For ulcerative lesions, measurements are made from the base of the ulcer crater to the maximal depth of invasion.[8] In cases of regressing melanomas, multiple sections are often required to substantiate the diagnosis and determine thickness accurately. Final assessment must await paraffin sections. Frozen section analysis is unreliable in the evaluation of melanoma.

The authors recommend first excising suspicious pigmented lesions with narrow margins (2 mm) oriented parallel to the course of lymphatic drainage. Within 1 to 2 months, elective re-excision of the scar is performed. This two-step approach allows adequate time for counseling the patient and planning definitive management. Time also is available for obtaining lymphoscintography if lymphatic drainage patterns are unclear.

Primary tumor margins

Much of the dogma concerning the adequacy of resection margins for localized cutaneous melanomas arose from Handley's 1907 Hunterian lectures.[63] However, Handley's recommendations for wide margins were based not on primary tumors but on a single autopsy study of the distribution of tumor in the lymphatics surrounding cutaneous metastases. Furthermore, Handley did not actually specify 5-cm margins, which had been the standard practice for many years, but rather that the resection should be performed about an inch from the edge of the tumor. In the head and neck, it is particularly important to preserve as much of the normal tissue as possible to minimize cosmetic or functional disability without compromising oncologic principles.

Recent studies using primary tumor thickness as a correlate of survival have shown that wide (3 to 5 cm) surgical margins have no effect on the incidence of local recurrence or mortality.[189] Although this question is still open to scientific debate, clearly the risk of recurrence correlates more closely with the thickness of the lesion than with the width of the resection margins.

The World Health Organization (WHO) reported that survival was not influenced by the size of the resection margin even after compensating for the expected higher mortality with thicker melanomas.[39] Of 593 patients with stage I disease in the WHO study, 36 had margins of less than 1 cm, and 60 had margins greater than 1 cm but less than 2 cm. No local recurrences occurred in any of these patients with thin lesions, and only four local recurrences were noted in those with lesions of intermediate thickness. Cosimi and others[52] reported similar data. Of 49 patients with level II or III melanomas, more than one half were treated with margins of less than 2 cm. No local recurrences were noted in any patient treated with limited excision. As a result of a retrospective review of 147 patients at the Lahey Clinic over 25 years, Bagley and others[6] recommended resection margins of clinically uninvolved skin measuring twice the diameter of the primary melanoma, although narrower margins might be used in low-risk melanomas. In that study, the risk of in-transit, nodal, or systemic metastases was shown to be independent of margins; it was only a function of the risk status of the melanoma.

In a recent study of 586 patients with head and neck melanoma, surgical margins of less than 2 cm were used in over 80% of the patients. The overall local recurrence rate was only 4%. It was believed that these local recurrences could be accounted for by factors other than margins, such as tumor thickness, ulceration, and patient age.[189]

One prospective randomized study[195] examined 1-cm versus 3-cm excision margins in patients with trunk and extremity melanoma measuring 2 mm or less in thickness. In 612 evaluated patients, no differences in overall or disease-free survival were found between groups according to resection margins. Only three local recurrences occurred, all in the narrow resection group. No local recurrences were reported in either group when the lesion measured less than 1.0 mm in thickness.

The recommended surgical margins are 1 cm for lesions less than 1-mm thick, 1 to 2 cm for lesions 1- to 2-mm thick, 2 cm for lesions 2- to 4-mm thick, and at least 3 cm for lesions measuring greater than 4 mm in thickness. Lentigo maligna melanoma (LMM) may require wider margins to clear the *in situ* peripheral components of the lesion. The excision should extend to, but not include the fascia. Removal of melanoma in the face may require some modification of the dermal margin because of cosmetic and surgical reconstruction.[106] Wood's lamp illumination is helpful in revealing subclinical pigmentary changes especially in LMM. Complete excision with lesions should be evaluated with Wood's lamp examination prior to excision.

Based on the body of clinical research on margins of resection in melanoma patients, the authors have established clinical guidelines for patient care at the University of Michigan Cancer Center Multidisciplinary Melanoma Clinic. Definitive management is based on patient-specific considerations, and these guidelines provide a framework for patient care. Narrower margins may be employed when a vital structure is placed at risk (Table 26-4).[106]

The limited surgical defects created by narrower margins around a primary melanoma permit most excisions to be closed primarily by local, pivotal, advancement, or hinged flaps, with excellent cosmetic results. The authors reserve skin grafting techniques to reconstruct deficits that are considered to be at high risk of recurrence. Such lesions may include those with a depth greater than 1.5 to 4.0 mm or with deep fascial, muscle, or bone involvement. A skin graft facilitates surveillance and detection of tumor recurrence at the primary site as compared with a local or regional flap. However, the closure method does not appear to alter overall prognosis.[6,52]

Regional lymph nodes

No topic in the management of head and neck melanoma is surrounded by more controversy than the management of the regional lymphatics. Regional lymph nodes are the most common site of metastases from cutaneous melanomas.[149] Concepts in the overall management of melanoma must therefore acknowledge the risk of occult metastases in patients with clinically localized disease and take into account the prognosis when clinically evident regional metastases exist.

Surgeons have little disagreement that a patient with melanoma of the head or neck and clinically involved regional nodes should have a regional lymph node dissection. Overall survival rates for these patients are dismal, because 70% to 85% of patients with clinically evident nodal disease die of disseminated melanoma. Although metastases to the lymph nodes of the neck alter the prognosis, therapeutic dissection improves local and regional tumor control and benefits those few patients who may never develop disseminated melanoma (i.e., those rare patients with regional lymph node metastases from an unknown primary).[191] Adequate resection may achieve a 25% 5-year survival rate, which is superior to the results of either radiotherapy or chemotherapy. Also, because unmanaged regional tumor growth can be disfiguring and emotionally disabling for the patient, resection of nodal disease even in the face of systemic dissemination can improve the patient's quality of life.

Confusion exists in the current literature, however, as to whether immediate (prophylactic or elective) or delayed (when nodes become positive) lymphadenectomy for occult lymph node metastases is more beneficial. This confusion is related to the fact that survival data for wide local excision (WLE) versus WLE with elective neck dissection are derived from retrospective reviews of small numbers of treated pa-

Table 26-4. Follow-up guidelines at the University of Michigan Clinic

	Follow-up	
Breslow depth, mm	Physical examination	Chest radiograph
<0.75 (stage I)	Every 6 months for 1 year; once a year thereafter	Initial
0.76 to 1.49 (stage I)	Every 4 months for 3 years; once a year thereafter	Initial
1.5 to 4.0 (stage II)	Every 4 months for 3 years; once a year thereafter	Yearly
>4.0 (stage II)	Every 4 months for 3 years; once a year thereafter	Yearly
Regional (stage III) or distant (stage IV) disease	Every 3 to 4 months for 5 years; once a year thereafter	Every other visit for 5 years; yearly thereafter; initial computed tomography scans head, chest, abdomen, pelvis

From Johnson TM, Smith JW, Nelson BR: Current therapy for cutaneous melanoma, *J Am Acad Dermatol* 32:689, 1995. By permission.

tients in which differences in important prognostic factors (such as lesion thickness, tumor site, and presence of ulceration) have not been adequately considered. Furthermore, most studies of the value of regional dissections involve patients with extremity melanomas, and those results may not be directly applicable to head and neck melanomas, where overall prognosis is poorer and lymphatic drainage is more variable.

The rationale for elective neck dissection is based on the assumption that the growth and natural history of melanoma is in some respects orderly and that microscopic metastases disseminate first to the regional lymph nodes, then to distant sites. Removal of micrometastases before the occurrence of distant dissemination is therefore beneficial, and the decision to perform an elective dissection is based on the risk of occult metastases being present in a given patient. There is an obvious theoretic advantage in removing occult metastases over waiting until metastases become evident. This conjecture is supported by the poor 5- and 10-year survival rates (less than 25%) reported for delayed lymph node dissection.[11,79,170] Furthermore, significantly poorer survival rates are reported as the number of involved lymph nodes increases.[11,61,79,146] Recent data both support[120] and refute[77] the benefits of elective node dissection in patients with head and neck cutaneous melanoma. Resolution of this controversy awaits completion of ongoing prospective randomized trials.[9,36]

The major disadvantage of elective neck dissection is that some patients are subjected to unnecessary surgery. There is also a theoretic concern that neck dissection may encourage the dissemination of melanoma cells. In addition, some surgeons think that because rates of distant dissemination are so high once regional metastases have occurred, immediate elective neck dissection is a palliative procedure at best, and should be withheld until the development of positive nodes identifies those patients who may need regional disease palliation. Regardless of surgical philosophy, accumulated experience and newer concepts of histologic microstaging have

provided data useful in the decision-making process relating to an elective neck dissection. Factors to be considered include lesion thickness, melanoma type, tumor site, and presence of ulceration as they relate to the risk of occult metastases.

Occult metastases occur with primary head and neck melanomas in 14% to 62% of cases.[83,146,179] The risk of occult metastases varies directly with the thickness of the primary lesion. For melanomas of all sites the risk of regional metastases varies from virtually no risk for lesions less than 0.75 mm, to 25% for lesions 0.76 to 1.49 mm, to 57% for lesions 1.5 to 3.99 mm, and to 62% for lesions greater than 4.0 mm in thickness.[7,91,170] Similar estimated risks have been reported for axial (head, neck, trunk) locations.[16] Therefore, for patients with thin melanomas (less than 0.75 mm) elective neck dissection offers no significant benefit. Similarly, occult nodal metastases are also unlikely in patients with LMM; elective neck dissection is not indicated for this type of melanoma, which is highly curable with local resection alone.

For superficial spreading or nodular melanomas in the head and neck, lesions of intermediate thickness (0.75 to 4.00 mm) have increasingly higher rates of occult metastases.[146,179] These rates have been determined by histologic analysis of elective neck dissection specimens. These figures may underestimate the actual metastatic rate, since they are less than the 50% to 60% rate at which subsequent clinical nodal metastases develop when elective dissections are not performed for intermediate-thickness lesions.[7] These observations argue for elective neck dissection in localized, intermediate-thickness melanomas if one believes that removal of microscopic metastases is beneficial.

A number of authors have suggested an improved survival with elective neck dissection for deeply invasive head and neck melanomas.[3,12,60,146,170] Others, however, have argued that 5-year survival rates are similar when regional metastases have occurred regardless if they are occult or clinically evident, and that immediate elective neck dissection offers no major advantage over dissections delayed until metastases become evident.[58] This has been supported by the results of two randomized trials of WLE alone compared with WLE with elective neck dissection of melanomas in sites other than the head and neck.[169,194] However, the follow-up period in these trials was short, and it has been shown in at least one large prospective trial that the risk of failure from a WLE of a localized melanoma persists even 5 to 10 years after management. Balch and others[16] have demonstrated significantly lower 10-year survival rates for axial melanoma (0.76- to 4.0-mm thick) managed with WLE alone, compared with WLE with regional node dissection. This analysis included 430 patients and showed an 80% survival rate for patients with node dissection compared with a 56% survival rate for patients with WLE alone for lesions 0.76- to 1.49-mm thick, and a 64% survival rate compared with 33% survival for patients with lesions 1.50- to 3.99-mm thick.

Day and others[61] also have suggested that a good prognosis (80% survival over 5 years) can be expected in a subgroup of patients with melanomas less than 3.5-mm thick in whom elective neck dissection shows less than 20% of the nodes involved with melanoma. Likewise, Olson and others[146] reported 5-year survival rates of more than 50%, which were similar among patients receiving elective neck dissection for a head or neck melanoma in whom the histologic findings were either negative or showed only one or two positive nodes. By comparison, a 15% survival rate was reported for those with three or more positive nodes. It should also be noted that most studies of patients with head and neck melanomas report dismal long-term survival rates for patients managed with delayed neck dissection for metachronous regional metastases.[49,77,79,101]

Therefore, strong theoretic rationale exists for considering elective neck dissection for patients with lesions of intermediate thickness. However, the quantitative risk of occult regional metastases is not the only factor that may influence the decision to perform END, since the metastasis rate may be low in relatively thin (0.75 to 1.50 mm) intermediate lesions and therefore does not justify the morbidity of dissection. Primary tumor location in localized melanomas is also an important prognostic variable. The combination of specific location and measurement of thickness predicts recurrence and death from melanoma better than any other known combination of two variables.

In studying prognostic variables in intermediate-thickness lesions, Day and others[62] reported that localized head and neck melanomas of 0.85 to 1.69 mm in thickness arising on the face and anterior neck have a survival rate greater than 95%, which is similar to that for thin melanomas. Ulcerated melanomas also have a poorer prognosis and higher metastatic rates. Balch and others[15] reported 10-year survival rates of 60% to 70% for nonulcerated axial melanomas, compared with 25% survival for ulcerated lesions. Neck dissec-

tion should be considered for thinner lesions (0.75 to 1.5 mm) that are ulcerated.

Perhaps the most important consideration is the likelihood that the patient will return for routine follow-up examination and perform reliable self examination after WLE of a localized melanoma. If follow-up care is uncertain, immediate node dissection may be advisable.

A corollary to the theoretic considerations in elective neck dissections is the concept that many lesions on the face, scalp, or neck may have ambiguous lymphatic drainage patterns. The boundaries of elective neck dissection should encompass all lymphatics at risk if the dissection is to beneficial. Traditional dissection approaches may underestimate lymphatic drainage patterns for specific lesions. Preoperative lymphoscintigraphy has proven to be beneficial in predicting lymphatic drainage patterns.[119,141] Norman and others[141] have shown that traditional lymph node dissections for trunk or head and neck primaries may be inadequate in up to 60% of cases. Unexpected drainage to anterior cervical nodes from shoulder posterior neck lesions and to posterior cervical nodes from the shoulder, back, and neck was noted. For the posterior base of the neck, drainage was possible to six separate nodal basins including axillary sites. Such scanning techniques should be considered in all patients undergoing preoperative assessment for elective node dissection where lymphatic drainage patterns are not certain. The studies by Norman[141] suggest that lymphatic drainage overlap is so frequent with head and neck sites that routine lymphoscintigraphy may be warranted.

Morton and others[133] developed a novel technique to identify occult microscopic nodal disease. At the time of WLE of a primary melanoma, an intradermal injection of a blue dye (patent blue-U or radiolabeled dye) is performed. The dye is avidly taken up by the lymphatic vessels at the site of the cutaneous melanoma. A small incision is made over the site of the expected lymphatic drainage. The "sentinel node" to which the dye has traveled is identified and excised for immediate histopathologic examination. With frozen section examination, 21% of the sentinel nodes in patients with clinically localized melanoma were found to contain metastatic disease. Skip metastases to nonsentinel nodes were found in 21% of patients. This technique may improve nodal staying and help clarify the role of elective neck dissection.

Positron emission tomography (PET) using 2-fluorine-18 fluoro-2-deoxy-D-glucose (FDG-PET) is an evolving imaging technique that may identify subclinical regional node and viseral metastases. FDG is avidly taken up by melanoma and other tumors that have an increased use of glucose relative to normal tissue. High tumor-to-nontumor uptake ratios of fluorine-18 can then be achieved with PET scanning. Ongoing work on this promising modality is in progress at a number of institutions.[86]

Some of the controversy surrounding elective neck dissection has been stimulated by concern on the part of surgeons and patients regarding the morbidity and deformity associated with classic radical neck dissection. Because of the increasing recent proof for the efficacy of modified neck dissection in control of regional micrometastases from head and neck squamous carcinomas[29,118] and selected melanomas,[34] complete lymphatic dissections that preserve nonlymphatic neck structures (such as the spinal accessory nerve, sternocleidomastoid muscle, and internal jugular vein) may be an alternative consideration. Such dissections offer the potential of securing a favorable functional and cosmetic result as well as eradicating microscopic tumor deposits that could jeopardize long-term prognosis.

A final consideration is the age and gender of the patient and the morbidity of neck dissection. For women with melanomas, overall prognosis is better and the risk of metastases is slightly less. Younger patients appear to have a modestly better prognosis than elderly patients. In all patients the overall benefit of dissection must be weighed against the morbidity of the procedure, taking into account the thickness of the lesion, type of melanoma, location, and other prognostic characteristics.

With these accumulated data, justification for elective neck dissection can be established in situations with a high risk of occult regional metastases in which the pattern of lymphatic drainage can be predicted. That includes patients with lesions 1.5 to 4.0 mm in thickness (T_3) arising from most sites in the head and neck. Consideration should be given to preoperative lymphoscintigraphy, particularly in scalp, ear, and facial lesions. The decision to perform an elective neck dissection for patients with lesions 0.75- to 1.5-mm thick (T_2) needs to be individualized, with dissection advisable in most situations if any one of the following conditions exist: thickness approaching 1.5 mm, ulceration, nodular type, or location at a high-risk site (Box 26-1). In general, for lesions less than 1.5 mm in thickness, the authors perform WLE. The authors perform elective neck dissection in concert with WLE for lesions measuring 1.5 to 4.0 mm in thickness. However, recent data suggests that there may be no survival advantage to elective neck dissection for any lesion thickness (see Box 26-1).[106]

For patients with thick (greater than 4.0 mm) melanomas of the head and neck, prognosis is poor because of the high rates of distant visceral metastases associated with these le-

sions. Balch and others[16] have estimated that the risk of occult distant and regional metastases approaches 80%. In these patients, elective neck dissection is unlikely to alter the overall prognosis but it does offer the opportunity to provide benefit in terms of local and regional tumor control and provide staging information that may be useful in planning adjuvant management strategies.

Reliable statistical data substantiating the benefit of elective neck dissection in head and neck melanomas are currently lacking. Such data can be derived only from prospective randomized trials comparing WLE alone with WLE with elective neck dissection, in which management groups are stratified with respect to tumor thickness and other known prognostic variables. Until the results of such trials are known, the role of elective neck dissection will undoubtedly remain controversial. Stone and Goodacre[178] recently provided a detailed analysis and review of the literature regarding the principles of elective neck dissection in cutaneous melanoma.

In-transit metastases

In-transit metastases result from melanoma cells trapped in lymphatics and represent subcutaneous or intracutaneous metastases. As such they are associated with regional lymph node involvement and have a similarly poor prognosis. This is reflected by the inclusion of in-transit metastases in the American Joint Committee (AJC) staging system classification for nodal involvement (see Table 26-2). Optimal management has not been defined but varies according to the number and location of the metastases. When feasible, local aggressive surgical resection is more effective than systemic chemotherapy. Surgical excision, either in continuity with primary resection and node dissection or as a separate procedure for recurrent lesions, should be considered when the number of metastases is small and their location is amenable to resection. Other methods of management used in the past have included radiotherapy, intralesional immunotherapy with agents such as bacillus Calmette-Guérin (BCG) or dinitrochlorobenzene (DNCB), cryotherapy, and systemic or regional chemotherapy infusions.

Selected sites

External ear

The auricle is an uncommon site for melanoma. Of the 399 patients with melanoma reported by Gussack and others,[89] only 11% exhibited primary melanoma of the auricle, which is similar to both the University of California Los Angeles (UCLA)[180] and the New York University experiences.[164] Conley has reported 16% incidence of auricle melanoma among 223 patients with head and neck melanoma.[46] Lesions of the helical rim are the most common. Prognosis is based on Breslow depth. Wedge or star-shaped excision is generally adequate for thin rim lesions and achieves a better cosmetic result than does auriculectomy.[180] Lesions

---

Box 26-1. Indications for elective neck dissection in patients with head and neck melanoma

Melanomas 1.5- to 4.0-mm thick in any site with predictable lymphatic drainage.

Thick melanomas (greater than 4.0 mm) for local and regional tumor control.

Melanoma greater than 0.75-mm thick when inadequate patient follow-up is expected.

greater than 1.5 mm in thickness are frequently nodular or ulcerated and generally require at least a partial auriculectomy. Partial auriculectomy defects may be reconstructed with composite grafts or helical rim advancement flaps. In near-total auriculectomy patients, preservation of at least a portion of the upper helix is beneficial in patients who wear eyeglasses. It also aids in the stabilization of a prosthesis, whereas a total auriculectomy allows the fitting of a cosmetically acceptable total auricular prosthesis. Central auricle lesions (canal, concha, tragus, and antitragus) carry a poorer prognosis probably because of the difficulty in achieving adequate resection margins.[89] Wide cartilage resection and skin grafting, or total auriculectomy and possible lateral temporal bone resection, are routinely performed on such lesions.

Decision making for therapeutic or elective dissection of the regional lymph nodes should take into consideration the regional lymphatic drainage of the various portions of the auricle and the prognostic risk associated with the lesion (Fig. 26-6). Lymphoscintigraphy should be used preoperatively for lesions with ambiguous drainage. The incidence of nodal metastases varies from 20% to 60%, depending on the lesion's thickness.[34] The lymphatics from the external auricle drain anteriorly to the preauricular and periparotid nodes, posteriorly to the postauricular lymph nodes, and inferiorly to the subdigastric lymph nodes. Dissection of these lymph node groups in continuity with neck dissection is recommended and generally involves a superficial parotidectomy with facial nerve preservation.[91] If involvement of par-

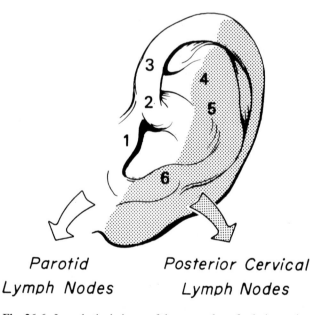

Fig. 26-6. Lymphatic drainage of the external ear for lesions arising on the helical rim anterior or posterior to Darwin's tubercle. Drainage patterns are based on development of the ear from six embryologic (numbered) hillocks derived from first and second branchial arches. (Modified from Macht SD: *Otolaryngol Clin North Am* 15:241, 1982.)

otid lymph nodes is evident, the deep lobe of the parotid should also be removed. In any case, if an elective neck dissection is performed, the periparotid lymph nodes should be included, because they are a primary nodal station. The accurate preoperative clinical assessment of parotid nodes is poor.[34]

Scalp

After the face, the scalp and neck are the most common areas for head and neck melanoma.[19,46,89] Tumors arising in the scalp are relatively aggressive and may go undetected for long periods of time, particularly in persons with abundant hair coverage. Scalp melanoma is associated with a high occult metastatic rate and poor prognosis. An elective neck dissection could be considered in melanomas 1.5 to 4.0 mm thick. For lesions larger than 4.0 mm, the risk of viseral spread is as high as for regional tumors. Conley[49] reported a 14% 5-year survival rate for patients with scalp melanoma who were managed with delayed neck dissection, compared with 25% survival for those managed with elective dissection.

The lymphatic drainage for scalp lesions arising anterior to a coronal plane drawn through the external auditory canals includes parotid, submandibular, submental, and upper jugular lymph nodes. Lesions posterior to this plane drain to occipital, suboccipital, postauricular, and posterior cervical or jugular nodes. The lymphatics do not pass through the pinna itself, and therefore auriculectomy is not required.[80]

Posterior scalp lesions are difficult to manage because lymphatic drainage can be either ipsilateral or bilateral.[78,82] Bilateral posterolateral neck dissection with WLE may be necessary for midline lesions. Thin (0.75 mm or less) temporal and parietal scalp lesions are managed like other areas with WLE alone. Temple lesions greater than 0.75 mm thick and intermediate thickness lesions may require wide excision in combination with superficial parotidectomy and in-continuity neck dissection.[91] Patients with melanoma arising from the posterior or lateral neck skin are also candidates for an elective neck dissection because their prognosis is poor and the neck lymphatics are immediately available for dissection at the time of primary excision. For scalp or neck lesions located near the midline, or those with ambiguous drainage, lymphoscintigraphy should be used to delineate regional nodal stations that drain the primary tumor.[22,141,198]

Face

Of over 800 patients with head and neck melanoma reported by Conley,[46] more than 30% had lesions arising on the face. Lesions of the face require adequate surgical and oncologic control while minimizing cosmetic deformity. WLE with primary closure is possible in many cases. Of significant importance is the recent observation that excessively wide margins may be unnecessary in most primary excisions. Margins of 1 to 2 cm are generally adequate and leave satisfactory cosmetic results. Regional node dissection can be considered for intermediate-thickness lesions (1.5 to 4.0 mm) when the lymphatic drainage can be predicted. In most cases node dissection is reserved for lesions more than 1.5-mm thick, with the addition of a superficial parotidectomy for preauricular and malar lesions.[89] Resection of the deep lobe of the parotid and in-continuity neck dissection are recommended if clinically obvious superficial parotid metastases exist.

O'Brien and others[143] evaluated 107 therapeutic and elective parotidectomies for cutaneous melanoma of the anterior scalp and upper two thirds of the face. Parotid involvement was found to be due to lymphatic metastases or direct invasion. Metastatic melanoma was found in only two clinically negative parotid glands. Following a histologically negative elective parotidectomy, however, no patients developed recurrence in the parotid bed. Complete superficial parotidectomy is suggested as a staging procedure to be performed with elective neck dissection for selected at-risk primary cutaneous sites. Skin flaps over the parotid bed should be kept thin because of lymphatics and superficial lymph nodes that are extraglaudular. Superficial parotidectomy will remove subfascial and intraparotid lymph node groups. Although a few lymph nodes may be found in the deep lobe of the parotid, most are located in the inferior portion in association with the deep parotid veins and do not drain the superficial skin region. These nodes can often be removed without completing a formal total parotidectomy. Therefore, routine total parotidectomy is not believed to be necessary. In most cases, adjuvant irradiation will be added if positive nodes are found. If large, clinically positive nodes are present in the parotid, intraglaudular lymphatic flow may be unpredictable and total parotidectomy may be justified. A lower recurrence rate was observed in patients who received postoperative radiotherapy on recognition of metastatic disease in the parotid gland. Barr and others[18] advocate superficial parotidectomy in the setting of locoregional disease in patients with cutaneous melanoma and evidence of preauricular disease. At-risk cutaneous sites with evidence of microscopic jugulodigastric metastatic disease are considered appropriate for in-continuity parotidectomy and neck dissection. Local flaps are generally used to reconstruct large facial defects because they provide better color and texture match than skin grafts, though skin grafts facilitate surveillance in worrisome or high-risk cases.

Nose

The nose is an uncommon site for a melanoma, making up only 2% to 5% of head and neck melanoma sites.[46] Metastases may spread bilaterally to facial, parotid, or cervical lymph nodes. Of 17 patients who were followed over a 34-year period, 29% survived 5 years.[33] Only 20% of the patients developed histologically positive lymph nodes, and all of those died of the disease. Lesions up to 1.5-mm thick require wide excision that may include the underlying perichondrium or cartilage, but leaves the inner lining intact.

Thicker lesions should be managed with full-thickness excision and local flap reconstruction. Because of unpredictable lymphatic drainage patterns, a neck dissection or superficial parotidectomy is reserved for subsequent nodal metastases.[33]

Eyelid

For all but thick lesions, excision of full-thickness skin down to the tarsal plate or orbital septum is recommended. Lid margins should be preserved (provided that they are not involved) and the defect repaired with a full-thickness graft.[91] Wedge excision with 1.0-cm skin margins is sufficient if the lid margin is involved. Lesions more than 1.5-mm thick require excision of the eyelid to the orbital rim. Extension through the full thickness of the eyelid into the periorbital fat is sometimes seen in advanced lesions and usually requires exenteration of the orbit.[91]

Mucosa

In general, the management of mucosal melanoma has not been uniform, therefore, results are difficult to interpret. Most published reports suggest a dismal 5-year survival rate of 10% to 15%.[47,102,177] The majority of head and neck melanoma patients seek management with ostensibly localized disease; however, 12% to 24% of patients have regional node metastases when they seek management.[102,177] The only clinical finding that has definite prognostic significance is the presence of distant metastases at the time of diagnosis.

The vast majority of patients with local disease undergo surgery as the initial management strategy. In the past, radiotherapy was used only in patients with uncertain surgical margins or with locally recurrent or unresectable disease. Historically, mucosal melanoma was characterized as radioresistant. Recent observations regarding the radiobiology and clinical response of cutaneous melanoma have suggested a role for radiotherapy in mucosal melanoma.[186] A critical review of radiotherapy alone in mucosal melanoma revealed a complete response rate of 50% to 75%. These data suggest a rationale for the use of combined surgery and postoperative radiotherapy to enhance local control. Patients with unresectable local disease or those who refuse surgery should be considered for radiotherapy alone as definitive management. It has also been documented that local control may be increased by adjuvant radiotherapy, especially in patients with questionable surgical margins.[172]

Not surprisingly, the issue of node dissection for the control of subclinical regional disease in cases of mucosal melanoma of the head and neck remains unclear. Because the status of the regional lymph nodes does not appear to affect survival, elective dissection of the neck is probably not warranted.[177] Surgery plus adjuvant radiotherapy provide the greatest benefit to patients with either regional metastases or large bulky primary disease. Chemotherapy has generally been reserved for patients with systemic disease and has not enhanced survival or locoregional control rates.

Patients with mucosal melanoma usually die of a combination of local recurrence and distant metastases.[102] Distant disease is associated with local recurrence in more than 90% of the cases.[27] The average time to first local recurrence is usually 9 to 12 months; once local disease recurs, distant metastases are usually diagnosed within 3 months.

FOLLOW-UP

The Multidisciplinary Melanoma Clinic of the University of Michigan Cancer Center has established a follow-up schedule that serves as a general guideline for patients with melanoma. Follow-up guidelines are based on the Breslow depth (in mm) of the primary tumor (Table 26-5). More frequent follow-up may be indicated in patients with multiple lesions, a large number of benign melanocytic nevi, evidence of atypical dysplastic nevi, family history of melanoma, or advanced stage of disease. The lifetime risk of a second melanoma is 1% to 8%. The mean duration until discovery of a second primary melanoma is 36 months. However, melanoma may recur and second primary melanoma may be discovered decades later. The Kaplan-Meier survival curve is long and shallow, suggesting a significant risk of recurrence up to 15 years after initial diagnosis.[106,171] These data reinforce the importance of lifetime surveillance.

A total body skin examination is performed including follow-up examination and inspection of the mucous membranes. The primary site and locoregional lymphatic groups are carefully examined. A review of systems is obtained with particular reference to potential metastatic sites such as bone, lung, gastrointestinal, and central nervous systems. Patient education with reinforcement of the importance of monthly self examination of the skin and regional lymph nodes, of the ABCDs of melanoma surveillance, and of the use of sunscreen is central to the postoperative care and management of melanoma patients.

OTHER MANAGEMENT MODALITIES

Data regarding adjuvant management approaches for melanoma are contradictory and difficult to interpret. Few studies have been prospective randomized trials, and management regimens consisting of chemotherapy, immunotherapy, or chemoimmunotherapy have varied greatly among studies. However, because histologic tumor thickness and pathologic staging of neck disease can identify groups of patients at high risk for recurrence, interest in adjuvant management strategies remains significant.

On the basis of recently completed clinical trials (Eastern Cooperative Oncology Group [ECOG], 1684) on the use of interferon-α2b in the postsurgical management of melanoma, the Food and Drug Administration (FDA) granted approval for the use of interferon-α2b in the care of selected melanoma patients. By virtue of the inadequacy of surgical therapy alone and the lack of effective alternative therapy, ECOG Study 1684 was undertaken to study the effects of interferon-α2b as adjuvant management to surgery in patients with no evidence of distant disease but with a high risk of systemic recurrence. The patient population was comprised of 280 patients with histologically confirmed deep primary (Breslow > 4 mm) or node-positive melanoma who underwent lymphadenectomy without evidence of residual or metastatic disease. Interferon-α2b was administered near the maximum tolerated dose. The majority of patients tolerated a full course of therapy. Relapse-free survival and overall survival were significantly improved in the management group.

Primary radiotherapy

Although surgical excision is considered the management of choice for melanoma and LMM, some elderly patients with large LMM lesions in the head and neck may not be suitable candidates for surgery. Similarly, it is accepted that surgical management of LMM is not indicated for extensive facial lesions where wide resection would lead to marked deformity and disability or would require extensive reconstruction.[4] Tsang and others[187] demonstrated that hyperfractionated radiotherapy with superficial x-rays is a simple and effective method of management for LMM of the head and neck. An actuarial tumor control rate of 86% was achieved at 5 years with acceptable late cosmetic appearance

Table 26-5. Surgical guidelines and prognosis for patients with stage I and II (localized) disease based on tumor thickness*

	Breslow's depth (mm)			
	<0.75	0.76–1.49	1.50–4.00	>4.00
Excision margin (cm)	1	1–2 (1 cm is adequate for lesions ≤1 mm)	1–2 (2 cm recommended for lesions >2 mm) ± END ± Adjuvant therapy	3 ± Adjuvant therapy
5-year survival rate (%)	95–99	80–95	60–75	< 50

* From Singluff and others: *Cancer* 70:1917, 1992. By permission.
END—Elective neck dissection.

in the majority of patients. Only 11% of patients demonstrated poor cosmesis at late follow-up (3 years) due to progressive skin pallor, atrophy, and telangiectasia in the treated area.

Beyond the management of selected primary cases of LMM, there is little role for definitive radiotherapy in the management of primary cutaneous melanoma of the head and neck.[181] In a retrospective review of the UCLA experience with head and neck melanoma from 1973 to 1992, Storper and others[181] demonstrated a 20% overall survival rate for patients managed with primary radiotherapy compared with 37% for the group overall. As discussed elsewhere in this chapter, the primary advantage of radiotherapy in the management of melanoma may be in its postoperative adjuvant capacity.

Adjuvant chemotherapy

The lack of effective drugs has limited the development of effective adjuvant chemotherapy. The most active drug has been dacarbazine, which has a response rate of only 20% to 30%. The use of other drugs such as the vinca alkaloids and the nitrosoureas in combination with dacarbazine has failed to improve response rates substantially.[122]

Initial trials of adjuvant chemotherapy or chemoimmunotherapy showed encouraging results in patients at high risk of relapse.[124,200] However, these trials either used historic control groups or consisted of too few patients to allow reliable interpretation. The results of adjuvant chemotherapy reported from large, prospective, randomized trials have been uniformly disappointing.[14,76,95,103,193] In fact, in a well-done randomized trial conducted by the Central Oncology Group, survival and disease-free intervals were significantly worse in patients receiving adjuvant dacarbazine compared with controls.[95] The lack of benefit from adjuvant chemotherapy reported in earlier trials has been consistent even when subgroups of patients categorized by various known prognostic variables were analyzed. Until newer drugs or regimens with higher rates of tumor response are developed, adjuvant chemotherapy approaches should be reserved for investigational protocols or carefully designed clinical trials. Current survival data do not support routine use in patients with limited resectable disease.

This viewpoint is further supported by the observation that resectable disease is frequently associated with relatively long disease-free intervals. The toxicity and morbidity that frequently accompany rigorous chemotherapy argue against prolonged adjuvant chemotherapy, since the potential benefit is doubtful and further impairment in quality of life is highly undesirable.

Chemotherapy for advanced disease

Once a melanoma has disseminated, the prognosis is dismal. If solitary metastases can be resected, a median survival of 8 months can be expected.[81] However, systemic dissemination or unresectable disease is associated with a survival of less than 6 months.[13,81]

The role of chemotherapy in the management of disseminated disease is limited. Because response rates with existing drugs and combination regimens are poor, a major consideration must be quality of life and palliation of symptoms. Outcome is not altered by intensive chemotherapy, and therefore decision making must take into account drug toxicity versus objective benefit. In general, asymptomatic patients do not need management, however, when symptoms occur, a trial of drug therapy may be warranted.

Several factors are useful in predicting tumor response to chemotherapy. The sites of metastases are important, since skin and soft tissue disease responds more favorably than visceral tumor involvement. Female gender and good patient performance status have also been suggested as favorable prognostic factors for response to chemotherapy, but a recent review indicates that these factors are more closely associated with survival than tumor response.[153] Prior management with chemotherapy significantly reduces the probability of subsequent tumor response. Although it has been reported that responders to chemotherapy survive longer than nonresponders,[50] the overall impact of chemotherapy on survival is minimal, and these differences probably reflect differences in tumor biology and other prognostic variables rather than an effect of chemotherapy. A major question has been whether any combination of drugs yields better results than the best single agent (dacarbazine) alone. Recently, the addition of tamoxifen to drug regimens, dose intensification, chemotherapy combined with hyperthermic perfusion, and combinations of chemotherapy with interferon-α and interleukin-2 have shown improved response rates, although duration of response has generally not increased substantially.

Because a great need exists for development of newer, more active drugs, and because standard drugs yield such poor results, some rationale exists for trials of new agents in previously managed patients. Patients with disseminated melanoma represent a valuable resource for new drug development, and this consideration, along with the patient's wishes and the clinical setting, may be important in deciding whether to use chemotherapy.

Adjuvant radiotherapy

Melanoma has traditionally been considered resistant to radiotherapy. However, much of the historic data supporting this opinion have lacked a scientific basis. In the late 1950s, Dickinson[65] reported increased survival rates with postoperative high-dose radiotherapy and the potential benefit of adjuvant therapy of melanoma was suggested.

Most of the prior data regarding the radioresistance of melanoma were based on management experiences with conventional fractionation schemes in patients with advanced disease. In fact, melanoma possesses a high degree of biologic heterogeneity and response to radiotherapy. In the early 1970s, work with melanoma cell lines in tissue culture indicated that the observed radioresistance of melanomas was the result of a broad shoulder on the cell survival curve.[92] It was subsequently shown that large-dose fraction radiotherapy could produce higher response rates than conventional 200-cGy daily fractions.[105] Furthermore, melanoma cells are believed to have a large capacity for repair of sublethal radiation damage, and this may partly explain earlier reports of radioresistance in these tumors.

In recent years a number of reports have demonstrated tumor regression with large-dose fraction radiotherapy for cutaneous and distant melanoma metastases.[30] Overgaard[147] reported increased response rates in patients with stage I and II melanomas using fraction sizes greater than 800 cGy compared with less than 400-cGy fractions. Responses, however, did not correlate with the total radiation dose. Doss and Memula[66] reviewed radiation response rates for stage III melanomas. Bone and cerebral metastases were the most common sites treated. Although the overall complete response rate was only 37%, a 67% response rate was noted with regimens of more than 400-cGy fraction. Harwood and Cummings managed 54 patients with high-dose fraction radiotherapy on days 0, 7, and 21, using a daily dose fraction of 800 cGy.[105] They divided their patient population into three clinical categories of disease: microscopic residual melanoma after surgery, gross residual melanoma after surgery, and recurrent melanoma. Local control rates were improved by irradiation; however, a high rate of systemic failure at other sites was noted, which emphasizes the need for more effective systemic therapy for melanoma.

Although recent reports of improved survival with radiotherapy for melanomas have been encouraging, most published trials of adjuvant radiotherapy report negative results. Creagan and others[54] showed no survival benefit for adjuvant radiotherapy after tumor resection in a retrospective study of patients with head and neck melanomas. Similarly, no benefit was demonstrated in patients with minimal residual melanomas, and furthermore, there were no survival differences between patients with gross residual tumor and those with no clinical evidence of disease at the start of radiotherapy. Unfortunately, in this study the dose per fraction of radiation was 200 cGy and the lack of benefit may have been related to the low-dose fractions used.

However, Ang and others[4] recently assessed the efficacy and toxicity of elective adjunctive radiotherapy given in five 6 cGy fractions to patients with cutaneous melanoma of the head and neck region at risk for locoregional relapse. This hypofractionated group of 174 patients was compared with an historic group and with that reported in the literature. The safety of hypofractonation was established in this study. In addition, the locoregional control rate of 88% with median follow-up of 35 months compares favorably with an historic-literature control rate of 50%. The survival rate of patients with lesion thickness of 1.5 to 4.0 mm was also higher than that observed in other studies. These findings led Ang and others[4] to conclude that adjuctive postoperative radiotherapy is indicated in patients with primary lesions measuring 1.5 to 4.0 mm in thickness.

Most reported studies consist of selected patients in whom the anatomic site, tumor extent, or risk of operation prohibited complete resection of the melanoma. In such instances local excision followed by adjuvant radiation management might be considered when wide excision is hazardous or grossly mutilating. However, because radioresistance of melanoma is an important clinical concern, surgical excision with appropriate margins and nodal dissection remain the mainstays in the appropriate care of the melanoma patient.

Radiotherapy has also been found to offer effective palliation for selected melanoma patients with distant metastases. Hilaris and others[94] reported 73 patients who received 139 courses of external radiotherapy for distant metastases. In their series, measurable responses were obtained in 57% of patients with osseous, cerebral, and visceral metastases. Equally favorable results were noted in patients with skin and lung metastases. A number of investigators have explored radiotherapy in combination with hyperbaric oxygen, hyperthermia, chemotherapy, immunotherapy, or neutron-beam irradiation. The results are encouraging but preliminary. Many of these experimental combined-treatment regimens are not widely available currently, and therefore are not as promising for study as simple alteration of the fractionation regimen.

Adjuvant immunotherapy

Immunology of melanoma

The immunologic aspects of melanoma have fascinated clinicians and scientists for decades. A number of observations have suggested that the immune system plays a role in the outcome of this disease. Spontaneous regressions of both primary and metastatic lesions have been well documented and imply that immunologic mechanisms are responsible.[73,183] Paradoxically, however, spontaneous regression of melanoma may portend an unfavorable prognosis. In addition, the long disease-free intervals that frequently characterize the natural history of melanoma suggest that host mechanisms may be operative in suppressing tumor growth. Melanoma also appears to be one of the more highly antigenic human malignancies, since host immune responses to tumor cells or extracts can be readily detected *in vivo* and *in vitro*. Evidence for this is based on demonstrations of complement-fixing antibodies to human melanoma antigens,[88] autologous serum cytotoxicity,[117] autologous antibodies to cultured melanoma cells,[37] delayed hypersensitive skin reactivity to tumor extracts,[28] and *in vitro* lymphocyte reactivity to melanoma extracts.[44,125] Taken together, these data indicate that tumor-associated melanoma antigens exist and that a patient's immune system can frequently recognize and respond to them.

In most studies, a decline in immune reactivity was noted with tumor dissemination. Other studies suggested that parameters of immunity correlated with clinical outcome after management;[26,68,114] however, such correlations have not been consistently demonstrated. The majority of evidence suggests that immune competence is relatively intact in early melanomas, and that depression in immune response is only regularly detected in advanced or disseminated disease. Although the cellular mechanisms responsible for tumor rejection or for the escape of tumor cells from immune recognition are not clearly understood, existing data on the immune response have prompted early optimism that nonspecific stimulation of the immune system may be of survival benefit in melanoma, particularly in those patients in whom immune competence can be demonstrated.

The recent discovery of regulating cytokines belonging to the class of interleukins has accelerated interest in the immunobiology of cell-mediated tumor immunity. In particular, interleukin-2 has been shown to stimulate the proliferation of cytotoxic lymphocytes termed *lymphokine activated killer cells* (LAK) and *natural killer* (NK cells). These cells believed to be critical in cell-mediated tumor cytotoxicity. With the use of recombinant human interleukin-2, autologous LAK cells can be grown in large numbers *in vitro* and can be administered to patients. It is well known that primary cutaneous melanoma is often infiltrated by lymphocytes. This phenomenon provides the opportunity to examine the local immunologic interaction between the tumor and its host. Lymphocyte infiltration has been characterized as brisk, nonbrisk, and absent. Clemente and others[43] recently demonstrated that a brisk infiltration response was associated with an improved 5- and 10-year survival in primary cutaneous melanoma compared with nonbrisk and absent tumor infiltrating lymphocytes. In addition, mitotic index was statistically significant. These discoveries have opened a new and exciting frontier of adoptive immunotherapy for patients with melanoma.

Adjuvant immunotherapy trials

Perhaps more than any other solid malignancy, the concepts of immunotherapy have held strong theoretic appeal for the melanoma patient. Early animal-model evidence of the efficacy of immunotherapeutic approaches for highly antigenic tumors, together with demonstrations of host immune reactivity to tumor-associated antigens in patients with melanoma, led to widespread clinical experimentation of immunotherapeutic and chemoimmunotherapeutic strategies. The rationale for these approaches was further supported by correlations of immune response with prognosis, which suggested that therapeutic benefit might be derived by immune stimulation in patients with localized disease who were at high risk of relapse from occult microscopic disease. Unfortunately, the interpretation and comparison of data from extensive clinical experiences with immunotherapy have been difficult because many trials were not adequately controlled

or consisted of small numbers of patients managed with a variety of immunotherapeutic agents and schedules.

The largest experience with nonspecific immunotherapy in melanoma has been with the bacterial immunostimulant, BCG. Of importance were early observations that the injection of BCG into intradermal melanoma nodules could cause regression of the injected nodule and distant noninjected cutaneous lesions.[134,135] However, injection of visceral or subcutaneous tumors was not equally effective. A large number of trials of systemic and regional BCG were subsequently undertaken. Benefit from BCG as a postsurgical adjuvant was suggested in regional node–positive patients with head and neck melanoma[69] and when used in combination with dacarbazine in disseminated disease.[90] However, the design of these trials suffered from the use of historic or nonrandomized controls in which comparability of tumor extent and other prognostic factors could not be ensured. The results of randomized trials of BCG immunotherapy for sites including the head and neck have uniformly shown no significant improvement in relapse rates or survival among management arms.[51,59,136,151,182] The various observations of tumor regression after intralesional BCG offer an additional form of therapy that is often overlooked for patients with recurrent metastatic disease. Best candidates for such management are those patients with intradermal metastases. Long-term remissions have been reported.[20] More recently, additional interest has been shown in intralesional α-interferon. A response rate of 45% for injected metastases and a rate of 21% for noninjected skin metastases have been reported in patients with advanced disease.[197] Although patients occasionally achieve complete regression of tumor, only a minority of patients benefit, and the results are temporary. Similar regression rates have also been achieved with the systemic administration of α-interferon.[55] Therefore, although responses are few, these forms of therapy show activity, occasionally result in prolonged remissions, and could be considered in selected patients.

Despite the negative results of most trials, great interest in the immunotherapy of melanoma persists. A variety of adjuvant immunotherapy strategies have been studied including use of levamisole, chemoimmunotherapy, and active specific immunotherapy. None have yet shown definite benefit in the adjuvant setting, although studies continue to test melanoma vaccines as adjuvant therapy.[35,197] Levamisole has been reported to be beneficial as an adjuvant, but study results have been controversial. Quirt and others[154] reported decreased death and recurrence rates with levamisole in a large four-arm trial comparing levamisole with BCG, BCG and levamisole, or observation. In contrast, Spitler[176] showed no differences in survival or recurrence in a randomized blind adjuvant study of levamisole versus placebo. Negative results with levamisole have also been reported in another small randomized study.[121]

Specific immune stimulation with melanoma antigens using either neuraminidase-treated tumor cells or partially purified antigens has not been thoroughly explored. Preliminary encouraging results have been reported but need to be confirmed in prospective randomized studies.[98,168] Some studies have reported tumor remissions with management strategies using autologous, irradiated tumor cell vaccines.[25] However, adjuvant management with viral oncolysates of human melanoma cell lines has failed to show significant disease-free survival benefit.[154] In some investigations, cyclophosphamide was added to increase the induction of the immune response by elimination of suppressor lymphocytes. This resulted in enhanced development of delayed hypersensitivity skin test responses to autologous melanoma cells.[24] Other studies have reported some remissions with the use of monoclonal antibodies directed against melanoma-associated cell surface glycoproteins (p97) or ganglioside antigens such as GD2, GD3, or GM2.[131,137,190] In all cases, these approaches are highly experimental and must be limited to well-designed research studies.

The development of specific *in vivo* imaging of melanomas using monoclonal antibodies is equally promising. Such imaging has been successfully performed in animal models and human subjects using radiolabeled monoclonal antibodies.[38,123] Highly selective binding of monoclonal antibodies to disseminated melanoma nodules also has been demonstrated in phase I clinical trials, as assessed after immunohistologic examination of biopsy specimens.[144] These preliminary observations offer encouraging evidence that such techniques may be useful not only for diagnostic imaging but for management approaches using antibodies labeled with therapeutic isotopes or cytotoxic agents conjugated to monoclonal antibodies. Further, improved diagnostic and prognostic information may be derived through immunohistologic studies of tumor sections using highly specific antisera or monoclonal antibodies.[5,139]

Adoptive immunotherapy

In 1976, Morgan, Rusetti, and Gallo[74] reported the isolation of a T-cell growth factor that was found to be important in the induction and proliferation of a subset of nonspecific lymphocytes. This lymphokine, later termed *interleukin*-2 (IL-2), is now known to be a member of a large family of related cytokines that modulate and regulate a variety of hematopoietic and immunologic cell functions. Interleukin-2 has been extensively characterized and is now produced in large, highly purified quantities through recombinant deoxyribonucleic acid (DNA) technology. Seminal *in vitro* and animal model studies using IL-2 by Rosenberg and others[158] and other investigators[113,130] demonstrated *in vitro* proliferation of LAK cells that when adoptively transferred to tumor-bearing animals, resulted in regression of established tumors and experimental metastases. In subsequent human trials in patients with advanced metastatic melanoma, therapy with *in vitro* cultivated autologous LAK cells combined with recombinant IL-2 or recombinant IL-2 alone resulted in significant tumor regression in 20% to 35% of patients.[159,161,175]

This management was associated with substantial toxicity and was generally reserved for younger patients without evidence of brain metastases. Durable complete response has been seen occasionally and has prompted investigations of other combinations of cytokines.[161] Trials of cultured autologous tumor infiltrating lymphocytes (TIL) were shown *in vitro* to be 50 to 100 times more potent than LAK cells.[160] With TIL cells, response rates as high as 60% have been reported in metastatic melanoma.[160] Recently, these efforts have been combined with gene therapy through the introduction of the gene coding for tumor necrosis factor into TIL.[108,162] Tumor necrosis factor secretion by these transduced TIL is increased 100-fold and results in enhanced effectiveness of these cells. Toxic side effects associated with high dosages of IL-2 therapy include fever, hypotension, malaise, nausea, vomiting, fluid retention, confusion, and liver and renal dysfunction. Despite these toxicities, biologic approaches to the management of advanced melanoma represent attractive alternatives to conventional palliative therapy. However, their usefulness is limited by the necessity for extensive immunologic research facilities and complex techniques for expanding and maintaining large numbers of cultured lymphocytes.

CYTOGENETICS

One of the most exciting frontiers of knowledge in melanoma is the exploration and discovery of those basic genetic changes that lead to malignant melanocyte behavior. Although some cytogenetic changes in cancer may be conserved across tumor types, many changes appear to be both tissue-specific and extremely variable. Our basic knowledge of the process of malignant transformation in melanoma has expanded to include ultraviolet light–induced changes that result in expansion of suppressor T cells, inactivation of Langerhans' cells, keratinocyte damage with release of cytokines that stimulate melanocytic growth and oncogene function, direct DNA damage, phenotypic changes in melanocytes, and ultimately clonal genetic changes. These concepts have led to an appreciation that malignant change is a continuously evolving process of accumulated genetic injury. Studies of chromosomal alterations in melanoma are important because alterations found consistently may represent locations of growth regulating genes and could have important diagnostic and prognostic implication. Recent cytogenetic analysis of premalignant and primary melanoma has implicated specific regions on chromosomes 9 and 10 (9p, 10q) as possibly associated with early malignant change.[53,148] However, very little other information exists about cytogenetic changes in common nevi, dysplastic nevi, or other atypical moles. More work has been directed at studies of metastatic melanoma where selected cytogenetic changes have been associated with prognosis.[184] Patients with melanomas showing abnormalities of chromosome 7 or 11 had significantly shorter survival rates compared with patients without these structural chromosome abnormalities. Numerous other chromosomal abnormalities were detected in over 95% of tumors studied (particularly on chromosomes 1, 6, 9, and 21), however, these other karotypic changes did not correlate with survival. The biologic relevance of these various specific chromosomal abnormalities is unclear, however certain consistently identified changes may correlate with regions known to affect cellular growth. A frequent finding in melanoma is the loss of the long arm of chromosome 6.[185] Studies to determine if a tumor suppressor gene might map to this region were performed by directly inserting a normal chromosome 6 into melanoma cell lines. This resulted in a dramatic change of *in vitro* morphology and suppressed tumorigenicity compared with parental lines. Tumorigenesis in columic carcinoma is believed to occur in a multistep genetic model. Evidence for a similar genetic progression in other malignancies has relied on findings in cultured lesion. Healy and others[93] examined autosomal arm loss in primary cutaneous melanoma and benign melanocytic nevi. Loss of heterozygosity in primary melanoma was identified most frequently on chromosomes 9p, 10q, 6q, and 18q. Loss of these chromosomal arms was related to the progression of melanoma. Although cytogenetic studies in melanoma are in their infancy, further evaluation of the basic genetics of melanoma should enhance our understanding of the progression of this cancer and will be useful in determining prognosis and therapy.

PREVENTION

The contrasting survival rates between patients with metastatic and patients with nonmetastatic melanoma and the nearly universal cure of patients with noninvasive (Clark's level I) or thin melanomas, underscore the importance of prevention and early detection in this malignancy. Because predisposing environmental factors, and in some cases genetic factors, have been clearly implicated, high-risk populations and individuals can be identified. Routine, noninvasive screening and increased public awareness should be widely promoted. The ABCDs of melanoma should be disseminated. Whether such interventions can affect survival rates is currently under study.[111,130,156] For screening to be effective, physicians need to be able to recognize the varied clinical presentations of melanoma. Prevention rather than early recognition also is an attractive goal. Avoidance of excessive sun exposure and routine surveillance skin examinations for patients with dysplastic nevi and early excision of atypical pigmented lesions are warranted. With increasing knowledge of cell biology, it may be possible in the near future to regulate on the genetic level those tumor initiators or promoters that are involved in melanoma carcinogenesis. As evidenced by tumor regression after adoptive immunotherapy, indirect approaches through manipulation of the immune system may also hold promise for prevention strategies.

SURVIVAL

It is clear that overall survival of patients with localized melanomas relates directly to tumor thickness and a number of other prognostic variables, such as melanoma type (nodu-

lar versus others), ulceration site (scalp and posterior neck versus others), and other less important variables, such as age, gender, and lymphocytic infiltration. Differences in survival rates tend to equalize after controlling for thickness at time of presentation. Therefore, the belief that LMM is inherently less ominous than other types of melanoma has been questioned.[2,110] The reported overall 5-year survival figures vary from 30% to 60%, depending on case mix. Emerging concepts have included observations that 5-year survival figures may not be as reliable as 10-year figures when estimating the risk of failure in patients with localized melanoma, and that the width of the resection margins is not as prognostically critical as was previously believed.

It has been consistently reported that the most important factor in survival is the presence of regional metastases. In localized melanomas, tumor thickness is directly related to occult regional metastatic rates. The prognostic importance of tumor thickness is certainly related to the association of thickness with occult regional metastatic rates, but it also may be independently associated with local and distant relapse rates. Some disagreement remains as to whether the level of invasion and the tumor thickness remain important to prognosis once regional metastases have occurred.[61,179] Regardless, it is clear that once clinically evident regional metastases have occurred, distant dissemination exists in 70% to 97% of patients, and 5-year survival is reduced to between 10% and 20%. Five-year survival rates for patients with localized melanoma are consistently reported as 70% to 80% when biopsy for neck nodes is negative and 15% to 25% when biopsy for neck nodes is positive.[17,34,89,169,179]

In most reports, the percentage of patients alive at 5 years who had occult, histologically positive nodes resected is slightly better (by 5% to 15%) than those with clinically and histologically positive nodes.[19,142] Statistical proof of better survival in the former group is lacking, however, because of the small numbers of patients in most reports and other problems inherent in retrospective comparisons of groups that might differ in important prognostic variables. Because truly effective treatment for disseminated disease is lacking, and clinically positive nodes portend distant dissemination, managing localized disease in an aggressive fashion appears justified when the risk of occult regional metastases is high. Finally, because of the documented prognostic information provided by accurate pathologic staging, it is of critical importance that trials of adjuvant management strategies in high-risk patients include histologic assessment of regional nodes to interpret survival end results reliably.

CONCLUSION

Melanoma is a capricious malignancy known for aggressive growth and dissemination. This characterization may be undeserved if the curability of early, thin lesions is considered. Advances in the management of melanomas have been made primarily because of a better understanding of the natural history of the disease and the improved definition of prognostic factors. Because the incidence of melanoma is increasing dramatically, it is crucial that lay and professional educational efforts be directed toward early recognition and diagnosis.

Accumulated data on the natural history of head and neck melanoma have provided reliable identifying characteristics for nevi that may be dysplastic or frankly malignant. Advances in histologic staging have allowed improved the prognosis of individual lesions, but the continued interest and cooperation of surgeons and pathologists are required. Significantly less disfiguring and debilitating local resections for head and neck melanomas are feasible in thin (<0.75 mm) lesions. Although controversy remains regarding the survival benefit of regional node dissections for intermediate-thickness localized melanomas, data suggest that a survival benefit is conferred by elective nodal dissection in such patients. Nevertheless, prognosis is enhanced by histologic determination of the presence of regional metastases and may in the future define a population of patients that could benefit from effective adjuvant therapy.

The results of current chemotherapy and immunotherapy regimens for patients with melanomas have been more promising than in recent years. Further basic research into the biologic mechanisms of melanocyte differentiation and growth regulation should enhance the further development of chemoprevention strategies. The development of sophisticated immunologic probes that use monoclonal antibodies, tumor vaccines, and new information regarding gene regulation offer the promise of new therapeutic approaches for melanomas in the future. For individual patients the diagnosis of melanoma still connotes a dreaded prognosis that demands sensitive, knowledgeable counseling and skilled management by a thoroughly informed multidisciplinary panel of cutaneous oncologists.

REFERENCES

1. Abrams J and others: Interferon alpha - 2b adjuvant therapy in postsurgical, high-risk melanoma, *Natl Cancer Inst Consensus Conf*, 1996.
2. Ackerman AB: Malignant melanoma: a unifying concept, *Am J Dermatopath* 2:309, 1980.
3. Ames FC, Sugarbaker EV, Ballantyne AS: Analogies of survival and disease control in stage I melanoma of head and neck, *Am J Surg* 132:484, 1976.
4. Ang KK and others: Post-operative radiotherapy for cutaneous melanoma of the head and neck region, *Int J Radiol Oncol Biol Phys* 30: 795, 1994.
5. Atkinson B and others: Identification of melanoma-associated antigens using fixed-tissue screening of antibodies, *Cancer Res* 44:2577, 1984.
6. Bagley FH and others: Changes in clinical presentation and management of malignant melanoma, *Cancer* 47:2126, 1981.
7. Balch CM: Surgical management of regional lymph nodes in cutaneous melanoma, *J Am Acad Dermatol* 3:511, 1980.
8. Balch CM: Pathology, prognostic factors and surgical treatment of cutaneous melanoma, *Curr Concepts Oncol* 4:8, 1982.
9. Balch CM: The role of elective lymph node dissection in melanoma: rationale, results and controversies, *J Clin Oncol* 6:163, 1988.
10. Balch CM, Soong SJ, Shaw HM: *A comparison of worldwide melanoma data*. In Balch CM and others, editors: *Cutaneous melanoma*, Philadelphia, 1985, JB Lippincott.
11. Balch CM and others: A multifactorial analysis of melanoma III: prognostic factors in melanoma patients with lymph node metastases (stage II), *Ann Surg* 193:377, 1981.
12. Balch CM and others: A comparison of prognostic factors and surgical results in 1786 patients with localized (stage I) melanoma treated in Alabama, USA, and New South Wales, Australia, *Ann Surg* 196:677, 1982.
13. Balch CM and others: A multifactorial analysis of melanoma IV: prognostic factors in 200 melanoma patients with distant metastases, *J Clin Oncol* 11:126, 1983.
14. Balch CM and others: Ineffectiveness of adjuvant chemotherapy using DTIC and cyclophosphamide in patients with resectable melanoma, *Surgery* 95:454, 1984.
15. Balch CM and others: *An analysis of prognostic factors in 4000 patients with cutaneous melanoma*. In Balch CM and others, editors: *Cutaneous melanoma*, Philadelphia, 1985, JB Lippincott.
16. Balch CM and others: *Elective lymph node dissection: pros and cons*. In Balch CM and others, editors: *Cutaneous melanoma*, Philadelphia, 1985, JB Lippincott.
17. Ballantyne AJ: Malignant melanoma of the skin of the head and neck, *Am J Surg* 120:425, 1970.
18. Barr LC and others: Superficial parotidectomy in the treatment of cutaneous melanoma of the head and neck, *Br J Surg* 81:64, 1994.
19. Batsakis JG: *Tumors of the head and neck: clinical and pathological considerations*, ed 2, Baltimore, 1979, Williams & Wilkins.
20. Bauer R and others: Long-term results of intralesional BCG for locally advanced recurrent melanoma, *Proc Am Soc Clin Oncol* 9:276, 1990.
21. Beahrs OH and others: *Melanoma of the skin (excluding eyelid)*. In Beahrs OH and others, editors: *Manual for staging of cancer*, ed 3, Philadelphia, 1988, JB Lippincott.
22. Bennett LR, Lago G: Cutaneous lymphoscintigraphy in malignant melanomas, *Semin Nucl Med* 13:61, 1983.
23. Beral V and others: Cutaneous factors related to the risk of malignant melanoma, *Br J Dermatol* 109:165, 1985.
24. Berd D, Mastrangelo MJ: Active immunotherapy of human melanoma exploiting the immunopotentiating effects of cyclophosphamide, *Cancer Invest* 6:337, 1988.
25. Berd D and others: Treatment of metastatic melanoma with an autologous tumor cell vaccine: clinical and immunological results in 64 patients, *J Clin Oncol* 8:1858, 1990.
26. Bernengo M and others: The prognostic value of T lymphocyte levels in malignant melanoma, *Cancer* 52:1841, 1983.
27. Blatchford SJ and others: Mucosal melanomas of the head and neck, *Laryngoscope* 96:929, 1986.
28. Bluming AZ and others: Delayed cutaneous sensitivity reactions to extracts of autologous malignant melanoma: a second look, *J Natl Cancer Inst* 48:17, 1972.
29. Bocca E and others: Functional neck dissection: an evaluation and review of 843 cases, *Laryngoscope* 94:942, 1984.
30. Brascho DJ: *Radiotherapy for metastatic melanoma*. In Balch CM and others, editors: *Cutaneous melanoma*, Philadelphia, 1985, JB Lippincott.
31. Breslow A: Thickness, cross-sectional areas, and depth of invasion in the prognosis of cutaneous melanoma, *Ann Surg* 172:902, 1970.
32. Breslow A: Tumor thickness, level of invasion and node dissection in stage I cutaneous melanoma, *Ann Surg* 182:572, 1975.
33. Byers RM, Smith L, DeWitty R: Malignant melanoma of the skin of the nose, *Am J Otolaryngol* 3:202, 1982.
34. Byers RM and others: Malignant melanoma of the external ear, *Am J Surg* 140:518, 1980.
35. Bystryn JC and others: Immunogenicity of a polyvalent melanoma antigen vaccine in humans, *Cancer* 61:1065, 1988.
36. Cady B: Prophylactic lymph node dissection in melanoma: does it help? *J Clin Oncol* 6:2, 1988.

37. Carey TE and others: Cell surface antigens of human malignant melanoma: mixed hemadsorption assays for humoral immunity to cultured autologous melanoma cells, *Proc Natl Acad Sci U S A* 73:3278, 1976.

38. Carrasquillo IA and others: Diagnosis of and therapy for solid tumors with radiolabeled antibodies and immune fragments, *Cancer Treat Rep* 68:317, 1984.

39. Cascinelli N and others: Stage I melanoma of the skin: the problem of resection margins, *Eur J Cancer* 16:1079, 1980.

40. Chang P, Knapper WH: Metastatic melanoma of unknown primary, *Cancer* 49:1106, 1982.

41. Clark WH and others: The developmental biology of primary human malignant melanoma, *Semin Oncol* 2:83, 1975.

42. Clark WH Jr and others: The histogenesis and biologic behavior of primary human malignant melanoma of the skin, *Cancer Res* 29:705, 1969.

43. Clemente CG and others: Prognostic value of tumor infiltrating lymphocytes in the vertical growth phase of primary cutaneous melanoma, *Cancer* 77:1303, 1996.

44. Cochran AJ, Jehn UW, Gothoskar BP: Cell mediated immunity in malignant melanoma, *Lancet* 1:1340, 1972.

45. Cohen LM: Lentigo maligna and lentigo malijne melanoma. *J Am Acad Dermatol* 33:923, 1995.

46. Conley JJ: Is melanoma changing? *Otolaryngol Head Neck Surg* 104:327, 1991.

47. Conley JJ: Melanomas of the mucous membranes of the head and neck, *Laryngoscope* 99:1248, 1989.

48. Conley JJ, Hamaker RC: Melanoma of the head and neck, *Laryngoscope* 87:760, 1977.

49. Conley JJ, Pack GT: Melanoma of the head and neck, *Surg Gynecol Obstet* 116:15, 1963.

50. Constanza ME and others: Results with methy-CCNU and DTIC in metastatic melanoma, *Cancer* 40:1010, 1977.

51. Constanzi JJ: *Chemotherapy and BCG in the treatment of disseminated malignant melanoma.* In Terry WD, Windhorst D, editors: *Immunotherapy of cancer: present status of trials in man*, New York, 1978, Raven.

52. Cosimi AB and others: Conservative surgical management of superficially invasive cutaneous melanoma, *Cancer* 53:1256, 1984.

53. Cowan JM, Halahan R, Francke U: Cytogenetic analysis of melanocytes from premalignant nevi and melanomas, *J Natl Cancer Inst* 80:1159, 1988.

54. Creagan ET and others: Radiation therapy for malignant melanoma of the head and neck, *Am J Surg* 138:604, 1979.

55. Creagan ET and others: Recombinant leukocyte A interferon in the treatment of disseminated malignant melanoma: analysis of complete and long-term responding patients, *Cancer* 58:2576, 1986.

56. Crombie IK: Racial differences in melanoma incidence, *Br J Cancer* 40:185, 1979.

57. Crombie IK: Variation of melanoma incidence with latitude in North America and Europe, *Br J Cancer* 40:774, 1979.

58. Crowley NJ, Seigler HF: The role of elective lymph node dissection in the management of patients with thick cutaneous melanomas, *Cancer* 66:2522, 1990.

59. Cunningham TJ and others: *A controlled study of adjuvant therapy in patients with stage I and II malignant melanoma.* In Terry WD, Windhorst D, editors: *Immunotherapy of cancer: present status of trials in man*, New York, 1978, Raven.

60. Das Gupta TK: Results of treatment of 769 patients with primary cutaneous melanoma: a five-year prospective study, *Ann Surg* 186:201, 1977.

61. Day CL and others: Malignant melanoma patients with positive nodes and relatively good prognosis: microstaging retains prognostic significance in clinical stage I melanoma patients with metastasis to regional nodes, *Cancer* 47:955, 1981.

62. Day CL and others: Cutaneous malignant melanoma: prognostic guidelines for physicians and patients, *Cancer* 32:113, 1982.

63. Day CL and others: Narrower margins for clinical stage I malignant melanomas, *N Engl J Med* 306:479, 1982.

64. Deresa SS, Silverman DT: Cancer incidence and mortality trends in the United States, 1935-74, *J Natl Cancer Inst* 60:545, 1978.

65. Dickinson RJ: Malignant melanoma: a combined surgical and radiotherapeutic approach, *Am J Roentgenol* 79:1063, 1958.

66. Doss LL, Memula N: The radioresponsiveness of melanoma, *Int J Radiat Oncol Biol Physiol* 8:1131, 1982.

67. Dorzewiecki KT: Survival with malignant melanoma, *Cancer* 49:2414, 1982.

68. Eilber FR, Morton DL: Impaired immunologic reactivity and recurrence following cancer surgery, *Cancer* 25:362, 1970.

69. Eilber FR and others: Adjuvant immunotherapy with BCG in treatment of regional lymph node metastases from malignant melanoma, *N Engl J Med* 294:237, 1976.

70. Eldh J: Excisional biopsy and delayed wide excision versus primary wide excision of malignant melanoma, *Scand J Plast Reconstr Surg* 13:341, 1979.

71. Elwood JM and others: Pigmentation and skin reaction to sun as risk factors for cutaneous melanoma Western Canada Melanoma Study, *BMJ* 288:99, 1984.

72. Epstein E: Effect of biopsy on the prognosis of melanoma, *J Surg Oncol* 3:251, 1971.

73. Everson TC: Spontaneous regression of cancer, *Ann NY Acad Sci* 114:721, 1964.

74. Farrar JJ and others: The biochemistry, biology and role of interleukin-2 in the induction of cytotoxic T-cell and antibody forming B cell responses, *Immunol Rev* 63:129, 1982.

75. Fears TR, Scotto J: Changes in skin cancer morbidity between 1971-72 and 1977-78, *J Natl Cancer Inst* 69:365, 1982.

76. Fisher RI and others: Adjuvant immunotherapy or chemotherapy for malignant melanoma, *Surg Clin North Am* 61:1267, 1981.

77. Fisher SR: Cutaneous malignant melanoma of the head and neck, *Laryngoscope* 99:822, 1989.

78. Fisher SR, Cole TB, Seigler HF: Application of posterior neck dissection in treating malignant melanoma of the posterior scalp, *Laryngoscope* 93:760, 1983.

79. Fortner JG and others: Biostatistical basis of elective node dissection for malignant melanoma, *Ann Surg* 186:101, 1977.

80. Franklin JD and others: Cutaneous melanoma of the head and neck, *Clin Plast Surg* 3:413, 1976.

81. Fuen LG and others: The natural history of resectable metastatic melanoma (stage IV A melanoma), *Cancer* 50:1675, 1982.

82. Goepfert H, Jesse RH, Ballantyne AJ: Posterolateral neck dissection, *Arch Otolaryngol* 106:618, 1980.

83. Goldsmith HS: Melanoma: an overview, *Cancer* 29:194, 1979.

84. Greene MH, Young T, Clark WH Jr: Malignant melanoma in renal transplant recipients, *Lancet* 1:1196, 1981.

85. Greene MH and others: Acquired precursors of cutaneous malignant melanoma, *N Engl J Med* 312:91, 1985.

86. Gritters LS, Francis IR, Zazadny KR: Initial assessment of positron emission tomography using 2-fluorine-18-fluoro-2-deoxy-D-glucos in the imaging of malignant melanoma, *J Nucl Med* 34:1420, 1993.

87. Gumport SL and others: The diagnosis and management of common skin cancers, *Cancer* 31:79, 1981.

88. Gupta RK, Morton DL: Suggestive evidence for *in vivo* binding of specific antitumor antibodies of human melanomas, *Cancer Res* 35:58, 1975.

89. Gussack GS and others: Cutaneous melanoma head and neck, *Arch Otolaryngol* 109:803, 1983.

90. Gutterman JU and others: Chemoimmunotherapy of disseminated malignant melanoma with DTIC and BCG, *N Engl J Med* 291:592, 1974.

91. Harris TJ, Hinckley DM: Melanoma of the head and neck in Queensland, *Head Neck Surg* 5:197, 1983.

92. Harwood AR, Cummings BJ: Radiotherapy for malignant melanoma: a reappraisal, *Cancer Treat Rev* 8:271, 1981.

93. Healy E and others: Allelotypes of primary cutaneous melanoma and benign melanogytic nevi, *Cancer Res* 56:589, 1996.

94. Hilaris BS and others: Value of radiotherapy for distant metastases from malignant melanoma, *Cancer* 16:765, 1963.

95. Hill GJ and others: DTIC and combination therapy for melanoma, *Cancer* 47:2556, 1981.

96. Hinds MW, Kolonel LN: Cutaneous malignant melanoma in Hawaii: an update, *West J Med* 138:50, 1983.

97. Hollinshead AC and others: Soluble membrane antigens of human malignant melanoma cells, *Cancer* 34:1235, 1974.

98. Hollinshead AC and others: Pilot studies using melanoma tumor associated antigens (TAA) in specific-active immunochemotherapy of malignant melanoma, *Cancer* 49:1387, 1982.

99. Holman CDJ, Armstrong BK: Pigmentary traits, ethnic origin, benign nevi and familial history as risk factors for cutaneous malignant melanoma. *J Natl Cancer Inst* 72:257, 1984.

100. Holman CDJ, Armstrong BK, Heenan PJ: Relationship of cutaneous malignant melanoma to individual sunlight exposure habits, *J Natl Cancer Inst* 76:403, 1986.

101. Hoyt DJ, Fisher SR: Survival following recurrent malignant melanoma of the head and neck, *Laryngoscope* 99:586, 1989.

102. Hoyt DJ and others: Mucosal melanomas of the head and neck, *Arch Otolaryngol* 115:1096, 1989.

103. Jacquillat C, Banzet P, Maral J: Clinical trial of chemotherapy and chemoimmunotherapy in primary malignant melanoma, *Recent Results Cancer Res* 80:254, 1982.

104. Jansen GT, Westbrook KC: *Cancer of the skin.* In Suen JY, Myers FN, editors: *Cancer of the head and neck*, New York, 1981, Churchill Livingstone.

105. Johanson CR and others: 0-7-21 Radiotherapy in nodular melanoma, *Cancer* 51:226, 1983.

106. Johnson TM and others: Current therapy for cutaneous melanoma, *J Am Acad Dermatol* 32:689, 1995.

107. Kaplan EN: The risk of malignancy in large congenital nevi, *Plast Reconstr Surg* 53:421, 1974.

108. Kasid A and others: Human gene transfer characterization of human tumor-infiltrating lymphocytes as vehicles for retroviral-mediated gene transfer in man, *Proc Natl Acad Sci U S A* 87:475, 1990.

109. Koh HK, Kligler BE, Lew RA: Sunlight and cutaneous malignant melanoma: evidence for and against causation, *Photo Chem Photo Biol* 51:765, 1990.

110. Koh HK and others: Lentigo maligna melanoma has no better prognosis than other types of melanoma, *J Clin Oncol* 2:994, 1984.

111. Koh HK and others: Evaluation of melanoma skin cancer screening in Massachusetts: preliminary results, *Cancer* 65:375, 1990.

112. Kraemer KH and others: Dysplastic nevi and cutaneous melanoma risk, *Lancet* 2:1076, 1983.

113. Lafreniere R, Rosenberg SA: Adoptive immunotherapy of immune hepatic metastases with lymphokine activated killer (LAK) cells and recombinant interleukin-2 can mediate the regression of both immunogenic and nonimmunogenic sarcoma and adenosarcoma, *J Immunol* 135:4273, 1985.

114. Lee ET and others: An analysis of skin tests and their relationship to recurrence ~and survival in stage III and stage IV melanoma patients, *Cancer* 49:2336, 1982.

115. Lee JAH: *The causation of melanoma.* In Balch CM and others, editors: *Cutaneous melanoma*, Philadelphia, 1985, JB Lippincott.

116. Lew RA and others: Sun exposure habits in patients with cutaneous melanoma: a case control study, *J Dermatol Surg Oncol* 9:981, 1983.

117. Lewis MG and others: Tumor-specific antibodies in human malignant melanoma and their relationship to the extent of disease, *BMJ* 3:547, 1969.

118. Lingeman RE and others: Neck dissection: radical or conservative, *Ann Otol* 86:737, 1977.

119. Lock-Anderson J and others: Preoperative cutaneous lymphoscintigraphy in malignant melanoma, *Cancer* 63:77, 1989.

120. Loree JR, Spiro RH: Cutaneous melanoma of the head and neck, *Am J Surg* 158:388, 1989.

121. Loutfi A and others: Double blind randomized prospective trial of levamisole placebo in stage I cutaneous malignant melanoma, *Clin Invest Med* 10:325, 1987.

122. Luce JK: Chemotherapy of melanoma, *Semin Oncol* 2:179, 1975.

123. Mann BD and others: Imaging of human tumor xenografts in nude mice with radiolabeled monoclonal antibodies, *Cancer* 54:1318, 1984.

124. Mastrangelo MJ and others: *Postsurgical adjuvant therapy.* In Clark WH and others, editors: *Human malignant melanoma*, New York, 1979, Grune & Stratton.

125. Mavligit G and others: Tumor-directed immune reactivity and immunotherapy in malignant melanoma: current status, *Prog Exp Tumor Res* 19:222, 1974.

126. McGovern VJ and others: Is malignant melanoma arising in a Hutchinson's melanotic freckle a separate disease entity? *Histopathology* 4:235, 1980.

127. McKinnon JG and others: Natural history and treatment of mucosal melanoma, *J Surg Oncol* 41:222, 1989.

128. McNeer G, Das Gupta TK: Prognosis in malignant melanoma, *Surgery* 56:512, 1964.

129. Medina J: Malignant melanoma of the head and neck, *Otolaryngol Clin North Am* 26:73, 1993.

130. Miller AB and others: Report on a workshop of the UICC project on evaluation of screening for cancer, *Int J Cancer* 46:761, 1990.

131. Mitchell MS and others: Active specific immunotherapy for melanoma, *J Clin Oncol* 8:856, 1990.

132. Molinari R and others: Retrospective comparison of conservative and radical neck dissection in laryngeal cancer, *Ann Otol* 89:578, 1980.

133. Morton DL and others: Intraoperative lymphatic mapping and selective cervical lymphadectomy for early stage melanoma of the head and neck, *J Clin Oncol* 11:1751, 1993.

134. Morton DL and others: Immunologic factors which influence response to immunotherapy in malignant melanoma, *Surgery* 68:158, 1970.

135. Morton DL and others: BCG immunotherapy of malignant melanoma: summary of a seven-year experience, *Ann Surg* 180:635, 1974.

136. Morton DL and others: *Adjuvant immunotherapy of malignant melanoma: preliminary results of a randomized trial in patients with lymph node metastases.* In Terry WD, Windhorst D, editors: *Immunotherapy of cancer: present status of trials in man*, New York, 1978, Raven.

137. Morton DL and others: Active specific immunotherapy with melanoma cell vaccine and immunomodulation in patients with metastatic melanoma, *Proc Am Soc Oncol* 10:295, 1991.

138. Mule JJ and others: Antitumor efficacy of lymphokine-activated killer cells and recombinant interleukin-2 *in vivo*: survival benefit and mechanisms of tumor relapse in mice undergoing immunotherapy, *Cancer Res* 46:676, 1986.

139. Nakajima T and others: Immunohistochemical demonstration of S100 protein in malignant melanoma and pigmented nevus and its diagnostic application, *Cancer* 50:912, 1982.

140. National Cancer Institute: *Cancer statistic review 1973-1987*, Bethesda, Department of Health and Human Services, 1990 (NIH publication no 90-2789).

141. Norman J: Redefinition of cutaneous lymphatic drainage with the use of lymphoscintigraphy for malignant melanoma, *Am J Surg* 162:432, 1991.

142. O'Brien CJ and others: Experience with 998 cutaneous melanomas of the head and neck over 30 years, *Am J Surg* 162:310, 1991.

143. O'Brien CJ and others: Evaluation of 107 therapeutic and elective parotidectomies for cutaneous melanoma, *Am J Surg* 168:400, 1994.

144. Oldham RK: Monoclonal antibodies as anticancer agents, *Adv Exp Med Biol* 166:45, 1983.

145. Oldham RK and others: Monoclonal antibodies in the treatment of cancer: preliminary observations and future prospects, *Med Oncol Tumor Pharmacother* 1:51, 1984.

146. Olson RM, Woods JE, Soule EH: Regional lymph node management

and outcome in 100 patients with head and neck melanoma, *Am J Surg* 142:470, 1981.

147. Overgaard J: Radiation treatment of malignant melanoma, *Int J Radiat Oncol Biol Phys* 6:41, 1980.

148. Parmiter AH and others: Possible involvement of the chromosome region 10q24 > q26 in early stages of melanocytic neoplasm, *Cancer Genet Cytogenet* 30:313, 1988.

149. Patel JK and others: Metastatic pattern of malignant melanoma: a study of 216 autopsy cases, *Am J Surg* 135:807, 1978.

150. Perzik SL: *Treatment of melanoma.* In Kagan AR, Miles JW, editors: *Head and neck oncology: controversies in cancer treatment*, Boston, 1981, Hall.

151. Pinsky CM and others: *Surgical adjuvant immunotherapy with BCG in patients with malignant melanoma: results of a prospective, randomized trial.* In Terry WD, Windhorst D, editors: *Immunotherapy of cancer: present status of trials in man*, New York, 1978, Raven.

152. Plager C and others: Adjuvant immunotherapy of MD Anderson Hospital (MDAH stage III-B malignant melanoma with Newcastle disease virus oncolysate), *Proc Am Soc Clin Oncol* 9:281, 1990.

153. Presant CA, Bartolucci AA: The southeastern cancer study group: prognostic factors in metastatic malignant melanoma, *Cancer* 49:2192, 1982.

154. Quirt IC and others: Improved survival in patients with poor prognosis malignant melanoma treated with adjuvant levamisole: a phase III study by the National Cancer Institute of Canada clinical trials group, *J Clin Oncol* 9:729, 1991.

155. Reiger E: Overall and site-specific risk of malignant melanoma associated with nevis counts at different body sites: a multicenter case control study of the German central malignant melanoma registry, *Intl J Cancer* 62:393, 1995.

156. Rigel DS and others: Importance of complete cutaneous examination for the detection of malignant melanoma, *J Am Acad Dermatol* 14:857, 1986.

157. Rogers GS and others: Effect of anatomic location on prognosis in patients with clinical stage I melanoma, *Arch Dermatol* 119:644, 1983.

158. Rosenberg SA and others: Regression of established pulmonary metastases and subcutaneous tumor mediated by the systemic administration of high dose recombinant interleukin-2, *J Exp Med* 161:1169, 1985.

159. Rosenberg SA and others: A progress report on the treatment of 157 patients with advanced cancer using lymphokine activated killer cells and interleukin-2 or high-dose-interleukin-2 alone, *N Engl J Med* 316:889, 1987.

160. Rosenberg SA and others: Use of tumor-infiltrating lymphocytes and interleukin-2 in the immunotherapy of patients with metastatic melanoma: a preliminary report, *N Engl J Med* 319:1676, 1988.

161. Rosenberg SA and others: Experience with the use of high-dose interleukin-2 in the treatment of 652 cancer patients, *Ann Surg* 210:474, 1989.

162. Rosenberg SA and others: Gene transfer into humans: immunotherapy of patients with advanced melanoma using tumor infiltrating lymphocytes modified by retroviral gene transduction, *N Engl J Med* 323:570, 1990.

163. Roses DF and others: Selective surgical management of cutaneous melanoma of the head and neck, *Ann Surg* 192:629, 1980.

164. Surveillance Epidemiology and End Results Program: Cancer statistics, *Cancer* 34:7, 1984.

165. Shafir R and others: Pitfalls in frozen section diagnosis of malignant melanoma, *Cancer* 51:1168, 1983.

166. Shafir R and others: The thin malignant melanoma: changing patterns of epidermiology and treatment, *Cancer* 50:817, 1982.

167. Shah JP, Huvos AG, Strong EW: Mucosal melanoma of head and neck, *Am J Surg* 134:531, 1977.

168. Siegler HJ and others: Specific active immunotherapy for melanoma, *Ann Surg* 190:366, 1979.

169. Sim FH and others: A prospective randomized study of the efficacy of routine elective lymphadenectomy in management of malignant melanoma: preliminary results, *Cancer* 41:948, 1978.

170. Simons JN: Malignant melanoma of the head and neck, *Am J Surg* 124:485, 1972.

171. Singluff CL Jr and others: The annual risk of melanoma progression: implications for the concept of cure, *Cancer* 70:1917, 1992.

172. Snow GB, VanDerEsch EP, VanSlooten EA: Mucosal melanoma of head and neck, *Head Neck Surg* 1:24, 1978.

173. Sober AJ: Solar exposure in the etiology of cutaneous melanoma, *Photoderm* 4:23, 1987.

174. Solomon AR, Ellis CN, Headington JR: An evaluation of vertical growth in thin superficial spreading melanomas by sequential serial sections, *Cancer* 52:7338, 1983.

175. Sondel PM and others: Clinical and immunological effects of recombinant interleukin-2 given by repetitive weekly cycles to patients with cancer, *Cancer Res* 48:2561, 1988.

176. Spitler LE: A randomized trial of levamisole versus placebo as adjuvant therapy in malignant melanoma, *J Clin Oncol* 9:736, 1991.

177. Stern JS and others: Mucosal melanoma of the head and neck, *Head Neck Surg* 1991.

178. Stone CA and others: Surgical management of regional lymph nodes in primary cutaneous malignant melanoma.

179. Storm FK, Eilber FR: *The value of lymphadenectomy in melanoma of the head and neck.* In Kagan AR, Miles JW, editors: *Head and neck oncology: controversies in cancer treatment*, Boston, 1981, Hall.

180. Storm FK and others: Malignant melanoma of the head and neck, *Head Neck Surg* 1:123, 1978.

181. Storper IS and others: The role of radiotherapy in the treatment of head and neck cutaneous melanoma, *Am J Otolaryngol* 14:426, 1993.

182. Strechi JM and others: A randomized trial of adjuvant chemotherapy and immunotherapy in stage I and stage II cutaneous melanoma, *Cancer* 55:707, 1985.

183. Summer WC: Spontaneous regression of human melanoma, *Cancer* 13:79, 1980.

184. Trent JM and others: Relation of cytogenetic abnormalities and clinical outcome in metastatic melanoma, *N Engl J Med* 322:1508, 1990.

185. Trent JM and others: Tumorigenicity in human melanoma cell lines controlled by introduction of human chromosome 6, *Science* 247:568, 1990.

186. Trotti A, Peters LJ: Role of radiotherapy in the primary management of mucosal melanoma of the head and neck, *Semin Surg Oncol* 9:246, 1993.

187. Tsang RW and others: Lentigo melanoma of the head and neck, *Arch Dermatol* 130:1008, 1994.

188. Tucker MA, Misfeldt D, Coleman CN: Cutaneous malignant melanoma after Hodgkins disease, *Ann Intern Med* 102:37, 1985.

189. Urist MM and others: The influence of surgical margins and prognostic factors predicting the risk of local recurrence in 3445 patients with primary cutaneous melanoma, *Cancer* 55:1398, 1985.

190. Vadhan-Raj S and others: Phase I trial of mouse monoclonal antibody against GD3 ganglioside in patients with melanoma: induction of inflammatory responses at tumor sites, *J Clin Oncol* 6:1636, 1988.

191. Velez A, Walsh D, Karakousis CP: Treatment of unknown primary melanoma, *Cancer* 68:2579, 1991.

192. Veronesi U, Cascinelli N: Narrow excision (1 cm margin), *Arch Surg* 126:438, 1991.

193. Veronesi U and others: A randomized trial of adjuvant chemotherapy and immunotherapy in cutaneous melanoma, *N Engl J Med* 307:913, 1982.

194. Veronesi U and others: Delayed regional lymph node dissection in stage I melanoma of the skin of the lower extremities, *Cancer* 49:2420, 1982.

195. Veronesi U and others: Thin stage I primary cutaneous malignant melanoma: comparison of excision with margins of 1 or 3 cm, *N Engl J Med* 318:1159, 1988.

196. VonWussaw P and others: Intralesional interferon-alpha therapy in advanced malignant melanoma, *Cancer* 61:1071, 1988.

197. Wallack MC, Bash J, Bartolucci A: Improvement in disease-free survival of melanoma patients in conjunction with serologic response in a phase Ia Ib southeastern cancer study group trial of vaccinia melanoma oncolysate, *Am J Surg* 55:243, 1989.

198. Wanebo HJ, Harpole D, Teates CD: Radionuclide lymphoscintigraphy with technetium 99m antimony sulfide colloid to identify lymphatic drainage of cutaneous melanoma at ambiguous sites in the head and neck and trunk, *Cancer* 55:1403, 1985.

199. Wick MM and others: Clinical characteristics of early cutaneous melanoma, *Cancer* 45:2684, 1980.

200. Wood WC and others: Randomized trial of adjuvant therapy for high-risk primary malignant melanoma, *Surgery* 83:677, 1978.

Chapter 27

Reconstruction of Facial Defects

Shan R. Baker

Skin cancer is the most common cancer of humans, and most skin cancers occur on the face. The incidence of squamous cell carcinoma, basal cell carcinoma, and melanoma is increasing, perhaps because of the depletion of the ozone layer or other environmental factors not yet determined. Most cutaneous malignancies are managed surgically, leaving skin defects that require reconstruction. Skin cancers, birth defects, and injuries as a result of trauma and burns, require that surgeons be skilled in the repair of facial defects. This chapter addresses the management of many types of facial defects, primarily those resulting from ablation of cutaneous malignancies. However, the principles of local flap design and tissue movement can be readily applied to the reconstruction of all forms of facial defects.

Most facial defects result from ablation of cutaneous malignancies, and most cases can be repaired by primary wound closure or with a local cutaneous or musculocutaneous flap. Because the topic of facial reconstruction is extremely broad and complex, this chapter discusses only local flaps and grafts in the repair of facial cutaneous defects with the occasional appropriate reference to the repair of skeletal deficiencies. Other publications better address the use of regional flaps in facial reconstruction.[5,7,12]

The face can be divided into aesthetic facial units, which include the forehead, cheeks, eyelids, nose, lips auricles, and sometimes the scalp. Reconstruction of some of these areas of the face are discussed elsewhere in this textbook. A multitude of different flaps and grafts can be used to repair a given facial defect; thus several techniques for repair of a given aesthetic facial unit are discussed. The algorithm in Figure 27-1 displays an approach for analyzing and developing a management plan for surface defects of the face and neck. The selection of a specific flap depends on the location and size of the defect and the intrinsic properties of the flap. Larger defects of the face and neck may be difficult to resurface with local flaps without considerable impairment in form or function. In such circumstances, the surgeon should select a regional flap or skin graft, which may be aesthetically less pleasing but will provide a functional repair. These decisions are determined by clinical judgment. The greater the experience of the surgeon, the better the clinical judgment.

CLASSIFICATION OF LOCAL FLAPS

Several methods are used to classify cutaneous flaps:[3,15] (1) by arrangement of their blood supply (e.g., random versus arterial); (2) by configuration (e.g., rhomboid, bilobe); (3) by location (e.g., local, regional, distant); and (4) by the method of transferring the flap. Local cutaneous flaps are designed immediately adjacent to or near the location of the defect. When classified by method of transfer (Box 27-1), local flaps are divided into pivotal, advancement, and hinged. A fourth method of tissue movement is microsurgical, although this method does not apply to local flaps. Most local flaps are moved, in reality, through a combination of pivoting and advancement. For example, most pivotal flaps are aided in tissue movement by using the intrinsic elasticity of the flap through stretching (advancement). Thus, surgeons often speak of combined mechanisms of tissue movement, such as advancement rotation flap. For classification purposes, however, the major mechanism of tissue transfer should dictate the term given to describe a particular flap, unless both mechanisms are of approximately equal importance, in which case the terms describing both mechanisms should be used.

PIVOTAL FLAPS

The three types of pivotal flaps are rotation, transposition, and interpolated (see Box 27-1). All pivotal flaps are moved toward the defect by rotating the base of the flap around a

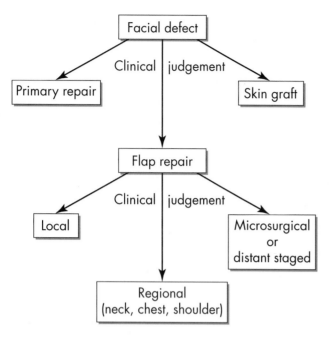

Fig. 27-1. Skin defect repair.

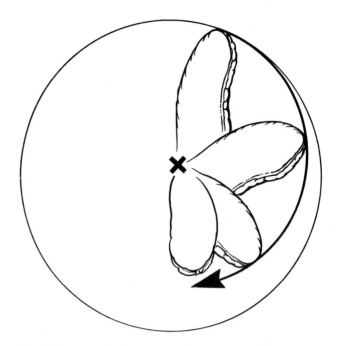

Fig. 27-2. The effective length of a pivotal flap moving through an arch of 180° is reduced 40%. (Adapted from Gorney M: *Tissue dynamics and surgical geometry.* In Kernakian DA, Vistnes LM, editors: *Basic concepts of reconstructive surgery,* Boston, 1977, Little, Brown.)

> **Box 27-1.** Local flaps classified by tissue movement
>
> Pivotal Flaps
> Rotation
> Transposition
> Interpolated
> Advancement Flaps
> Pedicle
> Bipedicle
> V-Y
> Hinged Flap

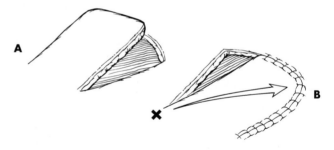

Fig. 27-3. **A,** Rotation flaps are pivotal flaps with curvilinear configuration. Removal of a Burow's triangle can facilitate repair of the donor site. **B,** Standing cutaneous deformity will form at the base of the flap. Triangle-shaped defects use a portion of this redundant tissue. (From Baker SR, Swanson N: *Local flaps in facial reconstruction,* St Louis, 1995, Mosby.)

---

pivotal point. Except with island axial flaps, which have been skeletonized to the level of the nutrient vessels, the greater the degree of pivot, the shorter is the effective length of the flap (Fig. 27-2). This is because the pivotal point is fixed in position and the base of the flap is restricted when pivoting around this point because of the development of a standing cutaneous deformity (dog ear). A pivotal flap should be designed to account for this reduction in effective length as it moves through the pivotal arc, which may be as much as 40% with an arc of 180°.

Rotation flaps

Rotation flaps are pivotal flaps that have a curvilinear configuration. They are designed immediately adjacent to the defect and are best used to close triangular defects (Fig. 27-3). Rotation flaps are usually random in their vascularity but, depending on the position of the base of the flap, may be axial. Because a rotation flap has a broad base, its vascularity tends to be reliable. When possible, the flap should be designed to be inferiorly based, which promotes lymphatic drainage and reduces flap edema. Rotation flaps are useful in repairing medial cheek defects located near the nasofacial sulcus or nasal sidewall. The curvilinear border of the flap can often be positioned along the infraorbital rim, which represents an important border of aesthetic units (eyelid and cheek). Positioning the incision for the flap along this border enhances scar camouflage.

Large rotation flaps are particularly useful for reconstruction of sizable posterior cheek and upper neck defects. Large medial, inferiorly based rotation flaps are a flexible means of transferring large amounts of tissue from the remaining cheek and upper cervical regions. Incisions for the flap are placed in a preauricular crease and can extend for some distance along the anterior border of the trapezius muscle to facilitate rotation of upper cervical skin toward the area of the posterior cheek. A Z-plasty at the base of the flap facilitates closure of the secondary defect. Chin reconstruction often can be readily accomplished with rotation flaps, occasionally using two flaps to optimize the use of the aesthetic border of the submental crease to camouflage incisions. Smaller rotation flaps may also be used for repair of defects located in the glabellar area. Because rotation flaps are less dependent than most on tissue elasticity for movement, they are particularly useful for scalp defects in which the skin is quite inelastic. In addition, curvilinear configuration of rotation flaps adapts well to the spherical shaped cranium. Thus, scalp defects in general are best reconstructed with one or more rotation flaps. A rotation scalp flap must be quite large relative to the size of the defect, with the width of the pedicle being twice the width of the defect.[18] Rotation flaps have relatively few disadvantages. The defect itself should be somewhat triangular or should be modified by removing additional tissue to create a triangular defect. The configuration of the flap creates a right angle at the distal tip, and the surgeon should take care in positioning the tip so that it is not subjected to excessive wound tension and vascular compromise. As with all pivotal flaps, a rotation flap may develop a standing cutaneous deformity at the base that may not be easily removed without compromising the vascularity of the flap. Thus, a second-stage removal of the deformity may be necessary.

Transposition flaps

In contrast to rotation flaps, transposition flaps have a linear axis (Fig. 27-4). Both are pivotal flaps moving around a pivotal point. A transposition flap can be designed similar to a rotation flap so that a border of the flap is also a border of the defect. However, it may also be designed with borders that are removed from the defect, with only the base of the flap contiguous with the defect. The ability to construct a flap at some distance from the defect with an axis that is independent of the linear axis of the defect is one of the greatest advantages of transposition flaps. This advantage enables the surgeon to recruit skin at variable distances from the defect, selecting areas of greater skin elasticity or redundancy. In addition, the ability to select variable sites for harvesting a flap ensures that the donor site scar by its location and orientation will best be camouflaged.

Transposition is the most common method of moving local flaps into skin defects of the head and neck. Transposition flaps, elevated in a multitude of sizes, shapes, and orientation, are usually of random blood supply, but may occasionally be axial or compound. A transposition flap is a

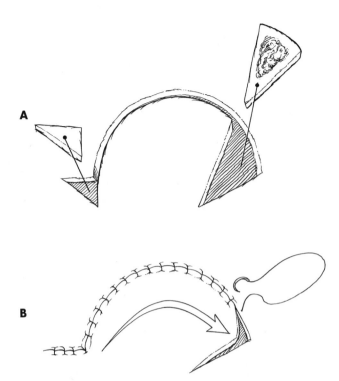

Fig. 27-4. A, Transposition flaps have a linear configuration. **B,** The greatest line of wound closure tension is between the pivotal point and the most peripheral point of the flap. (**A,** Adapted from Baker SR, Swanson N: *Local flaps in facial reconstruction*, St Louis, 1995, Mosby.)

reconstructive option for small to medium-sized defects in most configurations or locations, thus making it the most useful local flap in head and neck reconstruction. Although it is recommended that the length of random cutaneous transposition flaps not exceed three times their width, this ratio is not very applicable to such flaps designed on the face and scalp. More important than this ratio are the location and the specific orientation of a transposition flap. The abundant vascularity of the skin of the face and scalp often enables the development of flaps that exceed the 3 : 1 ratio. An example is the inferiorly or superiorly based melolabial transposition flap, in which its linear axis is directly above and parallel to the linear axis of the angular artery. Although the flap is rarely elevated as a true axial flap incorporating the angular artery, many small peripheral branches of the artery are probably included in the base of the melolabial flap, accounting for its dependability even when designed as a lengthy flap.

Interpolated flaps

The interpolated flap is a pivotal flap that has a linear configuration, but it differs from transposition flaps in that its base is located at some distance from the defect (Fig. 27-5). Thus, the pedicle should pass over or under intervening tissue. If the pedicle passes over intervening tissue, the flap should subsequently be detached in a second surgical

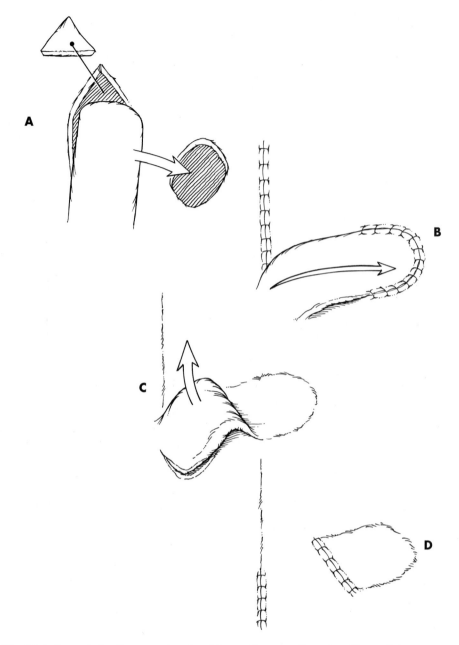

Fig. 27-5. Interpolation flaps are pivotal and have a linear configuration. The pedicle passes over intervening tissue and requires subsequent division.

procedure. This is perhaps the greatest disadvantage of these flaps. On occasion, the pedicle can be de-epithelialized or reduced to subcutaneous tissue only and brought under the intervening as an island flap to allow a single-stage reconstruction.

Common interpolated flaps used in the repair of facial defects are the vertically oriented midforehead flaps, which include median and perimedian flaps.[1] These flaps are highly effective in reconstruction of the midface because of their excellent vascularity and because their superb skin color and texture match the skin of the nose. The high success rate,

reliability, and popularity are primarily the result of a dependable axial blood supply. Based on the supratrochlear artery and its anastomoses to surrounding vessels, midforehead flaps are axial flaps with excellent vascularity that can be transferred without delay. The excellent vascularity allows for the incorporation of cartilage or tissue grafts, which can then act as support structures or lining tissue for nasal reconstruction. Careful removal of muscle and subcutaneous fat from the distal portion of a midforehead flap makes it thin, pliable, and easily contoured to fit any defect of the midface. The frontalis muscle and fascia are included with the distal flap when more stiffness and bulk are required to fit defects of greater depth.

The close proximity of forehead skin to the midface provides a source of skin with an excellent color and texture match to the central face. Modern use of the midforehead flap has been expanded beyond nasal reconstruction to include any soft-tissue defect of the midface that the flap can be designed to reach.[6] Defects of the medial canthal region, upper and lower eyelids, medial cheek, melolabial region, and upper lip may be repaired with midforehead flaps. These flaps may also be used in combination with other flaps for the reconstruction of complex facial defects, for example a midforehead flap can be combined with a scalping flap for total nasal reconstruction.

ADVANCEMENT FLAPS

Advancement flaps have a linear configuration and are moved into a defect by being stretched forward. These depend on the elasticity of the tissue of the flap (primary movement) and tissue adjacent to the defect (secondary movement) to achieve wound closure. Tissue transfer is achieved by moving the flap and its pedicle in a single vector. Advancement flaps can be categorized as pedicle, bipedicle, or V-Y. Bipedicle advancement flaps are used primarily for repair of large defects of the scalp; the flap is designed adjacent to the defect and advanced into the defect perpendicular to the linear axis of the flap. This leaves a secondary defect, which usually should be covered with a split-thickness skin graft. As a consequence, bipedicle flaps are rarely used for reconstruction of the face and neck.

Pedicle advancement flap

A pedicle advancement flap is created by parallel incisions, which allow the tissue to ''slide'' in a single vector toward a defect (Fig. 27-6). The movement is in one direction, and the flap advances directly over the defect. As a consequence, the flap should be developed adjacent to the defect, and one border of the defect becomes a border of the flap. Repair with an advancement flap involves primary and secondary tissue movement. In primary movement, the incised flap is pushed or pulled forward by stretching the skin. Secondary movement of surrounding skin and soft tissue immediately adjacent to the defect occurs in a direction opposite the movement of the advancing edge of the flap. This secondary movement may help in repair, by providing less wound closure tension, or may be detrimental, by displacing nearby facial structures.

Complete undermining of the advancement flap and of the skin and soft tissue around the pedicle is important to enhance tissue movement. Standing cutaneous deformities are created with all pedicle advancement flaps and may require excision. Excision of standing cutaneous deformities (Burow's triangles) may also facilitate movement of the flap. Unlike the pivotal flap, in which a single-standing cutaneous deformity should be dealt with at the base of the flap, de-

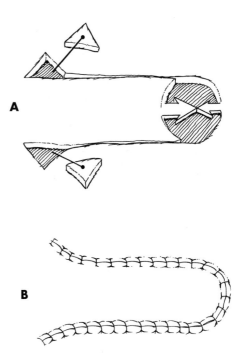

Fig. 27-6. A and **B,** A pedicle advancement flap is created by parallel incisions, which allow a tissue to slide in a single vector toward the defect. Secondary movement of surrounding skin immediately adjacent to the defect occurs in a direction opposite the direction of the flap. (Adapted from Baker SR, Swanson N: *Local flaps in facial reconstruction*, St Louis, 1995, Mosby.)

formities develop on both sides of the base. However, they may be excised anywhere along the length of the flap and not necessarily near the base. Selection of the best location for excising tissue is based on where it can be placed within relaxed skin tension lines or long aesthetic borders. Bilateral Z-plasties performed at the base of the flap often eliminate or reduce the need for excision of standing cutaneous deformities. Occasionally, if the flap is sufficiently long, standing cutaneous deformities can be subdivided into multiple smaller puckers of tissue that need not be excised but merely can be ''sewn out'' by sequentially suturing the flap lengths in one half. On the face, pedicle advancement flaps work particularly well in the forehead (particularly in the vicinity of the eyebrow), helical rim, upper and lower lips, and medial cheek. Mucosal advancement flaps are also useful for vermilion reconstruction. Bilateral advancement flaps are commonly used to close large defects, resulting in H- or T-shaped repairs depending on the configuration of the defect (Fig. 27-7). Repair in this manner is often referred to as an H-*plasty* or T-*plasty*. In both cases, advancement flaps are designed on opposite sides of a defect and advanced toward each other, each responsible for reconstructing a portion of the defect. In such cases, standing cutaneous deformities are often excised partly in the area of the defect and partly along the linear axis of the two flaps. The two flaps harvested from either side of the defect do not necessarily have to be of the

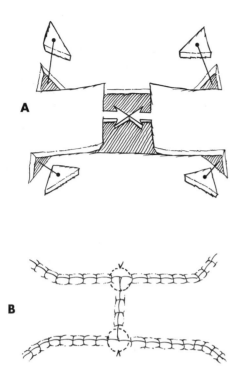

Fig. 27-7. A and **B,** Bilateral advancement flaps with excision of Burow's triangles.

same length. The length of each flap is determined primarily by the elasticity and redundancy of the donor resource.

A special type of pedicle advancement flap is the island advancement flap. A segment of skin is isolated as an island while protecting the subcutaneous tissue and blood supply. The geometric shape of the cutaneous island may vary but is frequently triangular. As the flap advances toward the recipient site, the donor area is closed in a simple V-Y manner. This flap is particularly useful in the repair of medium-sized defects of the medial cheek near the alar base.

V-Y advancement flap

The V-Y advancement flap is unique in that the V-shaped flap is not stretched toward the recipient site but advances by recoil or by being pushed rather than pulled toward the defect. Thus, the flap is allowed to move into the recipient site without any wound closure tension. The secondary triangular donor defect is then repaired by advancing the two edges of the remaining donor site wound toward each other. In so doing, the wound closure suture line assumes a Y configuration, with the common limb of the Y representing the suture line resulting from closure of the secondary defect.

V-Y advancement is useful when a structure or region requires lengthening or release from a contracted state. The technique is particularly effective in lengthening the columella in the repair of cleft lip nasal deformities in which a portion or all of the columella is underdeveloped (Fig.

27-8). A V-Y advancement flap is elevated, recruiting skin from the midportion of the lip between the philtral ridges. The length of the columella is augmented by advancing the flap upward into the base of the columella. The secondary donor defect is approximated by closing the remaining lip skin together in the midline. V-Y advancement is also helpful in releasing contracted scars that distort adjacent structures, such as the eyelid or vermilion. An example is the correction of an ectropion of the vermilion caused by scarring (Fig. 27-9). The segment of distorted vermilion is incorporated into the V-shaped flap and advanced toward the lip to restore the natural topography of the vermilion-cutaneous junction. The skin edges on both sides of the secondary defect are then advanced toward each other and sutured. The suture line becomes the vertical or common limb of the Y configuration.

Y-V advancement flaps

Y-V advancement flaps differ from V-Y advancement flaps by making a Y-shaped incision initially. In contrast to the V-Y design in which the V-shaped flap recoils or is pushed toward the area for supplementation, in the Y-V design, the flap is pulled or stretched toward the area for supplementation. The flap augments the area of the common limb, while reducing the triangular area. Y-V advancement flaps are indicated in circumstances in which the surgeon wants to decrease the redundancy of an area by moving tissue away from the site. Occasionally, relocating a free margin of a facial structure may be useful to improve symmetry.

HINGE FLAPS

Cutaneous hinge flaps, sometimes referred to as trap door, turn-in, or turn-down flaps, have a unique method of tissue movement. These flaps may be designed in a linear or curvilinear shape with the pedicle based on one border of the defect. The flap is dissected in the subcutaneous plane and turned over on to the defect like a page in a book. The epithelial surface of the flap is turned downward to provide internal lining for a facial defect that requires external and internal lining surfaces. The exposed subcutaneous surface of the hinge flap is covered by a second flap. Thus, hinge flaps are always used with another flap or graft that provides the external coverage of the defect. The vascular supply of hinge flaps is derived from the soft-tissue border of the defect that it is designed to repair. As a consequence, such flaps have limited and often restricted vascularity. Survival of hinge flaps can be improved if they are used when the wound margin of the defect is well healed rather than freshly created. Because the pedicle of the hinge flap is along a border of the defect, the flap should be elevated in such a way that as flap dissection proceeds toward the base of the flap, the plane of dissection becomes deeper; thus, the base is thicker than the distal portion of the flap. This technique enhances vascularity of the flap by increasing the likelihood of including within the pedicle more nutrient vessels.

Hinge flaps are commonly used for repair of full-thick-

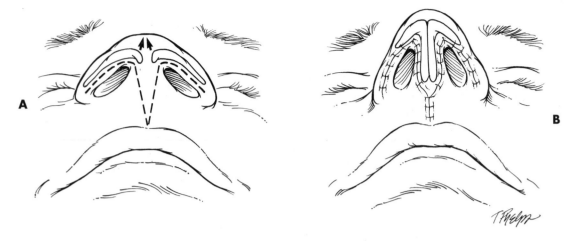

Fig. 27-8. A and **B,** A V-Y advancement flap augments columellar length.

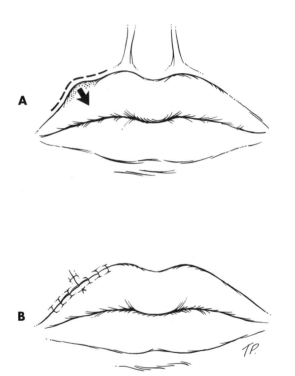

Fig. 27-9. A and **B,** A V-Y advancement flap corrects ectopian of vermilion. Adapted from Baker SR, Swanson N: *Local flaps in facial reconstruction*, St Louis, 1995, Mosby.)

ness nasal defects in which the remaining adjacent nasal skin is sufficient to develop a hinge flap for internal nasal lining. Hinge flaps may also be used to close mature sinofacial and salivary fistulas anywhere in the upper aerodigestive tract. Hinge flaps consisting of subcutaneous tissue and sometimes muscle without overlying skin can be used to fill in contour deficits.[16] Hinged flaps consisting of nasal mucosa with or without attached septal cartilage are frequently used for internal lining in the repair of full-thickness nasal defects.

These mucosal flaps are axial and do not require a thick base to ensure adequate vascularity.

DEFECTS OF THE NOSE

Skin cancer is most frequent on the nose; thus, reconstructive surgeons should be familiar with several methods for repairing nasal defects using local flaps. Burget and Menick[13] have elevated reconstructive rhinoplasty by emphasizing the importance of replacing deficient nasal tissue with similar tissue. For example, defects of the internal nasal lining are replaced with hinged or bipedicle advancement mucosal flaps harvested from the remaining nasal lining. Missing cartilage or fibrofatty tissue giving contour to the nose is replaced with septal or conchal cartilage, positioned and sculpted to replicate as closely as possible the missing skeletal support. Thinning and contouring the cartilage grafts should be emphasized so that they replicate the exact topography of the contralateral cartilage if present, or the form that may be expected in an ideally shaped nose. Burget and Menick[13] also emphasized the aesthetic advantages of isolating nasal defects as a separate entity from any extension of the defect onto the cheek or lip, repairing each aesthetic unit with independent flaps. This maintains scars in borders between major aesthetic units and prevents distortion or obliteration of these borders while maximizing scar camouflage. Within the nasal aesthetic units, subunits can be identified, including the dorsum, nasal sidewalls, ala, tip and columella (Fig. 27-10). When a surface defect involves greater than 50% of the surface area of the subunit, resurfacing of the entire subunit with a flap usually provides a better aesthetic result by hiding scars along borders of the subunits.[13]

The nasal ala is a common site of nasal defects resulting from removal of skin cancers. If not repaired properly, distortion of the alar margin and partial collapse of the external nasal valve occur with compromise of the airway. Too often in the past, the alar facial sulcus and nasal alar crease have

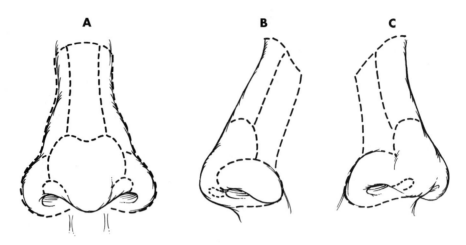

Fig. 27-10. A through **C,** Nasal topographic aesthetic units. (Adapted from Baker SR, Swanson N: *Local flaps in facial reconstruction*, St Louis, 1995, Mosby.)

been violated by transposition flaps harvested from the medial cheek to repair alar defects. When this occurs, a completely natural appearing border between the cheek and the ala and nasal sidewall is extremely difficult to restore. For this reason, the author prefers to use interpolated flaps from the cheek, the pedicle of which crosses over, but not through, the alar facial sulcus. The pedicle may consist of skin or subcutaneous tissue only and is detached from the cheek 3 weeks after the initial transfer to the nose.[8] This interval allows the surgeon to aggressively defat and sculpt the distal flap at the time of flap transfer and again at the time of pedicle detachment and flap inset. On detachment of the flap, the patient has a completely natural appearing alar facial sulcus and nasal alar crease (provided the defect does not extend into the crease) because no incisions or dissections have been made in these regions. Usually, resurfacing of the entire ala is preferred, removing any remaining skin. Full-thickness defects are reconstructed by restoring the internal nasal lining deficit with a vascularized vestibular skin or mucosal flap. Full-thickness defects of the ala with a vertical height of 1.5 cm or less can use a bipedicle mucosal flap for internal lining (Fig. 27-11). The flap is created by making an extended intercartilaginous incision from the nasal dome to the lateral floor of the vestibule. The vestibular skin is mobilized inferiorly, and the inferior edge is sutured to the inferior border of the nasal vestibular skin defect. If the vestibular skin defect extends to the alar rim, then the inferior aspect of the flap is sutured to the edge of the cutaneous flap to provide external coverage of the defect. The flap is attached to the overlying cartilage grafts to provide structural support by horizontal mattress sutures placed through the cartilage and bipedicle flap. The donor site for the flap is repaired with a thin full-thickness skin graft harvested from the standing cutaneous deformity removed when closing the donor site of the interpolated cheek flap.

After reconstruction of the internal nasal lining defect

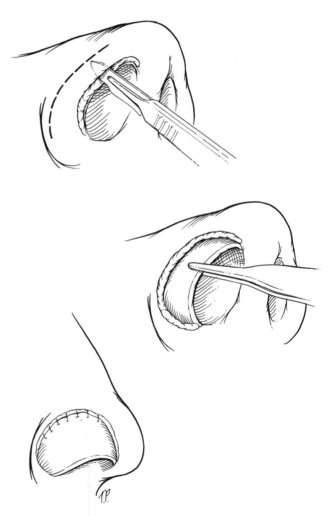

Fig. 27-11. For full-thickness defects of the ala with a vertical height of 1.5 cm or less one can use a bipedicle mucosal advancement flap for internal lining. The donor site is closed with a thin full-thickness skin graft. (Adapted from Baker SR, Swanson N: *Local flaps in facial reconstruction*, St Louis, 1995, Mosby.)

with a bipedicle mucosal flap, the next step is to completely replace all missing nasal cartilage with free cartilage grafts harvested from the nasal septum or preferably from the auricle. If the inferior edge of the lateral crura has been removed, the missing cartilage should be replaced with a free cartilage graft and additional grafts should be placed along the alar margin inferior to the position of the original lateral crus. This prevents notching or upper contraction of the alar rim. Likewise, when the fibrofatty tissue of the lateral portion of the alar lobule is missing, it should be replaced with free cartilage grafts because this tissue, although not rigid, provides structural support and contour to the lobule. If the surgeon depends strictly on a skin flap to replace the fibrofatty tissue in the alar lobule, less structural support is provided, and scar contracture causes an unnatural appearance, usually with some notching of the alar rim and partial collapse of the external nasal valve.

Once the structural support for the alar lobule has been secured, a cheek flap is planed to resurface the lobule and cover the restored skeletal support. A template is fashioned to exactly represent the size and shape of the surface defect. This template is used to design a superiorly based melolabial interpolated flap. The flap should be designed so that the medial border falls in the melolabial sulcus. The flap is elevated in a subcutaneous plane and may be lifted on a skin and subcutaneous fat pedicle or based on a subcutaneous pedicle only. A subcutaneous pedicle is preferred in nonsmokers because the flap can transpose more easily and reduces the amount of skin to be removed from the upper melolabial fold, thus maintaining better facial symmetry. The flap donor site is closed primarily by undermining the skin of the cheek. The standing cutaneous deformity that occurs with advancement of the cheek skin medially is excised, and a portion is used as a full-thickness skin graft to cover the donor site of the intranasal mucosal flap. The interpolated flap is transposed over the alar facial sulcus, and the distal two thirds of the flap is thinned appropriately so that the flap will drape over the cartilage grafts in a manner that replicates the contour of the alar lobule and alar nasal crease. This may require thinning of the flap to the level of the dermis in the area along the alar rim to restore the delicate topography of the rim. When the defect involves the alar rim and internal nasal vestibular skin, the inferior border of the flap is sutured to the inferior border of the bipedicle mucosal flap to replace the missing internal nasal lining. The proximal one third of the interpolated flap is left with an ample amount of subcutaneous tissue to enhance flap vascularity. At the time of pedicle detachment, the proximal portion of the flap to be inset is defatted and contoured.

The main advantage of the melolabial interpolated flap is that it does not violate the aesthetically important alar facial sulcus. It also minimizes distortion of the melolabial fold because the skin removed from the cheek is skin located at the inferior aspect of the fold where greater skin redundancy is present. Using a subcutaneous pedicle, only a small amount of skin from the upper melolabial fold is discarded as a result of a small-standing cutaneous deformity in that area during closure of the donor site.

When tissue defects extend into the alar facial sulcus, the task of restoring this area of complex topography to its natural appearance (i.e., symmetrical to its counterpart) is difficult. When confronted with this problem, the surgeon often prefers to reconstruct the medial cheek and alar facial sulcus component of the defect with an advancement cheek flap and reconstruct the alar lobule with a separate cheek or forehead interpolated flap (Fig. 27-12). This allows each flap to reconstruct the independent aesthetic units of the nose and cheek and places the junction of the borders of the two flaps along the restored alar facial sulcus. When such defects are reconstructed with a single transposition cheek flap, partial or complete obliteration of the alar facial sulcus occurs, and it should be restored through additional operations. This usually involves multiple surgical procedures and only limited success.

Surface defects of the nasal tip, columella, sidewalls, and dorsum are best repaired with paramedian forehead flaps, although partial loss of the columella may be repaired with a single or bilateral superiorly based melolabial interpolated flap. If the defect involves greater than 50% of the surface area of an aesthetic subunit, then the remaining skin should be removed and the entire subunit of the nose resurfaced. As with reconstruction of the ala, all missing cartilage should be replaced. Auricular cartilage is an excellent source for replacing missing lower lateral cartilage, whereas septal cartilage is most useful for replacing upper lateral cartilage. Full-thickness defects require pedicle or bipedicle septal mucosal flaps for repair of the internal lining (Fig. 27-13). Although small defects of the nasal tip lining can be repaired with a bipedicle vestibular skin flap, as discussed, Burget and Menick[13] showed that the entire mucosal lining of the nasal septum can be mobilized as a hinge flap based anteriorly on the caudal septum and nourished by the septal branch of the labial artery. This hinge flap is turned laterally across the nasal passage to provide lining to the lateral nasal wall. When greater lining deficits (e.g., the entire length of the sidewall) are present, a second mucosal flap from the contralateral side is developed. In contrast to the ipsilateral flap, the contralateral flap is hinged on the dorsal septum and is nourished by the anterior ethmoid artery (see Fig. 27-13). Thus, the lining for a heminasal defect is supplied inferiorly by an ipsilateral hinge septal mucosal flap based on the superior labial artery and superiorly by a contralateral septal mucosal hinge flap based on the anterior ethmoid artery. A permanent septal fistula remains. Although crusting may occur for several months, the large septal fistula is rarely symptomatic. The ipsilateral mucosal flap crosses the nasal passage in such a way that it blocks the airway and should be detached from the caudal septum to restore a patent nasal passage. This maneuver is accomplished using local anesthesia 3 weeks after initial transfer. The excellent vascular sup-

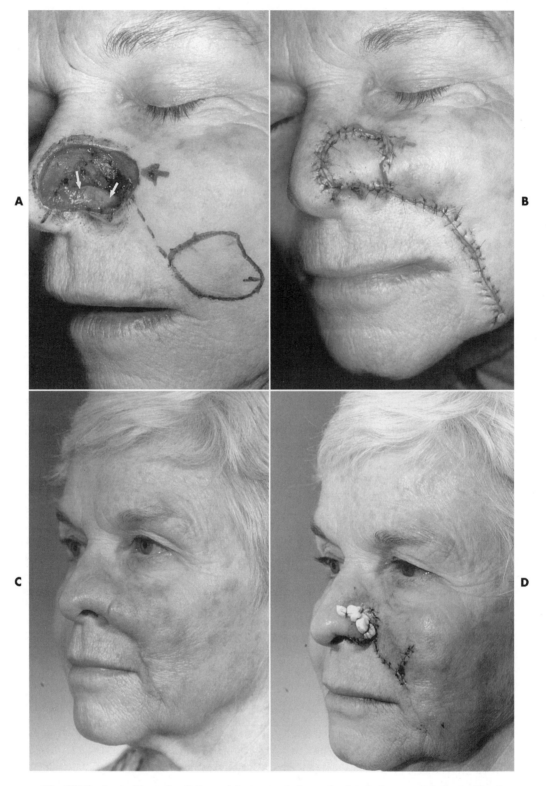

Fig. 27-12. A, A skin and soft-tissue defect extends from alar lobule into medial cheek. Cheek advancement flaps are designed to repair cheek defect. Separate subcutaneous pedicle interpolation flaps are designed to resurface the alar lobule after placement of auricular cartilage graft *(arrows)* along the missing alar margin. **B,** Two flaps are in position. **C** and **D,** Three weeks after transfer of interpolation flap, the pedicle is separated and the distal flap is sculptured to reconstitute the alar nasal crease. The standing cutaneous deformity from the cheek advancement flap is removed in the melolabial sulcus.   *Continued*

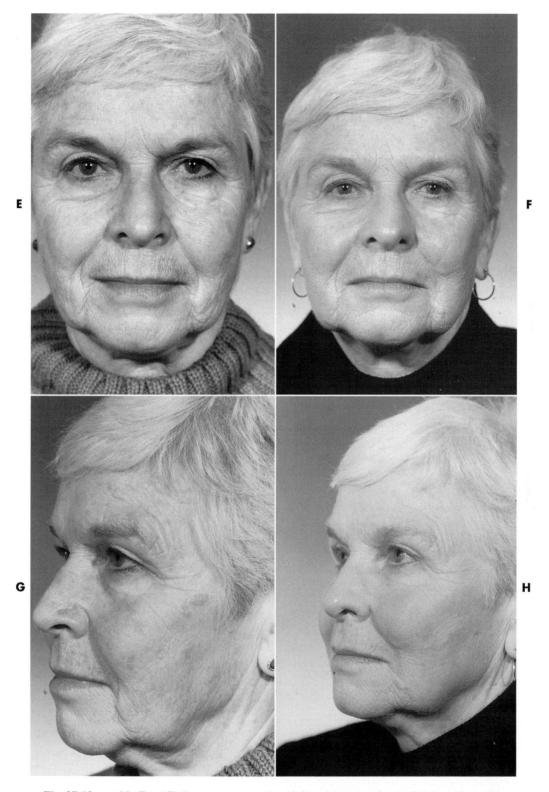

Fig. 27-12, cont'd. E and **F,** One-year preoperative *(left)* and postoperative *(right)* view. Harvesting the interpolation cheek flap from jowl area reduces asymmetric fullness of the melolabial folds. **G** and **H,** Preoperative *(Left)* and 1-year postoperative *(right)* view. The reconstituted alar nasal crease simulates original crease by aggressively debulking flap at the time of inset.

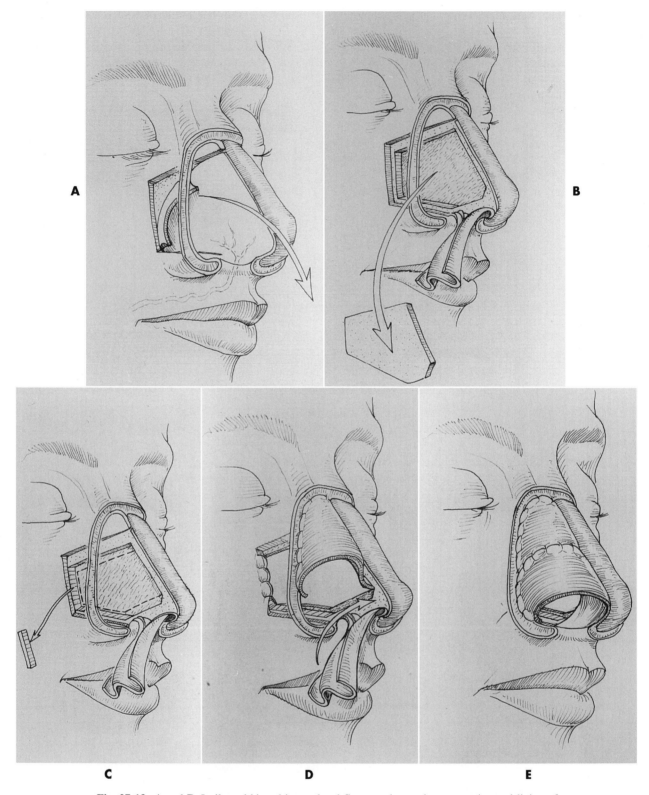

Fig. 27-13. A and **B,** Ipsilateral hinged interpolated flaps can be used to restore internal lining of full-thickness nasal sidwall defects with a vertical height of 2.5 cm or less. In such instances, exposed septal cartilage is removed to allow septum to heal by second intention. **C** through **E,** For defects greater than 2.5 cm in vertical height, a second contralateral septal mucosal hinged flap is required to supplement ipsilateral flap.

ply of these mucosal flaps provides a well-vascularized recipient site to support free cartilage grafts of all sizes. The grafts are sandwiched between the mucosal flap internally and the interpolated forehead or cheek flap externally and thus have a dual source of vascularization.

In repair of full-thickness central nasal defects of the tip or dorsum, a composite turnout flap consisting of septal cartilage with attached mucosa on either side is developed. Its base is centered in the region of the nasal spine and upper lip and contains both septal branches of the superior labial arteries. A flap of appropriate dimensions is outlined and incised with a right angle knife or scissors. Such flaps may include bone and extend from the nasal floor inferiorly to the level of the medial canthi cephalically and posteriorly

to include portions of the perpendicular plate. To allow rotation, the septal mucoperichondrial leaves are separated from the septal cartilage near the nasal spine and a triangular-shaped piece of septal cartilage at the level of the inferior septal angle is removed (Fig. 27-14). This maneuver permits the flap to rotate up and out to reach the tip and dorsum. The flap is designed overly wide and long to create an excess of mucosa and cartilage. As the flap pivots into position, its distal end passes over the exposed remnant of the nasal bones or missing dorsal septum and locks into position. The extra lining is peeled downward as bilateral hinge flaps, which extend laterally to line the dorsal nasal vault and tip. Cartilage grafts are placed on top of these flaps to restore missing dome cartilage in the case of central tip defects or to restore

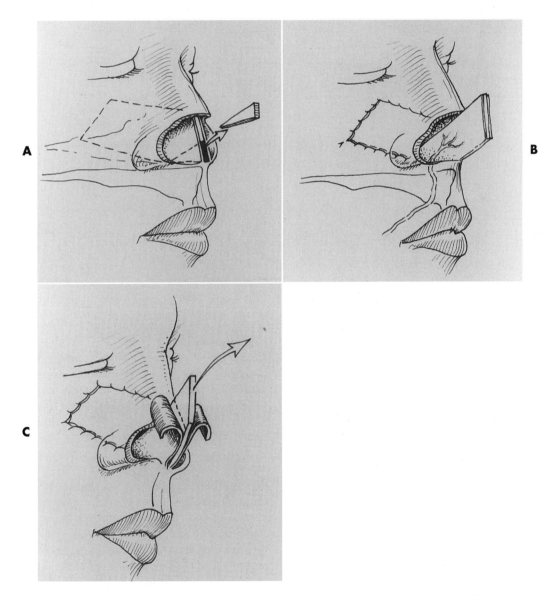

Fig. 27-14. A through **C,** A composite pivotal septal flap is used to replace structure and internal lining for central defects of the tip and dorsum.   *Continued*

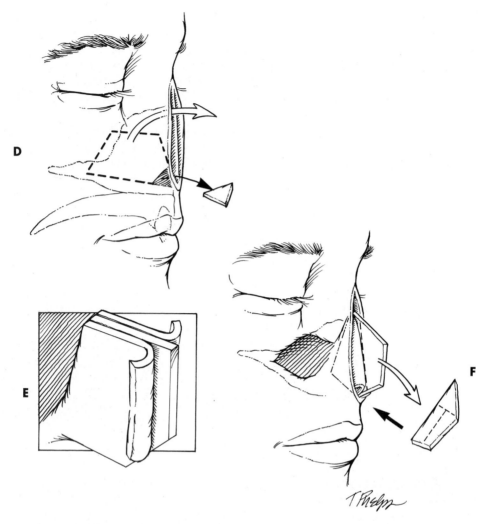

Fig. 27-14, cont'd. D through **F,** A similarly constructed composite flap may be used to reconstruct internal lining and skeletal support for the nasal dorsum. (Adapted from Baker SR, Swanson N: *Local flaps in facial reconstruction,* St Louis, 1995, Mosby.)

nasal bridge in the case of dorsal defects. A paramedian forehead flap provides the external surface cover to complete the reconstruction (Fig. 27-15).

Paramedian forehead flaps are the preferred local flap for resurfacing most large nasal defects. The flap may be dissected under local or general anesthesia. The base of the pedicle is placed in the glabellar region centered over the supratrochlear artery on the same side as most of the nasal defect. The origin of the supratrochlear artery is consistently found to be 1.7 to 2.2 cm lateral to the midline and corresponds usually to a vertical tangent of the medial aspect of the brow. The vessel exits the orbit by piercing the orbital septum and passing under the orbicularis oculi muscle and over the corrugator superciliary muscle. At the level of the eyebrow, the artery passes through orbicularis and frontalis muscle and continues upward in a vertical direction in a subcutaneous plane. The pedicle of the flap may be as narrow as 1.2 cm. A narrow pedicle provides greater effective length

with less standing cutaneous deformity than a broader pedicle (Fig. 27-16). An exact template of the defect is used to design the paramedian forehead flap, which is centered over the vertical axis of the supratrochlear artery. If adequate length necessitates extending the flap into hair-bearing scalp, turning the flap obliquely along the hairline will prevent transfer of hair-bearing skin to the nose. The flap is elevated in a plane just superficial to the periosteum of the frontal bone. To avoid injury to the arterial pedicle, blunt dissection near the brow separates the corrugator muscles from the flap and facilitates mobility. If necessary, incisions can be extended below the brow to enhance the length of the flap. Adequate flap mobilization usually requires complete sectioning of the corrugator superciliary muscle to achieve free movement of the flap. Before inset, the flap is sculptured and contoured to fit the depth, breadth, and height of the defect by removal of all or some of the muscle and subcutaneous tissues from the distal portion of the flap. When neces-

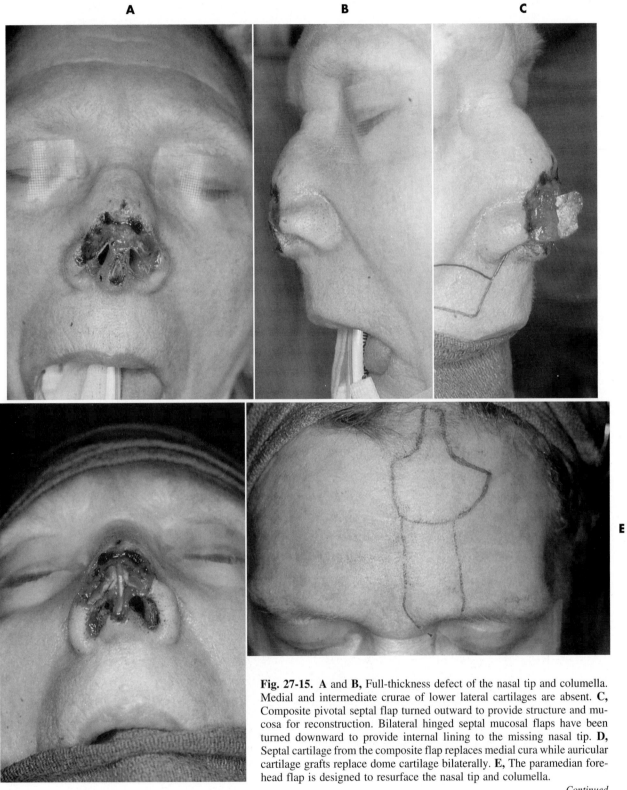

Fig. 27-15. A and **B,** Full-thickness defect of the nasal tip and columella. Medial and intermediate crurae of lower lateral cartilages are absent. **C,** Composite pivotal septal flap turned outward to provide structure and mucosa for reconstruction. Bilateral hinged septal mucosal flaps have been turned downward to provide internal lining to the missing nasal tip. **D,** Septal cartilage from the composite flap replaces medial cura while auricular cartilage grafts replace dome cartilage bilaterally. **E,** The paramedian forehead flap is designed to resurface the nasal tip and columella.

Continued

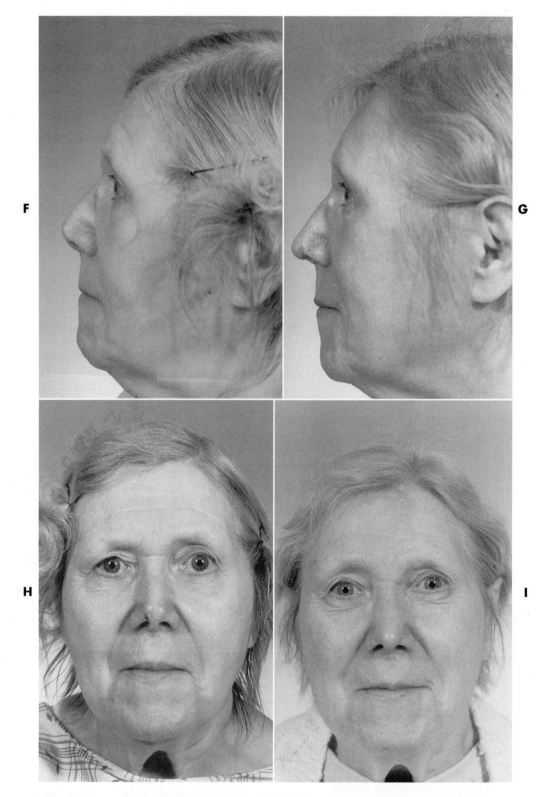

Fig. 27-15, cont'd. F and **G,** Preoperative *(left)* and 1-year postoperative *(right)* profiles show enhanced tip projection after reconstruction. **H** and **I,** Preoperative *(left)* and 1-year postoperative *(right)* views show restored tip definition and shape.

sary, all but 1 mm of the fat beneath the dermis may be removed. It may be necessary to resect a portion of the dermis along the edge of the flap so that the thickness of the skin flap matches the adjacent nasal skin. Only the distal three fourths of the flap required for reconstruction is sculptured; the proximal one fourth is left thick and is debulked at the time of pedicle detachment 3 weeks later. Donor site closure is accomplished by undermining the forehead skin in the subfascial plane from the anterior border of one temporalis muscle to the other. Several parallel vertical fasciotomies 2 to 3 cm apart may be necessary to achieve primary closure of the wound. Any portion of the donor site that cannot be closed primarily should be left to heal by second

intention, keeping the open wound moist at all times. Healing by second intention usually results in an acceptable scar but may take several weeks for complete healing. When necessary, the scar can be revised later. Three weeks after the initial flap transfer, the pedicle is divided under local anesthesia. The dorsal skin above the defect is undermined for approximately 1 cm. The portion of the transposed skin flap that was not thinned at the time of transposition is now thinned appropriately. For skin-only nasal defects that extend to the rhinion, the flap should be aggressively thinned to the level of the dermis to reduplicate the thin skin that is normally found in this area. Deep layer closure is not necessary because closure should not be under any tension. The

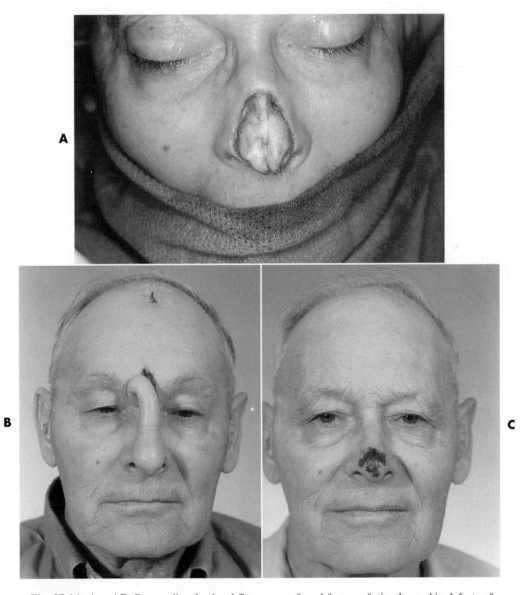

Fig. 27-16. A and **B,** Paramedian forehead flaps are preferred for resurfacing large skin defects of the nasal tip or dorsum. A narrow pedicle enhances effective flap length. **C** and **D,** Preoperative and 2-year postoperative view. Note symmetry of medial brows after detachment of the pedicle. **E** and **F,** Preoperative and 2-year postoperative view.

Continued

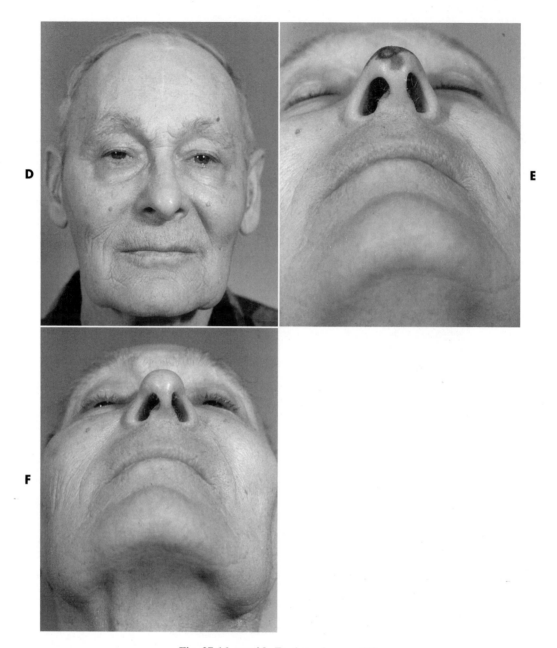

Fig. 27-16, cont'd. For legend see p. 543.

base of the pedicle is returned to the donor site in such a way as to create the normal intereyebrow distance (see Fig. 27-16). Care should be taken to maintain the muscular component of the proximal pedicle that is returned so that a depression between the eyebrows does not occur. Any excess pedicle should be discarded rather than returned to the forehead above the level of the eyebrows.

DEFECTS OF THE LIP

The lip plays a key role in deglutition, formation of speech, and facial expression. Reconstruction offers a unique challenge to the surgeon. Few other sites require such attention to precise details of form and function. Over the past several years, emphasis has been on reconstructing the aesthetic units of the lip or even the aesthetic subunits. For the upper lip, these are the filtrum and the two lateral segments. This principle can be applied in repairing smaller sized defects of the lip and frequently obviates the need to borrow tissue from the cheek.

Surgical procedures used to reconstruct the lip after tumor ablation may be classified as:[2] (1) those that use remaining lip tissue, (2) those that borrow tissue from the opposite lip, (3) those that use adjacent cheek tissue, and (4) those that use distant flaps. The first two categories enable the reconstruction to remain within the aesthetic units of the lips and when possible, are the preferred method of surgical manage-

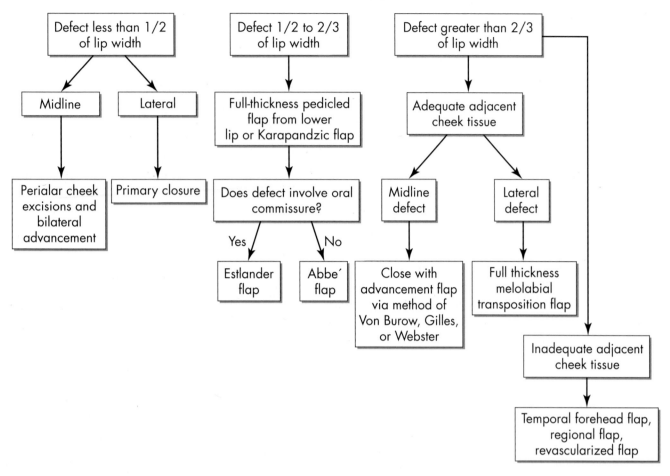

Fig. 27-17. Correction of lower lip defects.

ment. The algorithms displayed in Figures 27-17 and 27-18 provide a helpful approach to reconstruction of the lip for defects that are full thickness or represent loss of skin and muscle.[2] This approach categorizes the size of lip defects into those less than one half the width of the lip, those between one half and two thirds of the lip, and those greater than two thirds of the lip width. The edges of the defect immediately retract, so the defect size is measured *before* excising the lesion. Defects less than one half the lip width can usually be managed by primary wound closure or by using smaller local flaps confined to an aesthetic subunit of the lip (Fig. 27-19). In the lower lip, a wedge excision should not be carried below the mental line unless necessary for tumor removal. A W-plasty at the mental line allows for rectangular excision. Lateral advancement flaps may be required when the defect base is broad. The W-shaped configuration maximizes the conservation of tissue and prevents an unsightly pointed chin, which occurs when the incision is extended below the mental crease. Primary closure should be in four layers: mucosa, muscle, deep dermal, and skin. Care is taken to perform a precise approximation of the ''white line'' at the vermilion border on either side of the defect.

Primary wound closure of defects near the midline of the upper lip can be facilitated by excising a crescent of cheek skin in the perialar region to increase flap advancement. This method is similar to that described by Webster.[20] Perialar skin excision allows advancement of the remaining lip segments medially and lessens wound closure tension after primary wound repair.

Reconstruction of defects from one half to two thirds of the lip usually requires lip augmentation. Closure can be most readily achieved by a full-thickness pedicle flap from the opposite lip (lip switch flap) or from the adjacent cheek. The Karapendzic flap[17] may also be effective in closing medium-sized defects of the lip and, in some instances, may provide better functional results than other denervated flaps. This technique consists of circumoral incisions through the skin and sucutaneous tissue, encompassing the remaining portions of the upper and lower lips.[5] The orbicularis oris is mobilized and remains pedicled bilaterally on the superior and inferior labial arteries. Adequate mobilization enables primary closure of the defect by rotating portions of the remaining lip tissue into the defect. The advantage of the Karapendzic flap is that it restores a continuous circle of functioning orbicularis muscle to maintain oral competence.

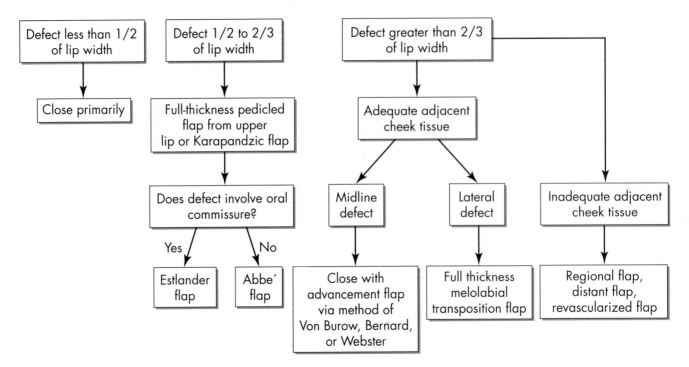

Fig. 27-18. Correction of upper lip defects.

However, because no new tissue is recruited to aid in the reconstruction of the lip, microstomia may be a problem. Also, the circumoral incisions can be unsightly. Patients 60 years of age or older often develop laxity of the oral stoma following a Karapendzic flap and do not require commissuroplasties to correct the microstomia.

Local flaps are preferable to regional flaps for closing defects of less than two thirds of the lip width because of the close skin color, the similar texture, and the availability of mucous membrane for internal lining. Defects located away from the commissure are best closed with an Abbé flap consisting of a full-thickness flap from the opposite lip pedicled on the vermilion border and containing the labial artery.[4] Estlander[14] devised an operation for closure of a lower lip defect near the commissure of the mouth.[14] Since the original description of the Abbé and Estlander flaps, the operations have been modified to accommodate surgical defects located anywhere in the upper or lower lip.

The Abbé and Estlander flaps should be constructed so that the height of the flap equals the height of the defect. The width of the flap should be approximately one half that of the defect to be reconstructed; however, when the entire filtrum is missing, the width of the flap should equal that of the filtrum. This will restore the total aesthetic subunit, which is preferable cosmetically and functionally. The pedicle should be made narrow to facilitate transposition and should be positioned near the center line of the recipient site. The secondary defect should be closed in four layers with accurate approximation of the vermilion border.

The pedicle of the Abbé flap crosses the oral stoma and

may be severed in 2 to 3 weeks. During the interval between transfer of the flap and division of the pedicle, the patient is maintained on a liquid or soft diet that does not require excessive chewing. Precise approximation of the vermilion border is essential to insure at the time of pedicle severance.

The superiorly based Estlander flap may be modified from its original description so that the flap lies within the melolabial sulcus (Fig. 27-20).[10] This provides better scar camouflage of the donor site and, at the same time, allows easy rotation of the flap into the lower lip defect. The Estlander flap causes oral commissure distortion, or microstomia, which may be corrected with a secondary commissuroplasty when desired.

Defects greater than two thirds of the width of the lip and some smaller lateral defects are best reconstructed by using adjacent cheek flaps in the form of advancement or transposition flaps. Massive or total lip defects are best reconstructed by using regional or distant flaps or vascularized microsurgical flaps. Large defects of the upper lip may be reconstructed by transferring bilateral crescent-shaped perialar cheek tissue downward and medially (Bruns flaps). If wound closure tension is excessive, an Abbé flap may be added in the midline.[10]

Similarly, midline lower lip defects may be closed by full-thickness advancement flaps as described by Bernard,[13a] Webster[20] or Gilles. These techniques may require excision of additional triangles in the melolabial sulcus to allow advancement of the cheek flaps. Triangular excision should follow the lines of the sulcus and should include only skin and subcutaneous tissues. The underlying muscle is mobi-

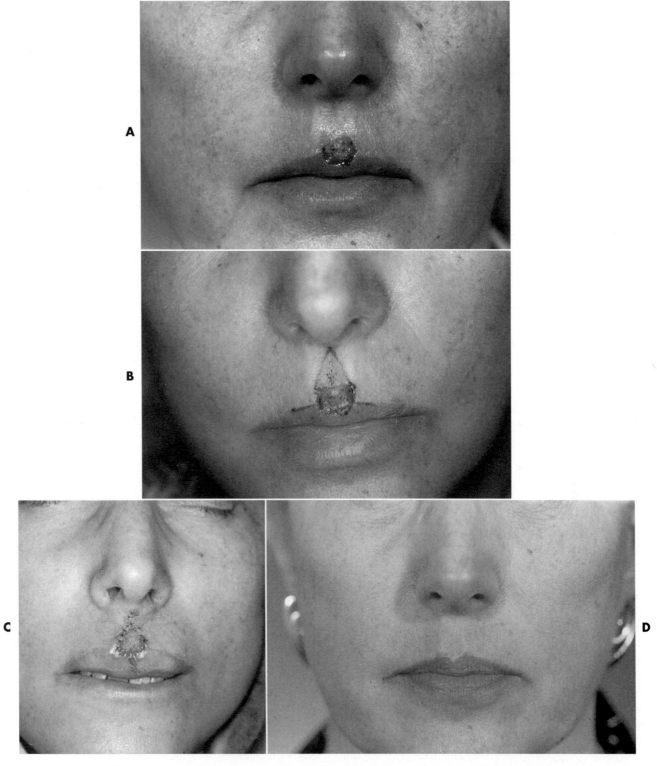

Fig. 27-19. A, A small skin defect confined to the philtral aesthetic subunit. **B,** A V-Y musculocutaneous island pedicle flap is designed within the subunit. **C,** Flap advancement. **D,** The 7-months postoperative view.

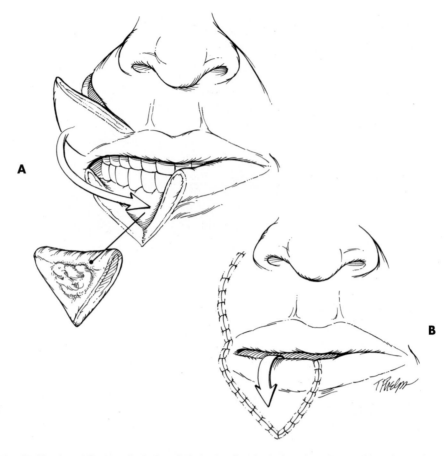

Fig. 27-20. A and **B,** Superiorly based Estlander flap is designed so the resulting donor site scar lies within or parallel to melolabial sulcus. Mucosal advancement assists in correcting discrepancies in vermilion vertical height of flap and recipient site. (Adapted from Baker SR, Swanson N: *Local flaps in facial reconstruction*, St Louis, 1995, Mosby.)

lized to form a new commissure. The mucous membrane is separated from the muscle and advanced outward to provide a vermilion border. Incisions are made in the gingival buccal sulcus as far posterior as the last molar tooth, if necessary, to allow proper approximation of the remaining lip segments without excessive wound closure tension.

Melolabial transposition flaps consisting of skin and subcutaneous tissue or full-thickness flaps consisting of skin, subcutaneous tissue, and mucosa can be useful in reconstructing lip defects as large as three fourths of the width of the lip.[11] Large skin-only defects of the lateral lip are repaired nicely with melolabial flaps; however, keeping with the principles of maintaining borders between aesthetic units, some surgeons prefer to repair defects that extend from the lip onto the cheek with two separate flaps (Fig. 27-21). A large rotation flap from the remaining lip segment is useful for repairing skin-only defects of the upper lip that extend into the cheek. The cheek component of the defect is then repaired by a separate transposition or advancement cheek flap. This places nearly all the scars in the melolabial sulcus while maintaining the integrity of the border between the lip and cheek aesthetic units.

Adjacent cheek tissue may not be applicable or sufficient for reconstruction of near-total defects of the lip. In such cases, regional flaps may be used for reconstruction. Excisions of the lower lip, chin, and anterior section of the mandible for carcinoma often require such flaps for reconstruction.

The temporal forehead flap designed as a bipedicle advancement or pedicle interpolation flap may be used for total upper lip reconstruction, but the unsightly secondary deformity precludes its common use. The flap may be lined with a split-thickness skin or mucosal graft. In males, hair-bearing scalp may be incorporated to provide hair growth for scar camouflage.

Several regional flaps are used for repair of large defects of the upper and lower lip. Other publications describe the use of regional flaps in lip reconstruction.[7]

RECONSTRUCTION OF CHEEK DEFECTS

Relative to the nose and lip, repair of cheek defects is less complex and is usually best accomplished with transposition or advancement flaps. Rhombic-shaped and other transposition flaps are very versatile and can be used anywhere in the cheek for small-to medium-sized defects. Par-

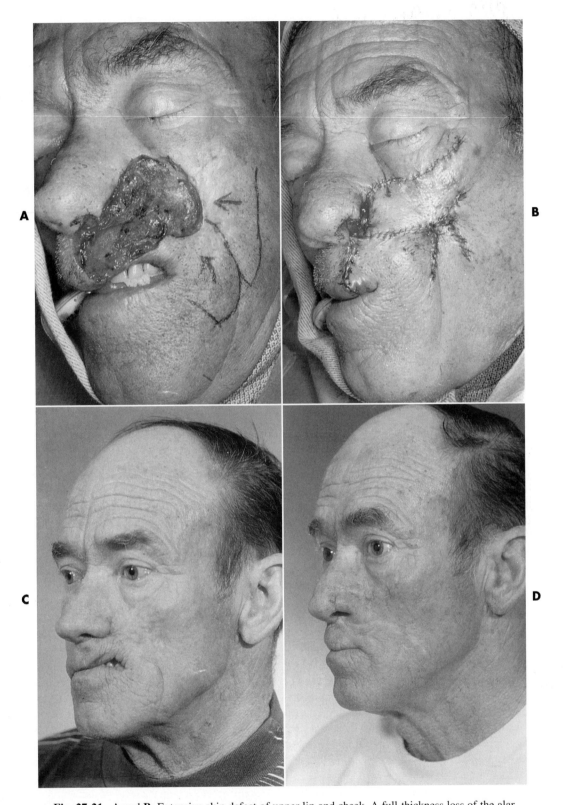

Fig. 27-21. A and **B,** Extensive skin defect of upper lip and cheek. A full-thickness loss of the alar lobule is present. Repair of cheek and lip defects are planned with flaps harvested from separate aesthetic units of the face. Repair of the alar defect is delayed. **C** and **D,** Preoperative *(left)* and 1-year postoperative view *(right)*. The alar lobule was reconstructed with a hinged septal mucosal flap, auricular cartilage graft, and paramedian forehead flap.

Continued

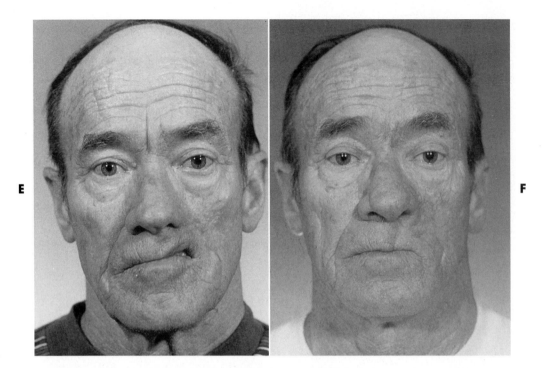

Fig. 27-21, cont'd. E and **F,** Preoperative *(left)* and 1-year postoperative view *(right).*

ticular attention should be placed in designing flaps for repair of defects near the lips or eyelids. For rhombic-shaped flaps, the orientation should be designed so that the area of greatest wound closure tension is away from these structures so as not to cause distortion. Rhombic-shaped flaps are a type of transposition advancement flap. This flap is useful when the defect has a shape of a rhombus with angles approximating 120° and 60°. Success of the flap depends on adjacent areas of redundant skin. These areas should lie adjacent to the 120° angle of the rhombus. The flap is designed by extending a line of the rhombus straight out from the point of the 120° angle. The length of this line should equal the length of the side of the rhombus. At the end of this line, a second line is extended parallel to the side of the defect and is of the same length. The flap is dissected in the subcutaneous plane and requires wide undermining of the entire area of the flap and defect. The flap is transposed and sutured into position. The donor site is closed primarily and represents the area of greatest wound closure tension. Usually a standing cutaneous deformity should be excised to complete the repair.

A bilobed flap represents a double transposition flap that has a single pivotal point and is useful in repairing larger cheek defects (Fig. 27-22). The axis of the two lobes is dependent on where the resource of tissue is located and as such, may be separated by a few degrees up to 180°. The greater the separation, the greater the standing cutaneous deformity between the two lobes. Large bilobed flaps are useful for repair of central and lateral cheek defects recruiting tissue from the remaining preauricular and infra-auricular areas. Depending on the location of the defect, the first

lobe may be designed as much as 20% smaller than the defect. It may be made even smaller when a great deal of advancement of the defect margins is possible or desirable. The second lobe that is used to repair the donor site of the first lobe is usually constructed 20% smaller than the first lobe. In general, the major advantage of a bilobed flap is the ability to recruit redundant tissue from two independent areas to assist in the repair of the defect. The major disadvantage of the flap is the extensive undermining that is required and the extensive linear scar that is created. When the incision lines do not fall within relaxed skin tension lines the scars may not be favorable. Bilobed flaps for repair of cheek defects should be based inferiorly, and the standing cutaneous deformities should be excised in such a way that the resulting scars are parallel to or lie within natural skin creases.

Rotation flaps are useful for repairing medial cheek defects in the vicinity of the border between the nasal sidewall and the cheek. The curvilinear border of the flap can often be positioned along the infraorbital rim, which represents an important aesthetic boundary. By positioning the incision for the flap along this border, the surgeon can enhance scar camouflage. When possible, the margin of the rotation flap should extend above the level of the lateral canthus to reduce the risk of lower lid retraction (Fig. 27-23). It may also be helpful to suspend the flap to the periosteum of the lateral orbital rim. Despite these precautions, lower lid retraction is not an uncommon sequela when a rotation flap is used to repair large medial cheek defects in elderly patients who frequently have lax lower eyelids. Large rotation flaps are

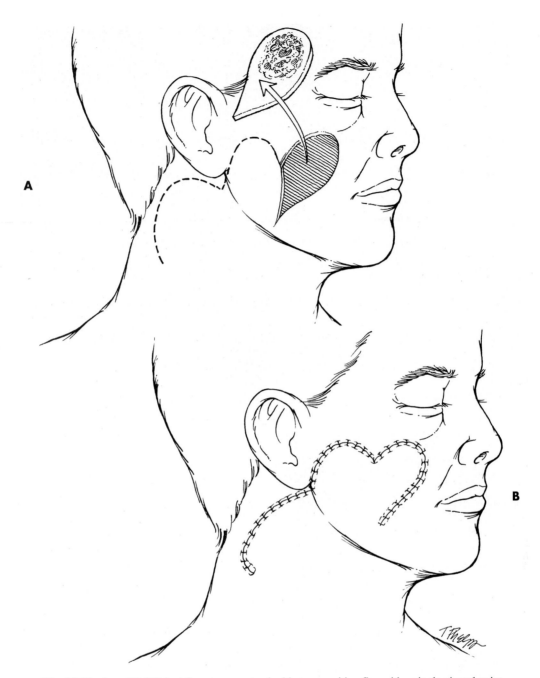

Fig. 27-22. A and **B,** Bilobed flaps represent a double transposition flap with a single pivotal point. (Adapted from Baker SR, Swanson N: *Local flaps in facial reconstruction*, St Louis, 1995, Mosby.)

particularly useful for reconstruction of sizable defects of the posterior cheek and upper neck. Large inferiorly based rotation flaps provide a flexible means for transfer of large amounts of skin from the remaining cheek and upper cervical skin.[3] Incisions for the flap are placed in a preauricular crease and can extend to the level of the clavicle or below along the anterior border of the trapezius muscle to facilitate rotation of the upper cervical skin toward the posterior cheek area. To enhance vascularity to such flaps, it is advantageous

to dissect the flap beneath the superficial musculoaponeurotic system in the cheek and beneath the platysmal muscle in the neck. A sub–superficial musculoaponeurotic system dissection in the face allows the placement of a great deal of tension on the flap without compromise of the skin vascularity. Care should be taken however, to not injure the mandibular branch of the facial nerve (Fig. 27-24).

Advancement flaps are dependent on the elasticity of the skin for successful repair. Many cheek defects can be closed

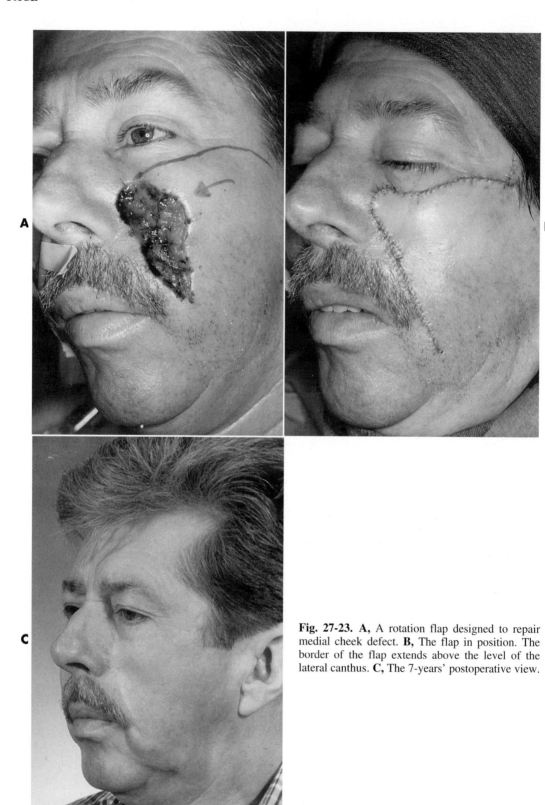

Fig. 27-23. **A,** A rotation flap designed to repair medial cheek defect. **B,** The flap in position. The border of the flap extends above the level of the lateral canthus. **C,** The 7-years' postoperative view.

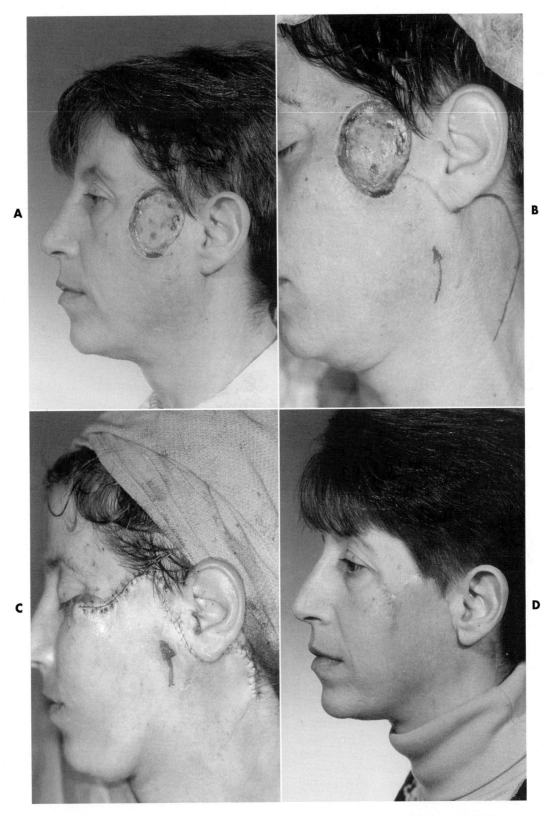

Fig. 27-24. A, A large cheek defect in a 40-year-old female smoker. No redundant cheek skin is available because of the patient's age. **B,** A bilobed cheek and neck flap designed for repair. **C,** The flap is transferred. The flap was dissected beneath the superficial musculoaponeurotic system, which allowed great wound closure tension without compromise of skin vascularity. **D,** The 3-months postoperative view.

or greatly reduced in size by simply advancing the defect margins and closing as much of the defect as possible within relaxed skin tension lines. Advancement flaps may be designed so that the incisions fall within natural skin creases of the cheek. To follow this principle, incisions used to form the border of the flap usually should diverge slightly rather than remain completely parallel. It is usually necessary to remove bilateral standing cutaneous deformities near the base of the flap. This should be accomplished in such a way that the resulting scar lies within relaxed skin tension lines. As an alternative, to bilateral Z-plasties at the base of the flap reduce or eliminate the standing cutaneous deformities. Advancement flaps work well for medial and central cheek defects.

V-Y advancement flaps are particularly useful for repair of small-and medium-sized skin defects of the medial cheek near the alar facial sulcus. This technique is useful for younger patients in whom there is a lack of redundant facial skin and in patients who have considerable subcutaneous facial fat (chipmunk cheeks) (Fig. 27-25). The flap is designed in a triangular configuration with the surface area of the flap 1.5 to 2 times the surface area of the defect. The skin of the flap is isolated as an island on a subcutaneous pedicle by incising through skin around the perimeter of the flap. The subcutaneous pedicle is then dissected flaring away from the margins of the flap. Incisions should be made through the fat down to the level of the facial musculature. This deep dissection provides the mobility of the flap, enabling it to be advanced 2 to 3 cm. This mobility is enhanced by undermining the proximal and distal one-fourth of the flap just deep to the skin. The peripheral margins of the donor and recipient site should also be undermined for 2 cm in the subcutaneous plane to provide for secondary tissue movement and easy closure of the donor site. The flap is advanced and sutured in the recipient site first, followed by layered closure of the donor site.

A disadvantage of the V-Y subcutaneous advancement flap is that not all of the incisions used to harvest the flap fall within relaxed skin tension lines. However, when appropriately selected, the flap has many advantages. A major advantage is the limited dissection required compared with other techniques. Thus, there is minimal dead space with a concomitant reduced risk of the development of hematoma and seroma. Another major advantage is that no standing cutaneous deformity develops and, therefore, no tissue is discarded. The flap is harvested from the jowl area, where facial skin is most redundant and, as a consequence, there is minimal or no deformity of the melolabial fold and sulcus.

Most skin defects of the cheek can be repaired with primary closure, transposition, or rotation flaps. Transposition flaps tend to be very useful and are usually harvested from adjacent cheek skin, but they can be developed in the upper neck to resurface larger defects in the lower cheek. Melolabial transposition flaps are best designed as a superiorly based flap (Fig. 27-26). This design allows the recruitment of re-dundant skin in the lower medial face for construction of the flap. Such flaps can be used for small- to moderate-sized defects of the upper, middle, and lower medial aspect of the cheek. Positioning the base of the flap near the alar facial sulcus enhances the vascularity of the flap by including the numerous perforating vessels that extend into the subcutaneous tissue from the facial artery. Superiorly based transposition flaps are excellent for repairing defects of the medial and lateral aspect of the cheek. The flap is designed so that the medial border of the flap lies in the melolabial sulcus whenever possible. The width of the flap is dependent on the size of the defect and the quantity of donor site resource. The larger the flap or the greater the arc of pivot, the larger the standing cutaneous deformity. Excision of standing cutaneous deformities of the cheek can be accomplished at the time of flap transfer or delayed for a second stage; however, some excision of the standing cutaneous deformity is nearly always necessary because it will not completely absorb by itself.

FOREHEAD DEFECTS

Reconstruction of defects of the forehead should accomplish the following goals:[19] (1) preservation of frontalis muscle function, (2) preservation of sensation of the forehead skin, and (3) placement of scars within aesthetic borders or the horizontal furrows of the forehead. The forehead aesthetic unit is defined by junctional lines with the frontal scalp superiorly, the temporal scalp and temple laterally, and the eyebrows and glabella inferiorly. The forehead can be divided into aesthetic subunits, which include median, paramedian, and lateral temple.[19] The median is in the midline of the forehead. The paramedian extends from midline to a vertical axis above the pupil, and the lateral temple extends from the paramedian border to the temporal hair line laterally. Siegle[19] noted that when planning repair of forehead defects aesthetic goals include (1) maintenance of eyebrow symmetry, (2) maintenance of natural appearing temporal and frontal hairlines, (3) the hiding of scars when possible along hairlines or eyebrows, (4) the creation of transverse instead of vertical scars whenever possible (except in the midline forehead), and (5) the avoidance of diagonal scars.

Primary wound repair of defects of forehead skin are often possible in older individuals and in those with sun-damaged skin. Deep horizontal furrows may provide extra skin for reconstruction. When primary closure is not possible, the use of single or multiple local flaps is preferred over skin grafts because of the poor aesthetic result from the use of skin grafts. When a local flap is not possible, healing by second intention is often less deforming than a skin graft. For midline forehead defects, healing by second intention often produces a very acceptable aesthetic result, particularly when the defect is located in the superior aspect of the forehead. Should the scar not be acceptable, a later scar revision usually provides an excellent result.

Defects of the central one third of the forehead can be

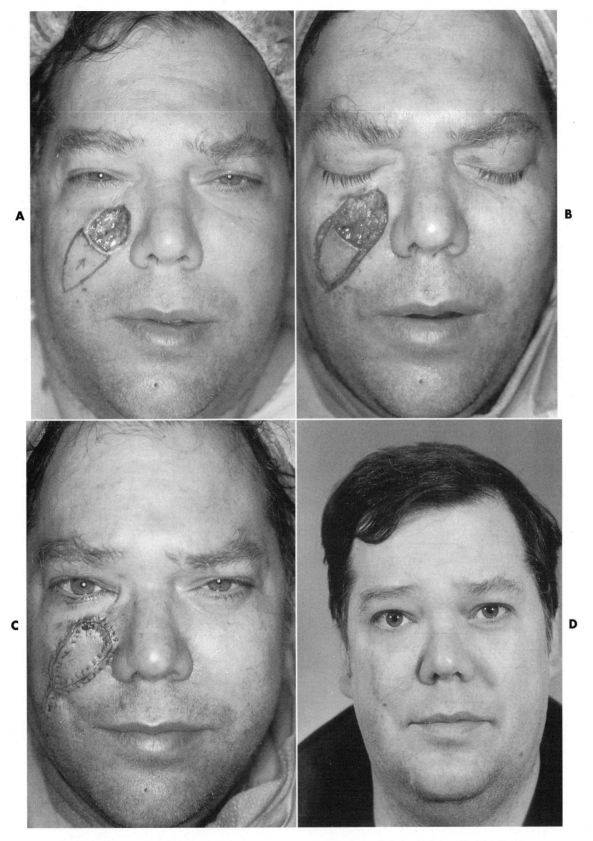

Fig. 27-25. A, The V-Y advancement flap designed to repair medial cheek defect. **B,** The flap is based on the subcutaneous pedicle. **C,** The flap is positioned in a recipient site. **D,** The 5-month's postoperative view.

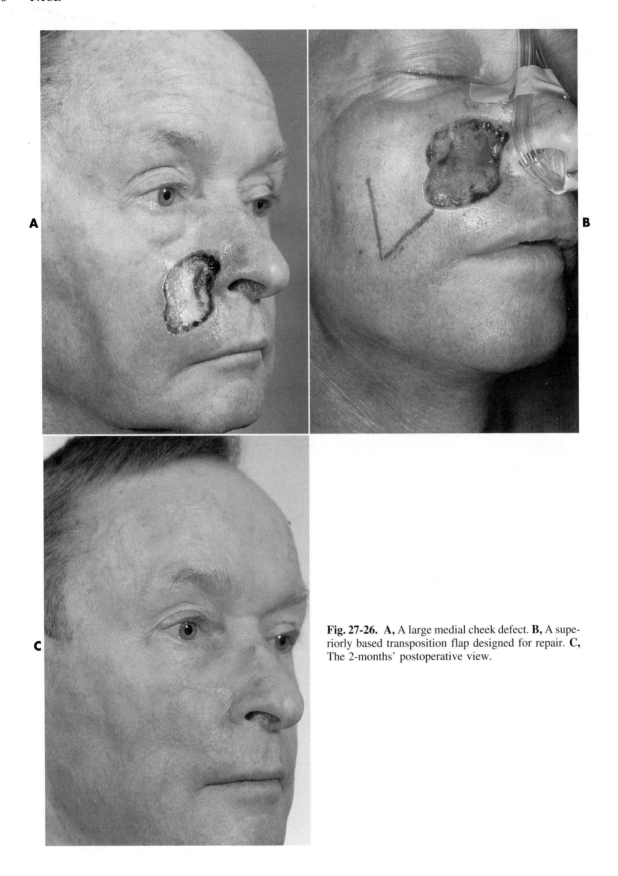

Fig. 27-26. A, A large medial cheek defect. **B,** A superiorly based transposition flap designed for repair. **C,** The 2-months' postoperative view.

repaired in a vertical axis with a predictably pleasant aesthetic result. This is probably caused by the natural dehiscence or attenuation of the frontalis muscle in this portion of the forehead. Larger midline defects closed in a vertical orientation may result in large standing cutaneous deformities, which may be excised with use of a W-plasty within glabellar creases (Fig. 27-27). An M-plasty superiorly may also be necessary to eliminate a standing cutaneous deformity at the hairline. M-plasty and W-plasty techniques reduce the overall vertical length of the closure scar. This type of repair allows extensive undermining in the subfascial plane to facilitate closure without compromise of motor or sensory function of the forehead.

In general, vertical oriented primary repairs, rotation flaps and transposition flaps are to be avoided in the repair of paramedian forehead defects because they often result in verticle scars.[19] Vertical scars in the lateral two thirds of the forehead on either side are usually wide and quite noticeable. Such scars should be avoided whenever possible and revised with a geometric closure when present. Median and par-

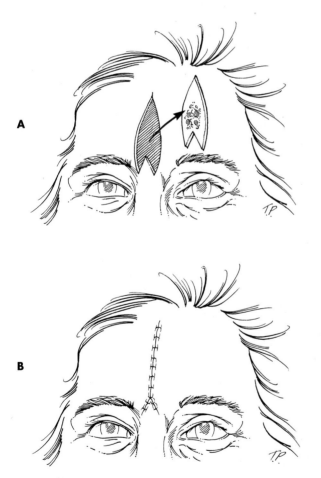

Fig. 27-27. A and **B,** Closure of large midline forehead defects are often facilitated by W-plasties inferior or M-plasties superior to the border of the defect. (Adapted from Baker SR, Swanson N: *Local flaps in facial reconstruction,* St Louis, 1995, Mosby.)

amedian forehead defects can be reconstructed with unilateral or bilateral advancement flaps, keeping most of the resulting scars oriented horizontally.

The lateral forehead represents a transition in topography from the convexity of the median and paramedian forehead to a flat lateral forehead, which continues into a slightly concave temple. The slightly concave nature of the temple makes this region of the forehead particularly good for healing by second intention. The enhanced elasticity of lateral forehead skin compared with more centrally located skin allows more reconstructive options. Primary wound closure is also often feasible with orientation of the repair parallel to the forehead skin creases, which become curvilinear as they arc downward toward the cheek. These lines are excellent locations for placement of incisions. The location of the temporal hairline and the brow dictate the orientation and size of advancement, rotation, and transposition flaps in this area. The surgeon should take particular care in the lateral forehead area when dissecting such flaps because of the vulnerability of the frontal branch of the facial nerve. Advancement and advancement rotation flaps are perhaps most useful for repair of lateral forehead defects (Fig. 27-28). Usually bilateral advancement flaps are preferred over single flaps, with the greatest advancement achieved from the more elastic laterally based flaps.

A variation of advancement flaps for repair of medium-sized defects of both the lateral and paramedian forehead is the O-T or A-T repair. This method consists of extending horizontal incisions along both sides of the defect within relaxed skin tension lines or along the border of the brow or temporal hairline. The two flaps are dissected in the subcutaneous plane and advanced toward the triangular or circular shaped defect (Fig. 27-29). Standing cutaneous deformities are resected when necessary from within the brow or are eliminated by the rule of halving the wound closure. If necessary, the standing cutaneous deformity that results from the pivotal portion of the flap movement may be removed by enlarging the defect itself. The final wound closure takes the configuration of a T-shaped repair. Thus, circular defects closed in this manner are referred to as an *O-T repair* and triangular defects (A-shaped) are referred to as an *A-T repair.* These techniques camouflage scars, except for those along the central vertical wound closure line.

Rotation flaps are very useful in reconstructing medium and large lateral forehead defects. A unilateral rotation flap based inferiorly and laterally and designed so that its curvilinear incision follows the margin of the temporal hairline is an excellent method of reconstructing lateral forehead defects that are close to the hairline. The curvilinear incision can be designed to incorporate hair-bearing scalp to bring hair into the reconstructed area if some of the temporal tuft has been lost.[19] The standing cutaneous deformity that inevitably forms with such a flap can be removed inferiorly in the crow's feet to camouflage the scar.

The most effective technique for reconstruction of the forehead usually involves one or more advancement flaps.

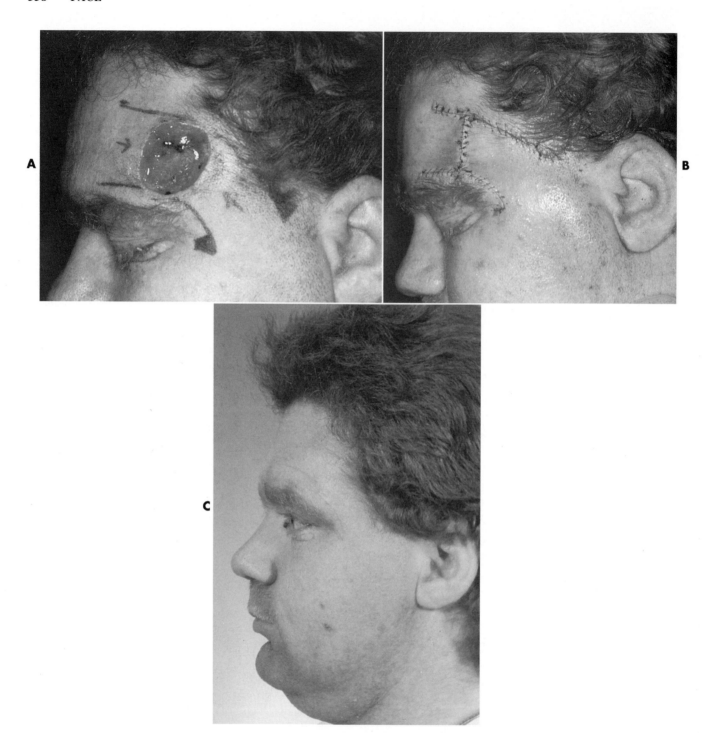

Fig. 27-28. A, The medially based advancement and laterally based advancement rotation flap designed to repair lateral forehead defect. **B,** The flaps advanced. A standing cutaneous deformity of the laterally based flap is removed in periocular rhytid. **C,** The 6-months' postoperative view.

Despite the relative inelasticity of forehead skin, the use of advancement flaps is preferred because they produce the most favorable cosmetic result. However, the surgeon should be aware that many skin defects of the forehead can be successfully managed by allowing the wound to heal by secondary intention. This often gives a cosmetic result that is comparable with that of flap repair when the appropriate forehead site is selected. An ideal location for healing by secondary intention is high on the forehead well away from the brow, in the central or lateral third of the forehead.

Tissue expansion enables the surgeon to reconstruct sizable forehead defects, which in the past could be repaired

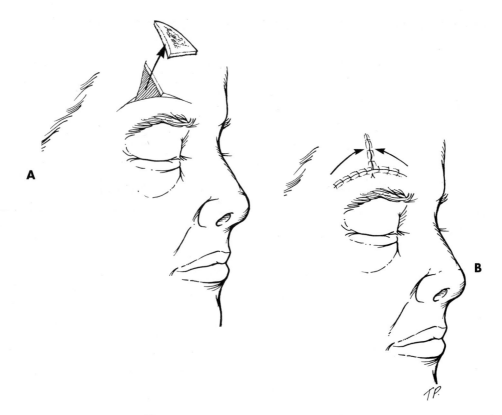

Fig. 27-29. A and **B,** A T-shaped repair of a lateral forehead defect. (Adapted from Baker SR, Swanson N: *Local flaps in facial reconstruction*, St Louis, 1995, Mosby.)

only with skin grafts. Controlled, prolonged tissue expansion can be used to reconstruct very large forehead defects by expansion of the remaining forehead skin over 6 to 12 weeks. Reconstruction is achieved by direct advancement of the expanded skin or used in combination with other scalp, cheek or temple skin flaps. The disadvantages of tissue expansion include the fact that it is a two-staged procedure and considerable deformity of the forehead is present during the expansion process. These disadvantages are far outweighed by the excellent results that can be achieved with tissue expansion in the repair of very large defects of the forehead.[9]

REFERENCES

1. Alford EL, Baker SR, Shumrick KA: *Midforehead flaps.* In Baker SR, Swanson NA, editors: *Local flaps in facial reconstruction*, St Louis, 1995, Mosby.

2. Baker SR: *Lip reconstruction.* In Holt GR, Gates GA, Mattox DE, editors: *Decision making in otolaryngology*, Burlington, Ontario, 1983, Mosby.

3. Baker SR: Local cutaneous flaps in soft tissue augmentation and reconstruction in the head and neck, *Otolaryngol Clin North Am* 27:139, 1994.

4. Baker SR: *Malignancy of the lip.* In Gluckman J, editor: *Otolaryngology*, ed 3, Philadelphia, 1988, WB Saunders.

5. Baker SR: *Options for reconstruction in head and neck surgery.* In Cummings CW and others, editors: *Otolaryngology—head and neck surgery: update 1*, St Louis, 1989, Mosby.

6. Baker SR: *The orbit and midface.* In Soutar DS, Tiwari R, editors: *Excision and reconstruction in head and neck cancer*, New York, 1994, Churchill Livingstone.

7. Baker SR: Regional flaps in facial reconstruction, *Facial Plast Surg* 23, 5, 925, 1990.

8. Baker SR, Johnson TM, Nelson BR: The importance of maintaining the alar facial sulcus in nasal reconstruction, *Arch Otolaryngol Head Neck Surg* 121:617, 1995.

9. Baker SR, Johnson TM, Nelson BR: Technical aspects of prolonged scalp expansion, *Arch Otolaryngol Head Neck Surg* 120:431, 1994.

10. Baker SR, Krause CJ: *Cancer of the lip.* In Suen JY, Myers EN, editor: *Cancer of the head and neck*, New York, 1981, Churchill Livingstone.

11. Baker SR, Krause CJ: Pedicle flaps in reconstruction of the lip, *Facial Plast Surg* 1:61, 1983.

12. Baker SR, Swanson NA: Regional and distant skin flaps in nasal reconstruction, *Facial Plast Surg* 2:33, 1984.

13. Burget GC, Menick FJ: *Aesthetic reconstruction of the nose*, St Louis, 1993, Mosby.

13a. Bernard C: Concer de la levre inferieure opéré par un procédé nouveau, *Bulletin et memoirs de la société de chirugic* 3:357, 1853.

14. Estlander JA: Eine methods aus der einen Lippe Substanzverlustre der Onderen zu Ersetzen, *Arch für Klin Chir* 14:622, 1872.

15. Grabb WC, Myers MB: *Skin flaps*, Boston, 1975, Little Brown.

16. Johnson TM and others: Utility of the subcutaneous hinge flap in nasal reconstruction, *Dermatol Surg* 3:459, 1994.

17. Karapandzic M: Reconstruction of lip defects by local arterial flaps, *Br J Plast Surg* 27:93, 1974.

18. Panje WR, Minor LB: *Reconstruction of the scalp.* In Baker SR, Swanson NA, editors: *Local flaps in facial reconstruction*, St Louis, 1995, Mosby.

19. Siegle RJ: *Reconstruction of the forehead.* In Baker SR, Swanson NA, editors: *Local flaps in facial reconstruction*, St Louis, 1995, Mosby.

20. Webster JP: Crescentic peri-alar cheek excision for upper lip flap advancement with a short history of upper lip repair, *Plast Reconstr Surg* 16:434, 1955.

Chapter 28

Local Anesthesia in Facial Plastic Surgery

Craig S. Murakami
Maurice Morad Khosh

Local anesthesia plays an important role in facial plastic and reconstructive surgery. The effectiveness of local anesthesia has allowed the development of procedures that require increasing precision and operative time. Often, the vital role of local anesthetics in the success of operations goes unnoticed. Infiltration of local anesthetic agents is frequently considered a task that precedes an operation. In reality, it should be considered as the step that begins the operation. Proper local anesthesia will significantly improve homostasis, decrease patient discomfort, and effectively reduce surgical morbidity. Therefore, administration of anesthesia should be attended to carefully. Surgeons who practice facial plastic and reconstructive surgery often find themselves performing the dual role of anesthesiologist. Because of this added responsibility, it is imperative that surgeons be familiar with basic information pertaining to local anesthesia and intravenous sedation and become proficient in their administration.

HISTORY

The use of local anesthetic agents probably began thousands of years ago in the Andes Mountains. The mountain villagers chewed the leaves of the *Erythroxylon coca* bush for its euphoric properties and its magical ability to increase endurance and strength.[2,30] Peruvian artifacts dating back to 2500 BC yield evidence of widespread cocaine use as an anesthetic agent. Peruvians with skull fractures, headaches, and mental illness underwent the religious rite of trephination by the village shaman, who spat cocaine-filled saliva into the wound. This ritual offered vital anesthesia and hemostasis to an otherwise painful and bloody procedure.

It was not until 1860 that Niemann[52] isolated the alkaloid cocaine from *E. coca* and documented its anesthetic effect on the tongue. Freud was a proponent of cocaine as a medicinal agent and studied the drug diligently. In 1884, he published the widely read *Cocaine Papers*, in which he recommended cocaine for multiple ailments (e.g., morphine addiction, fatigue, depression).[12] Koller,[39] a Viennese ophthalmologist, began using cocaine as a topical anesthetic agent for ophthalmologic surgery.[39] Soon thereafter cocaine was successfully used by surgeons as a topical anesthetic for laryngeal[63] and nasal surgery.[8,60] Sporadic reports described how to obtain anesthesia by direct injection of cocaine into the operative field using a hypodermic syringe.[53,59] In 1885, Halsted[32] reported the first peripheral nerve block using an injection of cocaine at the root of the nerve, a technique that led to the development and practice of regional anesthesia.

Throughout the late 1800s and the early 1900s, widespread use of cocaine led to an appreciation of its toxic and addictive properties. A search for less toxic local anesthetics resulted in synthesis of procaine (an ester derivative of *p*-aminobenzoic acid) by Einhorn[28] in 1899. Other ester derivatives, such as tetracaine and chloroprocaine, were subsequently developed. In 1948, Lofgren[45] synthesized lidocaine, the first amide anesthetic. Lidocaine caused fewer allergic reactions and adverse responses than the ester compounds, and its success led to a widespread search for other amide anesthetics.

MECHANISM OF ACTION

Electrical phenomena in nerve membranes depend on (1) differences in concentration of sodium and potassium in the nerve axonoplasm and the extracellular fluid and (2) the permeability of the nerve membrane to these ions. In the resting state, there is a -60- to -90-millivolt (mV) potential across the nerve cell membrane. Impulse conduction in neurons is primarily the result of a change in cell membrane permeability to sodium ions. Stimulation of a nerve triggers the activation of sodium channels and an influx of sodium ions into the cell, causing a membrane depolarization. Local anesthetics work by blocking sodium ion permeability, thus preventing the propagation of an action potential.

The exact mechanism by which local anesthetic agents block sodium influx and nerve conduction is not clear. Early investigators proposed a membrane expansion theory, which held that local anesthetic agents caused nonspecific expansion of the nerve cell membrane, constricting sodium channels. The membrane expansion blocked the influx of sodium ions, limiting membrane depolarization and thus preventing the subsequent conduction of action potentials in the nerve. Investigators now postulate that a specific membrane receptor in or near the sodium channel regulates sodium permeability.* The sodium channel is proposed to be a large polypeptide with four homologous regions, each containing six to eight amino acids. The homologous subunits form an α helical structure, which spans the cell membrane. The sodium channel is rendered open by a shift in configuration of the α helix, which creates a pore in the center of the α helix for passage of ions. It is suggested that local anesthetics inhibit membrane depolarization by binding to a region of the α helix and by preventing the configuration shift necessary for sodium channel activation.[11]

Local anesthetic effects vary according to the class of nerves that are involved. Nerves can be classified broadly into three major categories (A, B, C) based on their relative size. Cutaneous sensory nerves of the face are small, nonmyelinated C fibers that are rapidly blocked by a local anesthetic. The B fibers are small myelinated preganglionic sympathetic nerves that are slightly resistant to anesthetic blockade. Finally, A fibers are large myelinated fibers that conduct motor function, proprioception, pressure sensation, and to a lesser degree, pain and temperature. A fibers are the most resistant to anesthetic agents. Because of these differences, sequential nerve blockade begins with pain and temperature sensitivity, then proprioception, and lastly motor function. The usual concentrations of local anesthesia typically block pain fibers without affecting motor function.

CLASSIFICATION

An ideal local anesthetic agent would temporarily block sensory nerves with a short onset time, have excellent tissue penetration, exhibit minimal tissue reaction, and be painless

*Refs. 19, 20, 22, 35, 43, 57, 66.

to administer. To achieve these goals, various manipulations are made at distinct sites on the anesthetic molecule. Local anesthetics contain three distinct moieties: (1) a tertiary amine that is the hydrophilic portion, (2) an aromatic ring that is the hydrophobic portion, and (3) a connection that is an amide or ester linkage. Changes in the hydrophilic portion affect the anesthetic agent's solubility, whereas changes in the hydrophobic portion affect the agent's ability to penetrate nerve membranes. The tertiary amine portion of the agent is found in the protonated quaternary ammonium salt form and the unprotonated amine base form (Fig. 28-1). The uncharged form is capable of nerve membrane penetration, whereas the charged form is believed to enhance water solubility and possess the bioactivity that is responsible for blocking sodium channels and preventing nerve conduction. The distribution of these two forms of a particular anesthetic is dictated by the unique pKa (dissociation constant) of each agent. The pKa is the hydrogen ion concentration (pH) at which both forms are found in equal proportions. Most agents have a pKa of eight to nine, which indicates that 5% to 35% of the molecules are in the uncharged form at physiologic pH.[20]

An anesthetic compound falls under 1 of 2 broad categories depending on whether it has an ester or an amide linkage between the aromatic ring and the tertiary amine. Numerous local anesthetic agents from the ester and amide groups are currently available. This discussion is limited to the agents most commonly used in facial plastic surgery (Table 28-1).

Table 28-1. Local anesthetics

Drug	Class	Onset	Duration (hr)	Dose (mg/kg)
Cocaine	Ester	Rapid	1-2	3
Tetracaine	Ester	Delayed	2-3	1
Lidocaine	Amide	Rapid	1-2	3-5 plain
				5-7 with epinephrine
Bupivacaine	Amide	Delayed	2-4	3

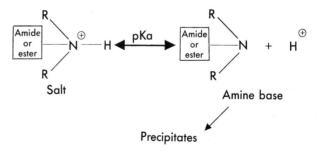

Fig. 28-1. Anesthetic dissociation. Note that a higher pH will promote formation of an amine base form and precipitate local anesthetics.

Esters

Cocaine is still the most frequently used ester anesthetic because of its rapid onset of action and excellent hemostatic effect. It is unique among the local anesthetic agents because of its vasoconstrictive and euphoric effects. Cocaine is a benzoic acid ester, whereas most other agents of the amino-ester category are derivatives of p-aminobenzoic acid. By preventing uptake of norepinephrine from terminal synapses, cocaine causes vasoconstriction, and sensitizes the patient to catecholamines. Excessive stimulation of the sympathetic system can result in multiple untoward cardiovascular responses (tachycardia, blood pressure changes, diaphoresis, vasospasm). Cocaine is administered topically with a maximum dose of 3 mg/kg[38] (approximately 200 mg for the average adult), although some sources allow even higher doses.[33,71] The drug is supplied as a 4% or 10% solution. Toxicity correlates with the total amount of drug administered not the concentration. In most cases, 4 to 5 ml of a 4% solution provides adequate anesthesia for an intranasal procedure. Current commercial preparations of cocaine are usually in 1-unit dose vials with an identifying dye marker to avoid overdosing or accidental infiltration. The combination of cocaine with 1:1000 epinephrine to form cocaine mud is dangerous and is no longer recommended because of the combined catecholamine effects of these ingredients.[33,48,56]

Unfortunately, systemic effects have been noted with cocaine use within the clinically safe dosage; (e.g., coronary artery vasospasm has been documented with intranasal doses as low as 2 mg/kg).[15,36,41,62] Thus, cocaine should be administered with great care and frugality. Pledgets should be vigorously squeezed to eliminate excess drug before application to minimize drainage into the pharynx. The pledgets should be removed after 5 to 10 minutes to prevent unnecessary absorption of cocaine. Many surgeons have abandoned cocaine because of its associated problems and adopted a less toxic combination of lidocaine with oxymetazoline or phenylepherine.

Tetracaine is another topical ester anesthetic used for head and neck anesthesia. This extremely potent anesthetic should be used judiciously to avoid complications. The maximum dose is 1 mg/kg[38] which makes this agent approximately six times more toxic than lidocaine with epinephrine. Tetracaine was at one time widely used as a topical agent in endoscopy and tonsillectomy, but there were frequent complications because of a lack of strict dosage monitoring.[48] Today, tetracaine is used in a limited number of ways with strict dosage schedules. Ophthalmic preparations are commonly used in occuloplastic surgery. Tetracaine with epinephrine and cocaine can be safely used topically to anesthetize small cutaneous wounds.[14,54] Absorption through cutaneous wounds is believed to be slower and safer than absorption through mucous membranes.[1,13] Therefore, tetracaine with epinephrine and cocaine is not recommended

---

> **Box 28-1.** TAC dosages
>
> 10 kg = 0.5 ml
> 20 kg = 1.0 ml
> 30 kg = 1.5 ml
> 40 kg = 2.0 ml
> Maximum dose of cocaine is 2.5 mg/kg.
> Maximum dose of tetracaine is 5 mg/kg.

TAC—0.5% tetracaine, 1:2000 epinephrine, 2% cocaine.

for use on nasal, oral, or mucosal lacerations. The usual concentration of tetracaine with epinephrine and cocaine is 0.5% tetracaine, 1:2000 (0.5 mg/ml) epinephrine, and 11.8% cocaine. However, a weaker solution (0.5% tetracaine, 1:2000 epinephrine, 2% cocaine) has been used with equal success. The dose schedule for this weaker solution is listed in Box 28-1. This needle-free anesthetic has become especially popular for treating pediatric lacerations, in which the administration of local anesthesia is often more difficult than the wound repair.[14,54,74] Although animal studies have demonstrated that tetracaine with epinephrine and cocaine diminishes the cellular defense to bacterial inoculations,[6] this has not been found to be of clinical significance in humans.[14]

Amides

The most frequently used anesthetic agent in soft-tissue surgery is lidocaine. This agent has a rapid onset, excellent tissue penetration, a 1- to 3-hour duration of action, and minimal local and systemic toxicity. In most circumstances, lidocaine is used with 1:100,000 or 1:200,000 epinephrine to provide hemostasis, increase anesthetic duration, and reduce systemic toxicity. The toxic dose is 3 mg/kg (approximately 200 mg in the average person) and 5 to 7 mg/kg (approximately 500 mg), respectively, without and with epinephrine.[38] Although it is usually administered by infiltration, lidocaine also is effective as a topical 4% solution when applied to mucosal membranes.

Eutectic lidocaine and prilocaine 5% cream is a topical preparation for cutaneous application. To be effective, the cream is applied to skin surface 30 to 60 minutes before a procedure. This results in superficial anesthesia, which can reduce the pain of needle sticks, cannula insertion, curettage, skin biopsies, and harvesting of skin grafts.[4,31,40,65] The potential for inducing methemoglobinemia, attributed to a metabolite of the prilocaine component of the formulation, prohibits its use in infants younger than 6 months.[10]

Bupivacaine is an amide agent used for longer procedures because of its extended duration of action of 2 to 4 hours. It is used in concentrations of 0.25% or 0.50% with or without 1:200,000 epinephrine and is generally safe and effective. Compared with lidocaine, it has a slower onset time but has an increased potency and toxicity. The recommended dose is 3.0 to 3.5 mg/kg or approximately 225 mg in an average adult.[21,38,75]

VASOCONSTRICTOR AGENTS

Vasoconstrictor agents are frequently combined with local anesthetics to minimize local bleeding, enhance the duration of action, and reduce plasma concentrations, thereby diminishing potential systemic toxicity. Epinephrine is the most commonly used vasoconstrictor. Norepinephrine, levonorfedrin, and phenylephrine are less commonly used. The addition of epinephrine increases the anesthetic duration by 30% to 50%. Epinephrine is an α- and a β-receptor stimulant but is primarily used for local α-receptor stimulation on vascular smooth muscle. With commercial epinephrine concentrations of 10 μg/ml (1:100,000) or 5 μg/ml (1:200,000), toxicity is rarely a problem as long as nontoxic doses of a local anesthetic agent are administered. However, other medications or medical conditions may sensitize patients to epinephrine, and these particular situations should be reviewed. Epinephrine concentrations of 1:100,000 or 1:200,000 are as effective in achieving hemostasis as more concentrated forms.[42,49,64] In most facial soft-tissue operations, the degree of vasoconstriction caused by these concentrations of epinephrine in the local anesthetic does not affect flap survival. The exception is in flaps that are delayed before transposition. In this situation, flap survival is adversely affected, and anesthetics without epinephrine are recommended.[55,77]

HYALURONIDASE

Hyaluronidase is an enzyme found in certain strains of streptococcal bacteria, snake venom, ox spleen, and the testicle of mammals. The clinical usefulness of this enzyme relates to its ability to cleave the bond between the moieties that form the ground substance in connective tissue. Commercially, hyaluronidase, which is of bovine testicular origin, is available as a lyopholized powder or in a stabilized solution containing 150 or 1500 units/ml United States Pharmacopela. The recommended total dose is 1500 units.

Adding, 1 to 2 ml of a local anesthetic to a vial of lyopholized hyaluronidase (1500 units), results in immediate dissolution of the hyaluronidase. This mixture is then added to the total volume of anesthetic to be used. Smaller amounts of hyaluronidase can be used, although 1500 units is the recommended dose regardless of the volume injected. Allergic reactions to hyaluronidase have been reported, and its use in atopic patients is cautioned.[72]

Duran-Reynolds[27] was the first to investigate the spreading ability of hyaluronidase combined with local anesthetics. When the tissue was massaged, the spread of the infiltrate greatly increased. This spreading ability also results in less tissue distortion when hyaluronidase is added to local anesthetics. Other reported benefits of hyaluronidase include rapid tissue infiltration and increased area of anesthesia.[18,44,69] Conflicting reports regarding onset and duration

of anesthesia exist.[12] Hyaluronidase is currently used by many surgeons in various cosmetic or reconstructive surgical procedures of the face.

METABOLISM

Esters and amides differ dramatically in their metabolic breakdown. The esters are hydrolyzed by plasma pseudocholinesterases.[20] Procaine and tetracaine hydrolysis results in p-aminobenzoic acid, which is excreted in the urine. This metabolite, and not the intact anesthetic molecule, accounts for the unwanted allergic reactions. Cocaine is different and undergoes degradation by plasma esterases to benzoylecgonine and ecgonine.[50]

Metabolism of amides is generally more complex than ester degradation and results in multiple metabolites that require excretion. Amides are primarily metabolized by the liver, and only small amounts are excreted unchanged in the urine. Therefore, patients with significant hepatic disease or taking drugs that affect hepatic metabolism may reach toxic blood levels of anesthetic after administration of nontoxic anesthetic dosages. Cimetidine is most notable among the drugs that alter hepatic degradation of amides. Lidocaine blood concentrations have been found to be significantly higher in patients concurrently taking cimetidine.

ADVERSE DRUG INTERACTIONS

Halogenated inhalation anesthetics used for general anesthesia sensitize the myocardium to epinephrine. Current recommendations are that under general anesthesia with halogenated agents the maximum doses of epinephrine to which patients should be exposed are 4 μg/kg with halothane; 6 μg/kg with isoflurane, and 8 μg/kg with enflurane.

Patients taking monoamine oxidase inhibitors (MAOIs) for treatment of depression should avoid epinephrine, which may incite a hypertensive crisis. These patients are especially sensitive to the narcotic meperidine. To a lesser degree, tricyclic antidepressants also sensitize patients to epinephrine. Patients taking these medications should seek recommendations from their physician as to the possibility of discontinuing the drug perioperatively.

Antihypertensive β-blockers were thought to adversely affect the administration of epinephrine by creating an unopposed α environment. Initial recommendations were to discontinue the use of β-blockers in the preoperative period. This led to rebound hypertension in some patients. Current recommendations are to continue the use of β-blockers through the preoperative period and into the immediate postoperative period.[17,46]

ADMINISTRATION TECHNIQUE

Most local anesthetic agents are relatively insoluble at physiologic pH and are made water-soluble by being dissolved in weak solutions of hydrochloric acid. In addition, anesthetics often contain epinephrine to promote vasoconstriction. Anesthetic solutions are typically stored at a low pH of 3.5 to 5 to prevent degradation of light-sensitive epinephrine to adenochrome.[23] A low pH solution is very painful when administered by infiltration. Adding an 8.4% sodium bicarbonate buffer to the anesthetic agent in a 1:10 ratio raises the pH to 7.2 to 7.4 (Fig. 28-2) and dramatically reduces the pain of injection.[3] If sodium bicarbonate is added immediately before injection, there is little precipitation of the anesthetic agent or degradation of the epinephrine.[51] A buffered solution will contain more anesthetic agent in the non-protonated, uncharged form. Theoretically, this promotes nerve penetration (Fig. 28-3) and quickens the onset of anesthesia without increasing the duration of nerve blockade.[9,12,24,34,67] This characteristic has been of benefit in regional spinal anesthesia, but this minor increase in nerve penetration appears to have little consequence in facial surgery. A low pH environment increases the protonated form of the local anesthetic and may inhibit nerve penetration and delay the onset of anesthesia. This partly explains the difficulty in anesthetizing infected tissue, which is usually acidic. Whether buffered anesthetics are more effective than unbuffered anesthetics in low pH environments remains unknown.

Administration of local anesthetics is generally simple and safe but is usually associated with temporary patient discomfort. This discomfort is attributed to the pain of skin puncture, the acidity of the local anesthetic, and the hydrostatic pressure of the anesthetic infiltration. These factors are further accentuated by the patient's anxiety and the sympathomimetic effects of epinephrine. Several simple maneuvers can diminish patient discomfort during anesthetic infiltration. For small procedures, the pain caused by the initial needle puncture can be blunted by applying ice or EMLA cream to the area to be treated. Use of a small-gauge needle further reduces the pain of skin puncture. The pain of infiltration is significantly reduced by neutralizing the local anesthetics with sodium bicarbonate,[3] and by infiltrating slowly to minimize hydrostatic pressure in the tissues. Five to 10 minutes should be allowed for adequate onset of anesthetic and hemostatic effects. During this period, skin preparation can be performed.

Smaller syringes exert more injection pressure and require less work than larger syringes. Using a 3-, 5-, or 10-ml syringe is therefore preferable to using larger syringes. Using a control type syringe allows for easy aspiration before injecting near large vessels of the head and neck. The anesthetic should be distributed evenly and precisely to avoid tissue distortion with unnecessary volumes. Advancing the needle to its full depth and injecting as the needle is withdrawn will place a thin line of anesthetic droplets that will only minimally distort the tissue; this practice will also reduce the possibility of intravascular injection. In most procedures a 27- or 30-gauge 1.5-inch needle is used. It is a common misconception that a short 0.5-inch needle is less painful. In fact, a short needle requires more puncture sites and often results in areas that are inadequately anesthetized.

The goal of anesthesia in the head and neck region is to temporarily block anatomic areas supplied by cranial nerve V and cervical nerves II and III (Fig. 28-4). The surgeon should be familiar with the foramina of these nerves and how they relate to the pupil, orbital rims, medial canthus, canine dentition, sternocleidomastoid muscle, and other anatomic landmarks.

Rhinoplasty

Once the patient is lightly sedated, the nasal cavity is topically anesthetized with approximately 3 ml of 4% or 10% cocaine. Alternatively, a 1:1 mixture of 4% lidocaine and 0.5% oxymetazoline can be used. Each pledget is vigorously squeezed to eliminate excess drug before application. Infiltration of nasal soft tissue using 1% lidocaine with 1:100,000 epinephrine is then initiated. Just before injec-

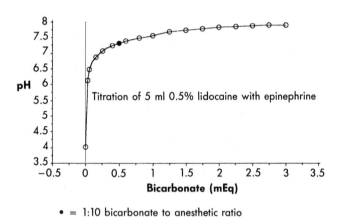

$\bullet$ = 1:10 bicarbonate to anesthetic ratio

Fig. 28-2. Titration. The addition of sodium bicarbonate to a local anesthetic in a 1:10 ratio achieves physiologic pH.

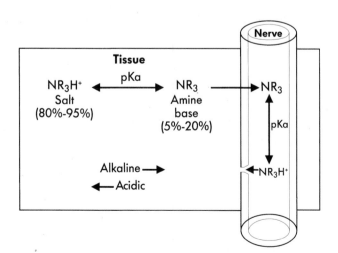

Fig. 28-3. Nerve penetration. The amine base can penetrate nerve membranes, but the salt form internally blocks sodium channels.

tion, a short-acting intravenous sedative (e.g., methohexital, or Propofol) may be administered.

First, the infraorbital nerves (Fig. 28-5, *A*) are anesthetized through an intranasal or percutaneous approach using approximately 0.5 ml per side. The nasal root and lateral nasal wall are infiltrated intranasally with 1 ml per side, keeping the depth of injection near the periosteum. Small amounts of anesthetic may also be injected on the internal surface of the nasal bones to improve anesthetic blockade and hemostasis. Next, 1 to 2 ml of anesthetic is used to anesthetize the nasal tip, columella, and alae (injection site 3) through a percutaneous injection. The percutaneous approach affords access to both sides of the nose under direct visualization. A single 1-ml injection is placed across the base of the nose (injection site 4), anesthetizing the remaining portions of the nasal spine, lateral alae, and inferior

columella. The average rhinoplasty requires 6 to 10 ml of anesthesia.[25,68]

If septal repair is necessary, the septum (injection site 5) is infiltrated with 2 to 3 ml in a submucoperichondrial plane (Fig. 28-5, *B*). This hydrostatic dissection allows easier elevation of septal flaps and supplies greater anesthesia over the maxillary crest, where manipulation of bone is extremely sensitive. This anesthetic technique should supply adequate anesthesia during osteotomies, although additional intravenous boluses of methohexital or propofol may be necessary to increase the amount of sedation.

Blepharoplasty

Blepharoplasty requires minimal amounts of local anesthetic. Most surgeons use 1% lidocaine with 1:100,000 epinephrine to anesthetize the eyelids and provide adequate he-

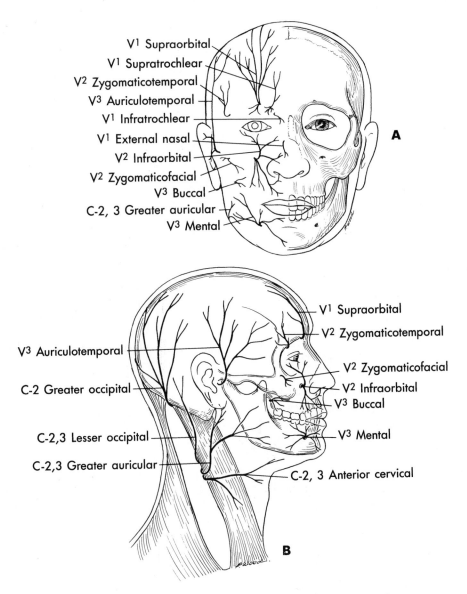

Fig. 28-4. A, Trigeminal nerve I, **B,** Trigeminal nerve II.

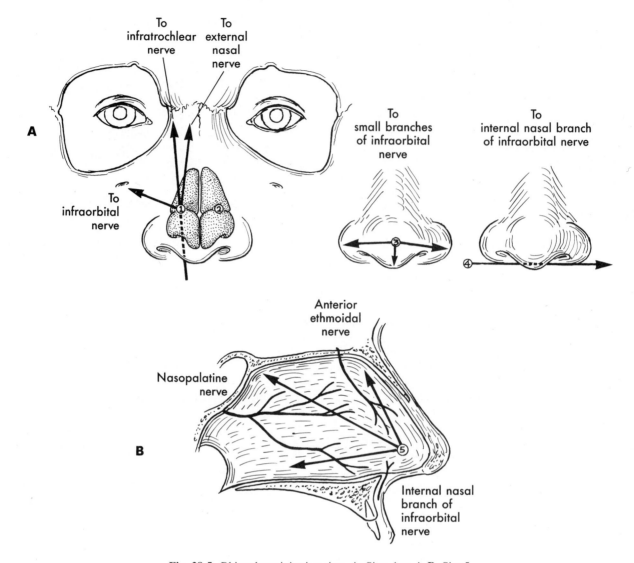

Fig. 28-5. Rhinoplasty injection sites. **A,** Sites 1 to 4. **B,** Site 5.

mostasis. To avoid unnecessary distortion of the delicate eyelid tissue, only 2 ml of anesthetic should be used in each lid. Incisions should be marked on the skin before local infiltration. Dissection, traction, and cauterization of postseptal orbital fat may require an additional 0.5 ml of anesthetic. This injection is placed at the base of the fat pedicle before clamping, resection, and cauterization.

If a transconjuctival approach for the lower blepharoplasty is chosen, the conjunctiva is first topically anesthetized with one to two drops of 0.5% tetracaine ophthalmic solution. The lower lid is then distracted from the globe, and the needle is inserted into the conjunctiva, inferior to the lower edge of the tarsus until the orbital rim is reached. The needle is then withdrawn slightly, and 1 to 2 ml of local anesthetic is deposited.

Rhytidectomy

The patient is preoperatively sedated with 5 to 10 mg of oral diazepam. Once in the operative suite, the patient is further sedated with midazolam and fentanyl until comfortable. It is important to remain in verbal contact with the patient to provide reassurance and to eliminate unnecessary anxiety. Verbal contact is also useful in monitoring the depth of sedation. A solution of 1% lidocaine with 1:100,000 epinephrine is mixed with 0.5% bupivacaine with 1:200,000 epinephrine in a 1:1 ratio. This mixture has a quick onset and a 2- to 3-hour duration of anesthesia. The anesthetic is injected with a 10-ml control syringe and a 25-gauge spinal needle. At the incision sites, a 27-gauge 1.5-inch needle is used.

The face is sequentially anesthetized in units as the opera-

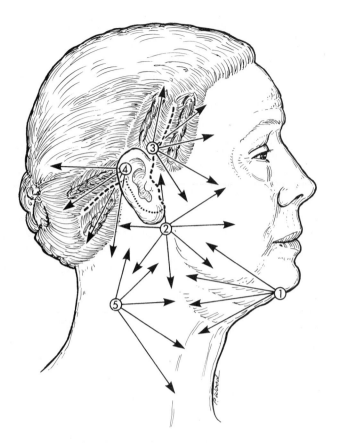

Fig. 28-6. Rhytidectomy injection sites.

tion progresses (Fig. 28-6). The first unit anesthetized is the submental triangle and the anterior neck. This initial series of injections, which requires approximately 10 to 20 ml of anesthetic, allows for liposuction and surgical access to the anterior platysma. The injection begins in the submentum and radiates across the anterior part of the neck to the level of the hyoid, over the angle of the mandible, and across to the sternocleidomastoid muscle.

After liposuction is performed and the anterior platysmal bands have been surgically addressed, one side of the face and neck is anesthetized in the following manner: Injections are begun in the periauricular region (injection site 2) and extended across the anterior part of the face in a subcutaneous plane. Deeper injection that could temporarily paralyze the facial nerve should be avoided. The temporal region is infiltrated from a site just superior to the root of the helix (injection site 3). The postauricular region is injected from a site posterior to the superior aspect of the conchal bowl (injection site 4). Finally, the posterior part of the neck is infiltrated from a site along the posterior margin of the sternocleidomastoid muscle (injection site 5). To anesthetize one side of the face, 20 to 30 ml of anesthetic is used. The contralateral side is anesthetized in an identical manner using another 20 to 30 ml of local anesthetic. A total of 40 to 60 ml of local anesthetic is used for the entire face.

COMPLICATIONS

Complications from local anesthetics vary from relatively minor and self limited ones to major life-threatening events. Both types should be expeditiously diagnosed and treated. Minor complications of local infiltration usually consist of local tissue injury secondary to bleeding, infection, or allergic reactions. Minor changes in wound healing have been shown in animal studies but do not appear to be a major problem in the clinical setting.[16] True allergic reactions to anesthetics are rare and usually caused by the ester class. These agents have *p*-aminobenzoic acid [PABA]–like metabolites that can be antigenic. Most allergic reactions to ester agents are mild and result in cutaneous hives, but a few patients may actually manifest severe anaphylaxis.[56] Allergic reactions to the amide class are much less common and tend to be less severe.

Patients with an unclear history of allergy to local anesthetics should avoid ester compounds. People suspected of having a mild allergy to both amide and ester compounds should avoid anesthetics that contain the preservative methylparaben, which can be allergenic. Local anesthetic skin-testing techniques are not reliable[5] but may offer reassurance when selecting an agent for minor procedures that only require minute amounts of anesthetic agent. Infiltration with an antihistamine such as diphenhydramine causes local anesthesia; this technique may be useful in patients who have had severe reactions to the usual anesthetics. Antihistamines can exhibit anesthetic effects because of structural similarity to local anesthetics.

The more dangerous complications of local anesthetics are caused by their effects on the central nervous system (CNS) and cardiovascular system. Systemic toxicity is unusual when nontoxic doses are administered. However, increased rate of absorption, elevated carbon dioxide pressure (PCO_2),[22] and the cardiopulmonary hemodynamics of the patient may affect the toxic threshold of a local anesthetic.

Most fatalities from local anesthetics result from drug overdose and poor anesthetic technique.[1,48] Direct injection of normally nontoxic doses into a large vessel can produce toxic symptoms, but this danger is easily avoided with careful infiltration. It should be the surgeon's responsibility to check all drug concentrations and dosages and not rely on the surgical staff for this important task.

Most anesthetics initially cause CNS stimulation, which is thought to occur by selective depression of inhibitory neurons.[29] Initial symptoms of toxicity include tinnitus, blurred vision, dizziness, slurred speech, shivering, muscle twitches, and tremor. Moderately toxic levels result in seizure activity, which is exacerbated by elevated levels of carbon dioxide and acidosis. Agents such as bupivacaine, cocaine, and tetracaine are more potent and consequently have lower seizure thresholds than lidocaine. Increasing anesthetic blood levels into higher toxic levels will result in CNS depression, severe respiratory depression, and death.

Local anesthetic agents can also affect the electrical conductivity of the myocardium. Nontoxic doses may show antiarrhythmic properties, but toxic doses can result in myocardial depression, decreased cardiac output, and circulatory collapse. The myocardium is also sensitive to epinephrine which can cause hypertension, tachycardia, ectopic beats, and other deleterious arrhythmias when toxic levels are reached. These signs and symptoms of systemic toxicity should be recognized immediately and treated appropriately to avoid major complications or life-threatening injury. Once a minor reaction is recognized, the surgical procedure is terminated, all intravenous sedatives are stopped, intranasal pledgets that contain anesthetics or epinephrine are removed, and the patient is given oxygen by mask. Verbal contact is maintained with the patient to encourage respiration and monitor the depth of sedation. In most circumstances, these measures are all that is necessary, and the procedure is continued after a brief waiting period to ensure the patient is stable and drugs have returned to nontoxic levels.

Elimination of hypoxia and hypercarbia not only prevents CNS injury but also reduces the risk of seizures. If seizures do occur, they are treated effectively with intravenous diazepam or barbiturate. Naloxone is given intravenously to reverse the respiratory depression and sedation caused by narcotics. If the airway is obstructed or respiration is dangerously depressed, the patient should be intubated and ventilated with assistance. Tachycardia and hypertension are treated with small doses of propranolol, whereas hypotension usually responds to intravenous fluids and Trendelenburg position. Once stabilized, the patient should continue to undergo close observation and cardiac monitoring until awake. If patients remain unstable or their conditions questionable, a decision should be made to immediately transfer the patient to an intensive care facility for closer monitoring and the appropriate consultation.

INTRAVENOUS SEDATION

Intravenous sedation has evolved over the past 50 years and is now used in the hospital operating rooms and outpatient procedure rooms for numerous minor surgical procedures. The goals of sedation in the patient undergoing minor surgical procedures under local anesthesia are (1) patient safety, (2) modification of patient behavior, (3) positive patient response to treatment, and (4) return to pretreatment level of consciousness by the time of discharge.

All local anesthetics are CNS depressants. There are potentially hazardous interactions between local anesthetic agents and sedative or narcotic drugs. The physician who uses sedation during surgical procedures should have proper personnel and equipment available to manage any reasonable emergency situation. An emergency cart should be readily accessible and should include the necessary drugs and equipment to resuscitate a nonbreathing and unconscious patient. This equipment should include a positive-pressure oxygen delivery system that can administer greater than 90% oxygen at a 5-L/min flow rate for at least 60 minutes.

Before the surgical procedure, the patient should undergo a thorough anesthetic history and physical examination. Particular attention should be paid to allergies, current medications, and troublesome cardiovascular or respiratory complaints. The physical examination should focus on the patient's airway: patency, obvious deformities, and ease of management or intubation. Patients should not undergo surgical procedures using a local anesthesia with intravenous sedation if the following conditions or similar problems are identified: history of severe sleep apnea, poorly controlled seizures, craniofacial anomalies with difficult airway access, cerebral palsy with abnormal swallowing, severe gastroesophageal reflux, chronic hypoxia, or poorly controlled hypertension.

Intravenous sedation can be categorized into deep or conscious sedation. Deep sedation is a controlled state of depressed consciousness or unconsciousness from which the patient is not easily aroused. This may be accompanied by a partial or complete loss of protective airway reflexes and the ability to respond to physical stimulation or verbal command. Conscious sedation is a minimally depressed level of consciousness that retains the patient's ability to maintain a patent airway independently and continuously and respond appropriately to physical stimulation or verbal command. The separation between these two types of sedation is often narrow; therefore, administration of intravenous sedation requires experience and close monitoring. For procedures that require deep sedation, it is recommended that sedation be administered by an anesthesiologist or trained nurse anesthetist.

During sedation the heart rate, respiratory rate, and blood pressure should be continuously monitored and recorded at specific intervals by the anesthesiologist or nurse anesthetist. At a minimum, patients should have continuous electrocardiography and pulse oximeter monitoring. The patient should be discharged only when the cardiovascular and airway stability are assured and the patient is alert and can ambulate safely with minimal assistance.

Potential serious complications cannot be ignored: e.g., idiosyncratic drug reactions, anaphylaxis, respiratory depression, airway obstruction, hypoxemia, aspiration, and cardiac arrhythmias. The risk of death from intravenous sedation is reported to be 1 in 314,000 cases. Proper drug selection and administration are paramount to a successful operation and should be reviewed by the operating surgeon on a regular basis.

Drugs for sedation

Four classes of intravenous agents for conscious sedation exist: benzodiazepines, barbiturates, opioids, and the newer alkylphenols (Table 28-2). The goals of conscious sedation are anxiolysis, amnesia, modified consciousness, and analgesia. The clinician should be familiar with the specific attri-

Table 28-2. Sedatives

Drug	Class	Water soluble	Pain	Analgesia	Amnestic	Duration (min)
Diazepam	Benzodiazepine	No	Yes (thrombophlebitis)	No	Yes	Long (60-120)
Midazolam	Benzodiazepine	Yes	No	No	Yes	Short (15-30)
Propofol	Alkylphenol	No	Yes	No	Minimal	Short (5-10)
Methohexital	Barbiturate	Yes	Slight	No	Yes	Short (5-10)
Fentanyl	Opiate	Yes	No	Yes	No	Short

butes of each class of drug to attain these objectives. For example, if anxiolysis or amnesia is desired, a benzodiazepine or similar agent is the drug of choice. If analgesia is desired, an opioid is chosen. In this situation, a barbiturate would be relatively contraindicated because barbiturates exhibit antianalgesic properties that might increase the patient's perception of pain.

Benzodiazepines are useful adjunctive drugs for minor surgical procedures under local anesthesia. Bensodiazepines possess antianxiety, sedative, amnestic, anticonvulsant, and skeletal muscle relaxant properties. However, possible idiosyncratic reactions such as increased anxiety, restlessness, and disinhibition may occur. Lorazepam, diazepam, and midazolam are the currently available benzodiazepines. The duration of lorazepam is too long for use in the ambulatory patients. Diazepam in 2.5- to 5-mg increments (up to 0.3 mg/kg) can produce conscious sedation adequate for outpatient procedures. Because diazepam is insoluble in water, it is commercially available in solutions of propylene glycol at a pH of 6.6 to 6.9. As a result of this acidity, intramuscular or intravenous injections are often painful. Dilution with water or saline decreases the irritation without altering the potency. Preceding the injection of diazepam with a small dose of lidocaine (1 ml, 20 mg) will also significantly reduce the irritation. Midazolam is an excellent sedative that is approximately four times more potent than diazepam. In doses of 1 to 2.5 mg (up to 0.1 mg/kg), midazolam can produce sedation appropriate for outpatient surgery. In the pediatric population, there has been reported success using intranasal midazolam that is absorbed through mucous membranes.[76] Midazolam is superior to diazepam because of its more rapid onset, shorter duration, and lack of venous irritation. Midazolam causes more amnesia than diazepam, with relatively light levels of sedation.

The analgesic properties of short-acting opioids such as fentanyl and alfentanil are especially useful in outpatient surgery. Because of the rapid onset and short duration, these drugs can be closely titrated to alleviate patient discomfort without oversedation. Fentanyl is the most widely used agent because of its relative potency[37] (80 times more potent than morphine). It is given in 12.5- to 25-μg doses every 3 to 5 minutes until pain is relieved. Alfentanil is an analog of fentanyl that is less potent (1/5 to 1/10) and has one third the duration of action. It also has less respiratory depression (1/13) than fentanyl.[61] Both of these drugs work well in combination with a benzodiazepine for outpatient sedation.[7]

Barbiturates are useful during procedures requiring conscious sedation. Thiopental is the most commonly used barbiturate in these types of procedures. It has a rapid onset, and its duration is short (5 to 6 minutes) because of rapid redistribution from the brain to muscle. However, detoxification is slow, and thiopental may cause prolonged postoperative sedation when multiple doses are given. Methohexital is similar to thiopental but appears to have a quicker recovery time, which makes it particularly useful if large or repeated doses of sedation are necessary. Doses should be carefully titrated to avoid apnea, and it should not be used in patients with asthma because of its tendency to induce histamine release and bronchospasm. Unfortunately, barbiturates do not contain analgesic properties and may actually be antianalgesic. For this reason, barbiturates are usually administered with an opioid.

The alkylphenols are the newest class of drugs for intravenous sedation. Propofol is the only agent in this group currently available. Propofol produces a dose-dependent CNS, cardiovascular, and ventilator depression very similar to that caused by the barbiturates. The onset of action of propofol is nearly identical to that of thiopental or methohexital; however, recovery is much faster and is associated with few postanesthetic side effects such as nausea, confusion, drowsiness, and restlessness.[26,47,58,70] Propofol appears to have cardiorespiratory depression effects similar to methohexital.[73] It has extremely poor water solubility and is mixed with a lecithin emulsion (10% intralipid) that causes local irritation. Side effects are rare but include thrombophlebitis, involuntary skeletal muscle movements, coughing, and hiccups. Because of propofol's short duration (5 to 10 minutes), prolonged sedation should be performed using an infusion pump and a continuous drip or by repeated boluses at regular intervals.

SUMMARY

Local anesthetics are an important part of facial surgery and have contributed to advances in the field. Anesthetic agents and techniques have progressively evolved over the past 100 years, and the search for safer, more effective agents and methods continues. Each new drug will have its own characteristic onset time, duration, penetration, and complications. Newer drugs will undoubtedly replace some of the more toxic ones currently in use. Otolaryngologists should remain abreast of changes in local anesthesia and continue to incorporate new drugs or techniques with higher degree of efficacy or safety.

REFERENCES

1. Adriani J, Campbell D: Fatalities following topical application of local anesthetics to mucous membranes, *JAMA* 162:1527, 1956.
2. Aldrich MR, Baker RW: *Historical aspects of cocaine use and abuse.* In *Cocaine: chemical, biological, clinical, social and treatment aspects,* Cleveland, 1976, CRC Press.
3. Arndt KA and others: Minimizing the pain of local anesthesia, *Plast Reconstr Surg* 72:676, 1983.
4. Arthur GR, Covino BG: What's new in local anesthetics? *Anesth Clin* 6:357, 1988.
5. Baker JD, Blackmon BB: Local anesthesia, *Clin Plast Surg* 1:25, 1985.
6. Barker W and others: Damage to tissue defenses by a topical anesthetic agent, *Ann Emerg Med* 11:307, 1982.
7. Ben-Shlomo I and others: Midazolam acts synergistically with fentanyl for induction of anesthesia, *Br J Anaesth* 64:45, 1990.
8. Bettman U: A case illustrating the applicability of muriate of cocaine in nasal surgery, *JAMA* 3:598, 1884.
9. Buckley FP and others: Acid and alkaline solutions of local anesthetics: duration of nerve block and tissue pH, *Anesth Analg* 64:477, 1985.
10. Buckley MM, Banfield P: Eutectic lidocaine/prilocaine cream: a review of the topical anesthetic/analgesic efficacy of a eutectic mixture of local anesthetics (EMLA), *Drugs* 46:126, 1993.
11. Butterworth J, Strichartz GR: Molecular mechanisms of local anesthesia: a review, *Anesthesiology* 72:711, 1990.
12. Byck R: *Cocaine papers by Sigmund Freud,* New York, 1974, Stonehill Publishing.
13. Campbell D, Adriani J: Absorption of local anesthetics, *JAMA* 168:873, 1958.
14. Cannon CR and others: Topically applied tetracaine, adrenaline, and cocaine in the repair of traumatic wounds of the head and neck, *Otolaryngol Head Neck Surg* 100:78, 1989.
15. Chiu YC and others: Myocardial infarction with topical cocaine anesthesia for nasal surgery, *Arch Otolaryngol Head Neck Surg* 112:988, 1986.
16. Chvapil M and others: Local anesthetics and wound healing, *J Surg Res* 27:367, 1979.
17. Cooke JE: Drug interactions in anesthesia, *Clin Plast Surg* 12:83, 1985.
18. Courtiss EH, Ransil BJ, and Russo J: The effects of hyaluronidase on local anesthesia: a prospective, randomized, controlled, double blinded study, *Plast Reconstr Surg* 95:876, 1995.
19. Covino BG: Pharmacology of local anesthetic agents, *Rational Drug Ther* 21:1, 1987.
20. Covino BG: Pharmacology of local anesthetic agents, *Surg Round* 1:44, 1978.
21. Covino BG: Ultralong-acting local anesthetic agents, *Anesthesiology* 54:263, 1981.
22. Covino BG, Vassallo HG: *Local anesthetics: mechanisms of action and clinical use,* New York, 1976, Grune & Stratton.
23. DeJong RH, Cullen SC: Buffer-demand and local anesthetic solutions containing epinephrine, *Anesthesiology* 24:801, 1963.
24. DiFazio CA and others: Comparison of pH-adjusted lidocaine solutions for epidural anesthesia, *Anesth Analg* 65:760, 1986.
25. Dingman RO: Local anesthesia for rhinoplasty and nasal septum in rhinoplastic surgery, *Plast Reconstr Surg* 28:251, 1961.
26. Doze VA and others: Comparison of propofol with methohexital for outpatient anesthesia, *Anesth Analg* 65:1189, 1986.
27. Duran-Reynolds F: Tissue permeability and the spreading factor in infections, *Bacteriol Rev* 6:197, 1942.
28. Einhorn A: Ueber die chemie der local anesthetica, *Munchen med wochenschr* 46:1218, 1899.
29. Frank GB, Saunders HD: A proposed common mechanism of action for general and local anesthetics in the central nervous system, *Br J Pharmacol* 21:1, 1963.
30. Gay GR and others: Cocaine in perspective: "gift from the sun god" to "rich man's drug", *Drug Forum* 2:409, 1973.
31. Gupta AK, Sibbald RG: Eutectic lidocaine/prilocaine 5% cream and patch may provide satisfactory analgesia for excisional biopsy or curettage with electrosurgery of cutaneous lesions: a randomized, controlled, parallel group study, *J Am Acad Dermatol* 35:419, 1996.
32. Halsted WS: Practical comments on the use and abuse of cocaine, suggested by its invariably successful employment in more than a thousand minor surgical operations, *N Y Med J* 42:294, 1885.
33. Henderson RL, Johns M: The clinical use of cocaine, *Drug Ther Bull* 7:31, 1977.
34. Hilgier M: Alkalinization of bupivacaine for brachial plexus block, *Reg Anaesth* 10:59, 1985.
35. Hille B and others: *Molecular mechanisms of anesthesia,* New York, 1975, Raven Press.
36. Isner JM, Chokshi SK: Cocaine and vasospasm, *N Engl J Med* 321:1604, 1989.
37. Reisine T, Pasternak G: *Opioid analgesics and antagonists.* In Hardman JG, Limbird LE, editors: *The pharmacological basis of therapeutics,* ed 9, New York, 1996, MacMillan Publishing.
38. Katz JD, Lee KJ: *Anesthesia for head and neck surgery.* In *Essential otolaryngology—head and neck surgery,* East Norwalk, Conn, 1991, Appleton & Lange.
39. Koller C: On the use of cocaine for producing anesthesia of the eye, *Lancet* 127:990, 1884.
40. Lander J and others: Determinants of success and failure of EMLA, *Pain* 64:89, 1996.
41. Lange RA and others: Cocaine-induced coronary artery vasoconstriction, *N Engl J Med* 321:1557, 1989.
42. Larrabee WF and others: Effect of epinephrine on local cutaneous blood flow, *Head Neck Surg* 9:287, 1987.
43. Lee AG: A consumer's guide to model of local anesthetic action, *Anesthesiology* 51:64, 1979.
44. Lewis-Smith PA: Adjunctive use of hyaluronidase in local anesthesia, *Br J Plast Surg* 39:554, 1986.
45. Lofgren N: *Studies on local anesthetics: xylocaine, a new synthetic drug,* Stockholm, 1948, Ivar Haeggstroms.
46. Lynch S: *Anesthesia.* In *Aesthetic plastic surgery,* Philadelphia, 1980, WB Saunders.
47. MacKenzie N, Grant IS: Propofol for intravenous sedation, *Anesthesia* 42:3, 1987.
48. Mayer E: The toxic effects following the use of local anesthetics: an analysis of the reports of forty-three deaths, *JAMA* 82:876, 1924.
49. Millay DJ and others. Vasoconstrictors in facial plastic surgery, *Arch Otolaryngol Head Neck Surg* 117:160, 1991.
50. Misra AL and others: Physiologic disposition and metabolism of ecgonine in the rat, *Res Commun Chem Pathol Pharmacol* 8:55, 1974.
51. Murakami CS, Ross B: Buffered local anesthesia and epinephrine degradation, *J Dermatol Surg Oncology* 20:192, 1994.
52. Niemann A: Ueber eine neue organsche base in den cocablattern, *Vierteljarhelsschrift fur Practische Pharmacie* 9:489, 1860.
53. Pritchard O: Cocaine as a local anesthetic, *Lancet* 2:1167, 1884.
54. Pryor G and others: Local anesthesia in minor lacerations: topical TAC versus lidocaine infiltration, *Ann Emerg Med* 9:568, 1980.
55. Reinisch J, Meyers B: The effect of local anesthesia with epinephrine on skin flap survival, *Plast Reconstr Surg* 54:324, 1974.

56. Ritchie JM, Greene NM: Local anesthetics: the pharmacological basis of therapeutics, New York, 1980, MacMillan Publishing.
57. Ritchie JM, Greengard P: On the mode of action of local anesthetics, *Annu Rev Pharmacol Toxicol* 6:405, 1966.
58. Rodrigo MRC, Jonsson E: Conscious sedation with propofol, *Br Dent J* 166:75, 1989.
59. Roe JO: The correction of angular deformities of the nose by subcutaneous operation, *Med Rec* 40:57, 1891.
60. Roe JO: The deformity termed ''pug nose'' and its correction by a simple operation, *Med Rec* 31:621, 1887.
61. Scamman FL and others: Ventilatory and mental effects of alfentanyl and fentanyl, *Acta Anaesthesiol Scand* 28:63, 1984.
62. Schenck NL: Cocaine: its use and misuse in otolaryngology, *Trans Am Acad Ophthalmol Otolaryngol* 80:343, 1975.
63. Semon F: Cocaine as a local anaesthetic in intra-laryngeal operations, *Lancet* 2:912, 1884.
64. Siegel RJR and others: Effective hemostasis with less epinephrine: an experimental and clinical study, *Plast Reconstr Surg* 51:129, 1973.
65. Slitter R, Goodacre ET: EMLA cream of the ears: is it effective? A prospective randomized control trial of the efficacy of topical anesthetic cream in reducing the pain of local anesthetic infiltration for prominent ear correction, *Br J Plast Surg* 48:150, 1995.
66. Strichartz G: Molecular mechanisms of nerve block by local anesthetics, *Anesthesiology* 45:421, 1976.
67. Strobel GE, Bianchi CP: The effects of pH gradients on the action of procaine and lidocaine in intact and desheathed sciatic nerves, *J Pharmacol Exp Ther* 172:1, 1970.
68. Tardy ME: *Rhinoplasty*, St Louis, 1986, Mosby.
69. Thale H: Use of lypholized hyaluronidase in cosmetic surgery about the face, *Plast Reconstr Surg* 10:260, 1952.
70. Valtonen M and others: Propofol infusion for sedation in outpatient oral surgery, *Anaesthesia* 44:730, 1989.
71. Verlander JM, Johns ME: The clinical use of cocaine, *Otolaryngol Clin North Am* 14:521, 1981.
72. Watson D: Hyaluronidase, *Br J Anaesth* 71:422, 1993.
73. White PF: What's new in intravenous anesthetics? *Anesthesiology* 6: 297, 1988.
74. White WEB and others: Topical anesthesia for laceration repair: tetracaine versus TAC (tetracaine, adrenaline, and cocaine), *Am J Emerg Med* 4:319, 1986.
75. Wilkinson TEA: *''Rule of 50'' to avoid overdosage with local anesthetics.* In *The art of aesthetic plastic surgery*, Boston, 1989, Little, Brown.
76. Wilton NC and others: Preanesthetic sedation of preschool children using intranasal midazolam, *Anesthesiology* 69:972, 1988.
77. Wu G and others: The hazards of injecting local anesthetic solutions with epinephrine into flaps, *Plast Reconstr Surg* 62:396, 1978.

SUGGESTED READINGS

Courtiss EH: Office surgery, *Clin Plast Surg* 10:223, 1983.
Dunbar RW: *Anesthesias in plastic surgery.* In Lewis J, editor: *The art of aesthetic plastic surgery*, Boston, 1989, Little, Brown.
Gordon HI: *Drugs for outpatient surgery.* In Regnault P, Daniels RK, editors: *Anesthetic plastic surgery*, Boston, 1984, Little, Brown.
Jonathan E, Benumuf L: New anesthetic drugs, *Anesth Clin North Am* 6: 251, 1988.

Chapter 29

Tissue Expansion of the Head and Neck

Gordon H. Sasaki

Joseph E. Berg

The head and neck surgeon should be concerned with the functional and aesthetic outcomes of a reconstructive procedure. To achieve these goals, surgeons have developed various operations that range from simple (skin grafts) to complex (composite free-tissue transfers). The surgeon's responsibility is to select a method that is reliable, safe, and effective and that satisfies the cosmetic needs of the patient.

Tissue expansion is an established technique that provides additional skin with the characteristics of near-perfect color, texture, sensation, and special adnexal elements (hair, sweat glands, and sebaceous glands) for the reconstructive site. Occasionally, tissues other than skin (muscle, fascia) may be included during the expansion process. In most cases, donor tissue for expansion is selected from adjacent to the defect. Regional and distant tissue rarely may be expanded to satisfy specific soft-tissue concerns. The hallmark of tissue expansion remains the production of a domed flap, which, after transfer, produces a minimal or hidden donor site scar.

Tissue expansion continues to be a labor-intensive procedure. Because of the silicone balloon, the surgeon is challenged by the possibility of infection caused by exposure and leakage throughout expansion. Tissue expansion demands that the surgeon comprehend its indications and contraindications, masters its technical aspects, conveys to the patient its benefits and limitations, and is competent to manage any complications. Not every defect needs to be managed by expansion (e.g., an infected or vascularly compromised defect that will not tolerate the presence of a buried foreign body). In addition, patients who cannot cope with the temporary deformity of the expanded flap should not participate in this two-staged reconstructive procedure.

HISTORY

The ability of human tissue to stretch gradually has been observed throughout history.

Physiologic expansion

During growth, human tissues adapt to physiologic expansion to maintain function and to prevent aesthetic deformities. The enlarging fetal brain stretches the skull at suture lines to respond to the rapid growth of the cerebral hemispheres. During pregnancy, primary breast tissue gradually enlarges from hormonal stimulation and stretches the skin envelope. During the later stages of pregnancy, the gravid uterus and fetus expand the abdominal soft tissues, producing stretch marks on the overlying skin (Fig. 29-1).

Pathologic expansion

The slow growth of benign tumors (cavernous hemangiomas, epithelial cysts) and the more rapid growth of malignant lesions (liposarcomas, retinoblastomas) readily stretch the surrounding tissues.

Artificially induced expansion

The cultural use of instruments and ornaments (e.g., plates or metal rings) to enlarge lips in Chadean women[52] and to lengthen the necks of Burmese women in the Paduang society[8] has been recorded by anthropologists since the nineteenth century (Fig. 29-2).

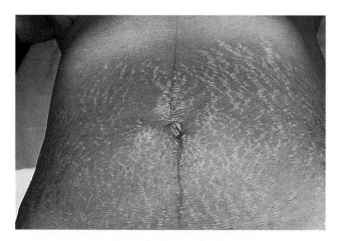

Fig. 29-1. Multiple pregnancies and large birth weights have gradually stretched the abdominal skin and deeper structures. Excess skin and fat persist with a diastasis of the rectus abdominus muscles. Striae formation represents scar deposition within the skin from hormonal and expansion stresses.

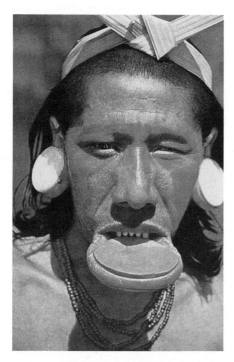

Fig. 29-2. The substitution of enlarging plates to the lips has been practiced in many cultures as an ornament for beautification, as depicted in this South American native.

Controlled clinical expansion

In 1905, Codvilla[10] published his early experiences of bone and soft-tissue lengthening in lower extremities that were shortened through congenital deformities. Magnuson[26] continued to evaluate bone-lengthening procedures in the lower extremities with his report in 1908. In 1921, Putti[37] concentrated on soft-tissue expansion (muscles, nerves, ves-

sels) during femoral lengthening with an external apparatus. In 1970, Matev[29] used the principles of gradual bone distraction with external skeletal traction to lengthen the thumb metacarpal after amputation at the joint level.

In 1957, Newmann,[31] a New York plastic surgeon, published a successful case of soft-tissue expansion with a buried subcutaneous balloon. The details of Newmann's technique and device form the basis of modern expansion methods, in particular, subcutaneous expansion with externalized tubing. Newmann was presented with the sequelae of a traumatic ear amputation that lacked available skin and cartilaginous structures. He inserted a balloon under the adjacent scalp and non–hair-bearing skin above and posterior to the deformity. For 2 months, the balloon was gradually expanded with saline through an attached tubing that exited from the skin. Newmann estimated that the balloon produced about a 50% increase in adjacent skin to cover a cartilaginous framework to complete the ear reconstruction. Unfortunately, the significance of Newmann's technique was not recognized for its reconstructive potential until almost 20 years later.

In 1975, Radovan[38,39] approached Schulte in Goleta, California, to discuss the merits of designing a silicone balloon with two remote valves that would be buried under the skin for expansion (Radovan, personal communication). In Radovan's original expander system, one valve removed saline while the other permitted only the addition of fluid. Radovan inserted his prototype expander device under healthy skin adjacent to a 7- × 11-cm tattoo on a patient's arm. The newly stretched skin was sufficient to replace the tattooed skin. Radovan published his first case and others from 1975 to 1978, initially unaware of the work of Newmann years before. In 1975, Austad and Rose[4] began animal and clinical research, unaware of Radovan's clinical endeavors, with an osmotically driven self-inflating expander system in the plastic surgery department at the University of Michigan. Austad and Rose contacted the Dow-Corning Medical Products Division to manufacture their early expanders in January 1976. A few weeks later Radovan reported his first clinical case. In 1980, Lapin and others[24] reported their findings with the use of an incorporated self-contained valve expander in primary breast reconstruction.

From 1980 to 1990, the concept and clinical experience with tissue expansion evolved at a rapid and proliferative rate. Application of tissue expansion focused on congenital (giant hairy nevus), developmental (male-patterned baldness, absence of breast formation in Poland's syndrome), acquired (tattoos), posttraumatic (scars, burn keloids, alopecia), and neoplastic (mastectomy, Mohs' defects) problems. Expansion techniques were also developed for elongating transected nerves, stretching shortened vessels, and expanding anophthalmic orbits for ocular prostheses. Long-term expansion of regional or distant tissues, then transposed to the recipient site by intact vascular pedicles or by microvascular anastomoses, represents a modification of the transfer method rather than a conceptional change. Common to all of these tissue-short challenges was the gradual stretching of adaptive tissues with a buried balloon. Variations on this expansion process have included external devices (sutures, skin applicators), shorter expansion periods, and disposable intraoperative balloons for immediate limited expansion.

Tissue expansion has evolved into an established reconstructive technique, taking its place among other time-tested procedures, such as skin grafts, skin flaps, and myocutaneous flaps, in the arsenal of the otolaryngologist. In a more limited fashion, intraoperative tissue expansion has made small inroads in aesthetic surgery (i.e., rhytidectomy, facial augmentation with silicone implants, breast augmentation). On the other hand, intraoperative tissue expansion has been more successfully applied to tissue-short complications after plastic surgery, such as elevated brows after open forehead-lifts, lower lid ectropion from excessive skin resection, and excessively high temporal sideburns after face-lift. Refinements in technique will continue to evolve and challenge the surgeon to satisfy the varied requirements of the defect and the patient.

PHYSIOLOGY OF EXPANSION

Structure of human skin

Healthy human skin contracts, stretches, and relaxes continually during growth, maturity, and aging. In fact, each area of a person's skin differs from other sites, depending on the structural requirements for which it was intended. For example, dermis of the eyelid skin remains the thinnest in the body with a paucity of adnexal structures. In contrast, dermis of scalp skin contains an abundance of hair follicles, sebaceous glands, and sweat glands contributing to its thickness and relative inflexibility. Epidermis on the palms and soles is thicker and more cornified than epidermis on other areas of the body because of frequent use and superficial trauma. Thus, the physical properties of dermis depend on the amount and distribution of adnexal structures within its borders and on the quantity and location of collagen, elastin, and ground substance within the same layer. On the other hand, the epidermis is the protective barrier of skin and plays a lesser role than the dermis in defining the skin's character.

A loose weave of type II collagen is located in the upper papillary layer of the dermis. The papillary layer is generally the same depth as the overlying epidermis and its basement membrane. In the thicker reticular layer of the dermis, the type II collagen fibers are more compact and aligned than those in the papillary dermis. Collagen fibers are convoluted and wavy in relaxed skin. When the skin is tautly stretched, the fibers become more parallel to the vector of force and lose a part of their twisted patterns. Further stretching of these newly oriented fibers resists additional skin extension.

The short elastin fibers are uniformly interspersed between the larger collagen fibers and are located in the papillary and reticular layers of the dermis. Unlike collagen fibers, elastin fibers are linked to one another by an intricate system of end-to-end side junctions. The primary function of elastin is to restore stretched collagen fibers to their natural, relaxed convoluted forms. Collagen fibers lack the ability to spring back to their original state. In fact, overly extended collagen may become permanently deformed when the limits of acceptable stretch or elastin recoil are exceeded. Striae formation is thought to represent fibrous scar tissue formed in response to microhemorrhage within disrupted collagen and elastic fibers.

Mucopolysaccharide ground substances (heparin sulfate, chondroitin sulfate, dermatan sulfate) and tissue fluid act as lubricants to permit the efficient multivectorial movements of collagen and elastin while stretching, recoiling, and relaxing as skin tension changes. The need for expansion of blood and lymphatic vessels along with neural fibers does not significantly retard expansion of skin. Conversely, injury to these delicate structures during aggressive expansion can lead to skin ischemia, sensory changes, and edema. Some studies[22,48] have emphasized the criteria for more rapid skin expansion to reduce the risk of injury of these delicate structures.

Viscoelastic properties of skin

Skin adapts to stress by two viscoelastic responses termed *stress-relaxation* and *creep*. Stress-relaxation occurs when skin is stretched to a given constant length. Over time, the force required to maintain this constant length gradually decreases. Gibson[14] first described the concept of stress-relaxation, which was later applied by Liang and others[25] in a presuturing technique. This method uses the intrinsic ability of skin to stretch and relax under suture tension. Sutures plicate the area of planned skin excision for 12 to 14 hours before surgery. Liang and others showed that less tension (up to 40%) was required to close a skin defect of standard size.

Creep is divided into biologic and mechanical phenomena. Pregnancy, morbid obesity, and lymphedema, are examples of biologic creep, in which gradual stress stretches skin, muscles, blood vessels, lymphatics, and nerves. All of these tissues expand by creep in part, increasing their lengths by cell division and synthesis of collagen and elastic fibers.[15]

Gibson and others[16] reported on the effects of mechanical creep by stretching skin with hooks at surgery. The beneficial effects of mechanical creep were attributed to the mechanisms of (1) relative dehydration of tissue by displacement of fluid and mucopolysaccharide ground substances, (2) parallel realignment of collagen fibers, (3) microfragmentation of elastic fibers, and (4) migration of undermined tissue into the field defect by the stretching force. Gibson[15] and Hirshowitz and others[19] emphasized that cyclic loading of skin is the most effective way to recruit extra tissue. If skin is load-cycled, the maximum stretching is achieved after three to four repetitive force tensions.

Sasaki[44,45] applied the concept of mechanical creep by

using a silicone balloon at surgery. Sasaki has performed this technique, referred to as *intraoperative sustained limited expansion* (ISLE), in more than 500 patients to gain up to 2.5 cm of extra tissue. Using ISLE, a small intraoperative balloon (1.5, 2.5, 5, 10, 20, or 50 ml) is selected on the basis of the area of the donor tissue needed (Fig. 29-3). The silicone balloon is buried subcutaneously adjacent to the defect with an externalized fast-fill valve (Fig. 29-4). The balloon is initially filled to tissue tolerance (ischemia) and left inflated for 1 to 3 minutes. After deflation, the second fill for 1 to 3 minutes will be more than that used during the first inflation because of tissue recruitment. A third cycle of maximal filling (more than the second volume), for the same period of time will complete the expansion process. Table 29-1 records the average amount of recruited tissue per expander from different anatomic regions. Because of the thicker and therefore less elastic nature of skin from the scalp, nasal tip, and back, the average amount of tissue

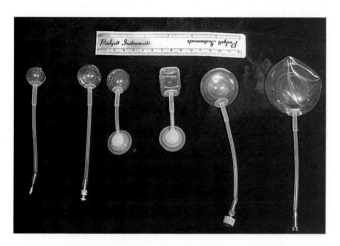

Fig. 29-3. An array of intraoperative expanders shows the variety of sizes (far left expander, 1 ml; far right expander, 25 ml) and shapes that may be used for intraoperative sustained limited expansion. These expanders usually have a two-way valve (fifth expander from the right) for ease of expansion and deflation. Larger volume implants may also be used for rapid immediate expansion of skin to resurface larger defects.

Table 29-1. Intraoperative sustained limited expansion technique and tissue gain

Anatomic site	Average tissue gain per 1.5- to 50-ml expander (cm)
Scalp	1.0-2.5
Forehead	1.0-2.5
Upper half of nose	1.0-1.5
Nasal tip	0.5-1.0
Midface	1.0-2.5
Neck	1.0-2.5

gained by ISLE in these areas is less than that anticipated from thinner areas of more elastic skin.

Physiologic changes during expansion

After a silicone tissue expander is inserted in the subcutaneous fatty plane under the skin and incremental saline fillings are begun, the intraluminal pressure remains low. As the saline volume approaches the stated capacity of the expander unit, the intraluminal pressure slowly begins to increase. The transient increase of pressure is caused by the resistance of the overlying tissue and by the elastic characteristics of the silicone envelope. As tissue creep occurs in response to the increased pressure within the implant, the overlying soft tissue expands with a concomitant decrease in pressure within the expander unit. The pressure decreases and tissue relaxation may occur 2 to 6 hours after filling (Fig. 29-5). Factors that may prolong the duration of tissue tension and increased intraluminal pressure include tissue fibrosis (radiation injury, scarring) and stiffer healthy tissue (galea aponeurotica, unyielding thicker back skin, skeletal muscle). Abrupt and prolonged intraluminal pressures have been associated with increased rates of balloon leakage[18,32] and with atrophy of surrounding tissues (fat, muscle, skin).

Tissue creep alone cannot account for the final amount of extra skin produced during serial expansion. Tissue migration inward from surrounding skin toward the apex of the expander may occur in skin from older patients. Tissue compression above and below the expander unit results in "more" skin when the expander is removed. Finally, Austad and others[3] observed that expanded skin responded by increasing the rate of epidermal mitoses and collagen syntheses.

Microcirculation during expansion

Tissue expansion traumatizes skin circulation during creation of the surgical pocket by transecting vascular perforators and injuring the delicate subdermal plexi. Added insult to the microcirculation occurs during serial expansion by mechanically narrowing vascular diameters, occluding the thin walls of veins and lymphatics and encouraging microthrombi formation by endothelial injury. The surgeon should rationally conclude that such vascular embarrassments may compromise the reliability of the expanded skin. Clinically, the surgeon recognizes skin ischemia during expansion by observations of skin blanching and tissue firmness and complaints of pain from the patient.

Sasaki's clinical experience in more than 1500 chronic expansion cases suggests that the vascular flow within expanded skin remains robust despite these concerns. Because chronic tissue expansion produces a series of vascular compromises, the blood supply increases as temporary ischemia is induced. Tissue expansion may be considered a variation of other delaying techniques that improve the circulation within nonexpanded skin flaps.

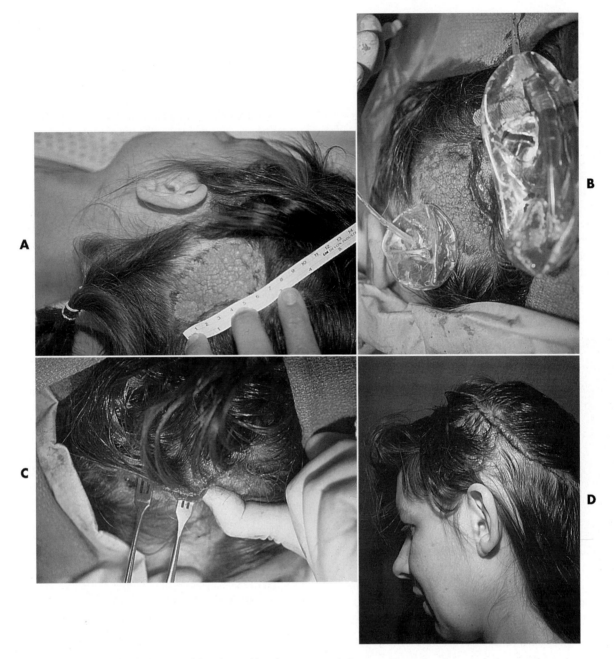

Fig. 29-4. A, 24-year-old patient with a large congenital nevus (4 × 7 cm) located above and posterior to the ear within the parieto-occipital scalp. Excision and immediate coverage was planned using intraoperative sustained limited expansion. **B** and **C,** A 160-ml rectangle expander (5 × 12 cm) and a 100-ml round expander (8 cm) were inserted under the galea aponeurotica of the adjacent healthy scalp. Through a 5-cm paralesional incision, serial expansion and relaxation over three cycles (1 to 3 minutes) provided sufficient tissue for coverage. Transverse galeotomies aided in the recruitment of tissue. **D,** The patient is shown 3 weeks after surgery with a single line of closure of stable hair-bearing scalp skin. A degree of scar widening is expected in the postoperative period.

Indirect measurement of blood flow

Sasaki indirectly quantitated skin blood flow in 56 patients before, during, and after expansion using five noninvasive methods. Dermafluorimetry proved to be the most reliable method to record gradual decreased uptake (arterial) and increased retention (venous) of fluorescein dye during expansion and relaxation. At the end of the inflation phase,

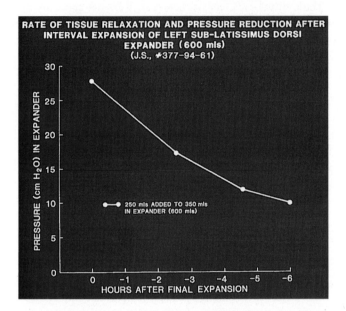

Fig. 29-5. The rate of tissue relaxation and pressure reduction is recorded after interval filling of an expander (600 ml) under the latissimus dorsi muscle. A rapid decrease in intraluminal pressure is measured after 250 ml of saline is added to 350 ml of silicone. An initial pressure of 28 cm H$_2$O decreases to 11 cm H$_2$O as muscle and skin creep occur within 6 hours of expansion.

a discrete area of low fluorescein uptake was present at the apex of the expander unit. Tissue relaxation occurred within minutes to hours; typical fluorescein entry and elimination patterns were determined by temperature monitoring, photoplethysmography, laser Doppler, and tissue oximetry during skin inflation and subsequent relaxation.

Intraluminal pressure-volume curves obtained immediately after each inflation period in softer tissue showed a direct relationship between expander volume and postexpansion pressure (Fig. 29-6). Manometric pressures as high as 60 to 140 cm H$_2$O (41 to 103 mm Hg) were recorded after saline filling as a consequence of the elasticity of silicone and tissue resistance. After a brief time (6 hours), however, the intraluminal pressure gradually decreased to less than 32 mm Hg. This decrease in intraluminal pressure was caused primarily by a "give" of the surrounding tissues (see Fig. 28-5). In contrast, intraluminal pressures remained increased for a prolonged time in scarred and irradiated tissues. Whenever the intraluminal pressure exceeds 32 mm Hg for more than 6 hours, irreversible skin ischemia and necrosis can occur because of diminished capillary flow. In these situations, smaller volumes of saline should be injected over longer intervals (2 weeks) to decrease skin ischemia. In clinical cases, monitoring of blood flow parameters by an indirect method is unnecessary. Clinical assessment of tissue tolerance during expansion (absence of skin pallor, firmness, elicited pain) predicts the eventual survival of expanded tissue.

Direct measurement of blood flow

Cherry and others[9] and Sasaki and Pang[47] reported independently that chronic expansion of porcine skin by subcutaneously positioned silicone balloons increased blood flow, as measured by the radioactive microsphere technique, and

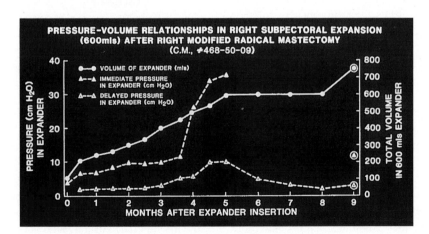

Fig. 29-6. Intraluminal pressure-volume curves obtained immediately before and after inflation in a breast expander under the pectoralis major muscle show a direct relationship between volume and pressure over 9 months of expansion. When the total volume of injected saline approaches the 600-ml capacity of the implant at 4 to 5 months *(solid circle line)*, the intraluminal pressures obtained immediately after 30 to 60 ml of saline injection at 2-week intervals rise abruptly between 10 to 37 cm H$_2$O *(solid triangle line)*. Intraluminal pressures obtained before saline fill remain low (2 to 10 cm H$_2$O) throughout the 9-month expansion period, indicating tissue creep and relaxation.

did not compromise hemodynamics within skin flaps constructed on expanded skin. Flap viability and capillary blood flow were compared among random acute skin flaps, delayed skin flaps (buried uninflated expander), and expanded tissue (inflated expander). Both flap viability and capillary blood flow were significantly greater in delayed flaps and identically designed flaps raised on expanded tissue than in acutely elevated flaps. Blood flow was also measured by microsphere technique within capsules encompassing nonexpanded and expanded flat and was not found to be significantly elevated in either one.

Epidermis

In most tissues examined throughout the expansion process, minimal histomorphic changes were observed within the epidermis. Occasionally, reactive hyperplasia, hyperkeratosis, parakeratosis, and spongiosis were seen after rapid and overfilled expansion. Other investigators[3,5,30] observed thickening of the epidermis and a threefold increase in mitotic activity. Melanocytic activity with melanin deposition increases slightly during expansion but returns to a normal pigment distribution and a normal amount a few months after flap advancement. This activity may be responsible for the slight hyperpigmentation observed in expanding tissues.

Dermal collagen and elastin

The dermis reacts most significantly to stretch forces during and after expansion.[51] Collagen fibers can support 10,000 times their own weight and constitute about 30% of the dermis.[12,53] Elastin fibers contribute only 1% of the dermis, returning the collagen fibers from their stretched pattern to their unstrained configurations. Austad and others[3] and Pasyk and others[35] reported that the dermis rapidly thins during the first 3 weeks of expansion. These investigators also observed increased fibroplasia (fibroblasts, collagen deposition and alignment) and thicker and more compact elastic fibers. They suggested that the greatest tissue yield after stretching is generated at low strains largely because of the reorientation of the collagen fibers in the direction of the applied stress.

Histologic observations by Sasaki confirm these changes in the collagen and elastic fibers. The reticular dermis became thinner (about 30%) after expansion. The reduced thickness was caused by, in part, increased compactness of collagen and ground substances in the papillary and reticular layers of the dermis. Trichome stains showed myofibroblasts within the reticular layer during expansion. In contrast, elastic fibers appear to lose their continuity and become more fragmented with expansion. This histologic finding may explain the reluctance of overly stretched tissues to retract after removal of the expander. Because most expanded tissue appears to contract immediately after removal of the silicone balloons, a significant number of uninjured elastic fibers probably exist within the stretched skin.

Dermal appendages and specialized organelles

In most human tissues analyzed before, during, and after judicious expansion, the dermal appendages and specialized organelles of the dermis showed minimal or no significant changes. These structures included hair follicles, sebaceous glands, sweat glands, sensory nerves and their end receptors, and blood and lymphatic vessels. The trauma of aggressive expansion caused fibrous replacement of these structures. These histologic changes, however, were not clinically apparent. For example, patients did not complain of excessive hair loss, dry skin, decreased perspiration, swelling, or ischemia after surgery. Some patients noticed, however, a degree of abnormal sensation within the expanded skin that returned to near-normal levels after 6 to 12 months. Discernible microscopic changes in sensory receptors and nerves in the expanded tissues were absent.

Adipose tissue

Fat cells within adipose tissue are extremely vulnerable to surgical trauma because of their intolerance to short ischemia, pressure, and expansion. The expander unit compresses fatty tissue above and below the balloon as filling occurs. The increasing duration of temporarily increased pressures within the expander produces ischemia in the subcutaneous fatty plane. Fat necrosis leads to an inflammatory response that resembles an infectious process and to a concave deformity. Although judicious expansion with low volumes and intraluminal pressures may preserve more fat cells, a significant degree of fat injury occurs during the insertion phase and at the second stage of excision and advancement of the flap.

Muscles

Facial muscles and larger striated muscles in the remainder of the body can resist the injuries that occur during the expansion process. In more than 300 cases of expansion in the upper and lower extremities, Sasaki observed the flattening of muscles covered by the posterior layer of the expander's capsule. Muscle strength was not compromised during the expansion process nor after the completed reconstruction. Although obvious functional disturbances were not observed in facial muscle animation, one patient could not elevate her eyebrow in the postoperative period. This patient may have experienced injury and replacement fibrosis of her frontalis muscle from rapid and aggressive expansion. Serial biopsy of the frontalis muscle after 3 years continued to show muscle fibrosis with brow ptosis. Inadvertent injury to the frontal branch of the facial nerve could not be excluded.

Blood vessels

Ruiz-Razura and others[41-43] have reported observations in intraoperative arterial expansion in experimental studies. Vein interposition grafts were compared with acute expansion and elongation in mongrel dogs. The created 2.5-cm arterial gaps, which could not be bridged by undermining alone, were directly approximated by intraoperative expansion with a 100% patency rate. The acutely stretched arteries showed minimal histologic changes and retained their inherent ability to contract. Ruiz-Razura and others used arterial expansion to provide additional vessel length to successfully bridge a traumatic arterial gap and a resected pseudoaneurysm.

Hong and others[21] postulated that additional vessel length observed in chronically expanded blood vessels may derive mostly from tissue gain rather than from tissue loan. These expanded vessels appeared to behave in a manner similar to unexpanded vessels after transection and microanastomosis during free-flap transfers. Expanded vessels in a pedicle flap permit an enlarged arc of rotation and advancement during reconstruction.

Nerves

Peripheral nerves have successfully undergone expansion to elongate them for a tension-free repair. Sciatic nerves in rats have been stretched 40% for more than 14 days and showed no significant changes in latency or conduction velocity. Long-term effects on expanded nerves have yet to be determined in extended studies.[17,27]

Capsules

The formation of scar capsules around tissue expanders represents an inflammatory response against a foreign body. A capsule barrier develops within 1 week of implantation of a smooth-wall silicone tissue expander or breast implant. The capsule is composed of collagen bundles that are parallel to the implant surface. Elongated fibroblasts, which produce the collagen fibers, are interspersed within the capsule. Occasional myofibroblasts (contractile cells that manufacture collagen fibers) are also found within the capsule. The capsules around smooth-wall silicone tissue expanders are generally thicker than those around smooth-wall silicone breast implants.

Sasaki studied capsules from 20 patients who completed expansion for breast reconstruction. Strips (5 × 30 mm) from fresh capsules were secured on a transducer and immersed in a water bath. Serotonin was added to the bath to stimulate any myofibroblast within the capsule, and myograph tracings were made of contractions. None of the capsules that were expanded for 12 to 20 weeks contracted with serotonin stimulation. In contrast, capsule strips from silicone implants that were stimulated for 6 to 36 months showed contractile activity. The significance of these findings remains unknown.

When a tissue expander is removed, the residual capsule gradually disappears over 12 months. The capsule has been used as a vascular flap to support a skin graft. Bengtson and others[7] observed a 100% survival of skin grafts over expansion capsules compared with a 28% survival over non-expanded capsular flaps.

PATIENT INFORMATION

Because tissue expansion gradually creates a hemispheric mound adjacent to the site of reconstruction, a temporary cosmetic or functional deformity usually develops. Therefore, before expansion is begun, patients should be informed that such changes may occur. Most patients will tolerate this inconvenience and attempt to camouflage the mound (e.g., by wearing a ski cap, hat, or scarf) during the later stages of expansion. In selected cases, the expander can be deflated before a social event and re-expanded thereafter.

Surgical planning

Preoperative planning is essential to ensure a safe and effective expansion process. The patient should be an acceptable candidate for this two-staged procedure, which is time-consuming, arduous, and physically or psychologically demanding. In addition, use of a silicone balloon may jeopardize the success of the reconstruction because of infection, exposure, and skin ischemia produced by the foreign body. Thus, optimal judgment of expander size and configuration, expander location, pocket size and depth, instillation of saline, and type of flap advancement minimizes complications while maximizing the amount of skin expansion.[46]

Expander number, size, and shape

The implantation of a single expander unit for a singular defect minimizes the risk of complications, reduces the visible deformity, and hopefully provides sufficient skin to cover the defect. A practical method of selecting the expander to be used is based on the width and length of the anticipated defect, the dimensions of conventional expanders, and the size of the adjacent donor site.

One expander may be adequate if it slightly exceeds the length of the defect. On the other hand, multiple expanders should be considered if the length of a defect extends beyond the length of the longest conventional expander.

The amount of flap advancement that may be anticipated after completion of judicious expansion with a single expander can be derived from either one half the base diameter of the expander unit or one half of the diameter of the expansion dome (Fig. 29-7). For example, if the diameter of a round expander or the width of a rectangle expander measures 8 cm, the generated flap will be advanced about 4 cm. Thus, in theory, if the defect's maximum width measures 10 cm, a single expander with a width of 20 cm should be selected. The largest conventional expanders available have a diameter up to 9 to 10 cm and thus produce only 5 cm of flap advancement. Any defect with a width greater than 5 to 6 cm may thus require the insertion of two expanders, one on either side of the defect. The combined length of flap advancement from the two expanders (10-cm base) should provide adequate coverage for a 10-cm wide defect. However, the decision of whether to place an expander unit on both sides of a defect is based on the availability of donor

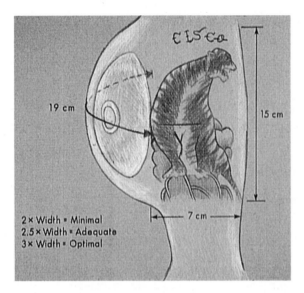

Fig. 29-7. The minimal amount of skin expansion that is required to resurface a forearm tattoo 7 cm wide should be two times the defect's width (14 cm). Because expanded tissue contracts by 2 to 3 cm after surgical release, the diameter of the domed flap should be two and a half to three times the defect's breadth to assure sufficient coverage (17.5 to 21 cm). The surgeon can anticipate that more expanded skin length will be regained when coverage occurs on a curved surface (e.g., the head).

tissue on both sides. When only one donor site is possible, serial expansion of the same donor site should be considered. This technique is referred to as the *leapfrog method.*

The shape of an expander is selected to best fit the configuration of the defect and donor tissue. Round expanders usually generate more flap length than rectangular or crescent-shaped expanders because a round expander possesses a wider base diameter than that in rectangular or crescent-shaped expanders of the same volume. Round expanders require a larger donor site and may not be able to reach the end zones of a defect. Rectangular expanders can accomodate narrower donor sites and usually approach the terminal portions of the defect. Crescent-shaped expanders provide more efficient use of expanded flaps to cover both the central and end portions of defects.

Expander location

Expanders should be inserted under optimal tissue to take advantage of simple advancement or transposition flaps. The expander should avoid tissue with scarring, atrophy, or irradiation injury. At times, however, the surgeon has little choice but to use such compromised tissue because it is the only available donor site. In the case of scalp or forehead expansion, the expander may be located under the periosteum or galea aponeurosis. In the midface area, the prosthesis is usually positioned under the skin and subcutaneous layers. In the neck, a pocket is usually dissected in the subcutaneous fatty layer but rarely beneath the platysma muscle.

Expanders are located under healthy skin adjacent to a defect. Occasionally, the expander may be positioned partially under the defect (skin graft) to minimize implant migration away from the lesion. Expanders may also be located directly under a stable benign lesion (large nevus) for a simple closure.

Expander incision

Incision for insertion of the expander unit may be made within the defect (intralesional), beside the defect (junctional), or away from the defect (distant). The advantage of a distant site is avoidance of a potential weak area during expansion. Whenever a paralesional or intralesional incision is used, wound healing at the entry site can be delayed. With such approaches, the presence of a thin or unstable closure, suture contamination or infection, or pressure knuckling from the underlying expander predicts a setback or a need to abort the procedure. Sasaki prefers to use a remote incision whenever possible to eliminate incisional problems that can abort the procedure. With experience, a distant crease line or scar can almost always be found away from the outlined expander pocket and can serve as a remote incision site. In the head and neck, favored incision locations include behind the earlobe (midface and neck pockets), postauricular (scalp and forehead pockets), and posterior to the hairline (midforehead and nasal pockets).

Distant incisions permit earlier and more rapid skin expansion because there is no direct force on the incision caused by the prosthesis. Thus, the surgeon may design the direction of the remote incision independent of the force vector of expansion and camouflage it to be parallel to the skin crease or scar axis. When no site remote from the balloon is convenient, the surgeon should place the incision at least 4 to 6 cm from the proposed leading edge of the expander. Such a maneuver reduces the probability of implant exposure at the incision site. In this case, the optimal direction for the incision is perpendicular to the expander's major axis. The location of any remote incision should consider the possibility of a need for secondary procedures.

The dissection of the pocket for the remote valve is made through the same incision as that of the expander, but it should be located a reasonable distance from the incision site. Injection ports should not be positioned under the thin hairless skin in the postauricular area because the skin can be easily eroded by the firm valve. After expansion is completed, the filling valve and its tubing may be easily retrieved along with the balloon through the original incision.

Preoperative considerations

The proposed outline of the expander, injection port, and incision line should be drawn on the patient's skin. An accurate outline of the anticipated defect should also be marked. Before the operative site is painted with a bacteriostatic soap, prophylactic systemic antibiotics are given. The expander unit is bathed in an antibiotic solution consisting of 1000 ml of saline and 50,000 units of bacitracin. This solution will also be used to irrigate the surgical pockets and to fill the expander unit. In the head and neck, the use of a metal in-line connector may be necessary to lengthen the distance between the balloon and its injection port.

Surgical technique

In most locations, dissection of the pockets for the tissue expander units may be safely performed under local anesthesia. Anesthesia and vasoconstriction are achieved with buffered 0.5% lidocaine and 1:200,000 epinephrine, which aid in dissection and hemostasis. In children and in most patients undergoing scalp insertion (regardless of age), general anesthesia is preferred because of reduced discomfort and bleeding.

After the incision is made, the desired plane of dissection is within the deep subcutaneous fat (midface, nose, neck) or under the subperiosteum (scalp, forehead). In the head and neck, a dissection plane is rarely made directly under any of the facial muscles (frontalis, procerus, platysma) because of possible injury to facial nerve branches. The pocket size for the balloon should be large enough to permit the base of the prosthesis to lie flat without folding or distorting. The pocket dimension should follow the external skin markings to prevent dissections under skin grafts or development of a too-large pocket, which permits the implant to migrate. Tissue elevation is facilitated by the use of long dissecting scissors, tissue spreaders, and curved dissectors. The pocket for the filling port should mimic the size of the valve to prevent migration or overturning. Occasionally, anchoring sutures are used to prevent the balloon or valve from migrating toward the incision line.

After the pockets are irrigated with the bacteriostatic solution, the partially filled expander is gently inserted with a finger or a large round tipped plastic suction device. The implant should be positioned upright with its base on the floor of the pocket. The valve is inserted through the same incision. The tubing is placed away from the incision line and fixed with a few absorbable sutures. It is very important to prevent curling of the tubing, which may obstruct expansion or, more commonly, erode through the skin. Thus, the tubing should lie taut between the balloon and valve.

Before skin closure, the filling solution diluted with a small amount of methylene blue dye is injected using a 23-gauge butterfly needle through the soft spot on the valve. The expander is filled to tissue tolerance to (1) obliterate dead space, (2) accurately position the expander within the confines of the pocket in an upright position, (3) reduce bleeding, and (4) check for unit integrity. The surgical team should scrutinize the implant unit before insertion to discover any imperfections. The incision is closed in layers, then covered with a steri-strip dressing on which an antibiotic ointment is applied. Oral antibiotics are continued for 3 days after surgery. Patients may shower and shampoo anytime after surgery. Sutures are removed in 2 to 3 weeks, or sooner, if suture infection or an abscess develops.

Postoperative management

Expansion begins after the second or third week to ensure that the incision has appropriately healed. By then, the opportunity for significant perioperative complications (infections, dehiscence, unstable skin, hematomas, seromas) has passed. Capsule formation is begun with a reduction of pain. A sterile setup with gloves, 23-gauge needles, and a 30-ml syringe is arranged for every expansion. The skin over the valve site may be anesthetized with a topical anesthetic cream applied 3 to 4 hours before needle insertion. The skin may also be temporarily anesthetized by freezing the skin with a spray or ice cubes. The skin is wiped with alcohol to remove oil and debris. Next, a poridone-iodine paint is applied over and beyond the skin outline of the valve. Gentamicin ophthalmic cream (1.0%) is then placed on the skin over the fill port in an attempt to prevent dragging in skin bacteria during the needle stick into the valve and sealing of the entry point after withdrawal of the needle. The saline is withdrawn with an 18-gauge needle from a 30-ml disposable bottle into the syringe. If additional saline is required during a single filling, the solution from a new bottle is drawn into the syringe. Serial withdrawals from a larger saline bottle or bag (especially for use in multiple patients or multiple expanders within a single patient) may increase the possibility of bacterial or fungal contamination. If a patient has more than one expander, a new syringe, 23-gauge needle, and saline vial are used for each expander system. The amount of saline fill depends on clinical assessment of the expanded tissue. Useful parameters include prolonged pallor of the overlying skin, firmness of the skin on palpation, and complaints of excessive pain or pressure by the patient. The use of manometric measurements as a means of avoiding overfilling is impractical and unnecessary in most situations. It is prudent to underfill rather than overfill at each expansion to reduce the chances of skin ischemia and necrosis. Patients will be inconvenienced (and surgeons embarrassed) if they need to return for fluid withdrawal because of overly aggressive expansion.

Serial expansion is usually conducted every week or every other week. Biweekly expansions may be performed but usually do not significantly reduce the total time required for the expansion process. In children, frequent expansions in an attempt to gain more tissue in a shorter time should be balanced with the degree of psychologic trauma and tissue intolerance produced by this approach.

Second surgical procedure

Expansion continues until sufficient tissue has been created to close the defect. The most reliable measure of tissue expansion and advancement is based on the circumference of the dome of the expanded skin (see Fig. 28-7). As described, the total length of expanded skin should be two and a half to three times the width of the defect. In general, 6 to 12 weeks are required to achieve maximum tissue expansion in the head and neck.

The second stage involves surgery for removal of the expander unit and completion of the reconstruction. After local or general anesthesia, the expanded site is acutely stretched using a technique referred to as *booster expansion*. Acute expansion appears to produce additional tissue for reconstruction without significantly injuring the surrounding tissue. The ISLE technique may provide up to 1 to 2 cm of additional tissue from each expander to contribute to the final reconstructive effort. After 5 to 10 minutes of hyperexpansion, the expander, valve, and tubing are removed through a generous incision made within the defect or at its junction with the balloon. The distant scar may be reopened to aid in the extraction of the remote valve system. After trial advancement of the expanded flaps over the defect, the surgeon determines whether the entire defect can be closed. Capsulotomy around the base of the capsule may allow further advancement of the flaps. Crisscrossing capsulotomies or a complete capsulectomy opens the expanded flap for further advancement. The decision to perform a crisscrossing capsulotomy or a complete capsulotomy over the flap's dome is determined at surgery. A complete capsulectomy may damage hair follicles in a scalp reconstruction or may create a thin skin flap that may not provide optimal tissue for the defect. In such cases, the entire capsule should be left intact or only a limited capsulotomy should be performed.

Tissue expansion often causes atrophy of the subcutaneous fat beneath the expander, producing a concave depression at the reconstructive site. Because of this possible problem, every effort should be made to save as much of the subcutaneous tissue at the defect. After removal of the lesion, the remaining tissue is used to fill the soft-tissue deficiency. Meticulous skin closure is performed in a layered fashion, usually over a surgical drain.

CLINICAL EXAMPLES OF HEAD AND NECK EXPANSION SURGERY

Scalp reconstruction

The goal of scalp reconstruction is to provide stable hair coverage for alopecia or diseased hair-bearing scalp.[28]

The two-staged procedure has been successfully applied to reconstruct congenital (giant hairy nevus), developmental (male-patterned baldness), traumatic (scar, burn hypertrophy), neoplastic (basal or squamous cell carcinomas), irradiated, and skin-grafted sites.

Expansion of the scalp is always performed beneath the periosteum, approached through a distant incision. Strategic placement of one or more expanders is almost always necessary for large lesions. Scalp expansion has been performed in neonates without permanent injury to the subjacent calvarium or brain tissue. However, the calvarium may show a temporary or permanent depression and the infant skin may develop pressure necrosis over the valve or balloon because of the thinness of the tissue.

Hair follicle retention within the expanded scalp will not be appreciably changed after reconstruction, but a decrease in hair density will be apparent because of the increased interfollicular distance. Sensation may slightly change after the flaps are advanced, and scar stretchback may occur to a variable degree that may require secondary scar revision.

Central defects are most expeditiously reconstructed by expanding healthy scalp in both temporal areas (Fig. 29-8). Large temporo-occipital defects may require two expanders placed along the edge of the defect (Fig. 29-9). As a rule, side-to-side advancements are more effective than moving tissue from a cephalic to caudad direction. Large defects in the occiput or anterior scalp may require two expansions to satisfy the reconstructive goals.

Since 1979, 20 aesthetic procedures for male-patterned baldness and 212 scalp reconstructions have been completed (Table 29-2). More than 50 of these procedures required two or three expansions. Expanders are positioned under the periosteum without a need for periosteal scoring. At the final stage, extensive capsulectomies and base capsulotomies may be needed to unfurl and advance the flaps. Scalp expansion may require more than 12 weeks of expansion with a typical biphasic progress curve. Initially, there will be resistance to expansion for 2 to 4 weeks until the periosteum is overcome. A more rapid expansion is observed thereafter as the scalp skin stretches. After expansion was completed, 32 minor (14%) and 14 major (6%) complications were observed (Table 29-3).

Table 29-2. Site distribution of 20 aesthetic and 212 reconstructive scalp surgeries

Site	Cases (n)
Aesthetic	
Male-patterned baldness	20
Reconstructive	
Right temporoparietalis scalp	59
Anterior central scalp	53
Posterior central scalp	19
Left temporoparietalis scalp	51
Occipital scalp	30

Table 29-3. Complications in 20 aesthetic and 212 reconstructive scalp surgeries

Minor (6%)		Major (6%)	
Complication	Cases (n)	Complication	Cases (n)
Malposition	2	Infection	13
Implant failure	4	Flap necrosis	1
Exposure	15		
Infection	11		

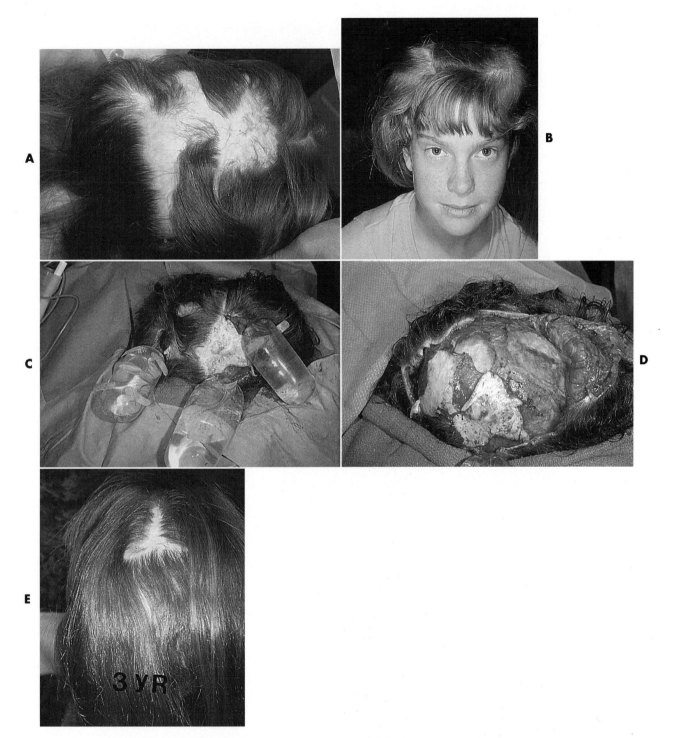

Fig. 29-8. A, A 12-year-old patient sustained burn trauma to the midposterior scalp at an early age. Multiple attempts to remove the skin graft with fractional reductions and rotational advancement scalp flaps resulted in an irregular pattern. **B,** Two 480-ml rectangle expanders (7 × 16 cm) were inserted along each temporal side of the defect, disregarding the presence of overlying scars from previous advancement flaps. A 640-ml rectangle expander was positioned under the galea across the occiput. All expanders were inserted through a 3-cm incision in the posterior sulcus of each ear. **C** and **D,** After "booster" expansion was performed, the three expanders were removed. Capsulectomy of the entire dome and peripheral base capsulotomy advanced the flaps over the defect. The elevated capsule formation or the calvarial surface was removed to create a smooth coverage. **E,** The resulting scar shows a small degree of widening 3 years postsurgery. The patient has not requested further scar revision. Scalp sensation and hair density remain excellent.

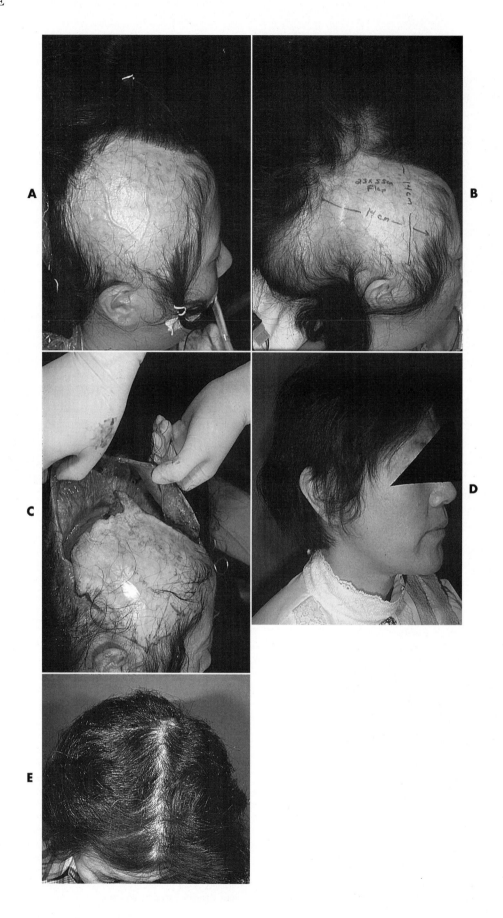

Forehead reconstruction

Traumatic forehead defects may result in a loss of all skin layers to the bone. Most congenital lesions (e.g., giant nevi) involve skin and underlying subcutaneous fat. Forehead reconstruction may require replacement of the frontal hairline, skin, subcutaneous fat, and the frontalis muscle. Expansion of adjacent tissue provides replacement of all the tissue structures with the exception of a functioning frontalis muscle unit (Fig. 29-10). Attempts to transpose an expanded frontalis muscle to the opposite side of the forehead often result in an adynamic unit because of direct injury to the muscle or nerve. Low fill volumes may prevent injury to this sensitive muscle unit. Medial advancement of an expanded frontalis muscle and skin unit for 1 to 2 cm can result in establishing the full width of this brow elevator. Expansion of brow depressors, such as the corrugators, procerus, and orbital portions of the orbicularis oculi muscles, has not successfully provided functional units for animation.

Since 1979, Sasaki has reconstructed 61 forehead defects involving re-establishment of the frontal hairline, skin, or skin and muscle units (Table 29-4). Most deformities were lateral or midline forehead defects. For myocutaneous defects, expansion of frontalis muscle and skin is performed with an expander under the periosteum or galea aponeurotica. This level of dissection is bloodless and rapid. For skin and subcutaneous problems, the expander is positioned only under the donor forehead skin and fat. Elevation of donor skin from the subjacent frontalis muscle is more apt to injure the skin compared with that during subperiosteal dissection.

Complications have been infrequent in the forehead region (Table 29-5).

Advancement of expanded tissue is more easily accomplished from side-to-side than from a cephalad to caudad direction. Defects as large as 50% of the forehead have been reconstructed by expansion of the contralateral forehead tissue. In these cases, extensive capsulotomies, capsulectomies, and judicious backcuts may be required to unfurl and advance the expanded tissue (Fig. 29-11).

Midface reconstructions

In clinical situations it is often impossible to limit discussion of tissue expansion to the midface area only. Because many clinical problems (burns and trauma, benign and malignant tumors, birthmarks) involve the entire face, a discussion of midface reconstruction almost always includes the forehead, eyebrows, eyelids, nose, ears, and neck regions. To aid the surgeon in planning expansion surgery however, the midface may be conveniently divided into seven anatomic zones. As in the forehead area, the advancement of expanded skin is most easily accomplished from side-to-side rather than from a cephalad to caudad direction.

The distribution of 119 cases of midface reconstruction is listed in Table 29-6. The lateral or preauricular area (zone I) is most easily reconstructed by expansion of donor skin from the central (zone II) and paranasal areas (zone III). Lesions located near the nose (zone III) are resurfaced by expansion of donor sites in zones I and II. The final incision closure lines should ideally follow the aesthetic lines along the subcilliary line, nasomaxillary junction, nasolabial fold,

---

Table 29-4. Site distribution of 61 forehead reconstructions

Site	Cases (n)
Right half of forehead	24
Central forehead	9
Left half of forehead	21
Transverse defect	7

Table 29-5. Complications in 63 forehead reconstructions

Minor (11%)		Major (4%)	
Complication	Cases (n)	Complication	Cases (n)
Exposure	6	Infection	2
Dehiscence	4		
Flap ischemia	1		

Fig. 29-9. A, A 47-year-old female sustained an avulsion scalp injury that required skin grafting. For many years a toupee was used to cover the right frontoparieto-occipital defect (14 × 14 cm). **B and C,** Two 640-ml rectangle expanders (8 × 19 cm) were inserted through a 3-cm incision in the left postauricular sulcus. The remote valve systems were located in the posterior neck. The expanders were positioned along the interface of the defect with healthy scalp skin. After serial expansion each week (20 to 30 ml per expander), sufficient tissue was developed (2.5 × 14 cm width of defect) in 4 months. At surgery, "booster" expansion, capsulectomy, and base capsulotomy provided sufficient coverage. **D and E,** The patient shows stable hair replacement with a scar along the frontal hair line, upper helical rim of the ear, postauricular sulcus, and occiput. Scalp sensation remains nearly normal. Hair density is sufficient to hide the scars. Frontalis muscle function was preserved for brow elevation and symmetry.

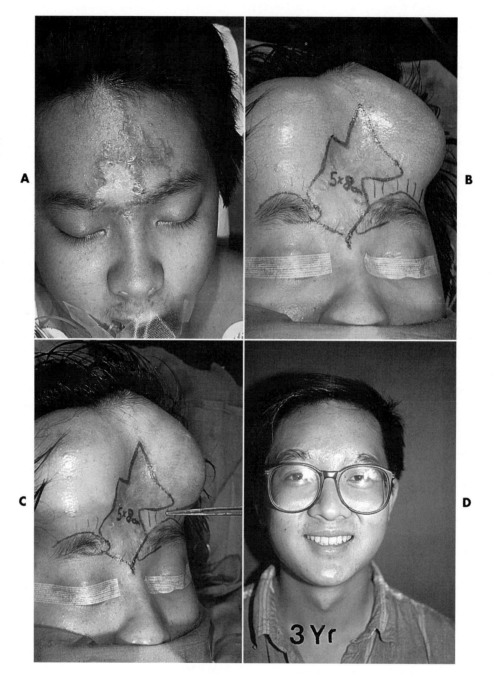

Fig. 29-10. A, A 23-year-old patient sustained a midforehead avulsion and multiple lacerations from a motor vehicle accident. Two full-thickness skin grafts were necessary to cover the interbrow-glabellar defect. Frontalis muscle function was present, but corrugator and procerus muscle activity was minimal. **B,** Two 100-ml round expanders (8 cm) were inserted through a 1.5-cm midsagittal scalp incision and positioned 5 cm posterior to the frontal hair line. The expanders were positioned under the frontalis galea aponeurotica adjacent to the central defect. **C,** "Booster" expansion is shown prior to excision of the 5- × 8-cm skin graft. The duration of the "booster" expansion was 5 to 10 minutes to gain 1 or 2 cm of additional tissue without further lateral undermining. **D,** The patient is shown 3 years after reconstruction with an acceptable vertical midline scar. The brow complexes are symmetric at rest and elevate evenly with frontalis muscle activity. Corrugator muscle activity has minimally returned. Sensation remains normal up to the scar complex.

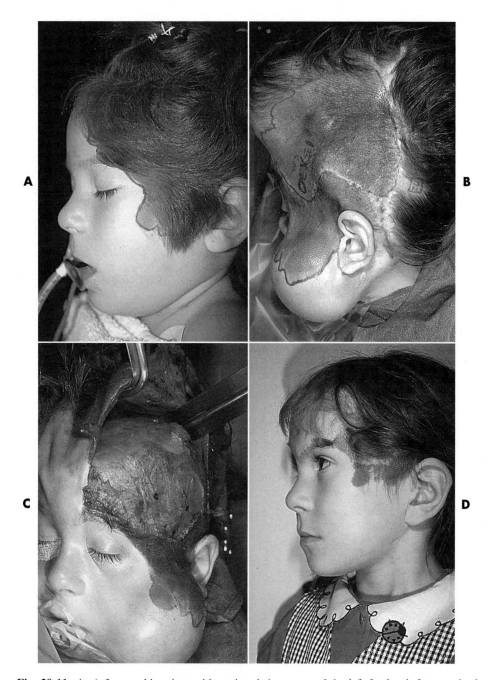

Fig. 29-11. A, A 3-year-old patient with a giant hairy nevus of the left forehead, frontoparietal scalp, and lateral upper cheek. Because of the cosmetic deformity and the malignant potential, expansion surgery was planned. **B,** Two rectangular expanders (1000 ml) were inserted under the healthy adjacent forehead and scalp tissue through a 2.5-cm incision in the right ear sulcus. Pockets were created in the subgaleal plane by dissecting from the opposite ear to the defect interface. The forehead extension of the anterior expander was positioned under the galea of the frontalis muscle unit. A third round expander (200 ml) was positioned in the subcutaneous fatty plane under a portion of cheek nevus and the healthy adjacent midface skin. This expander was inserted through a 1.5-cm incision in the retrolobular sulcus of the left ear lobe. **C** and **D,** After 4 months of serial expansion, almost the entire forehead and scalp nevus was replaced with expanded tissue. Slight paresis of the left frontalis muscle was observed 1 year after surgery. Most of the cheek nevus was excised with advancement of healthy midface skin up to the side burn area in front of the ear. Reconstruction will be completed in a few years with another expansion surgery.

marionette fold, and mandibular border. Zone II defects are effectively removed by expansion of donor tissues in zones I and III, but the resultant midcheek scar will be more visible (Fig. 29-12).

Expansion of donor tissue from the lower cheek and neck for replacement of large skin defects in the upper lip, lower lip, and chin is not recommended because the skin characteristics of the donor tissue often do not match the recipient skin. The final results of expansion in this area may produce significant distortion to these mobile structures (Fig. 29-13). Complications of midface expansion are more common than those observed in the forehead region (Table 29-7).

Neck reconstruction

Cervical skin has elasticity and movement, which is advantageous for tissue expansion. Expansion of neck skin has made reconstruction of difficult problems (e.g., burn scar contractures, congenital nevi, traumatic scars) possible. In the past, these entities were managed with relaxing incisions, Z-plasties, skin grafts, and local flaps. Expansion under the platysma muscle may lead to a gathering of the muscle under the mandible and to potential nerve injury during the insertion and expansion of implants.

The expanded neck skin may eventually be advanced in a transverse or vertical direction. However, expanded tissue advanced in a cephalad or caudad direction has a tendency to contract and shorten. This effect may result in a blunting of the acute cervicomandibular angle. In contrast, expanded skin transposed in a horizontal direction toward the midline or the sides of the neck tends to form hypertrophic scars. These shortcomings are related to the force vectors exerted by flexion-extension and lateral rotary movements. The underlying platysma muscle also plays a significant role in scar hypertrophy, which is observed commonly after burn trauma.

Vertical expanded skin advancement

When a defect involves the upper portion of the neck, donor skin in the lower aspect of the neck may be expanded. Cephalad advancement results in acceptable reconstruction with the scar located under the mandiblular margin. The cervicomandibular angle may be recreated with multiple permanent tacking sutures from the capsulodermal layer of the expanded neck flap to tissues along the neck angle.

Expansion of skin in the upper third of the neck to resurface a defect above the mandible may lead to several postsurgical sequelae. The native cervicomandibular sulcus may be lost because of increased skin tension during the cephalad advancement of tissue, or there may be a downward pull on the lip commissures caused by tethered skin. Thus, reconstruction of the lower third of the midface is usually better managed by expanding available cheek skin above the defect. Thirty-seven patients have undergone skin expansion of the neck with advancement of tissue in a vertical direction (Table 29-8).

Horizontal expanded skin advancement

When a lesion is primarily located in the midneck, two laterocervical expanders may be used to advanced tissue toward the midline with a Z-plasty closure (Fig. 29-14). Compression on the mandibular branch of the facial nerve or on the jugular veins has never resulted in facial muscle paresis or venous hypertension. When a defect exists on the lateral aspect of the neck, expansion of the adjacent donor neck skin with a single balloon results in adequate tissue for replacement. Twenty-six patients have had skin expansion of the neck with advancement in a horizontal direction (see Table 29-8). Complication rates have been low in this area (Table 29-9).

Table 29-6. Site distribution of 119 midface reconstructions

Site	Cases (n)
Zone I (preauricular)	33
Zone II (midcheek)	28
Zone III (paranasal)	58

Table 29-7. Complications in 109 midface reconstructions

Minor (12%)		Major (4%)	
Complication	Cases (n)	Complication	Cases (n)
Malposition	2	Infection	4
Implant failure	1		
Exposure	5		
Incision dehiscence	4		
Flap ischemia	1		

Table 29-8. Site distribution of 63 neck expansions

Site	Cases (n)
Vertical advancement	37
Horizontal advancement	26

Table 29-9. Complications in 63 neck expansions

Minor (5%)		Major (4%)	
Complication	Cases (n)	Complication	Cases (n)
Flap ischemia	3	Infection	2

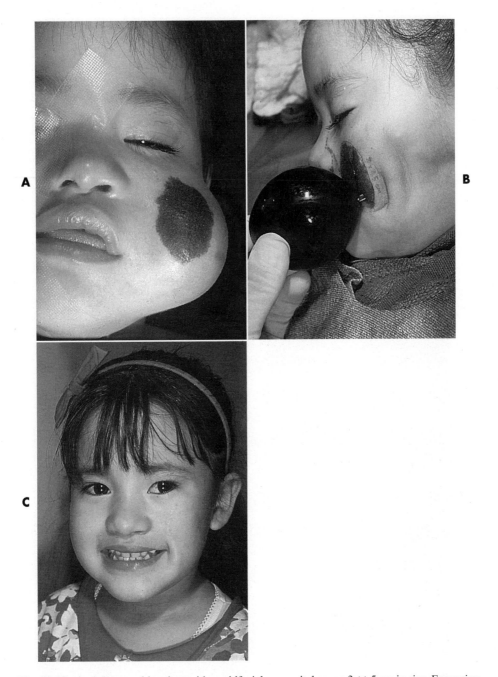

Fig. 29-12. A, A 3-year-old patient with a midfacial congenital nevus 3 × 5 cm in size. Expansion of zones I and III was accomplished by the insertion of a single 150-ml round expander under the nevus and the adjacent healthy tissue. The expander was inserted through a 1.5-cm incision behind the lobule of the left ear. **B,** Gradual expansion occurred over 6 weeks with weekly fillings. Measurement of the dome flap to 8 to 10 cm was necessary to remove the nevus with an oblique scar. **C,** The patient is shown 2 years after reconstruction with an acceptable scar, facial symmetry at rest, and animation. No midfacial muscle paresis was observed.

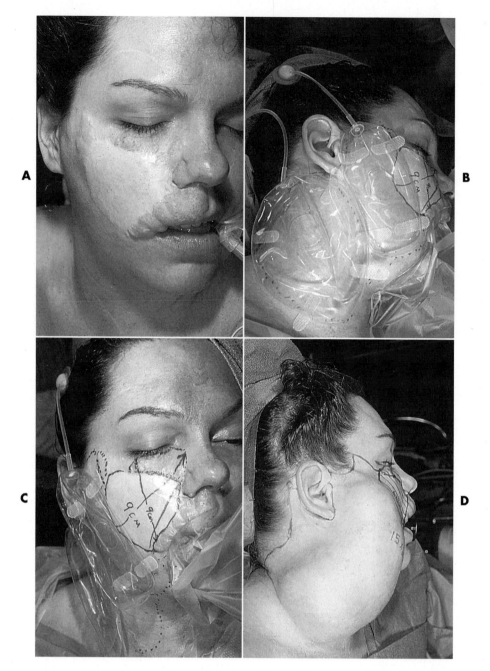

Fig. 29-13. A, A 32-year-old patient underwent a right midface excision of a hemangiosarcoma and coverage with a skin graft. The patient requested resurfacing that was similar to her cheek skin. **B,** A 160-ml rectangle expander (5 × 12 cm) was placed beneath the available healthy skin of the middle third of the patient's face. A 600-ml round expander (7 × 13 cm) was positioned below the mandibular border within the lateral neck. Both expanders were inserted through a 3-cm incision along the hairless border above the outline of the ear's helical rim. This incision would be distant from the edges of the expanders and permit insertion of the remote valves in the adjacent scalp. **C and D,** Serial expansion of the midface and neck skin occurred over 4 months to generate a large rotational advancement flap to replace the 9- × 9-cm graft.

Continued

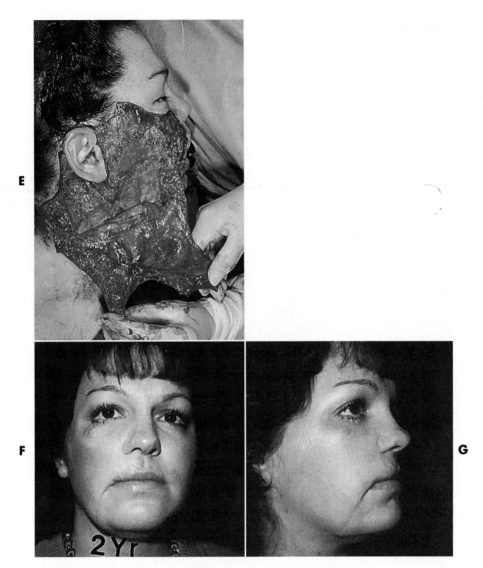

Fig. 29-13, cont'd. E, A large rotational advancement flap from the neck, postauricular area, and preauricular skin was required to complete an aesthetic reconstruction. Dome capsulectomy was performed to unfurl the flap and create a thin, supple cover. Retained portions of the de-epithelized skin graft accentuated the nasolabial fold and malar prominence. Suspension sutures elevated the flap from the neck to prevent sagging. Sutures were placed under the mandible to maintain the cervicomandibular contour. A portion of the expanded flap was inset around the right ala, nasal sill, philtral column, upper lip, and commissure. **F** and **G,** The patient is shown 2 years after surgery with functional and aesthetic midface-neck reconstruction. There was no problem with lower lid ectropion or commissure deformity.

Nasal reconstruction

Expansion of skin should be adequate to three-dimensional nasal reconstruction. The critical layers that should accompany such an effort include adequate skin, selected structural support, and sufficient lining. Mucosal lining can usually be obtained from turndown mucosal flaps. Mucosal expansion has been reported for closure of large nasoseptal perforations[40] and craniofacial clefts.[33,50] In the past, skin grafts have sufficed for a dry lining of the nose. Nasal support may be obtained from several sources, including cranial, rib, or iliac bone grafts and septal or conchal cartilaginous grafts. Skin coverage may come from expanded skin flaps in the central forehead region.

Subtotal reconstructions require replacement of a portion of the skin, bone, cartilage, and lining support (Fig. 29-15). Total nasal reconstruction implies that the entire nasal complex should be restored. This type of reconstruction involves skin coverage that may be obtained with the insertion of a subperiosteal expander in the midfrontal forehead. Serial expansion produces a dome flap with a diameter of 10 to

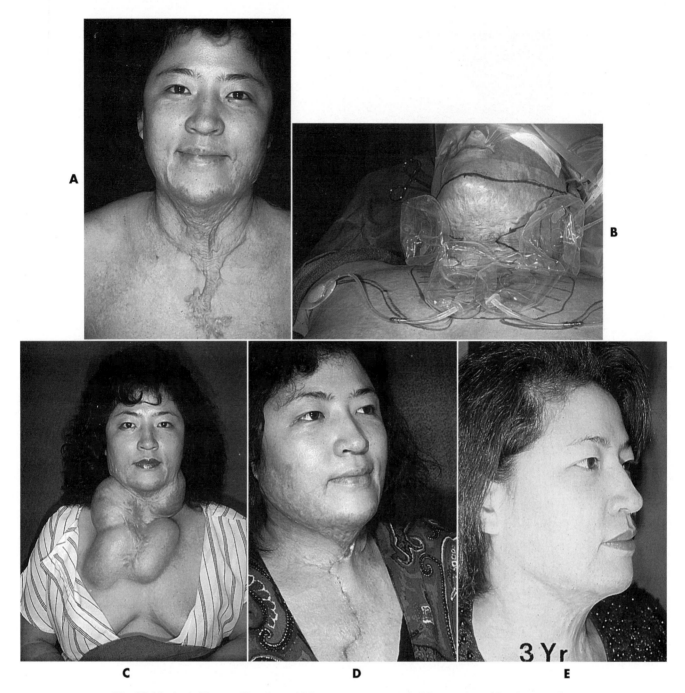

Fig. 29-14. A, A 47-year-old patient with burn scar contracture of the anterior midneck, extending down to the low midsternum. The patient requested improvement of the scar and a release of the cervicomandibular angle. **B,** Four 320-ml rectangular expanders (6 × 16 cm) were inserted around the scar from the neck to the sternum. The two neck expanders were placed into their subcutaneous pockets through a 2-cm incision behind each ear lobe. The two sternal expanders were positioned through a 2-cm incision behind each anterior axillary fold. **C,** Serial expansion on a weekly basis over 3 months produced sufficient tissues to replace the scars and the involved platysma muscle. Carotid insufficiency and venous stasis were not observed during the expansion process. **D** and **E,** The patient is shown 3 years and 6 weeks after surgery. The zig-zag scar has undergone minimal hypertrophy with pressure and silicone-sheeting dressings.

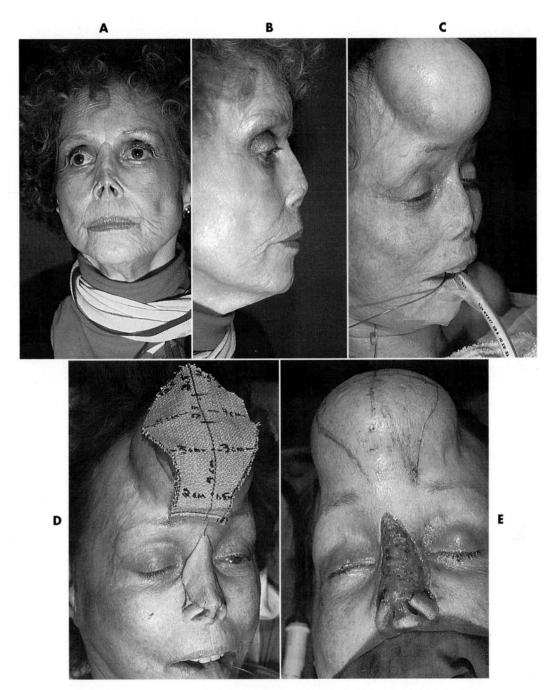

Fig. 29-15. A and **B**, A 54-year-old female with a markedly distorted columella, absent nasal tip, and dorsal nasal scars from an abbreviated glabellar flap. The patient had previously undergone Mohs' chemosurgery for advanced basal cell cancer of the nasal tip and columellar complex. **C**, A 100-ml round expander (8 cm) was inserted through a vertical 2-cm midsagittal scalp incision about 5 cm posterior to the frontal hairline. The expander was located in the subgaleal plane. **D**, Serial expansion was performed every 2 weeks until a 14- to 16-cm dome flap was created. The size of the dome permitted an 8-cm wide glabellar flap to be designed based on a right supraorbital and supratrochlear neurovascular supply. The remaining lateral portions of the expanded flap were sufficient for a midline forehead vertical closure. **E**, The small dorsal glabellar flap and scars were excised along with a release of both medial alar rims and columella. Cartilage grafts from the ear concha reconstructed missing portions of the alar domes and medial crurae.

Continued

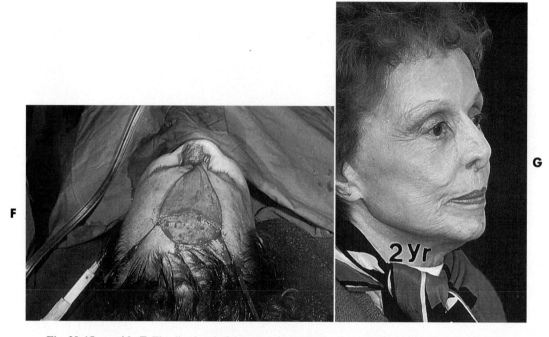

Fig. 29-15, cont'd. F, The distal end of the expanded glabellar flap was thinned to the subcutaneous layer to infold the tissue to resemble the skin of the nasal tip and columella. Infolding provided skin coverage and inner lining for the nasal vestibules. **G,** The patient is shown 2 years after reconstruction with sufficient tissue for the nasal tip, alae, and columella in addition to the dorsal skin.

12 cm, which permits design of a 4- to 5-cm wide midfrontal flap of adequate size for correction of the nasal dorsum and for direct closure of the forehead donor area. If the nasal alar and columellar areas require skin replacement, a dome flap with a diameter of 14 to 16 cm is recommended. This will provide a 7- to 8-cm wide midfrontal flap with enough length to reconstruct the columella, while allowing direct approximation of the donor site. The distal half of the midfrontal flap should be thinned of its muscle, capsule, and subcutaneous fat to create a thin pliable flap to cover the imported cartilage or bone grafts.

Ear reconstruction

Tissue expansion provides the surgeon with a technique for ear reconstruction. Its primary advantage is to create additional thin, pliable, vascularized non–hair-bearing skin to cover an autogenous cartilaginous framework. This method can produce enough skin to create an acceptable total or partial ear reconstruction, posterior sulcus, and closed donor site. Thirty-five ear reconstructions have been completed with an acceptable complication rate (Tables 29-10 and 29-11).

Reconstruction may be successful when adequate normal non–hair-bearing postauricular skin exists (Fig. 29-16). With expansion, the thin skin can be draped over the cartilaginous framework to highlight the outline of an ear. Usually,

Table 29-10. Site distribution of 35 ear reconstructions

Site	Cases (n)
Traumatic	
Helical rim	15
Helical rim and antehelix	10
Total loss	4
Congenital	
Microtia	5
Malrotation	1

Table 29-11. Complications in 35 ear reconstructions

Minor (15%)		Major (6%)	
Complication	Cases (n)	Complication	Cases (n)
Malposition	1	Infection	2
Implant exposure	8		

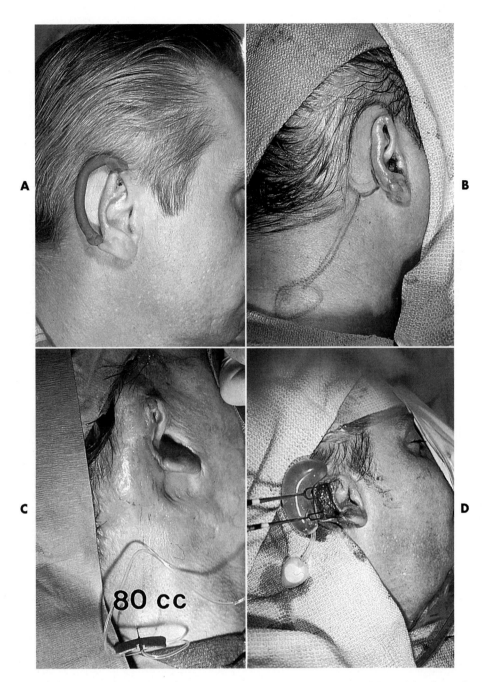

Fig. 29-16. A, A 48-year-old patient with loss of the helical rim of the right auricle after a dog bite. The limitation of reconstruction was the amount of available non–hair-bearing skin. **B,** A curvilinear 20-ml expander was inserted behind the ear at the level of the helical rim under the thin postauricular skin. The surgical approach was through a 2.5-cm horizontal incision at the base of the neck hairline posteriorly. **C,** Weekly serial expansion produced sufficient skin to cover an autogenous cartilage graft and provide a sulcus. **D** and **E,** The expander was removed at the scar interface. A portion of the eighth rib cartilage was carved to resemble the helical rim. The graft was inserted and spliced to the cephalic portion of the helical rim and the distal end tucked under the concha and antehelix. **F** and **G,** The patient shows a symmetrically shaped ear measuring about 6.5 cm in vertical height and 3 cm in width. The posterior sulcus is adequate for projection and a groove for glasses. *Continued*

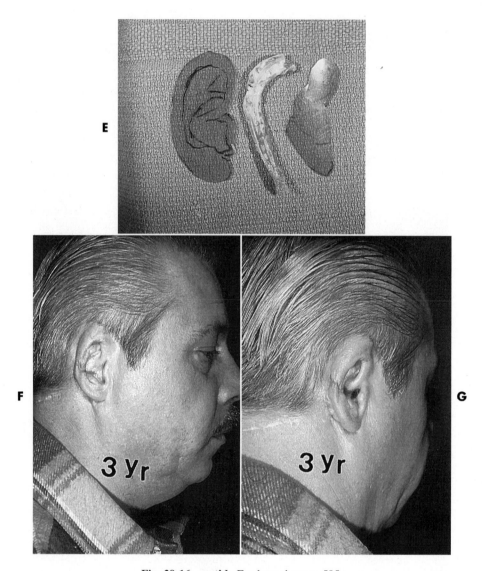

Fig. 29-16, cont'd. For legend see p. 595.

the final volume within the expander should be 100 to 150 ml of saline. With removal of the capsule, the extra skin is sufficient for both the ear and a deep postauricular sulcus reconstruction. The donor site for the cartilaginous framework is the synchondrosis of the 8th to 10th ribs.

COMPLICATIONS

The rate of major complications in the use of tissue expanders has decreased with improvement in technique, patient selection, and surgeon experience.

Infection

Infection of an expander in the head and neck is relatively uncommon because of the excellent blood supply in the region and the thickness of the skin. Infections still can occur on occasion. If an implant becomes infected shortly after placement or filling, an attempt can be made to salvage the case by instituting immediate antibiotic coverage, irrigation, drainage, and correction of the implant exposure. However, when the infectious process has advanced and invaded the capsule, it is more judicious to remove the implant and control the infection, while anticipating future replacement.

Implant failure

Inspecting and pretesting the implant should identify most material defects. The implant should be tested *in situ* for the ability to access the valve and to withdraw and inject the saline fluid.

Pressure ischemia and skin necrosis

Pressure ischemia of the implant can lead to tissue necrosis with exposure of the prosthetic system. Firmness of the valve, curling of the tube, and buckling of the balloon edges can slowly erode the overlying skin. Judicious placement of the valve deep within subcutaneous tissue should minimize the risk of this complication. A valve that becomes exposed can be moved into a new pocket to salvage the expansion process. An exposed valve also may be converted into an external port, which permits continuous drainage.[23] When an implant fold is encountered, a slower rate of expansion is often required and steri-strips can be used as external support for the skin to prevent skin necrosis. Massage or changes in deflation and reinflation of the prosthesis rarely resolve the fold.[2,6] If these measures are unsuccessful and overinflation does not smooth the fold, extreme vigilance should be practiced during expansion.

Bone erosion

A few patients have experienced outer table and full-thickness erosion of the skull secondary to tissue expansion for scalp reconstruction.[13,34,36] Bone thinning is temporary but is more severe in children than in adults.[11] Osteoclastic activity increases, and bone resorption and remodeling increase around the expander. At 9 months, bone normalization was observed by tomography.

SUMMARY

Tissue expansion is an innovative and established method to gain ideal tissue for reconstruction with a minimal secondary defect. Expansion satisfies the aesthetic and functional requirements for reconstruction.[46]

Skin is the most commonly available tissue for expansion. Muscle units have begun to be incorporated in the expansion process to provide an expanded myocutaneous flap. Nerves, tendons, and vessels may be stretched to obviate the need for intervening grafts.

Other applications for expansion in difficult clinical cases are being cautiously attempted to define the limitations of the technique. Intraoperative expansion of skin offers another alternative for coverage of small defects without the need of a buried expander.[45] By combining tissue expansion with other traditional methods, the surgeon has several reliable techniques to provide optimal tissue replacement.

REFERENCES

1. Argenta LC, Marks MW, Pasyk KA: Advances in tissue expansion, *Clin Plast Surg* 12:305, 1984.
2. Austad ED: Contraindications and complications in tissue expansion, *Facial Plast Surg* 5:4, 1988.
3. Austad ED and others: Histomorphologic evaluation of guinea pig skin and soft tissue after controlled tissue expansion, *Plast Reconstr Surg* 70:704, 1982.
4. Austad ED, Rose GL: A self-inflating tissue expander, *Plast Reconstr Surg* 70:107, 1982.
5. Austad ED, Thomas SB, Pasyk K: Tissue expansion: dividend or loan? *Plast Reconstr Surg* 78:63, 1986.
6. Baker SR, Neil AS: Tissue expansion of the head and neck, *Arch Otolaryngol Head Neck Surg* 116, 1990.
7. Bengtson and others: Capsular tissue: a new local flap, *Plast Reconstr Surg* 91:1073, 1993.
8. Burnett W: Yank meets native, *National Geographic* 88:124, 1945.
9. Cherry GW and others: Increased survival and vascularity of random

10. Codvilla A: On the means of lengthening in the lower limbs, the muscle and tissues which are shortened through deformity, *Am J Orthop Surg* 2:353, 1905.
11. Colonna M and others: The effects of scalp expansion on the cranial bone: a clinical, histological, and instrumental study, *Ann Plast Surg* 36:255, 1996.
12. Duffy JS, Shuter M: Evaluation of soft-tissue properties under controlled expansion for reconstructive surgical use, *Med Eng Phys* 16:304, 1994.
13. Fudem GM, Orgel MG: Full thickness erosion of the skull secondary to tissue expansion for scalp reconstruction, *Plast Reconstr Surg* 82:368, 1988.
14. Gibson T: Discussion: reconstruction of the tip of the nose and ala by load cycling of the nasal skin and harnessing of extra skin, *Plast Reconstr Surg* 77:320, 1986.
15. Gibson T: *The physical properties of the skin*. In Converse JM, editor: *Reconstructive plastic surgery*, Philadelphia, 1977, WB Saunders.
16. Gibson T, Kenedi RM, Craik JE: The mobile microarchitecture of dermal collagen: a bioengineering study, *Br J Surg* 522:751, 1965.
17. Hall GD and others: Peripheral nerve elongation with tissue expansion techniques, *J Trauma* 34:401, 1993.
18. Hallock GG: Maximum overinflation of tissue expanders, *Plast Reconstr Surg* 80:567, 1987.
19. Hirshowitz B, Kaufmann T, Ullman J: Reconstruction of the tip of the nose and ala by local cycling of the nasal skin and harnessing of extra skin, *Plast Reconstr Surg* 77:316, 1986.
20. Homma: Fascia-vascularized vs muscle-vascularized prefabricated flaps using tissue expanders: an experimental study in a rat mode, *J Reconstr Microsurg* 11, 1995.
21. Hong C, Stark B, Futrell W: Elongation of axial blood vessels with a tissue expander, *Clin Plast Surg* 14, 1987.
22. Iwahira Y, Muruyama: Combined tissue expansion clinical attempt to decrease pain and shorten placement time, *Plast Reconstr Surg* 91:408, 1993.
23. Jackson J: Use of external reservoirs in tissue expansion, *Plast Reconstr Surg* 80:266, 1987.
24. Lapin R and others: Primary breast reconstruction following mastectomy using a skin expander-prosthesis, *Breast* 6:97, 1980.
25. Liang MD and others: Presuturing: a new technique for closing large skin defects. Clinical and experimental studies, *Plast Reconstr Surg* 81:694, 1988.
26. Magnuson PS: Lengthening shortened bones of the leg by operation, *Univ Penn Med Bull* 103, 1908.
27. Manders EK, Sayyers GC: Elongation of peripheral nerve and viscera containing smooth muscle, *Clin Plast Surg* 14, 1987.
28. Manders EK and others: Skin expansion to eliminate large scalp defects, *Ann Plast Surg* 12:305, 1984.
29. Matev I: Thumb reconstruction after amputation at the metacarpophalangeal joint of bone lengthening, *J Bone Joint Surg Am* 52A:957, 1970.
30. Matturri L and others: Cell kinetics and DNA content (ploidy) of human skin under expansion, *Eur J Basic Appl Histochem* 35:73, 1991.
31. Newmann CG: The expansion of an area of skin by progressive distention of a subcutaneous balloon, *Plast Reconstr Surg* 19:124, 1957.
32. Nordstrom REA and others: Tissue expander injection dome leakage, *Plast Reconstr Surg* 81:26, 1988.
33. Ozgur FF, Gursu KG: Tissue expansion in median facial cleft reconstruction: a case report, *Int J Oral Maxillofac Surg* 23:137, 1994.
34. Paletta CE, Bass J, Shehadi: Outer table skull erosion causing rupture of scalp expander, *Ann Plast Surg* 23:538, 1989.
35. Pasyk KA, Austad ED, Cherry GW: Intracellular collagen fibers in the capsule around self-inflating silicone expanders in guinea pigs, *J Surg Res* 36:125, 1984.
36. Penoff J: Skin expansion: a sword that "stretches" two ways. Scalp expansion and bone erosion, *J Craniofacial Surgery* 1, 1990.

37. Putti V: The operative lengthening of the femur, *JAMA* 77:934, 1921.

38. Radovan C: Development of adjacent flaps and a temporary expander, *ASPRS Plast Surg Forum* 2:62, 1975.

39. Radovan C: Reconstruction of one breast after radical mastectomy using a temporary expander, *ASPRS Plast Surg Forum* 1:41, 1978.

40. Romo T, Jublanski RD: Long-term nasal mucosal tissue expansion: use in repair of large nasoseptal perforations, *Arch Otolaryngol Head Neck Surg* 121, 1995.

41. Ruiz-Razura A and others: Clinical applications of acute intraoperative arterial elongation, *J Reconstr Microsurg* 4:6, 1993.

42. Ruiz-Razura A and others: Comparative study between acute intraoperative arterial elongation and the use of the interpositional vein graft for arterial reconstruction. Presented at the 9th Annual Meeting, American Society for Reconstructive Microsurgery, Kansas City, M, September 26, 1993.

43. Ruiz-Razura A and others: Acute intraoperative arterial elongation: histological, morphologic, and vascular reactivity studies, *J Reconstr Microsurg* 10:367, 1994.

44. Sasaki GH: Intraoperative expansion as an immediate reconstructive technique, *Facial Plastic Surgery* 5:4, 362, 1988.

45. Sasaki GH: Intraoperative sustained limited expansion (ISLE) as an immediate reconstructive technique, *Clin Plast Surg* 14:563, 1987.

46. Sasaki GH: *Tissue expansion: guidelines and case analysis*, Arlington, Tenn, 1985, Dow Corning Wright.

47. Sasaki GH, Pang CY: Pathophysiology of skin flaps raised on expanded pig skin, *Plast Reconstr Surg* 74:59, 1984.

48. Schneider: Comparison of rapid versus slow tissue expansion on skin-flap viability, *Plast Reconstr Surg* 92:1126, 1993.

49. Timmerga EJ and others: The effects of mechanical stress on healing skin wounds: an experimental study in rabbits using tissue expansion, *Br J Plast Surg* 44:514, 1991.

50. Toth BA, Clufkides MC: The role of tissue expansion in the treatment of atypical facial clefting, *Plast Reconstr Surg* 86:119, 1990.

51. Versaci AD, Balkovich ME: *Tissue expansion*. In Habal M, editor: *Advances in plastic and reconstructive surgery*, Chicago, 1984, Mosby.

52. Weeks GS: Into the heart of Africa, *National Geographic* 100:257, 1956.

53. Wood EJ, Bladon PT: *The human skin*, London, 1985, Edward Arnold.

Chapter 30

Hair Restoration Surgery

Sheldon S. Kabaker
Michael R. Macdonald

Throughout history, powerful cultural symbolism has been associated with hair—its length and its loss.[40,51] Behavioral scientists have become interested in the effects of this physical trait on social attitudes, attributions, and action with a mixture of findings related to hair loss. Although some downplay its role in maintaining a positive body image,[79] many investigators offer evidence of substantial negative psychologic impact.[13-15,24] Neither gender escapes the difficulties associated with hair loss. Greater distress may be associated with even minimal loss in women because, for them, this is a less common and less familiar plight. Not surprisingly, the anxiety associated with hair loss is highest in those patients seeking treatment.

Scalp hair loss, or alopecia, may be a result of any number of causes, including trauma, radiation, and disease. Most commonly, it is a result of hereditary male-pattern baldness. This problem affects more than half of the male population.[29,56] Alopecia in women usually manifests as a diffuse thinning, but occasionally a male-pattern type of hair loss occurs.

In recent years, there has been an explosive growth in techniques for the management of alopecia. This area has attracted the participation of "hair restoration surgeons" from broadly varying fields of medicine, including otolaryngology, dermatology, plastic surgery, family medicine, psychiatry, and general surgery. The combined knowledge and experience of experts in these fields has produced a rapid evolution of approaches. New instrumentation and ideas have allowed surgeons to build on older techniques of hair transplantation, scalp reduction, and scalp-flap reconstruction. New drugs may offer some hope for future nonsurgical treatment alternatives that can be offered to patients not suited to surgical intervention.

In treating the most common type of alopecia surgeons should remember that aging and hair loss are dynamic processes. The goal is a look that appears natural when the patient is aged 35, 45, 55, and 65 years. Consistent with the varied presentation of these patients and the multiple treatment options available, a number of controversies have evolved: Should scalp reduction be performed or should it be avoided, particularly in the younger patient? Is there a role for flaps? Are "mega sessions" (greater than 800 grafts) the answer to hair transplantation, or does a multistep grafting approach produce a better result? The goal of this chapter is to provide an overview of the techniques available, with an emphasis on those that currently appear to be most popular.

PATHOPHYSIOLOGY

The average human scalp has approximately 100,000 hairs (slightly more for blondes and slightly less for redheads). The visible hair shaft is the dead protein end-product of the hair matrix, which lies deep in the subcutaneous fat at the base of the hair follicle canal. Living cells in the matrix multiply rapidly. Immediately above this multiplication area is the zone of keratinization where, by a process of dehydration and chemical change, the new cells die, creating the dense cohesive mass of keratinized cells called the *hair shaft.* As cells are added to the base of the follicle, the shaft moves out and "hair" grows. This growth is cyclic, rather than continuous, with approximately 90% of the hairs in the *anagen* (activity) phase, and 10% in the *telogen* (resting) phase at any given time. The growth cycle of scalp hair is approximately 1000 days (longer in women than in men), with subsequent shedding occurring randomly throughout the scalp. Certain events can alter this pattern. For example, during pregnancy, more follicles are maintained in the growing phase, and there is less shedding than usual. After delivery, approximately 30% of follicles go into the resting phase, causing a temporary, self-correcting shedding of hair, generally about 3 months postpartum. Prolonged febrile episodes induce an increase in telogen with noticeable shedding about 3 to 12 weeks afterward. The hair cycle also is subject to chronobiologic influences: In the northern temperate zones, daily hair shedding actually may double in the fall months with decreased shedding in the spring.[63]

Androgenic alopecia is the most frequent type of hair loss in both genders. Male-pattern baldness is the common name used for this process because it occurs much more frequently in men than in women. It eventually affects 60% to 80% of white men. Twenty percent of men notice initial hair loss shortly after puberty. By age 30, 30% of this population shows some baldness. The incidence increases to 50% to 60% by age 50.[29] In blacks, the incidence is approximately one quarter of that in whites.[70] In Japanese men, the incidence is one quarter of that of white men in early years, but increases to one third with advancing age.[76] In Chinese men, male-pattern baldness is rare before age 40.[29]

In the study of identical twins, Hamilton showed that the extent and development of male-pattern baldness depended on the interaction of three factors: androgens, genetic predisposition, and age.[29] It is thought to be controlled by a single sex-linked autosomal dominant gene. The expressivity of this trait is influenced by an interaction of several genes (polygenic) and certain environmental factors.[6,22] Although hereditary and aging influences operate at the genome level, no expression of baldness occurs in the absence of circulating androgens. Each hair follicle is genetically predisposed to respond or be immune to androgenic (and other) factors that inhibit its growth. This has been shown in auto-graft studies wherein full-thickness hair-bearing grafts from the occipital scalp were transplanted to the bald frontal scalp as the basis of early hair-graft transplantation technique.[62] Androgens variably affect different regions of hair growth. They produce increased growth of pubic, axillary, beard, and chest hair while retarding growth of scalp hair in genetically susceptible people.[65] Not all androgen-sensitive hair growth is controlled by the same hormone. Testosterone influences axillary and public hair growth, whereas dihydrotestosterone (DHT) affects beard growth and pattern baldness.[65]

The 5-α reductase enzyme is responsible for the metabolism of testosterone to DHT; the aromatase enzyme metabolizes androstenedione to estrone and testosterone to estridiol.[69] Both enzymes play a role in pattern baldness. Extensive hair loss in men is not necessarily a reflection of increased testosterone, but it may be a result of the lack of aromatase enzyme and increased 5-α reductase activity producing higher levels of DHT. Thus, male-pattern baldness is androgen-dependent, mediated by DHT through the 5-α reductase enzyme system. Inflammation also may play a role in some patients by stimulating cytokines and growth factors, which retard hair growth.[20,80]

The end result of this androgen-mediated process is miniaturization of susceptible hair follicles. The follicles become progressively smaller in size with shorter periods of growth so that the coarse "terminal" hairs progress through a thinner, more lightly pigmented intermediate phase before they are replaced by fine "vellus" hair. In women, this process frequently is modified. Their hair loss advances beyond the stage of vellus hairs to produce a bald scalp that is completely hair-free. In approximately 10% of these women with no signs of clinical hyperandrogenism (e.g., acne, hirsutism), chemical hyperandrogenism is detected.[49,36,27] As a result, women with advanced male-pattern baldness should be investigated for an underlying cause of possible hyperandrogenism.

CLASSIFICATION OF MALE-PATTERN BALDNESS

Hamilton published the first useful classification of male-pattern baldness in 1951.[29] A modification of this by Norwood[57] has become the standard system of classification used by hair restoration surgeons. This complete classification system includes seven categories plus a variant type, as seen in Figure 30-1.

Standards for classification of male-pattern baldness

Type I:	No recession or minimal recession along the anterior border of the hairline, in the fronto-temporal region.
Type II:	Triangulated areas of recession in the fronto-temporal region, usually symmetrical. Hair also is lost or sparse along the mid-frontal border of the scalp.
Type III:	Deep frontotemporal recessions, usually symmetrical and either bare or sparsely covered by hair. These recessions extend farther posteriorly than a point that lies approximately 2 cm anterior to a line drawn on the coronal plane between the external auditory meati.
Type III (vertex):	Hairs lost chiefly in the vertex. There may be some frontal recession, but it does not exceed that seen in Type III. This type of baldness is most common with advancing age.
Type IV:	Frontal and frontotemporal recessions, which are more severe than that seen in Type III, in addition to a sparseness or absence of hair in the vertex. These bald areas are extensive and separated from each other by a band of moderately dense hair that extends across the top of the scalp. This band joins the fully haired fringe on each side of the head.
Type V:	The vertex region of alopecia remains separated from the frontotemporal region by a band of hair that is narrow and sparser across the crown.
Type VI:	Frontotemporal and vertex regions of alopecia are confluent, and the entire area of alopecia is greater laterally and posteriorly than in type V. The bridge of hair across the crown in type V is absent.

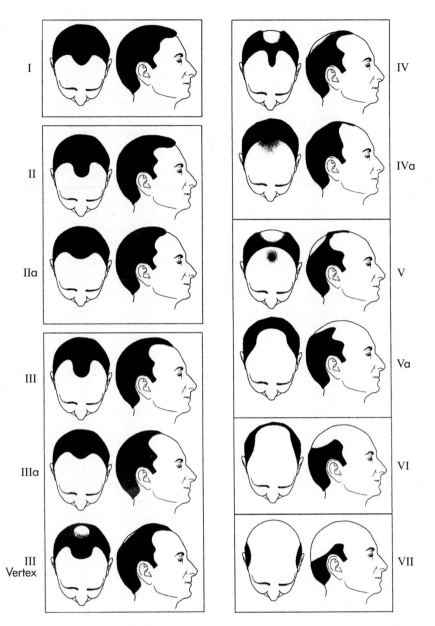

Fig. 30-1. The classification of male-pattern baldness. Common and type A variants. (From Norwood OT: *South Med J* 68:1359, 1975.)

Type VII: This type is the most severe form of male-pattern baldness. All that remains is a narrow horseshoe-shaped band of hair that begins laterally, just anterior to the ear, and extends posteriorly on the sides and low on the occiput. The hair usually is not dense and frequently is fine. The hair also is extremely sparse in the nape of the neck and in a semicircle over both ears. The anterior border of the band of hair on each side of the head extends to a region just in front of the ears.

Viewed from above, types V, VI, and VII are all characterized by areas of alopecia that are outlined by hair on the sides and back of the scalp, forming the shape of a horseshoe.

Standards for classification of type A variant male-pattern baldness

Type A variant classification of male-pattern baldness represents approximately 3% of men. It is distinguished by two major features and two minor features. The major features should be present. The minor features are not necessary for this classification, but frequently are present.

Major features

1. The entire anterior border of the hairline progresses posteriorly without the usual island or peninsula of hair in the mid-frontal region.

2.   There is no simultaneous development of a bald area on the vertex. Instead, the anterior recession just advances posteriorly toward the vertex.

Minor features

1.   Static sparse hairs frequently persist throughout the entire area of hair loss.
2.   The horseshoe-shaped fringe of hair that remains on the sides and back of the head tends to be wider and reach higher on the head than seen in types V, VI, and VII.

Type IIA: The entire anterior border of the hairline lies high on the forehead. The usual mid-frontal peninsula or island of hair is represented by only a few sparse hairs. The area of denudation extends no further than 2 cm from the mid-frontal line.

Type IIIA: The area of denudation approaches or may actually reach the mid-coronal line.

Type IVA: The area of hair loss extends beyond the mid-coronal line. There may be a considerable amount of thinning posterior to the actual hairline.

Type VA: The area of alopecia does not reach the vertex and is advanced in a posterior direction.

Other types of androgenic alopecia described by Norwood include diffuse, unpatterned alopecia, diffuse patterned alopecia, senile alopecia, and male-pattern baldness with persistent mid-frontal forelock. Simplified categorizations also have been introduced by Juri[32] and Mayer and Fleming.[47]

Female baldness patterns can be similar to those seen in men, and in these patients they can be categorized according to the Norwood classification system. More often, female alopecia consists of a diffuse thinning in an oval area on top of the scalp. In 1977, Ludwig[42] classified androgenic alopecia in females in three stages:

Grade I: Perceptible thinning of the hair on the crown. A thin band of higher density is retained at the hairline.

Grade II: More pronounced rarification of the hair within the crown area than seen in grade I.

Grade III: Total or almost total hair loss within the crown area.

Ludwig indicated that there always was a more dense area of hair, from 1 to 3 cm in width, at the hairline. This hairline region also thins with time.

Nonandrogenic alopecia also should be considered. Hair loss may be caused by injury to the hair root or keratinized hair shaft. If only the shaft is damaged, alopecia will be temporary because the underlying follicular apparatus will grow new hair. However, an inherently diseased root or toxic factors influencing the function of a follicle can stop hair growth and cause hair loss followed by: (1) immediate regrowth of hair; (2) temporary failure to regrow hair; or (3) the persistent inability to regrow hair. If the follicle is completely destroyed, there is permanent loss of hair. The etiology of the injury may be traumatic, hormonal, infectious, neurologic, nutritional, toxic, or factitious. Traumatic alope-

cias may occur as a result of externally applied traction with certain hairstyles or chronically applied pressure. This frequently is seen in black women. Internal pressure effects may originate with cysts or neoplasm. Hair loss may occur as a result of traumatic or iatrogenic surgical scars, thermal or radiation injury, and may be caused by bacterial or fungal infection. Patients with alopecia areata of unknown etiology or temporary hair loss associated with chemotherapy are not candidates for hair replacement surgery.

MEDICAL MANAGEMENT

Before considering a surgical approach to a patient's alopecia, any treatable etiologic factors should be eliminated. The aim of subsequent hair ''restoration techniques'' is to produce a positive, visible change that looks as natural as possible throughout the patient's lifetime. The full amount of hair is not restored. Instead, the patient's remaining hair should be rearranged to create an illusion of a net gain. The most commonly used methods of hair redistribution are based on variations or combinations of grafting or ''hair transplantation,'' scalp lifting or reduction, and scalp flaps. Each of these techniques depends on proper patient selection and counseling followed by careful short- and long-term planning.

PATIENT SELECTION AND COUNSELING

Hair restoration surgery is a calculated risk. Although family history and age at the time of presentation may give the surgeon some feel for the possible course of hair loss, these factors are by no means predictive. One thing that is certain and should be impressed on the patient is that the chronologic progression of male-pattern baldness is relentless and uncertain. Ideally, management should allow for changes in the hair pattern with an ever-increasing bald area and an uncertain supply of permanent hair as the patient ages. The law of reciprocal supply and demand dictates that greater baldness than anticipated always should mean less hair to remedy the baldness than anticipated. As a result, rather than minimizing and soothing the current concerns of the patient, the physician should amplify these factors by attempting to extrapolate the future progression of hair loss.

Unfortunately, the patient (especially the younger patient) often may view the problem as ''frozen and fixed'' in the present. The patient may request aggressive treatment now with the inappropriate belief that he or she does not care what it looks like when he or she is aged 50 or 60 years. However, any 50- or 60-year-old surgeon immediately recognizes the folly of this request.

A sobering and deliberate reorientation of the patient's goals often is required, which is one of the more important tasks faced by the hair-restoration surgeon, requiring a large amount of time, energy, and empathy. Fortunately, unlike the anxious younger patient with high expectations, balder patients and older patients generally are more reasonable. In patients with Norwood type VI or VII hair loss pattern or in patients with extensive hair loss at a young age and potential progression to this type of pattern, the availability of donor hair becomes a major consideration. Because of these issues of supply and demand, pretreatment goals should be developed carefully. These patients with extensive loss likely will have to settle for either a ''thinning look'' created by grafting large numbers of smaller grafts or the creation of a more densely grafted ''isolated frontal forelock'' as suggested by Marritt and Dzubow.[44]

MEDICAL THERAPY

Before considering a surgical approach, medical treatment occasionally may be considered. Endocrinopathies associated with hair loss can be helped by internal surgical correction or administration of hormones. Hair regrowth may not occur until many months after surgery or after the institution of appropriate drug therapy. In some patients, the correction of a hormonal imbalance, such as the adrenogenital syndrome, merely prevents further hair loss. The best treatment for fungal infections of the scalp is the administration of adequate oral doses of griseofulvin until results of fungal cultures, Wood's light fluorescence, and the microscopic examination of hairs are negative. Bacterial folliculitis of the scalp is treated with appropriate antibiotics and monitored by culture and sensitivity studies. Abcesses, furuncles, and carbuncles should be incised and drained. Most infections of the scalp are limited to the superficial parts of the hair follicle, sparing the critical deeper portions. After the infection is eradicated, if the papilla is viable, the follicle again is capable of growing hair. The ''trichotillo test'' was devised to differentiate between self-inflicted alopecia (often denied by the patient) and alopecia areata. The patient is advised not to touch a patch applied to the scalp and usually manages to comply, at least partially, because of the surgical adhesive used. By 3 weeks, the site will appear darker. At this time, removal of the patch reveals early regrowth of hair, confirming the diagnosis of trichotillomania. Response to corticosteroid therapy is often diagnostic of and therapeutic for alopecia areata. The regrown hair usually has the same texture and pigment as the patient's unaffected hair. Occasionally, and especially in patients with alopecia totalis, the new hair is temporarily white or darker and curlier than normal. The application of high-potency topical steroids (e.g., 0.5% triamcinolone acetonide cream) under impervious occlusion may help, especially with children unwilling to have injections. Those with cicatricial alopecia, such as pseudopelade, discoid lupus erythematosus, and lichen planus can benefit from intralesional corticosteroid injections during the early inflammatory stage. Topical and oral corticosteroids also may help.

Drug therapy for androgenic baldness

A number of topical and oral treatments for androgenic hair loss have been tried. Of these, only topical Minoxidil appears to have any trichogenic effect. This local vasodilator acts like a K^+ agonist to reduce cytoplasmic-free calcium.[48] The relevance of this unique cellular mechanism to hair growth is unclear,[18] although in large clinical trials involving 2326 men and 630 women, the non-vellus hair counts were somewhat higher in patients treated twice daily with Minoxidil than in control patients—nearly 20% over baseline.[50] The addition of topical tretinoin to topical Minoxidil showed a marginal increase in effectiveness over Minoxidil alone.[9,41] Unfortunately, in those male and female patients who respond, this response is only temporary. When the treatment is discontinued, the hair gained is lost, and the hair that should have been shed during the treatment period will follow within 3 to 4 months.[5,61,39] For those who continue its use, there is a peak effect at approximately 1 year with a slow decline in regrowth subsequently.[37,60]

Studies looking at several other agents are ongoing. These agents include finestaride (Proscar)—a 5-α reductase inhibitor;[19,77] cyproterone—an antigonadotropic for women with pattern hair loss[52]; spironolactone—an aldosterone antagonist that blocks testosterone production in the adrenal gland for female androgenic alopecia[12]; topical antiandrogens;[26] topical cyclosporine 1%;[28,68] and a Chinese herb extract called *Dabao*.[38] An electrostatic current device also has been tried based on experiences with wound healing and bone regrowth.[43] No large or well-controlled trials have been conducted on any of these treatments to provide adequate evidence to the hair restorative surgical community or the Food and Drug Administration to support their use.

SURGICAL MANAGEMENT

Planning the hairline

The most artistic components of hair restoration surgery involve the creation of the anterior hairline and determination of the direction and orientation of the transplanted hair. With flaps and scalp lifts or reductions, the luxury of planning normal hair direction is eliminated, which presents one of the disadvantages of these techniques with respect to future hairstyling. Regardless of which technique is used, the same principles of hairline design apply.

The anterior hairline balances the face and creates a focal region for the observer's attention. The location and design of this hairline also indelibly sets the stage for the future hair pattern and future restoration efforts. It should be emphasized that a hairline that is placed too far posteriorly may be moved forward with subsequent treatment. The reverse does not readily apply. The present and future constraints of donor hair volume and quality should be considered. Reinforcement should be given to the concept that, even though the patient may want the hairline of his or her youth, what really is needed is a hairline that looks natural and will age well.

General guidelines for hairline placement may be given but should be tailored to the patient. In those with mild-to-moderate baldness, the natural frontal hairline is lost. The temporal hairline recedes posteriorly, and the apex of the frontotemporal triangle recedes along a plane drawn vertically through the lateral canthus. In patients with extensive baldness, the frontal hairline is lost, and the temporal hairline recedes inferiorly and posteriorly so that the apex of the frontotemporal triangle is lost. Some general guidelines may be followed.

1. Design the hairline as far posteriorly as is aesthetically acceptable for the mature male hairline. Often, this is further back than patients initially request.
2. The frontal mid-point should never be placed lower than the superior border of the upper one third of the face—usually 6 to 7 cm from the mid-glabellar point (horizontal line drawn through the eyebrows).
3. A transplanted hairline should usually have a mid-point that is 7 to 9 cm above the mid-glabellar point if potential hair loss is mild to moderate. It could be 9 to 11 cm from the mid-glabellar point for those with extensive hair loss (Fig. 30-2).
4. In most patients, the hairline should be placed on the flat surface of the frontal scalp rather than on the vertical forehead areas.
5. The frontal hairline should look oval from the top and front views and horizontal from the profile view, and as an option gentle inward or concave curves in the area of the mid-pupillary line (Fig. 30-3).
6. Restoration of the frontotemporal angle should be performed with caution. This should be a distinct angle,

less than 90° (much less in whites; more obtuse in blacks). The apex of the temporal peak should lie 1 or 2 cm posterior to a pretragal vertical line, drawn at the anterior part of the sideburns, in the region of the lateral canthal line (vertically).

7. When creating a female anterior hairline, the rule of thirds and the full, rounded hairline concept should apply.
8. If the patient wears a parted hairstyle, an attempt should be made to keep grafts medial to this part. This may be an indication for a lateral scalp lift to pull the sides of the scalp up so that the part can be within the natural hair. The hair should be parted no further lateral than a line drawn cephalically from the lateral canthus.
9. The hairline itself frequently is restored only with micrografts to create a transition zone with gradually increasing density from front to back. This avoids an abrupt hairline. Micrografts may be used here with scalp flaps or lifts to camouflage any postoperative sequelae.

Special cases

Severe hair loss. In some patients with severe hair loss and inadequate hair to cover the entire balding region, an appropriate alternative may be required. Under these circumstances, Marritt and Dzubow[44] recommend limiting the recipient area to a "frontal forelock," which can be created

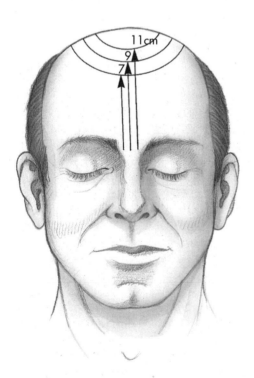

Fig. 30-2. Negotiating the hairline measured from the radix. The lowest points correspond to 7, 9, and 11 cm above the glabella.

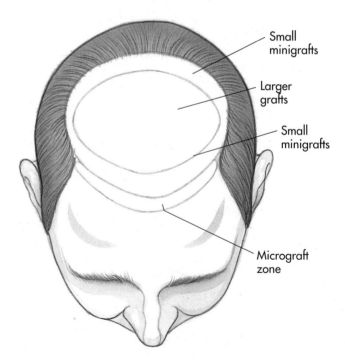

Fig. 30-3. The planning for placement of hair grafts. The highest one outlines the "isolated frontal forelock."

with excellent density to dramatically alter the appearance and to successfully frame the face (see Fig. 30-3).

Low forelock. Traditionally, a wispy low forelock would not be included in the newly designed hairline. The problem created here depends on how long the forelock persists—possibly for years. An acceptable alternative would be to maintain this characteristic portion of the patient's hairline by including the natural forelock in a slightly wider transition zone of transplanted micrografts.

SMALL GRAFT HAIR TRANSPLANTATION

Hair-bearing autografts for the correction of traumatic alopecia first were reported by Dunham in 1893.[21] Flaps and relatively large free grafts were used subsequent to this until 1939 when Okuda, a Japanese dermatologist, described the use of small 2- to 4-mm full-thickness autografts of hair-bearing skin to correct alopecia of the scalp, eyebrow, and mustache areas.[59] In 1943, Tamura[75] reported the use of single-hair grafts. Because of World War II, this work was not recognized until years later. Orentreich described a multiple punch-graft technique similar to that of Okuda in 1959.[62] He introduced the concept of "donor dominance": The ability of autografts to maintain the integrity and characteristics of the *donor* area after transplantation to a new site, rather than taking on the characteristics of the recipient site. He refuted the then-popular theory that common baldness was the result of ischemia. These findings have formed the basis of donor hair site selection from the permanent hair-bearing areas on the back and sides of the head, earning him recognition as the "father of modern hair transplant surgery."

Present techniques

Earlier grafting techniques depended on a donor graft diameter of 3 to 5 mm. After a number of years, 4 mm became the standard graft size. This size was thought to be optimal for transplanting the largest number of hairs without incurring loss as a result of central avascular necrosis. The principle problem with this has been related to the creation of a "corn-row," "toothbrush," or "tufted" effect, especially in darker-haired patients. More recently, the trend has been toward the use of smaller grafts. The smallest of these, referred to as a *micrograft*, contains only 1 or 2 hairs. *Minigraft* is the term used to describe any donor graft with a size between a traditional graft and a micrograft. The *strip graft* is a linear graft preferred by some authors to avoid compression of the transplanted hairs.[74,12] Figure 30-4 illustrates the various types of grafts most commonly in use, and Table 30-1 summarizes the terminology and essential characteristics of the various grafts.

With the larger traditional grafts, a round circular punch was used for harvesting the donor tissue. A slightly smaller punch was used to create the recipient site (Fig. 30-5). The donor areas were left to close by secondary intention. This harvesting technique rarely is used now. Instead, the donor

Table 30-1. Graft classification terminology and features

Class	Grafts	Recipient site	Number of hairs
Standard or traditional	Round or square, approximately 4 mm	Round, 0.3–0.5 mm smaller than donor size	15–25
Minigrafts	Round, square or rectangular, 1.25–2 mm	Holes or slits, < 2 mm	3–8
Micrografts	Taken from thinnest hair, lower in scalp	Slits, zone at anterior hairline	1–2

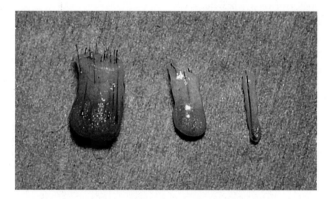

Fig. 30-4. A photograph showing standard 4-mm round graft (15 to 20 hairs), a six-hair minigraft, and a single-hair micrograft.

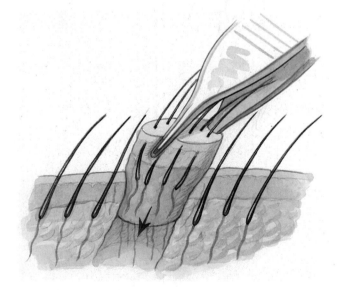

Fig. 30-5. The placement of a "standard" 4-mm graft into a 3.5-mm recipient site hole.

tissue generally is harvested in either parallel horizontal strips (Fig. 30-6) or a fusiform block from the permanent hair-bearing regions of the occipital or temporal scalp. The donor site is closed with staples or sutures with or preferably without undermining. This tissue then is cut into the desired number of minigrafts and micrografts. A trichoscope may be used before removal of the donor tissue to estimate the patient's hair density. This information allows the calculation of the appropriate length of strip(s) needed to obtain the desired number of grafts with appropriate numbers of hairs.

Micrografts are used to create a natural look at transition zones, such as in the creation of the anterior hairline, although they generally do not provide adequate density for a normal postoperative appearance in the bulk of transplanted regions. Instead, slightly larger minigrafts often are used as the "workhorse" grafts to provide the desirable density posterior to the hairline.

Some surgeons, including the authors, prefer to achieve the desired end result through three or four sessions of approximately 300 to 500 minigrafts and 100 to 200 micrografts. With each subsequent session, the bald spaces be-

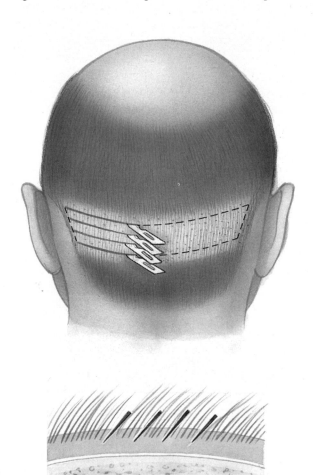

Fig. 30-6. A multibladed knife is used to cut long strips to be made into minigrafts and micrografts.

tween grafts are filled in with new hair-bearing graft tissue. Ideally, 3 to 6 months should be allowed between sessions for the initial transplant growth and healing, although this interval may be shortened to 4 to 6 weeks because at this time there is adequate healing of the scalp to support further transplantation, but the previous graft recipient sites are still visible. Between 6 weeks and initial growth, the grafted areas are difficult to identify clearly. During this interval, the creation of new recipient sites carries the risk of removal of previously transplanted grafts.

Recently, the concept of "mega transplant" sessions has become more popular. This involves the transfer of large numbers of small grafts (1 to 4 hairs) for coverage of bald areas in fewer sessions. The number of grafts in a mega session is not uniformly established. Rassman describes this as greater than 500 grafts per session but reports that it is possible to transplant as many as 4000 grafts (1 to 3 hairs each) in a single session.[67] Generally, a mega session involves more than 1000 grafts. This labor-intensive work uses 3 to 10 assistants.

Many different combinations of the previous may be used, depending on the patient's hair loss pattern, hair color, styling preferences, and treatment objectives. An overview of a typical procedure follows.

1. Consent is documented, pertinent history, physical finding, and laboratory work are reviewed. A series of photographs is taken to provide objective documentation preoperatively (and subsequently to follow the progress postoperatively).
2. In consultation with the patient, the anterior hairline is carefully planned and marked on the scalp. Other planned recipient regions also are marked out on the scalp (i.e., grid pattern).
3. The appropriate donor site is located, and the area is shaved with a mustache trimmer, leaving a few millimeters of hair growth over the strips of hair-bearing skin to be excised. The hair surrounding the donor area is kept away from the surgical field, either using tape or elastic bands.
4. A trichoscope may be used to estimate the patient's hair density so that the length and number of strips needed to obtain the appropriate number of grafts desired may be calculated.
5. The patient is placed in the prone position on the operating table or sitting up in a dental chair. The donor and recipient areas are cleansed with an antiseptic solution. The donor area is anesthetized with 10 to 20 ml of 1% lidocaine with 1:100,000 epinephrine. Inhaled nitrous oxide or intravenous sedation may be used to decrease the discomfort associated with this and other initial infiltrations of local anesthetic. 20 to 100 ml of saline solution is infiltrated in the same region to obtain firm turgor for improved tissue cutting.

6. The strips are harvested using a multibladed (usually four to seven blades) knife (Fig. 30-7). Care is taken to cut parallel to the hair shafts. Bleeding vessels are occasionally coagulated or sutured if needed, particularly if the occipital vessels are transected. The donor site is closed using wide staples. Undermining usually is not done. The donor strips then are cut into the desired size and number of grafts, while the recipient sites are prepared (Fig. 30-8).

7. With the patient placed in the supine position, bilateral supraorbital and supratrochlear blocks are performed, using 2% lidocaine with or without epinephrine. Local anesthesia then is infiltrated anterior to the anterior hairline. For the first session, 1% lidocaine with 1:100,000 epinephrine may be used. For subsequent sessions, 2% lidocaine with 1:100,000 epinephrine is used because these patients seem to be more resistant to anesthesia. A mixture of 1% or 2% lidocaine with 1:100,000 epinephrine and 0.5%

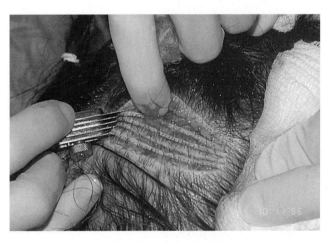

Fig. 30-7. A donor harvesting with a multibladed knife.

bupivicaine with 1:100,000 epinephrine then is infiltrated into the recipient areas posterior to the anterior hairline.

8. Graft recipient sites behind the anterior hairline region are made using 1-mm, 1.25-mm, 1.5-mm, or 1.8-mm punches. The size of the punches generally decreases as the anterior hairline is approached to create a finer, more natural look. Many surgeons prefer recipient slits made with a small knife blade, especially in areas that have natural or grafted hairs. Multiple recipient sites for single-hair grafts are created within a 5-mm zone along the planned anterior hairline using a 16- or 18-gauge needle or an Arnold Lightning Knife (A to Z, San Jose, Calif) (Fig. 30-9). Alternatively, a CO_2 laser can be used to make recipient slits or holes.

9. The recipient area is reinjected with 3 to 5 cc of 2% lidocaine with epinephrine, 1:20,000 to attain further hemostasis and anesthesia.

10. The hair grafts are placed into the recipient sites using Forster forceps (Figs. 30-10 and 30-11).

11. After the transplant session is completed, a dressing may be applied. Although many surgeons send the patients home without any dressing, the authors prefer to apply light dressing with a water-soluble gel between the dressing and the grafts to hold the grafts in position. This dressing may be removed either in the office on the first day after surgery or by the patient on the second day.

12. Donor-site staples are removed 7 to 10 days after surgery. Most patients resume full (but nonstrenuous) activity 2 days after surgery.

13. The procedure is repeated after 6 to 12 weeks, excising the old donor scar and placing grafts between previous ones.

14. The result after two or three sessions can be dramatic (Figs. 30-12 and 30-13).

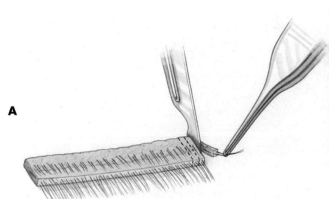

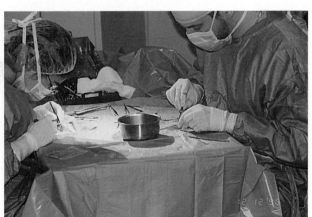

Fig. 30-8. A, Grafts being cut from donor strips. **B,** Assistants cutting grafts.

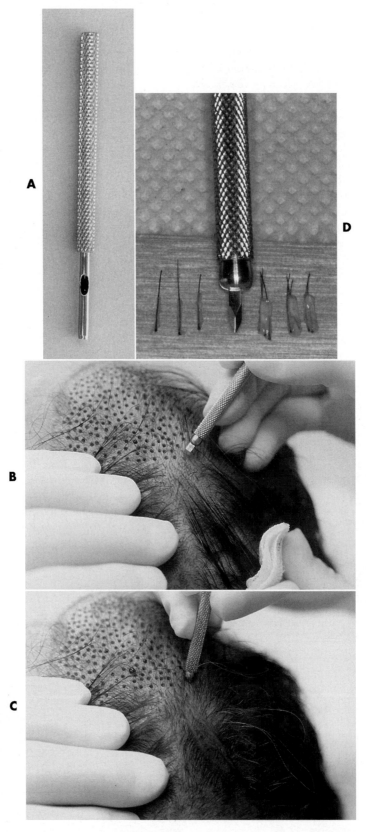

Fig. 30-9. The recipient site preparation. **A,** Super punch™ for making recipient holes. **B,** Holes made with punch. Lightning knife™ with chisel-shaped blade. Projection equal to height of donor minigrafts. **C,** Knife pushed into the hilt to create slits of uniform desired depth. Note angle of recipient site always parallels the natural hair direction. **D,** Knife with pointed narrow blade. Depth adjusted to equal the height of micrografts to be placed at anterior zone of hairline. (Photos courtesy of James Arnold, M.D.)

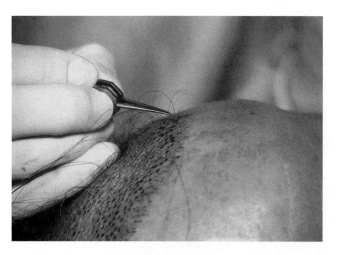

Fig. 30-10. The placement of grafts into recipient sites.

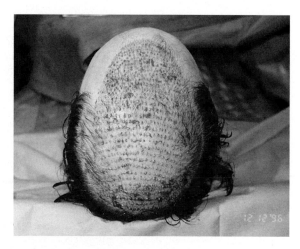

Fig. 30-11. The completion of placement of 1200 grafts (minigrafts and micrografts).

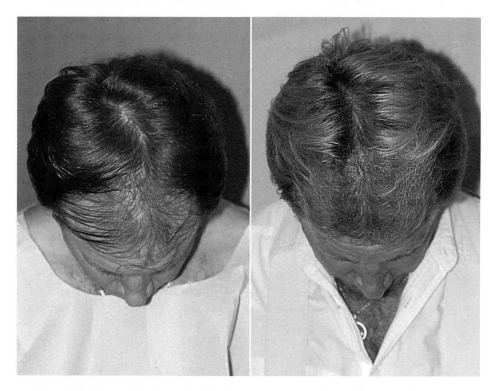

Fig. 30-12. The result after two sessions of minigrafts and micrografts (type IIA baldness).

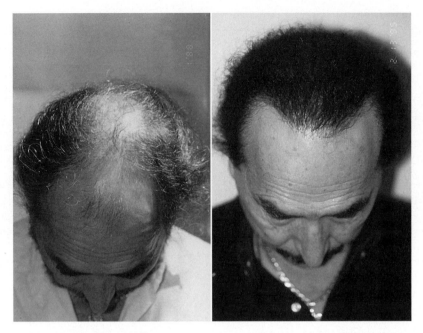

Fig. 30-13. The result after three sessions (12 of 500 grafts, type V baldness).

COMPLICATIONS

The complication, which frequently occurs but is easiest to avoid, is related to inappropriate hairline placement. The hairline placed too low usually is done in accordance with the patient's wishes, but it often produces less-than-pleasing cosmetic results. Unanticipated alopecia progression may expose other complications related to recipient site design and planning. Regressing hair may leave behind a halo of bald skin between grafted areas and the natural hairline, necessitating periodic "catch-up" procedures.

Complications related to the transplanted tissue most commonly include localized or regional edema and ecchymosis, which generally appears after the second postoperative day and can be minimized, or prevented, by applying pressure (e.g., sports headband, foam–rubber compression dressing) and ice compresses over the forehead region. Also, the use of small volumes of local anesthetic in the frontal zone (3 to 5 ml of 2% lidocaine with highly concentrated epinephrine, 1:20,000) is useful, along with steroid administration. Intramuscular or intravenous steroids may reduce this problem. Ridging may occur as a result of subcutaneous scar production in densely transplanted regions. Local steroid injection may improve this, but if the problem is severe, surgical excision of excess scar tissue may be required at a future sitting. Cysts may form where grafts are placed upside down, buried, or piggy-backed (two grafts in the same recipient site). This problem usually may be corrected by unroofing the cyst. "Telogen effluvium" refers to loss of hair adjacent to transplanted grafts. The patient may be reassured that this generally is temporary. Patients occasionally may be distressed by poor growth of grafted hairs, which often is

permanent. This may occur as a result of alcohol preservative in some saline preparations[73] or poor tissue handling. Transplanted hairs may regrow, if there is damage to the lower impermanent follicle, although regeneration appears to depend on the preservation of follicular stem cells in the perifollicular sheath around the mid-follicular isthmus.[16] Finally, in a small percentage of patients (0.5% to 1%), there is loss of follicles from causes that are not clearly identifiable.[71]

SCALP REDUCTION AND LIFTS

Bald scalp reduction was first reported by Blanchard and Blanchard.[7,8] Unless the patient had an unusually lax scalp, this often resulted in "stretchback"[55,56] so that, even after multiple procedures, the net result of alopecia reduction was less than satisfactory. However, many hair restoration surgeons continue to perform scalp reduction on selected patients (Figs. 30-14 and 30-15).

Techniques introduced to counteract the elastic forces of the skin have included prereduction scalp expansion[1,3,35,54] and scalp extension.[25] Expansion uses inflatable, saline-filled silicone bags, whereas scalp extension uses linear, stretchable silicone bands with metal fixation hooks (Fig. 30-16). Each of these implants are placed in the relatively avascular plane deep to the galea until adequate "permanent" skin stretch is obtained. They then are removed before the final reduction procedure (Figs. 30-17 and 30-18). Scalp lifting emerged as an alternative that used extensive undermining of the entire donor scalp, well below the level of the inferior hairline and into the skin of the neck.[10,11]

These solutions have been effective in producing skin

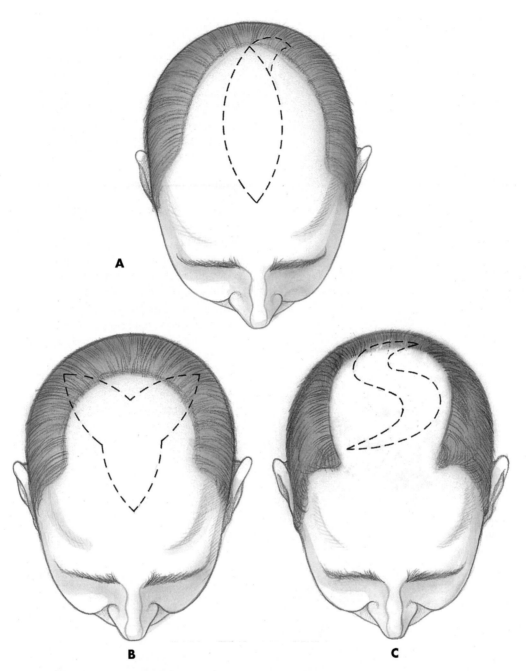

Fig. 30-14. Three commonly used patterns for scalp reduction. A horseshoe shape (not shown) often is used for the scalp-lift procedure.

stretch for dramatic skin redraping. Unfortunately, they have created their own set of problems: misdirected hair, severely decreased donor density, elevated inferior hairline, detectable halos, and, of course, surgical scars. Perhaps the most noticeable of these is related to the misdirected hair. Normally, temporoparietal hair points directly down toward the ears and exits the scalp at an acute, rather flat angle. Midscalp hair points in a frontal direction (a 90° shift) and has more elevation from the plane of the head. When both superior aspects of the fringe are brought in approximation with

a scalp reduction or lift, the hair direction becomes divergent in this region. This often is obvious to the observer. Consequently, limited or incomplete scalp lift and modified scalp-reduction techniques are best applied in conjunction with hair grafting (Fig. 30-19).[2,78]

FLAP PROCEDURES

A complete review of the techniques available for surgical hair replacement should include the scalp flap procedures, wherein unique pedicled hair-bearing scalp flaps can

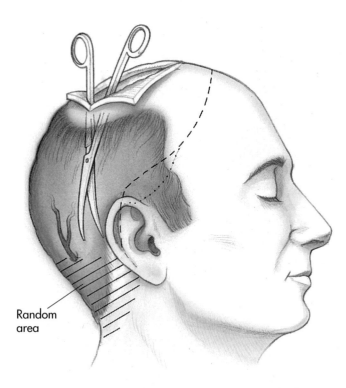

Fig. 30-15. Subgaleal undermining for scalp reduction. Additional subcutaneous undermining below the nuchal ridge and into the neck creates the scalp-lift operation.

be used to create complete hairlines or half hairlines that are of great density and are aesthetically acceptable. Although few hair transplant surgeons perform these, scalp flap procedures should be understood by any physician involved with hair transplantation. The large delayed temporoparietal-occipital (TPO) pedicle flaps devised by Jose Juri of Argentina[32] and the nondelayed flaps described by Elliott and others[23] have become important procedures in hair replacement surgery.

Anatomic considerations

The human scalp consists of a thick skin containing a tight pattern of hair follicles, glands, fat, fibrous tissue, lymphatic channels, and a vascular system. There is an abundance of interconnections of the blood supply that courses through the dermis and the subcutaneous layers of the scalp skin.[17] The only area of the scalp that is somewhat deficient in vascularity is in the mid-sagittal plane.

The vascular system consists of anatomosing arteries and arterioles feeding the plentiful capillaries of the deep dermal layers. Five pairs of major arteries nourish the scalp. The paired supraorbital and supratrochlear vessels are branches of the ophthalmic artery; the paired superficial temporal arteries, postauricular arteries, and occipital arteries are derived from the external carotid system.

Beneath the vascular components of the scalp is the fi-

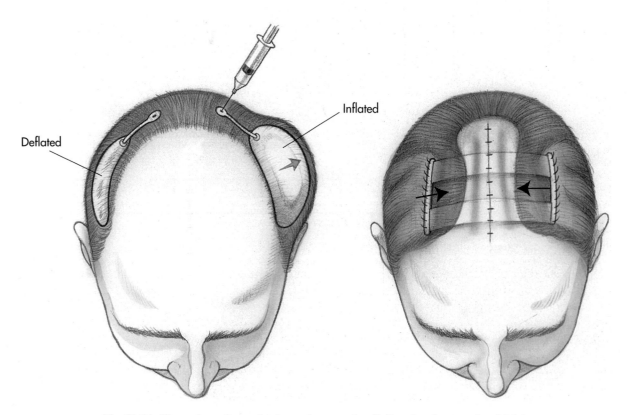

Fig. 30-16. Illustrations of prereduction scalp expansion *(left)* and scalp extension *(right)*.

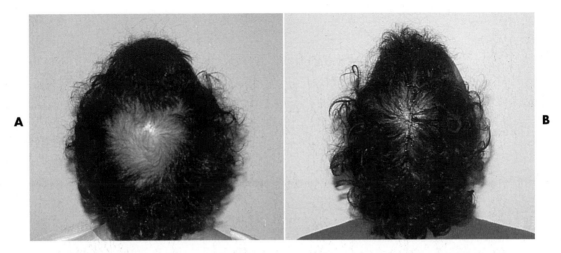

Fig. 30-17. A thirty-five-year-old patient shown **A,** before and **B,** after two scalp reductions for crown baldness.

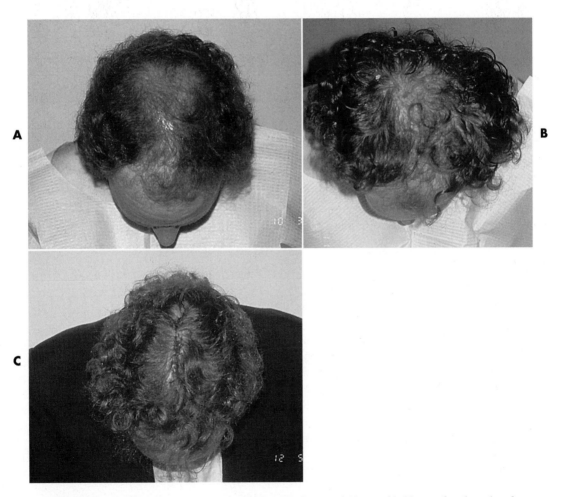

Fig. 30-18. A to **C,** A thirty-year-old patient with closure of 11 cm of baldness after 6 weeks of scalp expansion.

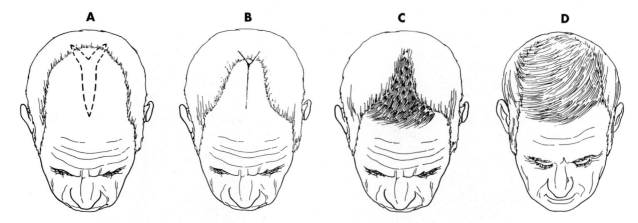

Fig. 30-19. A partially reduced scalp with frontal grafting. **A,** The skin is removed from within the dotted lines and the scalp edges are pulled upward and stitched in place. **B,** Potential results after one or two scalp reductions. Further reduction procedures may be done. **C,** The bald area has been reduced by scalp reductions. Hair grafts are shown filling in the remaining bald areas. **D,** An example of styling, with the completed result after multiple scalp reductions and hair grafts.

brous, tough galea aponeurotica, which anteriorly fuses with the frontalis muscle and posteriorly with the occipital muscle. Beneath the galea is a loose, fibroareolar layer overlying the pericranium. This loose fascial plane allows for the sliding phenomenon used in moving scalp tissue. The plane of separation and movement is not as distinct posteriorly as anteriorly where the galea is present.

Bald scalp usually is 30% to 60% thinner than hair-bearing scalp. The aging and balding scalp is less vascular than the youthful one. Scalp thickness and elasticity vary greatly. The variability of scalp elasticity has been found to be the most important factor relative to the ease or difficulty in performing scalp flap procedures. This factor especially applies to scalp reduction, which is an advancement flap procedure.

Patient selection

Patient motivation is perhaps the most important consideration in the selection of candidates for flap procedures. In addition to strong and consistent motivation, the ideal candidate should have a stable, somewhat limited balding pattern with good crown coverage and dense, thick donor hair. These usually are men who, for personal or professional reasons, wear hairpieces but who may prefer a permanent and reasonably aesthetic alternative solution to this prosthesis. They often have had some hair grafting, but desire greater density of hair than grafting alone can achieve (Table 30-2).

The older patient with frontal baldness and a flexible scalp is the ideal candidate for a pedicle flap operation. Those with a greater extent of baldness can be provided with dense frontal coverage using flaps, but they may require other types of coverage behind them. A tight scalp requires tissue expansion before flap procedures.

Table 30-2. Comparison of flaps and grafts

Grafts	Flaps
Patient selection: Most patients with male-pattern baldness of any degree with good donor hair	Best for frontal baldness with flexible scalp
Technical: Relatively simple technique; labor intensive	More difficulty; specific training in aesthetic scalp flap surgery
Results: Thinning, but ''natural'' look attainable; cosmetic results in 9-12 months; few serious complications	Cosmetic results as soon as 1 week after surgery; great density; backward/lateral hair direction; risk of necrosis ($< 8\%$)

LARGE DELAYED TEMPOROPARIETAL-OCCIPITAL PEDICLE FLAPS

The TPO flap is an exacting procedure with fine details and subtleties that require an efficient and imaginative operative technique. This operation (or series of operations) transfers the greatest amount of hair in the shortest period of time compared with other forms of surgical hair restoration. One TPO flap contains 8,000 to 10,000 hairs. The hair in the flap continues to grow, thereby bypassing the telogen phase of grafting. For instance, if the donor fringe hair were 4 inches long, it would be that long after flap surgery. Grafted hair would take 11 months to become 4 inches long and that would apply only to the grafts from the first session.

Design

As with other techniques, a hairline is first designed on the scalp. Some frontotemporal recession may be incorporated into the planned hairline, but if there is a desire for a

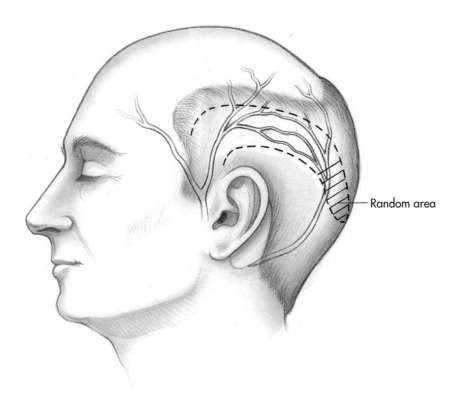

Random area

Fig. 30-20. The design of delayed temporoparietal-occipital flap.

large amount of recession and if the hairline is located in a relatively posterior location, a dog-ear may be anticipated when the flap eventually is turned. The dog-ear, however, can be treated later, and this can be incorporated into the surgical plan. This additional small procedure is the price paid for a more aesthetic hairline result.

After the hairline is designed, the posterior branch of the superficial temporal artery is located by palpation and confirmed by Doppler ultrasound. This vessel usually runs superiorly through the mid-portion of the sideburn and then curves in a posterior direction. It need only be identified in the proximal 3 to 4 cm of the flap design. The inferior edge of the flap should start at a point about 3 cm above the root of the helix and the superior origin of the flap should start 4 cm from the first point at an angle of 35° to 45° to a line drawn from the horizontal. The posterior branch of the superficial temporal artery should be in the center of the pedicle of the flap (Fig. 30-20).

Juri originally described the flap to be 4 cm wide, although a range of 3.25 to 4.5 cm may be safely used. An expanded flap can be up to 6 cm in width. The usual length of the flap is greater than the frontal hairline. A flap that is between 22 to 30 cm long often is required.

The peak of the frontal hairline usually is at the junction of the posterior and middle thirds of the flap. The anterior third of the flap is relocated within the temporal hairline during the surgical transfer. Therefore, it is the posterior two thirds of the flap design that becomes the frontal hairline.

Delays

Because of the mismatched flap length-to-width ratio and the random blood supply at the distal portion of the flap, Juri described two delay procedures for vascular preconditioning of the flap. The first delay procedure is essentially the creation of a bipedicled flap whose posterior circulation is provided by the perforating branches of the occipital artery (Fig. 30-21). The second delay operation is performed 1 week after the first delay. The distal 6 to 8 cm of the flap are cut around and then undercut (Fig. 30-22). The undercutting transects the occipital artery supply, which comes through the occipital musculature. The second delay usually requires ligature hemostasis of the large perforating[33,34] vessels before suturing the skin edges. In the senior author's modification of Juri's technique, the first procedure involves cutting around the flap design, except for a 4- to 5-cm bridge on the mid-superior edge of the flap. The distal end of the flap is undercut, accomplishing what is performed during the classical second delay described by Juri. One week later, the uncut bridge is transected and stapled closed. This second procedure takes 5 minutes and could even be done without local anesthesia, although local anesthesia with epinephrine is used for the hemostatic effect. A bipedicled flap is thus created and converted 1 week later to a unipedicled flap.

The need for delay in these large flaps of an 8:1 length-to-width ratio has been challenged, and the operation has been performed without delay. Also, it has been done with

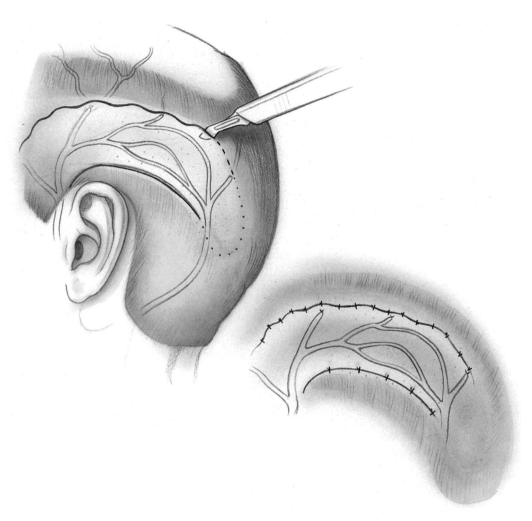

Fig. 30-21. The first delay of temporoparietal-occipital flap, step I.

one delay so that all of the steps in both delays of Juri's procedure were confined to one session. Ohmori's reports indicate that delays are not necessary for free flaps.[58] The free flap only needs definite proximal arterial blood supply and is sewn into the recipient bed without tension or torsion. Unfortunately, despite occasional successful cases of large flaps done without delay, not all scalp flaps have the favorable arterial directional anatomy for consistent results. Also, the fact that the pedicle of the flap often is sewn in place with some torsion, which causes some compromise in blood flow, justifies the usual practice of delaying this flap.

Flap transfer

The major procedure of transferring the flap is performed 1 week after the second delay. The flap is elevated by sharp and blunt dissection deep to the galea. The hairline incision is made with the knife tilted posteriorly at about a 45° angle to the scalp. Fleming and Mayer emphasized the need to design the new hairline in a slightly "wavy" irregular configuration, corresponding to that along the superior edge of

the flap. This beveled incision is made to a depth equal to the length of the hair follicles and is deepened in a more perpendicular direction beyond this, down to the subaponeurotic tissue. The incision in the hair-bearing temporal scalp is beveled parallel to the hair follicles to prevent trauma. The scalp above the hairline is undermined, and the leading edge of the flap is sutured to the forehead skin, which has been slightly undermined (Fig. 30-23). A dog-ear develops at the proximal suture site.

The parietal scalp is easily undermined in the subgaleal space. Posteriorly, the scalp is undermined in the supramuscular plane. Once the hairline is reached, undermining of the neck is continued in the subcutaneous plane, similar to the dissection used in a face-lift. The postauricular skin is undermined to the helical rim and into the lobule. The neck undermining may go as far as halfway between the hairline and the clavicle. Even with extensive undermining, there can be tension on the closure of the donor site. Often, a full-thickness skin graft from the excised bald scalp is needed to close a portion of the donor site to avoid excessive tension.

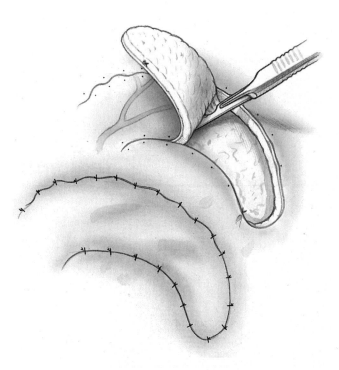

Fig. 30-22. The second delay of temporoparietal-occipital flap, one week later. Complete the incision, raise the flap, and resuture.

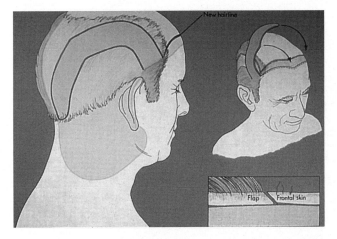

Fig. 30-23. The flap is rotated, and its leading edge deepithelialized and sutured in place.

Finally, the excess bald skin is trimmed away in segments at the closure line of the posterior edge of the flap. A large suction drain is placed under the dissected neck skin (Fig. 30-24).

The second temporoparietal-occipital flap

A second large flap procedure may be performed 3 to 4 months after the first procedure when the scalp has loosened somewhat. The design is similar to the frontline flap, but it may be taken higher or even at the edge of the fringe hair. The transfer procedure requires less meticulous suturing and

few dog-ear problems occur because the angle of rotation is less severe. The second flap is placed approximately 4 cm behind the frontal flap, except in patients with limited stable balding patterns in whom it may be placed immediately posterior to the first flap. Later, excision of intervening bald scalp and galeal removal beneath the flaps allows stretching of the flap in the anterior and posterior dimension to gain greater scalp coverage (Fig. 30-25).

Donor closure problems with a second flap occur more often because circulation to the superior segment of the donor closure site should traverse old and new incision lines. This is the area most distant from the axial blood supply.

Third temporoporietal-occipital flap

Juri[32] described using an occasional third flap for posterior coverage. The authors prefer to perform scalp reductions or punch grafting to cover the remaining cosmetic deficiency at the crown rather than offering a third flap procedure. A TPO flap can be used to correct isolated crown baldness in older patients.

Fleming and Mayer[46] often perform scalp reductions before flap rotations, except in patients with only frontal baldness and with no indication of future crown baldness. Lateral scalp expansion usually is necessary before flap surgery on patients with these reduced scalps (Fig. 30-26).

Morbidity

As with extensive front-line grafting, forehead and eyelid edema with ecchymosis can occur on the third or fourth postoperative day after any of these flap procedures, which presents no long-term problem and usually resolves within 10 days. Short-term steroid therapy (Decadron, 10 mg intramuscularly or intravenously), ice compresses, or a foam-rubber compression dressing on the forehead for the first 3 or 4 days after surgery may minimize these problems.

Dog-ears or bulges of the elevated forehead skin at the anterior proximal side of the flap resolve in 5 or 6 weeks. At this point, most of the patients require a minor adjustment procedure.

Occasionally, necrosis of the distal flap end or of the donor-closure site may occur, which usually does not become apparent before 10 days after surgery. By 6 weeks, the degree of full-thickness loss can be assessed. Treatment of this problem should be conservative initially to promote delayed healing. Broad-spectrum antibiotics, daily antibiotic ointment applications, and dressings may aid in this process. Granulation tissue develops, and epithelialization usually is completed after 12 weeks. Donor-closure defects, including widened scars, may require late revisional surgery 6 or more months postoperatively).

Nondelayed (lateral) flaps

In 1977, Elliott[23] published his description of nondelayed scalp flaps for the treatment of male-pattern baldness. He proposed a less formidable operation than that described by

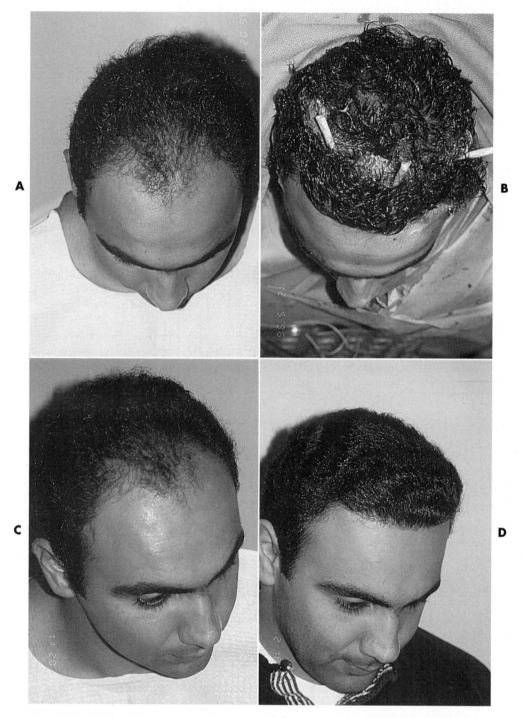

Fig. 30-24. A, The temporoparietal-occipital flap procedure on a 30-year-old (type II baldness) patient. **B,** Immediate postoperative view. Note complete coverage of bald area and proximal bulge (dog-ear). **C,** The preoperative three-quarter view. **D,** Ten weeks postoperative, three-quarter view.

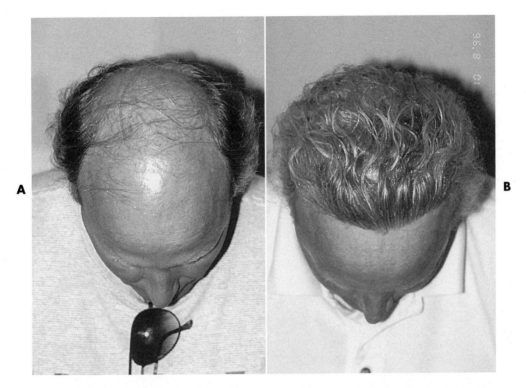

Fig. 30-25. A, A 40-year-old patient with class VI baldness. **B,** After two flaps and reduction between flaps.

Juri,[31] which involved a nondelayed, anteriorly based, TPO flap. This flap was much smaller than Juri's, so that after a transposition, it formed only one half of the hairline. A second, similar flap from the other side completed the hairline (Fig. 30-27). The flaps are 2.2 to 3.0 cm in width and taper slightly distally; the length is between 12 to 20 cm. The flaps are designed well within the assumed permanent fringe hair. Closure of the donor area and insetting of the flap into the planned hairline recipient site is performed in a manner similar to that described for the Juri flap.

A second small flap usually is performed 3 to 6 months after the first flap has been completed so that there is some return of laxity to the scalp. This is necessary to allow for donor closure on the second side. Two small flaps may rarely be performed simultaneously under selective conditions. If there is a strong frontal forelock and if the flap does not have to go to the mid-frontal scalp, the surgeon can transfer one of these nondelayed flaps and then, if the donor closure is without much tension, proceed to the second side in the same sitting. More commonly, each flap is designed long enough for some overlap in the mid-line, and the flaps are rotated in two separate sittings. The extra length in the mid-line is preserved to provide a greater amount of hair coverage in this region.[30,47]

The principal disadvantage of the small-flap technique is that it provides only a frontal hairline and largely eliminates the opportunity to have major vascular supply for further flap procedures. The main advantage and appeal of the small-flap technique is that it may seem to be a lesser procedure than a Juri flap.

The problems and complications, such as necrosis of the flaps, donor-closure problems, and hair loss, are seen more frequently than with the Juri flap procedure. Two flaps should be transposed and survive completely to create a hairline, but less hair is transferred than by one TPO flap operation alone. As a result, the authors no longer perform the small-flap procedures routinely.

Hairstyling

If proper techniques are used and no complications occur, the scarring at the anterior hairline should be equivalent to a pretrichial forehead lift. The direction of the hair in the rotated flap generally is posterior. This is in contrast to the anterior direction of the natural hairline. This directionality often may be corrected by styling. The most useful styles are permanents or back-combing of the flap hair. The black patient, who generally has naturally curly hair, does well with the flap techniques. In a straight-haired patient, a permanent will help spread the hair over a greater area so that it blends into the thinner remaining hair. Micrografts also may be added later to improve the flap hairline.

Preauricular and postauricular flaps

These narrow flaps, based superiorly, have been described by Nataf[53] to increase grafted hairlines and to provide partial crown coverage. Because the flap is made so

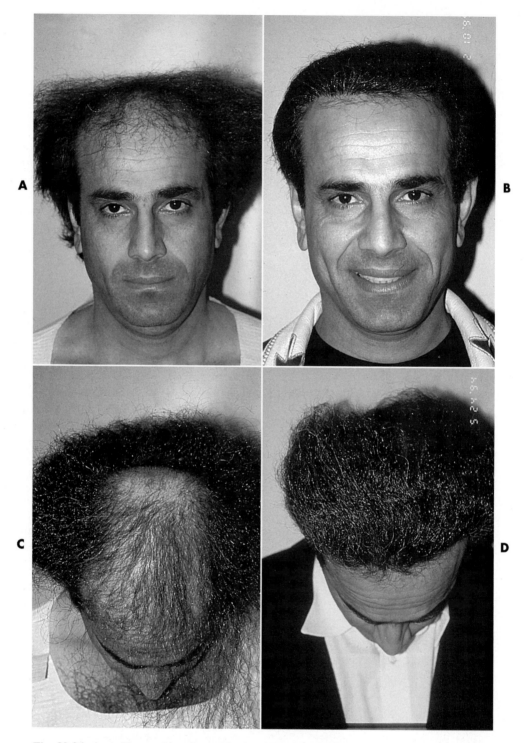

Fig. 30-26. A, A 38-year-old patient with class VI baldness. **B,** After scalp reduction, followed later by lateral scalp expansion and temporoparietal-occipital flaps. **C,** The top view, preoperative. **D,** The top view, postoperative.

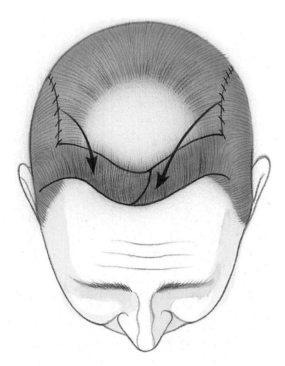

Fig. 30-27. A diagram of non-delayed lateral scalp flaps.

that the hair grows anteriorly, some theoretical cosmetic benefit is obtained, especially when combining this with punch grafts. These flaps are based opposite to the circulation of the scalp. As a result, delay procedures have been used, but predictable survival of these flaps is not consistent. The flaps rarely are long enough to produce half of a hairline. Marzola[45] has advocated the use of the preauricular flap in conjunction with extensive scalp reductions.

Free flaps

Ohmori[58] and Juri[31] report experiences with free TPO flaps using microsurgical anastomotic techniques. Although most patients had posttraumatic alopecia, free flaps also were successfully used in the treatment of male-pattern baldness. The flap design is similar to that of Juri's pedicled flap. Anastomoses are made to the superficial temporal artery and vein on the contralateral side without delay procedures. When successful, the free flap has anterior hair growth, most nearly approximating a natural hairline, although this single free flap can use up both superficial temporal artery systems, thereby precluding a second flap or a salvage flap in case of flap necrosis. Ohmori[58] has described an operation that anastomoses the ipsilateral occipital vessels to the superficial temporal vessels and, thereby, allows for a potential second flap on the other side. Using free flaps involves specific training, skills, and preparation. This technique has not yet been widely accepted or used and probably will only find appropriate application in isolated situations.

Expanded scalp flaps

As with scalp lift or reduction techniques, tissue expansion provides a major adjunct to flap procedures for hair replacement surgery. Expansion allows the surgeon to offer these procedures to patients whose scalps are inherently or postoperatively too tight to advance.[35,64,66]

With the addition of tissue expansion, lateral reduction procedures can be done with expanded flaps either before or after TPO flap rotation, and often complete closure of the crown and mid-scalp can be achieved. The major drawback of this procedure is the major deformity that occurs in the process of expanding the tissues. Therefore, scalp reduction using these expanded flaps for male-pattern baldness would only be indicated for the highly motivated and demanding patient who desires the ultimate in potential coverage and can stand the temporary deformity and the discomfort. Patients who have tight cicatricial alopecia that was previously deemed inoperable have been successfully treated with tissue-expansion techniques.

The expanded "Bilateral Advancement Transposition" and "Triple Advancement Transposition" flaps

Anderson introduced a new combination of expanded simultaneous transposition and advancement flaps in 1993.[4] Although these are somewhat complex and technically difficult procedures, as suggested in Figures 30-28, 30-29, and 30-30, they provide the advantages of avoiding temporal dog-ears and providing a desirable anterior–superior direction of hair growth. These procedures involve either bilateral advancement transposition (BAT) flaps or triple advancement transposition (TAT) flaps, with the goal of complete elimination of bald scalp.

Reconstructive scalp surgery

All the principles and procedures described in this chapter regarding aesthetic scalp surgery apply to reconstructive scalp work. Most posttraumatic alopecia can be treated by serial excision (scalp reduction), hair grafting, scalp expansion, and flaps, providing there is enough donor hair-bearing scalp.

With the advent of tissue expansion and free-flap surgery, most posttraumatic alopecias can be resurfaced with hair-bearing tissue or, at the least, full-thickness skin.

SUMMARY

Although there are many other causes of baldness to be considered for men and women, the most common type of baldness is androgenic or male-pattern baldness. If either a man or a woman has inherited the genetic susceptibility for male-pattern baldness from the maternal or paternal side of their family, baldness results, in genetically susceptible follicles. Although androgen levels may be normal, these follicles have increased levels of 5-α reductase, which is responsible for the conversion of testosterone to dihydrotes-

Text continued on p. 626

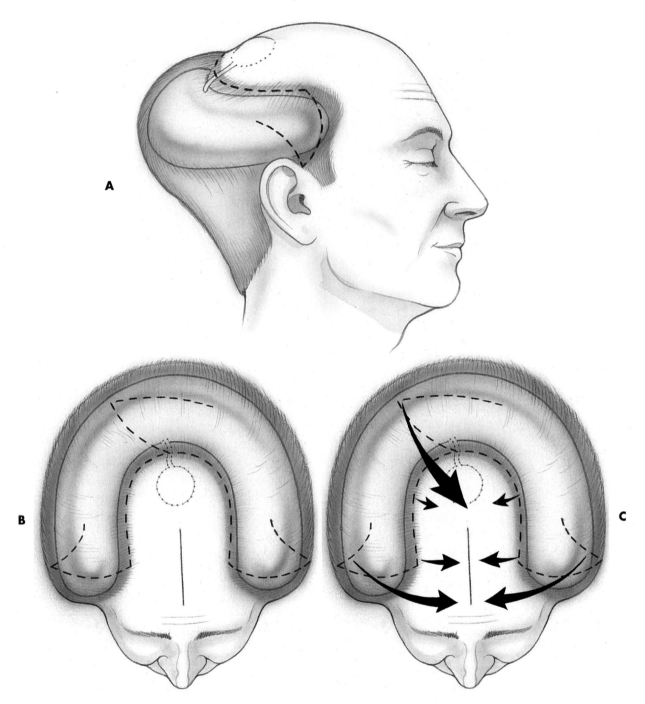

Fig. 30-28. A diagram of expanded triple advancement transposition flaps. Up to 3 months of expansion required. **A,** The lateral view, expander filled. Right flap shown. **B,** The top view showing outline of three superiorly based flaps. **C,** Flap advancement and rotation.

Continued

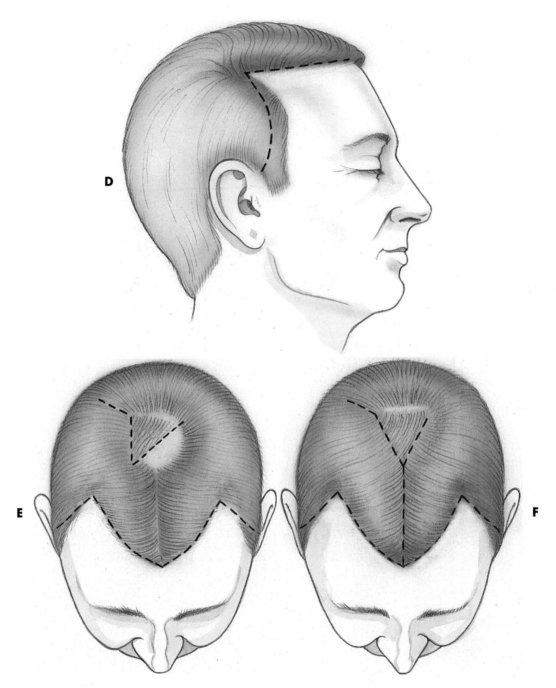

Fig. 30-28, cont'd. D, The lateral view of right flap in place and donor closure. **E,** Three flaps positioned with incomplete removal of baldness. **F,** Baldness completely removed after later scalp reduction.

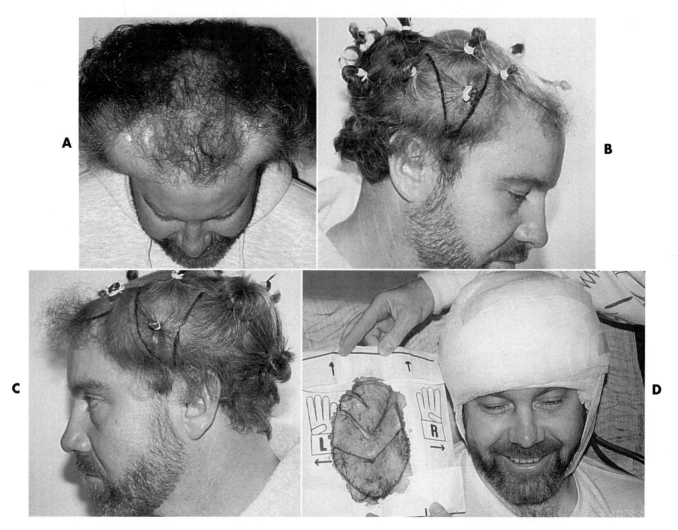

Fig. 30-29. A, The expansion of scalp with horseshoe-shaped expander before triple advancement transposition flap. **B** and **C,** The expanded flap design. **D,** Specimen of total bald scalp.

Continued

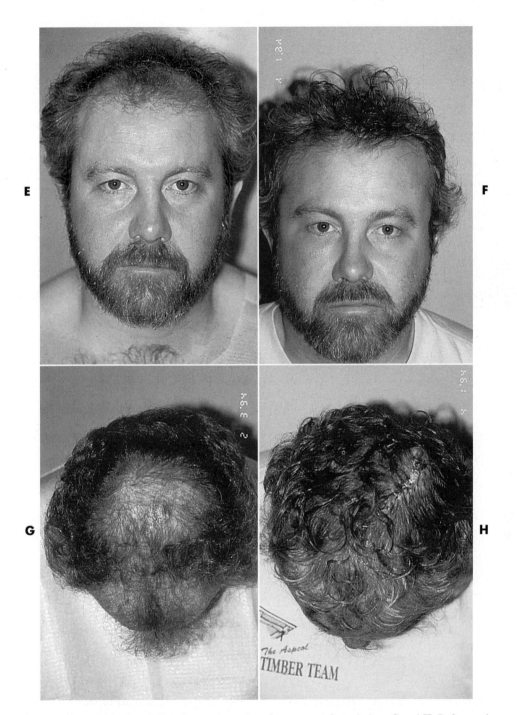

Fig. 30-29, cont'd. E and **F,** Before and one day after surgery, frontal view. **G** and **H,** Before and one day after surgery, top view.

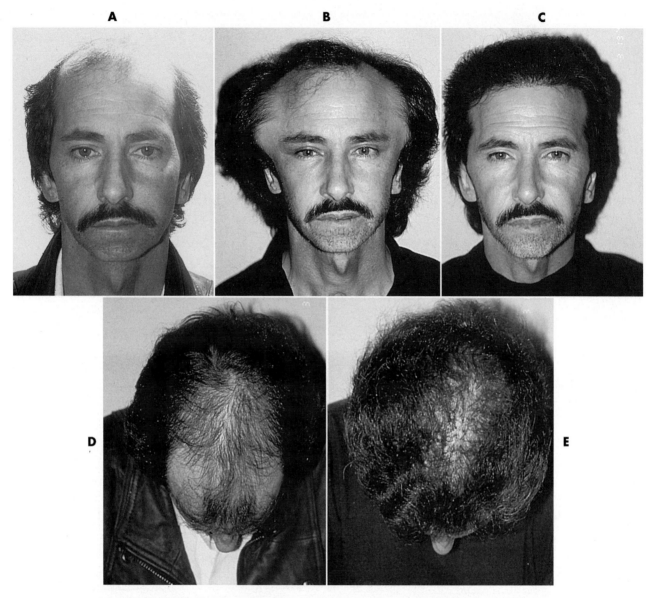

Fig. 30-30. A, Type Va baldness. **B,** After 10 weeks of expansion. **C,** The front view after bilateral advancement transposition flaps. **D** and **E,** The top view before and after bilateral advancement transposition flaps.

tosterone. It frequently is inevitable that baldness increases with age and that the earlier it begins, the more extensive it tends to be.

Although hair-restoration procedures do not truly give the patient a full head of hair, in many patients, they give the illusion of a full head of hair. To balance illusion and reality, it is necessary to blend art and science. The relationships between the various attributes of the patient's hair loss, character, density, bulk, and color should be carefully considered along with the patient's personality. An understanding of the patient's expected final hair-loss pattern and extensive preoperative counseling should be combined to create a long-term plan. Proper selection and execution of a single

technique or a combination of techniques with appropriate management of any complications ultimately produces results that closely approximate a ''natural-appearing'' hair pattern. In so doing, realistic expectations of the surgeon and patient frequently may be met.

REFERENCES

1. Adson MH, Anderson RD, Argenta LC: Scalp expansion in the treatment of male pattern baldness, *Plast Reconstr Surg* 79:906, 1987.
2. Alt TH: Scalp reduction as an adjunct to hair transplantation: review of relevant literature and presentation of an improved technique, *J Dermatol Surg Oncol* 6:1011, 1980.
3. Anderson RD: Expansion-assisted treatment of male pattern baldness, *Clin Plast Surg* 14:477, 1987.

4. Anderson RD: The expanded "BAT" flap for treatment of male pattern baldness, *Ann Plast Surg* 31:385, 1993.

5. Bamford JT: A falling out following Minoxidil: telogen effluvium, *J Am Acad Dermatol* 16:144, 1987.

6. Bergfield WF, Redmond GP: Androgenic alopecia, *Dermatol Clin* 5:491, 1987.

7. Blanchard G, Blanchard B: La reduction tonsurale (detonsuration): concept nouveao dans le traitement chirurgical de la calvitie, *Rev Chir Hir Esthet* 4:5, 1976.

8. Blanchard G, Blanchard B: Obliteration of alopecia by hair lifting: a new concept and technique, *J Natl Med Assoc* 69:639, 1977.

9. Bozzano GS, Terezakis N, Galen W: Topical tretinoin for hair-growth promotion, *J Am Acad Dermatol* 15:880, 1986.

10. Brandy DA: Extensive scalp-lifting, *J Dermatol Surg Oncol* 15:563, 1989 (letter).

11. Brandy DA: The bilateral occipital parietal flap, *J Dermatol Surg Oncol* 12:1062, 1986.

12. Burke BM, Cunliffe WJ: Oral spironolactone therapy for female patients with acne, hirsutism and androgenic alopecia, *Br J Dermatol* 112:124, 1985.

13. Cash TF: Physical attractiveness: an annotated bibliography of theory and research in the behavioral sciences, *Soc Behav Sci Doc* 11:2370, 1981.

14. Cash TF: The psychological effects of androgenic alopecia in men, *J Am Acad Dermatol* 26:926, 1992.

15. Cash TF, Price VH: Psychological effects of androgenic alopecia: comparisons with balding men and with female control subjects, *J Am Acad Dermatol* 29:568, 1993.

16. Choi Y-C, Kim J-C: Single-hair transplantation using Choi hair transplanter, *J Dermatol Surg Oncol* 18:945, 1992.

17. Conley J: *Regional flaps of the head and neck*, Stuttgart, 1976, George Thieme.

18. DeVillez RL: The therapeutic use of topical Minoxidil, *Dermatol Clin* 8:367, 1990.

19. Diani AR, and others: Hair growth effects of oral administration of finasteride, a steroid 5-α reductase inhibitor, alone and in combination with topical Minoxidil in the balding stumptail macaque, *J Clin Endocrinol Metab* 74:345, 1992.

20. Domnitz JN, Silvers DN: Giant cells in male pattern alopecia—a histologic marker and pathogenic clue, *J Cutan Pathol* 6:108, 1979.

21. Dunham T: A method for obtaining a skin flap from the scalp and a permanent buried vascular pedicle for covering defects of the face, *Ann Surg* 17:677, 1893.

22. Ebling FJ: The biology of hair, *Dermatol Clin* 5:467, 1987.

23. Elliott RA: Lateral scalp flaps for instant results in pattern baldness, *Plast Reconstr Surg* 60:699, 1977.

24. Franzoi SL, Anderson J, Frommelt S: Individual differences in men's perceptions of and reactions to thinning hair, *J Soc Psychol* 130:209, 1990.

25. Frechet P: Scalp extension, *J Dermatol Surg Oncol* 19:616, 1993.

26. Frieden IJ, Price VH: *Androgenic alopecia*. In Thiers BH, Dobson RL, editors: *Pathogenesis of skin disease*, New York, 1986, Churchill-Livingstone.

27. Georgala G, Papasotiriou V, Stavropoulos P: Serum testosterone and sex-hormone binding globulin levels in women with androgenic alopecia, *Acta Derm Venereol* 66:532, 1986.

28. Gilhar A, Pillar T, Etzioni A: Topical cyclosporin in male pattern alopecia, *J Am Acad Dermatol* 22:251, 1990.

29. Hamilton JB: Patterned loss of hair in men: types and incidence, *Ann N Y Acad Sci* 53:708, 1951.

30. Heimburger RA: Single-stage rotation of arteriolized scalp flaps for male pattern baldness: a case report, *Plast Reconstr Surg* 60:789, 1977.

31. Juri J, Juri C: The Juri flap, *Facial Plast Surg* II:269, 1985.

32. Juri J: Use of parieto-occipital flaps in the surgical treatment of baldness, *Plast Reconstr Surg* 55:456, 1975.

33. Kabaker SS: Experiences with parieto-occipital flaps in hair transplantation, *Laryngoscope* 88:73, 1978.

34. Kabaker SS: Juri flap procedure for the treatment of baldness, *Arch Otolaryngol* 105:509, 1979.

35. Kabaker SS and others: Tissue expansion in the treatment of alopecia, *Arch Otolaryngol* 112:720, 1986.

36. Kasick JM and others: Adrenal androgenic female-pattern alopecia: sex hormones and the balding woman, *Clev Clin Q* 50:111, 1983.

37. Katz HI and others: Long-term efficacy of topical Minoxidil in male pattern baldness, *J Am Acad Dermatol* 16:711, 1987.

38. Kessels AG and others: The effectiveness of the hair restorer "Dabao" in males with alopecia androgenetica: a clinical experiment, *J Clin Epidemiol* 44:439, 1991.

39. Kidwai BJ, George M: Hair loss with Minoxidil withdrawal, *Lancet* 340:609, 1992.

40. Klenhard W: *The bald book*, Santa Monica, Calif, 1986, Science Med Press.

41. London-Wong DM, Hart LL: Minoxidil with tretinoin in baldness, *DICP* 24:43, 1990.

42. Ludwig E: Classification of the types of androgenic alopecia (common baldness) occurring in the female sex, *Br J Dermatol* 97:247, 1977.

43. Maddin WS, Bell PW, James JH: The biological effects of a pulsed electrostatic field with specific reference to hair: electrotrichogenesis, *Int J Dermatol* 29:446, 1990.

44. Marritt E, Dzubow L: The isolated frontal forelock, *Dermatol Surg* 21:523, 1995.

45. Marzola M: *An alternative hair replacement method*. In *Hair transplant surgery*, ed 2, Springfield, Ill, 1984, Charles C Thomas.

46. Mayer TG, Fleming RW: *Aesthetic and reconstructive surgery of the scalp*, St Louis, 1991, Mosby.

47. Mayer TG, Fleming RW: Short flaps—their use and abuse in the treatment of male pattern baldness, *Ann Plast Surg* 8:296, 1982.

48. Meishiu KD, Cipkus LA: Biochemical mechanisms by which Minoxidil sulfate influences mammalian cells, *Dermatologica* 175(suppl 2):3, 1987.

49. Miller JA and others: Low sex-hormone binding globulin levels in young women with diffuse hair loss, *Br J Dermatol* 106:331, 1982.

50. Mitchell AD, DeVillez RL: Minoxidil for male pattern baldness, *Lancet* 1:1436, 1987.

51. Morris D: *Body watching: a field guide to the human species*, New York, 1985, Crown.

52. Nardi M and others: Cyprotrone acetate-ethinyl estridiol treatment of hirsutism, acne, seborrhea and alopecia, *Acta Eur Fertil* 6:153, 1975.

53. Nataf J: Surgical treatment for frontal baldness: the long temporal vertical flap, *Plast Reconstr Surg* 74:628, 1984.

54. Nordstrom RE, Pietila JP, Rantala E: Clinical experience with tissue expansion, *Facial Plast Surg* 5:317, 1988.

55. Nordstrom RE: "Stretch-back" in scalp reductions for male pattern baldness, *Plast Reconstr Surg* 73:422, 1984.

56. Norwood OT, Shiell RC, Morrison ID: Complications of scalp reductions, *J Dermatol Surg Oncol* 9:828, 1983.

57. Norwood OT, Shiell RC: *Hair transplant surgery*, Springfield, Ill, 1984, Charles C Thomas.

58. Ohmori K: Application of microvascular free flaps to scalp effects, *Clin Plast Surg* 9:263, 1982.

59. Okuda S: Clinical and experimental studies of transplantation of living hairs, *Jpn J Dermatol* (Japanese) 46:135, 1939.

60. Olsen EA and others: Five-year follow-up of men with androgenic alopecia treated with topical Minoxidil, *J Am Acad Dermatol* 22:643, 1990.

61. Olsen EA, Weiner MS: Topical Minoxidil in male pattern baldness: effects of discontinuation of treatment, *J Am Acad Dermatol* 17:97, 1987.

62. Orentreich N: Autografts in alopecias and other selected dermatological conditions, *Ann N Y Acad Sci* 83:463, 1959.

63. Orentreich M: *Scalp hair replacement in men.* In *Advances in biology of the skin*, vol 9, New York, 1969, Pergamon Press.

64. Pierce AG: Possible use of the Radovan tissue expander in hair replacement surgery, *J Dermatol Surg Oncol* 11:413, 1985.

65. Price VH: Hormonal control of baldness, *Int J Dermatol* 15:742, 1976.

66. Radovan C: Tissue expansion in soft tissue reconstruction, *Plast Reconstr Surg* 74:482, 1984.

67. Rassman WR: *The art and science of small graft hair transplantation.* In Stough DB, Harber RS, editors: *Hair replacement, surgical and medical*, St Louis, 1996, Mosby.

68. Roenigk HH Jr.: New topical agents for hair growth, *Clin Dermatol* 6:119, 1988.

69. Sawaya ME, Hordinsky MK: The anti-androgens: when and how they should be used, *Dermatol Clin* 11:65, 1993.

70. Setty LR: Hair patterns of the scalp of a white and negro male, *Am J Phys Anthropol* 33:49, 1970.

71. Shiell RC, Norwood OT: *Hair transplant surgery*, Springfield, Ill, 1984, Charles C Thomas.

72. Stough DB VI, Nelson BR, Stough DB III: Incisional slit grafting, *J Dermatol Surg Oncol* 17:53, 1991.

73. Straub P: The cause of poor hair growth? *Hair Transplant Forum* 3: 17, 1993.

74. Swinehart J, Griffin EI: Slit grafting, the use of serrated island grafts in male and female pattern alopecia, *J Dermatol Surg Oncol* 17:243, 1991.

75. Tamura H: Pubic hair transplantation, *Jpn J Dermatol (Japanese)* 53: 76, 1943.

76. Takashima M, Iju, Sudo M: *Alopecia androgenica—its incidence in Japanese and associated conditions.* In Orfanos CE, Montagna W, Studen G, editors: *Hair research status and feature aspects*, Berlin, 1981, Springer-Verlag.

77. Tenover JS: Prostates, pates and pimples: the potential medical uses of steroid 5-α reductase inhibitor, *Endocrin Metab Clin North Am* 20: 893, 1991.

78. Unger MG, Unger WP: Management of alopecia of the scalp by a combination of excisions and transplantations, *J Dermatol Surg Oncol* 4:670, 1978.

79. van der Donk J: Psychologic characteristics of men with alopecia androgenetica and their modification, *Int J Dermatol* 30:22, 1991.

80. Yung JW and others: Cutaneous immunopathology of androgenic alopecia, *J Am Osteopath Assoc* 91:765, 1991.

Chapter 31

Management of Aging Skin

Charles N. Ellis

AGING AND PHOTOAGING

Although every living organism grows older, the process of aging is not well understood. During aging, both physiologic and structural changes occur. The skin, as an organ, also undergoes aging (Fig. 31-1). However, unlike most organs, the skin is directly exposed to the elements. Environmental factors induce changes in the skin that result in an aged appearance.[12,39] Thus, the signs recognized as aging of the skin are a combination of intrinsic aging (the natural effects of time) and extrinsic aging.

Intrinsic aging

Intrinsic aging of the skin in its pure state occurs only in sun-protected areas. Because societal habits have changed, exposure to the sun now occurs over larger parts of the body; thus, many people have few areas of sun-protected skin. However, the buttocks and inner arms may generally be used to examine intrinsic aging. A history of low sun exposure can be helpful in selecting patients for research. Most of these patients can be recognized by the minimal stigmata of photodamage.

As a person ages, furrows and folds appear in the skin. Some of these furrows and folds are the result of distortions (called *lines of expression*) caused by repeated muscular movements. Positions of the skin that are often repeated (e.g., positions assumed during sleeping) probably also induce folds in the skin. The constant pull of gravity causes sagging, particularly in the jowls. With age, changed fat distribution in the face causes an older appearance. These changes are not typically responsive to medicinal therapies, and cosmetic surgery may be necessary to reverse them.

In addition to the sagging caused by gravity, mildly atrophic skin and fine wrinkling characterize intrinsic aging.

Intrinsically aging skin sometimes has a "cigarette paper" appearance. Extrinsic aging is primarily composed of the alterations caused by photodamage, although other environmental agents may play a role.

Photoaging

Photodamage is the effect of ultraviolet light on exposed skin. Inevitably, photodamage is superimposed on the normal changes of intrinsic aging. Whereas intrinsic aging is typically characterized by fine wrinkles on a generally smooth and pale surface, photodamaged skin has many coarse wrinkles (in addition to fine wrinkles) and a rough surface. Thus, the term *photoaging* means skin that has suffered both the ravages of time and ultraviolet exposure.

Photoaged skin typically has altered, irregular pigmentation. Actinic keratoses, premalignant precursors of nonmelanoma skin cancers, are often present. Telangiectasias may occur; however, genetic predisposition has a greater influence on telangiectasias than on the other changes of photodamage. Photodamage in its most severe form causes a lax, leathery appearance with deep furrows and wrinkles, which are often associated with working outdoors for many years. Telangiectasias and variable pigmentation are often present and are usually on a background of sallow skin. The surface texture typically changes, giving the skin a "cobblestone" appearance.

The cardinal signs of photodamage are wrinkles, brown spots (liver spots), and surface roughness. Coarse wrinkles tend to appear over the forehead and crow's foot area and on the back of the neck. A deep, coarse wrinkle cannot be totally effaced by stretching the skin. Fine wrinkling is more common over the cheeks and may occur on the entire face. These fine wrinkles can be made to disappear by stretching the skin. Wrinkling represents a spectrum of changes; there-

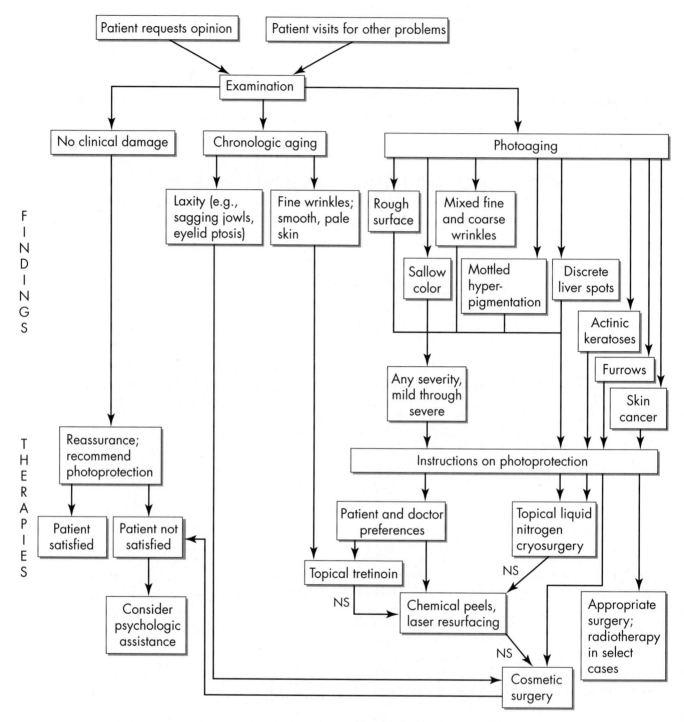

Fig. 31-1. Summary of diagnostic findings and management strategies.

fore, some wrinkles are not easily classified as coarse or fine. Wrinkles have no clear histologic correlate.

Smoking as an extrinsic factor

Cigarette smoking may have an important extrinsic influence on the appearance of skin.[9] Evidence strongly suggests that smokers have more wrinkles, particularly coarse wrinkles. These wrinkles are often prominent around the lateral corners of the eyes in the crow's-foot areas. The reasons for the changes in the skin are unknown; however, it has been hypothesized that cigarette smoking may induce changes in blood flow that cause undesirable alterations in the dermis. Another possibility is that toxins from cigarette smoke circulate through the bloodstream and alter fibroblast production of collagen or elastin.

Psychology of aging

The pursuit of ageless beauty is not distinctive of the late twentieth century but spans the millenia—from the animal oils, salt, and alabaster of ancient Egypt to the light exfoliation of Turkish fire and urine-bathed pumice stones of the Indian subcontinent.[5] Because patients may be psychologically reluctant to undergo surgery to manage aging skin, pharmaceutical approaches have substantial usefulness in medical practice. Many patients have psychologic challenges related to aging. For many people, a few wrinkles are merely undesirable but may eventually become intolerable. Additionally, brown spots are immediately recognized as signs of aging by the public. Many patients respond to management with an improved psychologic outlook that may extend beyond the mere satisfaction of therapy.[21] When their wrinkles and brown spots are managed, patients may select new hair or clothing styles or may undertake new activities.

Assessment of photodamage therapies

Several methods assess the effects of management on photodamaged skin. Clinical scales (which usually have ratings of absent, mild, moderate, or severe) have been used in all studies. With a scale, the investigator can assess the status of the skin at the time of evaluation and compare the change with the patient's pretherapy condition. Typically, photographs help the investigator recall the patient's appearance before therapy. Carefully controlled photography used at various times in a study can document the beneficial effects of the therapy and can provide a blinded approach for evaluators who are rating management.[2]

A series of pictures have been developed that grade degrees of photodamage on a scale from 0 to 8 (Fig. 31-2).[14] Such a scale promotes greater agreement among evaluators. Other researchers have suggested that photographs of patients taken before and after therapy may be randomly projected side-by-side so that evaluators can assess each patient's response to management. Whenever photographs are used, a professional setup is required, and extremely careful positioning of the patient is necessary.

To measure wrinkling, skin replicas have been widely used. In this technique, a silicone mold of the skin is made and sent to a laboratory for computerized image analysis. The most common method to assess the topography of these replicas is optical profilometry, a process in which an angled light is used to cast shadows across the mold. These shadows are then interpreted by computer.[20] Other image analysis methods have been used to assess close-up photographs of the skin and to evaluate the histologic condition of the skin. Electron microscopy of skin biopsy specimens yields extremely close-up topographic surfaces that can be analyzed by computer. To analyze the color of skin, color values may be determined with electronic colorimeters. The skin may also be recorded digitally, and a computer can assess the color levels within specified areas or lesions.

TRETINOIN THERAPY FOR PHOTODAMAGE

Tretinoin is the generic name for vitamin A acid (also called all-*trans*-retinoic acid or retinoic acid). Tretinoin in an emollient cream (Renova, Ortho Pharmaceutical Corporation, Raritan, NJ) is approved by the United States Food and Drug Administration (FDA) for use in reducing fine wrinkles, mottled hyperpigmentation, and roughness of facial skin (i.e., the major signs of photodamage). Nevertheless, more studies in this area have been performed with the original formulation of tretinoin, Retin-A (Ortho Pharmaceutical Corporation, Raritan, NJ). Retin-A has been widely used for more than 25 years for the management of acne, the indication for which it is marketed. Unless tretinoin is specifically stated to be in an emollient cream, this chapter is referring to the Retin-A formulation. The differences among all formulations of tretinoin are modest, and clinical differences in use are trivial, which is to be expected because the active ingredient is the same.

Original findings

A double-blind, vehicle-controlled investigation of topical tretinoin for photoaged skin was conducted in 30 patients.[38] By managing all patients with 0.1% tretinoin cream on one arm and a vehicle cream on the other, comparisons could be made to determine the efficacy of the active ingredient. After 16 weeks of therapy, 30% of the forearms that received the tretinoin were much improved, 40% were somewhat improved, and 30% were slightly improved. In contrast, the forearms treated with vehicle cream showed no improvement. Patients with fine wrinkling responded to tretinoin therapy, with 20% of the patients showing much improvement. Modest improvement in the color of the skin (as determined by its pinkness) was detected in the tretinoin-treated forearms. The smoothness of the skin (detected by feel) improved slightly with tretinoin management and coarse wrinkling showed a very slight change during the 16-week study. The forearms that received vehicle cream

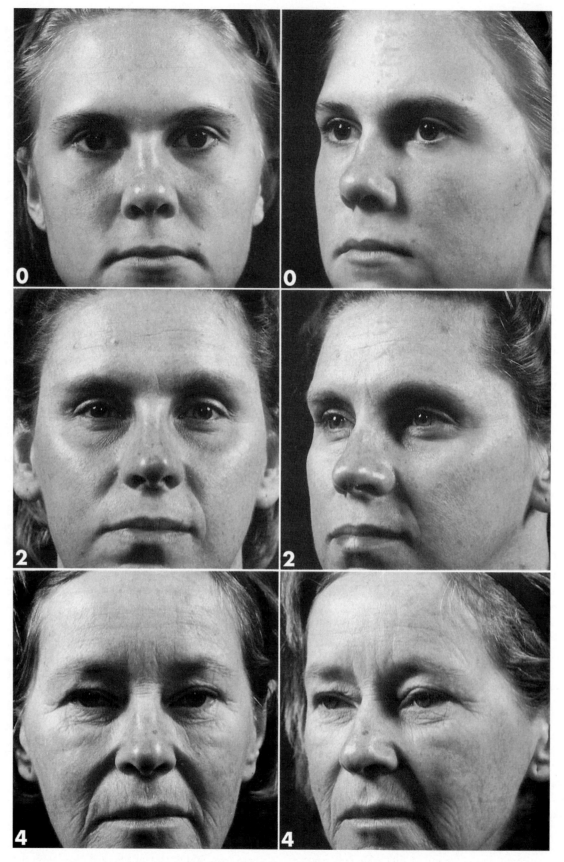

Fig. 31-2. For legend see opposite page.

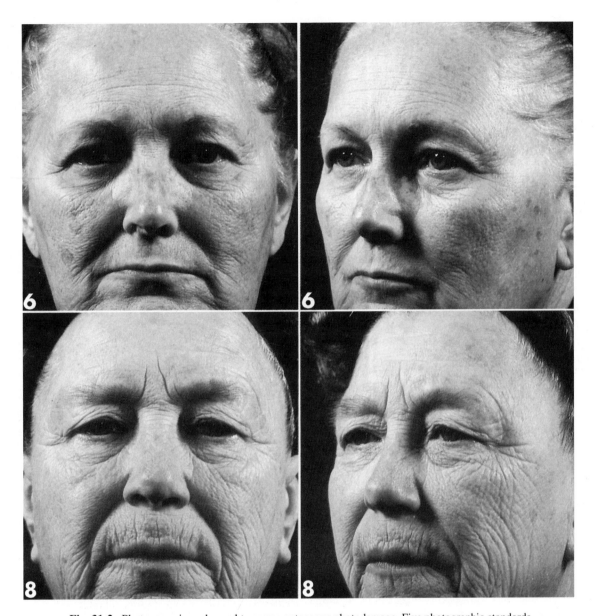

Fig. 31-2. Photonumeric scale used to assess cutaneous photodamage. Five photographic standards (*en face* and 45° oblique) illustrated the increasing severity of photodamage, where grade 0 represents no damage; grade 2, mild damage; grade 4, moderate damage; grade 6, moderate to severe damage; and grade 8, severe damage. (Copyright © 1991: Regents of the University of Michigan, Ann Arbor.)

showed no improvement in fine or coarse wrinkles, and less than 10% of patients had even slight improvement in color or smoothness.

Patients applied the same medicine that they used on their left forearms to their faces; thus, half of the patients used tretinoin, and half used only the vehicle cream on the face. Patient's faces were then compared in terms of the management received (in contrast, the forearms were compared in the same patient).

Whereas only 7% of the patients who used tretinoin on the face showed much improvement, 67% showed modest improvement, and 20% showed slight improvement. After 16 weeks, only one patient (7%) experienced no change as a result of the tretinoin management. The vehicle cream failed to improve any patient. Similar to in the forearms, fine wrinkling and color in the faces were improved more substantially by tretinoin management than were smoothness or coarse wrinkling. No improvement in any variable was detected on the faces that used the vehicle cream.

Histologic findings

Examination of skin biopsy samples from managed areas yielded significant histologic results. The mean epidermal thickness in the forearms increased by 82% with tretinoin, versus 8% with the vehicle cream. Similarly, the number of cells in the granular layer increased by 117% with tretinoin, versus 18% with the vehicle cream. The mitotic rate, as measured by the number of mitotic figures in the epidermis, increased after tretinoin therapy. In most patients, tretinoin induced a compaction in the stratum corneum epidermidis and an alteration from a basket-weave pattern of the stratum corneum to a more homogeneous appearance. A glycosaminoglycan-like material appeared in the intercellular spaces of the stratum spinosum epidermidis and in the lower portion of the stratum corneum epidermidis with tretinoin therapy; this material was not seen in sections from skin managed with the vehicle cream. Additionally, the tretinoin-managed areas showed wider vascular lumens.

Ultrastructural evaluation of the skin biopsy samples confirmed the light microscopy findings. For example, a fine granular material was present in the stratum corneum epidermidis. The appearance of this material is similar to that of a glycosaminoglycan and that found in skin after oral retinoid therapy.

Tretinoin therapy also decreased the number of melanosomes in basal cells and significantly decreased melanocyte activity. Additionally, after 16 weeks of tretinoin therapy, the number of anchoring filaments and anchoring fibrils at the dermal-epidermal junction substantially increased.[40] Under the basal lamina, the collagen of the papillary dermis substantially changed. New collagen was apparently generated and probably was produced by tretinoin-induced fibroblasts that appeared in greater numbers and showed greater activity than they did in the skin managed with the vehicle cream.

The rate of collagen I formation is slower in photodamaged skin than in sun-protected skin. Topical tretinoin therapy has been shown to partly restore collagen I levels in skin.[15]

Extended management of patients

The 30 patients who completed this original double-blind study continued in an open trial of tretinoin.[8] Despite a reduced dose of tretinoin in some patients and less frequent application in others, the improvements in fine and coarse wrinkling and skin texture that occurred during the original study were maintained. After 10 months of therapy, the number of lentigines was decreasing. Some patients remained in the study for 22 months of therapy and showed continued improvement throughout management (Fig. 31-3). The desirable pinkness of the face was maintained throughout therapy.

Kligman and others[26] evaluated the effects of 0.05% tretinoin cream on photodamaged forearm and facial skin in more than 400 patients who received daily 0.1% or 0.05% tretinoin cream in an uncontrolled fashion for 6 months to 3 years. Kligman and others[26] reported that patients showed minimal clinical changes after 3 months of 0.05% tretinoin. Other than mild irritation, the appearance of their skin was not substantially changed. However, encouraging evidence was detected in histologic preparations. Dysplasia and atypia, which are common in photodamaged skin, were essentially abolished with tretinoin therapy. Keratinocytes that would otherwise have shown a chaotic pattern showed resumption of normal polarity after tretinoin therapy. Tretinoin induced a thickened epidermis with a prominent granular layer and eliminated evidence of microscopic actinic keratoses. Although skin managed with emollient cream continued to show hyperkeratosis and an irregular surface of the stratum corneum epidermidis, skin managed with tretinoin developed a thinner horny layer with a smoother topography. Tretinoin therapy reduced the clumping of melanin induced by photodamage; instead, the melanin was dispersed throughout the epidermis.

Electron microscopy findings suggested increased metabolic activity of the keratinocytes, which is consistent with the light microscopy findings of acanthosis of the epidermis. The cells were found to be larger and more uniform when examined ultrastructurally. The epidermal thickness increased by an average of 40% with tretinoin versus 10% with emollient cream. Biochemical studies indicated an increased percentage of cells synthesizing deoxyribonucleic acid (DNA) in the epidermis. Although tonofilaments are thick in photoaged skin, tretinoin induced thinning and dispersion. The mucus-like substance that occurred with oral retinoid therapy also occurred with topical tretinoin therapy.

Although the dermis showed no substantial changes under light microscopy after 3 months of tretinoin therapy, electron micrographs indicated that dermal fibroblasts had become larger and more active. An increase in the numbers of small venules in the dermis was detected.

Blood flow was increased in tretinoin-managed forearms compared with those managed with emollient cream alone. Tretinoin induced an increase in transepidermal water loss that may be related to the thinning of the stratum corneum epidermidis. Although increased transepidermal water loss may occur with xerosis, patients had no complaints of dryness after tretinoin therapy. Electrical conductance of the skin surface measured by a skin-surface hydrometer showed no difference between the tretinoin- and emollient-managed forearms. Although assessments of the skin with various instruments have inherent inaccuracies, the overall pattern of the measurements was consistent with the histologic effects of tretinoin therapy.

Because of greater sun exposure, photodamage of facial skin is more pronounced than that of the forearms, and elastotic degeneration in the upper dermis of the face may be extreme. The histologic effects of tretinoin therapy as reported by Kligman and others[26] were more impressive on

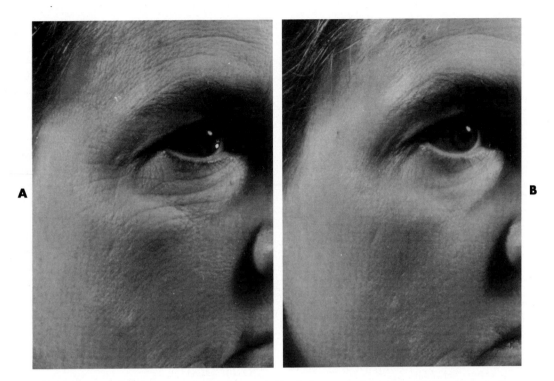

Fig. 31-3. A, Right cheek and periorbital wrinkles before tretinoin therapy. **B,** Wrinkles are decreased after daily applications of 0.1% tretinoin cream for 11 months. (From Cummings CW and others: *Otolaryngology—head and neck surgery, ed 2, Update I*, St Louis, 1995, Mosby.

the face than on the forearm. These findings were in part related to longer periods of management. Additionally, the severity of photodamage allowed the normalizing effects of tretinoin therapy to be even more apparent. After longer management, the papillary dermis increased in size, contained more active fibroblasts, and pushed down the elastotic, damaged tissue. New collagen was detected in elastotic areas. Similar findings were reported by Kligman[25] when tretinoin was applied to the skin of hairless mice that had been exposed to photoirradiation.

Additional studies of tretinoin

In a 48-week study, a lower concentration of tretinoin (0.025%) had comparable clinical efficacy with the 0.1% cream but a lower incidence of irritation.[19] Tretinoin is also effective in effacement of wrinkles in Asians.[13,18,29]

Large trials with an emollient form of tretinoin

Weinstein and others[37] and Olsen and others[30] reported the results of two multicenter trials. Each enrolled nearly 300 patients who used an emollient form of tretinoin for 24 weeks. A positive response was related to the concentration of tretinoin used: the 0.05% form yielded the best results, the 0.01% form had a weak clinical effect or no effect at all, and the 0.001% form was no different from the vehicle cream, which had a surprisingly good effect by itself. The new form did not eliminate the typical retinoid cutaneous

reactions, although on an anecdotal basis most patients preferred it to the original tretinoin vehicle (Retin-A). Bhawan and others[3] examined histologic specimens from the patients in the multicenter trials. Their data indicated that a dose-response relationship exists. There was no significant difference in the histologic condition after management with the 0.001% tretinoin form compared with that after management with the vehicle cream. The 0.01% and 0.05% concentrations induced typical retinoid-related histologic changes similar to those previously reported.

Actinic hyperpigmented lesions (brown spots)

Brown spots, or liver spots, are recognized as early signs of aging, and they may occur in patients who are as young as 30 years of age. Brown spots are commonly termed *actinic lentigines*, but similar brown spots may have different histologic causes and are probably pathogenically unrelated.[32] Indeed, only 60% of brown spots are actinic lentigines on biopsy. The rest are elastoses, seborrheic keratoses, spongiotic dermatitis, and other conditions. Surprisingly, tretinoin therapy appears to improve the appearance of all brown spots, and there has been no specific relationship of the histologic diagnosis to the efficacy of topical retinoid therapy.

In most early studies, brown spots were not carefully evaluated. The initial studies of tretinoin in the management of photodamaged skin were focused on wrinkles. The geneal appearance of the skin was also evaluated with specific attention to the erythema ("rosy glow") induced by retinoids, which was deemed desirable. Furthermore, the tired, sallow appearance to the skin was observed to become fresher and more youthful.

Tretinoin for brown spots

Because earlier findings suggested that lentigines may fade during treatinoin therapy[8,38] a careful double-blind trial was conducted to determine the effectiveness of tretinoin on brown spots associated with aging.[32] White patients with brown spots on their faces or hands were studied. All of the spots were initially diagnosed as actinic lentigines. After 10 months of tretinoin therapy, 42% of the facial brown spots became much lighter, and 42% were classified as lighter. Among patients using sunscreen and vehicle cream over the same period, only 7% of facial lesions became much lighter and 21% were classified as lighter. In patients who had excellent results and were followed-up for 6 months, the lentigines did not return, regardless of whether the patients continued with tretinoin or switched to a plain emollient. This result suggests that lentigines can be cured by tretinoin and that they do not recur. Not all brown spots completely regress with tretinoin therapy, but those that disappear are likely to remain absent.

On an anecdotal basis, many racial groups perceive their skins as substantially different. Some clinical differences do appear to be present. For example, aging facial skin of Asians in the Pacific basin is characterized more by the development of brown spots than by wrinkles. However, these brown spots represent the same spectrum of histologic diagnoses that occur in whites. Evidence continues to accumulate that tretinoin effectively resolves brown spots in Asians.[13,18,29]

Because the histologic diagnoses of the brown spots vary, tretinoin can likely be used to manage macular brown spots without regard to the specific diagnosis. Indeed, even if the diagnosis is thin seborrheic keratoses, tretinoin could be expected to have a beneficial effect. Although brown spots of all types are amenable to topical tretinoin, a desirable term for the hyperpigmented lesions is still lacking.

Actinic keratoses

Actinic keratoses are localized scaly patches on sun-exposed skin. They have slightly irregular margins and slight scales and feel like sandpaper to the examining finger. Because they tend to be flesh-colored, actinic keratoses are often more easily felt than seen; however, examination under an angled light sometimes reveals these sun-induced spots. They are more common in light-skinned people, who have less protection from the sun, and are prominent in patients who have had substantial sun exposure. Actinic keratoses are premalignant and are characterized by atypical keratinocytes that do not progress in the usual orientation to the skin surface.

When actinic keratoses are extensive and prominent, de-

structive techniques (cryosurgery, excision, electrodesiccation, curettage) are not practical or cosmetically acceptable. Patient-applied agents such as fluorouracil and masoprocol are often unsatisfactory because they lack efficacy or cause excessive irritation.

Tretinoin for actinic keratoses

Tretinoin therapy is effective in the management of actinic keratoses. A large, multicenter trial showed that actinic keratoses decrease after 10 months of tretinoin therapy. This study of 266 patients at 10 centers used 0.05% or 0.1% topical tretinoin once or twice daily for 6 to 12 consecutive months. Both lesion counts and lesion sizes decreased in a statistically significant manner during tretinoin therapy. Nevertheless, many actinic keratoses recurred after therapy was stopped. Although tretinoin may not be a first choice for management of actinic keratoses, most patients with photodamaged skin benefit from tretinoin during management for the other signs of photodamage. Similar findings have been reported for topical isotretinoin.[1]

OTHER CONDITIONS MANAGED WITH TRETINOIN

Modest improvements in the changes brought on by intrinsic aging are possible with topical tretinoin.[27] The histologic changes induced by tretinoin in the sun-protected skin of the elderly are more dramatic than the clinical findings.

Tretinoin may be useful in the management of melasma, a blotchy pigmentary change that usually occurs over the forehead and cheeks. Melasma is more common in women than in men, in part because it can be induced by the hormonal changes caused by oral contraceptives or pregnancy. Topical tretinoin is beneficial in the management of this condition in both whites and blacks.[16,24] Dark-skinned patients often have a problem with postinflammatory hyperpigmentation. For example, in many dark-skinned patients an acne lesion, on resolution, may leave a spot darker than the surrounding skin. Tretinoin helps these spots fade more quickly.[6] Tretinoin may be used with confidence in blacks because no evidence has shown that it is more irritating to black skin. Black patients may complain of an ashy appearance, which may be the result of mild peeling caused by tretinoin; adequate moisturization helps resolve this problem.

Topical tretinoin has also been introduced as a stimulus to hair growth in balding scalps. It has been suggested that although tretinoin has some efficacy as a monotherapy, it can be added to topical Minoxidil for a synergistic effect. Some physicians introduce tretinoin liquid to Minoxidil solution to achieve a solution with a concentration of about 0.025% tretinoin.

Striae, common stretch marks (e.g., occurring during pregnancy), improve when tretinoin is applied early when they still show signs of inflammation.[23] Striae in their final phase, when they are white, have not been shown to respond.

METHODS OF TRETINOIN USE

In the United States, topical tretinoin is available in a cream, gel, or solution (Retin-A) or in an emollient cream (Renova). Most patients with photodamaged skin prefer the emollient cream because their skin tends to be dry and the cream has a mild moisturizing effect. Only the Renova is labeled for use in managing certain signs of photodamage as part of a program that includes sun avoidance. At the time of FDA approval of Renova, it was controversial for what conditions the agent should be used and what claims could be made. The FDA-approved labeling reflects these uncertainties. Thus, the package insert for Renova is quite detailed, and the physician is advised to read it before prescribing. The information for patients specifically states that Renova is not a cosmetic preparation; it is a medical management to be used under a physician's supervision. Use of Retin-A for managing photodamaged skin is an off-label use.

The exact regimen is somewhat a matter of personal taste.[28] With proper advice and with the expectation of side effects, most patients with photodamaged skin can tolerate Renova.

Patients must receive proper information from the prescribing physician; printed information that outlines the expectations of the therapy is helpful. Because tretinoin should be used for several months before beneficial effects are seen, patients should be prepared. Also, side effects occur before improvement is noted, so proper patient instruction helps overcome this natural barrier to management. Tretinoin cream should be applied at bedtime, partly because the active ingredient degrades with exposure to ultraviolet light. Washing immediately before applying the tretinoin tends to make the skin more sensitive to the retinoid reaction and is thus unwise.

Although the medication should initially be applied sparingly, patients are encouraged to gradually increase the amount used. Typically, a patient applies a small dab of tretinoin cream in three or four places on the face and spreads the cream around into a thin film. The whole face should be managed, including the crow's-foot areas and the fine wrinkling on the upper cheeks. After patients have experience using the tretinoin on their faces, they may wish to apply it to the backs of their hands and even to their forearms. Application to the neck or intertriginous areas is not recommended, because this may cause excessive irritation. Application close to the eyes may cause a transient stinging sensation. Although it is important to warn the patient, this effect is not known to be harmful. This sensation probably indicates that the patient is applying the medicine close enough to the eyes to manage the adjacent skin.

Side effects

The retinoid reaction often occurs within the first week of therapy; however, some patients do not develop a reaction until the second month of management. The retinoid reaction, often termed *retinoid dermatitis*, is characterized by redness, dryness, and scaling of the skin. Patients complain of skin irritation. Over time, the reaction decreases, and patients should be encouraged to continue management through the duration of this side effect.

Pinkness of the skin may develop and is usually welcomed by the patient because it creates a healthy look. Despite its early onset, the rosy color may not be noticed during the time of the retinoid reaction. The rosy color persists throughout therapy and is not associated with feelings of irritation or burning sensations. Specific, discrete areas of skin that become inflamed may be actinic keratoses. Management of side effects usually entails reducing the frequency of application, the amount of cream applied, or the concentration of the cream. Occasionally, a mild topical corticosteroid is added for a few days.

Absorption of tretinoin through the skin is negligible, and there are no reports of retinoid-typical teratogenic findings in children whose mothers used topical tretinoin. Nevertheless, tretinoin should be used judiciously in women who are pregnant or who are trying to become pregnant.

ALPHA-HYDROXY ACIDS

Alpha-hydroxy acids are commonly referred to as fruit acids because they are found in fruits and certain foods. The α-hydroxy acids include glycolic acid (found in sugar cane), lactic acid (sour milk), malic acid (apples), tartaric acid (grapes), and citric acid (citrus fruits). Pyruvic acid and other α-keto acids are also used. Because they promote epidermal desquamation, these acids have been marketed in numerous nonprescription exfoliants, moisturizers, and cleansers that commonly contain 5% to 10% glycolic or lactic acids. Low-dose α-hydroxy and α-keto acids increase desquamation of corneocytes in the stratum corneum epidermidis. At high concentrations (70% to 100%), they promote epidermolysis and a full-thickness epidermal sloughing (i.e., a superficial chemical peel).

Most α-hydroxy acid products are cosmetics (e.g., moisturizers, night creams, day creams, hand lotions), according to FDA definition. As cosmetics, they are not required to undergo the rigorous clinical testing that is required for prescription agents such as tretinoin. Furthermore, cosmetics are not supposed to make claims that they alter the structure or function of skin, but the general population is unaware of these distinctions.

Studies have suggested that certain α-hydroxy acids are efficacious in decreasing signs of photodamage.[7,34,36] However, physicians often cannot control what product patients purchase at the pharmacy or grocery. Therefore, it is difficult to confidently recommend these nonprescription products as therapeutic agents. (Most of them are fine as moisturizers.) Pricing can vary widely by brand name. Similarly, the concentration of α-hydroxy acid in the product also varies. In addition, the effective concentration can be affected by the pH and the constituents of the vehicle. Thus, a 5% concentration can be mild to irritating depending on other factors (e.g., which acid is incorporated into the product). At high concentrations, some acids are used in chemical peels in physicians' offices. It is no wonder that physicians and the public are uncertain about α-hydroxy acids.

OTHER APPROACHES TO PHOTODAMAGE

The best management of photodamage is prevention. Although exposure to ultraviolet light during sunbathing and visits to tanning parlors are increasing, awareness of photoprotection is also increasing. Sunscreens, particularly those that block the ultraviolet B spectrum, are widely available. Broad-spectrum sunscreens that also block the ultraviolet A spectrum may be beneficial to many patients. Actinic keratoses may be reduced by regular sunscreen use and by reducing fats in the diet.[4,35] The concept of using biologic products such as melanin has been proposed and is undergoing testing in the United States. Topical isotretinoin (13-*cis*-retinoic acid, an isomer of tretinoin) is under investigation and has shown efficacy in improving signs of photodamage. Whether it will be commercially available is undetermined.

Other therapies for photodamage include liquid nitrogen cryotherapy for discrete lentigines and collagen injections for furrows. Chemical peels are discussed in Chapter 32. The use of topical tretinoin for 4 to 6 weeks before the chemical peel may provide a more even peel.[22] Similar in many respects to a chemical peel, laser resurfacing also manages photodamaged skin.

TRETINOIN'S MECHANISM OF ACTION

Retinoic acid enters the cell membrane readily and is bound to a cellular retinoic acid-binding protein. When it is transferred to the nucleus by mechanisms that are unknown, retinoic acid binds with a retinoic acid receptor. Retinoic acid and its receptor, along with another retinoid receptor (which binds with 9-*cis*-retinoic acid), activate retinoic acid response elements within DNA. These enhancing genes stimulate the production of retinoic acid–inducible target genes that lead to the production of specific messenger ribonucleic acid. Subsequent production of retinoic acid–inducible proteins leads to numerous alterations in the cell. These alterations are the result of new proteins that have a direct action and newly synthesized proteins that stimulate the expression of various other genes not directly regulated by retinoic acid.[31] In the skin, these changes lead to numerous histologic and biochemical findings.[11,33]

The extracellular matrix of the skin is composed largely of collagen and elastin. Ultraviolet irradiation is a principal cause of damage to the matrix at least in part by stimulating the production of matrix-degrading metalloproteinases.[10] The induction of these proteins can be inhibited by topical tretinoin applications.[10]

A rapid screening method would help determine which retinoids or other products might be useful in the management of photodamaged skin. A 4-day patch test provides information along these lines. Tretinoin has a dose-response relationship in this patch test, which measures spongiosis, epidermal thickness, and erythema in managed skin. The patch test has also been correlated with the clinical activity of different retinoids.[17]

REFERENCES

1. Alirezai M and others: Clinical evaluation of topical isotretinoin in the treatment of actinic keratoses, *J Am Acad Dermatol* 30:447, 1994.
2. Armstrong RB and others: Clinical panel assessment of photodamaged skin treated with isotretinoin using photographs, *Arch Dermatol* 128: 352, 1992.
3. Bhawan J and others: Effects of tretinoin on photodamaged skin: a histologic study, *Arch Dermatol* 127:666, 1991.
4. Black HS and others: Effect of a low-fat diet on the incidence of actinic keratosis, *N Engl J Med* 330:1272, 1994.
5. Brody HJ: *Chemical peeling*, St Louis, 1992, Mosby.
6. Bulengo-Ransby SM and others: Topical tretinoin (retinoic acid) therapy for hyperpigmented lesions caused by inflammation of the skin in black patients, *N Engl J Med* 328:1438, 1993.
7. Ditre CM and others: Effects of α-hydroxy acids on photoaged skin: a pilot clinical, histologic, and ultrastructural study, *J Am Acad Dermatol* 34:187, 1996.
8. Ellis CN and others: Sustained improvement with prolonged topical tretinoin (retinoic acid) for photoaged skin, *J Am Acad Dermatol* 23: 629, 1990.
9. Ernster VL and others: Facial wrinkling in men and women, by smoking status, *Am J Public Health* 85:78, 1995.
10. Fisher GJ and others: Molecular basis of sun-induced premature skin aging and retinoid antagonism, *Nature* 379:335, 1996.
11. Gendimenico GJ, Mezick JA: Pharmacological effects of retinoids on skin cells, *Skin Pharmacol* 6(suppl 1):24, 1993.
12. Gilchrest BA, Garmyn M, Yaar M: Aging and photoaging affect gene expression in cultured human keratinocytes, *Arch Dermatol* 130:82, 1994.
13. Goh SH: The treatment of visible signs of senescence: the Asian experience, *Br J Dermatol* 122(suppl 35):105, 1990.
14. Griffiths CEM and others: A photonumeric scale for the assessment of cutaneous photodamage, *Arch Dermatol* 128:347, 1992.
15. Griffiths CEM and others: Restoration of collagen formation in photodamaged human skin by tretinoin (retinoic acid), *N Engl J Med* 329: 530, 1993.
16. Griffiths CEM and others: Topical tretinoin (retinoic acid) improves melasma: a vehicle-controlled, clinical trial, *Br J Dermatol* 129:415, 1993.
17. Griffiths CEM and others: An in vivo experimental model for effects of topical retinoic acid in human skin, *Br J Dermatol* 129:389, 1993.
18. Griffiths CEM and others: Topical tretinoin (retinoic acid) treatment of hyperpigmented lesions associated with photoaging in Chinese and Japanese patients: a vehicle-controlled trial, *J Am Acad Dermatol* 30: 76, 1994.
19. Griffiths CEM and others: Two concentrations of topical tretinoin (retinoic acid) cause similar improvement of photoaging but different degrees of irritation: a double-blind vehicle-controlled comparison of tretinoin 0.1% and 0.025% creams, *Arch Dermatol* 131:1037, 1995.
20. Grove GL and others: Skin replica analysis of photodamaged skin after therapy with tretinoin emollient cream, *J Am Acad Dermatol* 25:231, 1991.
21. Gupta MA, Schork NJ, Ellis CN: Psychosocial correlates of the treatment of photodamaged skin with topical retinoic acid: a prospective controlled study, *J Am Acad Dermatol* 30:969, 1994.
22. Hevia O, Nemeth AJ, Taylor JR: Tretinoin accelerates healing after trichloroacetic acid chemical peel, *Arch Dermatol* 127:678, 1991.
23. Kang and others: Topical tretinoin (retinoic acid) improves early stretch marks, *Arch Dermatol* 132:519, 1996.

24. Kimbrough-Green CK and others: Topical retinoic acid (tretinoin) for melasma in black patients: a vehicle-controlled clinical trial, *Arch Dermatol* 130:727, 1994.

25. Kligman LH: Effects of all-trans-retinoic acid on the dermis of hairless mice, *J Am Acad Dermatol* 15:779, 1986.

26. Kligman AM and others: Topical tretinoin for photoaged skin, *J Am Acad Dermatol* 15:836, 1986.

27. Kligman AM and others: Effects of topical tretinoin on non–sun-exposed protected skin of the elderly, *J Am Acad Dermatol* 29:25, 1993.

28. Kligman AM: Topical retinoic acid (tretinoin) for photoaging: conceptions and misperceptions, *Cutis* 57:142, 1996.

29. Kotrajaras R, Kligman AM: The effect of topical tretinoin on photodamaged facial skin: the Thai experience, *Br J Dermatol* 129:302, 1993.

30. Olsen EA and others: Tretinoin emollient cream: a new therapy for photodamaged skin, *J Am Acad Dermatol* 26:215, 1992.

31. Pfahl M: Signal transduction by retinoid receptors, *Skin Pharmacol* 6(suppl 1):8, 1993.

32. Rafal ES and others: Topical tretinoin (retinoic acid) treatment for liver spots associated with photodamage, *N Engl J Med* 326:368, 1992.

33. Rosenthal DS and others: Changes in photo-aged human skin following topical application of all-trans retinoic acid, *J Invest Dermatol* 95:510, 1990.

34. Stiller MJ and others: Topical 8% glycolic acid and 8% L-lactic acid creams for the treatment of photodamaged skin, *Arch Dermatol* 132:631, 1996.

35. Thompson SC and others: Reduction of solar keratoses by regular sunscreen use, *N Engl J Med* 329:1147, 1993.

36. Van Scott EJ: Alpha-hydroxy acids: procedures for use in clinical practice, *Cutis* 43:222, 1989.

37. Weinstein GD and others: Topical tretinoin for treatment of photodamaged skin: a multicenter study, *Arch Dermatol* 127:659, 1991.

38. Weiss JS and others: Topical tretinoin improves photodamaged skin: double-blind vehicle-controlled study, *JAMA* 259:527, 1988.

39. West MD: The cellular and molecular biology of skin aging, *Arch Dermatol* 130:87, 1994.

40. Woodley DT and others: Treatment of photoaged skin with topical tretinoin increases epidermal-dermal anchoring fibrils: a preliminary report, *JAMA* 263:3057, 1990.

Chapter 32

Chemical Peel

Jennifer Parker Porter
Eugene L. Alford

Chemical peeling of the skin is a well-established method for improving or minimizing facial wrinkles, keratoses, age spots, freckles, dyschromias, and some scars. Chemical peeling is also known as chemo-exfoliation, chemical facial rejuvenation, chemabrasion, exodermology, and occasionally, chemical face-lifting. Chemical peeling of the face, when properly performed on appropriately selected patients, may bring about dramatic cosmetic improvement in facial appearance and eliminate dangerous solar damage to the skin. The results obtained using various techniques can greatly satisfy the patient and the physician.

Chemical peeling is a chemical process that has been used by facial plastic surgeons since Gillies used carbolic acid to reduce the increased elasticity of eyelid skin caused by aging.[16] Chemical peeling involves the application of an agent that deeply penetrates the upper layers of skin to bring about exfoliation by wounding the superficial skin layer, resulting in a slough. Nonspecific tissue regeneration results in a new layer of skin with a smoother, more youthful-looking appearance.

Historically, various agents have been used, including resorcinal, salicylic acid, trichloroacetic acid (TCA), napthal, and phenol. Ultraviolet light has also been used alone or in combination with a chemical agent to produce peeling of the skin. The most commonly used chemical peeling agents are TCA, α-hydroxy acids, and phenol-based agents. Each of these agents has distinctive characteristics and varies in the depth of penetration, method of action, and mode of use. To ensure the best opportunity for a successful chemical peel, the surgeon should be familiar with the histologic effects, depth of penetration, and proper mixing and application techniques for each agent. Errors in patient selection,

application technique, and postoperative care can lead to serious complications.

The tremendous growth of interest in cosmetic surgery through the 1970s, 1980s, and 1990s has made chemical peeling a frequently performed procedure. A study that surveyed the members of the American Academy of Facial Plastic and Reconstructive Surgery showed that 11,000 facial chemical peels were performed by Academy members in 1988 alone.[12] The American Society of Plastic and Reconstructive Surgeons reported 15,000 chemical peels performed by its members in 1986; and in a 1988 survery, the American Society of Dermatologic Surgery reported that 50% of its members performed chemical peels (compared with 13% in a 1984 survey). Therefore, chemical peeling has become an essential part of any cosmetic surgical practice.

HISTOLOGIC EFFECTS

To appreciate the histologic effects of chemical peeling requires understanding of the skin changes caused by chronic sun exposure and aging. Photoaged skin differs from chronologically aged skin, although both may have similar appearances. Photoaged skin has the following characteristics: elastosis, decreased collagen, and uneven melanocyte distribution.[11] Elastosis is moderate to severe, with densely tangled elastic fibers curled in amorphous masses. Collagen is decreased in the elastotic zones, and telangiectatic vessels are noted with a perivenular infiltrate of lymphocytes, histiocytes, and mast cells. An eosinophilic band of collagen lies just beneath the epidermis in the Grenz zone, and the dermal-epidermal junction is flat. The distribution of melanocytes is uneven with a variable amount of melanin granules in the keratinocytes, accounting for the mottled appearance of the skin.

Chronologically aged skin on the other hand shows a decrease in the amount of eosinophilic material in the dermis, the fibroblasts appear shrunken,[9] and melanocytes are decreased in number within the epidermis.

Histologic examination of the skin in patients who have undergone phenol chemical peel shows marked histologic changes.[11] The dermis becomes wider because of the reorientation of the collagen bundles parallel to the skin surface. This band of collagen lies just beneath the epidermis, and fine elastic fibers can be found coursing throughout the band of collagen. These changes have been noted to persist for up to 20 years. Histologic examination of the epidermis reveals an orderly arrangement of cells without microscopic evidence of actinic keratosis and a regular distribution of melanocytes.[11]

Similar histologic findings occur in skin treated with concentrations of 35% to 50% TCA. TCA at these concentrations causes necrosis and replacement of the epidermis and long-lasting dermal changes 0.4 to 0.5 mm thick, which results in a decrease in fine and medium wrinkles.[22] Concentrations of 80% TCA produce approximately 0.8 mm of dermal destruction, which may cause hypertrophic scarring. Therefore, the highest concentration of TCA that may be used safely is 50%.[22]

ETIOLOGY OF PHOTOAGED AND CHRONICALLY AGED SKIN

The development of wrinkles is multifactorial, including ultraviolet (UV) light, facial musculature, genetic make-up, gravity, wind, and aging. UV light plays a significant role in photoaging, particularly ultraviolet A (UVA) and ultraviolet B (UVB) light.[22] UVB (290 to 320 nm) contains the primary wavelengths that damage skin. UVA (320 to 400 nm) acts synergistically with UVB to increase the overall damage to the skin. Skin damaged by UV light appears thickened, leathery, and nodular, with many wrinkles that form a rhomboid pattern.[22] The skin may also exhibit lesions such as actinic keratoses and basal and squamous cell carcinomas. Repeated action of facial musculature may cause deep furrows, whereas genetic factors account for the skin thickness and ability to wrinkle.

Classification of skin

Several methods of patient classification have been developed to determine who is most likely to benefit from chemical peel. The most important use of a classification scheme is for guidance in selecting patients and planning individualized treatment. Two schemes that are commonly used are the Fitzpatrick Classification System of Sun Reactive Skin Types and the Glogau Scale of Photoaging. The Fitzpatrick system was originally designed to determine the dosage of psoralen ultraviolet A-range (PUVA) (photochemotherapy) needed to treat patients with psoriasis. Fitzpatrick developed the method to determine a patient's sunburn and suntan response, which estimates skin tolerance to UV exposure.[8] The

Table 32-1. Fitzpatrick classification system of sun reactive skin types

Unexposed skin color	Skin type	Sunburn	Tan
White	I	Yes	No
	II	Yes	Minimal
	III	Yes	Yes
	IV	No	Yes
Brown	V	No	Yes
Black	VI	No	Yes

From Fitzpatrick TB: The validity and practicality of sun reactive skin types I-VI, *Arch Dermatol* 124:869, 1988.

Fitzpatrick scale (Table 32-1) classifies skin based on the color of the unexposed skin and not race.[8] The scale is used in various clinical situations and in guidelines for sunscreen products. With respect to chemical peel, patients of Fitzpatrick types I to III have the best potential for a favorable outcome with minimal risk.

The Glogau classification scale (Box 32-1) is based on age and the amount of photodamage that has occurred[10] and serves as a reference point for physicians when discussing patient problems.

PATIENT SELECTION AND INDICATIONS

Chemical peeling involves the removal of the superficial skin layer and subsequent resurfacing as it heals. The peels have varied effects on the skin depending on the strength of the agent chosen. The characteristics of the skin to be treated also are important. Chemical peeling has multiple uses, including elimination of rhytids, removal of actinic keratoses, treatment of pigmentary dyschromias, and skin resurfacing for photoaging effects. For patients who present for facial rejuvenation, careful consideration should be given to the primary aspects that need improvement. For skin laxity and gravitational effects, a rhytidectomy is usually the procedure of choice. However, for patients with fine rhytids and minimal gravitational effects, a chemical peel may be appropriate. Optimal management may include a combination of surgical intervention and chemical rejuvenation. In this way, skin laxity, rhytids, skin pigmentary changes, scars, and actinic changes can all be addressed. Most patients who present for chemical peel desire rejuvenation or removal of rhytids. The depth of the skin pathology should be determined to select the proper agent to be used and to predict the likely benefit. The Fitzpatrick and Glogau skin classification schemes assist in choosing the patients most appropriate for a chemical peel. The Fitzpatrick classification stratifies the patients according to the amount of melanin in the skin and their skin response to solar exposure,[6] which helps to predict the likely response to peeling agents. For example, the patient who always burns and never tans is type I on the Fitzpatrick scale and a good candidate for chemical peel. Type II and III patients also are suitable candidates. Type V and VI patients are more likely to experience hyperpigmentation with most peels and are at significant risk for depigmentation with the deeper peels. Patients in these latter categories are generally not subject to the photodamage effects seen in fair-skinned patients and may only need a rhytidectomy for facial rejuvenation.

The Glogau classification scheme, which stratifies by photoaging changes, predicts patients likely to benefit from a chemical peel.[22] Type I and IV patients are usually not appropriate candidates for peeling. Type II and III patients are more appropriate candidates for chemical peeling, with superficial and medium depth peels for type II patients and medium to deep peels for type III patients.

Some patients will seek out chemical peel for removal of pigmentary changes of the skin, including freckling secondary to photodamage, postinflammatory pigmentary changes, and melasma. With any pigmentary disorder, however, examination with a Wood's lamp is especially helpful to assess the depth of the abnormality.[4] Epidermal lesions are enhanced by a Wood's lamp and in general are improved with a peel. Dermal changes do not enhance with Wood's lamp and are generally only minimally helped with a peel. Use of a chemical peel to treat deeper hyperpigmented lesions may only result in a lightened color. Chemical peel has been used successfully to remove seborrheic keratoses and precancerous lesions (e.g., actinic keratoses). Peels are especially useful for patients with multiple lesions about the face and chronic actinic changes of the intervening skin.

Contraindications

Chemical peels are not indicated for all types of skin lesions nor in all patients. Deep dermal scars rarely improve with a chemical peel, although results vary with superficial or medium depth scars.[6,13] Males are considered to be poor candidates for chemical peel because their thick facial skin prevents a good response to a chemical peel.[29] In addition, postoperative care requires the use of facial make-up, foundations, and other agents not generally acceptable to men.

Several relative and absolute contraindications to chemical peel exist (Table 32-2).[5] Hepatorenal disease may not allow for adequate clearance of phenol-based agents and is therefore an absolute contraindication.[5] Persons with heart disease should be evaluated and preapproved by a cardiologist for application of a phenol peel because of its potential arrhythmogenic side effects.[30] Patients with unstable psychiatric disease should not be considered for any type of chemical peel because patient cooperation is needed during and after the procedure. Peels are also contraindicated in any patient who is allergic to the reagent.

Relative contraindications to chemical peel include a physical inability to perform postoperative care, a history of radiotherapy to the face, a history of keloid formation, or a Fitzpatrick skin type IV to VI. Some physicians suggest that a chemical peel should be avoided in a patient who has a

---

Box 32-1. Glogau scale of photoaging

Type I

(No wrinkles)
Early Photoaging
  Mild pigmentary changes
  No keratoses
  Minimal wrinkles
Patient age: 20s or 30s
Minimal or no makeup

Type II

(Wrinkles in motion)
Early to moderate photoaging
  Early senile lentigines visible
  Keratoses palpable but not visible
  Parallel smile lines beginning to appear
Patient age: later 30s or 40s
Usually wears some foundation

Type III

(Wrinkles at rest)
Advanced photoaging
  Obvious dyschromia, telangiectasia
  Visible keratoses
  Wrinkles even when not moving
Patient age: 50 or older
Always wears heavy foundation

Type IV

(Only wrinkles)
Severe photoaging
  Yellow-gray skin
  Prior skin malignancies
  Wrinkled skin throughout, no healthy skin
Patient age: 50s or 60s
Cannot wear make-up because it cakes and cracks

From Glogau RG, Matarasso SL: Chemical peels: trichloroacetic and phenol, *Dermatol Clin* 13:263, 1995.

Table 32-2. Contraindications to chemical peel

Absolute	Relative
Hepatorenal disease	Physical restriction
Cardiac disease	Radiotherapy to face
Unstable psychiatric disease	Keloid former
Allergy	Fitzpatrick types IV to VI
Herpes simplex (active)	Herpes simplex (latent)
	Telangiectasias
	Medication use (estrogens, warfarin)
	Human immunodeficiency virus (low CD4)

past history of herpes simplex infections because a herpetic infection of the raw surface during the healing period can result in severe scarring. Antiviral medications such as acyclovir or valcyclovir should be used prophylactically in all such patients during the peripeel period. An active herpes infection would be a contraindication for chemical peel. Telangiectasias are often worsened by chemical peel.[20] A review of the patient's current medications is wise. Estrogen or a pregnancy within 6 months of the peel and oral contraceptives may enhance pigmentary changes.[5] Deep peels should be avoided in patients taking warfarin, while aspirin and nonsteroidal anti-inflammatory drugs have been administered without problem. Patients with human immunodeficiency virus (HIV) or immunosuppression may experience delayed healing and may be at an increased risk of infection. However, peels have been performed successfully in patients with HIV helper cell counts (CD4) only above 500.[4]

AVOIDANCE AND PREOPERATIVE TREATMENT

Avoidance of sun would prevent most the photodamage effects on the skin, although chronologic aging is a concomitant factor that leads to rhytid formation. For the aging patient who has already experienced significant UV exposure, appropriate counseling should be instituted so that further photo damage is avoided after the peel. Patients should be encouraged to wear sun protective clothing, wide-brimmed hats, and sunscreen with a sun protective factor (SPF) of 15 or greater. Sunscreen has been incorporated into many facial lotions and cosmetic products, including skin foundations and lipsticks. Although optimal, sunblocks are not cosmetically appealing for everyday use because of the appearance of zinc or titanium dioxide in a thick layer.

Retinoids

Tretinoin, (retinoic acid, Retin-A) has revolutionized the acceptability of chemical peeling. Retinoids work by thinning the stratum corneum, thickening the epidermis, and reversing the keratinocyte atypia.[14] In addition, tretinoin redistributes melanin throughout the epidermis and stimulates dermal collagen and glycosaminoglycan deposition.[32] The skin also becomes rosier because of neovascularization in the dermis.[32] Tretinoin may be used continuously for up to 6 months for various conditions including a reduction of rhytids, the removal of actinic keratosis, and the elimination of solar pigmentary changes.[11] Tretinoin is also a useful adjunct to chemical peel. Many recommend its use for 2 weeks before a peel to enhance the effects and depth of penetration of the peel.[23] Tretinoin appears to allow the absorption of the peeling solution more evenly and to promote quicker healing.[23]

Alpha-hydroxy acids

Alpha-hydroxy acids, the most popular of which is glycolic acid, come in various concentrations. In concentrations of 5% to 20%, the solution can be applied to the entire face to thin the stratum corneum and control dry skin, ichthyosis, and follicular hyperkeratosis. At concentrations greater than 70%, α-hydroxy acids cause epidermolysis below the level of the stratum corneum and can be used for spot treatment of seborrheic keratosis, actinic keratosis, and verruca vulgaris.[23] Application of concentrations of 50% to 70% has also been used for full-face chemical peeling.[18] The application is followed by the removal of the agent with water-soaked gauze after 1 to 2 minutes of skin contact. Examination of patients who have undergone glycolic acid peels at high concentrations reveals an improvement in the appearance of the rhytids. Glycolic acid can be applied often (every 1 to 6 weeks as needed) to obtain the desired effect. Daily use at a lower concentration is also recommended for a more gradual change or as a pretreatment regime before the use of a deep-peeling agent.[31]

Glycolic acid produces a superficial peel. When used in concentrations of 50% to 70%, glycolic acid peeling can be performed every 1 to 6 weeks. Increased collagen and elastin in the papillary dermis is noted, although epidermal necrosis is lacking. These changes revert to the original state when therapy is discontinued.[18] Lower concentrations are available for daily use. α-Hydroxy acids are safe for use in Asians, blacks, and Hispanics and can be used in other parts of the body without risk of scar formation.[18]

PEELING AGENTS

The depth of the chemical peel will depend on the type of agent chosen and more importantly on the concentration of the agent. Skin wounds generally occur in three distinct depths: Superficial peels include damage to the epidermis and superficial papillary dermis. Medium-depth peels injure the entire epidermis and the level of the papillary dermis and upper reticular dermis. Deep chemical peels injure the level of the midreticular dermis.[4] The depth of the injury is a general guideline to the type of long-term skin changes that will occur. The type of chemical agent used does not imply the depth of penetration, but the depth of the injury is determined by a combination of the agent chosen, the concentration of the agent, and the technique used. Table 32-3 delineates the predicted depth of wounding for several agents and concentrations.

The superficial peel is useful for the patient who desires a freshened appearance, and it may help decrease keratoses and dyschromias. Repeated applications can cause changes in the upper papillary dermis, similar to the changes seen with long-term use of tretinoin. These freshening peels have become popular and are good for eradicating fine wrinkling.[27] Superficial peels tend to produce little in the way of hyperpigmentation and rarely cause scarring. The medium-depth peel is useful in patients who have actinic keratoses, moderate rhytids, and dyschromias that lie in the epidermis and upper dermis.[24] These peels should be performed no less than 3 to 4 months apart. Deep chemical peels effec-

Table 32-3. Agents used in chemical peels

Depth of penetration	Peeling agent
Superficial	Jessner's solution
	10%-25% trichloroacetic acid
	α-hydroxy acid
	Tretinoin
	Unna's boot paste
Medium	35% trichloroacetic acid
	Carbon dioxide (hard) and 35% trichloroacetic acid
	Jessner's trichloroacetic acid
Deep	Baker's phenol

Table 32-4. Concentrations of trichloroacetic acid

10%-25%	Intraepidermal peel
30%-40%	Upper dermal peel
45%-50%	Upper or mid dermal peel

tively reduce heavy wrinkles, solar lentigines, lines secondary to photodamage, and superficial premalignant keratoses.[10] Some physicians use the deep peel to treat acne scars and melasma, but most often it is not helpful with these problems.

Factors that affect the outcome of a chemical peel include the preparation of the skin, the method of application, the concentration of the agent used, and the skin type of the patient. Application of the agent uniformly over the area to be treated is essential for good results.

APPLICATION OF THE PEELING AGENT

Preoperative management

Preoperative management of patients undergoing chemical peel should be uniform regardless of the peeling agent to be used. The following recommendations are guidelines for patient preparation. Preoperative management with tretinoin will enhance penetration of the peeling agent, promote rapid reepithelialization, and shorten the postoperative course.[14] No make-up should be worn for 24 hours before the application. During application, the head should be elevated 45° to 60° to minimize the amount of tissue edema. The administration of analgesics should be individualized to the needs of the patient. Cooling or fanning the face decreases the flushing sensation that is noted with TCA and other superficial peels. For patients undergoing phenol peel, hydration with a crystalloid solution to increase renal flow is essential and should begin preoperatively. Immediately before application of the peeling agent, the skin is cleansed. Various skin preparation regimens have been recommended with good results. No regimen is known to be the most effective. The surgeon should choose a routine that yields consistent results. Skin-cleansing solutions include septisol followed by acetone on gauze, alcohol on a cotton ball followed by 10% glycolic acid, or soap followed by diethyl ether.[15,22,24,29] Care should be taken not to use a skin preparation that is too abrasive, which may disrupt the stratum corneum and produce an uneven peel. Regardless of the regimen chosen, the primary goals are to cleanse the skin evenly and thoroughly and to remove all surface oils. After the skin is

cleansed, the peeling agent is applied. Many agents are available for peeling of the facial skin (see Table 32-3). A detailed discussion of the two most popular chemical peeling agents, TCA and phenol, follows.

Trichloroacetic acid

TCA is used for superficial, medium, and deep chemical peels by varying the concentration of the solution or by using enhancers. Pure TCA is more caustic than phenol; therefore, at concentrations of 50% or more TCA is prone to cause scarring.[24] TCA acts as a chemical cauterant by coagulating protein in the skin. As it penetrates the skin, TCA becomes neutralized by serum in the superficial dermal plexus.[24] The frosting that occurs at the time of application is caused by coagulation of proteins and deposition of salt on the surface of the skin. The intensity of the frost can be used to predict the depth of penetration and to ensure uniform application of the solution. A light frost is found in superficial peels and a heavy frost in deep peels. Deep peeling with TCA has no therapeutic advantage over the use of phenol and may cause more scarring; however, TCA causes less hypopigmentation and has no cardiotoxic effects.[23] For these reasons, TCA is the most commonly used medium-depth peel.

The concentrations of TCA commonly used to achieve the desired depth of penetration are listed in Table 32-4. A concentration of 10% to 25% produces a superficial peel, 30% to 40% a medium-depth peel, and 45% to 50% a deep peel. Histologic studies have confirmed a correlation between the chemical concentration and the depth of injury.[5] Skin preparation should follow a procedure similar to that outlined previously.

The formula for a TCA mixture uses a ratio of weight to volume,[23] so a 30% concentration uses 30 g of TCA crystals, United States Pharmacopeia (USP), and enough distilled water to make a total volume of 100 ml. This formula can be adjusted to make whatever concentration is desired.

TCA should be carefully applied in a systematic fashion within aesthetic units of the face, being careful not to overlap segments. Application of the agent is associated with a burning, stinging, and flushing sensation that becomes intense, usually lasting 1 or 2 minutes. Careful application prevents a pooling of agent in skin creases or depressions. Application is best performed using 2 × 2 gauze pad or cotton tip applicators. Because systemic toxicity is not associated with TCA, the agent can be applied to the entire face at a single time without untoward effects. The solution should be feathered into the hairline, vermilion, and across the lower edge of the jaw to avoid a visible line of demarcation. If the frost produced is uneven, a less concentrated solution may be reapplied to the less frosted areas.

TCA has several advantages compared with phenol (Box 32-2). TCA is less expensive and is stable for up to 6 months when stored at room temperature in amber or clear glass bottles.[24,25] TCA has no systemic side effects when used for cutaneous peels, and the concentration can be adjusted to create the desired depth of peel.[3,27] The peel is neutralized by serum in the dermis and need not be removed with an additional solution. The frosting and turgor of the skin can also be used to monitor the depth of the peel. Deeper peels are associated with an increased tissue edema and turgor of the skin.[24]

Phenol

Phenol is primarily used for deep peels and is preferred for fine and coarse facial rhytids (perioral and periorbital), spotty hyperpigmentation, actinic keratoses and other types of photodamage, superficial acne scars, and tightening of the skin after blepharoplasty.[15,29] Phenol acts as a keratocoagulant, which precipitates the surface proteins and prevents extension of tissue damage into the deep dermal layers.[15] Keratocoagulation occurs when the concentration of the phenol is greater than 80%. When the concentration of phenol is less than 50%, the effects are primarily keratolytic and will lead to deeper penetration, greater skin necrosis, and associated complications. The most common phenol formula is that of Baker, Gordon, and Seekinger:[1]

Phenol 88% (United States Pharmacopeia)	3 ml
Croton oil	3 drops
Septisol	8 drops
Distilled water	2 ml

Phenol solutions are not stable and therefore must be mixed fresh before each use.

Histologic changes present after a phenol peel include a flattening of the epidermis and increased density of the collagen bundles, which become arranged parallel to the epidermis. The horizontal arrangement of the collagen bundles may improve acne scars by causing elevation in the floor of the scar and exfoliation at the margin of the scar.[13]

The procedure itself involves skin preparation as outlined

above. Intraoperative cardiac and blood pressure should be monitored in all patients. Hydration with a crystalloid solution should be continued intraoperatively. Phenol should be applied to the skin after division of the face into six aesthetic subunits. The solution should be applied with a cotton-tipped applicator to each subunit, allowing 15 to 20 minutes between subunits for adequate elimination of the chemical from the systemic circulation. Uniform frosting of the skin indicates uniform penetration of the agent. To achieve safe, even application of the agent, applicators should be moist, but not dripping with solution. Cool compresses may be applied to lessen the postoperative discomfort. The solution may be applied to within 2 mm of the lid margins in the periorbital areas, and in the perioral region the peel should be carried just over the vermilion border to avoid a visible line of demarcation. The solution should be feathered into the hairline and carried below the lower edge of the mandible to hide the demarcation in the shadow. The entire procedure should take at least 60 to 90 minutes to avoid a systemic build-up of phenol and cardiotoxic effects.

POSTOPERATIVE CARE

Postoperative care of patients should follow certain basic principles that are common to the care of all wounded skin. Issues include occlusion versus nonocclusion, whether to apply ointments, when makeup can be used, and when the patient can return to regular activity. This treatment protocol applies to the TCA and phenol peels and can be modified to accommodate the more superficial peels.

Occlusion of the wounded skin with tape or semi-occlusive ointment dressings causes the phenol to penetrate more deeply.[28] Proponents of occlusive taping suggest that penetration of the agent is deeper with tape than with occlusive ointments. However, several studies indicate no clear difference in physical appearance of patients having occluded versus nonoccluded phenol peels.[2] For TCA peels, patients treated with occlusive tape have a reduced depth of wounding compared with patients treated with occlusive bacitracin ointment and Vigilon or nonocclusion.[3,19] If occlusive tape is used, waterproof tape should be applied in thin strips to the entire face. Some physicians only occlude areas with deep rhytids, such as the perioral, glabellar, or lateral orbital regions. The tape remains adherent for approximately 24 hours, after which time the natural responses to injury, edema, transudate, and bullae formation cause separation of the tape from the underlying skin. At this point, the tape is easily removed in the shower.[10]

On postoperative day 1, whether taping or ointment occlusion has been used, the patient is seen in the office and instructed to wash the facial skin five to six times daily with lukewarm water and a mild cleanser, followed by application of a moisturizing solution. The moisturizing solution will prevent drying and crust formation. Several moisturizing emollients have been used, including Crisco, aloe vera gel, polysporin ointment, and bacitracin ointment. Care also is taken not to pick at the crusts that form because this can cause deeper wounding.

The skin will take on a pinkish hue approximately 7 days after peeling. Makeup may be worn after 7 to 10 days. Water-based foundation can be used to cover the initial discoloration. The patient may usually return to work after 2 weeks.

TCA peels require similar care, with frequent cleansing and application of an emollient to prevent dryness. During the first 24 hours, soaks of 0.25% acetic acid should be applied four times per day, followed by application of a moisturizing solution.[17] Beginning on postoperative day 1, the face is cleansed with lukewarm water and a mild cleanser several times each day, followed by the application of a moisturizer. The use of makeup can begin on postoperative day 7 because the skin should be healed. A light pink color will be noted.

Sun exposure should be avoided for the first 6 months after the peel. If sun exposure becomes necessary, the patient will need to use a sunscreen of SPF 15 or more to protect the skin from further damage and hyperpigmentation.

IN CONJUNCTION WITH RHYTIDECTOMY

Preoperative evaluation for rhytidectomy should assess for actinic changes or fine wrinkling that will not be improved. These changes may best be addressed using a chemical peel. In rhytidectomy patients, chemical peel in areas that have been undermined should be postponed for 3 to 6 months to avoid possible sloughing of the skin.[15] In areas that have not been undermined, a peel can be performed the day after rhytidectomy.[15] An animal study using various peeling solutions on porcine flaps revealed that the best results (less shrinkage, minimal pigmentary changes) occurred when TCA was used.[7] As an adjunct to the same study, 35% TCA peels were applied to the skin of 35 patients who underwent simultaneous deep-plane face-lift; no complications were related to combined treatment. This combined simultaneous therapy can therefore be recommended, but only for deep-plane rhytidectomy.

COMPLICATIONS

Proper patient selection for chemical peels will help avoid most complications, which are usually associated with phenol-based peels because of their systemic absorption. However, some complications, such as pigmentary changes and infection, can occur with any type of peel. A discussion of the complications and the type of peel with which they are most often associated follows.

Cardiac toxicity

Cardiac monitoring is imperative when performing phenol peels because of the possibility of a cardiac rhythm disturbance. Phenol is known to be cardiotoxic when applied inappropriately.[30] Phenol application has been associated with cardiac arrhythmias, including premature atrial contractions, premature ventricular contractions, bigeminy, and trig-emeny. These cardiac arrhythmias can occur within minutes of beginning application of the solution but most often occur after application of the solution to more than one third of the face in 30 minutes. With onset of arrhythmia it is imperative that the peel solution be removed and followed by medical management. These problems can be avoided by dividing the face into five or six subunits for application of the solution, leaving 15 to 20 minutes between application to each subunit. Thus, a full-face peel should take at least 60 to 90 minutes to apply.[15] In addition, intravenous hydration before during and after the procedure is essential to avoid accumulation of the toxic by-products through enhancement of the excretion of the metabolite through the kidneys.

Pigmentary changes

Pigmentary changes of the skin can occur with any skin wounding agent, but occur more often with deeper peels. Fitzpatrick type I to III patients have fewer problems with pigmentary changes after a peel, whereas type IV to VI patients can undergo peeling with the understanding that they may need to allow 1 to 2 years for their skin to return to normal pigmentation. Type V skin is prone to irregular distribution of the pigmentation about the face.[23] The superficial and medium-depth peels (particularly TCA) are more prone to cause hyperpigmentation, whereas the deeper peels such as phenol are most commonly associated with hypopigmentation.[11] Treated skin will usually be of a different texture and color than the untreated adjacent skin (especially for phenol peels), so careful attention is necessary to feather the peel into the hairline and vermilion and along the mandibular line to avoid obvious lines of demarcation.[15] Hyperpigmentation may be treated with various quinolone-based lightening agents, such as Melanex. The addition of tretinoin or 1% hydrocortisone cream is advocated by some to enhance the quinolone effects. Pigmentary changes are more common if the patient is exposed during the first 6 months to sun exposure, pregnancy, or oral estrogens.[15]

Persistence of rhytids

An inappropriate choice of peeling depth may result in a persistence of rhytids, so an accurate assessment of the rhytid depth is essential. In addition, chemical peel is only effective for fine rhytids, whereas a rhytidectomy is necessary to treat skin sag.

Bacterial infection

Infection after chemical peel is uncommon,[23] in part because the agents themselves are bactericidal. However, postoperative application of ointments may promote folliculitis, which is readily managed with an antibiotic for penicillinase-resistant bacteria.[5] *Pseudomonas* infections may occasionally develop and are managed with ciprofloxacin. Such infections are rare when postpeel soaks are used.

Scarring

Scarring is very uncommon but is most often seen with high concentrations of TCA.[5] Chemical peels performed over the flaps during a standard rhytidectomy may have an increased chance of skin slough. When this occurs, the wound should be allowed to heal by secondary intention.[26] Patients with a history of hypertrophic scarring may be at an increased risk.

Milia

Milia are small epidermal inclusions found on the face in some patients after application of a peel. Milia may be caused by the occlusion of the pilosebaceous units resulting from application of the occlusive ointment. Milia usually resolve without any problems, but some recommend the use of a Buff-Puff to gently exfoliate the areas. Inclusions that persist for an extended time can be unroofed surgically.[22]

Reactivation of herpes simplex

A history of oral herpes simplex infection should be sought prior to application of a peeling agent. If the history is positive, the patient should begin acyclovir or valcyclovir treatment before surgery and continue treatment for 7 to 10 days after surgery. For prophylaxis, acyclovir may be given at a dose of 200 mg three times per day.[5] This prophylactic dose should be increased if an infection occurs. Even when an infection occurs, scarring is rare.[5,21]

Persistence of erythema

Erythema usually lasts about 7 to 14 days after a chemical peel but may occasionally last up to 3 months in some patients.[21] To hasten resolution of the erythema, the patient should be instructed to avoid sun exposure, to use sunscreen at all times, and to use makeup to hide the erythema. The preoperative use of tretinoin is thought to reduce the duration of erythema, and 1% hydrocortisone cream should be applied postoperatively when the erythema persists for more than 3 weeks.

REFERENCES

1. Baker TJ, Gordon HL, Seckinger DL: A second look at chemical face peeling, *Plast Reconstr Surg* 37:487, 1966.
2. Beeson WH, McCollough EG: Chemical face peeling without taping, *J Dermatol Surg Oncol* 11:985, 1985.
3. Brodland DG and others: Depths of chemoexfoliation induced by various concentrations and application techniques of tricholoraceitic acid in a porcine model, *J Dermatol Surg Oncol* 15:967, 1989.
4. Brody HJ: *Chemical peeling*, St Louis, 1992, Mosby.
5. Brody HJ: Complications of chemical peeling, *J Dermatol Surg Oncol* 15:1010, 1989.
6. Brody HJ, Hailey CW: Medium-depth chemical peeling of the skin: a variation of superficial chemosurgery, *J Dermatol Surg Oncol* 12:1268, 1986.
7. Dingman DL, Hartog J, Sieminow M: Simultaneous deep-plane face lift and tricholoroacetic acid peel, *Plast Reconstr Surg*, 93:86, 1994.
8. Fitzpatrick TB: The validity and practicality of sun reactive skin types I-VI, *Arch Dermatol* 124:869, 1988.
9. Gilchrest B and others: Chronologic and actinically induced aging in human facial skin, *J Invest Dermatol* 80:815, 1984.
10. Glogau RG, Matarasso SL: Chemical peels: trichloroacetic and phenol, *Dermatol Clin* 13:263, 1995.
11. Kligman AM, Baker TJ, Gordon HL: Long term histologic follow-up of phenol face peels, *Plast Reconstr Surg* 75:652, 1985.
12. Kotler R: *Chemical rejuvenation of the face*, New York, 1992, Mosby.
13. MacKee GM, Karp FL: The treatment of post-acne scars with phenol, *Br J Dermatol* 64:456, 1952.
14. Mandy SH: Tretinoin in the preoperative and postoperative management of dermabrasion, *J Am Acad Dermatol* 15:878, 1986.
15. McCollough EG, Hilliman RA Jr: Symposium on the aging face, *Otolaryngol Clin North Am* 13:353, 1980.
16. McCullough EG, Langdon PR: *Dermabrasion and chemical peel: a guide for the facial plastic surgeon*, New York, 1988, Thieme.
17. Monheit GD: The jessner's–trichloroacetic acid peel: an enhanced medium-depth chemical peel, *Dermatol Clin* 13:277, 1995.
18. Murad H, Shamban AT, Premo PS: The use of glycolic acid as a peeling agent, *Dermatol Clin* 13:285, 1995.
19. Peikert JM, Kaye VN, Zachary CB: A reevaluation of the effect of occlusion on the trichloroacetic acid peel, *J Dermatol Surg Oncol* 20:660, 1994.
20. Perkins SW: *Chemical peel*. In Cummings CW, editor: *Otolaryngology—head and neck surgery*, vol 1, St Louis, 1993, Mosby.
21. Resnik SS, Resnik BI: Complications of chemical peeling, *Dermatol Clin* 13:309, 1995.
22. Roenigk RK, Brodland DG: A primer of facial chemical peel, *Dermatol Clin* 13:349, 1993.
23. Rubin MG: *Manual of chemical peels*, Philadelphia, 1995, JB Lippincott.
24. Rubin MG: Trichloroacetic acid and other non-phenol peels, *Clin Plast Surg* 19:525, 1992.
25. Spinowitz AL, Rumsfield J: Stability-time profile of trichloroacetic acid at various concentrations and storage conditions, *J Dermatol Surg Oncol* 15:974, 1989.
26. Spira M, Gerow FJ, Hardy SB: Complications of chemical face peeling, *Plast Reconstr Surg* 54:397, 1974.
27. Stagnone JJ: Superficial peeling, *J Dermatol Surg Oncol* 15:924, 1989.
28. Stegman SJ: Medium-depth chemical peeling: digging beneath the surface, *J Dermatol Surg Oncol* 12:1245, 1986 (editorial).
29. Stuzin JM, Baker TJ, Gordon HL: Treatment of photoaging: facial chemical peeling (phenol and trichloroacetic acid) and dermabrasion, *Clin Plast Surg* 20:9, 1993.
30. Truppman F, Ellenberg J: The major electrocardiographic changes during chemical face peeling, *Plast Reconstr Surg* 63:44, 1979.
31. Van Scott EJ, Yu RJ: Alpha hydroxy acids: procedures for use in clinical practice, *Cutis* 43:222, 1989.
32. Weiss JS and others: Topical tretinoin improves photoaged skin: a double-blind vehicle controlled study, 259:527, 1988.

Chapter 33

Rhytidectomy

Mark S. Weinberger
Daniel G. Becker
Dean M. Toriumi

The post–World War II baby boomers are approaching the age of 50, thus heralding a dramatic shift in the demographic distribution of the U.S. population. The proportion of the population aged 65 or older is projected to increase from 1 in 8 today, to 1 in 5 by the year 2030.[24] Advances in healthcare and increasing emphasis on preventive care have improved the prospect of longer, healthier lives for aging individuals. These people desire a youthful look that is congruous with their good health and sense of well-being and therefore often seek plastic surgery. Increased media coverage of facial plastic surgery and advances in surgical training and technique have contributed significantly to growing patient awareness of and expectations for these procedures. It is not uncommon to hear patients discussing different techniques in plastic surgery and the purported advantages.

Rhytidectomy is a cosmetic surgical procedure of the face that is unique in that it has undergone many advances over the past decade. More advanced techniques enable surgeons to more closely approach the "ideal" surgical result, but unfortunately entail an increased risk of deformity or injury to the facial nerve. The procedure used will likely depend on the training and experience of the surgeon and the anatomy and expectations of the patient.

This chapter presents the time-tested philosophy and principles of rhytidectomy and an overview of state of the art facelift surgery. The preferred technique and several alternatives are described.

HISTORY

The earliest history of facelift is shrouded in secrecy. Because of post-Victorian Europe's disdain for vanity and the reluctance of early cosmetic surgeons to share their valuable "secrets" with others,[19] plastic surgery was usually performed at private facilities and was shunned by the medical community. Von Hollanden described the first procedure in 1912. The earliest procedures were by necessity conservative skin excisions with minimal undermining until the 1920s and 1930s, when more extensive procedures were described. In 1931, Lexer described a procedure that included skin excision and undermining. In 1925, Noel published a textbook that described cosmetic procedures and included pre- and postoperative photographs. Her work was extensive and seminal for its time, contributing to the early acceptance of these so-called "vanity" procedures.

As the facelift operation gradually gained acceptance, it could be performed at fully equipped hospitals and teaching institutions. Advances in anesthesia and refinements in surgical technique allowed for more extensive dissections. Also, several individuals, including Conley,[6] Skoog,[20] Webster and others,[25] Anderson,[2] and Rees,[19] advanced the science and dissipated the shroud of secrecy by sharing their techniques with others. These surgeons made major contributions to the understanding and teaching of rhytidectomy.

Until the 1970s, facelift essentially involved subcutaneous dissection with advancement and rotation of a skin flap only. Skoog[20] first described elevation of a skin and platysma flap in 1968. Although his technique did not gain widespread acceptance, it was significant in that it pointed to the necessity for deep-tissue repositioning. In 1976, Mitz and Peyronie[17] described the superficial musculo-aponeurotic system (SMAS), which led to the development of subcutaneous rhytidectomy with SMAS elevation and suspension. This procedure is the prototype for all rhytidectomy techniques, and it foreshadowed the current understanding of facelift as dissection and repositioning of the deeper tissues (SMAS-platysma complex) with incidental excess skin excision. The key element of this facelift procedure and others is that tension resides in the deeper tissue suspension, and the repositioning and suspension of these deeper tissues are responsible for favorable long-term results. Subsequent advances in the extent of dissection and resuspension include the deep-plane rhytidectomy and composite rhytidectomy described by Hamra.[8,10] Several authors have reported good long-term results and minimal complication rates with these procedures.[8,11]

ANATOMY

Aging is a continuous process involving anatomic changes in skin, soft tissue, and bone. The soft-tissue repositioning of facelift surgery can only temporarily counteract some of these progressive changes, namely the sagging and redundancy of cheek skin and soft tissue, the loss of cervicomental and mandibular definition, and laxity of the platysma and neck soft tissue.

The key to a successful and safe facelift operation is thorough understanding of the anatomy of the SMAS and its relationship to the facial nerve branches. The SMAS is a fibromuscular layer that represents the cephalad continuation of the superficial cervical fascia and forms a continuous sheath throughout the head and neck.[22] The thickness of this layer and its adherence to other structures vary considerably in different regions. The SMAS is thick and adherent to the underlying parotid fascia in the cheek. Beyond the anterior border of the parotid gland, the SMAS overlying the masseter and buccal fat pad is somewhat attenuated. More anteriorly, the SMAS surrounds the mimetic muscles of the face, which are innervated on their deep surfaces (except for the buccinator, levator anguli oris, and mentalis). Superiorly, overlying the zygomatic arch, the SMAS is densely adherent to the superficial layer of the deep temporal fascia, which forms the periosteum of the arch. Above the zygomatic arch, the SMAS is continuous with the temporoparietal fascia and is separated by a loose areolar layer from the deep temporal fascia. The SMAS continues superiorly as the galea aponeurotica and anteriorly invests the frontalis muscle. Inferiorly, the SMAS is continuous with and envelops the platysma muscle. Thus, the sub-SMAS plane could be elevated as a single continuous flap in the lateral cheek, temple, and neck, with the exception of the region over the zygomatic arch. The dense adherence to the periosteum of the arch and the fact that the temporal branch of the facial nerve lies on the immediate undersurface of the SMAS in this region preclude safe elevation of SMAS across the arch (Fig. 33-1).

The facial nerve emerges from its intratemporal course at the stylomastoid foramen and traces an anterolateral path through the parotid gland. Medially, the facial nerve branches emerge from deep to the parotidomasseteric fascia

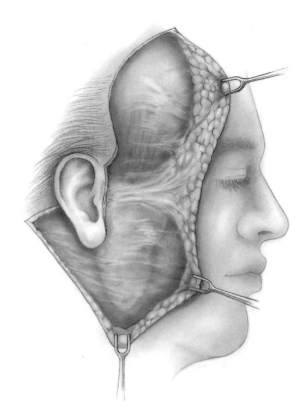

Fig. 33-1. The superficial musculo-aponeurotic system (SMAS) can be represented as a continuous sheath throughout the head and neck, although it varies greatly in consistency and adherence to underlying structures. The SMAS plane is overlying the temporalis fascia in the temple and the parotidomasseteric fascia in the cheek. Dense adherence to the periosteum of the zygomatic arch and the location of the frontal branch of the facial nerve on the immediate undersurface of the SMAS preclude its safe elevation over the arch.

to innervate the mimetic muscles on their deep surfaces. Dissection deep to the SMAS beyond the parotid gland presents a potential hazard to branches of the facial nerve. Each branch has a danger zone, the anatomy of which should be understood by the surgeon in exquisite detail.

The temporal branch emerges from the parotid gland just below the zygomatic arch and crosses the arch on the undersurface of the SMAS and temporoparietal fascia as several (three to five) rami, which run anterior to the superficial temporal vessels.[14] These branches are between points located 1.8 cm anterior to the root of the helix and 2 cm behind the anterior end of the zygomatic arch (Fig. 33-2). It should be emphasized that the nerve crosses the arch on the undersurface of a very sparse and adherent SMAS layer and lies over the periosteum of the zygoma (Fig. 33-3). This thin layer of protection over a bony prominence results in excessive vulnerability in this region. The nerve continues to run anterosuperiorly on the undersurface of the temporoparietal fascia to innervate the frontalis, entering the muscle from its deep surface 1.5 to 2 cm above the lateral margin of the eyebrow.

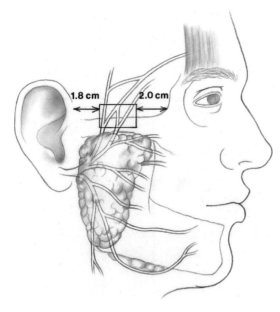

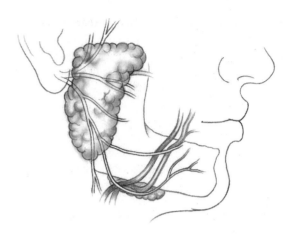

Fig. 33-2. The significant danger zone for the temporal branch of the facial nerve can be defined as the region overlying the zygomatic arch between 1.8 cm anterior to the helical root and 2 cm posterior to the anterior end of the arch. (Adapted from Larrabee WF Jr, Makielski KH: *Surgical anatomy of the face,* New York, 1992, Raven Press.)

Fig. 33-4. The marginal mandibular nerve loops below the mandible just anterior to the angle on the undersurface of the platysma muscle. It remains superficial to the facial vessels and crosses the mandible over the facial artery to enter the perioral musculature 2 cm from the oral commisure. In subcutaneous dissection, this nerve is protected by the platysma muscle. In superficial musculo-aponeurotic system dissection, this nerve is at risk anterior to the mandibular angle.

The zygomatic and buccal branches emerge from the parotid gland anteriorly and run deep to the parotidomasseteric fascia and superficial to the masseter and buccal fat pad. The buccal branch runs just below and parallel to Stensen's duct. These branches are at risk whenever dissection is carried deep to the SMAS anterior to the anterior border of the parotid gland. Care should be taken to remain superficial to the parotidomasseteric fascia when dissecting in this region.

The marginal mandibular branch is the most commonly injured facial nerve branch in facelift surgery. This branch loops inferiorly at or just anterior to the mandibular angle to run 1 to 2 cm below the inferior mandibular border until it crosses anterior to the facial vessels to innervate the perioral muscles on their deep surface 2 cm lateral to the oral commisure (Fig. 33-4). When dissection occurs in the subcutaneous plane, this nerve is protected by the platysma and facial musculature lateral to a point 2 cm lateral to the oral commissure. When dissecting in the sub-SMAS/platysma plane anterior to the mandibular angle, great care should be taken to avoid injuring this nerve, which lies on the immediate undersurface of the platysma muscle.

The great auricular nerve is the most common sensory nerve injured in facelift surgery. This nerve can be identified in the subcutaneous plane running perpendicular to and bisecting a line drawn from the mandibular angle to the mastoid tip.

DIAGNOSIS AND PATIENT SELECTION

A complex combination of physical and psychologic factors determines the best candidates for facelift surgery. The surgeon should spend as much or more time examining the patient's psychologic motivations than examining their

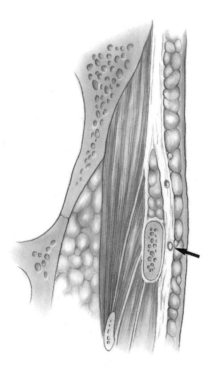

Fig. 33-3. In a coronal representation, the temporal branch of the facial nerve (*arrow*) can be seen to be applied to the immediate undersurface of the superficial musculo-aponeurotic system and the temporoparietal fascia layer, which is adherent to the periosteum of the zygomatic arch.

physical characteristics. The patient should understand the goals and limitations of the operation. Thus, the goals of the operation are to reposition ptotic facial and cervical soft tissues, counter the effects of aging, and achieve a natural, rejuvenated, nonoperated look. To achieve the best long-term results, the surgery should be supplemented every 5 to 10 years with minor "tuck-up" or ancillary procedures. A patient who understands that aging cannot be arrested or reversed but that certain anatomic components can be counteracted is most likely to be happy with the surgical result. Indeed, experienced surgeons have observed that two or more preoperative visits help the patient adequately understand the goals of surgery.

Facelifts are most successful in patients in whom aging has not yet taken an overwhelming toll on facial appearance.[23] However, chronologic age is of little significance in the selection of good candidates for facelift surgery. In general, a patient in good general health with favorable anatomic characteristics and appropriate psychologic motivations is a good candidate.

Physical characteristics that are particularly favorable include specific characteristics of bone, subcutaneous tissue, and skin. Because every patient does not meet all of these criteria, it is imperative to recognize the limitations that each of these factors may place on the surgical outcome. The optimal combination of attributes includes a strong, angular bony facial structure; thin skin with subcutaneous tissue that is mobile with respect to the underlying bone; a minimum of subcutaneous fat; a long, columnar neck with a cephalically positioned hyoid bone; a long, strong mandible; and a well-defined cervicomental angle approaching 90°. Favorable and unfavorable attributes should be pointed out to the patient to further emphasize the goals and limitations of the procedure. Any adjunctive procedures that may compensate for particular anatomic shortcomings may be discussed.

Further preoperative evaluation includes a complete history, review of systems, and physical examination. A history of any bleeding or bruising tendency or problems with prior surgical procedures or anesthetics should be elicited. The use of salicylates or nonsteroidal anti-inflammatory agents should be discontinued. The number of these products available in nonprescription analgesics and other combination preparations continues to increase and may be confusing to patients and physicians. Thus, the physician should carefully review all of the patient's medications and instruct the patient to take only acetaminophen for pain or inflammation in the 2 weeks before surgery. If a history of tobacco use is elicited, the patient should be advised to avoid tobacco 2 weeks before and 2 weeks after surgery because it has adverse effects on healing.[18]

Laboratory evaluation should include a complete blood count, coagulation profile, urinalysis, blood glucose, electrolytes, blood urea nitrogen (BUN), and creatinine. Chest radiograph and electrocardiography (ECG) are indicated in any patient with suspected cardiac or pulmonary disease or

patients older than 40 undergoing general anesthesia. Generally, a patient who is not a good candidate for general anesthesia also is not a good candidate for facelift surgery.

Standard preoperative facial photography is performed with a 90- to 105-mm macrolens. The patient's face is photographed in the standard frontal, lateral, oblique, and submental views. Also included are close-up views of both ears and views showing specific rhytids and platysmal banding brought into taut relief by a strong facial grimace.

At a second preoperative consultation, the photographs are reviewed, any facial asymmetries are carefully pointed out, and any specific limitations of the patient's facial anatomy are noted. The physician should review the incisions with the patient by drawing them on the photographs or on the patient's face with an eyebrow pencil.

PREOPERATIVE PREPARATION

Patients are instructed to wash their face and hair with hexachlorophene emulsion the night and morning before surgery. Shaving or trimming of hair is unnecessary because hair is easily controlled intraoperatively with bacitracin ointment and carefully parted along planned incision lines with small hemostats or rubber bands to stabilize hair tufts.

Before the administration of anesthesia, planned incisions and areas of fat excision are marked while the patient is in an upright position. The patient is then positioned on the operating table on a foam mattress with a pillow beneath the knees and the head elevated slightly. A narrow headrest facilitates access to the face and neck.

ANESTHESIA

Facelift surgery can be performed using general or local anesthesia with intravenous sedation. The choice of anesthetic technique is generally determined by the patient's and surgeon's preference and by the extent of the surgery to be performed. With either general or local anesthesia technique, a local anesthetic solution consisting of 0.5% lidocaine with 1:200,000 epinephrine is injected into the planned incision sites and infiltrated in the appropriate plane throughout the planned area of undermining to achieve hemostasis.

After administration of intravenous sedation, the local anesthetic should be injected in the region of the great auricular nerve to obtain a regional block and then in the planned incision sites and area of undermining (Fig. 33-5). The timing of this injection is critical because at least 15 minutes should elapse to achieve maximal hemostasis. Each side of the face should be injected separately with increments of time between injections to minimize the risk of toxicity and to optimize hemostasis. This procedure is conveniently accomplished by injecting the second side of the face just before closure of the first side is complete.

PREPARATION AND POSITIONING

Skin preparation beyond the preoperative facial wash and shampoo is not necessary. The head is draped to encompass all hair. When placed snugly along the hairline, this drape

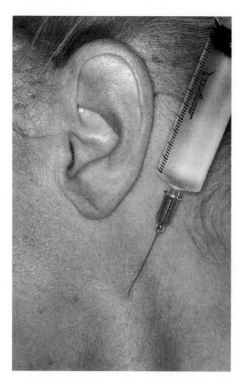

Fig. 33-5. The administration of local anesthetic is initiated with an auricular nerve block 2.5 cm below the earlobe. Only the first side is infiltrated, with infiltration of the contralateral side delayed 12 to 15 minutes before dissection ensues. This approach optimizes hemostasis and minimizes the risk of toxicity. (From Tardy ME, Thomas JR, Brown RJ: *Facial aesthetic surgery,* St Louis, 1995, Mosby. With permission.)

may be easily retracted to expose only the areas of the hairline where incisions are to be placed, thus controlling the remaining hair without further manipulation. A small amount of bacitracin ointment will smooth the hair back, and small hemostats are used to part the hair along the incision sites and control the hair tufts. A small foam sponge containing povidone-iodine is placed in the external auditory canal. A traction suture is placed along the posterior border of the helical rim to allow easy manipulation of the auricle.

The scrub nurse, operative assistants, anesthesiologist, and monitoring equipment are positioned as shown in Fig. 33-6. Management and coordination of the surgical team are vital to the smooth, fluid execution of facelift surgery. Operating time is reduced and technical safety is promoted when each team member participates in a well-orchestrated fashion by providing skin-flap countertraction during undermining, securing exacting hemostasis, ensuring facile instrument coordination, and avoiding unnecessarily repetitive or wasteful maneuvers.[23]

INCISIONS

Many incisions have been described for facelift surgery. There is no ''best'' incision; rather, the incision is determined by the anatomy of the patient and the procedure to

be performed. However, several principles apply when planning facelift surgery: optimal camouflage of scars in hairline, preauricular crease, retrotragal region, and infralobular region; preservation of normal lobular-facial attachment; and preservation of a normal contour of the hairline, including the beardline and sideburns in men.

The postauricular incision is planned for optimal camouflage and preservation of the occipital hairline. The cephalic extent of the incision is positioned where the posterior hairline intersects the margin of the helical rim. Posteriorly, the incision may be placed along the hairline or within the hair-bearing skin paralleling the hairline. In the former case, the hairline is preserved, with the possible drawback of a visible scar. This incision is useful when more than 2 cm of skin is to be removed. In the latter case, the posterior flap should be advanced somewhat anteriorly to avoid a stepoff at the hairline closure. As this incision continues anteriorly, it is irregularized as it crosses the auriculomastoid sulcus. This approach avoids any bowstring scar contracture across the concavity. The incision continues downward along the posterior surface of the auricle just above the auriculomastoid sulcus to the lobule-facial junction.

In the preauricular region, a posttragal incision is preferred in women along the posterolateral crest of the tragus. In men, the curvilinear incision follows a crease 3 to 5 mm anterior to the tragus to avoid displacement of the beardline onto the tragus. The incision continues superiorly to the root of the helix. Several variations of incisions into the temporal hairline exist. If the temporal unit requires lifting, the incision curves upward into the hair-bearing scalp in a gentle C-shaped configuration. If no temporal lifting is required, the incision continues from the root of the helix obliquely anteriorly within the temporal hair at an angle 30° above the horizontal. In men, the incision may follow the inferior edge of the sideburns to preserve its normal position (Fig. 33-7 *A, B*).

FLAP ELEVATION

After incisions have been marked and infiltrated with local anesthetic, a hook is placed in a small stab incision at the lobule-facial junction for traction and the auricle is retracted anteriorly with the traction suture. The lobule pedicle remains attached by a subcutaneous pedicle to avoid potential dislocation of normal lobular position. The posterior flap is incised and elevated in the subcutaneous plane. This dissection continues into the neck to the posterolateral border of the platysma (Fig. 33-8). Traction and countertraction on skin flaps are essential to ensure rapid uniform elevation in proper surgical planes. Dissection over the sternocleidomastoid muscle is difficult because the SMAS is fused with the muscular fascia in this region.[19] Care is necessary to avoid injury to the great auricular nerve branches and external jugular vein.

After the preauricular incisions are fashioned, dissection continues out onto the cheek in the subcutaneous plane just

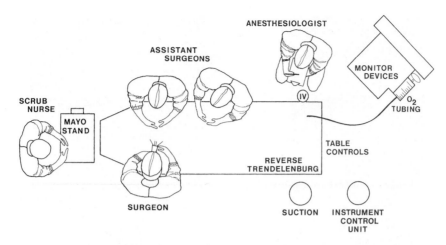

Fig. 33-6. Positioning of operative equipment, scrub nurse, and assistants for the smooth, fluid execution of the facelift procedure. (From Tardy ME, Thomas JR, Brown RJ: *Facial aesthetic surgery,* St Louis, 1995, Mosby. With permission.)

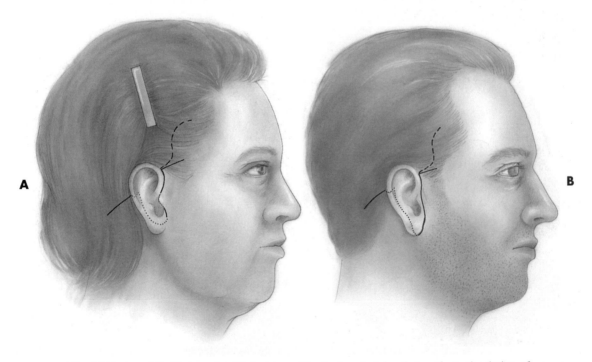

Fig. 33-7. A and **B,** Various facelift incisions. The basic principles that apply to the design of all facelift incisions include optimal camouflage of scars, preservation of normal auricular-facial relationship, and preservation of normal hairline.

superficial to the SMAS (Fig. 33-9). The extent of this dissection depends on the requirements and anatomy of the patient. Any dissection beyond the anterior border of the parotid gland potentially places the facial nerve branches at risk as the SMAS becomes more attenuated distally in the cheek. In the neck, as long as dissection is superficial to the platysma, the marginal mandibular nerve is protected beneath this muscle. This nerve branch becomes superficial 2 cm lateral to the oral commissure.

Elevation of the temporal flap proceeds in a plane just superficial to the temporalis fascia. This approach preserves the thin layer of SMAS and temporoparietal fascia over the zygomatic arch, in which the temporal branch of the facial nerve resides.

The extent of flap elevation may vary from short (4 to 6 cm) to long (cheek-neck flaps connected across the submentum) depending on the anatomy of the patient and the experience of the surgeon. The risk of facial nerve injury, hema-

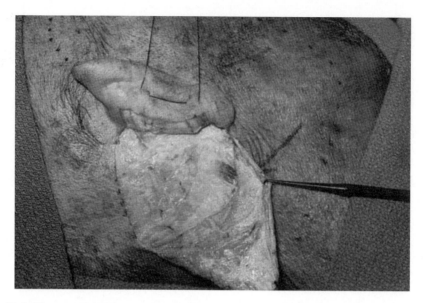

Fig. 33-8. The posterior flap is elevated in the subcutaneous plane to the posterolateral border of the platysma. (From Tardy ME, Thomas JR, Brown RJ: *Facial aesthetic surgery,* St Louis, 1995, Mosby. With permission.)

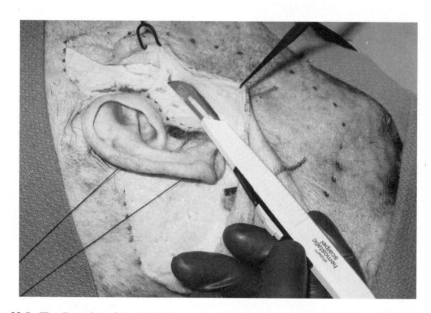

Fig. 33-9. The dissection of the cheek flap proceeds in the subcutaneous plane just superficial to the superficial musculo-aponeurotic system. (From Tardy ME, Thomas JR, Brown RJ: *Facial aesthetic surgery,* St Louis, 1995, Mosby. With permission.)

toma, and skin-flap necrosis is increased with long flaps. Mangat, McCollough, and Maack[15] have described a medium-length flap, which is elevated for 6 cm and then extended out several centimeters to the melolabial fold and oral commisure with a blunt dissection technique using a 4-mm liposuction cannula. According to the authors,[15] this "dry tunneling" technique reduces the risk of facial nerve injury.

MANAGEMENT OF THE SUPERFICIAL MUSCULO-APONEUROTIC SYSTEM/PLATYSMA COMPLEX

Proper management of the SMAS/platysma complex is debated among surgeons. However, general agreement exists that SMAS suspension maneuvers are responsible for favorable long-term results in rhytidectomy.

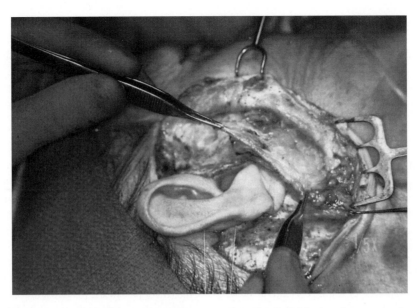

Fig. 33-10. The elevation and posterosuperior suspension of superficial musculo-aponeurotic system flap. (From Tardy ME, Thomas JR, Brown RJ: *Facial aesthetic surgery,* St Louis, 1995, Mosby. With permission.)

Before the anatomic description of the SMAS by Mitz and Peyronie[17] in 1976, Aufricht[3] advocated sutures deep to the superficial fat to achieve improved results in facelift surgery. Prior to the 1960s, other surgeons had been using various methods for suspending these deeper layers.[27] Webster, Smith, and Smith[26] showed improved results on the side of the face where SMAS plication sutures were placed compared with the contralateral nonplicated side. Since then, some form of SMAS suspension has gradually become accepted as a mainstay of facelift surgery.

Management of the SMAS/platysma complex ranges from the conservative plication to the more aggressive deep-plane dissections. Techniques include elevation and suspension of a SMAS flap, suture plication, imbrication, and various deep-plane and composite dissections. Plication or folding of the SMAS on itself in the preauricular and neck region is most appropriate in patients with a mobile SMAS and some pre-existing depressions in the lateral cheek, which are effaced by the redundant subcutaneous tissue fold created by the plication sutures. Otherwise, some form of imbrication or SMAS flap is the procedure of choice. One preferred method involves excising a strip of SMAS in the preauricular and infra-auricular region and then elevating an anterior flap of SMAS for 2 to 4 cm. Further flap elevation may be achieved with bloodless finger-sponge dissection.[23] This flap is secured with multiple nonabsorbable sutures with pull oriented in the posterosuperior direction (Fig. 33-10). Alternative methods include elevation of a SMAS flap with subsequent overlap and suspension. A SMAS flap can be elevated with safety beginning superiorly 1 cm below the zygomatic arch and extending inferiorly to 1 cm above the inferior

mandibular border and anteriorly to the anterior border of the parotid gland. Further dissection deep to the SMAS/platysma complex must proceed with caution due to potential risk to branches of the facial nerve.

DEEP-PLANE DISSECTIONS

The deep-plane rhytidectomy and composite rhytidectomy procedures described by Hamra[8,9] represent significant advances in facelift surgery. These procedures are based on the observation that conventional SMAS/platysma suspension techniques address only the aging neck and jawline and are inadequate to correct aging changes of the melolabial fold and malar area. According to Hamra, the increasing redundancy of the melolabial fold with age is caused by inferomedial descent of the cheek fat, whereas inferolateral descent of the ptotic orbicularis oculi muscle results in the descent of the malar crescent. To better address these regions, a composite flap is developed that is preplatysmal in the neck, suborbicularis in the malar region, and sub-SMAS in the face extending anteriorly to include the malar fat pad and developing the plane just superficial to the zygomaticus muscles. Once this composite flap is developed, these anatomic elements can be suspended in a direction opposite the vector of aging, using the skin as a vehicle for repositioning the deeper tissues. Hamra[8] and Kamer[11] reported excellent long-term results and minimal complication rates with this technique. Whether the improvement in results is worth the added risk is unsettled. Baker[4] has urged caution in adopting this technique, whereas Kamer[11] has presented 100 consecutive deep-plane facelifts with excellent results and minimal complications, concluding that "the surgical treatment of the aging face can be improved by entering the deeper planes of dissection.''

It has been asserted that as long as dissection stays superficial to the mimetic musculature of the face there is no risk to the facial nerve branches, which run deep to these muscles.[8,22] However, some authors have pointed out the potential risk to the zygomatic branch of the facial nerve when elevating the SMAS flap off of the zygomaticus muscles.[7,16] Any facial nerve branch innervating the inferior portion of orbicularis oculi from its deep surface is at risk in elevating orbicularis off of the malar fat pad. Because the SMAS is markedly attenuated in the region of the masseter and buccal fat pad, the anatomy of the facial nerve branches in this area must be understood in exquisite detail by any surgeon undertaking a deep-plane dissection.

A sub-SMAS or subplatysmal dissection beyond the parotid in the cheek and beyond the mandibular angle in the neck constitutes a potential risk of damage to facial nerve branches. For the patient and surgeon, this risk must be balanced with any possibility of a better cosmetic result.

SKIN REDRAPING AND CLOSURE

After repositioning of deep tissues is complete, the vector forces of skin-flap repositioning should be determined. These flaps should be positioned to provide the best lifting effect while preserving a natural unoperated look and providing optimal scar camouflage (Fig. 33-11). This goal is best accomplished with a posterosuperior direction of pull, which does not distort the hairline and preserves the normal relationship between the auricle and the face. The skin flaps are then positioned under no tension and incised to the limits of the scalp incision in two key positions: posteriorly at the

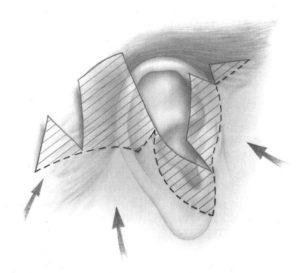

Fig. 33-11. The most favorable vector forces of skin repositioning to achieve maximum lifting and optimal scar camouflage are posterosuperior. Note that the direction of pull on the posterior flap is superior and slightly anterior at the occipital hairline to avoid any stepoff in this region. The direction of pull on the anterior flap is more posterior.

junction of the scalp hairline with the non–hair-bearing skin and anteriorly at the root of the helix.[23] These two points are secured with surgical staples, the redundant triangle of skin in the temporal hairline is excised, and this part of the incision is closed with surgical staples.

Next, the lobular-facial angle is recreated by dividing the skin flap along the lobular crease to the anterior aspect of the earlobe and then delivering the lobule to lie tension-free in the apex of this division. A single 6-0 prolene vertical mattress suture is placed at this junction.

The postauricular closure is accomplished by excising the overlapping skin so the flap edges oppose each other under no tension. The hair-bearing region is closed with surgical staples, and the postauricular region with 5-0 nylon suture. During closure, the postauricular flap is advanced somewhat anteriorly to realign the occipital hairline and to recreate the auriculomastoid sulcus. A small Penrose drain is placed in the lower part of the postauricular incision, or a suction drain is brought out through a small stab incision posteriorly in the hair-bearing skin.

The opposite side of the face is infiltrated with local anesthetic to allow adequate time for vasoconstriction, and finally, the preauricular flap is carefully tailored and sutured under no tension. The tragal region is meticulously fashioned and defatted to recreate the normal pretragal concavity. This incision is closed with a running 6-0 prolene suture.

The wound edges are cleaned, dexamethasone sodium phosphate ointment is applied, and the wound is dressed with adaptic, moist, fluffed gauze, and a circumferential 4-inch conform dressing. This bandage should apply light, even pressure and support.

POSTOPERATIVE CARE

For the first 24 hours, patients are prescribed limited bed rest with the head elevated to minimize edema. Control of blood pressure and nausea is critical in the early postoperative period. Pain is usually easily controlled with mild analgesics. Any complaint of severe pain should alert the physician to the possibility of an expanding hematoma.

The drain is removed and the dressing changed on the morning after surgery. A light dressing is continued for 48 to 72 hours for support and comfort. Incision lines are kept moist with ointment to avoid crusting. Oral antibiotics are prescribed for 5 to 7 days. Patients are allowed to gently shampoo the hair 48 to 72 hours postoperatively. Sutures are removed at 7 days, staples at 10 to 12 days.

ADJUNCTIVE PROCEDURES

Rhytidectomy alone often fails to adequately address the problems of the aging neck. Rejuvenation of the aging neck requires (1) an exacting diagnosis of the specific anatomic components of aging, which require correction, followed by (2) a surgical plan agreed on by patient and surgeon with realistic expectations for outcome. This approach usually includes some predetermined combination of a cervicofacial lifting procedure with SMAS suspension through plication or imbrication, submental lipectomy, excision or suturing of anterior platysmal bands, excision of subplatysmal submental fat, lateral-cervical lipectomy, and chin augmentation or repositioning.[23] This chapter describes the most common adjuncts to facelift surgery, submental lipectomy and platysmaplasty.

In the preoperative analysis of aging changes in the submental region, it is useful to classify patients into groups based on the presence of excessive skin, fat, and anterior platysmal bands.[12] This classification separates patients into surgical categories that are most likely to achieve a favorable outcome.

For patients with excess skin and little or no excess fat, a rhytidectomy with some form of suspension of the SMAS/platysma complex should be sufficient to correct the aging changes in the neck. Excessive fat in the submental or submandibular region may be addressed with open lipectomy through a submental incision, by defatting of the facelift flap as indicated, or with closed liposuction techniques. The use of a modified soft-tissue shaver for open lipectomy, which can also be used as a conventional liposuction cannula, has been described by Becker and others.[5]

If platysmal bands are present, they should be classified as minimal, moderate, or severe. Minimal banding may be corrected by sectioning through the lateral approach, and moderate to severe banding may be corrected by midline transection and plication through a submental incision, as described by Kamer and Lefkoff.[12] In patients with excess submental fat, lipectomy may unmask platysmal bands, resulting in a postoperative deformity. This possibility is best addressed at the time of primary surgery with transection and midline plication.[13]

COMPLICATIONS

The surgeon's best defense against complications is prevention. With strict adherence to the principles of appropriate patient selection, exacting anatomic analysis, careful preoperative preparation, meticulous surgical technique, and good postoperative care, the complication rate for facelift surgery should be very low. It also should be remembered that perfection does not exist in facelift surgery, and aggressive dissection to achieve a better result should be balanced with the potential risks to the patient. In purely cosmetic surgery, such as facelift, every surgeon should strive for a 0% complication rate.

It is important to distinguish between sequelae and complications because all sequelae should be understood by the patient to be a potential part of the postoperative course. Sequelae include postoperative bruising and swelling, temporary hypoesthesia in areas of incisions and undermining, and fine, well-camouflaged scars.

Hematomas are the most common complication after facelift surgery. Most are small, localized, benign hematomas that occur from several days to 2 weeks postoperatively.

Hematomas can usually be safely drained in the office with a large-gauge needle or a 2-mm liposuction cannula and managed with pressure dressings. Patients experiencing this complication may have persistent hyperpigmentation or soft-tissue irregularities.[15,23] Expanding or malignant hematomas are much less common and usually occur in the first 12 hours after surgery. Postoperative hypertension is thought to play a role in the development of this distressing complication.[21] Signs that herald the onset of an expanding hematoma include pain, nausea, agitation, swelling, and hypertension. Bluish discoloration and hardness of the buccal mucosa and lips indicate that rapid surgical intervention is necessary.[23] The patient should promptly undergo hematoma evacuation and control of bleeding to prevent flap compromise. Any delay in this definitive intervention jeopardizes the facelift flap. Hematomas that are adequately treated should have no serious long-term sequelae.

Skin-flap necrosis has a higher incidence in patients with longer and thinner flaps, in patients with hematomas, and in smokers.[1] If skin flaps of conservative length are elevated in the proper plane (leaving a layer of subdermal fat intact on the undersurface of the skin) are handled gently with fine-pointed instruments, and are closed under minimal tension, this complication should be preventable. Patients should be advised to stop smoking for 2 weeks preoperatively and 3 weeks postoperatively because the effects of nicotine on wound healing are well documented.[18] An area of skin slough that occurs should be managed conservatively with antibiotic ointment because a moist, nonocclusive environment promotes re-epithelialization.

Infection is a rare complication after facelift surgery. It is heralded by swelling, redness, pain, fluctuance, and drainage. Prompt drainage, culture, and appropriate antibiotic therapy should rapidly resolve infection. Possible predisposing factors include diabetes, external otitis, and undetected hematoma.[15]

Sensory nerve injury most commonly involves the great auricular nerve, which is usually easily identified when elevating the posterior flap. Great caution should be exercised when using electrocautery or placing suspension sutures in the region of the nerve because these procedures are likely sources of nerve injury.

Motor nerve injury may involve any branch of the facial nerve. The marginal mandibular is the most commonly injured, followed by the temporal branch. Detailed understanding of the anatomy of the danger areas for each of these nerves and meticulous surgical technique should prevent these complications.

Poor scars and deformities of the hairline and earlobe are entirely preventable based on the principles outlined. Some patients may develop hypertrophic scars despite a tension-free closure secondary to a genetic predisposition. These scars may be treated with intralesional corticosteroids. Hair loss may result from improper bevelling of incisions to pre-

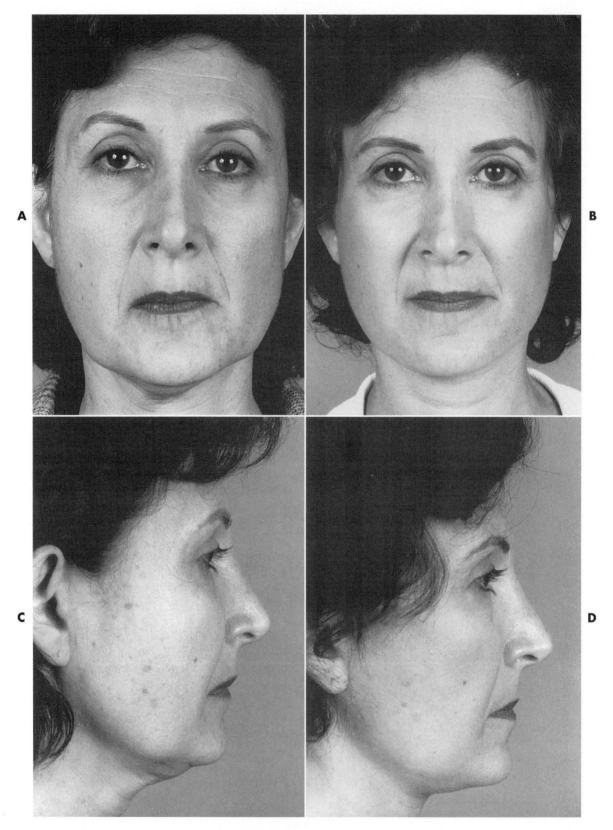

Fig. 33-12. A patient with favorable anatomic characteristics for facelift surgery shown **A** and **C,** preoperatively, and **B** and **D,** 8 months postoperatively.

serve hair follicles or excessive tension on flaps. Permanent hair loss can be treated with hair grafts.

Some patients will be dissatisfied despite an excellent aesthetic outcome. This dissatisfaction may be the result of unrealistic expectations or some deeper seated self-image problem. It is imperative that the surgeon acknowledge the patient's complaints and address them in a direct, respectful manner. Extensive psychologic support may be necessary because these patients may require more "hand-holding" than other cosmetic surgery patients. Plans should be made to correct any problems that are amenable to surgical correction at the appropriate time.

CONCLUSIONS

Facelift surgery will continue to grow in popularity as a youthful appearance is more sought after by an affluent, aging population. When this operation is performed by well-trained surgeons on properly selected patients, the aesthetic results should be a source of pride and satisfaction for patients and surgeons. More than any other plastic surgical procedure, rhytidectomy represents a balance between the ultimate aesthetic outcome and potential risk to the patient. Ultimately, the surgeon and patient are responsible for deciding which technique provides the appropriate balance between risk and the possibility of an improved result (Fig. 33-12 *A* to *D*).

REFERENCES

1. Adamson PA, Moran ML: Complications of cervicofacial rhytidectomy, *Fac Plast Surg Clin North Am* 1:257, 1993.
2. Anderson J: The tuck up operation: a new technique of secondary rhytidectomy, *Arch Otolaryngol Head Neck Surg* 101:739, 1975.
3. Aufricht G: Surgery for excessive skin of the face, Transactions 2nd International Congress of Plastic Surgery, Edinburgh, 1960, Churchill Livingstone.
4. Baker DC: Deep dissection rhytidectomy: a plea for caution, *Plast Reconstr Surg* 93:1498, 1994.
5. Becker DG and others: The liposhaver in facial plastic surgery: a multi-institutional experience, *Arch Otoloryngol Head Neck Surg* 122:1161, 1996.
6. Conley J: *Facelift operation*, Springfield, Ill, 1968, Charles C Thomas.
7. Furnas DW: Discussion of correction of the nasolabial fold: extended SMAS dissection with periosteal fixation, *Plast Reconstr Surg* 89:834, 1992.
8. Hamra ST: Composite rhytidectomy, *Plast Reconstr Surg* 90:1, 1992.
9. Hamra ST: *Deep plane rhytidectomy and browlift*. In Russell RC, editor: *Instructional courses*, vol 3, St Louis, 1990, Mosby.
10. Hamra ST: The deep-plane rhytidectomy, *Plast Reconstr Surg* 86:53, 1990.
11. Kamer FM: One hundred consecutive deep plane face lifts, *Arch Otolaryngol Head Neck Surg* 122:17, 1996.
12. Kamer FM, Lefkoff LA: Submental surgery: a graduated approach to the aging neck, *Arch Otolaryngol Head Neck Surg* 117:40, 1991.
13. Kamer FM, Minoli JJ: Postoperative platysmal band deformity, *Arch Otolaryngol Head Neck Surg* 119:193, 1993.
14. Larrabee WF Jr, Makielski KH: *Surgical anatomy of the face*, New York, 1992, Raven Press.
15. Mangat DS, McCollough EG, Maack RW: *Rhytidectomy*. In Cummings C and others, editors: *Otolaryngology—head and neck surgery*, ed 2, St Louis, 1992, Mosby.
16. Mendelson BC: Correction of the nasolabial fold: extended SMAS dissection with periosteal fixation, *Plast Reconstr Surg* 89:822, 1992.
17. Mitz V, Peyronie M: The superficial musculo-aponeurotic system (SMAS) in the parotid and cheek area, *Plast Reconstr Surg* 58:80, 1976.
18. Mosely LH, Finseth F, Goody M: Nicotine and its effect on wound healing, *Plast Reconstr Surg* 61:570, 1978.
19. Rees TD: *Aesthetic plastic surgery*, Philadelphia, 1980, WB Saunders.
20. Skoog T: *Plastic surgery: new methods and refinements*, Philadelphia, 1975, WB Saunders.
21. Strath R, Raju D, Hipps C: The study of hematomas in 500 conservative facelifts, *Plast Reconstr Surg* 59:694, 1983.
22. Stuzin JM, Baker TJ, Gordon HL: The relationship of the superficial and deep facial fascias: relevance to rhytidectomy and aging, *Plast Reconstr Surg* 89:441, 1992.
23. Tardy ME, Thomas JR, Brown RJ: *Facial aesthetic surgery*, St Louis, 1995, Mosby.
24. *The Wall Street Journal*. May 21, 1996.
25. Webster R and others: Conservative face-lift surgery, *Arch Otolaryngol Head Neck Surg* 102:657, 1976.
26. Webster RC, Smith RC, Smith KF: Face lift: part 3. Plication of the superficial musculoaponeurotic system, *Head Neck Surg* 6:696, 1983.
27. Webster RC, Smith RC, Smith KF: Face lift: part 4. Use of superficial musculoaponeurotic system suspending sutures, *Head Neck Surg* 6:780, 1984.

Chapter 34

Surgical Management of the Upper Third of the Aging Face

Ferdinand F. Becker
Calvin M. Johnson, Jr.
Lee M. Mandel

Although cervicofacial rhytidectomy has long enjoyed great attention among facial plastic surgeons, treatment of the upper third of the aging face was of only sporadic interest until approximately 20 years ago. In the late 1970s and early 1980s, research by Brennan[2-4] and Pitanguy[17] focused on the critical importance of this region in achieving the maximum cosmetic result for the aging-face patient. As the face ages, the skin loses elasticity, creating redundancy of skin in the neck and jowl areas. Deep and fine wrinkles develop in the cheeks and perioral areas caused by repeated contraction of the mimetic muscles of the face, with loss of the ability of the skin to spring back to its original condition. Blepharochalasis results in fine wrinkling of the eyelid skin, and crow's feet develop lateral to the lateral canthus. Laxity of the orbital septum causes protrusion of adipose tissue, creating bulges or bagginess in the eyelids. While slightly more resistant, the upper one third of the aging face is not immune to this process. As skin in the lateral brow region loses its elasticity and the orbicularis muscle loses its tone, the brow begins to fall. In an attempt to actively raise the brow, or because of excessive mimetic function, the frontalis muscle contracts. This action compresses the intervening skin and subcutaneous tissue over time, essentially forming a crease that eventually remains even after frontalis relaxation. Prolonged and continued squinting will similarly cause vertical and horizontal rhytids in the glabellar region secondary to action of the corrugator supercilius and procerus muscles, respectively. Ptosis of the forehead and brows often creates a tired, sad, or even angry look, depending on its degree and on gla-

bellar rhytidosis (Fig. 34-1). Although upper and lower eyelid blepharoplasties and cervicofacial rhytidectomies have been performed and written about for many years, surgical management of brow and forehead ptosis has only recently become an area of expanding interest. Failure to address the brow and forehead in a patient with significant ptosis of these areas will lead to an unsatisfactory aesthetic result.

Understanding the normal anatomic position of the eyebrow is important to surgically correct an abnormally positioned eyebrow (Fig. 34-2). Rafaty and Brennan[18] provided an excellent description of the ''ideal'' brow:

In women, the medial end of the eyebrow should begin at a vertical line drawn through the ala of the nose. The lateral end of the eyebrow should terminate at the oblique line drawn through the ala of the nose and the lateral canthus. The medial and lateral ends of the eyebrow should lie in a horizontal line. The medial end should have a club-head configuration that gradually tapers laterally. The maximum height of the brow should be at the lateral limbus (scleral-pupillary border). The brow should arch above the supraorbital rim. In men, the brow usually lies at the supraorbital rim.

Since the first part of this century, many procedures have been described to correct eyebrow and forehead ptosis. Brennan[2] published an excellent review of the literature on this subject. None of these procedures gained much popularity because of the scarring of the forehead that resulted from the direct procedures and the temporary benefits obtained from the limited forehead-lift procedures. The revival of the forehead-lift was brought about by the recognition of the

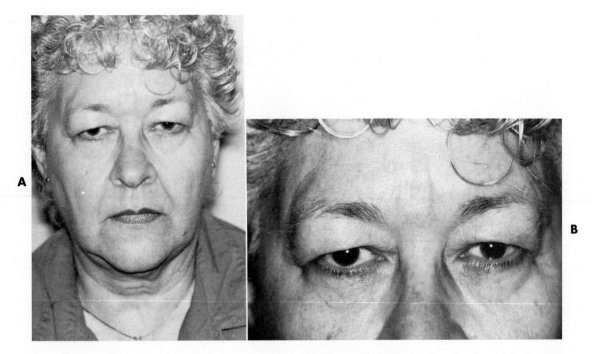

Fig. 34-1. A, A patient with severe forehead and brow ptosis who is not frowning but appears angry because of the severity of the ptosis. She also has generalized facial rhytidosis. **B,** Close-up of eyelid and eyebrow area.

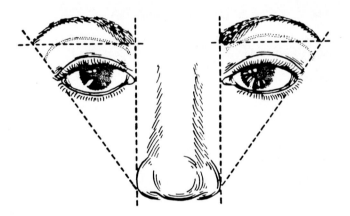

Fig. 34-2. The "ideal" eyebrow.

importance of an extensive dissection of the forehead down over the orbital rims and interrupting the corrugator and frontalis muscles. This evolutionary process was reviewed by Kaye,[10] who was instrumental in popularizing the procedure in the United States.

With the advent of endoscopy, aesthetic procedures can now be classified as open or closed. Endoscopic subperiosteal rhytidectomy and brow lifting are currently on the forefront of this technology; however, adequate long-term follow-up of these techniques is pending. These procedures essentially use orthopedic sutures to suspend the soft tissues from the skull or facial bones. Fundamentally, it is reasonable to assume that mere suspension and redistribution of

excess soft tissue would not yield the same longevity as excision. However, four "open" techniques of browplasty are available to effectively correct ptosis of the brows (Fig. 34-3): (1) direct browplasty with an incision of the skin immediately above the brow; (2) midforehead browplasty with an incision in a natural transverse forehead rhytid above the level of the brow; (3) midforehead rhytidectomy with an incision all the way across the forehead in a natural transverse rhytid; and (4) forehead rhytidectomy (coronal lift, forehead-lift, frontal lift) with an incision behind the temporofrontal hairline (classical coronal approach) or within the frontal hairline (trichophytic approach) (see Fig. 34-12). The transblepharoplasty browpexy procedure deserves mention, although this technique is considered minor and offers limited results compared with the other methods.[7] Transverse forehead rhytids and glabellar frown lines, along with eyebrow ptosis, may be treated with the forehead rhytidectomy and the midforehead rhytidectomy.

ANATOMY

The forehead receives its blood supply bilaterally from branches of the superficial temporal artery laterally and from the supraorbital and supratrochlear arteries medially. The superficial temporal artery lies in the plane of the temporoparietal fascia, whereas the supraorbital and supratrochlear arteries lie superficial to the pericranium as they exit their respective foramina.

Sensation to the forehead is supplied by branches of the

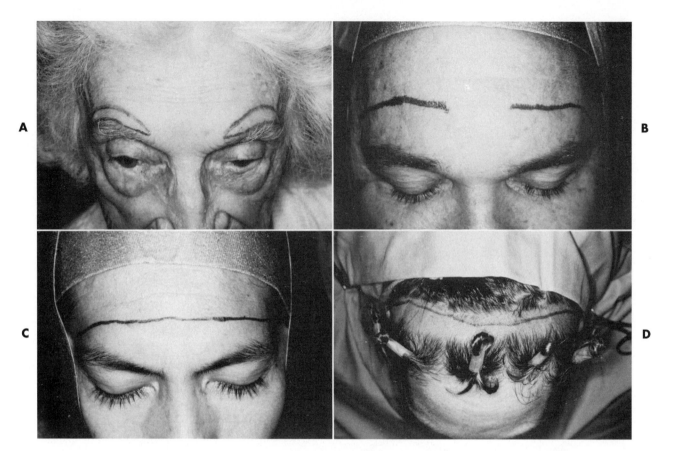

Fig. 34-3. A, Direct browplasty with excision of ellipse of skin immediately above the brow. **B,** Midforehead browplasty with incision in a natural transverse forehead rhytid above the level of the brow. **C,** Midforehead rhytidectomy with an incision across the forehead in a natural transverse rhytid. **D,** Forehead rhytidectomy (coronal lift, forehead-lift, frontal lift) with incision behind the temporofrontal hairline.

supratrochlear and supraorbital nerves (V1) medially and largely by branches of V2 laterally. Motor innervation is provided by the frontal branch of the facial nerve. This branch exits the parotid gland superiorly and travels diagonally across the zygomatic arch approximately one fingerbreadth (2 cm) behind the anteriormost aspect of the zygomatic arch at its junction with the lateral orbital rim. In the forehead region, the nerve usually runs beneath a line 2 cm above the brow, but this distance may be variable. In the temple region, the nerve lies in the plane of the temporoparietal fascia and enters the forehead musculature from the undersurface.[11]

DIRECT BROWPLASTY

The direct browplasty or brow-lift was first described by Passot[15] and was redescribed with modifications by Castanares.[5] The operation consists of excising an ellipse of skin from just above the eyebrow. Closure of the resultant wound raises the eyebrow, thereby decreasing the amount of excess skin of the upper eyelid. Anderson[1] and Rafaty, Goode, and Abramson[19] stressed the importance of suspending the brow

permanently by attaching the orbicularis muscle to the fascia of the frontalis muscle or periosteum of the frontal bone with nonabsorbable suture material to lend permanency to the ptosis correction (Fig. 34-4 *B, C*).

Technique

The face is prepared and draped in the usual sterile fashion. A marking pen is used to outline an elliptical excision of skin of the forehead with the lower limb of the ellipse placed at the upper brow margin (see Fig. 34-4). The amount of skin to be excised is determined by elevating the brow. Some surgeons prefer to do this with the patient in the sitting position. The high point of the elevated brow should be at the lateral limbus, and the ellipse should taper medially and laterally from this point. Local anesthetic with epinephrine is infiltrated into the skin and muscular layers. The incision is beveled cephalad to parallel the hair follicles, especially in the medial two thirds. The upper incision is beveled in the same fashion. The skin is excised in the plane just superficial to the orbicularis muscle. Care is taken not to penetrate the muscle and cause possible damage to sensory and motor

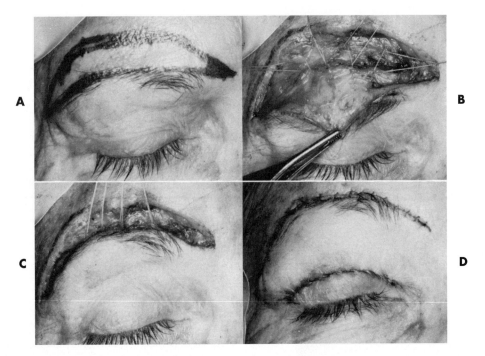

Fig. 34-4. A, Skin marking for direct browlift. **B,** Suspension sutures from orbicularis oculi muscle to frontalis muscle or periosteum. **C,** Suspension sutures tied. **D,** Skin closure completed; notice that upper blepharoplasty is always performed after the brow-lifting procedure.

nerve branches. Three to six permanent undyed sutures are used to suspend the orbicularis muscle to the frontalis fascia or periosteum above. When properly performed, this suspension will often approximate the wound. Symmetric elevation of the brows is critical. A dermal closure is carried out with interrupted slow-absorbing sutures, burying the knots. The brows should be slightly overcorrected. Blepharoplasty, when indicated, is carried out after the brow procedure. More conservative skin excision of the upper eyelids is indicated in this situation. The blepharoplasty also may be postponed 2 weeks or more to allow a more accurate assessment of the amount of skin to be excised. Antibiotic ointment and a light dressing are applied to the wound.

Discussion

Direct browplasty may be indicated in a patient with brow ptosis of any degree who has soft, nonoily skin that does not have a tendency for hypertrophic scarring and who does not object to using makeup to camouflage the scar. It is especially effective on patients with sagging of the lateral two thirds of the brows and little or no ptosis or furrowing of the glabella region. Forehead rhytids are not addressed in this procedure. Direct browplasty is effective for correction of unilateral brow ptosis associated with permanent unilateral facial or forehead paralysis from any cause (Fig. 34-5).

This operation is usually contraindicated in any patient with thick, oily Mediterranean-type skin or a history of abnormal scarring and in any patient who finds a facial scar unacceptable. This procedure may be contraindicated in a patient with an unusually low temporal hairline because the postoperative appearance of the brow located near the temporal hairline can create an unnatural appearance.

The advantages of the direct browplasty are it's speed, ease of performance, low morbidity, and considerably lower cost compared with more elaborate forehead operations. The procedure is very effective, and postoperative recurrence of brow ptosis is rare.

The major disadvantage of direct browplasty is the resulting scarring, the severity of which may be variable and could require ancillary procedures (i.e., dermabrasion, scar revision). The scars may require camouflage with cosmetics, and care should be taken to avoid sun exposure lest the scar become more apparent. Elimination of fine upper brow hairs occasionally results in an unnatural, sharply defined upper brow border that the patient may find objectionable.

Since the revival of the forehead rhytidectomy, direct browplasty is rarely used. It is most often performed on a female patient who does not want to be subjected to the morbidity of the more elaborate forehead-lifting procedures and is willing to accept a forehead scar. The procedure is rarely recommended to male patients unless they have smooth, nonwrinkled foreheads or unilateral permanent facial paralysis.

MIDFOREHEAD BROWPLASTY

The midforehead browplasty takes advantage of the natural transverse forehead rhytids that are usually present in men needing brow elevation (Fig. 34-6). By placing the inci-

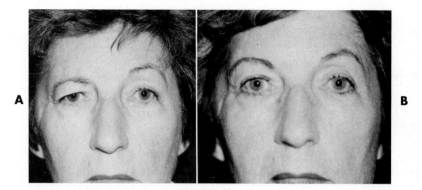

Fig. 34-5. A, A patient with unilateral brow ptosis secondary to paralysis of the frontal branch of the facial nerve. **B,** Postoperative view of the patient after direct browplasty and upper blepharoplasty.

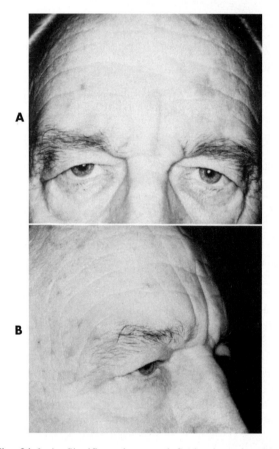

Fig. 34-6. A, Significant brow and forehead ptosis with glabellar rhytidosis, lateral hooding, and numerous transverse forehead rhytids: frontal view. **B,** The oblique view of the same patient.

sions in natural lines, the resulting scars are usually well hidden. Rafaty, Goode, and Fee[19] described their approach to this procedure and reviewed the literature on the subject. Patients should be informed before surgery that these scars take several months to mature.

Technique

After preparation and draping, the patient is asked to raise the eyebrows. A natural horizontal forehead rhytid above the brow is then selected on each side and marked out (see Fig. 34-7). Usually the first or second wrinkle above the brow is selected, depending on the amount to be excised. Often rhytids of unequal distance from the brows are selected (see Fig. 34-7, *A*), making the resultant scars less apparent than scars along the same horizontal. After infiltration of local anesthetic with epinephrine, the skin is incised along the previously marked line. Dissection is carried out inferiorly just superficial to the forehead musculature and carried down to the orbital rims. Again, care is taken not to violate the frontalis or orbicularis muscles to prevent injury to sensory or motor nerve branches. The orbicularis muscle is then suspended to the frontalis muscle or periosteum with permanent suture, as in the direct browplasty. An amount of skin is excised such that the wound can close without tension. The wound is closed in a similar manner to the previous procedure. If indicated, blepharoplasty is carried out after the brow procedure.

Discussion

Midforehead browplasty is most often indicated for the male patient with brow ptosis (Fig. 34-8). A female patient who is not a candidate for a forehead rhytidectomy and has deep horizontal forehead creases may occasionally be selected.

Midforehead browplasty is relatively contraindicated in anyone with smooth, nonwrinkled forehead skin and in most women. The operation is contraindicated in patients with histories of abnormal scarring or in patients who cannot accept facial scars.

As with the direct browplasty, midforehead browplasty has the advantages of speed, ease of performance, and low morbidity. The procedure is relatively inexpensive compared with more elaborate forehead procedures and is very effective with minimal postoperative recurrences.

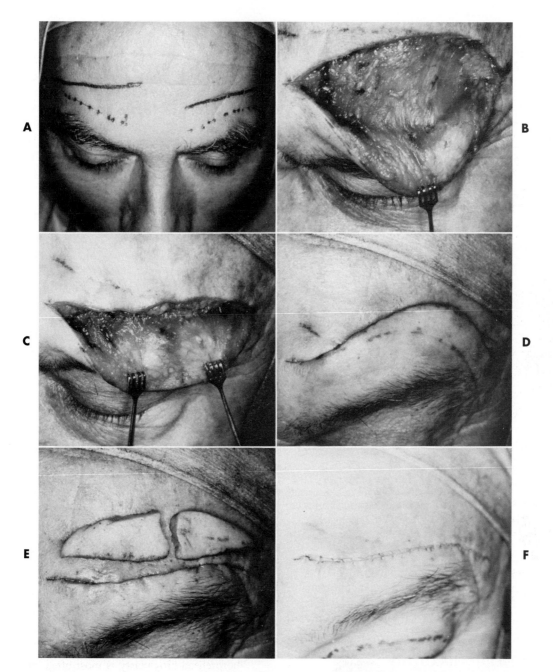

Fig. 34-7. A, Skin marking for midforehead browplasty in second transverse rhytid above the brow. The first transverse rhytid above the brow is marked with stippling. Note the unequal level of proposed brow incision. **B,** Skin elevation in deep subcutaneous plane just superficial to the muscular layer down over the orbital rims. **C,** Suspension sutures from orbicularis oculi muscle to frontalis muscle secured. **D,** Skin to be excised overlapped after suspension sutures in place. **E,** Dermal closure complete. Note excised skin. **F,** Skin closure complete. Note blepharoplasty marked only after browplasty has been completed.

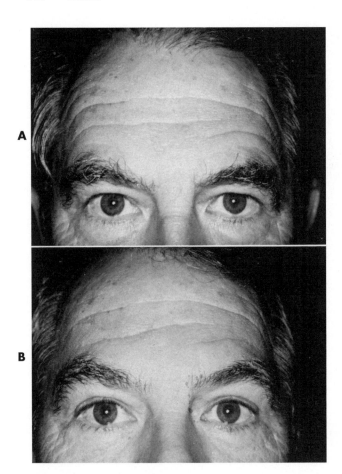

Fig. 34-8. A, A male patient with significant brow ptosis and blepharochalasis. **B,** Postoperative photograph of midforehead browplasty at unequal levels on forehead and upper and lower eyelid blepharoplasty.

The major disadvantage of midforehead browplasty, similar to direct browplasty, is the resulting scar. The patient should be willing to accept the fact that the scar will take several months to mature. A scar in a natural forehead rhytid in a male patient, however, is often not noticeable.

MIDFOREHEAD RHYTIDECTOMY

The mid forehead rhytidectomy, also known as the midforehead-lift, was described by Johnson and Waldman.[9] This operation is basically an extension of midforehead browplasty wherein the incisions above the brows are connected in a natural transverse forehead rhytid. Through this small increase of the incision in the forehead, the entire brow-glabella-forehead complex can be surgically explored and managed. As with midforehead browplasty, the midforehead rhytidectomy is carried out most often in men with deep transverse forehead rhytids and occasionally in older women with pronounced forehead creases. The incision should follow the natural creases precisely, although the resulting incision is often asymmetric and slightly irregular. The final scar mimics this crease and should not resemble a surgical scar. The operation is more versatile than midforehead browplasty because the vertical dimension of the skin incision can be varied. The excision of skin should be of uniform width across its length if the glabella-brow complex is to be raised equally as a unit. It may vary in width if some areas of the complex are to be elevated more than others. If relatively greater elevation of the glabellar area is desired, the excision of skin should be wider medially than over the lateral brows. As with all operations for brow ptosis, 0.5 to 1 cm of overcorrection is recommended.

Technique

After the skin is prepared and draped, the first or second natural horizontal forehead rhytid that goes all the way across the brow is marked out (Fig. 34-9). Local anesthesia with epinephrine is infiltrated across the entire forehead. The supraorbital notches are palpated, and their locations are marked on the overlying skin. The incision is made through the skin and subcutaneous tissue. Elevation is carried out in the same plane as in the midforehead browplasty. The dissection is carried down over the orbital rims in the plane superficial to the musculature. Care is taken to prevent damage to the supraorbital nerves. If glabellar rhytidosis and ptosis is a significant problem, a transverse incision can be made through the frontalis muscle above the nasal root. This incision does not extend laterally beyond the previously marked supraorbital notches. A muscle flap is then developed inferiorly in the plane just superficial to the periosteum. The medial limbs of the corrugator muscles are identified and isolated; injury to the supraorbital and supratrochlear nerves and vessels is avoided. A section of the corrugator and procerus muscles may then be excised. The superior flap may be dissected superiorly in the subgaleal plane bilaterally, medial to the supraorbital notches. The central portion of the frontalis muscle and fascia may be incised horizontally. These incisions are not extended laterally beyond the pupils to preserve lateral frontalis function. A segment of frontalis muscle and fascia may be excised and the edges sutured, elevating the glabellar and medial brow tissues. The orbicularis muscles are then suspended superiorly with permanent sutures to the fascia of the frontalis muscle or periosteum as in the previous procedures to ensure permanent correction of the brow ptosis. Although not usually necessary, a small drain may be placed in the incision and brought out through a separate stab incision in the lateral hairline. The skin incision is closed as previously, with a dermal layer of interrupted sutures with buried knots and a running locking 6-0 monofilament skin suture. A light pressure dressing is applied. If a drain is used, it is removed the following day; the pressure dressing should be uniform to avoid compromise of the skin flaps. In operations directly on the forehead and brow, sutures are usually removed 5 to 7 days after surgery and supportive tapes are applied for several days more.

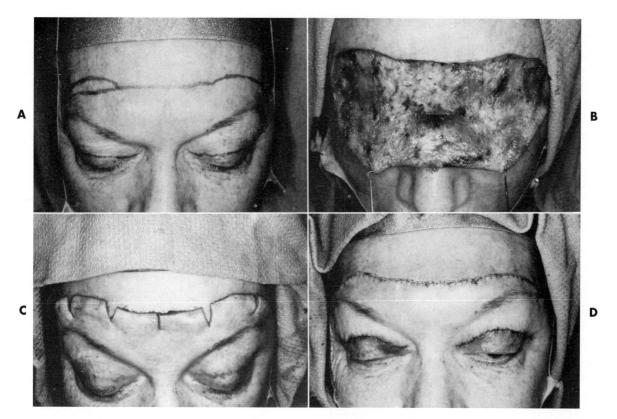

Fig. 34-9. A, Skin marking for midforehead rhytidectomy. Extra mark to patient's right was for a small proposed scar revision. **B,** Extent of skin undermining. **C,** Skin-splitting incisions made to estimate amount of skin to be excised. **D,** Skin closure complete. Note blepharoplasty is performed after the brow and forehead procedure.

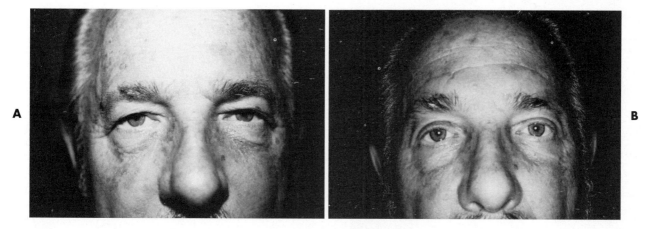

Fig. 34-10. A, A patient with significant forehead and brow ptosis and blepharochalasis. **B,** The status after midforehead lift and upper and lower blepharoplasty.

Discussion

The midforehead rhytidectomy may be indicated in the male patient with prominent forehead rhytids who has significant ptosis and rhytidosis of the glabellar complex in addition to ptosis of the brows (Fig. 34-10). Forehead rhytidectomy is most often indicated in female patients and is the preferred operation. Midforehead rhytidectomy, however, may be indicated occasionally in an older female patient with deep horizontal forehead rhytids and a high forehead or sparse, thin anterior scalp hair (Fig. 34-11).

Contraindications to the midforehead rhytidectomy include a history of abnormal scarring; smooth, nonwrinkled forehead skin; markedly sebaceous forehead skin (especially in males); and the patient's inability to accept a facial scar.

The advantages of the midforehead rhytidectomy are direct access to the glabellar region and the ability to correct brow ptosis.

The disadvantages of the midforehead rhytidectomy center on the resulting scar, which may require revision, dermabrasion, or camouflage with cosmetics. These outcomes and the fact that the scar will take several months to mature must be discussed with the patient before surgery.

FOREHEAD RHYTIDECTOMY

Over the past several years, treatment of eyebrow and forehead ptosis using forehead rhytidectomy (coronal lift) has become widely accepted as the gold standard. In the early part of this century several approaches to forehead-lifting involved excision of skin anterior and posterior to the hairline as well as resection of muscle. Brennan[3] published an excellent review of the literature on this subject. The

earlier operations, unfortunately, were limited, and the results were temporary and ineffective. Subsequently, galeal fasciotomy and frontalis myotomy were recognized as vital steps in the treatment of forehead rhytidosis. The expanded coronal approach to brow- and forehead-lifting with improvements and modifications has been described and popularized by Brennan,[3] Connell,[6] Kaye,[10] and Vinas, Caviglia, and Cortinas.[21] In addition to interruption of the galea-frontalis complex, it is important in the expanded coronal operation to carry the undermining and dissection down over the supraorbital rims and root of the nose and to the zygomatic arches. Dissection is carried deep to the galea and frontal layers, and therefore damage to the frontotemporal branch of the facial nerve is avoided. This plane of dissection is deeper than that used for the direct brow and midforehead operations previously described. A clear understanding of the anatomy of the temporal branch of the nerve is vital in this operation, and the reader is referred to the works of Liebman and others,[12] Pitanguy,[16] and Larrabee and Makielski.[11] The surgeon should be cautious to identify and protect the supraorbital neurovascular bundles as they emerge from

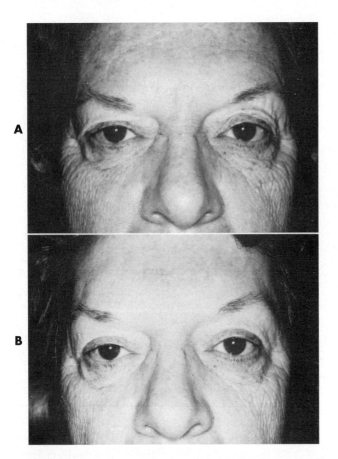

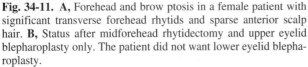

Fig. 34-11. A, Forehead and brow ptosis in a female patient with significant transverse forehead rhytids and sparse anterior scalp hair. B, Status after midforehead rhytidectomy and upper eyelid blepharoplasty only. The patient did not want lower eyelid blepharoplasty.

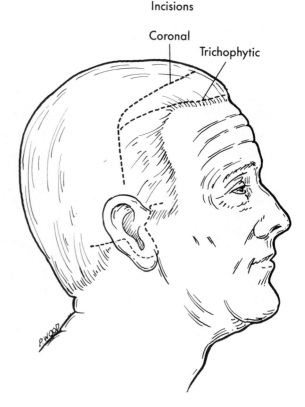

Fig. 34-12. Separation of the forehead rhytidectomy incision from the cervicofacial rhytidectomy incision. Coronal versus trichophytic incisions.

their foramina. When a facelift is performed with a forehead-lift, many surgeons recommend one continuous incision for the entire operation,[8,10] while these authors prefer to separate the two incisions and operative compartments completely (Fig. 34-12).[3,13] The frontal operation is performed in the deep subgaleal plane just superficial to the pericranium. The rhytidectomy is carried out in the more superficial subcutaneous plane of the temple and cheek to prevent damage to the underlying frontal branch of the facial nerve. This important nerve can be more easily protected by separating the two compartments. Also, if a complication were to develop (i.e., hematoma, infection), the problem would remain confined to the compartment in which it developed.

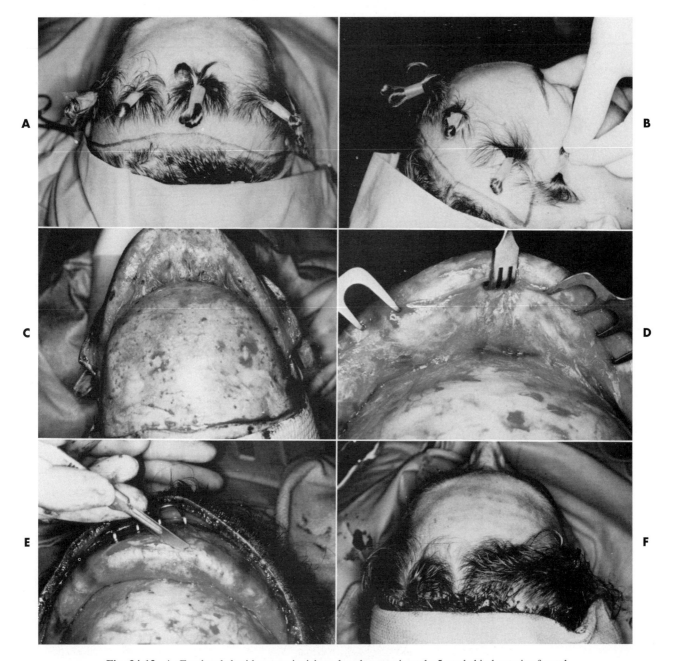

Fig. 34-13. A, Forehead rhytidectomy incision placed approximately 5 cm behind anterior frontal hairline and paralleling the same. One cm of hair anterior to incision trimmed. **B,** Lateral view. **C,** Coronal flap elevated in the subgaleal plane from above. **D,** Dissecting bluntly from lateral orbital rims medial and nasal area lateral to expose and preserve supraorbital pedicles. **E,** Galea and frontalis muscle incised. **F,** Closure of incision accomplished with several galeal sutures and stainless steel skin staples.

Technique

The patient is prepared by parting the hair 1 cm wide approximately 5 cm posterior to the hairline, beginning 2 cm above the ear on one side and extending across to the same location on the other side. The hair anterior to the part is braided (Fig. 34-13). Intravenous sedation or, if preferred, general anesthesia is provided. Local anesthesia with epinephrine is injected along the proposed incision, zygomatic arches, supraorbital rims, and root of the nose. Infiltration is also carried out in the subgaleal plane across the forehead. After allowing an adequate amount of time for vasoconstriction, the incision is made with a wide surgical blade, beveling the cut from anterior to posterior to parallel the hair follicles. The cut is carried through the galeal layer to the pericranium. The flap is dissected in a subgaleal plane just superficial to the pericranium medially and the temporalis fascia laterally. When the brows are approached, the dissection is carried down laterally over the orbital rims and medially to the root of the nose. Careful blunt dissection is used from the lateral orbital rims to the nasal root area until the supraorbital neurovascular bundles are identified and carefully preserved (see Fig. 34-13, *D*). After the flap has been completely raised, horizontal relaxing incisions are carried out in the galea and frontalis muscle between the midpupillary lines. These incisions are carried no further laterally to prevent any denervation of the forehead and to preserve forehead expression. The corrugator and procerus muscles are excised to eliminate glabellar frown lines. Hemostasis is secured throughout the procedure with bipolar electrocautery. The only major vessels encountered are the anterior

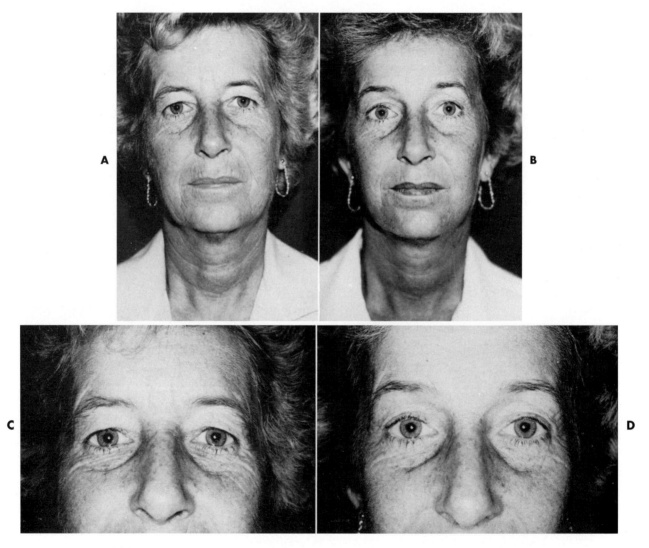

Fig. 34-14. A, Patient with eyebrow and forehead ptosis in addition to blepharochalasis and generalized facial rhytidosis. **B,** Postoperative status after forehead rhytidectomy, upper and lower blepharoplasty, cervicofacial rhytidectomy, and circumoral chemical peel,. **C,** Preoperative view. **D,** Postoperative view.

branches of the superficial temporal arteries, which are very carefully cauterized or ligated. The flap is returned to its original position and skin-splitting incisions are performed after the amount of excess skin to be excised is determined by upward pull on the flap. The flap is fixed superiorly with slow-absorbing suture, reapproximating the galeal layer at the sites of the skin-splitting incisions. Excess skin is then trimmed, beveling the cut from anterior to posterior. The rest of the galeal layer is reapproximated, and the scalp is closed with surgical skin staples. A drain may be placed before closure, but is usually not necessary. A light dressing is applied to the forehead and scalp. As noted, the brow ptosis is always overcorrected, and blepharoplasty is always performed secondary to the forehead-lift.

The primary indication for forehead rhytidectomy is significant brow ptosis (Fig. 34-14). Secondary indications include deep transverse forehead creases (forehead rhytidosis), lateral hooding (Fig. 34-15), glabellar frown lines, and crow's feet. This procedure is primarily performed on female patients, and is occasionally indicated in younger patients with significant brow ptosis who desire blepharoplasty (Fig. 34-16).

The primary contraindications to the classic forehead rhytidectomy are a high frontal hairline and thin, sparse anterior hair, which is why forehead rhytidectomies are performed less frequently on male than on female patients.

The main advantage of the forehead-lift is that the scar is camouflaged behind the hairline. The operation is very effective with long-lasting results and addresses all the problems associated with forehead aging (i.e., glabellar ptosis, rhytidosis).

The main disadvantage of the forehead-lift is that it is more extensive than the other operations mentioned and, therefore, carries a greater risk of complications. However, the attendant morbidity rate is low. The procedure requires more operating time, thereby increasing the expense over the other operations. Also, more experience and expertise is required on the part of the surgeon. The classic forehead-lift raises the frontal hairline, which may be a disadvantage in some patients.

For patients who have a high frontal hairline, the incision can be made 2 mm behind the hairline anteriorly (trichophytic approach) (Fig. 34-17). In this approach, the incision follows the hairline laterally to the temple where it is carried back into the hair-bearing scalp and downward above the ear as in the classic coronal incision (see Fig. 34-12). The incision behind the anterior hairline is beveled from posterior to anterior exactly opposite to that of the classic approach. This approach preserves hair follicles at the anterior aspect of the incision. As the skin is trimmed at the end of the operation, non–hair-bearing skin anteriorly is sutured to hair-bearing skin posteriorly. The remaining hair follicles under the anterior end of the incision will grow through the scar over the ensuing months and partially camouflage it (Fig. 34-18). After the incision is made, the procedure is carried out exactly as described for the classic forehead rhytidectomy. On closure, careful approximation of the dermis in the frontal area is performed with 4-0 polyglactin 910 sutures, and fine 6-0 Prolene suture is used to close the skin of the anterior hairline. The skin within the scalp laterally is closed as in the classic operation. This variation allows people with high hairlines to be eligible for the forehead-lift as long as they are willing to accept a partially visible scar at the anterior hairline. Often patients wear their hair down to cover this area, so this approach is acceptable to most patients. The trichophytic approach has more indications, and many more patients can enjoy the benefits of this procedure.

BOTULINUM TOXIN

Use of botulinum toxin type A (Botox, Allergan, Irvine, Calif) has recently come into vogue for the management of glabellar frown lines. This agent can be used solely, injected into the corrugator and procerus muscles, or in conjunction

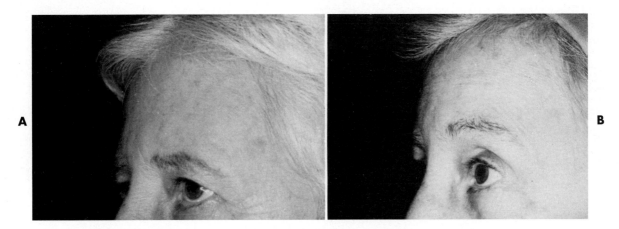

Fig. 34-15. A, Patient with significant brow and forehead ptosis with lateral hooding. **B,** Postoperative status after forehead rhytidectomy and blepharoplasty. Note marked improvement of lateral hooding.

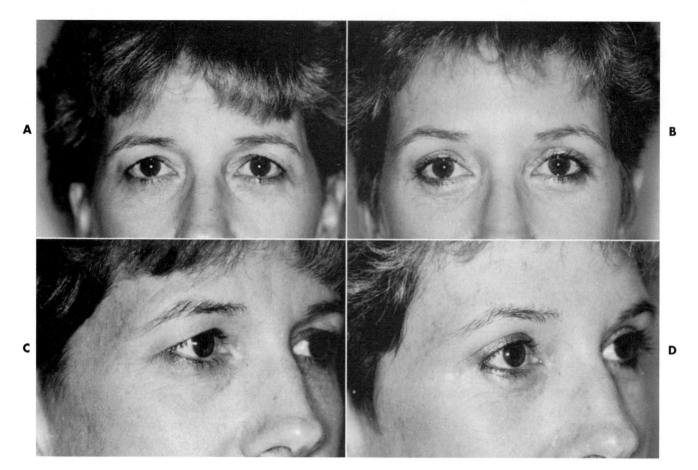

Fig. 34-16. A, Preoperative view of patient in her early 40s with significant brow ptosis in addition to blepharochalasis of the upper and lower eyelids. **B,** Postoperative view after forehead rhytidectomy and upper and lower eyelid blepharoplasty. **C,** Preoperative view. **D,** Postoperative view.

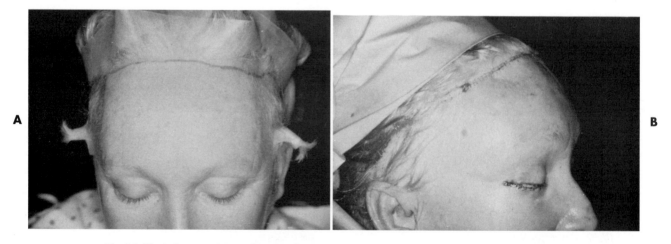

Fig. 34-17. A, Preoperative marking for trichophytic forehead rhytidectomy. **B,** Immediate postoperative view showing location of incision.

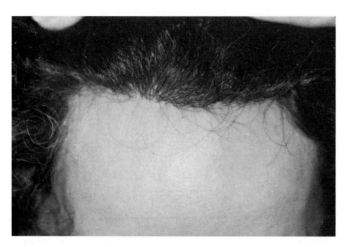

Fig. 34-18. Postoperative view after 6 months of trichophytic incision for forehead rhytidectomy showing hairs growing through incision line.

Table 34-1. Complications associated with brow-lifting operation

Complication	Procedure
Hematoma	Minor
	Direct browplasty
	Midforehead browplasty
	Midforehead rhytidectomy
	Major
	Forehead rhytidectomy
Infection	All
Numbness	Midforehead rhytidectomy
	Forehead rhytidectomy
Hair loss	Forehead rhytidectomy
Scarring	Direct browplasty
	Midforehead browplasty
	Midforehead rhytidectomy
Altered mimetic function	Midforehead rhytidectomy
	Forehead rhytidectomy

with direct and midforehead browplasty. Some surgeons inject the toxin into the frontalis muscle to treat forehead rhytidosis. The effects, which occur secondary to irreversible blockade at the neuromuscular motor end plate, last from 3 to 5 months at which time new nerve endings form synapses at distant sites in the muscle. The efficacy is currently being judged more by anecdotal reports than by prospective study; however, as experience is gained with its use, botulinum toxin type A (Botox, Allergan, Irvine, Calif) will undoubtedly become a valuable adjunct to facial aesthetic surgery.

COMPLICATIONS

As with any surgery, brow-lifting operations have a risk of complications (Table 34-1). Fortunately, infections are quite rare in the facial region secondary to an excellent blood supply. Patients should scrub the face, scalp, and neck for several days before surgery with an antibacterial soap to decrease the bacterial count of the skin, thereby minimizing the possibility of infection.

Hematomas can develop in any surgical procedure. Thorough intraoperative hemostasis with bipolar cautery is the best preventive measure. Careful preoperative evaluation will disclose patients with significant hypertension, bleeding disorders, and anticoagulant therapy, which can be managed before surgery. Hematoma is least likely to occur in direct browplasty, in which very little dissection is necessary. The risk increases progressively with midforehead browplasty, midforehead rhytidectomy, and forehead rhytidectomy (in that order). Particular care should be taken to control the cut edges of the superficial temporal artery in forehead rhytidectomy.

In direct browplasty, midforehead browplasty, and midforehead rhytidectomy, the dissection is carried out in the plane just superficial to the muscle. If this plane is respected, the supraorbital and supratrochlear nerves, and the temporal branch of the facial nerve will not be damaged. In forehead rhytidectomy, the dissection is carried out deep to the galeal layer. If this level of dissection is maintained and there is no significant stretch on the flap, these structures should not be injured. Numbness posterior to the coronal or pretrichial incision is caused by division of the distal ends of the supraorbital nerves. However, this complication does not seem to be of concern to most patients, and sensation usually returns by 3 to 6 months postoperatively. Rarely, a patient may develop transient hypesthesia or intermittent pain, probably secondary to a needle injury of the nerve.

Hair loss may be encountered with the forehead rhytidectomy procedures, particularly if widening of the scar takes place.[14] It is, therefore, imperative that undo tension not be placed on this closure by avoiding overresection of skin and reapproximating the galea. As mentioned, careful beveling of the skin incision in the direction of the hair follicles should be performed in the classic approach.

Alteration in facial mimetic function is an anticipated outcome of these procedures, owing to the modification of the frontalis or the corrugator and procerus muscles. If incision of the frontalis muscle is carried too far laterally, however, the forehead will be rendered expressionless and detract from the aesthetic result.

With the direct operations, the patient must be aware that scars may be visible in the forehead area. However, the scars in the midforehead area are usually camouflaged well in natural skin folds. Pigment changes of the skin are rare. If these surgical techniques and principles are carefully followed, the possibility of complications should be minimal.

SUMMARY

When evaluating a patient for the possibility of facial rejuvenation surgery (Fig. 34-19), attention to and careful evaluation of the aging changes of the upper third of the

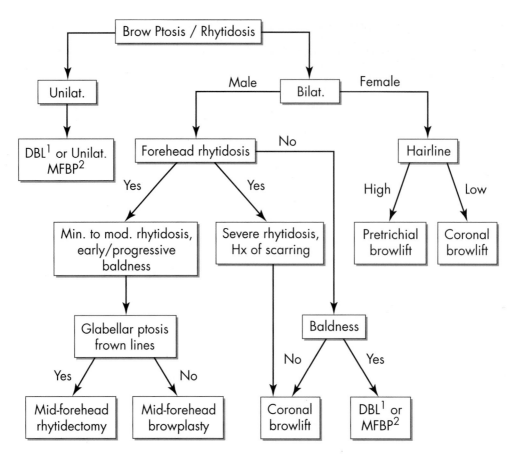

Fig. 34-19. Algorithm for the management of ageing changes of the forehead.

face are vital. If blepharoplasty and rhytidectomy only are carried out in a patient who has aging changes of the face, including significant ptosis of the brows and forehead, the results are likely to prove unsatisfactory. Ptosis of the forehead and brows results in a tired, sad look or even an angry look when medial brow ptosis and glabellar rhytidosis are significant. In such cases, a well-performed blepharoplasty and rhytidectomy can result in improvement. Of the four operations used to treat brow and forehead ptosis, forehead rhytidectomy and midforehead rhytidectomy can treat forehead and glabellar rhytidosis. Direct browplasty is rarely performed but is still useful for unilateral facial or forehead paralysis and in the female patient with isolated brow ptosis. In males with brow ptosis, the preferred operation is midforehead browplasty. If significant glabellar and medial brow ptosis and glabellar rhytidosis are present, the two incisions for the midforehead browplasty can be connected and a midforehead rhytidectomy performed. The latter operation is rarely performed on a female patient and only if forehead rhytidosis is significant. In the female with a high frontal hairline, the trichophytic approach to the forehead-lift is preferred.

Proper selection and application of direct browplasty, midforehead browplasty, midforehead rhytidectomy, and forehead rhytidectomy are invaluable to the surgical management of the aging face. This chapter offers some of the finer aspects necessary for a successful result.

REFERENCES

1. Anderson JR: *Surgical treatment of periorbital aging.* In Conley J, Dickinson JT, editors: Proceedings of first international symposium on plastic and reconstructive surgery of the face and neck, New York, 1972, Grune & Stratton.
2. Brennan HG: Correction of the ptotic brow, *Otolaryngol Clin North Am* 13:265, 1980a.
3. Brennan HG: The forehead lift, *Otolaryngol Clin North Am* 13:209, 1980.
4. Brennan HG: The frontal lift, *Arch Otolaryngol Head Neck Surg* 104:26, 1978.
5. Castaneres S: Forehead wrinkles, glabellar frown, and ptosis of the eyebrows, *Plast Reconstr Surg* 34:406, 1964.
6. Connell BF: Eyebrow, face and neck lifts for males, *Clin Plast Surg* 5:15, 1978.
7. Doxanas MT, McCord CD: Browplasty and browpexy: an adjunct to blepharoplasty, *Plast Reconstr Surg* 86:248, 1990.
8. Gonzalez-Ulloa M: Facial wrinkles, integral elimination, *Plast Reconstr Surg* 29:658, 1962.

9. Johnson CM, Waldman SR: Midforehead lift, *Arch Otolaryngol Head Neck Surg* 109:155, 1983.

10. Kaye BL: The forehead lift: a useful adjunct to facelift and blepharoplasty, *Plast Reconstr Surg* 60:161, 1977.

11. Larrabee WF Jr, Makielski KH: *Surgical anatomy of the face,* New York, 1992, Raven Press.

12. Liebman EP and others: The frontalis nerve in the temporal brow lift, *Arch Otolaryngol Head Neck Surg* 108:232, 1982.

13. Ortiz-Monasterio F, Barrera G, Olmedo A: The coronal incision in rhytidectomy: the brow lift, *Clin Plast Surg* 5:167, 1978.

14. Papel ID: *Complications of brow lift.* In Eisle DW, editor: *Complications in head and neck surgery,* St Louis, 1993, Mosby.

15. Passot R: *Chirugie esthetique pure: techniques et resultats,* Paris, 1930, Gaston Doin & Cie.

16. Pitanguy I: The frontal branch of the facial nerve: the importance of its variations in facelifting, *Plast Reconstr Surg* 38:352, 1966.

17. Pitanguy I: Indications for treatment of frontal and glabellar wrinkles in an analysis of 3404 consecutive cases of rhytidectomy, *Plast Reconstr Surg* 67:157, 1981.

18. Rafaty FM, Brennan HG: Current concepts of browpexy, *Arch Otolaryngol Head Neck Surg* 109:152, 1983.

19. Rafaty FM, Goode RL, Abramson NR: The brow-lift operation in a man, *Arch Otolaryngol Head Neck Surg* 104:69, 1978.

20. Rafaty FM, Goode RL, Fee WE: The brow-lift operation, *Arch Otolaryngol Head Neck Surg* 101:467, 1975.

21. Vinas JC, Caviglia C, Cortinas JL: Forehead rhytidectomy and brow lifting, *Plast Reconstr Surg* 57:445, 1976.

Chapter 35

Blepharoplasty

Jeffrey J. Colton
G. Jan Beekhuis

The eyes play a primary role in human communication. When introduced to a person, one usually notices the other person's eyes first, and during conversation, the participants' eyes are focused on each other for a major part of the time. The eyes are capable of expressing the full range of human emotion—from anger to happiness, from hatred to love. The contour and movement of the skin, muscles, soft tissue, brow, and lashes, rather than the globe, allow the eyes to convey these expressions.

Abnormalities of the eyelid can occur in any age group and for a variety of reasons. In adolescents and young adults, an overabundance or pseudoherniation of orbital fat may cause severe bagginess of the upper or lower lids. Many young women exhibit ''bags'' of the lower lids at an early age. This condition causes a sleepy, heavy, or full look to the eyes and generally is hereditary. These abnormalities appear as early as during the late teen years or early 20s and often progress to become obvious in patients in their early 30s (Fig. 35-1).

The aging process can affect all of the tissues surrounding the eye. Many consider these changes normal and acceptable, and in certain patients, the changes are considered attractive. In most people, these signs of aging are a focus of concern (Fig. 35-2). Changes that can occur in the upper and lower lids include (1) a progressive loss of elastic fibers and collagen in the eyelid skin, (2) skin changes caused by repeated sun exposure and gravitational forces, and (3) hypertrophy or age-related weakening of the orbicularis occuli muscle. With advancing age, characteristic changes occur, producing extra skin folds and wrinkles, a weakening of the orbital septum, and ptosis of the brow.

Blepharoplasty is a surgical procedure that is performed to modify these conditions. Although the procedures have been designed for the correction of aging effects, they are well suited to younger women for the correction of hereditary abnormalities. Eyelid surgery can dramatically improve the appearance of women in this younger age group.

HISTORY OF BLEPHAROPLASTY

Like many surgical techniques, blepharoplasty has roots in ancient times. The first mention of the technique was made by Aulus Cornelius Celsus, a first-century Roman. He described the excision of skin for ''relaxed upper eyelids'' in *De Re Medica* (25-35 AD). As early as the tenth century, surgeons in Arabia devised ways to excise excess skin folds in the upper lids that caused visual impairment.

Von Graefe first used the word *blepharoplasty* in 1817 to describe a technique for repairing deformities caused by resection of cancer in the eyelids. In the nineteenth century, Europeans such as Beer, Mackenzie, Albert, Graft, and Dupuytren advocated excision of excess upper eyelid skin. In 1844, Sichel provided the first accurate description of herniated orbital fat.

In the early 1900s, surgeons in the United States began to write about eyelid surgery. In 1907, Conrad Miller wrote *Cosmetic Surgery and the Correction of Featural Imperfections*, the first book on cosmetic surgery. His 1924 edition contains diagrams of incisions for upper and lower eyelid surgery that are similar to those used today. In the late 1920s, French surgeons began advocating the removal of herniated orbital fat for cosmetic reasons. Fat removal has been included as an integral part of blepharoplasty since the 1940s.

In the early 1950s, Castenares described in detail the fat

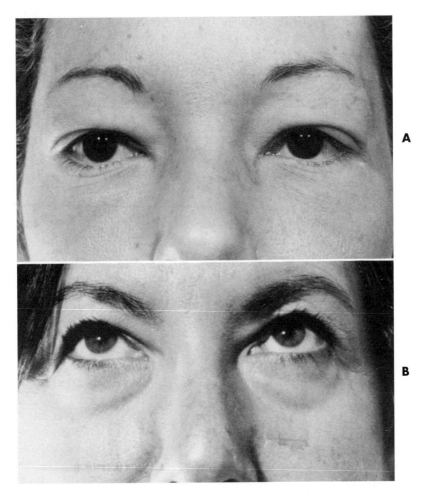

Fig. 35-1. A, The hereditary fullness of upper lids in a young woman caused by excessive skin, soft tissue, muscle, and herniation of fat. **B,** The bagginess of lower lids in a young woman caused by hereditary herniation of fat pads.

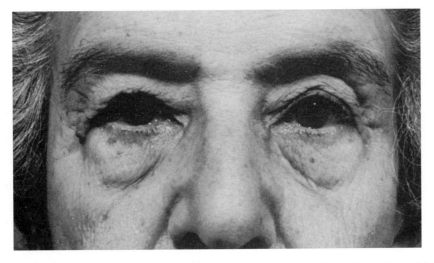

Fig. 35-2. The redundancy of skin, soft tissue, and muscle in upper lids and herniation of fat in both lids are characteristic of the aging process and its effects on tissues of eyelids. A patient, who is aged slightly more than 70 years, also has brow ptosis and probably atonic lower lids.

compartments of the upper and lower eyelids, although his work has been disputed in the past several years based on dye studies in cadavers.[1] In the 1970s, many refinements in technique were made, including methods of creating a supratarsal fold, a refinement in the crease line, and fixation and suspension techniques for lower lid blepharoplasty. The importance of careful evaluation of the hypertrophied orbicularis occuli muscle and its excision in blepharoplasty also has been recognized.[2]

ANATOMY OF THE ORBIT

The facial plastic surgeon should have a good working knowledge of the structures of the orbit.

Bony anatomy

The orbit is formed by seven bones of the skull: the frontal, zygomatic, maxillary, greater and lesser wings of the sphenoid, palatine, lacrimal, and ethmoid. In this bony compartment sits the globe and its contents: the first, third, fourth, fifth, and sixth cranial nerves (CN) and their associated vessels; the periorbital fat; the muscles that control movement of the globe and lids; and the lacrimal apparatus and drainage system.

Surface anatomy

The *lid crease* is the line created by the insertion of levator aponeurosis and the orbital septum into the orbicularis occuli muscle and subcutaneous tissue. This crease lies at the level of the upper edge of the tarsal plate, usually 9 to 11 mm from the lash line (Fig. 35-3). This line and its location are aesthetically important. When the lid crease is significantly closer to the lash line, the eye takes on a heavy, full, or sleepy appearance. In women, a smooth exposed area from the lash line to the lid crease allows for the easy use of eye makeup. This crease is part of the focus of the blepharoplasty procedure. In Asians, this crease should be created if a more occidental appearance of the eye is desired.

The *lid fold* is that tissue above the lid crease that may protrude and prolapse over the lid crease, obscuring it (Fig. 35-4) and even covering the lashes. The lid fold may extend the entire horizontal length of the upper lid, or it may be apparent only laterally or centrally. The fold may be composed of excess skin, hypertrophied orbicularis occuli muscle, redundant soft tissue, prolapsed lacrimal gland, herniated orbital fat, or any combination of these. Understanding the anatomy of a baggy eyelid preoperatively is important so that the surgeon can design procedures to correct the abnormality. For example, removing only skin from an upper eyelid that has hypertrophied orbicularis occuli muscle and redundant soft tissue will not result in the most effective correction. The successful blepharoplasty is designed to keep the lid fold from prolapsing to obscure the lid crease. The focus of the procedure should be on that area where reshaping and resculpturing of the tissues will give the best surgical result.

The *skin* of the upper lid is extremely thin, loose, and mobile over the deeper structures, characteristics which are essential for normal lid function and appearance. Because eyelid skin is well nourished, healing occurs quickly, and scar formation is favorable. The skin becomes thicker, coarser, and more sebaceous lateral to the bony orbital margins. Blacks (even those who form keloids elsewhere) do not form keloids on the upper lids if the incisions are not carried into this thicker skin laterally.

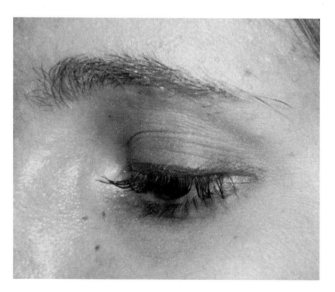

Fig. 35-3. A lid crease.

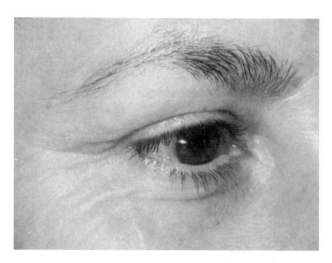

Fig. 35-4. A lid fold may protrude and prolapse over the lid crease, obscuring it. The fold may be composed of skin, soft tissue, hypertrophied orbicular muscle, and herniated fat.

Orbicularis occuli muscle

Beneath the skin and the thin subcutaneous tissue lie the fibers of the orbicularis occuli muscle, forming three distinct bands that end in the medial and lateral canthal tendons (Fig. 35-5).

The *pretarsal muscle* lies directly over the tarsus. The muscle, which lies over the orbital septum, is often modified in blepharoplasty. The *orbicularis occuli muscle* is beyond the bony margins of the orbit, blending superiorly with the frontal and corrugator muscles.

The heads of the pretarsal muscle form the medial canthal tendon, attaching to the anterior lacrimal crest and the lateral canthus, which inserts at the orbital tubercle just behind the orbital rim to form the lateral palpebral raphe. The orbicularis occuli muscle, which closes the lid, is strong. It may become hypertrophied and redundant, causing an excessive fullness of the upper or lower lid. The muscle receives innervation from the seventh cranial nerve (CN VII).

Partial resection of the orbicularis occuli muscle may be accomplished during blepharoplasty, although care should be taken not to injure underlying structures. Conservative resection maintains good apposition of the lids at rest and correct movement of the tear film.

Just deep to the orbicularis occuli muscle lies the *orbital septum* (Fig. 35-6). This is a thin sheet of fibrous tissue that originates along the superior orbital rim and hangs like a curtain across the lid. It joins the levator aponeurosis by interdigitating fibers at the level of the upper edge of the tarsal plate. The septum can be identified by placing slight traction on the lid margin and noting the tension transmitted to the brow. This septum keeps the orbital fat in its posterior position. Weakening of the septum from aging, hereditary predisposition, or trauma may cause protusion of the orbital fat.

Orbital fat

The orbital fat lies deep to the orbital septum (see Figs. 35-6 and 35-7), providing a cushion and flotation for the structures of the orbit. It is lobulated and loosely supported,

containing many small blood vessels and nerves. The fat separates the orbital septum from the levator aponeurosis and muscle. The upper lid has two fat compartments: central and nasal. The central compartment is the larger, and its fat is yellower than the light-colored more dense fat of the nasal compartment. The lower lid is believed to have three fat compartments: a small medial, a small temporal, and a fairly large central compartment. The fat in the medial compartment is lighter in color and more dense than the fat in the other compartments. This orbital fat does not seem to be related to other body fat because the quantity remains relatively constant regardless of obesity or weight loss. The fat is a static structure, and once removed, it does not regenerate. Castanares described these compartments in the early 1950s, although some of his findings have been disputed in recent years. The surgeon will find it helpful to think of fat distribution in a compartmentalized fashion while planning the operation. The orbital septum lies anterior to the fat pocket, and the levator aponeurosis lies posterior to it.

Levator muscle

The primary elevator of the eyelid is the levator muscle (see Fig. 35-6). Problems with the proper function of this muscle produce ptosis. The muscle originates from the orbital periosteum and passes forward above the superior rectus muscle, gradually forming a tendon that fans out to form the levator aponeurosis. This extends the full width of the lid at the level of the upper tarsus wherein the tendon fuses with the orbital septum to insert in the anterior third of the tarsus. Fibers from the aponeurosis blend with those of the orbital septum at the level of the tarsus and insert into the orbicularis occuli muscle, subcutaneous tissue, and skin to produce the lid crease. CN III supplies the levator muscle.

Müller's muscle

Müller's muscle originates from the belly of the levator aponeurosis and inserts at the retrotarsal margin (see Fig. 35-6). It receives innervation from the sympathetic system. Because of its extremely friable nature and its adherence to the levator muscle, few surgeons are able to isolate it as a distinct entity.

Lacrimal gland

The lacrimal gland is divided into two lobes that lie in the lacrimal fossa of the upper temporal portion of the bony orbit (see Fig. 35-7). The secreting ducts empty into the lateral aspect of the superior conjunctival fornix, moving across the cornea to empty into the lacrimal drainage system.

Tarsal plate

The tarsus often is called the skeleton of the eyelid (see Fig. 35-6). It is a fibrous plate that is approximately 10 mm wide in the central upper lid, narrowing medially and laterally. The tarsus of the lower lid is a bit narrower, from 4 to 5 mm at its center. The tarsal plates extend from the lateral

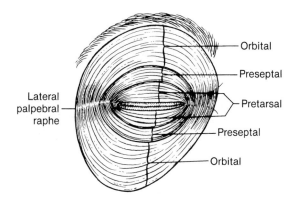

Fig. 35-5. The divisions of the orbicular eye muscle.

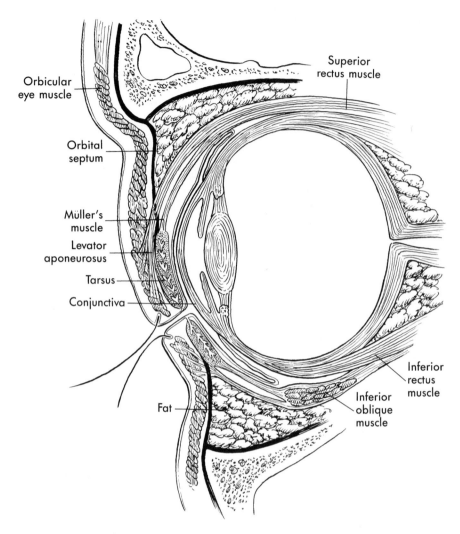

Orbicular eye muscle

Orbital septum

Müller's muscle

Levator aponeurosus

Tarsus

Conjunctiva

Fat

Superior rectus muscle

Inferior rectus muscle

Inferior oblique muscle

Fig. 35-6. The cross-section of the orbit and eyelids.

commissure to the punctum, containing numerous meibomian glands that empty into the ciliary border. The tarsus and conjunctiva form the inner lining of the lids.

Conjunctiva

The conjunctiva, which is a mucous membrane containing mucus-secreting goblet cells, is firmly attached to the posterior aspect of the tarsus. It covers the tarsus and Müeller's muscle, reflecting on itself in the upper fornix. It then extends down onto the globe as far as the limbus. As the levator muscle contracts, the tarsus is pulled upward and backward, and the retrotarsal margin closely follows the globe.

On the lower lid is a fine *gray line* (similar to the vermilion-cutaneous border of the lip) that separates the anterior from the posterior part of the lid (Fig. 35-8). Anteriorly, the surface is covered by stratified squamous epithelium containing the eyelashes and the sweat and sebaceous glands. Posterior to the gray line, the surface epithelium is low strati-

fied columnar epithelium containing meibomian glands. The gray line is an important surgical landmark in lid reconstruction and shortening. Sensory innervation of the lids comes from branches of the first (upper lid) and second (lower lid) divisions of the trigeminal nerve.

TERMINOLOGY

A certain amount of confusion has existed regarding the term *blepharochalasis*, having been used to describe virtually any degree of excess skin or fat of the eyelids. This term should be reserved for a rare disorder that may occur in young women, associated with swelling and edema of the lids with progressive tissue breakdown. This causes prolapse of the orbital fat (and perhaps the lacrimal gland), resulting in drooping of the lid. *Dermachalasis* means relaxation of skin (baggy skin). It is associated with the aging process and variable amounts of fat herniation and prolapse. *Blepharoptosis* (drooping eyelid) is caused by a malfunction of the levator muscles.

remembering that only herniated fat is corrected. The technique will not address hypertrophied muscle or excess skin. In approaching the procedure the surgeon may choose to sit at the patient's head rather than at the side. The conjunctiva can be anesthetized topically with tetracaine, 0.25%. The

lower lid is retracted and infiltrated with xylocaine, 1%, with epinephrine, and is then retracted caudally with a suture or small retractor (Fig. 35-40). The globe may be protected with a corneal shield or retractor. The surgeon then palpates the infraorbital rim, and the incision is made a couple of millimeters above that line. The electrosurgical knife can be used to make this incision. The orbital fat compartment is immediately encountered. Gentle pressure on the globe causes herniation of the fat through the incision line (Fig. 35-41). The fat compartments then are injected with lidocaine without epinephrine as in the standard lower-lid approach. The fat is dissected from each lower-lid compartment as

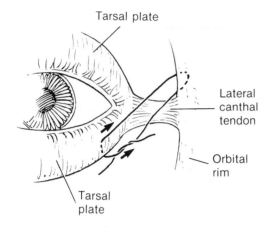

Fig. 35-38. Permanent suture may be passed from tarsal plate just inferior to the lateral canthus to periosteum inside and just deep to the orbital rim to create extra support for lower lid.

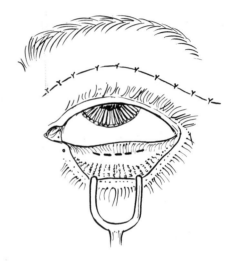

Fig. 35-40. The lower eyelid is retracted inferiorly to expose the conjunctiva. The incision is made 1 or 2 mm above the bony orbital rim.

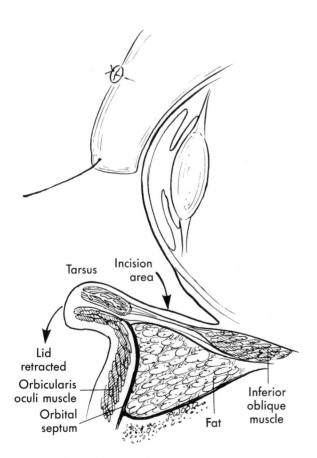

Fig. 35-39. An incision may be made through the lower eyelid conjunctiva to expose lower eyelid fat.

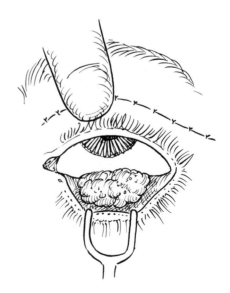

Fig. 35-41. After the incision is made, gentle pressure on the globe helps expose the herniated orbital fat.

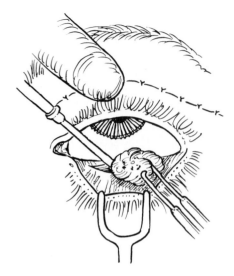

Fig. 35-42. After the fat has been clearly identified, it is dissected and removed.

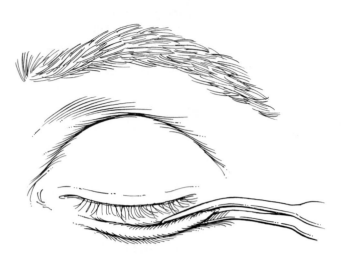

Fig. 35-43. The lower eyelid skin is grasped with a forceps and compressed with a hemostat. This is done until the skin surface is smooth without pulling the lid away from the globe. Skin lateral to the lateral canthus may be included.

determined by preoperative assessment (Fig. 35-42). The authors prefer direct dissection of the fat with the electrosurgical knife as described previously. After the fat has been resected, the procedure is concluded. The lower lid should be stretched cephalically to release any small adhesions. The incision may be closed with one or two sutures made of fast-absorbing gut although many surgeons prefer to leave the incision open. Either way, the incision heals quickly without difficulty. Some ophthalmic ointment may be placed in the cul-de-sac of the lower lid to assist healing. It has been the authors' experience that this is an efficient way to deal with selected patients.

Pinch technique

The transconjunctival blepharoplasty will not address the problems of excess skin or fine wrinkling of the lower lid. The authors have found that if their assessment indicates redundant skin and fine wrinkling, the pinch technique may be useful.

The pinch technique was described by Parkes, Fein, and Brennen in the early 1970s, involving picking up excess skin immediately below the lower eyelid lashes and compressing it with a small hemostat (Fig. 35-43). The resulting ridge of skin can be removed with a scissor, and the incision closed with 6-0 fast-absorbing gut suture. The pinch technique can be carried medially and laterally beyond the canthi to remove redundant skin. Two to four mm of skin may be safely removed in this way. Because the orbicularis muscle has not been disturbed, the chance of lower-lid ectropion or rounding is greatly decreased. Also, if an insufficient amount of skin was removed at the initial procedure, the same technique may be applied 3 or 4 months later to successfully remove additional skin. The authors have found this technique to be quick, efficient, and safe.

Skin resurfacing of the lower lid

If your clinical evaluation indicates excessive darkness of the lower lids or fine wrinkling, consideration should be given to resurfacing the eyelid skin. This can be done at the same time as the lower eyelid blepharoplasty. The authors have found that the use of trichloroacetic acid, 35%, placed on the lower eyelid and out into the crow's feet area at the time of lower eyelid surgery (which may include transconjunctival removal of fat and pinch excision of eyelid skin) is an effective way to help smooth the eyelid skin and lighten the dark discoloration. Patients experience about 5 to 10 minutes of burning after application but no discomfort thereafter. Postoperatively, the patient keeps the lower eyelid skin well lubricated with a vaseline-like product, and the peeling of the skin usually is complete by 1 week. A weak hydrocortisone cream (such as Locoid) may be used to help resolve the redness after completion of the peeling process. Patients may use makeup at this point. The authors have found that the redness usually persists for 2 to 4 weeks after the peel.

An alternative to chemical peeling is the use of the carbon dioxide laser for eyelid skin resurfacing, with the laser at reduced power (as compared with the rest of the face). Generally, one or two passes are adequate for acceptable resurfacing. The postoperative management is similar to that for a peel. The redness persists a bit longer than after a peel but not much longer. This technique may be used at the time of lower eyelid blepharoplasty.

The authors have found that their standard technique has evolved over the past decade and now involves: (1) transconjunctival removal of fat, (2) tightening the skin using the pinch technique when necessary, and (3) simultaneous resurfacing of the lower lid with trichloroacetic acid or carbon

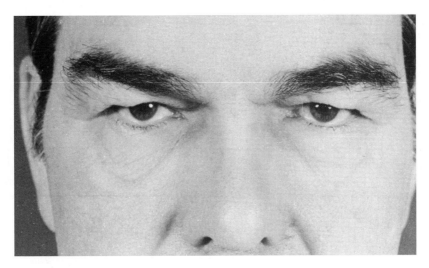

Fig. 35-44. A middle-aged man with ptosis of brow and baggy eyelids.

dioxide laser. The authors have found that the combination of these three techniques gives a nice improvement with small risk of lower-lid rounding or ectropion.

Brow ptosis

Careful consideration should be given to the position of the brow when planning blepharoplasty. In older patients, a combination of brow ptosis and excess upper eyelid skin often exists, causing the aesthetic problem the patient wants to have corrected. This condition should be accurately diagnosed preoperatively and discussed with the patient. If the brow is ptotic, surgery of the upper lid alone will not give a maximally satisfactory result (Fig. 35-44).

Correction of the ptotic brow may be accomplished using a direct approach. An incision is made along the cephalic edge of the eyebrow, and the deep surface of the brow is sutured to pericranium in the proper position above the supraorbital rim. An appropriate amount of skin is excised above the brow, and the incision is closed. If the patient has a prominent horizontal forehead crease, it may be used rather than the incision above the eyebrow itself. Both these techniques are easy to perform and control. They cause little postoperative discomfort or disability. The disadvantage of both is that the scar is visible. For women, it is more acceptable because it can be covered with eyebrow pencil or makeup. This presents a more difficult challenge in men. However, with careful attention, the scars may be completely acceptable.

Elevation of the brow also may be accomplished with a forehead lift. A coronal incision is used to lift the entire forehead, improving deep horizontal forehead creases and glabellar lines as well. The scar is placed in hairbearing tissue, which covers it nicely. The browlift techniques should be considered at the time of blepharoplasty because elevating the brows reduces the amount of skin to be removed from the upper lids.

POSTOPERATIVE CARE

Immediately after the surgical procedure, the patient is taken to the recovery room to be monitored for the next few hours. Cool, moist compresses are applied to the eyes. These are soothing and may decrease the postoperative edema and ecchymosis. Large compression dressings should be avoided because they tend to obscure any postoperative bleeding and are generally uncomfortable for the patient. Recovery room personnel should be carefully trained to observe closely for any signs of rapid swelling that may indicate postoperative bleeding. If any unusual swelling takes place, the physician should be notified immediately. If hematoma is confirmed, the patient should be returned to the operating room for evacuation of and control of bleeding. The onset of proptosis, pain, or visual disturbance requires immediate examination and appropriate action to resolve the problem.

Patients leave the ambulatory surgery center in a few hours and return home. They are able to eat normally and care for themselves in the usual way. They often are sleepy for the first 24 hours after surgery, and many prefer to continue the cool, moist compresses. The authors recommend that the patient sleep with the head slightly elevated for the first 48 hours. Patients are given prescriptions for an analgesic and sleeping preparation, although few use more than one or two pain pills or sleeping pills, and the majority use none at all. Patients apply an ophthalmic ointment to the incisions, which reduces crust formation and ensures easy, painless suture removal.

The patient is seen in the office 3 or 4 days after surgery, at which time the sutures are removed. After 1 week, the patient may wash the eyes normally, apply makeup, and follow normal personal routines.

COMPLICATIONS

Careful preoperative evaluation and adherence to safe, sound surgical technique help to maximize the favorable results and minimize complications. A variety of temporary sequelae may occur postoperatively that will resolve over time. Although serious complications are uncommon, it is imperative that the surgeon be familiar with the management of all potential problems.

Immediate postoperative period

Hematomas and *swelling of the orbit* may occur immediately after surgery despite meticulous hemostasis during the procedure. Often the onset of bleeding is related to coughing spasms, retching, or vomiting. In patients with hematoma or swelling in the orbit, the risk of visual loss caused by compression of the vascular supply of the optic nerve and globe increases dramatically. Hematoma without any signs of change or diminution in vision is best treated by returning the patient to the operating room, opening the incision, evacuating the clots, and controlling the bleeding.

If any loss of vision occurs, aggressive management should be instituted, including the previously mentioned procedures and intravenous administration of mannitol and steroids to decrease ocular pressure. If this does not relieve the pressure, a lateral canthotomy with lysis of the canthal tendon should be performed. If this is insufficient to relieve the pressure, bony decompression of the orbit should be performed. Such treatment is rarely needed, but the surgeon should be prepared to do whatever is necessary to protect the patient's vision. Emergency consultation with an ophthalmologist is appropriate.

Blindness after blepharoplasty is an exceedingly rare occurrence, although it is certainly one of the most feared complications. Fifty-eight cases have been reported with an incidence of approximately 0.04% or 1 in 2500 operations. Exhaustive investigations have failed to reveal an explanation for vision loss after blepharoplasty, although this complication has never been reported in the absence of periorbital fat removal.

Blepharoplasty rarely causes much pain, so severe pain postoperatively is a cause for concern because it may indicate a developing orbital hematoma, a corneal abrasion, or an attack of angle-closure glaucoma. If severe pain develops, these diagnoses should be eliminated.

First 2 weeks after surgery

A variety of minor problems may occur in the first 2 weeks after blepharoplasty. These are nearly always temporary and usually resolve without serious sequelae. Most patients experience *eyelid swelling* and *ecchymosis* that resolve over the first week or so. Occasionally patients experience ecchymosis in the lower lids that lasts for a longer time.

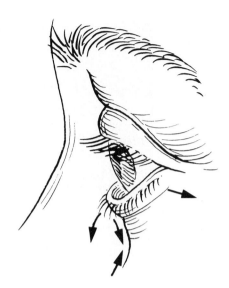

Fig. 35-45. Excessive skin removal from lower lid causes lid margin to pull away from globe and downward, resulting in ectropion.

Subconjunctival hemorrhage usually clears quickly. *Tearing* and a *burning* sensation may be noticed in the first or second week after blepharoplasty. The use of artificial tears before retiring and taping the eyes closed at bedtime may be advisable if the symptoms are severe. Most patients report some difficulty with the use of contact lenses immediately after surgery. Some women report *decreased sensitivity* of the upper lids when applying makeup. Full sensation nearly always returns. Patients may report discomfort in the lower lid areas if suspension sutures have been used.

A small amount of lagophthalmos or ptosis soon after surgery is not unusual. This generally resolves as the swelling of the upper lids decreases. If this persists, the patient may complain of a foreign body sensation. Lubricants during the day and at night should be part of the treatment of these patients, and the eyes should be taped closed at night. Severe lagophthalmos may require a removal of scar tissue and skin grafting of the upper lid, but mild cases essentially always clear with time.

Over the next several weeks, the patients may notice that the incision lines will be somewhat red and have occasional lumps and bumps, which may be slightly tender. These irregularities usually correspond to the sites of electrocoagulation and almost always subside totally. If there is prolongation of these indurated areas or widening or thickening of the scars, a solution of triamcinolone (10 mg/cc) may be injected to facilitate resolution.

Late complications

Most of the later complications are related to problems of lid position, scar formation, or unresolved aesthetic problems.

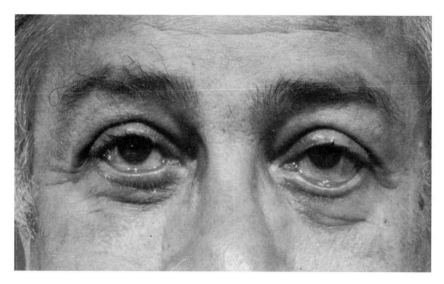

Fig. 35-46. A middle-aged man with bilateral ectropion after lower eyelid surgery.

Minimal *scleral show* may be noticeable after skin or lower lid blepharoplasty. Often this will improve with time, and massage may speed its resolution. Moderate scleral show may be the patient's major focus of concern. If the lower lid margin is in contact with the globe, one may elect a conservative course of massage and reassurance. If after several weeks the situation has not improved significantly or the patient is still dissatisfied, an additional procedure such as muscle suspension or lid shortening may be required.

Ectropion occurs when the lid margin is rotated inferiorly with separation from the globe. This condition is a serious complication (Figs. 35-45 and 35-46). It almost always will require further surgical intervention, such as horizontal lid shortening, muscle suspension, or skin grafting.

Occasionally *scars* may present a problem. Keloids in eyelid surgery are unusual, even in patients who form keloids elsewhere. Problems are minimized if the incisions are not carried laterally to the lateral orbital rim. Occasionally scars will web, especially those in the medial portion of the upper lid. This may require a Z-plasty at a later date. Suture tunnels and milia may be simply treated by evacuation of the contents with a needle or No. 11 blade.

Persistence of some aesthetic problem occasionally concerns the patient. Persistent *fat hernias* indicate either insufficient removal or inattention to specific compartments during the operation. These hernias may be removed at a second operation if they persist after several months. *Redundant skin* may exist in the upper lid, or an insufficient amount of soft tissue and muscle may have been removed. A prominent *orbicular ridge* beneath the lower lid also may be present. Most of these conditions result from errors in surgical judgment and may be corrected with secondary procedures later.

REVISION BLEPHAROPLASTY

It should not be necessary to repeat a well-done blepharoplasty. The patient who returns 7 to 10 years after initial surgery complaining of excess skin in the upper lids usually has ptosis of the brow. As the brow drops, the skin of the upper lid becomes redundant. This issue should be addressed if any further surgery is considered.

Revision surgery should be approached cautiously. The initial operating surgeon usually removed sufficient amounts of skin, and only very rarely should additional skin be removed from either the upper or lower lids. If persistent fat herniation or hypertrophied muscle is present, the operation should be designed to improve those specific problems. Overzealous removal of skin at secondary operation may lead to lagophthalmos and ectropion, which are serious problems.

SUMMARY

Blepharoplasty is a technique that may benefit all age groups. The procedure may be used to repair the effects of aging or to modify inherited abnormalities. An accurate and thorough diagnosis combined with meticulous surgical technique results in a well-done procedure and a pleased, satisfied patient.

REFERENCES

1. Barker DE: Dye injection studies of orbital fat compartments, *Plast Reconstr Surg* 59:82, 1977.
2. Castenares S: Classification of baggy eyelids deformity, *Plast Reconstr Surg* 59:629, 1977.
3. Rees TD: *Aesthetic plastic surgery,* Philadelphia, 1980, WB Saunders.
4. Tobin H: Electrosurgical blepharoplasty: a technique that questions conventional concepts of fat compartmentalization, *Ann Plast Surg* 14:59, 1985.
5. Reference deleted in pages.

SUGGESTED READINGS

Beekhuis GJ: Anesthesia for facial cosmetic surgery: low dosage ketamine-diazepam anesthesia, *Laryngoscope* 88:1709, 1978.

Beekhuis GJ: Blepharoplasty, *Otolaryngol Clin North Am* 3:225, 1980.

Dedo DD: *The atlas of aesthetic facial surgery,* New York, 1984, Grune & Stratton.

Iliff CE and others: *Oculoplastic surgery,* Philadelphia, 1979, WB Saunders.

Kaye BL, Grandinger G, editors: Symposium on problems and complications in aesthetic plastic surgery of the face, St Louis, 1984, Mosby.

Pastorek N: *Blepharoplasty,* Washington DC, 1983, American Academy of Otolaryngology Head and Neck Surgery Foundation.

Putterman A: *Cosmetic oculoplastic surgery,* New York, 1982, Grune & Stratton.

Spira M: Lower blepharoplasty: a clinical study, *Plast Reconstr Surg* 59:35, 1977.

Chapter 36

Endoscopic Rhytidectomy

H. Devon Graham, III

As aesthetic facial rejuvenation has become increasingly popular, surgeons and patients alike have searched for techniques that provide longer lasting natural-appearing results as well as decreased morbidity and recovery time. Endoscopic techniques have for some time used in general surgery, gynecology, orthopedics, otolaryngology, and thoracic surgery. Only in the past 2 to 3 years, however, have these techniques been widely accepted in the plastic and facial plastic surgery communities. Due to the efforts of several early pioneers in these fields, endoscopic procedures have become well refined and are now relatively standard techniques available in the armamentarium of most aesthetic surgeons. Although these techniques will never replace the more traditional open procedures, they have a definite role in facial plastic surgery because of decreased morbidity and excellent patient satisfaction.

The endoscope has been used in many areas of the body yet it has enjoyed it's widest application in facial aesthetic surgery. Endoscopic sinus procedures are well established, and early application of the techniques for the management of facial fractures has been promising.[8] In the head and neck area, the endoscopic forehead and brow-lift was the first clinical application of aesthetic endoscopy and is by far the most common endoscopic procedure performed today. Other aesthetic applications in the head and neck region include face-lift, malar fat pad–lift, and neck-lift.

THE FACE

Two very different approaches have been advocated for facial rejuvenation of the lower face and neck using minimal incisions and endoscopic assistance. In addition, endoscopic suspension of the malar fat pad to manage isolated mid-face ptosis used alone or in combination with a standard face-lift has also recently been described.[5] This technique has also been used by the author in selected cases and has been found to be quite useful given the proper indications. Most surgeons agree that the indication for minimal incision endoscopic lower face- and neck-lift is a relatively young patient with mild laxity of soft tissues around the chin and jaw line. These patients typically desire facial rejuvenation yet do not wish to undergo a standard incision face-lift procedure. The subperiosteal approach advocated by Ramirez[12] involves no skin resection and requires a subperiosteal dissection of the chin and mandible through a submental incision along with a cervicoplasty using lipectomy and platysma modification. This lower face and neck approach is typically combined with a forehead and/or temporal zygomatic dissection via small temporal, skin-muscle blepharoplasty and Caldwell-Luc incisions. Suspension sutures of 2-0 polyglactin 910 are placed in the periosteum and suborbicularis oculi fat (SOOF) pad as well as the periosteum just above the origin of the zygomaticus major muscles bilaterally. These stitches are then tunneled temporally and sutured to the deep temporal fascia. It is purported that the upward traction of these suspension sutures in the midface and temporal region will be transmitted to the lower face after the extensive subperiosteal dissection. The only visible redundant skin reportedly occurs in the preauricular area, which apparently redrapes and shrinks over 6 to 8 weeks.

In the subcutaneous approach advocated by Aiache,[1] dissection is performed through temporal incisions in the plane between the temporoparietal fascia and the deep temporal fascia over the zygomatic arch, along the orbital rim and malar bone, and inferiorly along the masseteric fascia for approximately 2 to 3 cm. Suspension sutures are then placed transcutaneously and are visualized with the endoscope from above through the temporal incisions. Those sutures are then secured to the deep temporal fascia. This technique differs markedly from that of Ramirez by shifting to a subcutaneous plane to elevate the remainder of the lower and midface in a manner similar to subcutaneous face-lifts. Temporal incisions are used with two mastoid region incisions located 2 and 5 cm below the ear, respectively. While the superficial musculoaponeurotic system (SMAS) is plicated posteriorly and superiorly, redundant skin may become apparent, and this is suture plicated in the form of a pleat in the hairline or in the postauricular area. This pleat is reported to smooth out and settle over a matter of weeks.

In the endoscopic malar fat pad–lift technique proposed by Freeman,[5] the ptotic malar pad is elevated and suture suspended either to orbital periosteum or deep temporal fascia if performed along with a temporal lift. This technique is a variation of that originally described by Owsley.[11] As an isolated procedure, it involves making an incision in a lateral crow's-foot crease extending medially in a subciliary position for a variable length depending on the length of the crease and the need for concomitant blepharoplasty. The incision is carried through skin and orbicularis muscle with dissection proceeding inferiorly to the insertion of the zygomaticus major muscle on the malar bone. This insertion should be previously identified and marked by having the patient smile widely while palpating the inferior border of the malar bone. This insertion will typically be found just lateral to the lateral canthus on the inferior aspect of the malar eminence. Dissection is carried deep to the orbicularis oculi towards the zygomaticus major muscle using blunt dissection. At this point, the endoscope is inserted and used to identify the head of the zygomaticus muscle. Dissection is carried superficial to the zygomaticus muscle fascia medially and superficially towards the melolabial fold. The fibro-fatty tissue of the malar pad is identified medial to the dissection pocket and is then grasped and suture suspended to the periosteum of the lateral orbital rim using 4-0 polydioxanone suture or nylon. The disadvantages of this procedure include the need for an external incision in a lateral crow's-foot crease and a minor-to-moderate amount of swelling lateral to the orbit, which can persist for 4 to 6 weeks. In addition, some redundancy of the lower lid skin may occur, which can be managed with blepharoplasty at the time of the procedure or with carbon dioxide laser skin resurfacing 6 to 8 weeks after the procedure. This procedure is applicable in patients with isolated midface elongation and malar pad ptosis either primarily or after a standard SMAS face-lift. This technique of repositioning the malar pad to a more youthful position over the malar eminence is also useful in patients who could benefit from malar or submalar implants yet are hesitant to have any synthetic material implanted.

When this technique is compared with midface suspension in the subperiosteal plan, the malar fat pad suspension procedure provides a more anatomic approach with superior results. In the subperiosteal technique the plane of dissection is beneath the superficial muscles of facial expression and the fat pad that comprises the melolabial fold. These muscles of facial expression, including the zygomaticus muscles, attach to the melolabial fold via the fibrous connections from the surrounding SMAS to the dermis. By dissecting deep to the muscles and applying superolateral traction to the subperiosteal layer, these fibrous connections will pull the fold and the rest of the cheek upward with, at best, no net gain and possibly even a worsened depth of the melolabial crease. By undergoing dissection above the muscles of facial expression and direct suspension of the fibro-fatty malar pad, the patient can achieve a more youthful fullness of the malar region along with a flattening of the melolabial fold and smoothing of the melolabial crease.

THE FOREHEAD

The forehead- or brow-lift is the most common application for the minimal incision endoscopic technique in facial plastic surgery. Because an excellent optic cavity can be created between the frontal bone and the soft tissues of the forehead and brow region, this area is ideally suited to the endoscopic technique. The surgery is designed to minimize the length of incisions, thus preventing the common sequelae of the open approach (i.e., scar alopecia, persistent forehead and scalp numbness) as well as decreasing postoperative discomfort and recovery time. In the evolution of the endoscopic forehead-lift procedure, debate was raised among surgeons as to what the best plane of dissection should be. Some surgeons favored the subgaleal approach used in the open coronal technique. Others preferred the subperiosteal approach because suspension could be achieved without skin stretch, decreasing the stress relaxation. As the technique evolved, most surgeons became proponents of the subperiosteal plane of dissection. This is an easier dissection, which affords a relatively avascular field. The procedure is, in fact, entirely different from the subgaleal approach, allowing repositioning of the brow, forehead, and hairline as a single unit rather than stretching the skin, which causes the relationship between the brows and the anterior hairline to elongate.

Indications

Endoscopic brow- and forehead-lifting, is designed to correct tissue ptosis, eliminate rhytids, and weaken any hyperdynamic action of the underlying musculature without creating additional deformities. Because the upper third of the aging face, especially the brow and glabellar complex, is one of the areas that first shows signs of aging, it is imperative that the facial plastic surgeon understand the aesthetic importance as well as the anatomy of the forehead region to achieve overall facial rejuvenation. The indications for endoscopic brow- and forehead-lifting are the same as those for the open technique, with only a few specific exceptions. Well-suited patients have generalized asymmetric brow ptosis as well as horizontal and vertical forehead and glabellar rhytids. Less favorable patients have relatively thick sebaceous skin and marked brow ptosis where skin excision may be required. Patients with loss of frontalis muscle function on one or both sides resulting from facial nerve paralysis are also poor candidates. In addition, patients with very high frontal hairlines would probably be better served using a pretricheal or trichophytic technique, though all patients should be evaluated on a case-by-case basis to determine the best approach to their particular problem.

Surgical anatomy

To achieve a successful outcome, the facial plastic surgeon should have an intimate knowledge of the functional and static anatomy of the forehead and face. Excellent descriptions and demonstrations of facial anatomic structures and the important relationships to open and endoscopic procedures are available.[3,9,13]

Surgical technique

The surgical technique has gone through many evolutionary changes from the original procedure in 1992 to the present technique. Much has been learned from early experiences in terms of planes of dissection and methods of fixation. The techniques used today are reliable and predictable methods of performing the endoscopic forehead- or brow-lift.[7]

Before proceeding to the operative suite, the surgeon should mark the desired vectors of pull on the forehead or brow complex in the holding area with the patient seated upright. Intravenous analgesics are administered followed by infiltrative local anesthesia using nerve and field blocks.[6] After intravenous sedation has been achieved and the area has been localized, three small 1- to 2-cm incisions are made in a vertical fashion approximately 1.5 cm posterior to the hairline. These three incisions are located in the midline and in the two paramedian areas corresponding to the desired vectors of pull (Fig. 36-1). The incisions are made with a No. 15 blade through skin, subcutaneous tissue, and periosteum. Dissection beneath the periosteum is then begun using a cottle elevator. It is important to maintain the integrity of the periosteum in the area of the incision for later suture suspension. The central optic cavity is then created in the subperiosteal plane using a large endoscopic elevator in a blind dissection to a level approximately 1.5 to 2 cm above the orbital rims. The 30° endoscope with sheath is then introduced through one of the incisions while the elevation continues through another under endoscopic visualization (Fig. 36-2 *A, B*). The suprabrow region should be carefully dissected using endoscopic visualization to identify and preserve the supraorbital neurovascular bundles. In 10% of patients, this neurovascular bundle will exit through a true foramen (located superior to the orbital rim through the frontal bone) rather than through a notch (Fig. 36-3 *A, B*). Posterior to the hairline incisions, the dissection is performed blindly in the subperiosteal plane to a level several centimeters beyond the coronal suture line (Fig. 36-4). After both supraorbital neurovascular bundles have been identified, dissection is carried inferiorly over the orbital rims at which point the periosteum is released at the arcus marginalis (Fig.

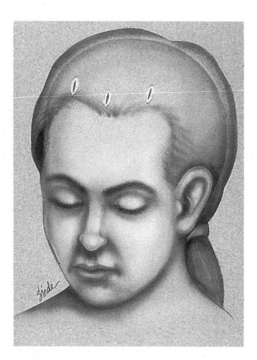

Fig. 36-1. Three central incisions are created corresponding to the desired vectors of pull.

36-5). As the periosteum is released and it separates, the overlying brow fat pad or retro orbicularis oculi fat (ROOF) becomes easily visible (Fig. 36-6). As the periosteum is separated medial to the supraorbital nerves, the fibers of the corrugator muscle will become apparent, oriented obliquely from the medial orbit to the soft tissue of the brow (Fig. 36-7). After complete inferior release of the periosteum in the central optic cavity, the musculature of the glabellar region should be addressed. In patients exhibiting noticeable vertical glabellar rhytids, the fibers of the corrugator muscles are isolated and divided, and a portion excised. Supratrochlear nerve fascicles will be encountered running through the fibers of the corrugator muscles and one should attempt to isolate and preserve as many of these as possible. If horizontal creases are a problem, the procerus muscle is divided. After the depressor musculature of the glabellar region has been addressed, the central portion of the procedure is complete. Next, in the temporal areas, the temporal pockets will be elevated bilaterally and connected to the central optic cavity. The temporal pocket is located over the temporalis muscle and is bounded by the cephalic edge of the zygomatic arch inferiorly, the orbital rim anteriorly, and the temporal line superiorly. A proper dissection plane in the temporal pocket is critical because this region contains the frontal branch of the facial nerve, and care should be taken to preserve this structure. The surgical anatomy of this area is shown in Figure 36-8.

The temporal pocket dissection is begun by creating a 1- to 1.5-cm incision within the hairline of the temporal tuft corresponding to the superior and lateral vector of pull de-

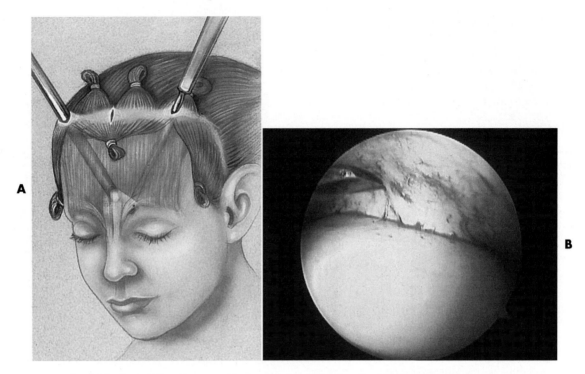

Fig. 36-2. A, A 30° endoscope with sheath is used for visualization through one incision while elevation continues through another. **B,** An endoscopic view of elevation in the subperiosteal plane.

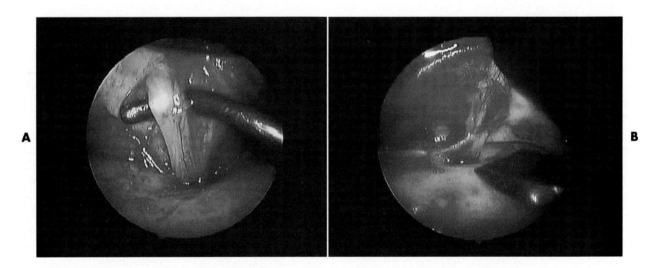

Fig. 36-3. A, An endoscopic view of the supraorbital neurovascular bundle exiting the supraorbital notch. **B,** An endoscopic view of the supraorbital bundle exiting through a true foramen.

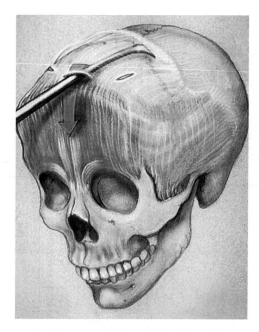

Fig. 36-4. Posterior dissection is performed blindly in the sub-periosteal plane.

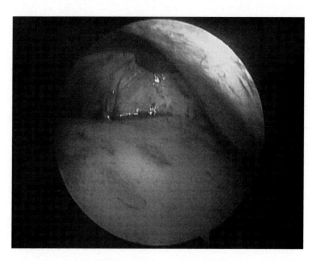

Fig. 36-6. As the periosteum is released at the arcus marginalis, the yellow-appearing retro orbicularis oculus fat becomes readily apparent.

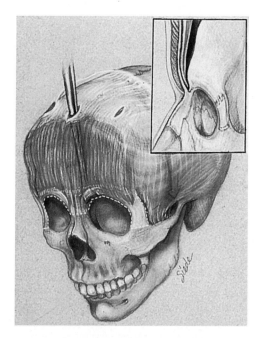

Fig. 36-5. The position of periosteal release at the arcus marginalis, which is critical to adequate repositioning of the forehead-brow complex.

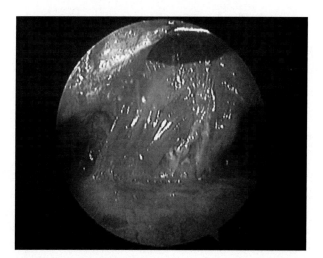

Fig. 36-7. The obliquely oriented fibers of the corrugator muscle can be seen medial to the supraorbital neurovascular bundles.

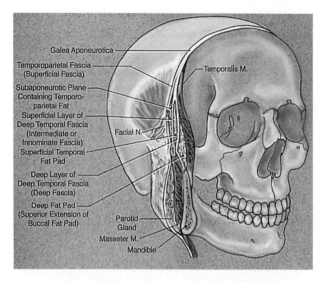

Fig. 36-8. The regional anatomy of the temporal area.

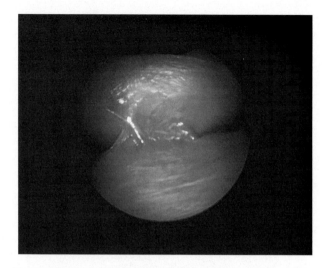

Fig. 36-10. Inferior lateral dissection is complete when the sentinel vein is encountered (this example exhibits twin veins).

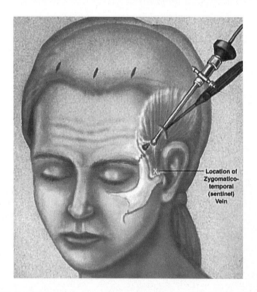

Fig. 36-9. Dissection of the temporal pocket using a 0° endoscope and endoscopic elevator.

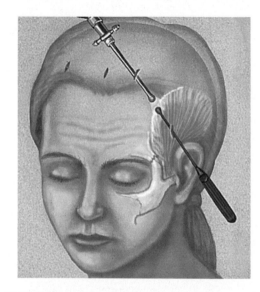

Fig. 36-11. The temporal pocket is joined with the central pocket under direct vision laterally to medially.

sired for the brow. The incision is carried through the skin and subcutaneous tissue and through the temporoparietal fascia. Dissection then proceeds inferiorly in the plane below the temporoparietal fascia and above the deep temporal fascia covering the temporalis muscle. Dissection should be advanced carefully and under direct vision using the 0° endoscope because the temporoparietal layer contains the frontal branch of the facial nerve (Fig. 36-9). Typically, the inferior dissection is complete when the sentinel vein is encountered at a level approximately corresponding to a horizontal line from the lateral canthus (Fig. 36-10). Under direct vision, the temporal pocket is joined with the central pocket superiorly by sharp and blunt dissection of the temporal line attachments of the periosteum, galea, and temporal fascias (Fig.

36-11). This dissection should proceed laterally to medially to maintain the proper plane. Once the two pockets have been joined, the dissection proceeds inferiorly using the fine beveled edge of the endoscopic elevator to elevate the temporal attachments. In the region of the fronto-orbital suture line, the fascial attachments become dense, and sharp dissection is often necessary to free the fascia from the underlying bone (Fig. 36-12). Once this dissection has been completed, the contralateral side is approached in the same manner. When this is completed, the entire forehead-brow complex will be quite mobile and can be slid inferiorly and superiorly over the underlying bone. Next, the fixation portion of the procedure is begun. Many techniques have been developed and used for fixation of the mobilized brow-fore-

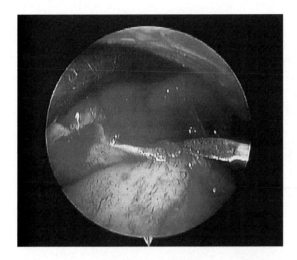

Fig. 36-12. Sharp dissection is often necessary to free the fascia from the underlying bone in the region of the fronto-orbital suture line.

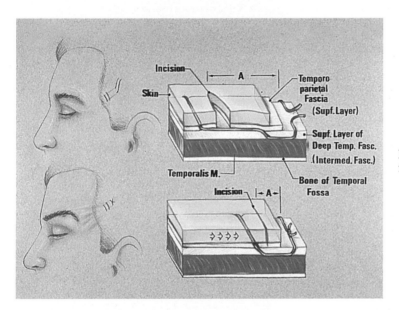

Fig. 36-13. Lateral suspension of the temporoparietal fascia to the underlying temporal fascia.

head complex to the underlying bone. These techniques include scalp plication, skin excision and advancement, external taping, and compression and suture fixation to microscrews, plates, bone anchors, or bone bars.*

After the entire elevation has been completed, the temporoparietal fascia is secured in the temporal region to the deep temporal fascia using 3-0 polydioxanone suture. This region cannot be overcorrected, and maximum support in this area is desired (Fig. 36-13). After this has been completed bilaterally, the central pocket suspension is started. Sutures of 2-0 nylon are placed approximately 1 cm anterior to the three hairline portals encompassing the periosteum, galea, and frontalis muscle. This provides a strong, solid purchase of tissue to suspend the brow-forehead complex superiorly

(Fig. 36-14). A separate incision is created approximately 6 to 8 cm posterior to the central portal slightly off the midline. A five-holed T-shaped microplate is affixed to the cranium with two 3-mm screws (Fig. 36-15). The suspension sutures are then passed from the anterior portals under the intact scalp flap and loosely secured to the horizontal bar of the T-shaped plate (Fig. 36-16). The patient, whose anesthetic plane has been lightened, is then raised on the operating table to a sitting position and brow height is evaluated. Final adjustments are made, and the sutures are secured (Fig. 36-17).

Long term results as evaluated objectively by our computerized measurement system have been gratifying, and this technique appears to stand up to the test of time (Figs. 36-18 *A, B*; 36-19 *A, B*; and 36-20 *A, B*). Few complications have been encountered compared with the open coronal tech-

* Refs. 1, 2, 4, 7, 10, 12.

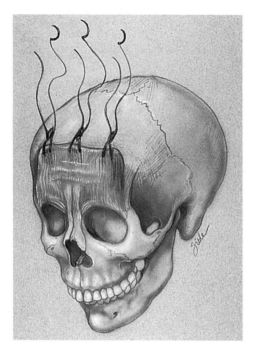

Fig. 36-14. Sutures are placed via the three central portals encompassing the periosteum galea and frontalis muscle.

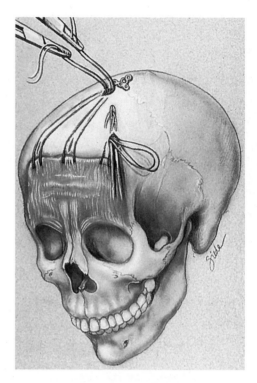

Fig. 36-16. The central suspension sutures are passed from the anterior portals under the scalp flap and loosely secured to the horizontal bar of the T-shaped plate.

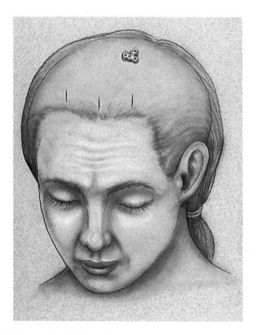

Fig. 36-15. A T-shaped microplate is placed through a separate incision slightly off the midline using two 3-mm screws.

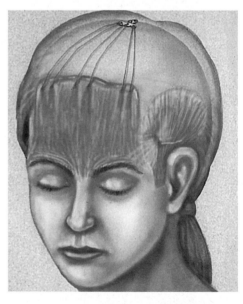

Fig. 36-17. Final adjustments are made with the patient in the upright position, and the sutures are secured.

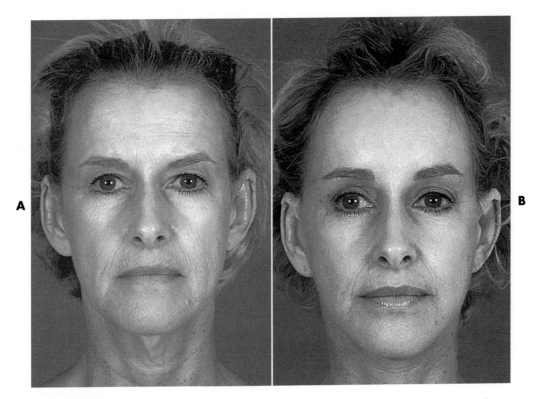

Fig. 36-18. A, Preoperative view of a patient with predominant medial brow ptosis as well as vertical glabellar and horizontal forehead rhytids. **B,** 1-year postoperative view of the same patient after endoscopic forehead-brow-lift, upper blepharoplasty, and rhytidectomy.

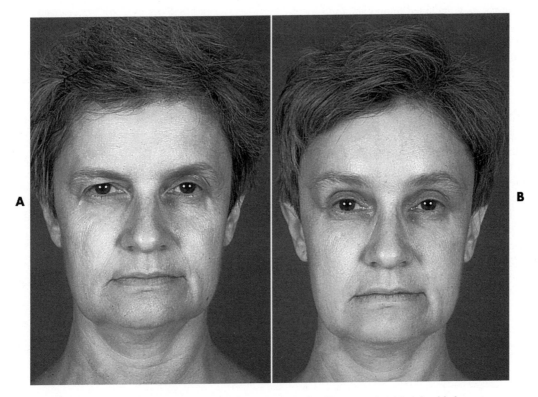

Fig. 36-19. A, Preoperative view of a patient with generalized brow ptosis with right-sided asymmetry **B,** 1-year postoperative view of the same patient after endoscopic forehead-brow-lift.

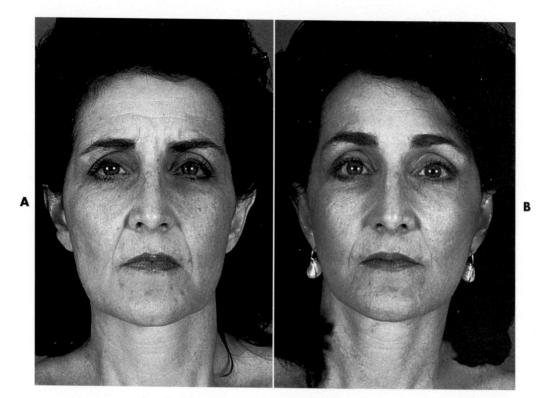

Fig. 36-20. A, Preoperative view of a patient with predominant lateral brow ptosis with vertical, glabellar, and horizontal forehead rhytids. **B,** 1-year postoperative view of the same patient after endoscopic forehead-brow-lift, endoscopic midface-lift, and rhytidectomy.

nique. Complications have included temporary mild localized paresthesias and some forehead and scalp itching. Two cases of temporary paresis of the frontalis muscle unilaterally were encountered in the more than 100 temporal dissections performed to date. These complications lasted for 1 week and 1 month, respectively.

CONCLUSION

The endoscope is a new tool for the facial plastic surgeon to dissect the tissues of the face through minimal incisional access. In certain applications, including the brow, forehead, and midface, the endoscopic techniques present clear advantages over the open technique, including avoidance of long incisions and the secondary sequelae associated with them. Additionally, improved magnification and visualization of small structures allow precise dissection in a compact area. As innovation continues, new techniques will continue to evolve and improve. Long-term studies are needed to determine the future role these techniques will play in managing the aging face.

REFERENCES

1. Aiache AE: Endoscopic facelift: paper presented at Endoscopy in Plastic Surgery: a consensus multi disciplinary symposium, Birmingham, Ala, July 20–24, 1994, *Aesthetic Plast Surg* 18:275, 1994.

2. Bostwick J III, Eaves FF, Nahai F: *Foreheadlift and glabellar frown lines: endoscopic plastic surgery,* St Louis, 1995, Quality Medical Publishing.

3. Duchenne GB: *The mechanism of human facial expression.* Cambridge, England, 1864, Cambridge University Press.

4. Freeman MS: The role of endoscopy in facial plastic surgery, *Curr Opin Otolaryngol Head Neck Surg* 4:223, 1996.

5. Freeman S: Malar fat pad lift, *Clin Facial Plast Surg* (in press).

6. Graham HD: *Anesthesia in facial plastic surgery.* In Walder SR, Willit JM, editors: *Practical aspects of facial surgery,* Norwalk, Conn, Appleton & Lang (in press).

7. Graham HD, Core GB: *Endoscopic forehead lifting using fixation sutures: endoscopic facial surgery,* St Louis, 1997, Mosby.

8. Graham HD, Spring P: Endoscopic repair of frontal sinus fracture, *Journal of Cranio-maxillofacial Trauma* 2:52, 1996.

9. Larabee WF, McKalskey KH: *Surgical anatomy of the face,* New York, 1993, Raven.

10. Newman JP, LaFerriere KL, Nishioka GA: Transcalaverial suture fixation for endoscopic brow and forehead lift, *Arch Otolaryngol Head Neck Surg* (in press).

11. Owsley JQ: Lifting the malar fat pad for connection of prominent nasolabial folds, *Plast Reconstr Surg* 91:463, 1993.

12. Ramirez OM: Endoscopic full face lift: paper presented at Endoscopy in Plastic Surgery: a consensus multi disciplinary symposium, Birmingham, Ala, July 20–24, 1994, *Aesthetic Plast Surg* 18:363, 1994.

13. Saski GH: Facial anatomy for the endoscopic surgeon: paper presented at Endoscopy in Plastic Surgery: a consensus multi disciplinary symposium, Birmingham, Ala, July 20–24, 1994.

Chapter 37

Suction Assisted Lipocontouring

Edward H. Farrior
Stephen S. Park

Having long been a part of cosmetic surgery, lipocontouring has continued to progress with the ever-changing technology of cosmetic surgery. Initially, lipocontouring was accomplished with the direct excision of fat through an open surgical approach; it now includes: suction lipectomy, small cannula lipectomy, and most recently, liposhaving. The goal of these procedures is to change the contour of the face or neck through the removal of localized fat deposits.

Suction lipectomy is an effective means of recontouring the face that has been popularized and refined over the past 30 years.[3-6,9] As with all cosmetic surgery, understanding the anatomy, physiology, and changes affected by the aging process is imperative. Based on these differences, a logical approach to the integration of suction-assisted lipocontouring into the practice of facial plastic and reconstructive surgery is possible (Fig. 37-1).

The distribution of body fat is a consequence of genetics and is influenced by hormones, diet, exercise, medications, and patient age. It has become apparent through tissue culture studies that, after a critical mass within an adipocyte has been reached, hyperplasia can occur.[11] Although the mechanism of adipocyte hyperplasia has not yet been determined, the consensus remains that any significant change in fat deposition occurs through the enlargement rather than the addition of cells.[7] Diet-resistant localized fat deposits, which are ideal for lipocontouring, may represent localized adipocyte hyperplasia. Liposuction reduces the number of adipocytes regardless of their size and therefore should yield a lasting result unless excessive weight gain occurs. The liposuctioned regions of hypertrophy should respond to weight gain in a fashion similar to adipocytes in other regions of the body and, therefore should be resistant to significant contour changes out of proportion to overall weight fluctuation.

Liposuction involves the application of negative pressure through a hollow cannula with a 3- to 6-mm lumen in the subcutaneous plane. Fat is then avulsed as atraumatically as possible. Because of the loose intercellular connections, fat cells are more easily aspirated than tissues with more structural integrity (e.g., muscle, vessels, nerves). Because the standard suction cannula has no cutting surface, structures with more integrity are protected. Liposhaving has recently been advocated as an alternative to liposuction. In this technique, a soft-tissue shaver is used with minimal suction to gently shave adipocytes.[4] The safety of this technique is of concern, and further investigation is under way. With liposuction and liposhaving, preserving important structures and maintaining bridges of uninterrupted tissue between the deep and superficial layers in an effort to maintain a healthier skin flap are the principles to be followed.

PATIENT SELECTION

One of the greatest challenges with facial plastic surgery is the art of proper patient selection, and lipocontouring is no exception. Patient selection begins with an informal interview to get a sense of the patient's motivation, expectation, and cooperation. The patient's motivation for pursuing a cosmetic procedure should be investigated. Some patients expect a change in external appearance to significantly impact on their personal or professional lives (e.g., to get a promotion at work, to dissuade a spouse's infidelity). These patients are bound to be disappointed. A patient's expectations should be precise and realistic. Lipocontouring allows for the removal of a particular area of subcutaneous fullness, and although it will not directly impact other areas, the change in contour may create the illusion of affecting surrounding areas and thereby influence the overall balance of

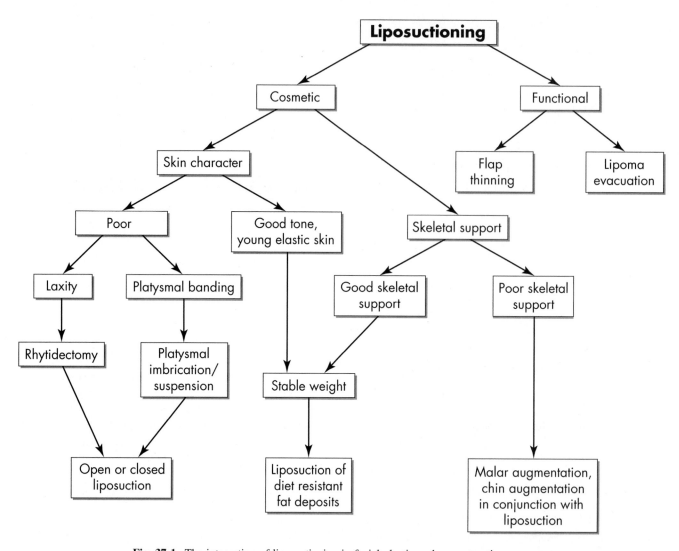

Fig. 37-1. The integration of liposuctioning in facial plastic and reconstructive surgery.

the face. For example, a submental lipectomy may appear to enhance chin projection (Fig. 37-2), shorten vertical height of the face, and create a wider and more cherubic appearing face. Likewise, facial and jaw lipocontouring may create a more angular facial contour (Fig. 37-3) but will not increase malar projection and could create a wasted appearance. The patient's expectations should be communicated preoperatively. Computer imaging can aid in communication, but it can also be misleading if not used prudently. Cooperation is imperative during the postoperative phase. A patient who cannot avoid the sun or continue with a pressure dressing postoperatively is a poor candidate for lipocontouring and should be dissuaded from pursuing surgery.

The ideal patient

The ideal patient is not particularly overweight and has a localized fullness that is secondary to an isolated pocket of subcutaneous adipose tissue refractory to weight loss. A patient who reports a familial pattern or who has had a dou-

ble chin since childhood is a good candidate. The submental, melolabial, submandibular, and buccal areas lend themselves well to lipocontouring. Younger patients tend to have greater skin elasticity, which contracts better on the new subcutaneous contour. These candidates are ideal for isolated lipocontouring. Conversely, the loss of skin elasticity and tugor in older patients will necessitate a skin-tightening procedure (see Fig. 36-1). Obese patients have excess adipose tissue in multiple layers and do not respond well to lipocontouring. Moreover, this procedure is not intended to replace general weight control.

Common pitfalls

Patient evaluation may yield common pitfalls that lead to untoward effects: (1) Significant ptosis of facial skin may appear accentuated after lipocontouring, creating a more aged appearance. These problems are best addressed with a formal face-lift.[8] (2) Lipocontouring depends on the skin's ability to contract and adhere to the new subcutaneous bed,

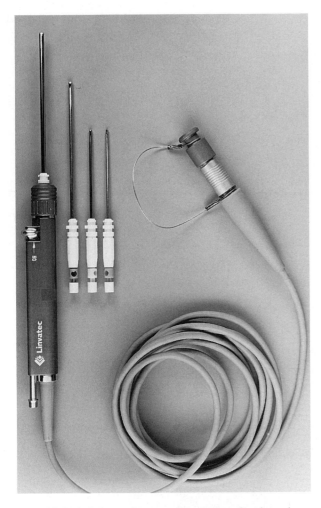

Fig. 37-5. Soft-tissue shavers and cannulas of various sizes.

(e.g., the angle of mandible, the anterior border of the sterno-cleidomastoid muscle, the hyoid bone and thyroid notch) may also be marked (see Fig. 37-6). After marking has been completed, the patient is taken to the operative suite where sedation and infiltration are carried out before preparing and draping the patient. This approach allows additional time for vasoconstriction to occur before surgery.

Anesthesia

Cosmetic procedures (alone or in conjunction with other cosmetic procedures) are performed under intravenous sedation and infiltration anesthesia. Sedation is administered by an anesthetist with close monitoring of the patient, allowing for the virtually painless infiltration and nerve block. Submental and submandibular sculpturing are done with a block of the cervical plexus and mental nerve and with direct infiltration. Facial and melolabial contouring is accomplished with mental and infraorbital nerve block with infiltration. Block and infiltration are achieved using 0.5% lidocaine with 1:200,000 epinephrine. Long-acting agents are unnecessary in these patients.

Adequate sedation is paramount but generally needs to be heavy only during nerve block and infiltration of the local anesthetic. Midazolam, fentanyl, and propofol are short-acting and combine sedation with analgesia and amnesia. When necessary, these procedures are performed under general anesthetia. In this case, infiltration without nerve block is sufficient to obtain vasoconstriction and improve hemostasis.

Surgery

The location of incisions depends on the site to be contoured. Marking and infiltration are done accordingly. Incisions are limited to 5 to 10 mm and are made within relaxed

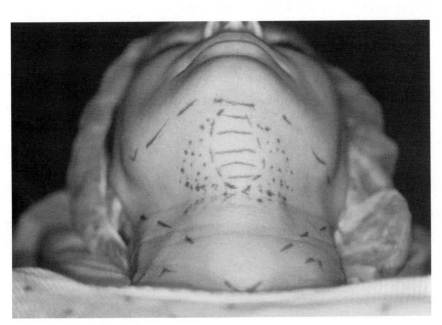

Fig. 37-6. Preoperative marking of anatomic structures, including margin of the mandible, sternocleidomastoid muscle, and hyoid bone with stippling of lateral feathered regions and vertical line through prominent submental fat pad.

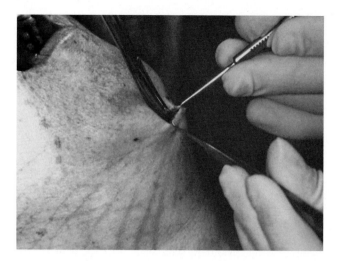

Fig. 37-7. Identification of the plane of dissection using Metzenbaum scissors.

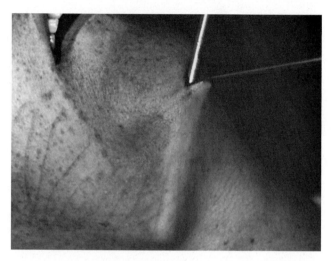

Fig. 37-8. Use of the suction cannula to develop subcutaneous tunnels while stabilizing the skin with a skin hook.

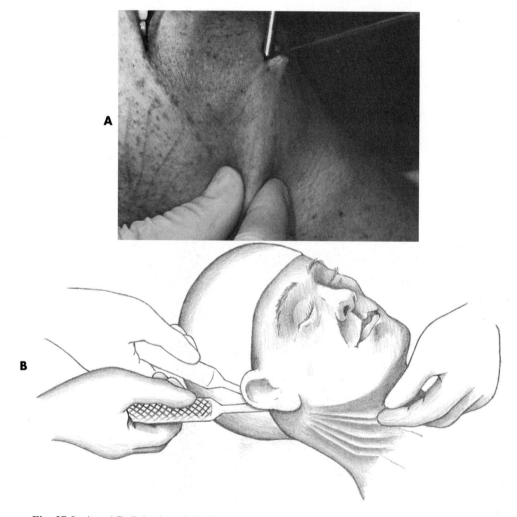

Fig. 37-9. A and **B,** Palpation of the distal cannula to ensure the depth of dissection and location of the distal cannula lumen.

skin tension lines. The submental region will usually be done first, then the jaw and posterior cervical areas, followed by the region of the melolabial fold as indicated. Flaps are then elevated starting with a small cannula and graduating to the cannula size to be used for the lipectomy. A 5-mm cannula is usually used in the submandibular, submental, and jowl areas and a 3-mm cannula is used for the melolabial fold. A nonaspirative cannula is used to make multiple interconnecting tunnels throughout the region to be aspirated. During the nonaspirative phase of flap elevation, it is important to follow the same technique that would be followed when aspirating. The aspiration port should be kept on the deep surface. The skin incision is stabilized with countertraction using a skin hook, and the correct plane is identified with scissors (Fig. 37-7). Graduating cannula sizes are used to develop the tunneling once in the correct plane (Fig. 37-8). The free hand is used to palpate the cannula tip and determine the depth of dissection (Fig. 37-9 *A, B*). Dissection is carried out in a spoke-like fashion from the incision. Multiple distal pseudopods from each spoke are used to ensure that lateral aspiration with feathering is executed thoroughly (Fig. 37-10). Additionally, nonaspiration tunneling is performed beyond the margins of the area to be aspirated to

allow complete redraping. The surgeon should concentrate on distal aspiration because each repetitive motion (Fig. 37-11) of the cannula will cross over the proximal adipose tissue in the region adjacent to the original insertion and may result in a hollowed appearance at that point. Hollowing and inconsistent flap elevation can also be avoided by palpating the cannula tip and preserving some fat on the undersurface of the flap. After complete nonaspiration elevation has been accomplished, the suction is applied at 1 atmosphere of negative pressure and multiple passes re-executed. Assessment of evacuated fat may require the release of the vacuum so that any fat in the cannula and tube may be drawn into the canister. This approach may be necessary when the volume removed is small. Aspiration from the postauricular incision includes the jowl, posterior cervical, and submandibular regions (Fig. 37-12). Crosshatching occurs with the submandibular portions aspirated from the submental incision. In aspiration of the jowl, it is imperative to release suction when withdrawing the cannula over the posterior facial soft tissue and masseter because this area may not require aspiration and a groove may be created in the posterior face. The margins can be tapered with a smaller cannula or with fewer passes. Liposuction of the melolabial fold or, more appropri-

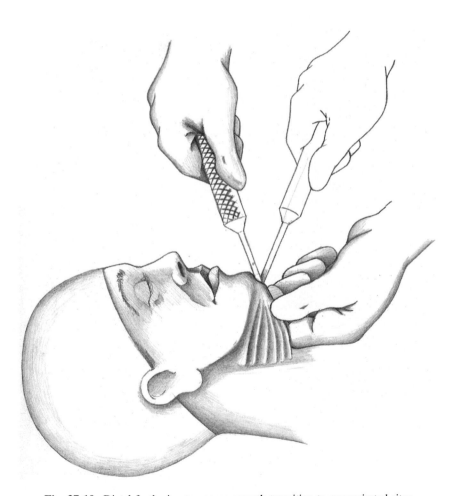

Fig. 37-10. Distal feathering to ensure smooth transition to nonaspirated sites.

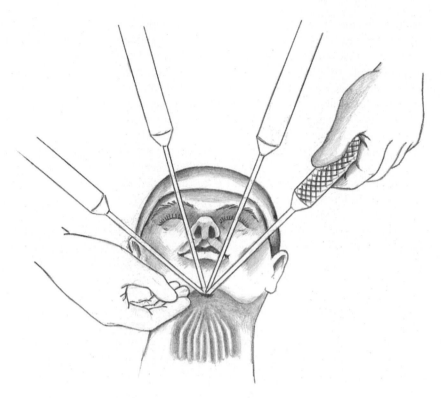

Fig. 37-11. Multiple distal tunneling to ensure smooth transition in all regions and to avoid overreduction of the immediate submental adiposity.

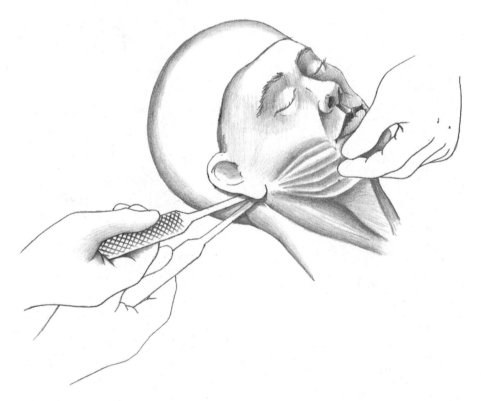

Fig. 37-12. Suction lipectomy of the jowl, posterior cervical, and submandibular region, which can be approached through the postauricular incision.

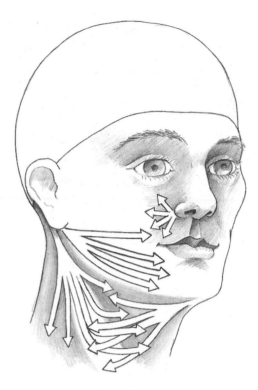

Fig. 37-13. Sites that can be approached through the submental, postauricular, and vestibular incisions.

ately, of the superior border of the fold is performed with a small cannula through an incision in the nasal vestibule (Fig. 37-13).

Submental lipectomy should extend inferiorly to the level of the thyroid cartilage, posteriorly to the anterior border of the sternocleidomastoid muscle with feathering over the muscle, and superiorly to the margin of the mandible. Lipectomy directed from the postauricular incision can extend anteriorly in the submandibular area to the anterior border of the platysmus muscle and superiorly to the margin of the mandible. In the jowl, the specific deposit is aspirated and feathering should be extended to the oral commissure and inferiorly to the margin of the mandible.

With liposhaving (Fig. 37-14 *A, B*), flap elevation is done in a similar fashion. The cannula is inserted with the blade inactive. Once the blade is activated, extreme care should be exercised at the incision to avoid damage to the skin margins. The cannula is passed in a more delicate fashion at a slower rate than with liposuction because shaving rather than avulsion is occurring. Minimal amounts of suction are applied, and the cannula must remain in motion when the blade is active because it will shave progressively deeper, jeopardizing other structures.

Lipocontouring can augment other cosmetic procedures. In conjunction with cervicofacial rhytidectomy, the cannula

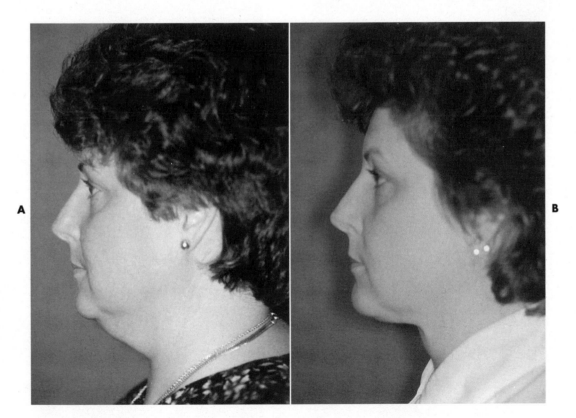

Fig. 37-14. A, Preoperative and **B,** postoperative photographs show a patient undergoing submental liposhaving with the illusion of enhanced chin projection caused by augmentation of the cervicomental angle.

can be used to elevate the flap while sculpturing the fatty tissue. The authors prefer to perform open liposuction for sculpturing after flap elevation. This approach frequently requires extension of liposuction tunnels beyond the limits of skin flap elevation. Open liposuction with cervicofacial rhytidectomy allows the surgeon to completely crosshatch each area, thereby reducing the risk of banding. Additionally, uniform flap thickness can be assured at the time of sharp elevation, reducing the risk of dimpling of the skin. In combining lipocontouring with mentoplasty, the surgeon need only extend the submental incision to about 3 cm to allow placement of the implant. All wounds are closed in a layered fashion.

Dressing

Postoperatively, all patients require a pressure dressing circumferentially around the head and neck. Antibiotic ointment is first applied to the incision and then covered with a nonadhesive dressing. Fluffs are then placed over the region aspirated, and a rolled cotton gauze is used to hold these fluffs in place. Coban R (3M, St. Paul, Minn) dressing is applied using light but continuous pressure (Fig. 37-15). The dressing is left undisturbed for 2 to 3 days and is then removed. After this, an elastic dressing is used at night and when indoors and changed by the patient as needed (Fig. 37-16). Antibiotics are used in all elective surgeries. Drains are not routinely used. Liposuction is usually not painful, but the circumferential dressing can be uncomfortable and anxiety-producing for some patients. For this reason, mild analgesics are helpful. Elevation of the head and continuous use of ice packs minimize swelling.

Recovery phase

Diligent patient education regarding the recovery phase can be very comforting to all those involved. Some degree of bruising and facial edema are to be expected and may last 1 week. The elevated skin may be numb for 3 to 9 weeks. As the facial skin scars and adheres to the new underlying contour, patients often note some firmness and tightness that diminishes over months. Pain is usually minimal and sufficiently relieved with acetaminophen. When larger volumes of fat are removed, shallow dimpling and wrinkling from excess skin can occur as the skin adheres. Diligent massage and patience will lead to a smoother final contour. Exercise

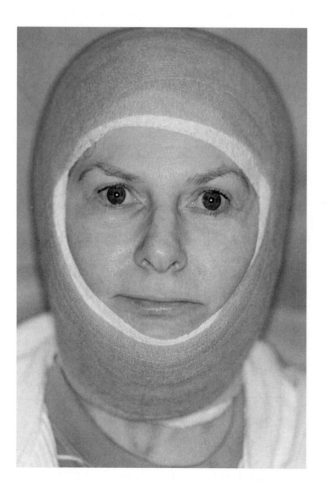

Fig. 37-15. Immediate postsurgical dressing.

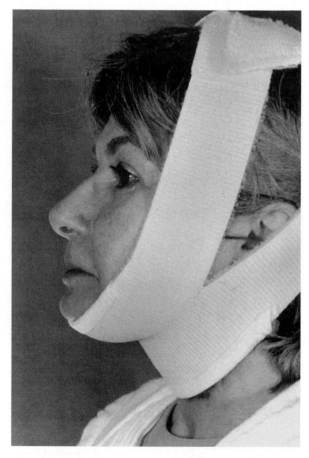

Fig. 37-16. A light dressing can be applied by the patient after the immediate postsurgical dressing is removed.

is to be avoided for 3 weeks after surgery and should be resumed gradually, beginning with aerobic activities and progressing to more strenuous exercise.

COMPLICATIONS

Complications from lipocontouring are uncommon but may be dramatic. The most frequent complication is hematoma or seroma, which is evacuated by needle aspiration and a pressure dressing reapplied. If a hematoma accumulates acutely, one should have a low threshold for drainage and exploration in the operating room. Infections or cellulitis usually arise from a preexisting hematoma and should be managed aggressively to reduce the risk of skin-flap necrosis or scarring. Pigment changes can follow an undiagnosed hematoma and result from a breakdown in hemoglobin products. Contour irregularities and asymmetries may manifest after all swelling has subsided and are more likely to occur as residual fullness on the right neck area because most surgeons are right-handed, making the left neck more accessible than the right side. If significant, this complication is best repaired with minor touchup procedures using the hand-held syringe technique, but not before 6 months postoperative to allow the full skin flap to soften as much as possible. For subtle areas, small quantities of corticosteroids can be injected to induce fat atrophy. This approach should be used conservatively because its effects continue for many months and are not reversible. Minor depressions can be remedied with autologous fat injection, but the longevity of the procedure is unknown. Motor or sensorineural injury are more serious but rare, usually representing a transient neuropraxia. Cardiovascular instability is associated with total body liposuction and results from massive fluid shifts. This complication does not occur from lipectomy in the head and neck areas. Pulmonary fat embolism can theoretically occur during any surgical procedure but has not been reported after liposuction alone.

SUMMARY

Lipocontouring is a necessary adjunct to a facial plastic and reconstructive practice. Multiple tools are available and should be judged individually. Patient selection and education are paramount to achieving satisfaction. The judicious use of liposuction in conjunction with other cosmetic procedures will enhance the results and the satisfaction of the patient and surgeon.

REFERENCES

1. Becker D, Park SS, Gross CW: *Results from current investigation*, 1995, University of Virginia.
2. Cueva R, Thomas JR, Davidson M: Liposuction to debulk the pectoralis major myocutaneous flap, *J Otolaryngol* 9:106, 1988.
3. Fournier PF: Why the syringe and not the suction machine? *J Dermatol Surg Oncol* 14:1062, 1988.
4. Gross CW and others: The soft-tissue shaving procedure for removal of adipose tissue: a new, less traumatic approach than liposuction, *Arch Otolaryngol Head Neck Surg* 121:1117, 1995.
5. Illouz YG: Body contouring by lipolysis: a 5 year experience with over 3000 cases, *Plast Reconstr Surg* 72:591, 1983.
6. Kesselring UK, Meyer R: A suction curette for removal of excessive local deposits of subcutaneous fat, *Plast Reconstr Surg* 63:305, 1978.
7. Markman B: Anatomy and physiology of adipose tissue, *Clin Plast Surg* 16:235, 1989.
8. Mladick RA: Lipoplasty: an ideal adjunctive procedure for the face lift, *Clin Plast Surg* 16:333, 1989.
9. Schrudde J: *Lipexeresis as a means of eliminating local adiposity.* In *International Society of Aesthetic Plastic Surgery*, New York, 1980, Springer-Verlag.
10. Setliff RC: The hummer, *Otolaryngol Clin North Am* 29:93, 1996.
11. Van R: *The adipocyte precursor cell.* In Cryer A, Van R, editors: *New perspectives in adipose tissue*, London, 1985, Butterworths.

Chapter 38

Facial Implants

Nabil S. Fuleihan

Autogenous tissue has always been considered the best implantation material. However, there are situations in which autogenous tissues are not available or will not give a good result. Implantation of autogenous tissue for major contouring is associated with morbidity from the donor site, prolongation of the surgery, and a possibility of absorption if the tissue is not vascularized. Insufficient amounts of autogenous material and difficulties in contouring of grafts may necessitate the use of alloplastic material for facial augmentation.

Among the first alloplastic materials used successfully were certain nonreactive metals including stainless steel, tantalum, and Vitallium. Since heat-cured acrylics were introduced and commonly used for contouring of the forehead and different areas of the skull during World War II, multiple plastic polymers have been used for facial contouring, including cold-curing methylmethacrylate, polyvinyl alcohol, polyisobutylene, polyvinyl chloride, polytetrafluoroethylene, polyethylene, tricalcium phosphate (bioabsorbable ceramic), dimethylpolysiloxane,[39,51] polyamide, and polyethylene terephthalate.

Scales[50] defined the properties of an ideal implant as follows:

1. Not physically modified by soft tissue
2. Not capable of inciting an inflammatory or foreign body reaction
3. Not capable of producing a state of allergy or hypersensitivity
4. Chemically inert
5. Noncarcinogenic
6. Capable of resisting strain
7. Capable of fabrication in the form desired
8. Capable of sterilization

The quality of tissues surrounding implants plays an important role in decreasing the rejection rate. The ideal host bed is one that is covered by well-vascularized thick skin and subcutaneous tissue that is not subjected to the stresses of trauma or motion.

CHEMICAL COMPOSITION

The chemical composition of an implant predicts its compliance to the ideal properties required for its use in soft-tissue contouring. Also, the chemical composition of an implanted material determines its *biocompatibility*, which is a term used to describe "the state of affairs in which a material exists within a physiologic environment without either the material adversely and significantly affecting the body, or the environment of the body adversely affecting the material."[67]

Biocompatibility is monitored by testing the tissue reactions, which are categorized as localized or systemic. The localized tissue reaction is the response of the adjacent tissue to the implant and its biodegradable products. The systemic reaction is due to a response to biodegradable substances or molecules that may migrate throughout the body, potentially resulting in immunologic, carcinogenic, or metabolic effects. *Toxicity* is the term used to describe the response to these effects. Toxicity of implants is usually caused by biodegradation or oxidation of implant material, resulting in the release of potentially bioactive substances.[18] The degree of localized inflammatory reaction induced by the implant is an indirect reflection of its degree of toxicity.[25] This is usually histologically assessed by the numbers of macrophages and giant cells adjacent to the implant.

Because "all of the common implant metals corrode at some finite rate in the human body,"[56] the ultimate success of the implant may depend on the potential reaction to these corrosion products. The interaction of implanted material with the immune system is an important aspect of the toxicity. This reaction depends on the size of the implant used and the degree of corrosion and biodegradation induced. The usual reaction associated with biomaterials is a T-cell–mediated response that may be systemic and not easily recognized.[20]

Hueper[23] and Oppenheimer, Oppenheimer, and Stout[38] report the formation of cancer in cancer-prone laboratory animals in conjunction with many implant materials. Malignant tumors have been reported in patients with implants, but a cause-and-effect relationship between alloplastic implants and cancer development has never been proven in humans. The number of persons living with different synthetic materials implanted is increasing every day.[17] The subject of metal implant–related carcinogenicity also has been studied. Of the 13 cases of cancer associated with a metal implant reported in humans, four have been reported in association with trauma devices made from cobalt-chromium alloy. However, a direct association between the metal implants and malignant changes have been difficult to establish. In consideration of the 120 million devices implanted during the 60-year history of contemporary orthopedic procedures, "the number of reported cases of sarcoma is so minute that no surgeon or patient would feel undue concern on this account."[16]

METALS

Biocompatibility of metals depends on their resistance to corrosion, as well as local and systemic tissue reactions to corrosion products. Hoar and Mears[19] reported that cobalt-chromium alloys should be relatively stable in the body. Vitallium, titanium, and stainless steel corrode at some finite rate in the human body.[56] The minimal localized reaction found indicated that these implants are extremely well tolerated by bony and periosteal tissues. Corrosion is controlled by the formation of an oxide film. Both titanium and chromium naturally form an oxide film, making them useful as alloys because of improved corrosion resistance. Corrosion products of stainless steel also have been associated with local tissue changes and potential systemic effects that can be carcinogenic,[24] metabolic,[60,66] immunologic,[13] and bacteriologic.[64] Osteointegrated implants produce a minimal tissue reaction that decreases the development of a fibrous layer around the implanted material, allowing a direct structural and functional connection between bone and implant.

Systemically, there is transport of the metal ions around the body, resulting in accumulation in certain organs, but the levels are not thought to be unduly high. Indeed, the changes in ion concentrations are described as minimal.[68]

The use of metals has been limited to skeletal applications (Figs. 38-1 through 38-3). Since the introduction of stainless steel in the 1920s, raw materials have been developed that will decrease the corrosive reaction around the implanted material (Table 38-1). Vitallium, formed mainly

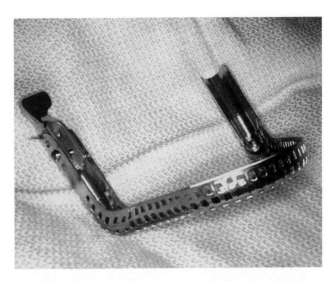

Fig. 38-1. Vitallium mesh implants with condyle extension.

from cobalt and chromium, was introduced later in the 1920s. This material showed an increased corrosion resistance. Titanium implants are widely used today because of their light weight, strength, and resistance to corrosion. They were shown to be less corrosive than both Vitallium and stainless steel.[21,32]

POLYMERS

Whereas metallic implants have been used for skeletal fixation and bony augmentation, polymers have been used for soft-tissue augmentation and contouring. The number of polymers used for this purpose has progressively increased over the past decade.

A polymer is an aggregate of atoms usually based on carbon and linked together to form chains by a process called *polymerization*.[2] Molecular weight depends on the number of repeating units. With increases in the degree of polymerization and cross-linking between polymer units, there is transformation of the polymer from a liquid to a more viscous state and finally to a solid form. The composition, molecular weight, and the degree of cross-linking have a profound effect on the properties of the polymer and its biocompatibility.

Polymers implanted in subcutaneous tissue produce an inflammatory reaction that results in the deposition of connective tissue around the implant. A fibrous capsule ultimately surrounds the implant. Liquid polymers, such as dimethylsiloxane, produce many small capsules that will surround the material injected, resulting in a honeycomb appearance.

Over the past decade, the most commonly used polymers for soft-tissue contouring of the face are poly(dimethylsiloxane), poly(amide), poly(methylmethacrylate), and poly(tetrafluoroethylene) (Fig. 38-4).

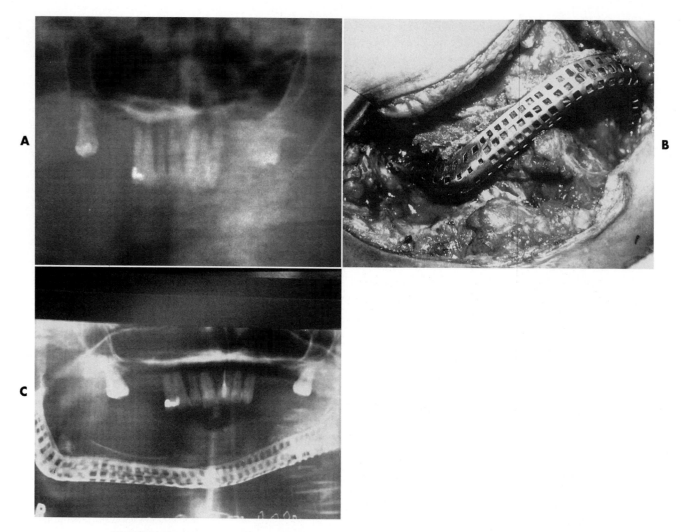

Fig. 38-2. A, A panoramic view of the mandible. Segment of mandible resected from right ramus to left body of the mandible. **B,** Vitallium mesh interposed between remaining left body of the mandible and right ramus. Mesh filled with multiple fragments of bone from iliac crest. **C,** A panoramic view of Vitallium mesh in place.

Continued

Poly(dimethylsiloxane)

The silicone polymers are the most widely used implants for facial contouring. They are composed of long chains of dimethylsiloxane units based on the element silicon, which is among the most abundant elements on earth. The element silicon is naturally present in human tissue as a component of mucopolysaccharides and may contribute to connective tissue structure by bridging or linking polysaccharides to protein.[42]

Siloxane is an acronym derived from sil (icon), ox (ygen), and (meth) ane. The viscosity of the dimethylsiloxane polymers depends on the degree of polymerization.[46] Cross-linking is used to produce a rubber or gel. Silicone polymers have been used in different forms for facial contouring. Medical-grade injectable silicone with a viscosity of 200 to 350 centistokes is a clear, oily, colorless, and odorless material with a high degree of chemical stability, allowing prolonged storage at room temperature and repeated steam autoclaving. Animal experiments showed that following intradermal, subcutaneous, intramuscular, and intraperitoneal injections there was an early migration of polymorphonuclear leukocytes to the area followed by a local and mild round cell reaction that subsided within 6 months. Within time, the silicone became encapsulated by the animal's own collagen. After massive subcutaneous doses of silicone were injected into rats, droplets of vacuoles were present in the reticuloendothelial system.[2,45]

Injectable silicone, introduced for restoration of facial contour in patients with hemifacial atrophy,[44] also was used for correction of certain depressed scars, glabella frown lines, malar and melolabial grooves, and certain postrhinoplastic deformities.[62,63] The use of injectable silicone was recently addressed by the US Food and Drug Administration (FDA). The FDA does not approve the use of this material.

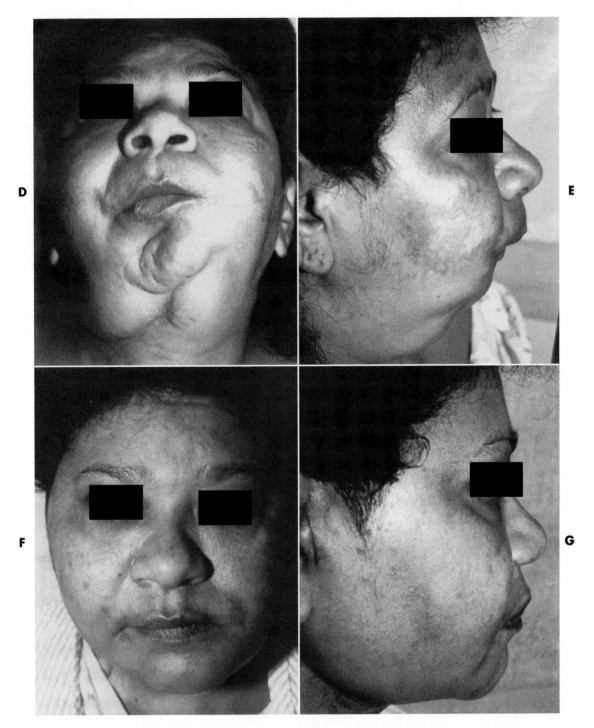

Fig. 38-2, cont'd. D, Preoperative basal view. **E,** Preoperative right profile. **F,** Face view with good contour of chin and lower third of face. **G,** Lateral view showing good contouring of area of body of the mandible with restoration of chin projection.

Liquid silicone is widely employed by the medical industry to coat certain suture materials and as an internal lubricant in some disposable syringes.[52]

When silicone rubber (Silastic) is implanted, a fibrous capsule is formed. This capsule does not adhere to the implant. Host tissues outside the capsule are not affected. Gradual deterioration of the silicone rubber can occur,[14] producing some postoperative failure. When silicone implants are used in joints, a giant cell reaction can be seen locally in connective tissue and synovium with no focal necrosis.[57] Preformed silicone implants are used for augmentation of different areas of the face including malar, submalar, nose,

Table 38-1. Composition of metallic implants

	Chromium weight, %	Nickel weight, %	Molybdenum weight, %	Carbon weight, %	Manganese weight, %	Phosphorus weight, %	Sulfur weight, %	Silicon weight, %	Nitrogen	Copper	Iron	Oxygen	Cobalt	Aluminum	Titanium	Vanadium
Stainless steel, wrought (ASTM-F55)	17-20	12.7	2-4	0.03 max	2.00 max	0.03 max	0.03 max	0.75 max	0.10 max	0.50 max	Balance	—	—	—	—	—
Co-Cr alloy: Vitallium, cast (ASTM-F90)	27-30	2.5 max	5-7	0.35 max	1.00 max	—	—	1.00 max	—	—	0.75 max	—	Balance	—	—	—
Titanium, pure (ASTM-F67)	—	—	—	0.10 max	—	—	—	—	—	—	0.5 max	0.45 max	—	—	Balance	—
Titanium, alloy (ASTM-F136)	—	—	—	0.08 max	—	—	—	—	—	—	0.25 max	0.13 max	—	5.5-6.5	Balance	3.5-4.5

ASTM—American Society for Testing and Materials.

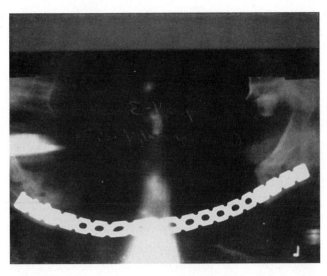

Fig. 38-3. Stainless steel plate positioned to bridge anterior mandibular defects, with lateral segments in position. Insertion of these implants around the chin area has been associated with higher extrusion rates.

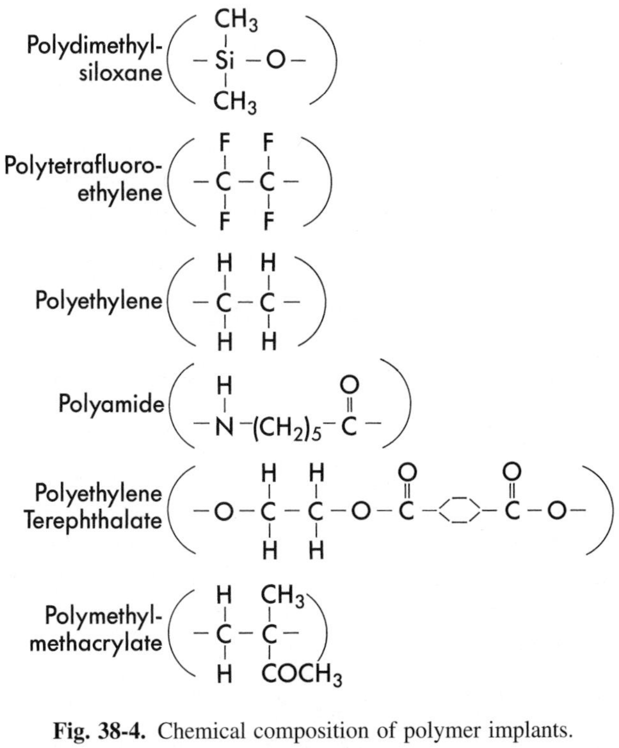

Polydimethyl-siloxane $\left(\begin{array}{c} CH_3 \\ | \\ -Si-O- \\ | \\ CH_3 \end{array} \right)$

Polytetrafluoro-ethylene $\left(\begin{array}{cc} F & F \\ | & | \\ -C-C- \\ | & | \\ F & F \end{array} \right)$

Polyethylene $\left(\begin{array}{cc} H & H \\ | & | \\ -C-C- \\ | & | \\ H & H \end{array} \right)$

Polyamide $\left(\begin{array}{cc} H & O \\ | & \| \\ -N-(CH_2)_5-C- \end{array} \right)$

Polyethylene Terephthalate $\left(\begin{array}{c} H \; H \quad O \qquad\quad O \\ | \; | \quad\; \| \qquad\quad \| \\ -O-C-C-O-C-\!\!\!\langle\bigcirc\rangle\!\!\!-C-O- \\ | \; | \\ H \; H \end{array} \right)$

Polymethyl-methacrylate $\left(\begin{array}{cc} H & CH_3 \\ | & | \\ -C-C- \\ | & | \\ H & COCH_3 \end{array} \right)$

Fig. 38-4. Chemical composition of polymer implants.

chin, and mandible regions. The use of silicone rubber in nasal augmentation has been associated with a high extrusion rate, especially when used in revision rhinoplasty cases, usually because of the necrosis of overlying skin. However, huge numbers of Asian patients have had successful primary nasal augmentation with silicone dorsal implants.

Poly(tetrafluoroethylene)

Proplast is a highly porous material prepared from Teflon (a fluorocarbon polymer) and carbon fibers, giving it a black color. This type of material is given the name Proplast I to differentiate it from Proplast II, which is white in color and formed of an aluminum oxide–coated Teflon. The space between the cross-linked polymer particles provides a porosity of the implant.[20] The size of the pores is usually between 200 and 500 μm. The pore volume of Proplast implant material constitutes 70% to 90% of the total volume.[29]

Proplast I is easily shaped or carved with a knife or scissors. Proplast II is firmer and more difficult to carve. Proplast has a low rejection rate. In an experimental study by Kasperbauer, Kern, and Neel,[28] Proplast was implanted in 17 rabbit ears. Although the black color of the implant was clearly visible beneath the skin at 1 year, only one partial implant exposure without obvious rejection was noted. A marked granulomatous reaction with many histiocytes and giant cells occurred within the implant. A similar reaction was present when Proplast was implanted in the subcutaneous tissue of the face of a rabbit.

Although tissue ingrowth provides a dependable fixation with a decreased chance of extrusion, it makes removal of these implants more difficult than with solid Silastic implants. The porosity allows loading the implant with antibiotic solution at the time of the surgery. Proplast has been associated with less bone resorption than was found with other firm implants.[53] When implanted adjacent to osseous surfaces, Proplast I and Proplast II cause the formation of osteoid tissue with or without a fibrous tissue zone between the outer surface of the implant and the osseous tissue.[22]

Silver[53] used Proplast to augment several different sites around the face and stressed strict guidelines for a successful implantation. Although this implant material is stable at temperatures greater than 392° F, it should be sterilized with a slow wet-steam autoclave at 250° F for 30 minutes. Steam autoclaving should not be performed more than three times on the same material. Proplast should be impregnated with an antibiotic saline solution (600 mg lincomycin [Lincocin]/30 ml saline) at the time of implantation. Infusion of the Proplast with antibiotic solution does not seem to affect tissue ingrowth. It is advisable to carve the material before the surgical procedure and handle it with powder-free gloves.

Proplast was used successfully for facial contouring procedures including chin augmentation, nasal dorsal augmentation, and correction of traumatic prominence loss and frontal bone defects. The manufacturer states that Proplast is not indicated as an implant (1) by itself in weight-bearing or articulating bony surfaces where compressive loading is likely (temporomandibular joint [TMJ]), (2) over sinus cavities, (3) where there is insufficient underlying bone or soft tissue to prevent collapse in the event of external pressure, (4) in patients with systemic disorders that may compromise tissue ingrowth or normal wound healing, (5) in recent areas of infection, (6) in patients with a phobia of implant material, or (7) in gas or cold sterilization.[29] Proplast implants have been removed from the market due to complications that include bony destruction in the condylar fossa as a result of exuberant foreign body giant cell reaction. Spagnoli and Kent[54] presented their experience in 680 implants in the TMJ area. They concluded that the long-term performance and survival of these implants is doubtful.

Gore-Tex

Gore-Tex is a fibrillated porous tetrafluoroethylene. It was introduced in facial reconstructive surgery in 1983.[37] It is chemically a stable polymer with high tissue biocompatibility as reflected in the prolonged use of this material in vascular surgery. The size of the pores in this polymer is approximately 30 microns, allowing tissue ingrowth and stabilization. This limited fibrous tissue ingrowth permits easy extraction of the Gore-Tex implant. The texture of the implant simulates that of dermis.

Its use in facial plastic surgery as a volume filler in the region of the cheeks, nose, and lips is increasing. Owsley and Taylor[40] described their experience with Gore-Tex in 106 patients over a 5-year period. Their conclusion is that this is a stable material.

This material also has been used as a suspender of the cheeks, brow, and platysma (Fig. 38-5). The patient in Figure 38-5 had complete right facial paralysis. Suspension of the cheek-lip region with Gore-Tex material allowed an improved suspension of the middle third of the face. This implant does not disintegrate or relax with time, thereby maintaining a stable tensile strength.

Poly(ethylene)

Polyethylene polymers consist of a large number of ethylene units linked together to form a highly branched micromolecule. Three types of polyethylenes are available. The low-density polyethylenes have approximately 10 to 30 branches per 1000 carbon atoms. This branching results in low yield strength and lower stiffness.[20] High-density polyethylene is a substantially linear molecule with minimal branching and with higher density, tensile strength, and stiffness. The ultra high–molecular weight polyethylene, with a molecular weight of approximately 4 million atomic mass units (AMU), is a component of total hip prostheses. The composition allows weight bearing. Low-density polyethylenes may be formed into porous sponge implants for reconstruction of nonload-bearing areas. Total ossicular replacement prostheses (TORP) and partial ossicular replacement prostheses (PORP) are polyethylene implants used for middle ear reconstruction. The implant becomes embedded in a connective tissue network with no chronic or acute inflammation. However, these implants have not proved to be ideal for middle ear reconstruction because of the high incidence of extrusion.

High-density polyethylene is frequently used in facial reconstruction. Different forms of high-density polyethylene are available to the facial plastic surgeon. Among these are Porecron (Effner GmbH, Berlin, Germany), Medpore (Porex, Fairburn, Ga), and Plastipore (Richards Manufacturing Company, Memphis, Tenn).[3,4] Porecron is a porous high-density polyethylene with a pore size of approximately 150 μm permitting ingrowth of connective tissue that is supplied by capillary vessels.

Canine studies using porous, high-density polyethylene have shown tissue ingrowth of osteoprogenitor mesenchyme within the first week. A few bone spicules within a soft-tissue matrix were present in the second week. Bone trabeculae with an active osteoblastic front were formed by the fourth week. Mature bone ingrowth into the surface of the pore was documented at the end of 1 year.[4,49] Proplast does not allow such bony ingrowth, possibly because Proplast pores do not have a sufficiently large diameter. Polyethylene implants retain their shape and do not undergo resorption after implantation. Proplast, on the other hand, gradually fragments, and parts of the synthetic material appear in medullary spaces.[3] Long-term studies with Proplast used in chin and zygomatic maxillary augmentations revealed an overall loss of bone and soft tissue thickness of approximately 57%.[30] In the case of high-density polyethylene, limited studies have showed evidence of soft-tissue loss without bony resorption.[4]

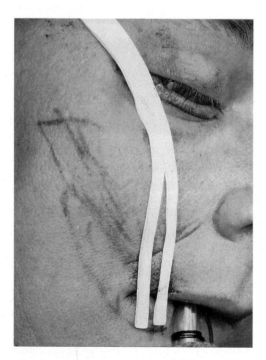

Fig. 38-5. GoreTex sheet positioned around the area of labial commissure for a patient with right facial paralysis.

Poly(amide)

Polyamide, known generically as nylon, was among the first commercial polymers introduced in the 1930s. Where nylon is implanted, hydrolysis of some of the 15 amide groups occurs in time. This is a reversal of the polymerization reaction and results in loss of approximately 25% of the tensile strength of nylon sutures.[20] After implantation, a moderate foreign body reaction is seen, which is slowly replaced by the ingrowth of fibrous tissue.[11] Stucker, Hirokawa, and Pruet[55] introduced the "auto-alloplast" concept to polyamide mesh (Supramid) implantation. The material is implanted in a secure area for a period of 6 weeks and then harvested and reimplanted in the area that needs augmentation. This process has decreased the extrusion rate.

Brown, Neal, and Kern[7] have shown that Supramid strands appear to disintegrate at 6 to 12 months in the rabbit face and ear.

Poly(ethylene terephthalate)

Polyethylene terephthalate polyester fibers are used as woven or knitted fabric configurations in implant applications. Mersilene mesh is a polyethylene terephthalate product. It is knitted so that it can be rolled, folded, or molded into any shape. This design allows an ingrowth of fibrous tissue. The mesh is available in sheets that are 0.25-mm thick. This polyester mesh does not undergo enzymatic degradation after implantation. Colton and Beekhuis[8] reported the use of Mersilene mesh for facial augmentation in 113 cases with a 4- to 5-year follow-up. The infection rate was around 7%. Removal of the implant after fibrous ingrowth has taken place is difficult, because the lack of capsulation around the implant makes it difficult to know whether complete removal was achieved. Polyethylene terephthalate (Dacron) has been used as a vascular replacement material. Dacron mesh (Osteo Mesh, Xomed, Inc. Gainesville, Fla) has been successfully used for reconstruction of craniofacial and mandibular defects.

Poly(methylmethacrylate)

The use of acrylic in reconstruction of cranial defects was started by Zander during World War II.[41] The medical-grade acrylic resin has two components: a powder of small polymethylmethacrylate spheres and beads 10 to 20 μm in diameter to which benzoyl peroxide has been added, and a liquid monomer in which the amino accelerator has been dissolved. The monomer polymerizes and links together the preexisting polymer. The polymerization reaction is exothermic with maximal temperatures reaching 120° C. After mixing, a moldable dough is formed that cures in about 10 minutes. The monomer is usually lost by evaporation; around 4% residual monomer remains. The reaction of the host to implantable acrylic may include toxicity, hypersensitivity, and systemic effects. Although uncommon, these reactions may be due to the exothermic reaction of polymerization or to the direct toxicity of the monomer. However, polymethyl-methacrylate has shown a high degree of tissue compatibility.

Hydroxyapatite

Calcium hydroxyapatite (Ca_{10} [PO4]$_6$ [OH]$_2$) is formed of crystals that have a similar composition to the inorganic components of osseous and dental tissues. This allows the implant to become an integral part of bony tissue. The material is composed of 39.9% Ca, 18.5% P, and 3.5% OH with Ca:P ratio of 1.67.[26] These crystals are fused together at temperatures of 1100° to 1300° C by a process called "sintering."[43,47] Depending on the conditions of the sintering process and composition, a range of degree of porosity and mechanical properties is achieved. In thin, porous, or dense forms, hydroxyapatites (HA) can serve as permanent bone implants with no tendency to resorption *in vivo*.[27] HA implants are quite brittle and have a relatively low tensile strength, which does not allow them to withstand bending and torsional forces.

The main advantage of HA implants is their ability to become directly integrated into bony tissue. HA implants have been shown to stimulate osteogenesis when placed against bone,[15] but implantation of HA in soft tissue did not result in bone formation.[6] HA has had wide application in the augmentation of the facial skeleton, including augmentation of the alveolar ridge, orbital floor reconstruction, and spacers for orthognathic and craniofacial procedures.[10] Salyer and Hall[48] compared the use of HA and autogenous bone grafts as onlays for facial augmentation. Their 3-year study shows that "porous hydroxyapatite as an onlay has a greater potential for movement than bone, and it may not become totally adherent for 4 months." This problem necessitated suture fixation of the HA. The HA became incorporated with 20% to 30% bone ingrowth and appeared to become fully established and stable by 12 to 16 months. Because of soft tissue thinning over HA onlays and the potential for late exposure, the authors recommend limiting the use of this material to maxillary and malar augmentation, thereby "avoiding potential reaction problems with mandibular and temporal positioning or when used in the forehead and lateral orbital regions."

Costantino[9] presented results of the experimental use of HA in 45 patients with craniofacial defects. They report a 5% infection rate. In cases where the HA implant was exposed to the paranasal sinuses, the infection rate was more than 93%.

Injectable collagen

Injectable Zyderm and Zyplast collagen are prepared from cowhide by purification, sterilization, and depyrogenation. Ninety-five percent of the product is type I collagen. Injectable collagen, used mainly for augmentation and contouring of skin defects, comes in three forms: Zyderm I, Zyderm II, and Zyplast. Zyderm I has a concentration of 35 mg/ml, whereas Zyderm II has a concentration of 65 mg/ml. Zyplast, a more cross-linked collagen, has more resistance to digestion by local tissue.

Zyderm injected into human skin and studied histologically was found to intersperse with human skin with no evidence of colonization of the implant by either connective tissue or blood vessels. There is progressive disappearance of the implant without a significant fibrous tissue reaction. Zyplast has a different histologic response. At 1 to 3 months, the implant forms a deposit that displaces the dermal collagen rather than dispersing along its fibers. This implant tends to induce a response from the surrounding tissue and new collagen formation adjacent to the implant. Early studies have shown that the Zyplast implant loses its integrity after 6 to 9 months.

Approximately 3% of patients tested for allergy to collagen develop a positive intradermal test. Patients with positive skin testing should not be treated with Zyderm or Zyplast injection. Previous studies have stressed that patients might develop an allergic response to injectable collagen during treatment despite a negative primary intradermal test. The arguments against any systemic autoimmune disease stress the fact that Zyderm is predominantly type I and type III bovine collagen, and there are no vascular diseases directed to this type of collagen. Goodpasture's disease involves type IV collagen.

Fat

The introduction of liposuction resulted in a renewed interest in fat transplantation. Material suctioned from one site of the body was readily available for insertion into other sites. The survival of fat transplants depends mainly on the techniques of harvesting, handling of graft fat tissue, the size of the needle used for injection, the volume injected, and the type of recipient site. Using a 14- to 16-gauge canula attached to a 20-ml syringe allows easy extraction of fat tissue. Different techniques have been used to prepare the collected fat including centrifuging the contents of the syringe, filtering, or washing with normal saline solution. The size of the needle used for insertion is an important factor in survival of the fat transplant. An 18-gauge needle seems to be the smallest size through which fat can be injected without serious damage to the integrity of the fat cell membrane.

Fat has been used in the augmentation of different areas of the face including cheek-lip groove region, lips, malar and submalar area, chin, glabella region, and areas of localized hemiatrophy (Fig. 38-6). Transplanted fat is rarely associated with any significant tissue reaction. Marques and others[34] found that after 180 days of injecting fat into auricles of New Zealand rabbits, adipose tissue was surrounded by a discrete layer of connective tissue and the graft was populated by many fat cells with preserved architecture. The inflammatory reaction consisted mainly of macrophages and giant cells containing large vacuoles filled with lipid. After 360 days the percentage volume of fat cells found was 14% to 45%, depending on the technique.[34]

Irradiated cartilage homograft

Irradiated homografts of costal cartilage were obtained from young human donors who were treated for possible transmitted diseases. Exposing the specimens to a radiation

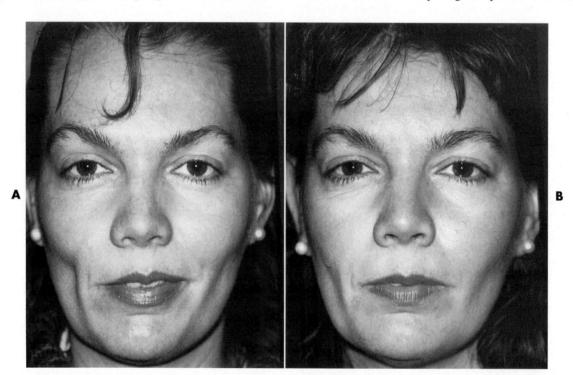

Fig. 38-6. A, Patient with history of atrophy of right buccal region after injection of absorbable implant. **B,** Seven months after fat transfer. Note the natural correction of her depression.

dose ranging from 30,000 to 60,000 Gy results in destruction of tissue antigenicity.[31] Insertion of such grafts in subdermal layers results in a minimal inflammatory reaction. Conflicting reports about the degree of resorption are present. The main use of irradiated homografts has been for augmentation rhinoplasty. Dingman and Grabb[12] reported 600 cases with an 11-year follow-up. Their conclusion was that minimal resorption occurs. Welling[65] reported 65% resorption after 9 years and 100% resorption after 15 years. The main disadvantages of this material include potential transmission of viral disorders, possibility of graft warping, lack of adherence of this graft to some of the underlying skeletal tissue resulting in mobility, and the risk of infection. Irradiated cartilage homograft is readily available, provides good structural support, and can be easily carved.

CLINICAL APPLICATIONS

Table 38-2 summarizes current trends in choices of material for facial contouring.

Forehead

Bony defects of the forehead may be caused by a congenital anomaly, traumatic loss of the frontal bone, resection of the frontal bone, or frontal sinusitis with loss of anterior or posterior table caused by osteomyelitis.

The choice of an implant material for forehead reconstruction is highly individualized. The location of the frontal sinus, degree of pneumatization, relation of the mucosa to the current defect, and history of previous infection should

Table 38-2. Current trends in facial augmentation

Part of face	Material used to augment
Forehead	Bone
	Methylmethacrylate
	Hydroxyapatite
Cheek	
Skeletal	Bone
	Silastic
	Hydroxyapatite
Soft tissue	Fat
	Collagen
	GoreTex
Orbit	Bone
	Titanium mesh
Auricle	Rib cartilage
Nose	Cartilage
	Bone
	GoreTex
	Silastic
Lips	Fat
	Collagen
	GoreTex
Chin	Silastic
Mandible	

be considered and carefully analyzed before attempting to reconstruct a forehead defect. Separation of the mucosal lining from the site of reconstruction is an essential part of the surgical planning. Insertion of bone grafts or implants into a bed containing mucosal elements predisposes the area to infection (Fig. 38-7).

If the defect to be reconstructed includes the posterior table of the frontal sinus, it is preferable to remove all mucosal elements using a burr and a microscope. Attempts are usually made to plug the frontonasal duct with bone chips, muscle, or fascia grafts. Fat obliteration is usually helpful in maintaining the separation from the nasal cavity. If the size of the defect is small and does not allow for good visualization of all portions of the sinuses, an osteoplastic anterior flap to open the entire anterior wall should be performed.

When the defect to be reconstructed involves the anterior table only, obliteration of the frontal sinus and plugging of the frontonasal duct is not usually necessary. In these cases it is best to maintain the patency of the duct and reconstruct the defect with an onlay bone graft.[33]

Merville, Brunet, and Derome[35] recommended a two-stage procedure in patients with histories of extensive infection and loss of frontal bone. These recommendations were (1) the removal of all sinus elements and isolation of the nasal cavity, with iliac cancellous bone grafts used to reconstruct the supraorbital area; and (2) later reconstruction of the frontal bone with irradiated bank bone graft.

The use of autogenous bone grafts has been associated with a significant incidence of resorption and subsequent recurrence of the defect. According to Marchac,[33] "alloplastic materials are considered for an overlay on a deformed bone and for cranial vault cranioplasties in carefully selected cases."

Munro and Guyron[36] believe that "there is no place for alloplastic materials." Their first choice is autogenous bone. They state that alloplastic material is contraindicated if the defect is adjacent to or involves the nose or paranasal sinuses, if there is a history of infection, and in cases where there is deficient soft tissue coverage. Acrylic (methylmethacrylate) is the most commonly used alloplastic material by neurosurgeons. Berghaus, Muleh, and Handrock[3] used Porecron, a porous polyethylene implant, for certain forehead reconstructions. This material is porous with a pore size of approximately 150 μm, allowing ingrowth of fibrous tissue.

Malar and submalar region

The contours of the malar and submalar regions dominate the middle third of the face. Surgeons who deal with facial contouring realize the importance of these defining elements of the middle of the face. This definition is usually a balance between the dimensions of the zygoma, malar eminence, and the overlying soft tissue. Perhaps the most important feature of the cheek is a malar highlight, noted on the skull as a

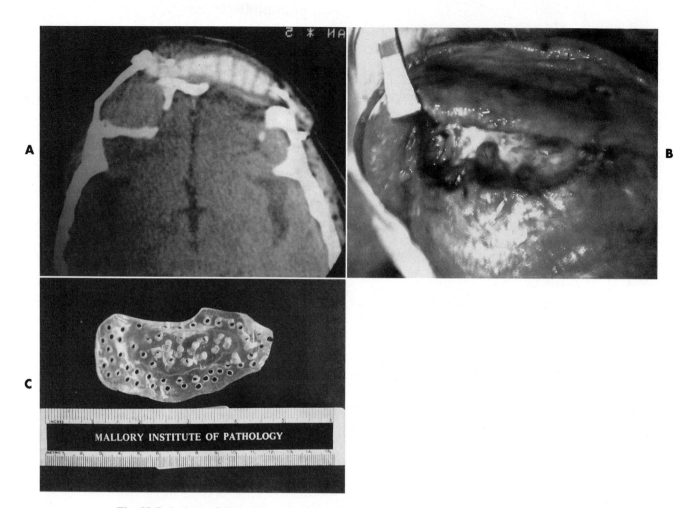

Fig. 38-7. Patient referred with recurrence of frontal sinus mucocele around acrylic implant that was positioned to fill defects in the frontal sinus. **A,** Computed tomography scan showing recurrence of infection around implant. **B,** Site of implant bed after evaluation of mucocele. View through bicoronal approach. **C,** Acrylic implant after removal.

long triangle with its base corresponding to the zygomatico-maxillary suture.[59] The transition from the zygomatic to the maxillary bony components is acute. This transition is not reflected on the outside facial contour of the thick soft tissue coverage in the central portion of the face. During the aging process, subcutaneous atrophy predisposes to grooving of the central portion because of lack of adequate bony support. Terino[58] discusses the use of a "zonal anatomy" when planning a malar augmentation. Careful examination of the bony structure of the middle third of the face shows that it is divided into two areas: (1) the malar and zygomatic complex, consisting of the area between the zygomaticomaxillary suture line and the zygomaticotemporal suture line; and (2) the infraorbital complex, consisting of the space between the medial and lateral buttresses.

Terino uses the term *malar space,* which he divides into five architectural and functional zones: (1) zone 3 corresponds to the area of the cheek medial to the perpendicular line drawn at the level of the infraorbital foramen; (2) zone 4 corresponds to the posterior third of the zygomatic arch; (3) zone 1 corresponds to the major surface of the malar bone, including the first third of the zygomatic arch; (4) zone 2 represents the middle third of the zygomatic arch; and (5) zone 5 represents the submalar region.

Augmentation in zone 3 is rarely needed unless the patient has a posttraumatic deformity. Zone 4 is a dangerous zone to perform surgery on because of its proximity to the frontal branch of the facial nerve and the capsule of the temporomandibular joint. Zone 2 augmentation increases the width of the upper third of the face. Zone 1 augmentation increases the projection of the malar eminence area (Fig. 38-8). Extension of the augmentation to involve zone 5 or the "submalar" zone results in a fuller cheek in the inferior projection.

The method of placing an implant in the cheek region depends on the deformity to be corrected. A careful analysis

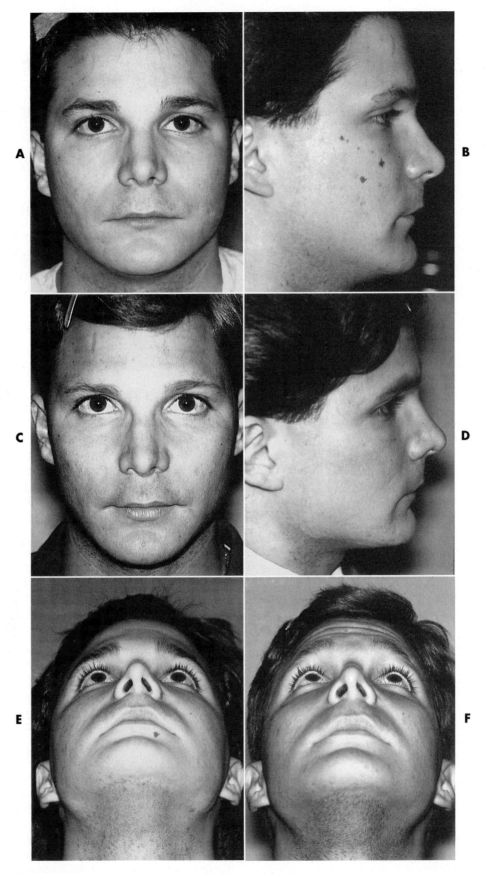

Fig. 38-8. Malar augmentation. **A,** Preoperative face view. **B,** Preoperative right profile with marking delineating anterior and posterior points of implant placement. **C,** Postoperative face view. **D,** Postoperative right profile. **E,** Preoperative base view. **F,** Postoperative base view.

731

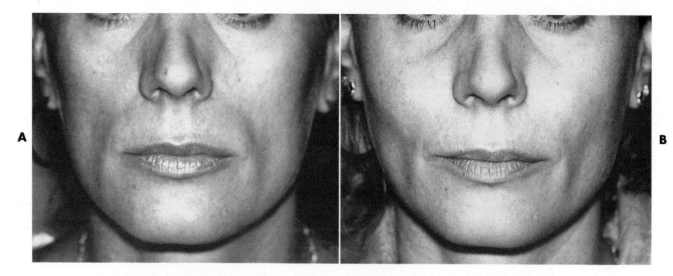

Fig. 38-9. A, Marked hollowing with flattening of submalar area. **B,** View after submalar augmentation.

of implant shapes and the contour of the cheek region, as well as the patient's expectations, need to be addressed. Different types of implants have been developed. The choice of the implant depends on the deformity to be corrected as well as the cheek contour that is desired. The presence of deep malar grooving or midfacial depression necessitates the use of an implant type that will address this deformity since augmentation of the malar eminence area might only result in exaggeration of the deformity (Fig. 38-9).

By using submalar augmentation as stressed by Binder,[5] the appearance of hollowing in the midface is improved. The author prefers the placement of these implants in a more posterolateral position to decrease the prominence of the cheek mound since the area of maximal projection in the central portion of the cheek is posterolateral to the cheek mound area.

Different surgical approaches are used for insertion of cheek implants. The author most often uses the intraoral approach. Occasionally the author uses the transconjunctival or blepharoplasty approach for the correction of cheek asymmetries caused by facial fractures associated with floor-of-orbit injuries. The author rarely uses the rhytidectomy approach because of the increased possibility of injury to facial nerve branches.

Chin implants

Establishing a balanced profile between the nose and chin improves facial harmony. A well-defined inferior border of the chin, with a smooth contour between the parasymphysis and body of the mandible, is an essential part of chin augmentation. This requires the use of implants that provide increased projection not only in the symphysis and parasym-

physeal areas but also in the anteroinferior third of the body of the mandible.

The size of the implant is determined with the patient's face positioned so that Frankfort's plane is horizontal. The patient is asked to close the mouth until the teeth are in their most comfortable occlusion and the lips are gently touching each other. The most practical guide for judging the amount of anteroposterior projection desired is the number of millimeters of implant material required to move the retruding chin pad forward until it sits just behind a vertical line dropped from the vermilion border of the lower lip. Obviously, sex, height, and the general facial features of the patient play important roles in the judgment. In women the chin profile is put 2 to 4 mm posterior to the vertical line dropped from the vermilion border.[61]

Once the anteroposterior dimension has been selected, the patient is evaluated from the front. A decision is then made as to how far laterally the implant must go to allow a gradual blending of the augmented chin into the cheeks. The mental nerve foramen is usually located 27 mm or more from the midline. If the implant is to extend over 25 mm, attention should be made to position the implant along the inferior border of the mandible and inferior to the mental foramen.

The incision for introduction of the implant may be made intraorally or externally at the junction of the chin and submental regions. The external incision rarely needs to be longer than 15 to 20 mm. Intraoral incisions are usually made on the posterior surface of the lip, 4 mm from the inferior labial fornix.

The author commonly uses the external or submental approach. After exposure of periosteum anteriorly, vertical in-

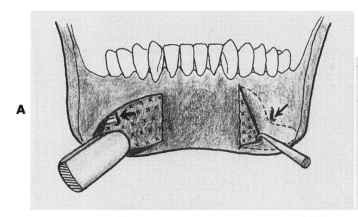

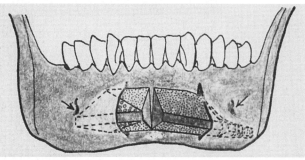

Fig. 38-10. A, Midline periosteum not elevated. Vertical incisions lateral to midline (*X*). **B,** Positioning of implant in periosteal pocket laterally and overlying periosteum in midline. (From Webster RC and others: Chin augmentation: subperiosteal and supraperiosteal implants, *Aesthetic Plast Surg* 1:149, 1977.© New York, 1977, Springer-Verlag. By permission.)

cisions are made through periosteum 10 to 18 mm from the midline (Fig. 38-10). With the surgeon using direct vision, an elevator lifts the periosteum lateral to the incisions along the inferior border of the mandible, avoiding the mental nerve. The size of the subperiosteal pockets created depends on the dimensions of the implant. After placement of the implants in the created pockets, they are fixed to the periosteum in the midline using a permanent long-lasting suture. The central portions of the implants rest anterior to the periosteum, and the lateral portions rest deep to it. The author believes that insertion of the central portion of the implant anterior to periosteum might decrease the rate of bone erosion (Fig. 38-11). Preformed implants can be inserted in a similar fashion into pockets prepared as described. The more flexible implants can be folded through the same incisions in such a way as to slip between the roof above and the shelf below and deep to the periosteum laterally. The author finds carving to be a simple procedure that allows precise tailoring of the implants to the aesthetic need (Figs. 38-12 and 38-13). Gel implants have been associated with distortion and asymmetry secondary to capsular contractures (Fig. 38-14).

Nasal implants

The use of alloplastic material for nasal augmentation is popular in the Far East and Japan.[1] Different shapes of Silastic implants have been used to provide dorsal and tip projections. Such alloplastic materials are associated with complications such as extrusion, displacement, and infection, particularly when used under scarred tissues as in revision or when used as ''pushers'' or projectors of the tip. The author prefers the use of autogenous cartilage or bone grafts for augmentation of the nasal dorsum and tip, especially in revisional rhinoplasties. Many recent reports have described the use of GoreTex for augmentation of the nasal dorsum.

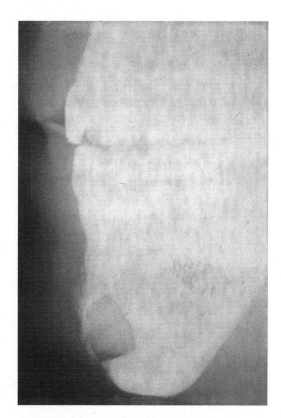

Fig. 38-11. Resorption secondary to chin augmentation. Note the degree of erosion of implant into mandible.

The incidence of infection of this implant has been less than 4% in different series. The use of this type of implant for dorsal augmentation is relatively safe, especially when compared with complications of nasal Silastic implants.

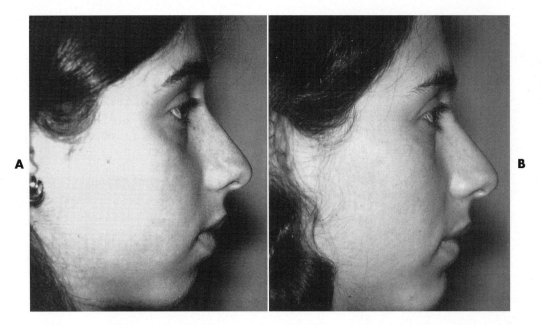

Fig. 38-12. A, Micrognathia with chin retrusion. **B,** Six months after insertion of chin implant.

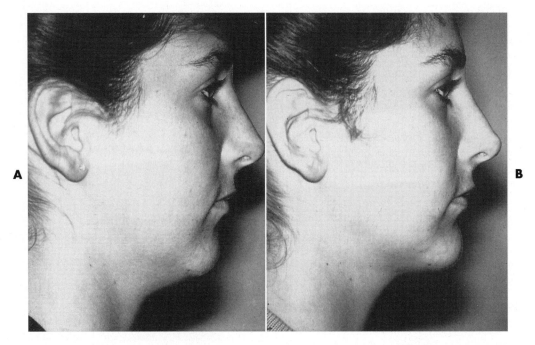

Fig. 38-13. A, Microgenia with excess fat deposition in neck. **B,** The view after chin augmentation and liposuction to submental and submandibular area.

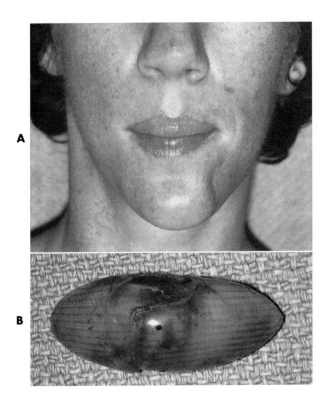

Fig. 38-14. A, Gel chin implant with associated asymmetry and distortion. **B,** Note the shape of implant removed.

REFERENCES

1. Adams JS: Grafts and implants in nasal augmentation: a rational approach to material selection, *Otolaryngol Clin North Am* 20:913, 1987.
2. Ashley FL and others: The present status of silicone fluid in soft tissue augmentation, *Plast Reconstr Surg* 39:411, 1967.
3. Berghaus A, Muleh G, Handrock M: Porous polyethylene and proplast: their behaviour in a bony implant bed, *Arch Oto Rhino Laryngology* 240:115, 1984.
4. Bikhazi HB, VanAntwerp R: The use of Medpor in cosmetic reconstructive surgery: experimental and clinical evidence. In Stucker F, editor: Plastic and reconstructive surgery of the head and neck. Proceedings of the Fifth International Symposium, Philadelphia, 1991, Mosby.
5. Binder WJ: Submaler augmentation, *Arch Otolaryngol Head Neck Surg* 115:797, 1989.
6. Boyne PJ and others: Evaluation of a ceramic hydroxyapatite in femoral defects, *J Dent Res* 57:108, 1978.
7. Brown BL, Neal HB, Kern SB: Implants of superficial Proplast, Plastipore, and Silastic, *Arch Otolaryngol Head Neck Surg* 105:605, 1979.
8. Colton J, Beekhuis GJ: Mersilene mesh in nasal and facial augmentation. In Stucker F, editor: Plastic and reconstructive surgery of the head and neck. Proceedings of the Fifth International Symposium, Philadelphia, 1991, Mosby.
9. Costantino PD, Freidman CD, Lane A: Synthetic biomaterial in facial plastic surgery, *Plast Reconstr Surg* 9:1, 1993.
10. Cullum PE, Frost DE, Newland TB: Evaluation of hydroxyapatite in repair of alveolar clefts in dogs, *J Maxillofacial Surg* 46:290, 1988.
11. Dickinson JT, Jaquiss GW: Alloplastic implants 1972, *Otolaryngol Clin North Am* 5:441, 1972.
12. Dingman RO, Grabb WC: Costal cartilage homografts preserved by irradiation, *Plast Reconstr Surg* 28:562, 1961.
13. Foussereau J, Laugier P: Allergic eczemas from metallic foreign bodies, *Transactions of the St John Hospital Dermatological Society* 52:220, 1966.
14. Frisch EE, Langley NR: *Biodurability evaluation of medical-grade high performance silicone elastomer.* In Fraker AC, Griffin CD, editors: Corrosion and degradation of implant materials: Second symposium ASTM, STP859, Philadelphia, 1985, American Society for Testing and Materials.
15. Grower MF and others: Bone inductive potential of biogradable ceramic Millipore filter chambers, *J Dent Res* 57:108, 1978.
16. Hamblen DL, Carter RL: Sarcoma and joint replacement, *Am J Bone Joint Surg* 66:625, 1984.
17. Harris HI: Survey of breast implants from the point of view of carcinogenesis, *Plast Reconstr Surg* 28:81, 1961.
18. Hayes AW: *Principles and methods of toxicology,* New York, 1982, Raven Press.
19. Hoar TB, Mears DC: Corrosion resistant alloys in chloride solutions: materials for surgical implants, *Proc R Soc Lond*, series A, 1966.
20. Holmes R: *Alloplastic implants.* In McCarthy JG, editor: *Plastic surgery,* vol 1, Philadelphia, 1990, WB Saunders.
21. Holt GR, Parel S, Branemark PI: Osteointegrated titanium implants, *Facial Plast Surg* 3:113–124, 1986.
22. Homsy LA, Anderson MS: *Functional stabilization of soft tissue and bone prosthesis with a porous low modulus materials system.* In Biocompatibility of implant materials, Tunbridge Wells, Kent, England, 1976, Sector Publishing.
23. Hueper WC: Cancer induction by polyurethane and polysiloxane plastics, *J Natl Cancer Inst* 33:1005, 1965.
24. Hueper WC: Experimental studies in metal carcinogenesis. I. Nickel careers in rats, *Tex Rep Biol Med* 10:167, 1952.
25. Hurley JV: *Acute inflammation,* ed 2, Edinburgh, 1983, Churchill Livingstone.
26. Jaffe HL: *Metabolic, degenerative and inflammatory diseases of bones and joints,* Philadelphia, 1972, Lea & Febiger.
27. Jaicho M: Calcium phosphate ceramics as hand tissue prosthetics, *Clin Orthop* 157:259, 1981.
28. Kasperbauer JF, Kern EB, Neel B: Grafts and implants in rhinologic surgery: laboratory findings and clinical considerations, *Facial Plast Surg* 3:125, 1983.
29. Kent JN, Misiek DJ: *Biomaterials for cranial, facial, mandibular and TMJ reconstruction.* In Fonesca RJ, Walker RV, editors: *Oral and maxillofacial trauma,* Philadelphia, 1991, WB Saunders.
30. Kent JN, Westfall RL, Carlton DM: Chin and zygomatic-maxillary augmentation with Proplast: long term follow-up, *J Oral Surg* 39:912, 1981.
31. Kridel RWH, Homin RJ: Irradiated cartilage grafts in the nose, *Arch Otolaryngol Head Neck Surg* 119:24, 1993.
32. Luckey HA, Kubli F, editors: *Titanium alloys in surgical implants. ASTM Special Technical Publication 796,* Philadelphia, 1983, American Society for Testing and Materials.
33. Marchac D: *Deformities of the forehead, scalp, and cranial vault.* In McCarthy JG, editor: *Plastic surgery,* vol 1, Philadelphia, 1990, WB Saunders.
34. Marques A and others: Autologous fat grafts: a quantitative and morphometric study in rabbits, *Scand J Plast Reconstr Hand Surg* 28:241, 1994.
35. Merville L, Brunet C, Derome P: Reconstructive frontale et des sinus frontaux, *Ann Clin Plast* 27:205, 1982.
36. Munro IR, Guyron B: Split-rib cranioplasty, *Ann Plast Surg* 7:341, 1981.
37. Neel HB: Implants of Gore-Tex, *Arch Otolaryngol Head Neck Surg* 109:427, 1983.
38. Oppenheimer BS, Oppenheimer E, Stout AP: Sarcomas induced in rodents by embedding various plastic films, *Proc Soc Exp Biol Med* 79:366, 1952.
39. O'Quinn B, Thomas JR: The role of Silastic in malar augmentation, *Facial Plast Surg* 3:99, 1986.
40. Owsley TG, Taylor CO: The use of Goretex for nasal reconstruction:

a retrospective study using 106 patients, *Plast Reconst Surg* 2:241, 1994.

41. Penhale KW: Acrylic resin as implant for correction for facial deformities, *Arch Surg* 50:233, 1945.

42. Ptersdorf RG and others, editors: *Harrison's principles of internal medicine*, ed 10, New York, 1983, McGraw-Hill.

43. Rao WR, Boehm RF: A study of sintered apatites, *J Dent Res* 53:1351, 1974.

44. Rees TD, Ashley FL: Treatment of facial atrophy with liquid silicone, *Am J Surg* 111:531, 1966.

45. Rees TD, Ballantyne DL, Hawthorne GA: Silicone fluid research, *Plast Reconstr Surg* 46:50, 1970.

46. Rees TD, Plott J, Ballantyne DL: An investigation of cutaneous response to dimethyl polysyloxane (silicone liquid) in animals and humans: a preliminary report, *Plast Reconstr Surg* 39:411, 1967.

47. Rejda BU, Peelen JGJ, deGroot K: Tricalcium phosphate as a bone substitute, *J Bioengineering* 1:93, 1977.

48. Salyer KE, Hall CD: Porous hydroxyapatite as an onlay bone graft substitute for maxillofacial surgery, *Plast Reconstr Surg* 84:236, 1989.

49. Sauer BW, Weinstein MA, Klawitter JJ: The role of porous polmeric material in prosthetic attachment, *J Biomed Mater Res* 5 (1):145, 1974.

50. Scales JT: Discussion on metals and synthetic materials in relation to soft tissue: tissue reaction to synthetic material, *Proc R Soc Med* 45:647, 1953.

51. Schultz RC: Facial reconstruction with alloplastic material, *Surg Ann* 12:351, 1980.

52. Selmanowitz VJ, Orentrich N: Medical grade fluid silicone, *J Dermatol Surg Oncol* 3:597, 1977.

53. Silver WE: The use of alloplastic material in contouring the face, *Facial Plast Surg* 3:81, 1983.

54. Spagnoli D, Kent JN: Multicenter evaluation of temporomandibular joint Proplast-Teflon disk implant, *Oral Surg Oral Med Oral Path Oral Radiol Endod* 74(4):411, 1992.

55. Stucker FJ, Hirokawa RH, Pruet CW: The autoalloplast: an alternative in facial implantation, *Otolaryngol Clin North Am* 15:161, 1982.

56. Sutow EJ, Pollack SR: *The biocompatibility of certain stainless steels.* In Williams DF, editor: *Biocompatibility of clinical implant materials,* vol 1, Boca Raton, Fla, 1981, CRC Press.

57. Swanson AB and others: *Host reaction to silicone implants: a long-term clinical and histological study.* In Fraker AC, Griffin CD, editors: Corrosion and degradation of implant material. Second symposium, ASTM, STP859, Philadelphia, 1985, American Society for Testing and Materials.

58. Terino ED: *Malar, mandible, and chin augmentation by alioplastic techniques.* In: Ousterhout D, editor: *Aesthetic contouring of the cranial facial skeleton,* Boston, 1991, Little, Brown.

59. Tolleth K: Concepts for the plastic surgeon from art and sculpture, *Clin Plast Surg* 14:585, 1987.

60. Underwood EJ: *Trace elements in human and animal nutrition,* ed 3, New York, 1971, Academic Press.

61. Webster RC and others: Chin augmentation: subperiosteal and supraperiosteal implants, *Aesthet Plast Surg* 1:149, 1970.

62. Webster RC and others: Injectable silicone for small augmentations: twenty year experience in humans, *Am J Cosmet Surg* 1:1, 1984.

63. Webster RC and others: Rhinoplastic revisions with injectable silicone, *Arch Otolaryngol Head Neck Surg* 112:269, 1986.

64. Weinberg ED: Iron and susceptibility to infectious disease, *Science* 184:952, 1974.

65. Welling DB and others: Irradiated homologous cartilage grafts, *Arch Otolaryngol Head Neck Surg* 114:291, 1988.

66 . Williams DF: *The response of the body environments to implants.* In Williams DF, Roaf R, editors: *Implants in surgery,* London, 1973, WB Saunders.

67. Williams DF: *Preface.* In Williams DF, editor: *Biocompatibility of clinical implant materials,* vol 1, Boca Raton, Fla, 1981, CRC Press.

68. Williams DF: *The properties and clinical uses of cobalt-chromium alloys.* In Williams DF, editor: *Biocompatibility of clinical implant materials,* vol 1, Boca Raton, Fla, 1981, CRC Press.

Chapter 39

Mentoplasty

Jonathan M. Sykes
John L. Frodel

The chin prominence is not present in any four-legged mammal.[5] During evolution, with the adoption of an upright posture and with verticalization of the face, the chin became an important facial feature. The events contributing to the evolutionary development of the chin in humans are open to speculation; however, the importance of the chin in the overall appearance of the face cannot be overstated.

In general, when patients inquire about improving their facial appearance, they rarely ask about surgical correction of the chin. More commonly, requests focus on seemingly more obvious problems, such as reduction of a large nose or correction of sagging skin of the neck and jowls. However, recognition, evaluation, and treatment of chin abnormalities often has a great impact on facial appearance. It is clear that all attractive faces have an underlying balance and structural symmetry to their facial skeletons.[9] Proper balance of the facial skeleton requires harmony and proportion of all bones of the face in all three planes of space. The chin should therefore be evaluated as it relates to important adjacent structures, such as the lips, teeth, and nose.[17] Appropriate treatment of aesthetic deformities of the chin will contribute to facial harmony and will often improve the appearance of the mouth, the lips, and the nose. It is for these reasons that every face should be carefully studied in order to determine why the chin appears unattractive. This will enable the surgeon to correct the deformity and improve facial proportion.

Surgical correction of aesthetic deformities of the chin can be performed by either chin augmentation with an implant, or by osteotomy and advancement (or reduction) of the bony mentum. Augmentation using alloplastic implants can camouflage a horizontal (anterior-posterior [A-P]) bony deficiency.[19] However, this technique is not effective in correcting vertical (superior-inferior) or transverse deformities of the lower face and chin. Horizontal bony osteotomy of the chin (osseous genioplasty) is a simple and versatile procedure. This technique allows horizontal advancement or reduction of the chin, vertical lengthening or shortening of the chin, and correction of transverse deformities of the chin. The procedure chosen to correct the specific aesthetic problem is based on the type and extent of the deformity[17] (Table 39-1). If carefully evaluated and planned, aesthetic correction of chin deformities can provide significant improvement in the overall balance and proportion of the face.

PATIENT EVALUATION

In order to precisely correct any chin deformity, careful preoperative analysis of the deformity is essential.[17,18] Specifically, the chin should be evaluated as it relates to other skeletal and soft-tissue structures, including the lips, teeth, nose, and soft tissues of the neck. A detailed history of past trauma, orthodontic treatment, or prior oral surgery is essential. This is important because many patients with dental malocclusion and underlying facial skeletal abnormalities are treated with orthodontics. This method of dental compensation may correct the malocclusion, but fails to improve the underlying skeletal deformity. It is therefore important to discuss prior therapy, including orthodontics, with the patient.

Physical examination should include inspection and palpation of the chin, lips, nose, and teeth. The entire face should be observed at rest and during animation to evaluate the mentalis soft-tissue mound and its support. With aging, patients may develop ptosis of the soft-tissue pad of the chin. In patients with open bite deformities and lip incompetence, hyperactivity of the mentalis muscles (''mentalis strain'') may occur (Fig. 39-1 *A, B*). For this reason, the dental occlusion should be carefully examined to determine if orthodontics or orthognathic surgery is needed.

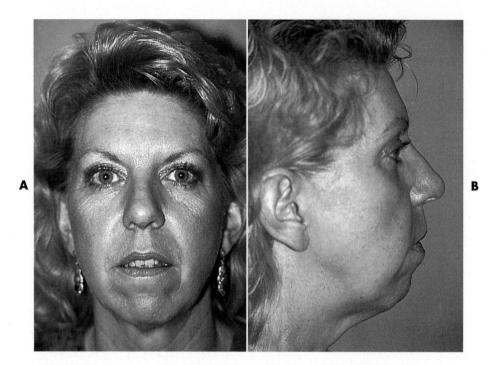

Fig. 39-1. A and **B,** Anterior-posterior and lateral photograph of a patient with posterior vertical maxillary access and an open bite deformity. Note the mentalis strain caused by the patient trying to close her lips at rest.

Table 39-1. Mentoplasty procedures

Horizontal (anterior-posterior)	Deformity **Vertical**	**Transverse**	**Procedure**
D	N or sl D	N	Chin implant or genioplasty
D	E	N	Genioplasty (advancement with possible ostectomy if significant vertical excess)
D	D	N	Bony advancement (with downgrafting for chin lengthening)
N	N	Asymmetric	Bony osteotomy (with resection of downgrafting)
E	N	N	Bony osteotomy (with setback)
E	E	N	Bony osteotomy (with ostectomy)

Modified from Sykes J, Frodel J: Genioplasty, *Op Tech Otolaryng* 6:319.
D—Deficient; E—Excessive; N—Normal; sl—Slight.

The evaluation of all patients for possible chin surgery should include consistent and reproducible clinical photographs in three views: A-P (frontal), lateral (profile), and oblique. These photographs allow analysis of the contour and projection of the chin as it relates to the lips, nose, labiomental groove, and soft tissues of the neck. If the physical evaluation and clinical photographs show a minor deformity requiring augmentation with an alloplast, radiographs of the chin are usually not necessary. However, if the deformity is more complex, (e.g., vertical chin excess with horizontal deficiency or transverse bony asymmetry), radiographic analysis is essential.

Radiographic evaluation of the chin routinely includes a panoramic radiograph (Panorex) and cephalometric radiographs in the A-P and lateral views. The panoramic radiograph shows the cortical outline of the mandible and the vertical mandibular height (Fig. 39-2). The Panorex also delineates the position of the tooth roots and of the inferior alveolar canals and mental foramina. The exact position of the mental foramen and canal are important to know preoperatively, in order to prevent intraoperative damage to the mental nerve. The inferior alveolar nerve, a branch of the third division of the fifth (trigeminal) cranial nerve, travels through the mandibular canal and exits the mental foramen

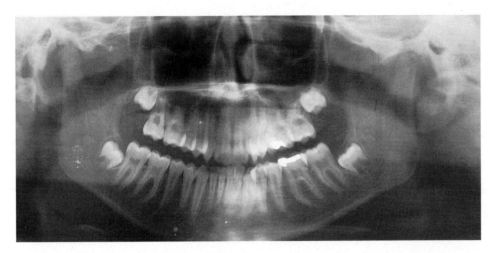

Fig. 39-2. Panoramic radiograph.

as the mental nerve. The mental nerve supplies sensation to the skin and mucous membranes of the lower lip and chin. The mandibular canal is often located 2 to 3 mm below the level of the mental foramen.[5] Bony osteotomies should therefore be performed at least 5 mm below the mental foramen, to avoid injury to the neurovascular bundle.

If bony genioplasty is considered, A-P and lateral cephalometric radiographs should be performed (Fig. 39-3). A-P views allow detection and evaluation of transverse skeletal asymmetries of the chin. Transverse asymmetries are common in patients with Goldenhar's syndrome or hemifacial microsomia, but are also commonly seen in nonsyndromic patients considering aesthetic surgery. When transverse bony or soft-tissue asymmetries are overlooked preoperatively in the patient with microgenia, augmentation with an alloplastic chin implant may accentuate the deformity.[17]

Lateral cephalometric radiographs allow detailed analysis of both the soft tissues and the facial skeleton. The cephalogram should be obtained at a standard distance with the head positioned so that the Frankfort horizontal line is parallel to the floor.[13] From this standardized lateral radiograph, a series of soft tissue and skeletal points can be identified. This allows various analyses of the chin as described by Ricketts,[14] Steiner,[16] Burstone,[2] Gonzalez-Ulloa and Stevens,[4] and others. Ricketts' analysis (Fig. 39-4) uses a tangent connecting the soft-tissue pogonion (most projecting point) of the chin with the most projecting point of the nasal tip.[14] In this system, the upper lip should lie about 4 mm behind the line, while the lower lip is ideally located 2 mm behind the line. While the Ricketts analysis correctly evaluates the lower face in profile, it places great importance on the projection of the nasal tip. The Steiner analysis uses the columellar inflection point *(s)* to identify the correct position for the chin point.[16] This method places importance on the lip position. The Holdaway "H" angle (Fig. 39-5) relates the position of the soft-tissue pogonion with important skeletal points on the mid- and lower face. No single analysis is

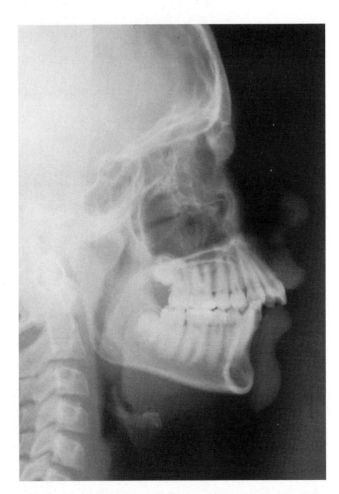

Fig. 39-3. Lateral cephalometric radiograph showing the bony and soft-tissue outline of a patient with a class II malocclusion and mild open bite deformity.

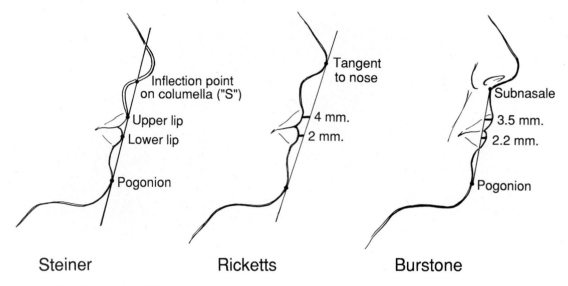

Fig. 39-4. Steiner, Ricketts, and Burstone analysis of the ideal relationship of the chin as it relates to the lips and other lower facial structures.

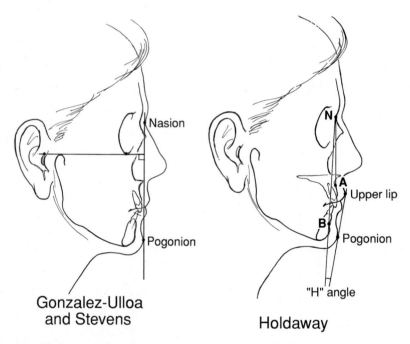

Fig. 39-5. The Gonzalez-Ulloa and Stevens and the Holdaway analyses of the chin and lower third of the face.

ideal, but each method attempts to determine the "ideal" positions for the soft tissues and skeleton of the chin, as these structures relate to the remainder of the face.

An accurate chin analysis using the lateral cephalogram involves dropping a vertical line from the Frankfort horizontal (porion-infraorbitale) through the soft tissue subnasale.[7] With ideal horizontal chin projection, the soft-tissue pogonion should lie approximately 4 mm behind this line (Fig.

39-6). The most frequently used evaluation of the chin drops a perpendicular line from the vermillion border of the lower lip and compares the A-P position of this line with the soft-tissue pogonion (the anterior-most projecting chin point) (Fig. 39-7). A general guideline for aesthetic chin position in this method is for the pogonion in a male patient to be positioned at the level of this vertical line, and for the pogonion in a female patient to be just posterior to the line. If the

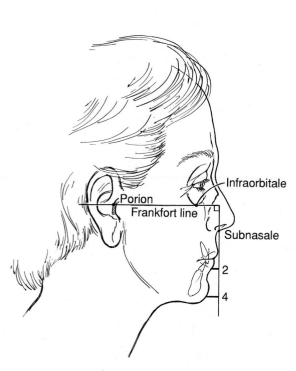

Fig. 39-6. Horizontal relationships of the chin and upper and lower lips as they relate to the nasale perpendicular line.

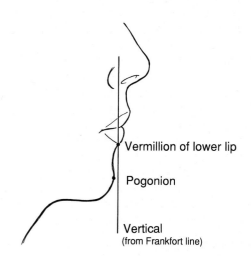

Fig. 39-7. The relationship of the chin position to a perpendicular passing through the vermillion border of the lower lip.

position of the soft-tissue pogonion is anterior to the proposed line, horizontal *macrogenia* is diagnosed, while *microgenia* is present if the chin is positioned posterior to the ideal line. Although this method is effective for A-P deformities (microgenia or macrogenia), it does not account for vertical or transverse discrepancies. Since many surgeons primarily use this evaluation method, vertical or transverse chin problems are often overlooked.

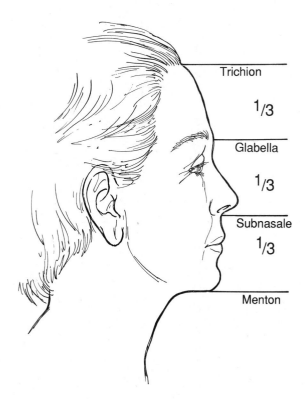

Fig. 39-8. Vertical heights (thirds) of the face.

Analysis of vertical facial heights also is essential in determining the appropriate heights of the lower facial third and the chin. Various methods for evaluating vertical facial heights have been used. The simplest technique involves division of the face into three equal thirds: the upper third, from the frontal hairline to the glabella; the middle third, from the glabella to the soft-tissue subnasale; and the lower third, from the subnasale to the menton (the lowest point of the chin) (Fig. 39-8). Because frontal hairline may vary significantly, an alternate method described by Powell and Humphreys[11] more accurately analyzes the vertical heights of the lower two thirds of the face. This method describes the middle third as the distance from the nasion to the subnasale, and the lower third as the distance from the subnasale to the menton (Fig. 39-9). The middle third distance in this analysis ideally represents 43% of the total height of the lower two thirds of the face,

$$\text{i.e.,} \quad \frac{\text{nasion-subnasale}}{\text{nasion-menton}} = .43,$$

while the lower third distance should approximate 57% of the total vertical height.

Other analyses of the vertical dimensions of the face have been described. One method includes inspection of the face in repose, when the maxillary incisor teeth should show 0 to 3 mm (Fig. 39-10). If more than 3 mm of the maxillary incisors are visible at rest, excessive facial length (usually in the midface) is sometimes present. Additional analysis of

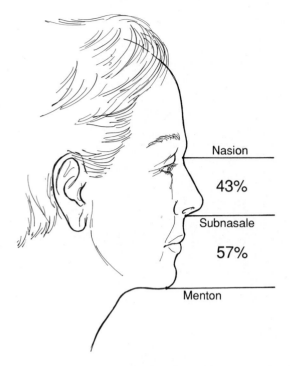

Fig. 39-9. Vertical relationship of the face without accounting for the upper facial one third.

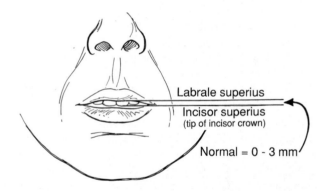

Fig. 39-10. Schematic diagram of incisor show of the maxillary teeth. A normal relationship would be 0 to 3 mm of central incisor visible.

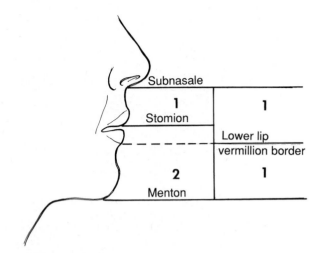

Fig. 39-11. Vertical relationships of the lower one third of the face.

the lower face includes subdividing the lower one third of the face. Two methods exist for subdivision of lower facial heights. The first includes a vertical third from subnasale to upper lip stomion and two thirds from upper lip stomion to the menton (Fig. 39-11). The second method divides the lower third into two equal parts, from the subnasale to the vermillion border of the lower lip and from the lower lip vermillion border to the menton. All of these analyses relate the height of the chin and lower face to the total facial height. In complex chin deformities, a vertical discrepancy as well as a horizontal deficiency or excess may often be present.

Another parameter that should be assessed is symmetry in the sagittal plane. Transverse asymmetries of the chin exist in many patients with congenital anomalies (Goldenhar's syndrome, hemifacial microsomia) or in patients who have had significant skeletal facial trauma. However, many patients with only aesthetic concerns have minor, but definite transverse asymmetries of the chin. In patients with assymetry of the facial midline, chin augmentation with an implant may correct the horizontal deficiency but accentuate the skeletal asymmetry. A-P cephalometric radiographs allow a comparison of the bony midline of the chin with the dental midlines of the maxilla and the mandible. If the skeletal and soft-tissue midline of the chin are not aligned with the dental midlines and with the upper facial skeletal midline (e.g., nasion), an asymmetric bony genioplasty or chin implant may be performed.

Each of the systems of analysis relates the soft-tissue pogonion with other facial structures. No single method provides comprehensive evaluation of the chin, but each allows a reference for assessing the bony and soft tissues of the chin and lower face. Using a variety of methods, appropriate evaluation of chin deformities can be achieved.

CHIN DEFORMITIES

Deformities of the chin and lower face may be related to either bony abnormalities or to soft-tissue malposition. The chin should be analyzed in all three planes of space: horizontal (A-P), vertical (superior-inferior), and transverse. The horizontal and vertical dimensions may each be deficient, normal, or excessive. Simple deformities such as mild horizontal chin deficiency (microgenia), are easily corrected using either an implant or bony advancement. More complex deformities, such as a patient with horizontal deficiency and vertical excess, usually require horizontal osteotomy for adequate correction.[12]

Soft-tissue deformities of the chin and submental region

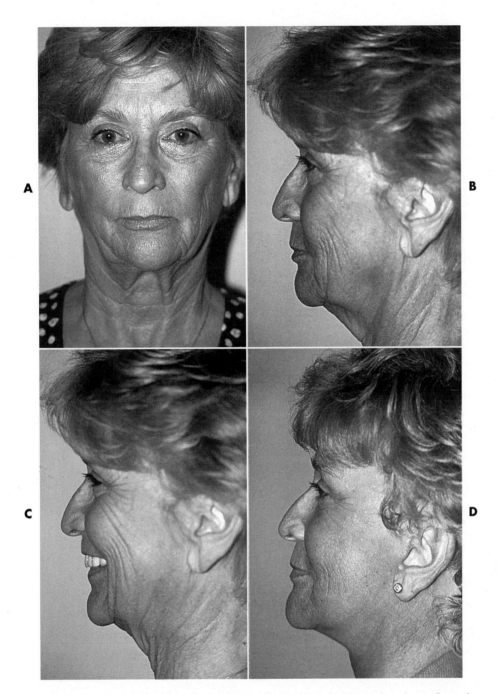

Fig. 39-12. **A** to **C,** Anterior-posterior lateral and smiling lateral preoperative views of a patient with senile ptosis of the chin. Note the deepened submental crease when smiling. **D,** Postoperative lateral view after deep plane facelift and soft-tissue correction of the ptotic mentalis pad.

also exist. Ptosis of the soft tissues of the chin often accompanies other signs of facial aging. This condition, commonly called a *witch's chin* or *senile chin deformity*, is caused by a weakening of the muscular attachments of the mentalis and depressor labii inferioris muscles. In this deformity, the soft-tissue pad of the chin falls below the mandibular line, and a deep horizontal crease develops in the submental region. Descent of the soft tissue chin pad is accentuated with smiling (Fig. 39-12 *A* to *C*). This deformity can be inadvert-

ently created or worsened surgically if the mentalis muscles are not reapproximated while inserting a chin implant (Fig. 39-12, *D*).

PROCEDURE SELECTION

The selection of the best procedure to correct a given deformity of the chin should be based on the type and extent of the deformity (see Table 39-1). Augmentation of the chin with an alloplastic implant is a simple and effective method of correcting a horizontal chin deficiency. This technique is limited by the availability of various sizes and shapes of alloplastic implants. An infinite number of shapes and sizes of implants may be required. However, most implants are manufactured in only three or four sizes and one or two shapes. Additionally, chin augmentation with implants is less effective in patients with significant vertical discrepancies (vertical excess or deficiency). Placement of an implant in such a patient may exacerbate the vertical excess and make the chin appear longer. For these reasons, implant augmentation is an effective method of camouflage for minor chin deformities, but may not be satisfactory for complex deformities.

Osteotomy of the bony mentum (osseous genioplasty) is a versatile and reliable procedure for correcting a variety of skeletal chin deformities. First described by Hofer in 1942,[6] this technique involves horizontal osteotomy and downfracture of the chin, with repositioning and fixation of the distal segment. Osseous genioplasty allows advancement or retrusion in the A-P direction, as well as lengthening or shortening in the vertical direction.[3,15,20] Additionally, the genioplasty procedure provides an approach for correction of transverse asymmetries of the chin. Although customized chin implants can be made to correct chin asymmetries, preformed implants are usually symmetrical.

Correction of soft-tissue ptosis has been described by Peterson[10] and other authors. The technique involves the removal of an ellipse of submental skin, creation of a flap of chin soft tissue, and advancement and plication of the soft-tissue flap inferiorly. This technique tightens the soft-tissue pad and obliterates the horizontal submental crease. However, the soft-tissue pogonion is effectively moved posteriorly, and some form of simultaneous augmentation (implant or bony advancement) is usually required.

SURGICAL TECHNIQUE: CHIN IMPLANT

In order to assure precise midline placement of the chin implant, the midline of the chin, lower lip, and neck (thyroid cartilage) are marked externally prior to the infiltration of local anesthesia. A mental nerve block is then performed using xylocaine 1% with epinephrine 1:100,000. Additional infiltration of anesthesia into the submental region, the gingivolabial sulcus, and the central portion of the lower lip and chin is performed to assure adequate anesthesia and vasoconstriction.

Either an intraoral or external (submental) incision and approach may be used to place a chin implant. If an extraoral approach is used, an incision (approximately 2 to 3 cm) is made in the submental crease and carried through the dermis and subcutaneous fat (Fig. 39-13 A, B). The mentalis muscles are then divided to enter a dissection plane just superficial to the periosteum of the anterior face of the mandible. The chin implant may be placed in either the subperiosteal or the supraperiosteal plane. The advantage of placing an implant beneath the periosteum is improved fixation of the

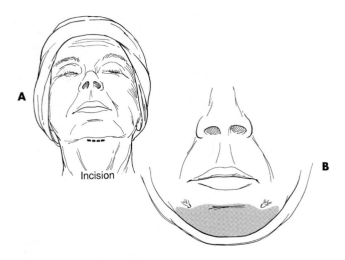

Fig. 39-13. A, Horizontal submental incision in the crease for placement of a chin implant. **B,** Schematic diagram indicating the extent of dissection (*stippled area*) for placement of a chin implant.

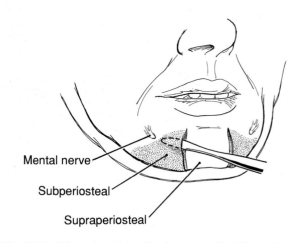

Fig. 39-14. Dissection planes for placement of a chin implant with the central dissection being supraperiosteal and the lateral pockets in the subperiosteal plane.

implant. However, subperiosteal placement has been shown to result in some erosion of the anterior mandible. For these reasons, most surgeons advocate dissection in the supraperiosteal plane centrally, with subperiosteal placement laterally (Fig. 39-14). This will theoretically minimize mandibular erosion, while maximally fixing the implant.

Many sizes, shapes, and types of implants have been used for chin augmentation. In general, the two shapes of implants are the central "button" implant, or the extended "anatomical" implant. Longer tapered implants have the advantages of being able to be placed in the subperiosteal plane laterally and they allow for lateral mandibular augmentation (Fig. 39-15). Most importantly, extended implants have the advantage of not being as apparent, if 1 to 2 mm of displacement occurs. Smaller central implants are more obvious, if slight postoperative displacement of the implant occurs.

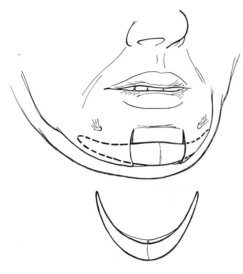

Fig. 39-15. Lateral subperiosteal placement of an extended alloplastic chin implant.

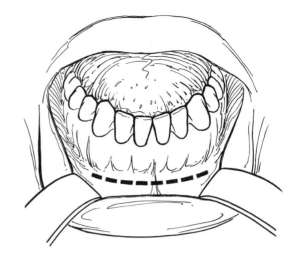

Fig. 39-16. Schematic diagram of a horizontal gingivolabial incision for bony genioplasty.

During the lateral subperiosteal dissection, the mental nerves should be identified and preserved. The implant should be placed along the inferior border of the mandible. If the implant extends laterally beyond the mental foramina, it should be positioned below the exit of the mental nerve (see Fig. 39-15). After placement of the implant, the mentalis muscles should be reapproximated and the soft tissue resuspended meticulously. If the mentalis muscle is not carefully realigned, postoperative ptosis of the soft tissues of the chin may occur. Closure of the mentalis muscle is performed with a No. 4.0 braided absorbable suture. The subcutaneous tissues and dermis are reapproximated with a No. 5.0 chromic suture, followed by skin closure with interrupted No. 6.0 monofilament nonabsorbable suture. A secure chin strap dressing is placed for 3 days to assure immobility of the implant. Perioperative antibiotics are used for 48 hours.

If an intraoral approach is used, the gingivolabial incision may be either horizontal or vertical. In either case, dissection through the mentalis muscles again occurs with placement of the implant in a supraperiosteal plane centrally and a subperiosteal pocket laterally. Closure is accomplished in two layers with the muscle closure achieving soft-tissue resuspension. A chin strap dressing is used for 3 days to secure the position of the implant.

SURGICAL TECHNIQUE: OSSEOUS GENIOPLASTY

Horizontal bony osteotomy of the chin (osseous genioplasty) is a versatile procedure that can be performed under general anesthesia or intravenous sedation with mentalis nerve block. If general anesthesia is used, nasotracheal intubation is preferred; however, if rhinoplasty is to be performed with the genioplasty, orotracheal intubation should be used.

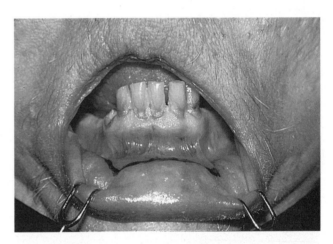

Fig. 39-17. Marking on cadaver illustrating the gingivolabial incision not in the crease to facilitate later closure.

A gingivolabial incision is made from one canine tooth to the other (Figs. 39-16 and 39-17). The incision is made on the labial side of the gingivolabial sulcus to allow an adequate mucoperiosteal soft-tissue cuff for wound closure. Dissection is then carried through the soft tissues and mandibular periosteum. Subperiosteal dissection is performed laterally with identification and preservation of both mental nerves (Figs. 39-18 and 39-19). A small inferior segment of soft tissue is preserved over the central segment (bony mentum) of the mandible to provide vascular supply to the distal segment after osteotomy.[1]

After the lateral subperiosteal dissection is completed, the proposed osteotomy is carefully measured and marked (Figs. 39-20 and 39-21). The bony midline is vertically inscribed with a side-cutting burr (Fig. 39-22) to allow the proximal and distal segments to be precisely aligned after osteotomy and repositioning. The osteotomy site is then measured and

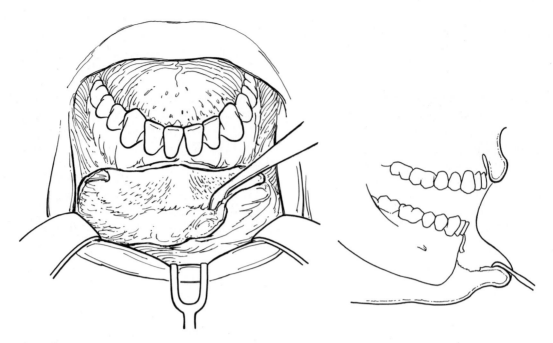

Fig. 39-18. Schematic illustration of the subperiosteal plane of dissection for genioplasty. Note the mental nerves are isolated, identified, and preserved and an inferior cuff of central soft tissue is maintained on the distal segment of the chin to increase vascularity.

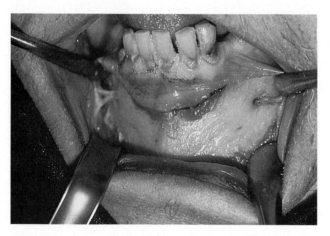

Fig. 39-19. The cadaver dissection of the subperiosteal plane of dissection for genioplasty.

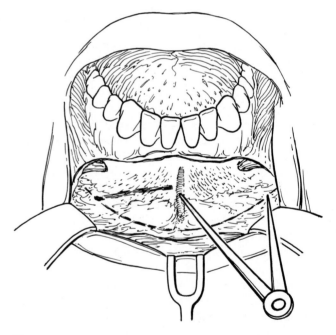

Fig. 39-20. Schematic illustration indicating measurement of the osteotomy site from the middle line to ensure symmetry.

marked with calipers to ensure a symmetrical osteotomy. The horizontal osteotomy should be placed below the level of the tooth roots to prevent dental injury.

During the preoperative assessment, a decision is made on the three-dimensional movement of the chin that is required. This treatment plan will affect the orientation of the osteotomy, as well as the actual movement after the osteotomy. If only A-P advancement is needed, the osteotomy is made with a horizontal orientation. If vertical movement (shortening) is needed in addition, the osteotomy is made in a more oblique orientation. An oblique osteotomy allows some vertical shortening as the distal segment is advanced.

If the chin length is excessive and significant shortening is planned, two oblique osteotomies are made and the intervening bone is removed.

After the osteotomy is marked, the bone cut is created with a reciprocating saw blade in a lateral-to-medial direc-

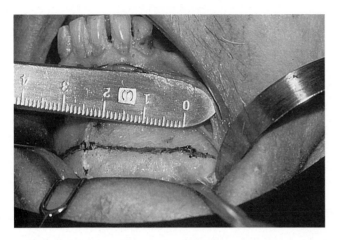

Fig. 39-21. The cadaver dissection indicating measurement of the osteotomy site from the middle line to ensure symmetry.

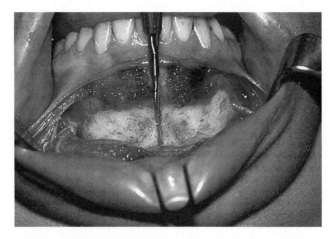

Fig. 39-22. Inscription of the bony midline with a sidecutting burr to facilitate later accurate approximation after osteotomy.

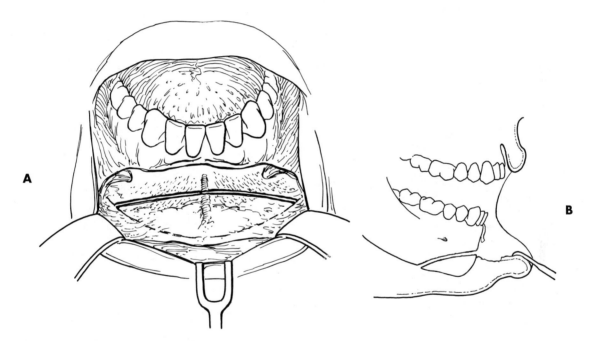

Fig. 39-23. **A,** Anterior-posterior and **B,** lateral schematic illustrations showing the horizontal mandibular osteotomy of the mentum well below the mental foramena.

tion (Fig. 39-23 *A, B*). The lateral extent of the osteotomy should be made at least 5 mm below the mental foramen, to avoid injury to the mental nerve. Gentle digital pressure is used to down-fracture the bony segment. A small amount of soft tissue must usually be separated from the posterior aspect of the distal segment to facilitate movement.

Repositioning of the distal segment is performed according to the preoperative treatment plan. If vertical lengthening is required, grafts are placed using autogenous bone or allogenic bone (Fig. 39-24). If vertical shortening is planned, a second parallel osteotomy is made above the first, or the intervening bone is burred away (Fig. 39-25).

After the segment is repositioned, it is fixed in position using adaptation plates, positional screws, or interosseous wires (Figs. 39-26 and 39-27). Adaptation plates may be preshaped and provide excellent fixation. The soft tissues of the chin and lips are then replaced, and the new contour is assessed.

The wound is closed in two layers with care taken to resuspend the soft tissues of the chin. Interrupted No. 3-0 catgut is used for the mentalis muscle and a running locking stitch of No. 3-0 chromic catgut is used for the mucosa. A pressure chinstrap dressing is applied for 5 days and the patient should eat a soft diet for 2 weeks.

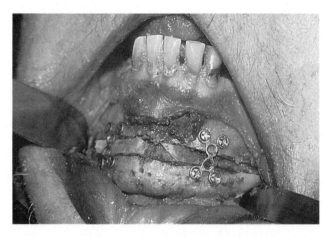

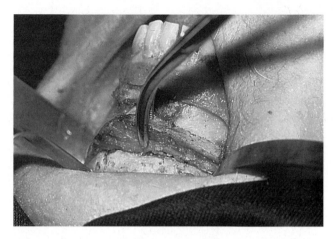

Fig. 39-24. Vertical lengthening of the chin by inserting bonegrafts into the down grafted osteotomy site.

Fig. 39-25. Bony ostectomy for shortening of the chin with removal of a segment of bone from the osteotomy site.

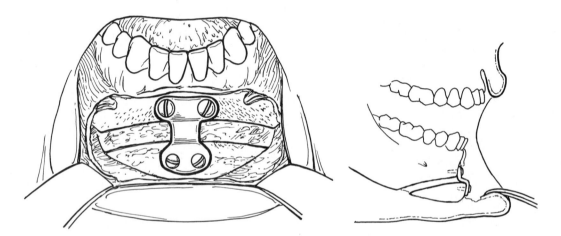

Fig. 39-26. Horizontal bony advancement of the chin with fixation with a prebent genioplasty plate. If bony contact is good, a single plate may be used.

Fig. 39-27. Intraoperative photograph of the preformed rigid genioplasty plate. Note that two small wires are used in this patient to insure stability of the bony movement.

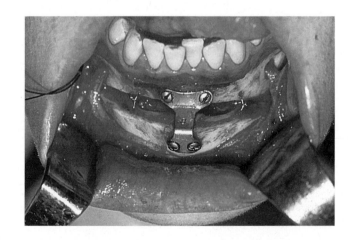

CLINICAL EXAMPLES

Case 1: A 22-year-old woman presented for rhinoplasty. She had had orthodontic treatment to correct a class II malocclusion. She desired chin augmentation, but refused bony genioplasty. At the time of rhinoplasty, chin augmentation was accomplished using an extended anatomical implant (Fig. 39-28 *A* to *D*).

Case 2: A 42-year-old woman with a nasal deformity and significant microgenia underwent advancement genioplasty and open rhinoplasty (Fig. 39-29 *A* to *F*).

Case 3: A 25-year-old woman with class III malocclu-

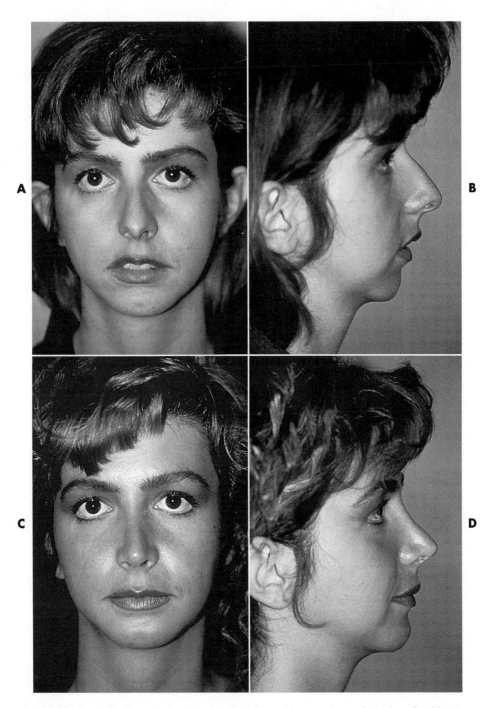

Fig. 39-28. A and **B,** Preoperative anterior-posterior and lateral views of a patient for rhinoplasty and chin augmentation. **C** and **D,** Six-month postoperative photograph of a patient after open rhinoplasty and chin augmentation with alloplastic implant.

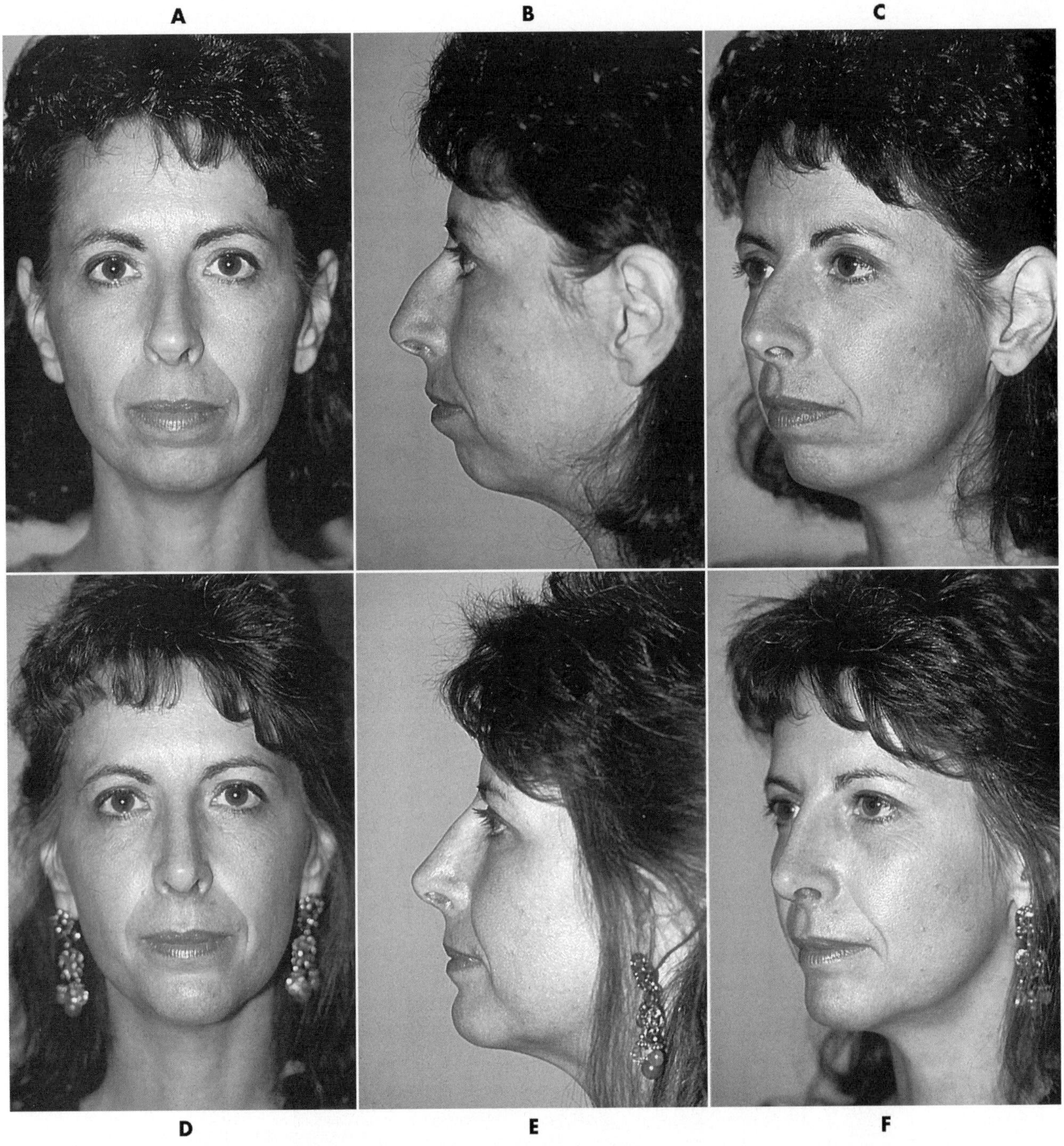

Fig. 39-29. A to **C,** Preoperative anterior-posterior, lateral, and oblique views of a patient for rhinoplasty and sliding advancement genioplasty. **D** to **F,** Six-month postoperative views of the patient after open rhinoplasty and advancement genioplasty.

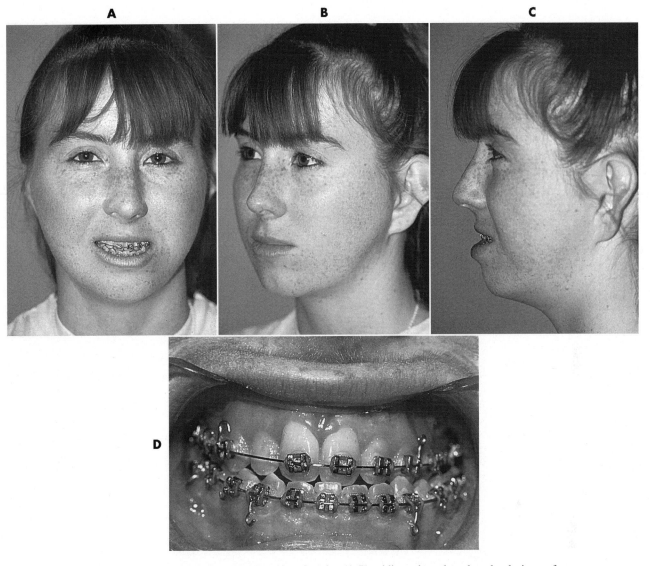

Fig. 39-30. A to **D,** Preoperative anterior-posterior (A-P), oblique, lateral, and occlusal views of a patient with significant congenital asymmetry, class III malocclusion, bilateral crossbite, and microgenia.

Continued

sion, bilateral crossbite, chin asymmetry, and temporomandibular dysfunction underwent Le fort's I maxillary osteotomy with advancement, bilateral sagittal split ramus osteotomy of the mandible with setback and rotation, and asymmetric advancement genioplasty (Fig. 39-30 *A* to *H*).

COMPLICATIONS

Complications after mentoplasty are uncommon. Chin implants may become malpositioned and occasionally are bothersome to patients with a thin overlying soft tissue pad. Infections are infrequent with either the intraoral or the submental approach. There have been reports of anterior mandible resorption with subperiosteal implant placement, occasionally causing secondary chin deformities.[8]

Complications after genioplasty include mental nerve injury and malunion or nonunion of the bony segments. Nerve damage is extremely uncommon with careful dissection. Malunion of the bone segments can occur, but the excellent vascularity and the lack of direct force on the osteotomy site make this an infrequent problem.

SUMMARY

Aesthetic surgery of the chin is extremely rewarding when performed in the carefully selected patient. Chin augmentation with alloplasts is a simple and effective means to correct mild to moderate horizontal microgenia. Horizontal osteotomy of the bony mentum (genioplasty) is a more flexible and versatile procedure that can correct chin deformities

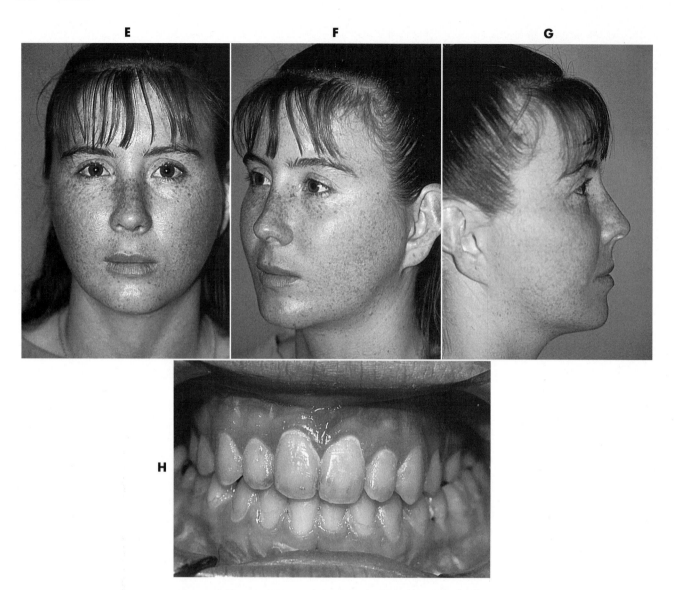

Fig. 39-30, cont'd. E to **H,** One-year postoperative A-P, oblique, lateral, and occlusal views of the patient after Le Fort's I maxillary osteotomy with advancement bilateral sagittal split, ramus osteotomy of the mandible with setback and rotation, and advancement genioplasty with rotation of the chin point.

in all three planes of space. When properly planned and executed, either procedure provides an important adjunct for the facial plastic surgeon.

REFERENCES

1. Bell WH, Gallagher DM: The versatility of genioplasty using a broad pedicle, *J Oral Maxillofac Surg* 41:763, 1983.
2. Burstone CJ: Lip osture and its significance in treatment planning, *Am J Orthod* 53:262, 1967.
3. Converse JM, Wood-Smith D: Horizontal osteotomy of the mandible, *Plast Reconstr Surg* 34:464, 1964.
4. Gonzalez-Ulloa M, Stevens E: Role of chin correction in profileplasty, *Plast Reconstr Surg* 41:477, 1968.
5. Guyuron B: *Genioplasty*, Boston, 1993, Little, Brown.
6. Hofer O: Operation der prognathie und mikrogenie, *Deutsche Zahnarztl Mund Kief* 9:121, 1942.
7. Lehman JA: Soft-tissue manifestations of aesthetic defects of the jaws: diagnosis and treatment, *Clin Plast Surg* 14:767, 1987.
8. Li K, Cheney M: The use of sliding genioplasty for treatment of failed chin implants, *Laryngoscope* 106:363, 1996.
9. McCarthy JG, Ruff G: The chin, *Clin Plast Surg* 15:125, 1988.
10. Peterson RA: Correction of the senile chin deformity in face lift, *Clin Plast Surg* 19:433, 1992.
11. Powell N, Humphreys B: *Proportions of the aesthetic face,* New York, 1984, Thieme-Stratton.
12. Precious DS, Delaire J: Correction of anterior mandibular vertical excess: the functional genioplasty, *Oral Med* 59:229, 1985.
13. Rakosi T: *An atlas and manual of cephalometry radiography*, Philadelphia, 1982, Lea & Febiger.

14. Ricketts RM: Esthetics, environment and the law of lip relation, *Am J Orthod* 54:272, 1968.

15. Spear SL, Kassan M: Genioplasty, *Clin Plast Surg* 16:695, 1989.

16. Steiner CC: Cephalometrics in clinical practice, *Angle Orthod* 29:8, 1959.

17. Sykes J, Frodel JL: Genioplasty, *Op Tech Otolaryngol*, 6:319, 1995.

18. Sykes J, Donald PJ: *Orthognathic surgery*. In Papel I, Nachlas NE, editors: *Facial plastic and reconstructive surgery*, St Louis, 1992, Mosby.

19. Wolfe A: *The genioplasty: an essential tool in the correction of chin deformities*. In Ousterhout DK, editor: *Aesthetic contouring of the craniofacial skeleton*, Boston, 1991, Little, Brown.

20. Wolff SA: *The chin*. In Wolfe SA, Berkowitz S, editors: *Plastic surgery of facial skeleton*, Boston, 1989, Little, Brown.

Index

Note: Page numbers set in italic indicate figures; those followed by *t* indicate tables; those preceded by *P* indicate material found in the Pediatric volume.